CLINICAL PROCEDURES FOR MEDICAL ASSISTANTS

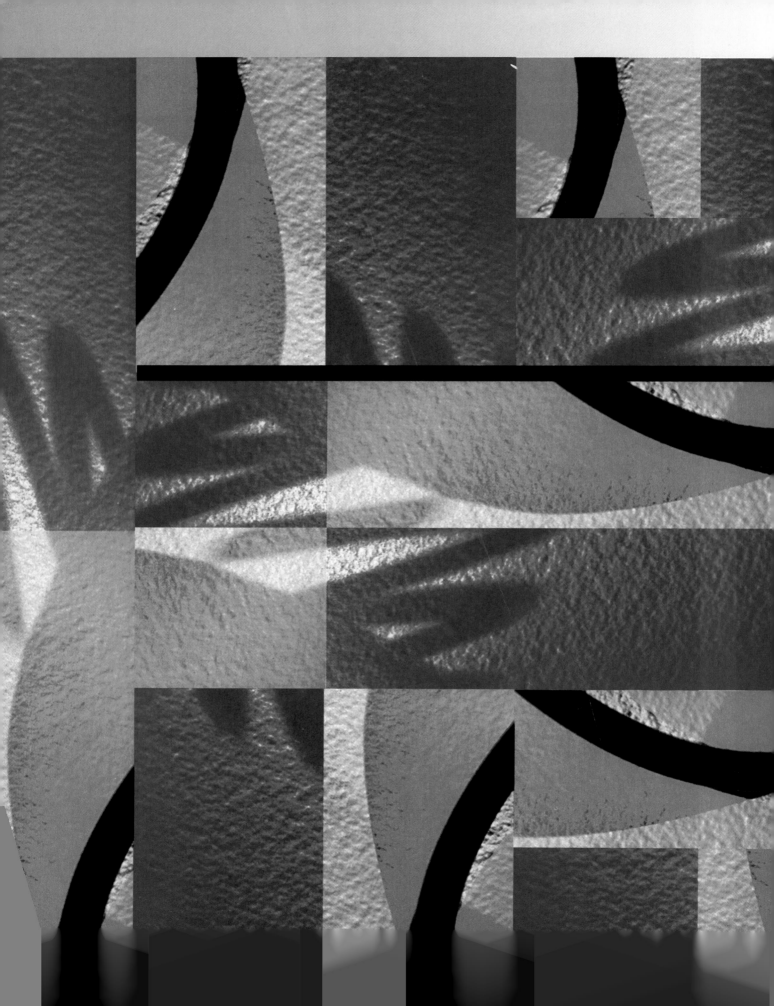

third edition

CLINICAL PROCEDURES FOR MEDICAL ASSISTANTS

Sharron M. Zakus, RN, BA, MS, CMA

Educator, Health Science Department,
City College of San Francisco, San Francisco, California
Formerly Director and Instructor, Medical Assistant Program,
College of California Medical Affiliates, San Francisco, California

with 772 illustrations

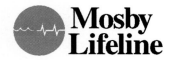

Publisher: David T. Culverwell
Acquisitions Editor: Eric Duchinsky
Developmental Editor: Julie Scardiglia
Assistant Editors: Christine H. Ambrose
                     Emerson John Probst, III
Project Manager: Gayle May Morris
Production Editor: Mary Cusick Drone
Manufacturing Supervisor: Betty Richmond
Designer: Studio Montage
Cover Image: © Pierre-Yzes Goavec/The Image Bank
Electronic Production: Joan Herron

THIRD EDITION

Printed in the United States of America

Composition by Mosby Electronic Production, St. Louis
Color Separation by Accu • color
Printing/Binding by Von Hoffman Press, Inc.

Mosby-Year Book, Inc.
11830 Westline Industrial Drive
St. Louis, Missouri 63146

International Standard Book Number 0-8016-6983-9

95 96 97 98 99 2000/9 8 7 6 5 4 3 2 1

To

Mom and **Dad**

Donn, Joseph, and **Jude**

and to the memory of **Nana**

Thank you for so much—
small words, but filled with meaning and feeling

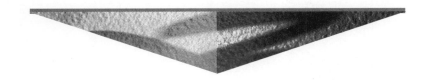

Preface

New techniques and developments in the medical field have a direct influence on the medical assistant's professional duties and responsibilities. Because the educational standards of each medically oriented professional career continue to escalate, each assumes new functions, roles, and responsibilities. With the increasing demands of modern medical practice on members of the medical profession, physicians are turning more and more to trained medical assistants to help administer their offices and perform routine clinical duties.

The intent of this book is to help medical assistants attain the knowledge and skills required to meet the increasing demands of their profession and enable them to function as major contributing individuals in the health care field.

A textbook should expose the student to new ideas, thoughts, and concepts. It should motivate the student or reader, and above all, it should teach. To achieve these goals, this book presents in a concise, clear, and readable style up-to-date, accurate information about clinical assisting and skills, theory, and related medical information that the medical assistant must understand in order to contribute to quality health care services for patients.

The chief objective is to aid the student and the teacher in the learning/teaching process. I have attempted to create a book that students will want to pick up and enjoy because it stimulates them, and thus a book from which they will learn eagerly and easily. I have also tried to make this book one that will excite teachers and in turn help make their teaching tasks easier (an instructor's manual, a video series, and a student workbook to accompany the third edition are available).

This book is designed to provide knowledge of effective and efficient techniques in contemporary patient care and assisting for beginning medical assistants. Moreover, it supplies current reference material for those assistants actively employed in a medical setting and serves as an information source for the principles and techniques underlying clinical assisting for individuals who wish to reenter the employment field. Actively employed medical assistants who have the first and/or the second edition of this book in their office and/or home library say that they refer to it frequently when performing their daily work duties. The objectives at the beginning of each unit and the case studies, vocabulary reviews, review questions, and performance tests given as a study guide at the end of each unit are particularly helpful for individuals preparing to take the national certification examination administered by the American Association of Medical Assistants.

The scope of this book meets the growing need for a comprehensive and effective textbook that deals with:

- Routine clinical skills and assisting techniques with related information required of the medical assistant.
- Patient procedures that may be performed satisfactorily by the medical assistant.
- Patient procedures in which the medical assistant may be required to assist the physician.
- Tests and procedures that the medical assistant must know to provide the patient with accurate preparatory information.
- Information necessary to understand the procedures, the medical techniques and their underlying principles, and the functions of other professionals who provide health care.
- Quality patient care as the medical assistant's primary goal based on the development of a positive attitude toward individual responsibilities and a commitment to the other members of the health care team.
- The most current theoretic information available, with an emphasis on practical application.

Acquiring clinical skills and assisting techniques is best accomplished when learning experiences are organized and the learner is provided with opportunities to acquire knowledge and to practice with professionals in settings that enhance learning. For example, in a skills laboratory, which is a simulation of a joblike environment, learners can practice new skills with each other; or in a clinical setting, which is a working experience, the learners may work under direct supervision.

This book also introduces the medical assistant to the nature and purpose of many procedures, both diagnostic and therapeutic, used by the various medical specialties and related medical fields, such as the changing and ever-expanding specialties of nuclear medicine, radiology, physical therapy, and laboratory technology, so that the medical assistant can anticipate and prepare the patient for procedures in these fields. Although the medical assistant is only indirectly involved with these specialties, it is essential to become knowledgable of these fields of medical practice.

The *third edition* of this book has been expanded from sixteen to nineteen units; some of the units have been renumbered. The depth of the text remains, but *every unit* incorporates new and the most up-to-date information available on clinical procedures and related theory.

More new and updated color photographs and illustrations have been added to reinforce content, to keep the text lively and engaging, and to enhance the student's visualization and understanding of the theory, procedures, and equipment presented. A glossary of the vocabulary terms from each unit and Appendixes A, B, and C remain. The Patient Bill of Rights is on page xxi in edition 3. These are valuable assets and reference sources for the student. Emphasis is on helping the students learn to perform the tasks, acquire the skills of their profession, use the related basic scientific and technical knowledge, acquire the capabilities for critical thinking and problem-solving (i.e., making reliable decisions related to their tasks and adapting to new situation), and treat the patient as a whole individual and not merely as a condition or as a diseased body part.

The organization in the units of the third edition remains the same as that of the first and second editions, as this has proven to be educationally effective for the learning and teaching process. Each unit contains the following:

- Cognitive and competency-based terminal performance objectives
- Vocabulary lists with pronunciation keys
- Specific procedures and related information

To help reinforce learning, each unit also includes:

- Reviews of vocabulary (most of which use medical reports as examples)
- Case studies
- Thought-provoking review questions relating to both theory and skills mastered, many with practical application to an on-the-job situation
- Performance tests

MAJOR CONTENT REVISION FOR THE THIRD EDITION

The major content changes are summarized as follows:

- *New:* Unit One—Universal Blood and Body Substance Precautions. This unit includes the latest federal regulations for Universal Precautions and discussion of HIV disease and the various types of hepatitis.
- *New:* Unit Eighteen—Anatomy and Physiology. This is particularly useful as a reference for students who have studied anatomy and physiology and for programs of study that must include these areas as part of the clinical aspect of the program.
- *New:* Unit Nineteen—Nutrition. This unit focuses on the contemporary issues of nutrition for everyone and also includes special diets.

- *New:* Appendix D—Latest immunization information.
- *New:* Tables have been added in many units.
- *New:* Infrared tympanic thermometry discussion and procedure.
- *New:* Medical record management, documentation, and retention.
- *New:* Cancer facts—How cancer works, cancer prevention and early detection, major cancer sites, warning signs and treatment.
- *New:* Vision tests.
- *New:* Pediatric examinations and pediatric visits.
- *New:* Section on the immune system.
- *New:* Procedures for suture removal and cast applications and care.
- *New:* Procedures for using the Safety-Lok and Monojet safety syringes.
- *New:* Insulin injections.
- *New:* Selected laboratory tests and handling and transport of specimens.
- *New:* Procedures for measuring a patient for crutches and a cane.
- *New:* Ambulatory cardiac monitoring (Holter monitoring).
- *Expanded:* Coverage on vocabulary, blood pressure, obstetric examination, Pap smears, physical examinations, eye examinations, immunizations, care of instruments and sterilization procedures, minor surgical procedures, drug administration, drug classifications, drug dosages and calculations, testing for tuberculosis, quality control for laboratory procedures, laboratory tests, physical therapy modalities, common heart rhythms and electrocardiograms, common emergencies and first aid, and various diseases and disorders, including sexually transmitted diseases.

The organization and careful selection ensure a relevant and complete resource for students, teachers, and practicing medical assistants, enhancing the competency level in each responsibility.

The reading level of the text was given special attention. Improved readability has resulted without compromising high educational standards and professionalism.

Textbook supplements for this edition include a new student workbook, a new series of twelve video cassettes addressing specific units and procedures, and an updated instructor's manual.

This is more than just a how-to book, it is also a why, when, where, who, and what book.

Included are explanations of the physician's actions during a patient examination or a procedure in which the medical assistant is participating. In addition, this book contains:

- A table of common blood tests with normal values and the significance of the results.
- A table of urine examinations with the type of specimen required and the normal values for the results.
- Tables of x-ray and nuclear medicine procedures, with the time period required for each, an indication of when special patient preparation is required, and samples of patient preparation.

• A table of patient conditions that benefit from physical therapy and the common modalities used.

• Guidelines for assisting with the patient history/interview.

• Complete unit dedicated to Universal Precautions, Nutrition, and Anatomy and Physiology.

• Expanded coverage on the health care and examinations for the obstetric and the hypertensive patient.

• Actual forms such as medical reports, case histories, and discharge summaries to allow the student to see how the vocabulary terms presented in the unit are used in an actual report, how the contents of the unit relate to medical reports, and how health care providers document information obtained about a patient.

• A summary of studies used for diagnosing conditions affecting body organs and systems.

• Performance tests and checklists that may be used by the students and adapted for teacher use in the instructor's manual and student workbook.

• Charting examples for the assistant to use when recording the completion and results of procedures and tests.

To aid the learning process for beginning students, vocabulary boxes are included with pronunciation of difficult terms as they are introduced. It will be helpful for the teacher to give the correct pronunciation of the term and then have the students repeat it.

In the unit on physical therapy, students are given the opportunity to design procedural steps; performance checklists and instructions to be given to the patient to use at home are included.

Information offered in each unit is written with the assumption that the medical assistant student has a background in or is currently studying basic anatomy, physiology, and microbiology. Thus detailed explanations pertaining to these subjects are omitted in the units. Unit Eighteen has been added to cover anatomy and physiology in more detail. The teacher of the class for clinical procedures is encouraged to review the theoretic aspects pertaining to these subjects as they relate to each skill the student will be expected to perform.

All procedures (skills and tasks) are presented in a concise, step-by-step format. When necessary, explanations of the physician's role, specific notes on patient care, and notes stressing the rationale behind a step are offered. The procedures are written to assist the student in the learning process. Sometimes the ideas or procedure steps are included in another procedure or unit to reinforce the ideas presented. The student should analyze the facts and try to place them in a meaningful order.

It should be remembered that frequently different methods and techniques may be used in a medical procedure. *This book presents one method of performing a procedure.* When there are regional differences of opinion, teachers are encouraged to teach the skill in the fashion most suitable for their area of practice.

This book is written with procedures that may be performed by medical assistants nationwide as identified by the American Association of Medical Assistants, although, because of various state laws, some procedures may not be considered a duty of the medical assistant. Nevertheless, it is hoped that the information provided helps medical assistants understand the nature and purpose of all procedures presented.

With these facets in mind, it is my hope that educators, students, and medical assistants will use this textbook with the enthusiasm and thirst for knowledge equal to my own as I researched, compiled, and wrote it. I also hope that this book challenges the student to develop a permanent interest in the medical field and a desire for continued growth and knowledge.

ACKNOWLEDGMENTS

This book could not have been compiled without the encouragement, support, inspiration, and assistance of many friends, colleagues, and other specialists in the medical field. I am deeply indebted to each one of them.

The completion of the third edition of this book also gives me the opportunity to thank all the educators and students who responded so positively to the first and second editions.

My very special gratitude is extended to Donn R. Harris for his unlimited support, understanding, faith, and encouragement throughout the writing of the complete manuscript and for his valuable assistance in various stages of preparation.

I am especially grateful for the dedicated and invaluable assistance of Ann A. Gunderson, RN, California Pacific Medical Center, Pacific Campus, San Francisco, for continuous consultations and review of numerous areas in this book, and for a valued friendship.

With pleasure, I gratefully acknowledge the following practicing professionals who offered special area consultations and reviews. I am deeply indebted to each of them for the time, energy, and knowledge that he or she so willingly contributed:

• Marlene Bonham, RPT, Physical Therapy, Education Coordinator, Pacific Presbyterian Medical Center, San Francisco, California

• Louise Brown, LVN, Pediatric Services, Kaiser Foundation Hospital, San Francisco, California

• Ruth Berry Hanley Bultman, RN, Kaiser Hospital Clinic, San Francisco, California

• Cecile M. Dawydiak, RN, MA, Department Chair, RN Nursing Dept., City College of San Francisco, California

• William Delameter, MT(ASCP), Children's Hospital of San Francisco, San Francisco, California

• Helen Archer-Dusté, RN, MS, CNA, Director, Pediatric Services, Kaiser Foundation Hospital, San Francisco, California

• Anne Emmons, MA, Gynecology, Obstetric, and Neurology Clinic Specialties, California Pacific Medical Center, California Campus, San Francisco, California

• Fred Schalit, BS, RP, MS (Pharmacology), San Francisco, California

• Elise Stone, MS, Health Education Coordinator, San Francisco Regional Poison Control Center, San Francisco General Hospital, San Francisco, California

- Patricia Suminski, Instructor/Coordinator, Milwaukee Area Technical College, Milwaukee, Wisconsin
- Barbara Willhite, Nursing Assistant Instructor, Southeastern Career Center, Versailles, Illinois
- William B. Wolfe, CRT, San Francisco, California
- Alisa Wright, Coordinator Pre-Allied Health Science, Pre-Allied Health Science Program, Housatonic Community College, Bridgeport, Connecticut
- Pat Zachary, RN, Pediatric Services, Unit Manager, Kaiser Foundation Hospital, San Francisco, California

I am indebted to the following professionals, who have provided continuing support and expertise:

- Julia Ender, MT (ASCP), San Francisco, California
- John M.Gunning, Mobile Intensive Care Paramedic, San Francisco, California
- Richard A. Jones, Branch Manager, California Medical Supply, San Francisco, California
- Marilyn Jordan, RN, MPH, Nurse Epidemiologist, Hospital Infection Control Unit, Medical Center at The University of California, San Franciso, California
- Elizabeth C. Lee, CRT, San Francisco, California
- Deborah Leeds, PharmD, Director of Pharmacy Services, Shield Healthcare Center, Berkeley, California
- Louisa Lo, RPT, Senior Physical Therapist, Outpatient Services, Pacific Presbyterian Medical Center, San Francisco, California
- Betty J. Mattea, BA, RT(R), Chairperson, Radiology Department, City College of San Francisco, San Francisco, California
- Ann McCabe, MT, BA, Microbiology, SmithKline Beecham Clinical Laboratory, San Francisco, California
- Tom McCarthy, Medico Supply Company, Inc., San Francisco, California
- Dennis McDevitt, Mobile Intensive Care Paramedic, San Francisco, California
- William C. McDill, RPT, Director, Physical Therapy Services, San Francisco, California
- Michelle Mendoza, RPT, Physical Therapy, California Pacific Medical Center, California Campus, San Francisco, California
- Bonnie Miller, DSN, OB-GYN Clinic RN, Children's Hospital of San Francisco, San Francisco, California
- James Mochizuki, CNMT, Nuclear Medicine Technologist, Pacific Presbyterian Medical Center, San Francisco, California
- Joseph I. Musallam, BSc, Senior Medical Technologist, California Pacific Medical Center, California Campus, San Franciso, California
- Robert Navarro, Mobile Intensive Care Paramedic, San Francisco, California
- James Pritchard, MT(ASCP), Laboratory Manager, Presbyterian Hospital of Pacific Medical Center, San Francisco, California

I thank the authors and publishers for their kind permission to use some of the illustrations from their books and all the firms and their representatives who cooperated with me in supplying illustrations and descriptive literature of their products. They are given appropriate credit throughout the book.

I am particularly grateful to Rick Brady, professional photographer, for his work in taking numerous photographs for this third edition and to Nancy Bauer and Donald O'Connor for their attractive and innovative illustrations.

I also thank Judith Werderitsch, Neila J. Burrows, and Ross Learning, Inc., of Oak Park, Mich., for their valuable input as consultants and contributors.

Many physicians; other laboratory, pharmaceutical, and medical personnel; and hospitals contributed medical reports and other special reference material and provided the facilities for taking many photographs.

I thank the Mosby production team for their assistance in the production of this book, especially Richard A. Weimer, Executive Editor; Eric Duchinsky, Acquisitions Editor; Julie Dusty Scardiglia, Development Editor; Christine H. Myers Ambrose, Emerson John Probst III, and Mary Beth Ryan Warthen, Assistant Editors; Gayle May Morris, Project Manager; Mary Cusick Drone, Senior Production Editor; Susan Lane, Senior Book Designer; and Joan Herron, Desktop Publisher.

Finally, I acknowledge all my past and present students and many other colleagues, friends, and family for their continued interest and support.

Sharron M. Zakus

To the Student

You are about the enter the professional area of clinical medical assisting, an interesting and challenging field. When you have mastered the knowledge and skills presented in this book, you will be able to enhance patient care, and increase your value to the physician, co-workers, and related health specialists.

Always keep in mind that you are an important member of the medical team and it is only through dedicated professional teamwork that quality and appropriate medical care can be provided and accomplished. Never underestimate your value in the field of medical care.

Points to keep in mind as you are studying and practicing procedures and assisting the physician include the following:

- The importance of being exact (precise) in all that you do
- The great service that you are rendering to the patient and to the physician/employer
- The influence that your attitude (positive or negative) can have on your performance and subsequent relationship with patients
- The legal implications of your actions
- That the career you are learning can be extremely rewarding and intellectually stimulating when you apply yourself and continually strive for improvement and continuing educational endeavors

For each unit in this book, read and master the objectives and vocabulary listed. Test yourself and a study companion with the review questions and performance checklists provided. When you think that you can perform a particular skill, have your instructor give you the performance test. Written and oral testing may also be given to you at the discretion of your instructor.

Samples of patients' records are provided for vocabulary review in the units and to allow you to see how medical personnel record information for a patient's permanent medical record. These records will stimulate your interest, enhance learning, and help you relate your studies to actual on-the-job experiences. Read each report carefully and relate its contents to the current and previous units of study.

Inherent in the performance of all clinical skills are basic principles that you should recall and integrate:

1. Use and understand the standards and techniques of the federal guidelines for Universal Precautions at *all* times.
2. Always check and follow the physician's orders.
3. Obtain and prepare the equipment necessary for the procedure. This involves knowledge of the procedure.
4. Thoroughly wash your hands before and after each procedure and patient contact.
5. Prepare and assist the patient both mentally and physically.

   Mental preparation involves an adequate but simple explanation of the situation. Patients are more relaxed and cooperative when they know what to expect during an examination or procedure. To explain effectively, you must know medical terminology and be prepared to translate that language into terms that the patient can readily understand. Provide reassurance and support while maintaining a supportive, empathetic (not sympathetic) attitude.

   Physical preparation involves positioning the patient correctly for the procedure, draping appropriately, and offering assistance as needed. always providing for the patient's comfort and safety.
6. Perform or assist the physician with the procedure.
7. Record the procedure and findings accurately.
8. Dispose of waste and used equipment correctly.
9. Clean and ready the treatment room and equipment for reuse.

As you begin your studies, I wish you success and happiness in a most rewarding professional career and share with you a poem (see page xii) that I have shared with many of my former students and graduates. Think about it as you begin this program of study and periodically throughout your new career.

Sharron M. Zakus

TAKE TIME

Take time to think—thoughts are the source of power.

Take time to play—play is the secret of perpetual youth.

Take time to read—reading is the fountain of wisdom.

Take time to pray—prayer can be a rock of strength in time of trouble.

Take time to love—loving is what makes living worthwhile.

Take time to be friendly—friendships give life a delicious flavor.

Take time to laugh—laughter is the music of the soul.

Take time to give—any day of the year is too short for selfishness.

Take time to do your work well—pride in your work, no matter what it is, nourishes the ego and the spirit.

Take time to show appreciation—"thanks" is the frosting on the cake of life.

Author unknown

Contents

unit one **U**niversal Blood and Body Substance Precautions, 1

Uniforms and clothing, 4
Laundry, 4
Communications of hazards to employees, 4
Compliance, 5
Infection control systems, 5
Barrier precautions, 6
Personal protective equipment, 7
Handling of equipment, supplies, and waste, 9
Employee health issues, 11
HIV infection and disease/AIDS, 13
Hepatitis, 15

unit two **P**hysical Measurements: Vital Signs, Height, and Weight, 18

Vital signs, 19
Physical measurements of height
and weight, 41

unit three **H**ealth History and Physical Examinations, 53

The medical record, 53
History and physical examination, 54
Summary of positive findings, 61
Diagnostic data, 61
Impression, 61
Care plans and suggested further study, 62
Progress notes, 62
Discharge summary, 62
Problem-oriented medical record, 62
Records management, 64
Special vocabulary, 65
Medical abbreviations, 66

unit four Preparing for and Assisting with Routine and Special Physical Examinations, 76

Preparing for and Assisting with Physical Examinations, 77

Gowning, Positioning, and Draping the Patient
for Physical Examinations, 84

Gynecologic Examination, 91

Pelvic Examination and a Pap Smear, 98

Rectal Examination, 99

Endoscopic Examination: Proctoscopy and Sigmoidoscopy, 99

Neurologic Examination, 118

Hearing Examination, 119

Eye Examination, 120

Obstetric Examinations and Record, 126

Pediatric Examinations, 134

unit five Infection Control: Practices of Medical Asepsis and Sterilization, 168

Basic Concepts and Goals, 169

Infectious Process and Causative Agents, 169

The Body's Defenses Against Disease and Infection, 173

Diagnostic Data, 177

Infection Control, 177

Methods to Control Microscopic Agents, 186

Ultrasonic Cleaning and Sterilization Procedures, 198

Summary, 200

unit six Surgical Asepsis and Minor Surgery, 202

Background of Sterile Technique, 203

Principles and Practices of Surgical Asepsis, 203

Handling Sterile Supplies, 204

Minor Surgery, 207

Wounds, 224

Dressings and Bandages, 227

Casts, 240

unit seven | Principles of Pharmacology and Drug Administration, 247

Pharmacology and Drugs, 248
Prescriptions, 252
Administer, Dispense, Prescribe, 258
Pharmaceutical Preparations, 258
Professional Responsibilities, 258
Oxygen Administration, 264
Routes and Methods of Drug Administration, 265
Factors Influencing Dosage and Drug Action, 270
Patient Education, 272
Injections, 273

unit eight | Diagnositc Allergy Tests and Intradermal Skin Tests, 299

Allergies, 299
Tuberculosis, 305

unit nine | Instillations and Irrigations of the Ear and Eye, 310

Ear Instillation, 310
Ear Irrigation, 310
Eye Instillation, 311
Eye Irrigation, 311

unit
ten # Laboratory Orientation, 322

The Typical Laboratory, 323
Liaison and Responsibilities of the Medical Assistant
with Laboratories, 324
Diagnostic and Therapeutic Procedures, 325
Collecting, Handling, Transporting, and Storing Specimens, 328
Quality Control and Laboratory Safety, 328
The Microscope, 330
Centrifuges, 334

unit
eleven # Collecting and Handling Specimens, 337

Specimens, 339
Urine Specimen Collection, 342
Stool Specimen Collection, 346
Respiratory Tract Specimens, 353
Wound Culture, 358
Smears for Cytology Studies, 358
Smears for Bacteriology Studies, 361
Gram Stain, 361
Bacterial Culture and Sensitivity (C&S) Testing, 363
Culture Media, 363
Vaginal Smears and Culture Collection, 363
Chlamydia Trachomatis:: the Direct Specimen Test, 370
Herpes Simplex Viruses: Diseases, Diagnosis, and Typing, 371
Lumbar Puncture, 373

unit
twelve # Urinalysis, 380

Urinary System: Formation and Components of Normal Urine, 380
Routine Urinalysis, 381
Detection and Semiquantitation of Bacteriuria, 403
Other Urine Tests, 408
Pregnancy Test, 408
Phenylketonuria, 408
Multiple-Glass Test, 409
Other Tests, 409

unit thirteen Hematology, 415

Blood Components, Functions, and Formation, 416
Obtaining Blood Samples, 418
Blood Tests, 433
Blood Chemistries, 437
Complete Blood Count: Hematology Test, 449
Blood Groups and Types, 452
Automation in the Clinical Laboratory, 452
Quality Control and Laboratory Safety, 467

unit fourteen Diagnostic Radiology, Radiation Therapy, and Nuclear Medicine, 470

Radiologic Procedures , 470
X-Rays, 471
Position of Patient for X-Ray Studies, 482
Radiologic Dangers, Hazards, and Safety Precautions, 485
Medical Assistant Responsibilities, 486
Processing X-Ray Film, 490
Storage and Management in the Office, 491

unit fifteen Physical Therapy, 496

Ultraviolet Light, 497
Diathermy, 497
Ultrasound, 498
Local Applications of Heat (Thermotherapy) and Cold (Cryotherapy), 498
Hydrotherapy, 503
Paraffin Wax Hand Bath, 504
Traction, 504
Massage, 505
Exercises, 505
Body Mechanics, 510
Wheelchairs, 512
Crutches, 513
Canes, 517
Walkers, 518
Electrotherapy Using Galvanic and Faradic Currents, 518
Electrodiagnostic Examinations, 519
Disabilities and Therapy, 519

unit sixteen Electrocardiography, 524

The Cardiac Cycle and EKG Cycle, 527
Electrocardiogram, 529
Phone-a-Gram: the Computerized EKG, 538
Automatic Electrocardiographs, 538
Digital Electrocardiograph Facsimile, 538
Automatic Cardiac Monitoring (Monitoring), 538
Treadmill Stress Test, 543

unit seventeen Common Emergencies and First Aid, 547

Cardiopumonary Resuscitation for Cardiac Arrest, 549
Emergency Medical Services System, 553
Heart attack: Signals and Actions for Survival, 554
Shock, 554
Abdominal Pain, 556
Allergic Reaction (Anaphylactic Reaction) Drugs, 556
Asphyxia, 556
Human, Animal, Snake, and Insect Bites and Stings, 556
Severe Bleeding (Hemorrhage), 557
Burns, 560
Cerebral Vascular Accident (Stroke), 563
Chest Pain, 564
Convulsions, 564
Epistaxis (Nosebleed), 565
Fainting (Syncope), 565
Foreign Bodies in the Ear, Eye, and Nose, 565
Fractures, 566
Head Injuries, 567
Hyperventilation, 567
Hypoglycemia—Diabetes (Insulin Reaction) and Hyperglycemia (Diabetic Coma), 568
Open Wounds, 569
Poisoning, 570
Poison Control Centers, 571

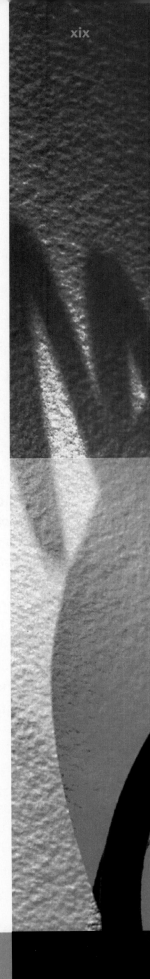

unit eighteen **Anatomy and Physiology, 577**

Body Planes, 579
Body Cavities, 579
Body Regions, 581
The Cellular Basis of Humans, 581
The Skeletal System, 582
The Muscular System, 588
The Circulatory System, 591
The Cardiovascular System, 594
The Nervous System, 596
The Digestive System, 605
The Respiratory System, 609
The Urinary System, 612
The Reproductive System, 615
The Endocrine System, 622
The Sensory System, 625
The Integumentary System, 629

unit nineteen **Nutrition, 634**

Nutrition and Your Health, 634
Digestion, 635
Metabolism, 635
Nutrients, 635
Fiber, 650
Salt and Sodium, 651
Alcohol, 653
Calories, 653
Dietary Guidelines for Americans, 655
Food Labeling, 656
BRAT, 660
Patient Teaching, 660

appendixes

A Special Vocabulary, 662
B Summary of Studies Used for Diagnosing Conditions
  Affecting Body Organs and Systems, 667
C Common Medical Terminology Combining Word Parts, 670
D Immunizations, 677

Glossary, 683

Patient Bill of Rights

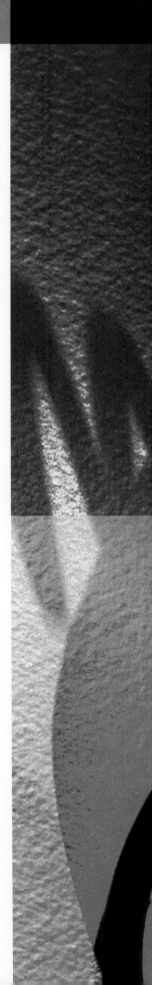

1. The patient has the right to considerate and respectful care.

2. The patient has the right to obtain from his physician complete current information concerning his diagnosis, treatment, and prognosis in terms the patient can be reasonably expected to understand.

3. The patient has the right to receive from his physician information necessary to give informed consent prior to the start of any procedure and/or treatment. . . . Where medically significant alternatives for care or treatment exist, or when the patient requests information concerning medical alternatives, the patient has the right to such information [and] to know the name of the person responsible for the procedures and/or treatment.

4. The patient has the right to refuse treatment to the extent permitted by law, and to be informed of the medical consequences of his action.

5. The patient has the right to every consideration of his privacy concerning his own medical care program.

6. The patient has the right to expect that all communications and records pertaining to his care be treated as confidential.

7. The patient has the right to expect that, within its capacity, a hospital must make reasonable response to the request of a patient for services.

8. The patient has the right to obtain information concerning any relationship of his hospital to other health care and educational institutions insofar as his care is concerned [and] any professional relationships among individuals, by name, who are treating him.

9. The patient has the right to be advised if the hospital proposes to engage in or perform human experimentation affecting his care or treatment [and] has the right to refuse to participate.

10. The patient has the right to expect reasonable continuity of care.

11. The patient has the right to examine and receive an explanation of his bill, regardless of source of payment.

12. The patient has the right to know what hospital rules and regulations apply to his conduct as a patient.

Adapted from American Hospital Association: *Nurs. Outlook* 24:29, 1976.

CLINICAL PROCEDURES FOR MEDICAL ASSISTANTS

Universal Blood and Body Substance Precautions

COGNITIVE OBJECTIVES

On completion of Unit One, the medical assistant student should be able to:

1. Define and pronounce the vocabulary terms.
2. State the primary purpose of infection control systems.
3. State why Body Substance Precautions (BSP) or Universal Precautions provide protection for all patients and health care workers.
4. List at least 12 situations when handwashing must occur.
5. State the most important function of handwashing.
6. State the purpose of wearing gloves. List at least seven situations when masks or face shields and protective eyewear should be worn by the health care provider.
7. Discuss the steps to follow if the glove(s) you are wearing is/are accidently torn or damaged.
8. Describe situations when masks or face shields and protective eyewear should be worn by the health care provider.
9. List three situations when a health care provider should wear a gown or a long-sleeved laboratory coat. State the reason why it would be worn in these situations.
10. Describe 12 procedures recommended for discarding and disposing of used needles and other sharps.
11. Describe and discuss eight procedures and techniques to follow for handling and transporting laboratory specimens. Include a description of how these specimens should be labeled.
12. Explain what to do with reusable equipment after use.
13. Explain how to dispose of broken glassware.
14. List at least five substances and/or items that should be treated as infectious waste. Discuss how these substances should be handled for disposal.
15. Describe how you should dispose of other waste materials such as paper towels and moist waste materials.
16. Explain how work and environmental surfaces should be cleaned and/or decontaminated.
17. Discuss what should be done with clothing and laundry that has been soiled with body secretions.
18. State the types of labels and signs that must be used to indicate areas and materials that would contain potentially infectious materials.
19. State the cause, signs and symptoms, stages of infection, diseases that may develop, means of transmission, diagnostic tests, and therapy used for HIV disease.
20. Differentiate between being HIV positive and having AIDS.
21. Become familiar with agencies that can provide up-to-date information on HIV disease.
22. State the cause and signs and symptoms of hepatitis.
23. Differentiate among the five types of hepatitis.
24. Discuss the vaccination for hepatitis B stating for whom it is recommended and how many doses are given.

TERMINAL PERFORMANCE OBJECTIVES

On completion of Unit One, the medical assistant student should be able to:

1. Demonstrate the correct procedures for following and adhering to the federal standards and Universal Precautions as outlined in this unit.
2. Dispose of equipment and specimens according to federal, state, and local standards.
3. Use equipment according to federal, state, and local standards.

The nature and severity of certain infectious diseases (namely, HIV, AIDS, and HBV) have led to the formulation and adoption by medical personnel of what are commonly referred to as the Universal Precautions (also known as the BSP). These standards, first recommended by the CDC, are a vital component and responsibility of many health care workers' everyday activities. The key to Universal Precautions is to handle all blood and body fluids as if known to be infected.

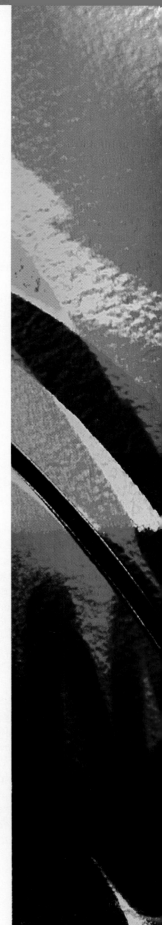

For the purposes of this unit, the following definitions apply according to the Centers For Disease Control and Prevention (CDC) and the Occupational Safety and Health Administration (OSHA).

Aerosol—Dispersion of fine particles into the air.

AIDS—Acquired (not born with) immune (body's defense system) deficiency (not working properly) syndrome (a group of signs and symptoms).

Bloodborne pathogens—Pathogenic microorganisms that are present in human blood and can cause disease in humans. These pathogens include, but are not limited to, hepatitis B virus (HBV) and human immunodeficiency virus (HIV).

Body substance—Any fluid or substance produced by the body that can carry infectious agents (for example, blood, urine, sputum, and stool).

Body Substance Precautions (BSP)—Same as, and used interchangeably with, Universal Precautions. A system focusing on the cautious handling of potentially infectious body substances by using barrier precautions (for example, gloves, masks).

Clinical laboratory—A workplace where diagnostic or other screening procedures are performed on blood or other potentially infectious materials.

Contaminated—The presence or reasonably anticipated presence of blood or other potentially infectious materials on an item or surface.

Contaminated laundry—Laundry that has been soiled with blood or other potentially infectious materials or may contain sharps.

Contaminated sharps—Any contaminated object that can penetrate the skin, including but not limited to needles, scalpels, broken glass, and broken capillary tubes.

Decontamination—The use of physical or chemical means to remove, inactivate, or destroy bloodborne pathogens on a surface or item to the point at which they are no longer capable of transmitting infectious particles and the surface or item is rendered safe for handling, use, or disposal.

Detergents—Chemicals used for cleaning purposes, sometimes used in combination with germicides (for example, LpH and Staphene).

Engineering controls—Controls (for example, sharps disposal containers, self-sheathing needles) that isolate or remove the bloodborne pathogens hazard from the workplace.

Exposure incident—A specific eye, mouth, other mucous membrane, nonintact skin, or parenteral contact with blood or other potentially infectious materials that results from the performance of an employee's duties.

HBV—Hepatitis B virus.

HIV—Human immunodeficiency virus.

Occupational exposure—Reasonably anticipated skin, eye, mucous membrane, or parenteral contact with blood or other potentially infectious materials that may result from the performance of an employee's duties.

Potentially infectious materials
1. Blood—human blood, human blood components, and products made from human blood.
2. The following human body fluids: semen, vaginal secretions, cerebrospinal fluid, synovial fluid, pleural fluid, pericardial fluid, peritoneal fluid, amniotic fluid, saliva in dental procedures, any body fluid that is visibly contaminated with blood, and all body fluids in situations in which it is difficult or impossible to differentiate between body fluids.
3. Any unfixed tissue or organ (other than intact skin) from a human (living or dead).
4. HIV-containing cell or tissue cultures, organ cultures, and HIV- or HBV-containing culture medium or other solutions.

Regulated waste—Liquid or semi-liquid blood or other potentially infectious materials, contaminated items that would release blood or other potentially infectious materials in a liquid or semi-liquid state if compressed, items that are caked with dried blood or other potentially infectious materials and capable of releasing these materials during handling, contaminated sharps, and pathologic and microbiologic wastes containing blood or other potentially infectious materials.

Sterilize—The use of a physical or chemical procedure to destroy all microbial life, including highly resistant bacterial endospores.

Universal Precautions—Same as, and used interchangeably with, Body Substance Precautions (BSP). An approach to infection control. According to the concept of Universal Precautions, all human blood and certain human body fluids are treated as if known to be infectious for HIV, HBV, and other bloodborne pathogens. Also, use of uniform infection control procedures with all patients and in all work situations, on the basis of the degree of exposure risk to body substances, not diagnosis (see page 5).

Waste
1. *Medical waste* (formerly referred to as infectious waste).
   NOTE: The terminology may vary from state-to-state and even from county to county. Check with your local agencies for the terms that they use most frequently.
   a. Laboratory wastes, including cultures of etiologic agents, (disease-producing microorganisms) that pose a substantial threat to health because of volume and virulence.

b. Pathologic specimens, including human tissue, blood elements, excrement, and secretions that contain etiologic agents, and attendant disposable fomites (disposable substances that can absorb and transport infectious microorganisms).

c. Surgical specimens, including human parts and tissue removed surgically or at autopsy, which in the opinion of the attending physician contain etiologic agents and attendant disposable fomites.

d. Sharps (needles, sharp disposable instruments, and glass slides). Sharps means any device having acute rigid corners, edges, or protuberances capable of cutting or piercing.

e. Liquid body substances such as blood, urine, bile, vomitus, or other secretions/excretions, and stool.

NOTE: The Environmental Protection Agency (EPA) estimates that about 15% of all medical waste is infectious. Infectious waste is defined as any waste capable of producing an infectious disease.

2. *Contaminated waste* is all moist waste, including products that have been in contact with the patient's body fluids or wastes that might attract vermin (for example, tongue blades; diapers; urine cups; moist, blood-stained dressings; nonsharp disposable instruments; and good wastes).

3. *Other wastes* are paper material and other office materials.

OR

4. *Nonmedical waste.* Waste not defined as "medical/biohazardous" (items such as paper towels, paper products, articles containing nonfluid blood, and other medical solid waste products commonly found in medical facilities.

a. Most patient care clinic and surgery waste such as dressings, disposable diapers, intravenous tubing and bags, surgical drapes, and ventilator circuits

b. Office and nonpatient care department waste

c. Kitchen waste

Spills should be cleaned up promptly. Large spills should be cleaned up by a gloved employee, using paper towels, which should be placed in an infectious waste container (Figure 1-1). Then 5.25% sodium hypochlorite (household bleach) diluted 1:10 should be used to disinfect the area. Sodium hypochlorite should not be placed directly on large amounts of protein matter (for example, urine, stool, blood, sputum) to protect the employee from noxious fumes. A 1:10 dilution of bleach may be ordered for the office or clinic from a hospital pharmacy.

- Laboratory work surfaces should be decontaminated with a disinfectant such as a 1:10 dilution of sodium hypochlorite or Staphene germicide solution at the completion of work activities or in the event of a specimen spill.
- Regular cleaning of diapering areas is recommended because of the potential for fecal or orally transmitted agents.
- Environmental surfaces in patient care areas should be cleaned with an approved disinfectant weekly and as needed.
- Periodic cleaning of the clinic or office environment is good housekeeping rather than an infection control concern.
- Materials used for cleanup should be disposed of in a covered, moist infectious waste container.
- Covers on examination tables and Mayo stands must be changed after each patient.
- At the end of the day, examination tables, counters, Mayo stands, and other equipment should be decontaminated with a disinfectant solution (for example, LpH solution).

- Supply closets should be dusted and cleaned at least monthly, using a rag saturated with 70% alcohol to wipe the shelves, then allowing the shelves to air dry. The door to the room should be left open while this procedure is in progress to avoid any side effects from fumes.
- Janitorial staff must be taught how to handle and dispose of ordinary, contaminated, and infectious waste.

Figure 1-1 *Spills of body fluids must be cleaned up by a gloved employee, using paper towels, which should then be placed in an infectious waste container. Afterwards, 5.25% sodium hypochlorite (household bleach) diluted 1:10 should be used to disinfect the area.*

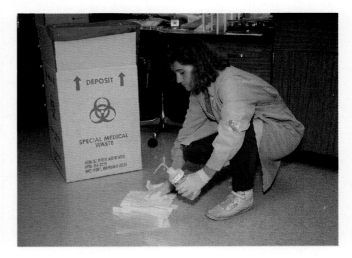

UNIFORMS AND CLOTHING

Uniforms and clothing that are soiled with body secretions should be cleaned with soap and cool water and washed, following normal laundering procedures. Clothing with large amounts of contaminates or that has been penetrated should be changed immediately or as soon as possible.

LAUNDRY

1. Contaminated laundry should be handled as little as possible, with a minimum of agitation.
   a. Contaminated laundry should be bagged or containerized without sorting or rinsing it at the location where it was used.
   b. Contaminated laundry should be placed and transported in bags or containers labeled or color-coded (Figure 1-2). When a facility uses Universal Precautions in the handling of all soiled laundry, alternative labeling or color-coding may be used if all employees recognize the containers as requiring compliance with Universal Precautions.
   c. Whenever contaminated laundry is wet and presents a reasonable likelihood of soaking through or leaking from the bag or container, the laundry should be placed and transported in bags or containers that prevent leakage.
2. The employer must ensure that employees who have contact with contaminated laundry wear protective gloves and other appropriate personal protective equipment.
3. When a facility ships contaminated laundry off-site to a second facility that does not use Universal Precautions in all laundry handling, the facility generating the contaminated laundry must place such laundry in labeled or color-coded bags or containers.

Figure 1-2 *Contaminated laundry should be placed and transported in bags or containers labeled or color-coded.*

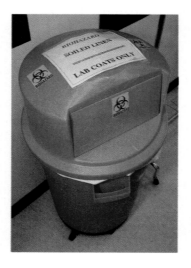

COMMUNICATIONS OF HAZARDS TO EMPLOYEES

LABELS
- Warning labels must be affixed to containers of regulated waste; refrigerators and freezers containing blood or other potentially infectious material; and other containers used to store, transport, or ship blood or other potentially infectious materials, except as stated below.
- Labels required by this standard must include the legend "BIOHAZARD" (Figure 1-3).
- The labels must be fluorescent orange or orange-red or predominantly so, with lettering or symbols in a contrasting color.
- Labels required must be affixed as close as feasible to the container by string, wire, adhesive, or other method that prevents their loss or unintentional removal.
- Red bags or red containers may be substituted for labels.
- Individual containers of blood or other potentially infectious materials that are placed in a labeled container during storage, transport, shipment, or disposal are exempt from the labeling requirement.
- Labels required for contaminated equipment must be in accordance with this paragraph and must also state which portion of the equipment remains contaminated.
- Regulated waste that has been decontaminated does not need to be labeled or color-coded.

SIGNS
- The employer must post signs at the entrance of work areas specified as HIV and HBV Research Laboratory and Production Facilities. These signs must bear the legend "BIOHAZARD" and state the name of the infectious agent; the special requirements for entering the area; and the name and telephone number of the laboratory director or other responsible person.
- These signs must be fluorescent orange-red or predominately so, with lettering or symbols in a contrasting color.

Figure 1-3 *Biohazard label.*

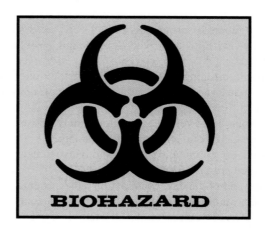

DISPOSAL

In the physician's office or clinic, a registered hazardous waste company picks up waste containers for proper disposal according to the standards set by the law. A qualified company can be found by asking another employee or looking in the yellow pages of your telephone book under "WASTE DISPOSAL—MEDICAL AND INFECTIOUS." Methods of treatment of medical waste are specified by law. Biohazardous waste cannot be disposed of without prior treatment, which is both costly and complicated.

COMPLIANCE

Universal Precautions must be observed to prevent contact with blood or other potentially infectious materials. Under circumstances in which it is difficult or impossible to differente between body fluid types, all body fluids must be considered potentially infectious materials.

Universal Precautions against transmission of blood-borne pathogens in the health care workplace are no longer just recommended—**they are law**. OSHA issued a federal standard on December 2, 1991.

The regulations covered by this standard apply to employees of facilities where a worker could be "reasonably anticipated" to come in contact with blood or other potentially infectious materials, including body fluids, saliva, and tissue. When it is difficult or impossible to differentiate between body fluid types, all body fluids shall be considered potentially infectious materials.

All health care facilities had to comply with the new blood-borne pathogen standard by July 6, 1992.

Each state must develop its own law, using these standards as guidelines. The federal regulation requires the following:

- A written infection control plan with a policies and procedure manual must be developed by every health care facility. It must be updated annually and made accessible to employees. This exposure control plan must also describe workplace risks, workers at risk, and how workers are trained and protected.
- Training and education in Universal Precautions must be provided annually for employees.
- Hepatitis B vaccinations must be offered within 10 days of employment to all employees who have occupational exposure at no cost to the employee. If employees decline the vaccinations, they must sign a form that indicates this decision. The vaccination must be made available to the employees at no cost if they decide to receive it at a later date.
- Records must be kept on each employee's training, occupational injuries, and vaccinations for at least 30 years.
- Personal protective equipment must be provided at no cost to the employee. Examples of protective equipment include gloves, masks and gowns.
- Engineering controls such as puncture-resistant containers for used needles must be in place.

- Work practice controls such as handwashing must be enforced.
- Biohazard signs must be posted.
- Warning labels must be used.
- Medical treatment and counseling must be made available to exposed employees.

Everyone has a responsibility to make these regulations work. The employer must provide the information and equipment, and the employee must use it.

The Universal Precautions, standards, and guidelines are presented in the beginning of this textbook because they are an integral part of many procedures and activities that you will study in other units. It is vital that you understand these principles, adhere to them at all times, and practice them until they become second nature. The Universal Precautions, or BSP, are to protect you and the patient against infectious conditions that could prove fatal. Their importance to you as a member of the health care team cannot be overemphasized.

Read this unit *very carefully,* make sure that you understand it completely, and practice and follow these guidelines diligently throughout your program of study and in your future career. There is an old saying: "The life you save may be your own." Keep this in mind as you practice these principles and precautions. It may help you realize the significance and role they play in combatting the spread of infectious disease. It may also influence your habits and techniques if you are ever tempted to take short cuts or use easier, less time-consuming techniques.

The spread and nature of infectious disease, the causative microorganisms, the body's defenses against disease and infection, immunity, immunizations, infection control, and the principles and techniques of medical asepsis and sterilization procedures are discussed in Unit Five. It is hoped that presenting the BSP at the beginning of this book will help you relate to the principles and rationales for many of the procedures in other units.

INFECTION CONTROL SYSTEMS

Infection control systems are designed to prevent health care workers from transferring infections to patients and from acquiring infections themselves. Infection precautions previously used were based on diagnosis. Universal Precautions improve on the traditional systems because they protect workers during the period before a patient's diagnosis is known. Sometimes it is not possible to tell by looking if a patient is infectious; and it is not practical to test all patients for all possible infections, nor is it timely because exposure would occur before test results are obtained. Pathologic agents may be present in body substances, even if they are not known to be present, and they may be transmitted from ostensibly clinically healthy individuals.

Universal Precautions are designed for use with all patients, not just those who are identified as infected. They are based on the knowledge of how diseases are transmitted and how disease transmission is prevented and on degree of exposure risk to blood and other body substances rather than on diagnosis, and precautions should be based on the degree of risk.

Universal Precautions should always include routine use of appropriate barrier precautions to prevent skin and mucous membrane exposure when contact with the patient's blood or other body substances is anticipated. Because all patients and laboratory specimens are considered possibly infected, Universal Precautions provide protection not only from known infected cases but also from unrecognized cases, therefore protecting patients and health care workers alike.

Health care workers who have weeping dermatitis or exudative lesions should not take part in direct patient care and should not handle patient-care equipment until the condition is resolved.

The following is in accordance with recommendations from the U.S. Public Health Service, CDC, and OSHA.

BARRIER PRECAUTIONS

The following barrier precautions should be used (Figure 1-4).

HANDWASHING

Body substances that may contain disease microorganisms easily contaminate health care givers' hands. If these microorganisms enter an opening in the body (for example, the mouth), infection can occur. Handwashing is one of the most effective means of infection control.

Handwashing should occur:
* Before eating or preparing food, drinking, smoking, applying cosmetics or lip balm, or handling contact lenses.
* Before performing clean or sterile invasive procedures.
* Before and after performing a clinical procedure.
* Before and after assisting a physician with a clinical procedure.
* Before and after touching wounds or other drainage.
* After coming in contact with blood or body fluids, mucous membranes, secretions, or excretions such as saliva, urine, and feces.
* After handling soiled linen or waste.
* After handling devices or equipment soiled with body substances (for example, urine collection containers).
* After removing gloves or other personal protective equipment such as masks, goggles, face shields, gowns, aprons, and caps.
* After using the toilet.
* After nose-blowing or coughing into the hands.
* Between each patient contact.

The most important function of handwashing is to remove infectious organisms. No handwashing product on the market kills all disease-causing organisms. Physical removal (that is, washing soil and organisms down the drain) is the most effective practice for removing infectious organisms. Soap-impregnated towelettes should be used *only* in the field, where handwashing facilities are not available; towelettes

Figure 1-4 *Category-specific precautions.* **A,** *Blood/body fluid precautions;* **B,** *drainage/secretion precautions;* **C,** *enteric precautions.*
A to C Courtesy Brevis Corp., SLC, UT.

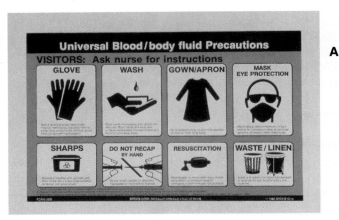

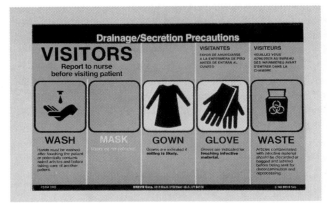

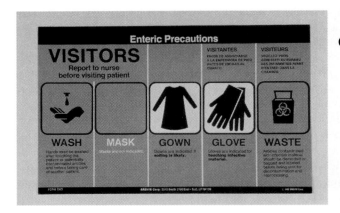

should not be substituted for soap and water in the office or clinic except during an internal disaster. Other chemicals such as alcohol or bleach should not be used for handwashing; they may damage skin and cause open or chapped areas, which are more easily infected.

Skin can become dry and chapped with frequent handwashing. Lotion used after handwashing helps replace the oils removed during handwashing. Hands must always be washed before using lotion. Using a lotion bottle while hands are dirty is likely to contaminate the lotion container and thereafter each user's hands. Claims that medicated lotions control this problem have proven less than satisfactory in test data. Each health care giver should use his or her own bottle of lotion, which can be left in a locker or other convenient location, and the user should be aware if the lotion becomes contaminated. Community lotion bottles should not be left in staff bathrooms (see the procedure for handwashing on page 184).

OSHA's federal regulations state that employers must provide handwashing facilities that are readily accessible to the employees. They must also ensure that employees wash their hands and any other skin with soap and water or flush mucous membranes with water immediately or as soon as feasible after contact of body areas with blood or other potentially infectious materials.

PERSONAL PROTECTIVE EQUIPMENT

GLOVES

Gloves give the health care provider additional protection beyond that of intact skin and handwashing. Gloves should be worn whenever contact with blood or other body fluids or tissue is expected. Both vinyl and latex gloves are suitable for patient care activities, and each has a 95% effectiveness rate. All gloves tear with heavy or prolonged use. Torn gloves should be replaced as soon as patient safety permits.

Hypoallergenic gloves, glove liners, powderless gloves, or other similar alternatives must be readily accessible for employees who are allergic to the gloves normally provided.

According to the FDA, an alarming number of health care workers (approximately 6% to 14%) have developed latex sensitivity or allergies as a result of the increased use of latex products in health care settings. Health care workers should be told that wearing latex gloves agrees with most people, but that some people have a reaction to them. Hypersensitive persons may experience local reactions such as contact dermatitis or contact urticarial syndrome (hives). Some develop more severe contact and systemic reactions and may react anaphylactically. (Anaphylactic shock is a severe and sometimes fatal systemic hypersensitivity reaction to a sensitizing substance. It is commonly marked by vascular collapse and respiratory distress, which can occur seconds or minutes after exposure to the allergen. Other symptoms may include nausea, diarrhea, hypotension, laryngeal edemas, arrhythmia, respiratory congestion, and shock.) If the health care worker experiences any of these symptoms, vinyl gloves should be worn. Some hypoallergenic gloves on the market still have a moderate amount of antigen content, which could cause a reaction in a person. If the health care worker starts to have a reaction, he or she must see the Employee Health Practitioner or the physician in the medical office or clinic, who will give advice on how to proceed. A physician from the Mayo clinic in Rochester, Minn., advises that any person who has a severe hypersensitivity to latex wear a medical identification tag indicating this fact, because in emergency situations rescue personnel wear latex gloves. Determining what component of latex triggers the allergy is a problem. Additional studies are being conducted by the CDC in Atlanta.

Gloves should be worn for the following procedures:
* When touching blood and body fluids, mucous membranes, or nonintact skin of all patients
* When handling items or surfaces moist with blood or body fluids and substances
* When performing venipuncture or other vascular access procedures
* When working with blood or specimens containing blood, body fluids, excretions, and secretions
* When cleansing reusable instruments and equipment; wear heavy rubber gloves over disposable gloves, a plastic apron or gown, and safety glasses, goggles, or personal glasses with solid side shields added when involved in decontamination activities of instruments and equipment
* When decontaminating areas contaminated with body substances
* When cleaning up blood spills and other contaminated areas; small spills should be wiped up with disposable absorbent towels; any broken glass should be scooped up with several paper towels and disposed of in a red sharps container; finally, the area should be mopped with a disinfectant; large blood spills also should be mopped up with a disinfectant
* *Sterile gloves* should be worn for all sterile procedures to protect both the patient and the care provider.
* *Nonsterile* gloves can be worn for nonsterile patient care procedures when worker protection is needed.
* *Finger cots or gloves* should be worn while working to cover cuts, abrasions, rashes, or minor infections on the hands.
* If a glove is torn or punctured by a needlestick or other accident, the damaged glove should be removed, hands rewashed, and a new glove put on as promptly as patient safety permits.
* If gloves are contaminated, the care provider should not touch telephone receivers, other uncontaminated surfaces, or other areas of the same patient's body that may be uncontaminated.
* **Care providers must change gloves between patients and wash hands immediately after glove removal.**
* Gloves always should be removed when answering the telephone, opening a door or drawer, handling a record book or worksheet, and performing other clean procedures.
* Handwashing remains the most effective infection control procedure. Glove use, as described, is used to augment the barrier provided by intact skin against infectious agents. But gloves can transport infectious agents from one person to another or to the mouth as easily as ungloved hands; therefore these policies are not to be interpreted as replacing the need for handwashing.

- Disposable gloves (single-use gloves) must not be washed or decontaminated for re-use.
- Utility gloves may be decontaminated for re-use if the integrity of the glove is not compromised. However, they must be discarded if they are cracked, peeling, torn, or punctured; if they exhibit other signs of deterioration; or when their ability to function as a barrier is compromised.

MASKS AND PROTECTIVE EYEWEAR

Masks and protective eyewear should be worn (1) to prevent exposure of the care provider's mucous membranes of the mouth, nose, and eyes during procedures that are likely to generate aerosol droplets or splashes of blood or other body fluids, and (2) when cleaning equipment that may have disease-producing microorganisms on it. Masks should cover both the nose and the mouth and fit close to the face so that air can be breathed only through the mask. Care providers should not loosen the mask. Over time, a mask becomes impregnated with moisture from the breath, and it is harder to breathe through the mask. When this occurs, the mask should be changed—not loosened. Masks should be discarded after each use or when they become damp. They are treated as regular, not infectious, waste.

Protective eyewear such as personal glasses (with solid side shields added), goggles, safety glasses, or face shields, should be worn to protect the face from any splashes (Figure 1-5). Procedures in which eyewear might be needed include certain diagnostic procedures such as endoscopies or any invasive surgical procedure, and when cleaning and decontaminating reusable instruments and equipment. Face shields are best suited for nonpatient care activities such as sorting laundry. After use, undamaged eyewear must be washed with soap and water and then dried before it is used again.

GOWNS, APRONS, AND LABORATORY COATS

A gown, apron, or laboratory coat should be worn to protect the arms and clothes during all procedures that are likely to generate splashes or soiling from blood or body fluids. The care provider should wear a gown when cleaning noncontaminated equipment, when cleaning and decontaminating reusable instruments and equipment, and when performing procedures involving contact with large amounts of patient substances. When performing laboratory procedures, the care provider should wear either a long-sleeved gown with a closed front or a long-sleeved laboratory coat buttoned shut. The gown or laboratory coat should be removed when leaving the laboratory area. Care providers should change a gown or laboratory coat immediately if it becomes contaminated with blood or body fluids and at other appropriate periods to ensure cleanliness. Contaminated gowns and laboratory coats

Figure 1-5 *Wearing protective eyewear and face masks.* **A,** *Goggles;* **B,** *safety glasses;* **C,** *face shields;* **D,** *face mask.*

A

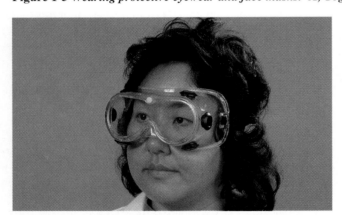

B

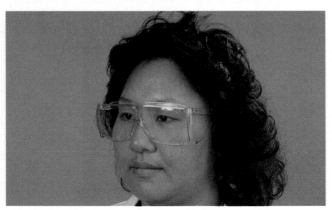

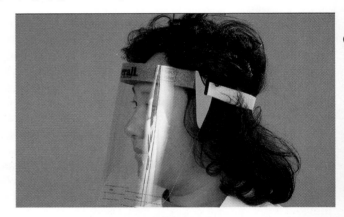

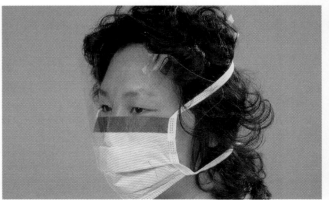

should be placed in a biohazard bag for sending to the appropriate laundry as arranged by the facility. If laboratory gowns or coats are contaminated with a microbiologic agent because of a laboratory accident, the gown or coat should be sterilized in the steam sterilizer before it is sent to the laundry.

Disposable plastic aprons should be worn if there is a significant probability that blood or body fluids may be splashed. After the task is completed, the disposable apron, if contaminated, should be discarded in a biohazard container or sterilized in the steam sterilizer before it is discarded as ordinary waste. Used laboratory wear should never be stored with street clothes.

VENTILATION DEVICES

Mouthpieces, resuscitation bags, pocket masks, or other ventilation devices should be available to use in areas where the need for resuscitation is predictable. Use these devices instead of mouth-to-mouth resuscitation on all patients.

HANDLING OF EQUIPMENT, SUPPLIES, AND WASTE

There are specific procedures for handling equipment, supplies, and waste taken from patient care areas and the laboratory and for caring for environmental surfaces.

NEEDLES AND OTHER SHARPS

Needles, scalpel blades, and any other sharps that can easily puncture the skin must be handled with extreme caution to prevent infection with HIV and hepatitis. Most needlesticks happen when used needles are not handled properly. Broken skin or mucous membrane contact and a needlestick or other blood-to-blood accident can transmit infection. The following procedures must be adhered to prevent any undue infection.

1. Place used disposable needles and syringes, scalpel blades, and other sharp items in a rigid, puncture-resistant disposable container with a lid (needle container) that is easily recognized (for example, a red container) and clearly marked as a biohazard (Figure 1-6). Preferably, the container should be made of rigid plastic and must be leakproof on the sides and bottom. Do not use cardboard or paper containers. Never put needles or sharps in the trash or linen. This is dangerous to others.

2. Locate puncture-resistant containers as close as practical to the area where needles and other sharps are used. The sharps containers should be located in each treatment room, at each laboratory table, and at any other area where syringes, needles, and slides are used in the office or clinic.

3. Keep needle containers upright throughout use and at a level where the top opening can be seen. Needles should not project from the top of the container.

4. *Never* try to take anything out of a needle box. If a needle will not go in easily and the box is not full, use a large syringe to dislodge it. Do not push or force items with your hands. If the box is full, arrange to have it replaced.

5. Place the cover to close, seal the sharps container when it is three-fourths full and dispose of the container as infectious waste. No additional protective garb is necessary for handling these containers. One method of disposing of full sharps containers is to place the full container in a brown cardboard box labeled "Infectious Waste and Biohazard" and marked with the biohazard symbol. This box is lined with plastic sheating or a strong, red plastic bag marked "Biohazardous Material." The disposal box should be located in a centralized, authorized area. A contract scavenger company should then pick up the sealed boxes and deliver them to an incineration company on a weekly basis.

6. Pick up improperly discarded needles with extreme caution and dispose of them in the nearest sharps container. Do not attempt to cap the needle. Wash your hands after you dispose of the needle. Use tongs or forceps to pick up the sharps.

7. *Never* purposely bend or break by hand a used needle. *Never* recap a used needle unless absolutely necessary or in approved special circumstances (for example, in drawing blood for blood gases). To recap vacutainer needles, put the cap on the table and slide the needle into it without holding the cap. Then tighten the cap at the needle hub.

8. *Never* remove a used needle from a used disposable syringe (*except* as discussed in No. 10).

9. *Never* put a used needle into your pocket.

10. Wear gloves when doing laboratory work in which a needle needs to be removed from a syringe. Discard the gloves immediately if they become contaminated with blood. It is preferable to use a needle disposal container that has an integral device for removing needles without necessitating touching the needles with your hands.

11. Discard vacutainer sleeves in the sharps container at the end of each day or when they are soiled with blood.

Figure 1-6 *Samples of easily recognized, rigid, puncture-resistant disposable containers with a lid and clearly marked as a biohazard.*

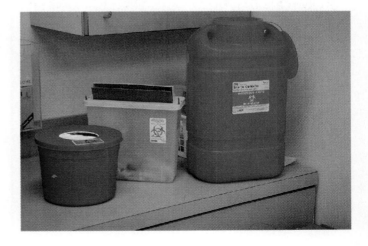

12. Place *reusable sharps* in a suitable puncture-resistant container after use and take them to the decontamination area, where they are cleaned and disinfected or sterilized. Wear protective garb such as gowns, aprons, gloves, and face protection while cleaning up.

LABORATORY SPECIMENS

To control the spread of infection and to protect the health of employees, patients, and the public, all laboratory specimens should be handled and transported according to the following procedures:

1. Specimens of blood or other potentially infectious materials must be placed in a container that prevents leakage during collection, handling processing, storage, transport, or shipping.

2. Laboratory specimens should be contained for transport. Special secure, stiff, impermeable containers such as the igloo-type containers should be used by messenger service personnel when transporting blood and other body fluids from the office or clinic to a laboratory. Specimen containers may be placed in test tube racks, then in the secure transport container. Some facilities also require that the specimen be placed in a Ziploc or other band-sealed plastic bag and sealed shut before being placed in the secure transport container for delivery to the laboratory. If the specimen container is too large to fit in a sealable plastic bag, the cap can be secured with tape and the entire item enclosed in a plastic bag with a twist tie. The laboratory work slip should be attached by rubber band or tape to the outside of the bag.

    Specimen mailers must have a metal inner container and a rigid outer container to comply with CDC regulations (see Figures 11-1 and 11-2).

3. The container for storage, transport, or shipping must be labeled or color-coded according to federal standards and closed before being stored, transported, or shipped.

4. If outside contamination of the primary container occurs, the primary container must be placed within a second container that prevents leakage during handling, processing, storage, transport, or shipping and is labeled or color-coded according to the requirements of OSHA standards.

5. All blood or body fluid specimens must be centrifuged in carriers with safety domes. The carrier and dome must be decontaminated according to the manufacturer's direction. Human tissue, blood, body secretions and excretions, or other specimens and cultures should be autoclaved before they are disposed of in a sanitary landfill.

6. Gloves should be used for handling laboratory specimens when contamination of the hands is anticipated. Care must be taken when collecting specimens to avoid contamination of the outside of the container or the laboratory slip. Put on disposable gloves and dispose of urine specimens in a toilet or utility sink and feces into toilets that empty into a sewer system.

Sinks should then be rinsed thoroughly and toilets flushed. (To avoid cross-contamination, this sink should *not* be used for other activities such as preparing clean supplies or supplying drinking water. Other sinks should be used for routine handwashing.) Dispose of specimen containers and gloves in a closed waste container lined with a strong plastic or vinyl bag marked "Biohazardous Waste."

7. Hands must be washed after handling all specimens and after removing gloves. Hands and other skin surfaces contaminated with blood or other body fluids must be washed immediately and thoroughly. When procedures have been completed or if a specimen is spilled, laboratory work surfaces must be decontaminated with a disinfectant such as a 1:10 dilution of sodium hypochlorite (household bleach) or Staphene germicide solution.

8. All potentially contaminated materials used in laboratory tests should be decontaminated, preferably by steam sterilization, before disposal or reprocessing. All infectious laboratory waste should be treated by steam sterilization, incineration, or disinfection before disposal to render the waste harmless. Promptly contact your supervisor when you have been exposed to blood or other body fluids.

REUSABLE EQUIPMENT

As soon as possible, if appropriate, all reusable equipment not classified as sharps should be placed in an EPA-approved detergent such as Hemosol or Coleo and transported to the decontamination area. Items that require sterilization or high-level disinfection first must be thoroughly cleaned and decontaminated. Cleaning and decontamination should be done by personnel wearing gloves, gown, and face protection. Each facility must develop cleaning and decontamination procedures appropriate to its needs.

Blood pressure equipment, scales, and other reusable room equipment should be decontaminated with a disinfectant solution at the end of each day. Stethoscope earpieces must be cleaned after each use with an alcohol swab. Tonometers must be disinfected with alcohol swabs, rinsed thoroughly in clean water, and then left to air dry or be dried with a clean nonlint material after *each* use. When visibly soiled or at least weekly, centrifuges should be cleaned with 70% alcohol swabs or disposable cloths soaked in 70% alcohol or LpH solution mixed according to the product's directions. Tourniquets can be soaked in a 1:10 dilution of 5% sodium hypochlorite solution for 15 minutes. Bloodstained tourniquets must be discarded. After each use, goggles and heavy rubber gloves used during decontamination procedures must be decontaminated with a detergent solution, rinsed, and then placed in an area specifically designated for such supplies. This equipment should be sterilized weekly.

BROKEN GLASSWARE

Broken glassware that might be contaminated must not be picked up directly with the hands. It must be cleaned up, using mechanical means such as a brush and dust pan, tongs, or forceps and then disposed of in a puncture-resistant container that is labeled or color-coded to indicate that it is for contaminated sharps.

TISSUES, BODY FLUIDS, AND CULTURES

- Patient specimens and the containers that hold them should be collected and treated as infectious waste.
- Cultures and the containers that hold them should be collected and treated as infectious waste.
- Human tissues or body parts should be treated as infectious waste.
- Large volumes of blood or drainage such as that from suction machines should be flushed down the sewer or disposed of in collection containers and treated as infectious waste.
- Used disposable dialysis equipment should be treated as infectious waste.
- Large volumes of urine, stool, or dialysate should be flushed down the sewer with appropriate precautions to guard against spillage.

While awaiting transport for disposal, infectious waste must be held in covered or bagged, leakproof waste containers. It must be collected in identifiable containers or bags for transportation to a separate disposal site. If disposal cans without working lids are used, moist trash must be bagged before it is placed in an open can. All trash containers must have a liner thick enough to withstand necessary handling, and they must be tied closed when disposed of. Waste containers should be cleaned weekly with a disinfectant solution.

OTHER WASTE

All other waste such as paper towels and packaging materials should be placed in regular waste containers lined with plastic or vinyl liners strong or thick enough to withstand necessary handling. For convenience, small items such as contaminated cotton balls may be disposed of in the sharps container. Other disposable, moist waste generated by clinics or offices should be collected in *covered* foot-operated cans that are lined with moisture-proof bags. When removed, the bags should be closed, not emptied, and disposed of as ordinary waste.

Each waste container liner must be removed as a single unit and tied shut without turning the container upside down to consolidate waste. Waste containers must be strong enough to resist tears and leaks under normal handling. Final disposal of waste is by approval of the local health officers and includes incineration, autoclaving, sewer system, or sanitary landfill.

SURFACES

- When body fluids are spilled, the visible material should be removed from surfaces followed by decontamination processes with an approved disinfectant such as a 1:10 dilution of sodium hypochlorite (household bleach) or Bytech solution. Gloves must be worn for this process.

UNIVERSAL SPILLS

Blood and body substances and rebag or collection vessels containing potentially virulent body fluids spilled on floors or work surfaces need quick action. A universal spill kit or treatment system gives medical assistants quick access to protection and containment of the spill. It should contain fog-free goggles and clear safety glasses with sideshields, gowns, masks, antimicrobial towels, and disposal bags. Liquid treatment systems may use microencapsulated technology that converts the liquid spill into a solid treated waste product that can be incinerated or disposed of in landfills. They are biodegradable, nontoxic, and nonflammable. All supplies should be in a readily accessible location and replenished promptly after use.

MERCURY SPILLS

Uncontained mercury (Hg) emits dangerous mercury vapors. A broken sphygmomanometer or thermometer must be quickly and safely cleaned up to prevent toxic vapor contamination. A mercury spill kit includes sponges, towels, liquid, or wipes containing a powder coating that consumes its own weight in mercury and is used to decontaminate an area after a mercury spill and amalgamate small mercury droplets. The resulting amalgam won't emit dangerous mercury vapors. The powder also converts elemental mercury on work surfaces, cracks, and other hard-to-reach areas in a mercury amalgam. For suspected mercury presence, a mercury indicator powder changes color overnight (for example, yellow to brown), when it comes in contact with mercury metal or vapor. It is sprinkled over surfaces suspected to contain mercury droplets and reduces the concentration of mercury vapor remaining in inaccessible areas after cleanup of spills. Gloves, eye wear, and personal protection equipment, including a mercury vapor chlorine respirator to protect against mercury vapor concentrations are other important considerations to ensure proper handling of mercury. A mercury recovery disposal bag safely contains the mercury and everything used to safely clean up mercury spills.

To avoid possible hazardous mercury spills, electric digital clinical thermometers or aeronoidal sphygmomanometers can replace the mercurial type.

EMPLOYEE HEALTH ISSUES

NEEDLESTICKS, MUCOUS MEMBRANE, OR CONJUNCTIVAL EXPOSURE TO BODY FLUIDS FROM AIDS PATIENTS

All needlesticks and other exposures to body fluids from AIDS patients must be reported to the physician and to the Employee Health Service if working at a hospital clinic. An accident report should be filled out. The employee is evaluated as for hepatitis B exposure and treated accordingly. Gamma globulin is given as a part of this protocol. An employee with exposure must receive counseling by the physician or Employee Health Service and information regarding the availability of antibody testing for those who wish it.

INDIVIDUALS WITH IMMUNOSUPPRESSION

Individuals with immunosuppression as a result of disease or therapy should evaluate, with their personal physicians, their own risk of work in a hospital environment. If these individuals think they are at risk, they should provide a letter from their physician to their supervisor indicating their ability to work and outlining any patient care areas in which they should not work.

EMPLOYEES WITH AIDS

Employees with AIDS should be handled on a case-by-case basis by an Employee Health physician in consultation with an AIDS Clinic physician. The final decision regarding work assignment is made by the Infection Control Committee using advice from Employee Health and AIDS Clinic physicians on a case-by-case basis, taking into account the safety of all employees and patients. Generally, asymptomatic office, clinic, or hospital employees with AIDS who have recovered from an intercurrent illness may return to work. They would be instructed about health care precautions such as handwashing and wearing gloves for contact with mucous

membranes or nonintact skin of patients. Any employee with exudative or weeping (that is, moist) skin lesions should be reassigned to nonpatient care areas. Evaluation of such employees is by the physician or the Employee Health Service of the hospital.

In situations in which it is not advisable for employees with AIDS to return to their clinical assignment, reassignment to another area should be coordinated with their supervisors.

CARDIOPULMONARY RESUSCITATION

Devices to protect employees from mucous membrane contact with blood and other secretions during any resuscitation should be made readily available. Ambu bags (Figure 1-7) should be on all crash carts and are to be used in preference to mouth-to-mouth resuscitation on all patients.

Cardiopulmonary resuscitation (CPR) recertification standards should be maintained. Since the AIDS agent is in saliva and since blood may be present in saliva, employees with AIDS should not participate in manikin CPR training. For the protection of all CPR participants in two-person CPR, the second rescuer simulates ventilation, and a solution of bleach is used to decontaminate the manikin's face and mouth between all participants.

NOTE: Precautions beyond those recommended should be avoided because their use does not afford additional protection and may interfere with patient care. Health care workers

OTHER DISEASES IN AIDS PATIENTS

PRECAUTIONS	RATIONALE
Cytomegalovirus (CMV) 1. Pregnant women should not give direct care to excretors of CMV. Women trying to become pregnant should use very good personal hygiene (handwashing and gloves) with any body secretions from any patient.	*Many AIDS patients excrete CMV. Because CMV may cause birth defects, it is advisable for pregnant women not to have direct contact with known excretors. Although proper hygiene has been shown to prevent acquisition of CMV, the standard community practice is for pregnant women to be excused from the care of any known CMV excretor. Pregnant women should be extremely cautious in the care of any patient, because not all CMV excretors are identified. Handwashing is extremely important after any patient or body fluid contact.*
Opportunistic and Other Infections 1. Masks (worn by others in the room when the patient cannot wear a mask) when the patient has an undiagnosed pulmonary process and is coughing, and when others have sustained close contact (until tuberculosis is excluded)	*Until the patient's respiratory illness is diagnosed, others need to be protected from diseases spread by the respiratory route. Immunocompetent persons need protection from Mycobacterium avium and Pneumocystis. Although some AIDS patients have CMV in their lungs, it is not known if CMV can be transmitted by the respiratory route.*
2. Other precautions should be as usual for the particular disease. See an Infection Control Manual for guidance.	*There is no evidence that the AIDS virus is spread by the respiratory route. However, since tuberculosis is a cause of pulmonary disease in a small percentage of cases, masks are a prudent precaution until tuberculosis is excluded.*

Figure 1-7 *An Ambu bag should be on all crash carts. The Ambu bag should be used in preference to mouth-to-mouth resuscitation on all patients.*

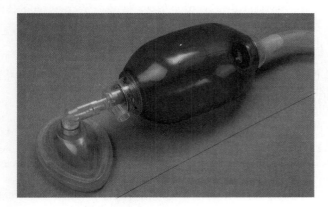

should be well informed about the ways in which HIV and other infectious diseases are transmitted and follow precautions appropriate for their protection. Use of excessive precautions by health care workers conveys misinformation to patients and other employees about the mode of transmission and appropriate precautions.

HIV INFECTION AND DISEASE/AIDS

CDC first defined AIDS in 1982. With incomplete scientific understanding at the time, AIDS was thought of as an immune disorder of unknown origin that led to the development of certain life-threatening opportunistic diseases. As time went on, other diseases were added to the initial list, and a distinction was made between the more and less severe conditions. As research continued, the HIV was isolated, and researchers described the life cycle of the virus, including the latency period during which infection caused by the HIV progresses silently. This led to a critical change in how the scientific community thought of and referred to AIDS. AIDS is now referred to as *HIV disease*; the designations *asymptomatic seropositive, AIDS-related complex (ARC),* and *AIDS* are stages of HIV infection and *not* totally different entities. The new definition of AIDS is clearly associated to the direct role of the HIV in the development of disease(s). Attention is now on the direct effects of the virus on the immune system health rather than on the physical manifestations of these effects. Disease starts at the time of infection, and the virus is active, even if symptoms are not apparent. Because viral activity is better understood, medical treatment can be started earlier. Early intervention has been shown to slow viral activity and disease progression. Early intervention is defined as starting therapy before the onset of AIDS. This prolongs survival and *quality*, disease-free time.

HIV DISEASE

HIV disease is caused by the virus known as human immunodeficiency virus. When the virus gets into a person's bloodstream, the person is HIV infected. The body produces anti-

bodies in response to this invasion and then can be referred to as HIV antibody positive. HIV disease attacks several types of cells in a person's immune system, especially the T cells. The immune system is the body system that helps protect the body against disease by producing antibodies against foreign substances (antigens) (see also Figure 5-3, page 175). When the immune system is weakened, the body loses its ability to fight common infections. Some illnesses can become life-threatening and may even be fatal.

HIV disease refers to all stages of HIV infection.

1. *Asymptomatic HIV disease.* This is the earliest stage of infection. The only indication of this stage of HIV infection is a positive HIV antibody blood test. Antibodies to the HIV can be found in the bloodstream usually from 3 to 6 months from the time the person was infected with the HIV. The person is presumed to be infected with the virus when antibodies are present. It is also assumed that the person can pass the virus on to others through the usual routes of transmission. Most people show no signs of illness at this time.

2. *Symptomatic HIV disease.* This is the middle stage of infection. Many people in this stage experience mild to severe physical symptoms that can't be explained by any other illness. Examples include swollen lymph glands at two or more sites in the body, persistent fever, diarrhea, and/or skin problems.

3. *AIDS.* This is the later stages of the disease when the immune system has been severely damaged by the HIV and can no longer fight some infections. People in this stage may develop one or more opportunistic infections, life-threatening diseases, or other diseases listed in the following paragraphs.

It is very important to understand the difference between being HIV antibody positive and having AIDS. The *incubation period for both stages 2 and 3* could be from several months to 10 years and as long as 13 years.

BROADENED DEFINITION OF AIDS

CDC revised the definition of AIDS in 1985 and 1987 and now again to include the following:

1. People who are HIV positive

2. People who are HIV positive and who have at least one of the 26 reportable opportunistic diseases or other serious diseases. These diseases include:
   a. Kaposi's sarcoma (KS): A sarcoma (cancer) affecting tissues beneath the skin and the mucous-secreting surfaces of the gastrointestinal tract, lymph nodes, and lungs.
   b. *Pneumocystis carinii* pneumonia (PCP): A pneumonia caused by a protozoan.
   c. Cryptococcosis: A fungal infection that may attack the brain, lungs, liver, intestinal tract, and skin.
   d. Non-Hodgkins lymphoma: A cancer affecting the lymph nodes.
   e. Candidiasis: A yeast infection that may be seen in the mouth, anus, genital region, and other areas of the body.

   f. Herpes simplex: A viral infection that may cause blisters or eruptions on the face, buttocks, anus, or genitals.

   g. CMV: A viral infection that frequently has symptoms similar to infectious mononucleosis or may produce no symptoms at all. In the person with AIDS, it can lead to serious infections, including pneumonia.

   h. Toxoplasmosis: A parasitic infection that may involve the brain and cause central nervous system disorders. It frequently shows symptoms of malaise and the flu.

   i. HIV dementia: HIV infection of the brain that may cause personality disintegration, confusion, disorientation, deterioration of intellectual capacity and function, and impairment of memory and judgment.

   j. Progressive multifocal leukoencephalopathy (PLM): This affects the coating of the nerve cells in the brain.

   k. *M. avium* complex (MAC): A bacterial infection.

   l. HIV-related wasting syndrome

   m. Pulmonary tuberculosis: An infection of the lung(s).

   n. Recurrent pneumonia: An infection in the lung(s).

   o. Invasive cervical cancer: Seen in females.

3. *ALL* people who are HIV positive with fewer than 200 T cells per cubic millimeter of blood *even if they do not have an opportunistic infection.*

Physicians consider a T-cell level of less than 200 to be a danger sign for getting AIDS-related disease. This is why it is included in the definition of AIDS. The T cells (also called a T4 cell, a CD4 cell, or a helper cell) help the body fight infections. In a person who is HIV positive, the HIV virus gets into the person's T cells and destroys them. The normal range for T cells is thought to be above 500 cells per cubic millimeter of blood. A *T cell count* is only one of several important tests that can help the physician determine the health of a person who has been diagnosed as HIV positive. Three other tests are available to help measure immune health or reflect the progress of HIV infection. One is the *beta-2 microglobulin test*, which measures the rate at which cells are dying and being replaced by new ones. The higher the number, the greater the degree of cell death. As HIV disease progresses to AIDS, this number goes up. A normal beta-2 number is around 2. A beta-2 number of 4 or 5 is typical of a person who is nearing or already has the diagnosis of AIDS.

A second test is the *p24 antigen test*, which measures the level of the protein p24. This protein is produced by the HIV. People who have been infected for a long period of time usually have significant levels of p24 and are thought to be at a greater risk of progressing to AIDS, but this is not always the case. Some people with AIDS never test positive to p24; thus this test does not always predict what will occur to an individual.

A third test that can be used to determine immune health is the *p24 antibody test.* Having a considerable level of p24 antibody is considered a good sign that the virus is more or less under control, thereby slowing down the action of the HIV. When levels of the p24 antibody drop, it is thought to be a sign that the person is moving closer to AIDS and the virus is becoming more active.

Despite the new broadened definition of AIDS, many believe that it still *does not* give us a total picture of the size of the epidemic because it still does not include some of the serious diseases that HIV-positive women and children can get.

HIV TRANSMISSION

A person can become infected with the HIV in the following ways:

1. Having unprotected vaginal, anal, or oral sexual intercourse with a person infected with HIV. The virus can be transmitted through semen or vaginal fluids.

2. Sharing an intravenous drug needle with an HIV-infected person. The virus can be transmitted to the needle user, injecting infected blood into the bloodstream.

3. Mother-to-child transmission. An HIV woman can transmit the virus to the unborn baby through the placenta; to the baby during birth; or after birth, through infected breast milk.

4. Transfusions with infected blood or blood products. However, since late spring 1985 all blood donations have been screened for HIV antibodies, and donors are also screened for risk factors to ensure that this method of transmission does not occur. **No one can get HIV by donating blood.**

5. Accidental contact with HIV-contaminated blood or body fluids by health care workers as discussed on the preceding pages of this unit.

HIV DISEASE IS NOT TRANSMITTED THROUGH CASUAL CONTACT SUCH AS CLOSE PROXIMITY, TOUCHING, OR SNEEZING.

SIGNS AND SYMPTOMS OF HIV DISEASE

The following are signs and symptoms that an HIV-positive person may experience, *but* they also could be signs and symptoms of diseases totally unrelated to HIV disease. Therefore it is imperative that a person see a physician for an accurate diagnosis and treatment for any troublesome condition.

A person can experience some or all of these signs and symptoms in any order:

1. Easy bruising, bleeding gums, or nose bleeds

2. Fevers greater than 100° F for 10 or more days

3. Dry cough

4. Memory, concentration, speech and/or coordination problems

5. Painful, swollen lymph glands

6. Persistent diarrhea

7. Persistent headaches, numbness, or tingling in the feet or hands

8. Persistent skin problems

9. Persistent vaginal infections

10. Recurrent, drenching night sweats

11. Shortness of breath

12. Sores or unusual blemishes or patches on the tongue or in the mouth

13. Unexplained fatigue that interferes with normal activities

14. Unintentional weight loss greater than 10 pounds

DIAGNOSIS OF HIV INFECTION

A blood test commonly referred to the *HIV or AIDS Antibody test* is used to determine if a person has been infected with the HIV. The technical name for this test is the *ELISA test* (Enzyme-Linked ImmunoSorbent Assay). It is used as the screening test. If the test results are positive, the person is said to be HIV positive or HIV antibody positive. A person who is HIV positive has HIV disease. Another test, the *Western Blot test,* can be performed to confirm the results of the ELISA test.

DRUG THERAPY

Two drugs currently being used for HIV-positive people are AZT (zidovudine) and ddC (HIVID) (zalcitabine). They are not a cure; but they work in similar ways to slow down the progression of HIV in the body. Studies have also shown that, by combining these drugs, the T cell count of the person increases. At this time it is unknown if people receiving both drugs will live longer or get fewer opportunistic diseases.

WORLD AIDS DAY

In 1988 the World Health Organization (WHO) established an annual event to take place on December 1 worldwide. On this special day, called "World AIDS Day," people around the world take special note of the AIDS pandemic. The purpose of this event is to increase public awareness of AIDS, promote participation in prevention efforts, and to disseminate information about the disease. According to the American Association for World Health, at least 10 to 12 million people have been infected with the HIV since the pandemic began. *Each person must fight this disease and the ignorance surrounding it by becoming an informational and educational resource for his or her own community.* Information can be obtained from the following agencies.

- Association of Nurses in AIDS Care, 704 Stony Hill Rd., Ste. 106, Yardley, Pa. 19067
- National AIDS hot line: (800) 342-AIDS
- Spanish AIDS hot line: (800) 344-SIDA
- Hearing-impaired AIDS hot line: (800) 243-7889
- National AIDS Information Clearinghouse: (800) 458-5231
- AIDS Clinical Trials Information Center: (800) TRIALS-A
- Project Inform (information on experimental AIDS drugs): (800) 822-7422
- Drug abuse hot line: (800) 662-HELP
- National Centers for Disease Control and Prevention voice information system: (404) 332-4555

HEPATITIS

Hepatitis is an inflammatory process and infection of the liver caused by a **virus**. There are several forms of this disease because new strains of the virus have appeared in the past 10 years.

HEPATITIS A

Hepatitis A, the less serious form, is usually transmitted by fecal contamination of food and water. The incubation period is 3 to 4 weeks. Gamma globulin is generally used to provide passive immunity. See "Immunity" in Unit Five.

HEPATITIS B

HBV, a potentially fatal disease, is transmitted through contaminated blood, contaminated needles, and also by other body fluids, including semen, saliva, and breast milk. It is of particular concern because of its association with the spread of the HIV infection leading to AIDS. The incubation period averages 60 to 90 days.

Signs and symptoms for both hepatitis A and hepatitis B are similar, but they are more severe for hepatitis B. They may include fever, chills, headache, generalized aches, loss of appetite, nausea, vomiting, dark yellow urine that may have a brownish tinge, diarrhea, clay-colored stools, enlarged and tender liver, and jaundice. If jaundice develops, it is usually first seen in the whites of the eyes and then in the skin.

Diagnosis is based on identifying the virus or the antibodies to the virus or through liver biopsy.

Treatment generally consists of rest and a high-protein diet until the disease runs its course. Treatment is more difficult for hepatitis B, which generally has a more serious prognosis and increased potential for relapse and remission.

Two types of vaccines are available for use in the *prevention* of hepatitis B. One vaccine made from human serum products was developed in 1981, and a synthetic version was developed a few years later. Both are considered safe and effective. Immunization against hepatitis B is recommended for those individuals considered to be at a high risk for the disease (for example, health care practitioners, intravenous drug abusers, people who have many sexual partners, people who require regular blood transfusions, and kidney dialysis patients). A series of three doses is given, the second and third doses given 1 to $1^1/_2$ and 6 months after the first dose. Dosage used varies with the age of the person and the type of vaccine. Many health officials and the CDC suggest that all infants and adolescents be vaccinated for hepatitis B to prevent the disease in the future, which is 100 times more contagious than HIV. The recommendation states that infants receive the first dose of HBV vaccine at birth and the next two doses during their regular immunization schedules. At this time no one knows how long the immunization lasts since the vaccine is relatively new. A booster dose *may* be required for immunized children at a later date. The CDC estimates that approximately 300,000 Americans are infected with HBV each year. Some may develop acute hepatitis and even die from it; about 10% become chronically infected carriers who can pass the disease to others; some develop liver cancer or cirrhosis and die many years after first becoming infected. It is also estimated that over one million people in the United States are carriers of the HBV.

HEPATITIS C

Hepatitis C, traditionally called *non-A, non-B hepatitis,* is the third type of hepatitis identified to date. Symptoms and treatment follow similar patterns to the other forms of the disease. This form of hepatitis accounts for 85% to 90% of the new cases of hepatitis each year.

HEPATITIS D

Hepatitis D or *"delta" hepatitis* is the newest form of the disease. It infects only people who have hepatitis B. Experts believe that this type of hepatitis may have more serious health consequences than any other type. The symptoms are usually more severe than those seen in the other forms of hepatitis. Hepatitis D is most frequently spread through intimate contact with intravenous drug users. Again, treatment consists of rest and a high-protein diet. Antibiotics may be used to resist bacterial infections that could cause additional problems. Vaccines *do not* appear to be effective for hepatitis D.

HEPATITIS E

Hepatitis E is transmitted by ingesting food or water that is contaminated with human feces. Hepatitis E is among the leading causes of acute viral hepatitis in young to middle-aged adults in developing countries. People at greatest risk for acquiring hepatitis E are those exposed to unsanitary conditions in which they may eat and drink contaminated food and water. Epidemics of hepatitis E have been reported in Asia, India, the Middle East, North Africa, and Mexico.

CONCLUSION

The importance of understanding and always adhering to the standards and guidelines given cannot be overemphasized. These standards *must* be used in all aspects of work and practice. Refer to this unit often for review and as a reminder of the significance of disease prevention and precautions. See also Unit Five on Infection Control.

CASE STUDY

The following is an excerpt from a Bloodborne Pathogen Exposure Control Plan for employee training. Read and discuss the italicized terminology.

TRAINING

Training for all employees will be conducted according to *EPA* and *OSHA* guidelines before initial assignment to tasks where *occupational exposure* may occur. Information includes but is not limited to:
1. The *Bloodborne Pathogen Standard*
2. *Epidemiology* and symptoms of bloodborne diseases
3. *Modes* of transmission of bloodborne pathogens
4. *Exposure Control Plan* and its location
5. Methods for recognizing tasks and other activities that may involve exposure to blood and other potentially *infectious materials*
6. Explanation of the use and limitations of methods that will prevent or reduce exposure
7. Information on the types, proper use and location of **Personal Protective Equipment (PPE)**

8. Information on the *Hepatitis B vaccine*, including its efficacy, safety, method of administration, benefits of being vaccinated, and the fact that the vaccine is provided free of charge from *CDC*
9. Information on the appropriate actions to take and whom to contact in an emergency involving blood or other potentially infectious materials
10. An explanation of the procedure to follow if an *exposure incident* occurs, including the method of reporting the incident and the medical follow-up that is made available
11. Information on the *postexposure evaluation* follow-up that is provided to the employee following an exposure incident
12. Explanation of the labels and color coding used to identify a *biohazardous waste*

REVIEW QUESTIONS

1. State why infection control systems were designed.
2. On what are the Body Substance Precautions (BSP) based?
3. What is the most important function of handwashing?
4. State when disposable single-use exam gloves should be worn at your job.
5. State when and why masks and protective eyewear should be worn.

6. State when and why a health care provider should wear a gown or a disposable plastic apron.
7. List ten procedures that must be followed to prevent infection with sharps or needles.
8. Differentiate between being HIV positive and having AIDS.
9. State the cause of HIV disease.
10. List 10 signs and symptoms of hepatitis.

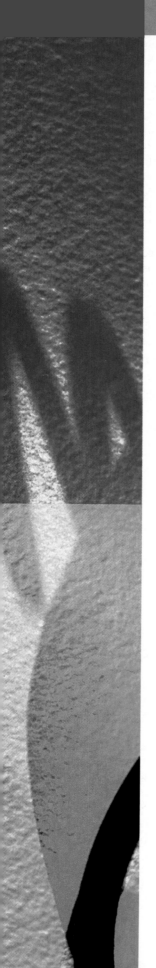

Physical Measurements: Vital Signs, Height, and Weight

COGNITIVE OBJECTIVES

On completion of Unit II, the medical assistant student should be able to:

1. Define the terms vital signs, temperature, pulse, apical heartbeat, respiration rate, and blood pressure and list the normal average values for each.
2. Define and pronounce the listed vocabulary terms that relate to temperature, pulse, respiration, and blood pressure and state verbally or in writing examples of each.
3. List the required equipment for taking a patient's vital signs and the general care for his or her equipment.
4. Recall and state the *general* instructions for taking temperature, pulse, respirations, and blood pressure.
5. Describe briefly the methods used to obtain and record a patient's vital signs.
6. When given hourly recordings of patient's temperatures, determine if these sets indicate normal or abnormal variations in daily body temperature.
7. When given the results of 25 patients' vital signs, state which results fall within normal ranges and which do not. State the reasons for the answers given.
8. List five situations in which taking an oral body temperature should be avoided or delayed.
9. For each, list two situations in which to avoid taking rectal and axillary temperatures.
10. Discuss the advantages of tympanic thermometry (infrared radiation temperature measurement).
11. State why the tympanic membrane and surrounding tissue are accurate indicators of true body core temperature.
12. List 10 situations that cause variations in a person's pulse rate.
13. List and locate the seven arteries in the body from which the pulse rate can be obtained with relative ease.
14. Describe what is meant by (a) the rate, rhythm, and volume of the pulse rate; and (b) the rate, rhythm, and depth of respirations.
15. List five situations that increase a person's respiratory rate and five that cause this rate to decrease.
16. List five situations that increase a person's blood pressure and five that cause this rate to decrease.
17. List and explain five factors that determine arterial blood pressure.
18. List five methods that may be used to control high blood pressure.
19. List four medical problems that could result if high blood pressure is not treated.
20. State six reasons for measuring a patient's height and weight.

TERMINAL PERFORMANCE OBJECTIVES

On completion of Unit Two, the medical assistant student should be able to:

1. Demonstrate the correct procedures for obtaining a patient's oral, axillary, rectal, and ear (tympanic) temperature using various types of equipment.
2. Identify and locate pulsations on the seven major arteries used to measure a patient's pulse rate; identify and locate the apical heartbeat.
3. Demonstrate the correct procedure for taking a patient's pulse rate and apical heartbeat.
4. Demonstrate the correct procedure for measuring a patient's respiratory rate.
5. Demonstrate the correct procedure for taking the systolic and diastolic blood pressures of a patient's brachial and popliteal arteries using various types of equipment.
6. Demonstrate the correct procedure for taking a patient's blood pressure by use of the palpation method.
7. Demonstrate the correct procedure for taking a patient's orthostatic blood pressure.
8. Convert 20 temperature results recorded in Celsius (centigrade) degrees to Fahrenheit degrees.
9. Convert 20 temperature results recorded in Fahrenheit degrees to Celsius (centigrade) degrees.
10. Demonstrate the correct procedures for measuring a patient's weight and height.

11. Convert 20 weight and height results recorded in kilograms and inches to pounds and feet (and inches if applicable).
12. Convert 20 weights recorded in pounds to kilograms.
13. Demonstrate the proper methods for caring for stethoscopes, sphygmomanometers, and thermometers after use.

The consistent use of universal precautions is required by all health care professionals in all health care settings as a method of infection control. It is assumed that these precautions are used in all of the following procedures. Review Unit One if you have any question on methods to use, as the methods/techniques will not be repeated in detail in each procedure presented in the unit.

Be sure to consult the latest guidelines issued by the Centers for Disease Control and Prevention and consult with infection control practitioners when needed to identify specific precautions that pertain to your particular work situation.

The student is expected to perform these objectives with 100% accuracy. Results obtained for pulse and respiratory rates are acceptable if within two beats or respirations, as determined by the instructor. Results for blood pressures are acceptable if within 2 to 4 mm Hg, as determined by the instructor.

Among the medical assistant's most routine clinical duties are the taking and recording of the patient's physical measurements, which include vital signs, height, and weight. Therefore the medical assistant must know and understand these measurements and be able to correctly obtain and record the values for each. This unit discusses these six measurements along with procedures and related vocabulary.

It is assumed that the medical assistant student has completed or is currently studying anatomy and physiology. Therefore detailed explanations of how the body produces vital signs are not included. See also Unit Eighteen, which is a brief overview of anatomy and physiology.

VITAL SIGNS

Vital signs are measurable, concrete indicators that pertain to and are essential for life. The four vital signs are temperature, pulse, respiration (tpr), and blood pressure (bp). These signs are routinely measured in each physical examination. Vital signs provide the physician with information that help:

- Determine the patient's condition by comparing the patient's body temperature, pulse, respiration, and blood pressure with normal values.
- Determine a diagnosis, the course, and the prognosis of the patient's condition.
- Designate the treatment that will be instituted.

TEMPERATURE

Body temperature, the degree of body heat, is a result of the balance maintained between heat produced and heat lost by the body. This is regulated by a central heat-regulating center located in a portion of the brain, the hypothalamus, that initiates the various mechanisms to increase or decrease heat loss.

Heat is produced by oxidation of foods in all body cells, especially those in the skeletal muscles and liver. The blood and blood vessels distribute it to other parts of the body. Eighty-five percent of body heat is lost through the skin by radiation, convection, and evaporation of perspiration. The remainder is lost through the respiratory tract and mouth and through feces and urine.

A variation from the normal range of a patient's temperature may be the first warning of an illness or a change in the patient's condition. As such, it is an important part of the diagnosis and treatment plan for a patient.

Normal Temperature Readings

Body temperature is measured by a thermometer placed under the tongue, in the rectum, in the axilla, or in the ear (tympanic membrane), because large blood vessels are near the surface at these points. The normal temperature values for these sites based on a statistical average are as follows:

- Oral: 98.6° F or 37° C
- Rectal: 99.6° F or 37.6° C
- Axillary: 97.6° F or 36.4° C
- Ear: The thermometer converts the temperature to an oral or rectal equivalent

Accurate rectal temperatures register approximately 1° F or 0.6° C higher than accurate oral temperatures. Accurate axillary temperatures register approximately 1° F or 0.6° C lower than accurate oral temperatures. The rectal temperature is considered to be the most reliable and accurate reading. The mucous membrane lining of the rectum, with which the thermometer comes into contact, is not exposed to the air, and the conditions do not vary as do those of the mouth or axilla.

Variations in Body Temperature

Normal body temperature varies from person to person and occurs at different times in each person.

- The daily average oral temperature of a healthy person may vary from 97.6° to 99.6° F (36.4° to 37.3° C).
- The lowest body temperature occurs in the early morning (2 to 6 a.m.)
- The highest body temperature occurs in the evening (5 to 8 p.m.)
- In a woman, body temperature may increase *slightly* during the menstrual cycle at the time of ovulation.
- Body temperature is slightly higher during and immediately after eating, exercise, or emotional excitement.
- Body temperature may vary more and is generally higher in an infant or young child than in an adult.

Abnormal temperatures occur when the body's temperature-regulating system is upset by disease or other physical disturbances.

Constant fever—High fever with a variation not exceeding 1 or 2° Fahrenheit [F] (0.6° or 1.2° Celsius or centigrade [C]) between morning and evening temperatures.

Convection—Transfer of heat by the automatic circulation of body fluids

Crisis—Sudden drop of a high temperature to normal or below; generally occurs within 24 hours.

Evaporation—Disappearance; loss.

Fever—Pyrexia, or elevation of body temperature above normal (98.6° F) or 37° C (centigrade or Celsius) registered orally. Some classify it as:

    Low: 99° to 101° F (37.2° to 38.3° C)
    Moderate: 101° to 103° F (38.3° to 39.5° C)
    High: 103° to 105° F (39.5° to 40.6° C)

Intermittent fever—Variations with alternate rises and falls, with the lowest measurement often dropping below 98.6° F (37° C). An intermittent fever reaches the normal line at intervals during the course of an illness (for example, a.m.: 98° F (36.7° C); p.m.: 100° F (37.8° C); a.m.: 98.6° F (37° C), p.m.: 101° F (38.4° C).

Lysis—Gradual decline of a fever.

Onset—Beginning of a fever.

Oxidation—Combining with oxygen.

Radiation—Sending out rays in the form of waves or particles

Remittent fever—Variations in temperature, but always above 98.6° F (37° C); a persistent fever that has a daytime variation of 2° F (1.2° C) or more (for example, a.m.: 100° F (37.8° C), p.m.: 103° F (39.5° C); a.m.: 99° F, p.m.: 102.4° F (39.1° C) (Figure 2-1).

Body temperature *decreases* in some illnesses; if a patient faints, collapses, or hemorrhages; or if the patient is in a fasting state, is dehydrated, or has sustained a central nervous system (CNS) injury. Subnormal temperatures, below 96° F (35.6° C), may occur in cases of collapse.

Body temperature *increases* are caused by the following:

• An infectious process
• Following a chill (the muscular activity that occurs in shivering (chills) releases heat and thus increases heat production in the body)
• Activity
• Emotions
• Environmental changes
• Age (the aged and infants show 1° F higher)
• Reactions to certain drugs
• Amount and type of food eaten (an increase in metabolic rate increases heat production in the body)

Fever usually accompanies infection and many other disease processes. Fever is present when the oral temperature is 100° F (38.8° C) or higher. Temperatures of 104° F (40° C) or higher are common in serious illnesses.

Thermometers

A thermometer calibrated in Fahrenheit or centigrade (Celsius) degrees is the instrument used to measure body temperature. Various models made of glass or special disposable materials are available. Newer models are electronic or the infrared tympanic thermometers. All good thermometers must pass a rigid inspection for proper calibration according to the standards set by the U.S. National Bureau of Standards.

The frequently used *glass thermometers* vary in shape. The rounded, short bulb is used when taking rectal temperatures because it is held better by the rectal muscles and does not traumatize the mucosa. It may also be used when taking an

axillary temperature. The slender bulb is considered more effective for oral temperatures. There are also rounded, short-bulb thermometers for both oral and rectal use. These are usually color-coded for easy identification (that is, oral thermometers have a blue identification mark at the end, and rectal thermometers have a red mark). All register the same temperature, although the "normal" temperature arrow is on the 98.6° F (37° C) mark for the oral thermometer and may be on the 99.6° F (37.6° C) mark for the rectal thermometer (Figure 2-2).

Clear plastic, disposable covers called **thermometer sheaths** are available to fit over the stem and bulb of all glass thermometers (Figure 2-3). These can be used when taking the temperature by any method. The rectal sheath is generally prelubricated for easier insertion. The sheath is placed on the thermometer according to the manufacturer's directions before the thermometer is used and removed before the temperature is read. When the sheath is removed from the thermometer, it turns in on itself, enclosing the area that has been in contact with the patient's body part, thereby helping to prevent the spread of any infectious agent that is present.

Safe and easy-to-use, battery-operated **electronic thermometers** work rapidly (within 10 to 45 seconds) and are accurately calibrated to within two tenths of a degree. They have disposable covers and interchangeable color-coded probes for both oral and rectal use. The temperature is registered on a dial or on a digital display on the equipment (Figure 2-4).

The IVAC is an example of an electronic thermometer currently used in many hospital settings (Figure 2-4).

The newest technology now makes it possible to measure body temperature in the ear in 1 to 2 seconds. This method is referred to as "*infrared tympanic thermometry*" and is thought to be the most accurate method of measuring body tempera-

Figure 2-1 *Temperature graph demonstrating the defined terms.*

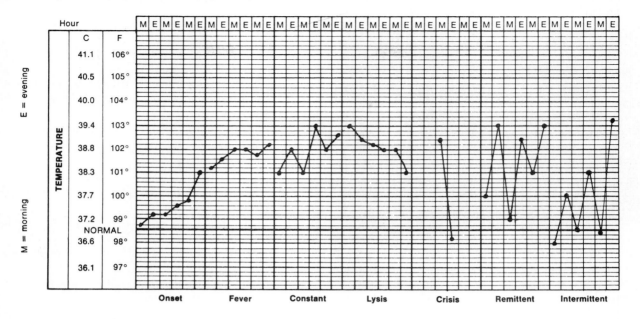

Figure 2-2 A, *Reusable glass thermometers. The slender bulb is best for oral temperatures; the rounded bulb is best for rectal temperatures and may also be used for axillary temperatures.* B, *One type of disposable thermometer. The last dot to turn dark indicates the temperature reading.*

Figure 2-3 *Disposable thermometer sheath.* A, *Apply the sheath to the thermometer according to the manufacturer's instructions.* B, *Remove the sheath before the temperature is read. The sheath folds back on itself to enclose patient's secretions.*

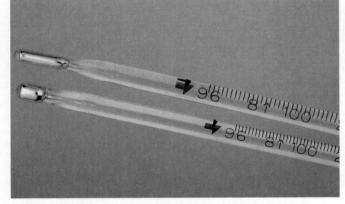

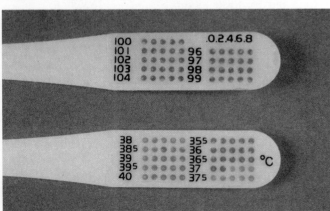

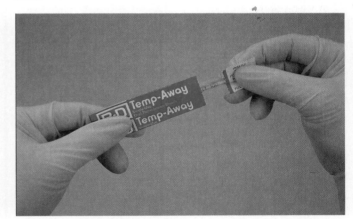

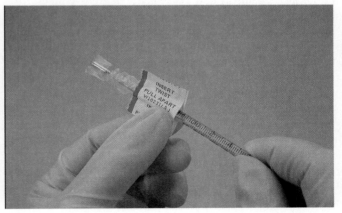

Figure 2-4 *The IVAC thermometer is an electronically operated device for taking both oral and rectal temperature safely and accurately.*

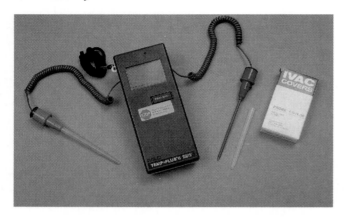

ture. Various models of these thermometers with disposable ear probe covers are available. The thermometer calculates the body temperature, converts it to an oral or rectal equivalent, and displays it on a digital screen (see Figure 2-10, page 32).

Advantages of the electronic and tympanic thermometers over the glass thermometers are that they are quick and provide protection from infection and the possibility of breakage and mercury spillage. There are some differences between the models available; therefore the manufacturer's directions must be followed for each thermometer.

How to Read a Glass Thermometer

When reading a thermometer, hold it between your thumb and the index finger of your right hand at the stem (the end away from the bulb.) Rotate the thermometer until you see the center clear (silver) line of mercury toward the bulb. Follow this line up until it ends. Sometimes you can see this line better by changing the direction of the light source. Fahrenheit thermometers are marked off in degrees, with intermediate marks at two tenths of a degree. When the mercury line ends between the two-tenths mark, read the temperature at the next highest two-tenths of a degree. Centigrade thermometers are marked off in degrees, with intermediate marks at one tenth of a degree. Centigrade readings can be converted to Fahrenheit readings and Fahrenheit degrees converted to centigrade degrees using the following formulas. Since the metric system is being used more frequently, you should know how to convert Fahrenheit degrees to centigrade degrees. The formula for this is:

$$C° = (F° - 32 × 5/9)$$

If the Fahrenheit temperature is 98.6°, then:

$$C° = (98.6° - 32) × 5/9$$
$$C° = 66.6° × 5/9$$
$$C° = 333/9$$
$$C° = 37°$$

To convert centigrade to Fahrenheit degrees, the formula is

$$F° = (C° × 9/5) + 32 \text{ (Table 2-1)}$$

Methods and Procedures for Taking a Temperaure

Use the following guidelines to determine which method to use:

1. *Oral* temperature should *never* be taken on the following:
   a. Children who are not old enough to know how to hold the thermometer in the mouth (4 years old and younger)
   b. Patients with a nasal obstruction, dyspnea, coughing, weakness, a sore mouth, mouth diseases, or oral surgery
   c. Patients receiving oxygen
   d. Uncooperative, delirious, unconscious, or intoxicated patients
2. *Axillary* temperatures should *never* be taken on the following:
   a. Thin patients who cannot make the hollow under the arm airtight
   b. Perspiring patients whose axilla cannot be kept dry for the required 10 minutes
3. *Rectal* temperatures should *never* be taken on the following:
   a. Rectal surgery patients
   b. Children or other patients whose body movements cannot be controlled for the required 3 to 5 minutes (time varies with agency policy)
4. *Tympanic* temperatures are the easiest and most reliable method. Use this method if a tympanic thermometer is available.

Equipment

- Thermometer
- Oral: Glass thermometers may be stored in a small, covered container with a small pad of cotton in the bottom and labeled *clean oral thermometer* or in individual, clean, labeled envelopes stored in a drawer
- Rectal: Glass thermometers may be stored in a small, covered container with a small pad of cotton in the bottom and labeled *clean rectal thermometers* or in individual, clean, labeled envelopes stored in a drawer
- Box of tissues or small cotton squares
- Container for waste
- Containers labeled "soiled oral thermometers" or "soiled rectal thermometers"
- Water-soluble lubricant such as K-Y jelly or Lubafax if taking a rectal temperature
- Disposable single-use exam gloves if taking a rectal or infant's temperature

General Instructions

1. Handle the thermometer with great care because it is a very delicate instrument.
2. Keep rectal thermometers separate from oral thermometers.

Text continues on page 27.

TABLE 2-1

Comparison of Centigrade and Fahrenheit Readings

C	F	C	F	C	F
34.0	93.2	36.5	97.7	39.0	102.2
34.1	93.4	36.6	97.9	39.1	102.4
34.2	93.6	36.7	98.1	39.2	102.6
34.3	93.7	36.8	98.2	39.3	102.7
34.4	93.9	36.9	98.4	39.4	102.9
34.5	94.1	37.0*	98.6*	39.5	103.1
34.6	94.3	37.1	98.8	39.6	103.3
34.7	94.5	37.2	98.9	39.7	103.5
34.8	94.6	37.3	99.1	39.8	103.6
34.9	94.8	37.4	99.3	39.9	103.0
35.0	95.0	37.5	99.5	40.0	104.0
35.1	95.2	37.6	99.7	40.1	104.2
35.2	95.4	37.7	99.9	40.2	104.4
35.3	95.5	37.8	100.0	40.3	104.5
35.4	95.7	37.9	100.2	40.4	104.7
35.5	95.9	38.0	100.4	40.5	104.9
35.6	96.1	38.1	100.6	40.6	105.1
35.7	96.3	38.2	100.8	40.7	105.3
35.8	96.4	38.3	100.9	40.8	105.0
35.9	96.6	38.4	101.1	40.9	105.6
36.0	96.8	38.5	101.3	41.0	105.8
36.1	97.0	38.6	101.5	41.1	106.0
36.2	97.2	38.7	101.7	41.5	106.7
36.3	97.3	38.8	101.8	42.0	107.6
36.4	97.5	38.9	102.0	42.5	108.5

*Normal oral temperature.

ORAL TEMPERATURE

PROCEDURE

1. Identify and evaluate the patient.

2. Wash your hands. **Use appropriate personal protective equipment (PPE) as indicated by facility.**

3. Assemble equipment.

4. Instruct the patient to assume a sitting position and explain the procedure.

5. Remove clean thermometer from the container.

6. If just removing the thermometer from the disinfectant solution, rinse with *cold* running water, and wipe dry from the stem downward to the bulb in a rotating manner with a tissue or cotton square. Discard cotton square.

RATIONALE

To avoid any accident or false reading, defer taking for 15 to 20 minutes if the patient has just finished eating, drinking, or smoking. Do not leave a patient alone unless he or she is absolutely responsible.

Complete explanations help gain the patient's cooperation and help the patient relax. Provide for the patient's comfort and safety.

This removes any disinfectant that may be irritating to the patient. You must use cold water because hot water may cause mercury to expand too much and break the bulb.

ORAL TEMPERATURE—cont'd

PROCEDURE	RATIONALE
7. Firmly holding the end of the thermometer, shake it down to 96° F (35.5° C) or lower. Do this by giving the wrist several quick snaps as though cracking a whip. Be careful to avoid contact with nearby objects. (If you are using a disposable plastic sheath to cover the thermometer, apply it now.)	*Constricting the mercury prevents it from going down, unless forced, and ensures an accurate temperature reading.*
8. Place the thermometer well under the patient's tongue into the sublingual pocket (see Figure 2-4, page 22).	*Temperature reading is produced from heat from superficial blood vessels under the tongue.*
9. Instruct the patient to keep lips closed, to breathe through the nose, and not to touch the thermometer with the teeth.	*Keeping the mouth closed prevents cooler air from the outside from affecting the temperature reading. Keeping teeth off of the thermometer prevents biting down and possibly breaking it.*
10. Leave the thermometer in place for 3 minutes.	
11. The pulse and respirations may be taken while the thermometer is registering.	
12. Remove the thermometer and wipe it from the stem toward the bulb, using a rotating motion. Never place pressure on the mercury bulb end of the thermometer, or remove the disposable plastic sheath if used and dispose of according to agency policy.	*Wiping removes any secretions and makes it easier to read the temperature. Wiping from stem to bulb also prevents contact of microorganisms from the patient's mouth with your fingers.*
13. Read the thermometer. Hold it horizontally in your right hand and rotate it slowly until you see the point at which the mercury column stops (Figure 2-5).	
14. Record the reading.	

15. Shake the mercury down to 96° F (35.5° C) or below and place the thermometer in the container for used oral thermometers or into a container of cool soap solutions.	*Charting example:*
	    March 2, 19••, 9 a.m.
	      Oral temp 98.8° F
	            or
	      Temp 98.8° F
	        J. Sublett, CMA

16. If retaking a questionable temperature, the medical assistant should check that the thermometer is shaken down to 96° F (35.5° C) or below, or use another thermometer or use another method, either rectal or axillary. If the temperature is found to be remarkably high or low for no apparent reason, take it again.	
17. Wash your hands.	

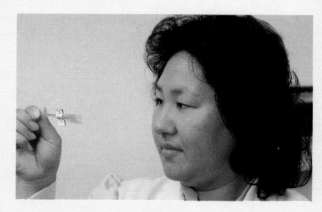

Figure 2-5 *Read the thermometer by holding it horizontally and rotating it slowly until you see the point at which the mercury stops.*

AXILLARY TEMPERATURE

PROCEDURE

1. Perform steps 1 through 7 as for temperature technique, using a rounded, short bulb thermometer.

2. Blot the axillary region dry with tissue or a cotton square.

3. Place the bulb end of the thermometer in the hollow of the axillary region with the end of the thermometer slanting towards the patient's chest (Figure 2-6).

4. Have the patient cross the arms over the chest. It may be more comfortable to hold the opposite shoulder.

5. Leave the thermometer in place for 10 minutes (time may vary according to agency policy).

6. The pulse and respirations may be taken while the thermometer is registering.

7. Remove and wipe the thermometer from the stem toward the bulb and read it. Hold a glass thermometer in your right hand to read it.

8. Record reading

9. Shake the mercury down to 96° F (35.5° C) or below and place the thermometer in the container for used thermometers.

10. Wash your hands.

RATIONALE

Avoid rubbing, as friction increases the blood supply in the area, thus increasing the temperature of the skin.

Ensure that the thermometer is in direct contact with the skin surface, not touching clothing or exposed to the air. Maintain proper position of the thermometer against blood vessels in the axilla.

This prevents as little air as possible from coming into contact with the thermometer. When the patient is unable to put his or her hand on the opposite shoulder, place it there gently and hold it with your own hand, or hold the patient's arm close to his or her side. When taking a child's axillary temperature, hold the thermometer in place for the entire time.

This ensures accurate registration of the temperature. A longer time is needed for the temperature to register than when taking an oral temperature because the axilla is more subject to the influence of air currents.

Never place pressure on the bulb end of the thermometer.

Charting example:
January 30, 19___, 11 a.m.
Axillary temp 97.6° F
or
Temp 97.6° F A or Ax.
M. Kubiak, CMA

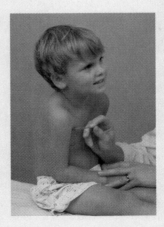

Figure 2-6 *Placing a thermometer for taking an axillary temperature.*

RECTAL TEMPERATURE

<table>
<tr><th>PROCEDURE</th><th>RATIONALE</th></tr>
<tr><td>

1. Perform steps 1 through 7 as for oral temperature, using a rectal thermometer.

</td><td>

Never use an oral thermometer for a rectal temperature.

</td></tr>
<tr><td>

2. Have the patient turn on the side with the upper leg flexed, if possible.

</td><td>

Do not expose the patient unnecessarily.

</td></tr>
<tr><td>

3. Don disposable single-use exam gloves.

</td><td></td></tr>
<tr><td>

4. Apply a water-soluble lubricant to the thermometer. (If you are using a disposable sheath over the thermometer, put it on and then apply the lubricant) (Figure 2-7).

</td><td>

Lubricant allows for easier insertion of the thermometer. Some disposable plastic sheaths are prelubricated.

</td></tr>
<tr><td>

5. Separate buttocks so that anus is exposed.

</td><td></td></tr>
<tr><td>

6. Gently insert thermometer approximately 1 to 1½ inches into the anal canal and instruct the patient to remain still.

</td><td>

Forceful insertion beyond 1 to 1½ inches may cause damage to the tissues involved. Movement could cause the thermometer to go farther into the rectum and possibly cause tissue damage, or the thermometer could slip out of the rectum. The thermometer could also slip out of the rectum if it is not inserted far enough.

</td></tr>
<tr><td>

7. Hold thermometer in place for 3 to 5 minutes (time may vary with agency policy.) You may take an adult's pulse and respiration while the thermometer is registering.

</td><td>

Never leave the patient alone when taking a rectal temperature.

</td></tr>
<tr><td>

8. Remove the thermometer. Remove the sheath covering if used. Wipe the thermometer in a rotating motion going only from the stem toward the bulb to remove any secretions.

Wipe the patient's anal area with a tissue to remove any lubricant. Wipe in the direction going toward the back.

</td><td>

Lubricant and any fecal material must be removed from the thermometer to allow for ease in reading the temperature.

Provide for the patient's comfort.

</td></tr>
<tr><td>

9. Read the temperature accurately. Hold the thermometer horizontally in the right hand and rotate it slowly until you see the point at which the mercury column stops.

</td><td>

Never place pressure on the bulb end of the thermometer. Be certain all fecal material is removed.

</td></tr>
<tr><td>

10. Record the reading, noting that a rectal temperature was taken.

</td><td>

Charting example:
May 19, 19__, 10 a.m.
  Rectal temp 99.6° F
    or
  Temp 99.6° F R
    Josh Burns, CMA

</td></tr>
<tr><td>

11. Shake the mercury down to below 96° F (35.5° C).

</td><td></td></tr>
<tr><td>

12. Place the thermometer in the container for used rectal thermometers.

</td><td></td></tr>
<tr><td>

13. Remove and dispose of gloves.

</td><td></td></tr>
<tr><td>

14. Wash your hands.

</td><td></td></tr>
<tr><td>

15. Assist the patient as needed.

</td><td>

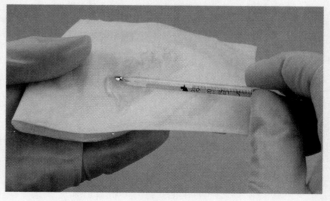

</td></tr>
</table>

Figure 2-7 *Lubricating thermometer for taking a rectal temperature. Put some lubricant on a tissue or paper; then put the thermometer into the lubricant so that the first inch of the thermometer is covered with lubricant.*

3. Wash your hands before and after handling a thermometer or taking a patient's temperature.
4. Wear disposable, single-use exam gloves when taking a rectal temperature.
5. Read the thermometer with great care to ensure accuracy.
6. Record the reading and indicate if it was other than oral. This notation must be made because of the differences in temperatures when taken in either the axilla or rectum.

Care of Glass Thermometers After Each Use

1. Shake mercury down to below 95° F (36° C).
2. Wash with soap and cold water, and then rinse with cold running water.
3. Dry the thermometer.
4. Place in a disinfectant solution such as glutaraldehyde (Cidex) or 70% alcohol; then rinse with *cold* running water and dry with a small piece of cotton before the next use.
5. If the thermometer is not to be reused after being disinfected, dry it and place in a covered container that has cotton in the bottom to protect the bulb. Store in dry containers or individual clean envelopes.

Taking an Infant's Temperature

1. Don disposable single-use exam gloves.
2. Lay the infant on the abdomen on a firm surface.
3. With your left hand, spread the cheeks of the buttocks so that you can see the rectum.
4. With your right hand, insert the lubricated bulb end of the rectal thermometer into the rectum approximately $1/2$ to 1 inch.
5. Place your right hand on the infant's buttocks, hold the buttocks firmly, and pinch the thermometer firmly between your fingers.
6. Place your other hand in the small of the infant's back, with your arm straight, and lean on the infant slightly. This helps hold the infant still (Figure 2-8).
7. Hold the thermometer in place for 3 to 5 minutes (time may vary with agency policy).

8. Remove the thermometer and place it out of reach of the infant.
9. Support the infant. Wipe the anal area to remove excess lubricant.
10. Wipe the thermometer with a tissue, read the temperature registered, and record it promptly.
11. Remove and dispose of gloves.
12. Wash your hands.

Infrared Radiation Temperature Measurement (Infrared Tympanic Thermometry)

All material objects give off electromagnetic waves from their surface. The cooler the object, the less energy these waves carry. The hotter the object, the more energy the waves carry. These waves vary in length, and the longest waves we can see are red. The energy of the radiation given off from our bodies is lower than these red waves, hence the term infrared, meaning below red. Infrared tympanic thermometers are based on the detection of thermal infrared radiation (heat).

Broad scientific research from around the world shows the tympanic membrane (eardrum) and its surrounding tissue to be *the most* accurate indicator of true core body temperature because the eardrum shares blood supply and is near the hypothalamus, the body's thermostat or the temperature control center of the brain (Figure 2-9).

One of the tympanic thermometers available, the hand-held Thermoscan (Figure 2-10, *A* and *B*) is like a camera in that it takes a snapshot of infrared heat given off of the eardrum and surrounding tissue and registers it on a sensitive surface. Instead of a lens, a gold-plated wave guide covered by a protective window is used; and instead of film, an infrared sensor is used. A shutter is used as it is in a camera. The thermometer then calculates the body temperature, converts it to an oral or rectal equivalent, and displays it on the digital screen—all within 1 second.

Figure 2-9   *The eardrum is an excellent site to measure body temperature because it is near the hypothalamus, which is the body's temperature control center.*

Figure 2-8   *Position for holding a thermometer and infant while taking the rectal temperature.*

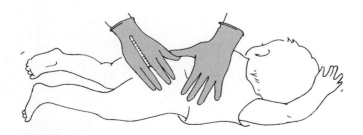

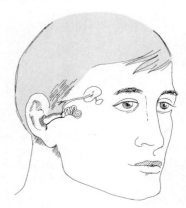

Advantages. Tympanic thermometry offers many benefits and advantages over traditional glass mercury, electronic, and digital thermometers (specifically accuracy, safety, speed, comfort, cleanliness, and user convenience). Therefore it is quickly becoming the preferred site for taking body temperature. Different models are available for both professional and home use.

Accuracy. Clinical studies show that the eardrum is an accurate indicator of true core body temperature because it shares blood supply and is near the hypothalamus, the body's "thermostat." The ear canal is a protected cavity, unaffected by environmental factors. Unlike traditional thermometers, tympanic thermometers do not have to be in place for an extended length of time; they are not affected by external factors such as eating, chewing gum, drinking, smoking, and breathing through the mouth—all of which affect oral thermometers; and, as with oral electronic thermometers, they do not depend on where they are placed in the mouth (for example, too far forward in the mouth and away from the sublingual artery). Reading the temperature from a tympanic thermometer is easy because it is displayed as a clear digital readout, thus eliminating the need to visually interpret the mercury column). In addition, the infrared tympanic technique is faster and more accurate than other methods because it measures the patient's temperature as it naturally radiates, not the thermometer's own temperature after extended patient contact. Presence of any form of otitis media (inflammation of the middle ear) does not affect the temperature measurement. Also, cerumen (ear wax) does not affect the tympanic membrane thermometer readings because cerumen is transparent to infrared energy. Finally, tympanic thermometers can be used when temperatures are difficult or impossible to obtain with conventional contact thermometers.

Safety, cleanliness and infection control. Infrared tympanic thermometers eliminate potential risks such as bowel perforation, breakage of glass thermometers, and mercury ingestion or contamination. Because they are placed in the ear, which is a dry, nonmucous membrane cavity, tympanic thermometers virtually eliminate the possibility of cross-contamination. The ear canal harbors fewer pathogens than the mouth or rectum. The probe tip is covered with a disposable cover which is changed for each patient. The disposable probe cover is ejected after use without having to be touched. These thermometers measure temperatures without touching the tympanic membrane (that is, there is not membrane contact). The probe tip has been designed to make it impossible to cause damage to the eardrum, regardless of the age of the patient.

Speed. Traditional thermometers may take as long as 5 minutes to display an accurate temperature. In contrast, tympanic thermometers take and display temperatures on an easy-to-read display in 1 second. Since infrared waves travel at the speed of light, readings can be taken almost instantaneously.

Comfort. Tympanic thermometers make temperature taking a fast, painless, noninvasive procedure. Because it is not physically or emotionally threatening, it does not add to the discomfort of any patient, especially a sick child or a nervous or elderly patient. No active cooperation is required; thus it can be used without disturbing a sleeping child or on an unconscious patient. In terms of ease of access and accuracy of core temperature, the tympanic site is superior to all others.

PULSE

The pulse is defined as the beat of the heart as felt through the walls of the arteries. It is produced by the wave of blood that

---

Figure 2-10 A, *Thermoscan PRO-1 Instant Thermometer, an infrared tympanic (ear) thermometer designed to display the temperature in less than 1 second. Disposable probe covers are used over the ear probe for each patient. B, The Thermoscan Instant Thermometer takes a snapshot of the heat given off by the eardrum and surrounding tissue.*

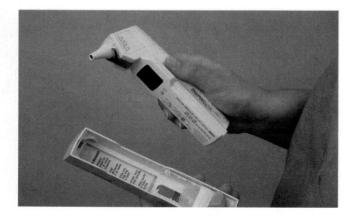

A

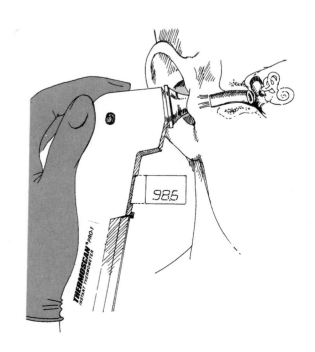

B

travels along the arteries with each contraction of the left ventricle of the heart.

The pulse can also be described as a throbbing caused by the alternate expansion and recoil of an artery. It is felt best when a superficial artery is pressed against a firm, underlying anatomic structure such as bone.

Apical Pulse

The apical rate is the rate per minute of the heartbeat as determined by auscultation of the apex of the heart. This is the most accurate pulse site. An apical pulse is taken on all children under 2 years of age and on patients with possible heart problems, regardless of age. It may also be taken when the radial pulse is inaccessible because of a cast or dressing. The *normal range* is 70 to 90 beats per minute; the *average rate* is 80 beats per minute.

To count the apical beat, place the chestpiece of a stethoscope over the apex of the heart and count the number of heartbeats for 1 minute.

The apex of the heart is located in the left fifth intercostal space on the midclavicular line (that is, between the fifth and sixth ribs on a line with the midpoint of the left clavicle). This position is usually just below the nipple.

When recording the results, you must indicate that it was the apical rate that was taken. On completion, wipe the earpiece and diaphragm of the stethoscope with an alcohol sponge and return it to the proper storage area.

Characteristics of the Pulse

When you are taking a pulse, the four important characteristics to note are the rate, rhythm, and volume of the pulse and the condition of the arterial wall, all of which vary with the size and the elasticity of the artery, the strength of contraction of the heart, and the tissues surrounding the artery.

The **rate** (frequency) of the pulse is the number of pulsations (beats) in a given minute. Normal (average) rates are outlined in the following section. Abnormal rates are those above or below the range of norms, and can be described as bradycardia (slow) or tachycardia (rapid).

The **rhythm** of the pulse pertains to the time interval between each pulse. Normal rhythm is described as regular (that is, intervals between pulsations are of equal length). Abnormal rhythm may be described as irregular, arrhythmic, bigeminal, skipping beats, or intermittent. Skipping an occasional beat occurs in all normal individuals, especially during exercise or after ingesting certain stimulants such as coffee. Most of these irregularities go unnoticed, but they may concern a patient enough to cause him or her to seek medical advice. When frequent beats are skipped or if the beats are highly irregular, the physician should be alerted, because this could be a sign of heart disease. In such cases, it is sometimes useful for one person to take the radial pulse for 1 minute and the other person to take the apical pulse by listening over the heart simultaneously (see page 34). The findings are recorded and compared. If the apical rate is greater, the difference is referred to as the **pulse deficit**. This could indicate inadequate blood circulation to the arms and legs when the heart contracts.

The pulse deficit is important in the examination of the patient with atrial fibrillation, one of the more common causes of a very irregular pulse. Atrial fibrillation is an irregular heartbeat marked by rapid, inefficient, random contractions of the atria in the heart.

The **volume** (also known as "intensity," "force", "character," or "quality") of the pulse is an indication of the general condition of the heart and the circulatory system. It pertains to the strength of the pulsations and may be described as full, strong, bounding, weak, feeble, thready, febrile, hard, or soft. Volume depends on the force of the heartbeat and the condition of the arterial wall, the the beat may vary in volume in association with irregularities of rhythm. If a pulse varies only in intensity but is otherwise perfectly regular, it is often a manifestation of heart disease.

The **condition of the arterial wall** pertains to the texture of the artery that you feel through the skin surface when palpating the pulse. A normal arterial wall is described as soft and elastic; abnormal conditions include hard, ropy, knotty, and wiry.

Variations in Pulse Rate

Individual pulse rates *normally vary* as a result of a person's sex, age, body size, posture, activity level, and health status, as well as functions of the nervous system and the volume and chemical composition of the blood.

In general, the pulse rate is faster in women (70 to 80 beats per minute) than in men (60 to 70 beats per minute) and is usually higher in short people than in tall people. Infants' and children's pulse rates are also more rapid than an adult's. When one is sitting, the rate is more rapid (for example, 70 beats per minute) than when lying down (for example, 66 beats per minute); and it increases when standing, walking, or running (for example, 80, 86, and 90 beats per minute, respectively). During sleep or rest, especially in athletes, the pulse rate may be as low as 45 to 50 beats per minute. The following list indicates some of the common causes of increases or decreases in the pulse.

Increase
- Fear or excitement
- Physical activity, exercise
- Fever
- Certain types of heart disease
- Hyperthyroidism
- Shock
- Pain
- Certain drugs
- Many infections

Decrease
- Mental depression
- Certain types of heart disease
- Chronic illness
- Hypothyroidism
- Certain brain injuries that cause intracranial pressure
- Certain drugs, such as digitalis

TYMPANIC MEMBRANE TEMPERATURE (EAR TEMPERATURE)

Equipment

Tympanic thermometer with battery (for example, Thermoscan PRO-1 instant thermometer)
Disposable probe cover

NOTE: Accurate measurements depend on correct technique. The following procedure is for the Thermoscan thermometer. Other brands (Ototemp, FirstTemp Genius 3000A) require slightly different techniques. *Follow the manufacturer's instructions.*

PROCEDURE

1. Wash your hands. **Use appropriate personal protective equipment (PPE) as indicated by facility.**

2. Assembly equipment.

3. Identify and evaluate the patient.

4. Instruct the patient to assume a sitting position and explain the procedure.

5. Apply a disposable cover to the probe tip (Figure 2-11).

6. Select oral or rectal equivalent and press "ON."

7. For adults, gently pull the ear up and back. For children, gently pull the ear back.

8. Gently insert the probe tip in the patient's ear until the tip fully "seals off" the ear canal. DO NOT apply pressure (Figure 2-12).

9. Depress and hold the activation button for 1 second.

10. Remove from the ear. Read the temperature and record promptly. The Thermoscan PRO-1 is programmed to display the actual ear temperature, as well as the oral, rectal, or core equivalents (see Figure 2-10, page 28).

11. Discard the disposable probe cover in the designated waste container.

12. Return the equipment to the designated area.

13. Wash your hands.

14. Attend to the patient as needed.

RATIONALE

Explanations help the patient to relax and cooperate. Also, many people have never heard of taking a temperature in the ear. Provide for the patient's comfort and safety.

Make sure that the thermometer is locked in the mode that you prefer.

This straightens the ear canal to get a clear view of the eardrum (See Figure 9-1).

The probe is positioned snugly in the ear canal to get a view of the eardrum and its surrounding tissue, just as a photographic camera is aimed at an object. It does not touch the eardrum.

This allows the unit to measure the infrared heat generated by the eardrum and surrounding tissue. This measurement is then converted into either an oral or rectal equivalent in either Centigrade or Fahrenheit degrees. The resulting temperature is displayed in 1 second.

Charting example:
August 1, 19___ 4 p.m.
Tympanic oral temp 98.6° F
J. Lee, CMA

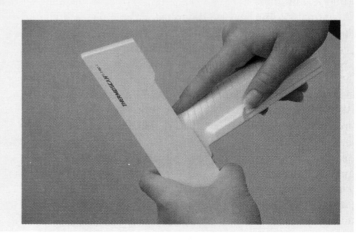

Figure 2-11 *Applying a disposable cover to the ear probe tip.*

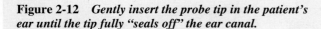

TYMPANIC MEMBRANE TEMPERATURE (EAR TEMPERATURE) —cont'd

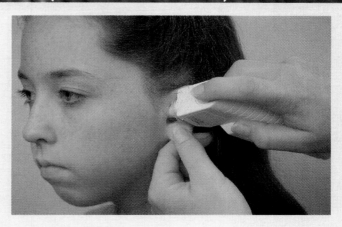

Figure 2-12 *Gently insert the probe tip in the patient's ear until the tip fully "seals off" the ear canal.*

VOCABULARY

Abdominal pulse—Abdominal aorta pulse.

Alternating pulse—Alternating weak and strong pulsations.

Arrhythmia (a-rith´ mi-a)—Irregularities in pulse or rhythm.

Bigeminal pulse (bi-jem´ in-al)—Two regular beats followed by a longer pause. It has the same significance as an irregular pulse.

Bradycardia (brad-i-kar´ di-a)—Slow heart action; extremely slow pulse, generally below 60 beats per minute.

Febrile pulse (feb´ rile)—A full, bounding pulse at the onset of a fever, becoming feeble and weak when the fever subsides.

Formicant pulse (for-mi-kant)—A small, feeble pulse.

Intermittent pulse—A pulse in which occasional beats are skipped.

Irregular pulse—A pulse with variation in force and frequency; may be caused by an excess of tea, coffee, tobacco, or exercise.

Pulse deficit—The apical rate is greater than the radial pulse rate.

Pulse pressure—The difference between the systolic and the diastolic blood pressure.

Example: If BP is 120/80,

$$\begin{array}{r} 120 = \text{systolic pressure} \\ -\underline{80} = \text{diastolic pressure} \\ 40 = \text{pulse pressure} \end{array}$$

A pulse pressure consistently over 50 points or under 30 points is considered abnormal

Regular pulse—The rhythm of the pulse rate is regular.

Slow pulse—A pulse between 40 and 60 beats per minute, often found among the aged and among athletes at rest.

Tachycardia (tak´´y-kar´ di-a)—A pulse of 100 or more beats per minute when the person is at rest; abnormal rapidity of heart action.

Thready pulse—A pulse that is very fine and scarcely perceptible, as seen in syncope (fainting).

Unequal pulse—A pulse in which some beats are strong and others are weak; pulse in which rates are different in symmetric arteries.

Venous pulse—A pulse in a vein, especially one of the large veins near the heart such as the internal and external jugular. Venous pulse is undulating and scarcely palpable.

RESPIRATION

Respiration is the act of breathing and consists of one inspiration or inhalation (that is, the taking of air containing oxygen into the lungs) and one expiration or exhalation (that is, the expelling of air containing carbon dioxide from the lungs). More technically, respiration is the taking in of oxygen (O_2) and its use in the tissues, and the giving off of carbon dioxide (CO_2). For this reason, respiration may be classified as external and internal. External respiration is the interchange of gases that takes place in the lungs between the alveoli and the blood; internal respiration is the interchange of gasses that takes place in the tissues between the body cells and blood.

Breathing is controlled spontaneously (autonomically) by the respiratory center in the medulla oblongata in the lower portion of the brain stem. A buildup of carbon dioxide in the blood stimulates respirations to occur automatically.

In the human body a relationship exists among the body temperature, pulse, and respiratory rates. The usual ratio of respiration to pulse is one to four (1:4). Respiration and pulse

VOCABULARY

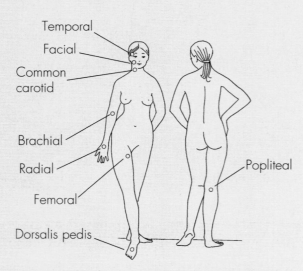

Brachial—Over the inner aspect at the bend of the elbow.
Common carotid—At right and left sides of the neck, at the anterior edge of the sternocleidomastoid muscle.
Dorsalis pedis—On the upper surface of the foot between ankle and toes.
Facial—Along the lower margin of the mandible.
Femoral—The anterior side of the pelvic bone, in the middle of the groin region.
Popliteal—At the back of the knee.
Radial—Over the inner aspect of the wrist area, on the thumb side. This site is the one most frequently used and accessible in most cases.
Temporal—At the temple, on the side of the forehead.

Figure 2-13 shows the body position of these arteries.

Figure 2-13 *Common arteries for determining pulse rates.*

Normal Pulse Rates (Average Number of Pulsation [Beats] in 1 Minute)

At birth	130 to 160 beats per minute
Infants	110 to 130 beats per minute
Children from 1 to 7 years	80 to 120 beats per minute
Children over 7 years	80 to 90 beats per minute
Adults	60 to 80 beats per minute

ordinarily rise proportionally to each degree rise in temperature because of increased metabolism in the tissue cells and the need for more rapid heat dissipation.

Characteristics of Respirations

When you are taking the respiratory rate of a patient, the three important characteristics to note are the rate, rhythm, and depth.

The **rate** of respirations refers to the number of respirations per minute and is best described as normal, rapid, or slow. In adults, normal rates are between 14 and 20 per minute; subnormal rates are 12 per minute and below and should be considered a serious symptom; above-normal rates are between 34 and 35 per minute; rapid rates are between 36 and 50 per minute. Any rate above 40 should also be considered a serious symptom. Rates of 60 per minute and above are dangerously rapid. Usually rapid respirations are also shallow and are seen in some diseases of the lungs. Deep respirations are characteristically slow, dependent on oxygen exchange, and common in conditions affecting intracranial pressure and in some forms of coma, including diabetic coma.

The **rhythm** may be described as regular or irregular. Regular breathing or respiration is characterized by inhalations and exhalations that are the same in depth and rate, whereas in irregular breathing, the inhalations and exhalations may vary in the amount of air inhaled and exhaled and in the rate of respirations per minute.

The **depth** of respirations depends on the amount of air inhaled and exhaled and is best described as either shallow or deep. In shallow respirations, small amounts of air are inhaled; they are often rapid. In deep respirations, larger amounts of air are inhaled, as in a "deep breath." These breaths are often slower.

Normal Respiratory Rates

At birth	30 to 60 respirations/minute
Infants	30 to 38 respirations/minute
Children	20 to 26 respirations/minute
Adults	14 to 20 respirations/minute

Abdominal respirations—The inspiration and expiration of air by the lungs accomplished primarily by the abdominal muscles and diaphragm.

Accelerated respirations—More than 25 respirations per minute, after 15 years of age.

Apnea (ap-ne´ ah)—Cessation or absence of breathing.

Artificial respiration—Artificial methods to restore respiration in cases of suspended breathing.

Biot's respiration—Irregularly alternating periods of apnea and hyperpnea; occurs in meningitis and disorders of the brain.

Cheyne-Stokes respiration (chan-stoks)—Respirations gradually increasing in rapidity and volume until they reach a climax, and then gradually subsiding and ceasing entirely for from 5 to 50 seconds, when they begin again. These are often a sign of impending death. Cheyne-Stokes respirations *may* be observed in normal persons (especially the aged) during sleep or during visits to higher altitudes.

Diaphragmatic respiration—Performed mainly by the diaphragm.

Dyspnea (dis-pne´ah)—Labored or difficult breathing.

Eupnea (up-ne´ah)—Easy or normal respiration.

Forced respiration—Voluntary hyperpnea.

Hyperpnea (hy″perp-ne´ah)—Increase in rate and depth of breathing.

Hyperventilation—Increase of air in the lungs above the normal amount; abnormally prolonged, rapid, and deep breathing, usually associated with acute anxiety or emotional tensions. Excessive intake of oxygen and the blowing off of carbon dioxide occurs. Decreased levels of carbon dioxide in the blood (hypocapnia) result. Immediate treatment consists of rebreathing into a paper bag to replace the carbon dioxide "blow off" while hyperventilating. Also see Unit Seventeen.

Hypoxia (hi-pok´se-ah)—Reduced amounts of oxygen to the body tissues.

Labored breathing—Dyspnea or difficult breathing; respiration that involves active participation of accessory inspiratory and expiratory muscles.

Orthopnea (or″thop-ne´-ah)—Severe dyspnea in which breathing is possible only when the patient sits or stands in an erect position.

Rales (rahls)—An abnormal bubbling sound heard on auscultation of the chest; often classified as either moist or crackling and dry.

Stertorous (ster´to-rus)—Characterized by a deep snoring sound with each inspiration.

Variations in the Respiratory Rate

Certain situations, both in health or in diseased states, cause variations in the normal respiratory rates.

Increased respiratory rate

- Excitement
- Nervousness
- Any strong emotion
- Increased muscular activity such as running or exercising
- Certain drugs such as ephedrine
- Diseases of the lungs
- Diseases of the circulatory system
- Fever
- Pain
- Shock
- Hemorrhage
- Gas Poisoning
- High altitudes
- Obstructions of the air passages

An increase in the carbon dioxide levels in arterial blood, which in turn stimulates the respiratory center

Decreased respiratory rate

- Sleep
- Certain drugs, such as morphine

- Certain diseases of the kidneys in which there is a coma
- Diseases and injuries that cause pressure on the brain tissue (for example, a stroke or skull fracture)
- Decrease of the carbon dioxide level in arterial blood (causes the respiratory centers to be depressed, causing decreased respiration rates)

BLOOD PRESSURE

Blood pressure (BP) is the pressure of the blood against the walls of the blood vessels. The pressure inside the arteries results from the pumping action of the heart muscle and varies with the contracting and the relaxing phases of the heart beat cycle. Systole is the phase when the heart contracts, forcing blood through the arteries, and diastole is the phase when the heart relaxes between contractions. Thus, when you are measuring a person's BP, there are two readings that you will need to take: systolic pressure and diastolic pressure (systole and diastole).

Systolic pressure, measured in millimeters of mercury (mm Hg), represents the force with which blood is pushing against the artery walls when the ventricles of the heart are in a state of contraction. During systole, blood is forced out of the heart into the aorta and pulmonary artery, and the pressure within the arteries is the highest.

Diastolic pressure, also measured in millimeters of mercury, represents the force of the blood in the arterial system

TAKING A RADIAL PULSE

Equipment

Watch with a sweep secondhand
Paper or graphic sheet to record pulse
Pen

General Instructions

1. Have the patient assume a comfortable position either sitting or lying down, with the arm supported.
Explanations help gain the cooperation and relaxation of the patient.

2. Do not take a pulse immediately after the patient has been emotionally upset or after exertion, unless so ordered.

3. Never use your thumb to take a pulse, because its own pulse is likely to be confused with the one being taken.

4. Always count any unusual pulse for a full minute, and repeat if uncertain.

5. When the pulse feels normal and is regular, count the number of pulsations for 30 seconds. Multiply this number by 2 to obtain the pulse rate for 1 minute.

PROCEDURE

1. Identify the patient and explain the procedure.

2. Wash your hands. **Use appropriate personal protective equipment (PPE) as indicated by facility.**

3. Position the patient with the arm supported and at rest.

4. Take a firm hold of the patient's wristbone just over the radial artery, with sufficient pressure to feel the pulsation distinctly. (Pulse rates at other locations previously noted are taken in similar fashion) (Figure 2-14).

5. Count the pulse for 60 seconds. Also see No. 5 under General Instructions.

6. Note the rate, rhythm, volume, and condition of the arterial wall.

7. Write the pulse rate down immediately.

8. Record accurately on the patient's chart.

RATIONALE

A firm hold inspires the patient's confidence. Excess pressure prevents the pulse from being felt. Never use your thumb to take a pulse, because the pulse in your thumb can be confused with that of the patient.

This gives the total beats per minute and provides adequate time to assess the rate, rhythm, and volume of the pulse. Always report any deviation from normal. If deviations are noted, always count the pulse rate for 1 full minute, and repeat if uncertain.

Do not trust it to memory.

Charting example:
July 9, 19 ___, 2 p.m.
   Pulse 78
      or
   Radial pulse, right arm —78
   Regular and strong pulsation
      Rae Evans, CMA

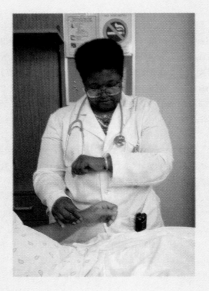

Figure 2-14 *Taking a patient's pulse. Correct position and technique are very important.*

TAKING THE RESPIRATORY RATE

Equipment

A watch with a sweep second hand
Paper or graphic sheet to record respiration rate
Pen

General Instructions

1. Have the patient assume a comfortable position.

2. Do not take the respiratory rate immediately after the patient has been emotionally upset or after exertion, unless so ordered.

3. Count any unusual respiratory rate for an additional minute.

4. Regular respirations may be counted for 30 seconds. This number is then multiplied by 2 to obtain the rate per minute.

PROCEDURE

1. Wash your hands. **Use appropriate personal protective equipment (PPE) as indicated by facility.**

2. Do *not* explain procedure to the patient.

3. Place your fingers on the patient's wrist as though counting the pulse.

4. Count each breathing cycle (inhalation and exhalation) as one breath by watching the rise and fall of the chest or upper abdomen.

5. Count for 1 full minute.

6. Record rate on paper immediately.

7. Record on patient's chart. Note (a) any abnormality if present; (b) any pain associated with breathing; and (c) the position the patient assumes because in some cases it may be significant (for example, when the patient can breathe easier when sitting up or when lying on one side or the other).

RATIONALE

The rate of respirations should be counted and their depth, rate, and rhythm studied without the patient's knowledge. The consciousness of being watched causes an involuntary change in the rate of respiration. A patient can control respirations if he or she wishes to.

When these movements are scarcely perceptible, place the patient's hand gently but firmly on his or her chest, keeping your fingers on the wrist or have the patient lie on his or her back and monitor the rise and fall of the stomach.

Do not trust it to memory.

Charting example:
January 15, 19_____, 2 pm
   Respirations 22 and regular
      L. Quarry, CMA

---

when the ventricles of the heart are in a state of relaxation. During diastole blood flows into the two ventricles of the heart and dilates them, and the pressure within the arteries is at its lowest point.

These measurements provide the physician with valuable information about a patient's cardiovascular system. Systolic pressure provides information about the force of the left ventricular contraction, and diastolic pressure provides information about the resistance of the blood vessels.

Clinically, diastolic pressure is more important than systolic pressure because diastolic pressure indicates the strain or pressure to which the blood vessel walls are constantly subjected. Since diastolic pressure rises or falls with peripheral resistance, it also reflects the condition of the peripheral vessels. For example, if a patient's arteries are sclerosed (hardened), both the peripheral resistance and the diastolic pressure increase.

BP is recorded and discussed as the systolic pressure over the diastolic pressure. A typical BP is expressed as 120/80 (mm Hg) *or* 120 over 80. The numeric difference between these two readings (in this case, 40 points) is called the *pulse pressure*, which may indicate the tone of the arterial walls. A normal pulse pressure is about 40; if consistently over 50 points or under 30 points, it is considered abnormal. You may see an increase in pulse pressure in arteriosclerosis mainly because of an increase in the systolic pressure, or in aortic valve insufficiency because of both a rise in systolic and a fall in diastolic pressure.

Factors that Determine Blood Pressure

A number of factors, acting in dynamic equilibrium and united through the central nervous system, determine the arterial BP:

1. *The pumping action of the heart and cardiac output*— How hard the heart pumps the blood, or the force of the heartbeat; how much blood it pumps and how efficiently it does the job
2. *The volume of blood within the blood vessels*—How much blood the heart pumps into the arterial system
3. *The peripheral resistance of blood vessels to the flow of blood*—The size of the lumen (that is, the central core or channel of the arteries, directly influences the resistance to the blood flow. When the lumen is narrow, the BP is higher; with a wider lumen, the BP is lower.
4. *The elasticity of the walls of the main arteries*—The main arteries leading from the heart have walls with strong elastic fibers capable of expanding and absorbing the pulsations generated by the heart. At each pulsation, the arteries expand and absorb the momentary increase in BP. As the heart relaxes in preparation for another beat, the aortic and pulmonary valves close to prevent blood from flowing back to the ventricles of the heart, and the artery walls spring back, forcing the blood through the body between contractions. In this way the arteries act as dampers on the pulsation and thus provide a steady flow of blood through the blood vessels. This elasticity of the arterial walls lessens with age, and because the arterial wall is less flexible, the BP is higher.
5. *The blood's viscosity, or thickness*—BP increases as the viscosity of blood increases. Polycythemia, an increase in red blood cells, causes this.

How much each factor contributes is not known, but it is generally thought that peripheral resistance and cardiac output have the greatest influence on BP.

Normal Readings and Values for Blood Pressure

At birth the systolic pressure is about 80 mm Hg. *At age 10* (young people), systolic BP varies normally from 100 to 120 mm Hg and diastolic from 60 to 80 mm Hg. *In adults* the *average* BP is 120/80. The *average ranges* are 90 to 140 mm Hg for systolic pressure and 60 to 90 mm Hg for diastolic pressure. As age increases, the BP gradually increases. In *older people* (around 60 years) the systolic BP normally varies from 140 to about 170 mm Hg, and diastolic varies from 92 to 100 mm Hg because of loss of resilience in the vascular tree and the physiologic changes of aging.

Variations in Normal Blood Pressure

BP can vary between the sexes (with women usually having a lower pressure than men), between different age groups, and even between individuals of the same age and sex. At birth it is the lowest; it continues to increase with age, usually reaching its peak in advancing age. Variations are also seen at different times of day and during different activities. BP is higher when a person is standing or sitting than when he or she is lying down. It is normally lowest just before awakening in the morning.

VOCABULARY

Benign hypertension (be-nin)—Hypertension of slow onset that is usually without symptoms.
Essential hypertension (idiopathic or primary hypertension)—Hypertension that develops in the absence of kidney disease. Its cause is unknown. About 85% to 90% of the cases of hypertension are in this category. Frequently, high BP runs in families and may be genetically determined.
Hypertension (hi´ per-ten´ shun)—High BP; a condition in which a patient has a higher BP than normal for his or her age, (for example, systolic pressure consistently above 160 mm Hg and diastolic pressure above 90 mm Hg). Mild or borderline hypertension is 140/90 to 160/95.
Hypotension (hi´ po-ten´ shun)—A decrease of systolic and diastolic BP to below normal (for example, below 90/50 is considered low BP).
Malignant hypertension (mah-lig´ nant)—Hypertension that differs from other types in that it is a rapidly developing hypertension and may prove fatal if not treated immediately after symptoms develop, before the blood vessels are damaged. This type occurs most often in persons in their twenties or thirties.

Orthostatic BP (or´tho-stat´ ik)—BP measured when the patient is in an erect, standing position.
Orthostatic hypotension—Hypotension occurring when a patient assumes an erect position.
Postural hypotension—Hypotension occurring on suddenly arising from a recumbent position or when standing still for a long period of time.
Renal hypertension—Hypertension resulting from kidney disease.
Secondary hypertension—Hypertension that is traceable to known causes such as a pheochromocytoma (tumor of the adrenal gland), hardening of the arteries, kidney disease, or obstructions to the kidney blood flow. Approximately 10% to 15% of the cases of hypertension are secondary. Patients with secondary hypertension can often be cured *if* the underlying cause can be eliminated.

There are many other situations that produce changes in the BP. The following lists indicate some of the common causes of an increase or decrease in a person's pressure.

Increased or elevated
- Exercise
- Stress, anxiety, excitement
- Conditions in which blood vessels become more rigid and lose some of their elasticity (for example, old age)
- Increased peripheral resistance caused vasoconstriction or narrowing or peripheral blood vessels
- Endocrine disorders such as hyperthyroidism and acromegaly
- Increased weight
- Smoking
- Pain
- Renal disease and diseases of the liver and heart
- Certain drug therapy
- Increased intracranial pressure
- Increased arterial blood volume

NOTE: In the right arm, it is about 3 to 4 mm Hg higher than in the left arm

Decreased or lowered
- Cardiac failure
- Massive heart attack
- Decreased arterial blood volume (such as in hemorrhage)
- Shock and collapse
- Dehydration
- Drug treatment
- Disorders of the nervous system
- Adrenal insufficiency
- Hypothyroidism
- Sleep
- Infections, fevers
- Cancer
- Anemia
- Neurasthenia
- Approaching death

Abnormal Readings

Hypertension is commonly referred to as the "silent killer" because patients frequently exhibit *no* symptoms. In children around age 10, upper limits of normal are 140/100; systolic pressure greater than 140 mm Hg are generally recognized as being abnormal. In adults a systolic pressure consistently above 150 mm Hg and a diastolic pressure consistently above 90 mm Hg are generally recognized as being abnormal. **Definite hypertension** is systolic pressure consistently over 160 mm Hg or diastolic pressure over 90 mm Hg. If the BP is consistently above this level, it could, if not treated, damage the heart, eyes, kidneys, and even the arteries. It can also be fatal. *Some specialists consider a BP in excess of 140/90 for people under the age of 60 as abnormal.* Diagnosis of hypertension is never based on only one reading. It is based on at least three consecutive daily or weekly pressure readings. Appropriate treatment of hypertension can markedly reduce the untoward effects such as heart failure, blindness, kidney failure, and stroke.

Hypotension is systolic pressure consistently under 90 with the diastolic pressure in proportion. In the absence of other signs or symptoms, hypotension is generally innocent. An extremely low BP is occasionally a symptom of a serious condition such as shock and *may* be associated with Addison's disease (underfunctioning of the adrenal glands) and severe iron-deficient anemia.

Detection and Evaluation of High Blood Pressure

The Joint National Committee on Detection, Evaluation, and Treatment of High Blood Pressure has recommended that all adults with *diastolic* BPs of 120 mm Hg or above should be referred promptly to a source of medical care. All persons with BPs of 160/95 mm Hg or above should have the BP elevation confirmed within 1 month. All persons *under the age of 50* with a BP between 140/90 mm Hg and 160/95 mm Hg should be checked every 2 to 3 months. All persons *over 50 years* of age with a BP between 140/90 mm Hg and 160/95 mm Hg should be checked every 6 to 9 months. All adults with *diastolic* BPs below 90 mm Hg should have their BP checked yearly.

The *purpose* of the BP recheck is to separate persons with initially elevated BP into (1) those whose diastolic BPs have returned to normal and who therefore require only annual BP remeasurement, and (2) those with sustained elevation in pressure that warrants treatment or further diagnostic study.

At each repeat visit, the person's BP should be taken two or more times, and the average pressure obtained should be used as the value for the visit. BP measurements should be obtained on at least *two* occasions before specific therapy is prescribed, unless the initial diastolic BP is greater than 120 mm Hg.

Patient education begins at the same time the BP is initially measured. Without alarming the patient, the person taking the pressure must carefully communicate the importance of following the recommended action.

The physician frequently includes the following when evaluating the patient's condition.

1. History

The medical history consists of any previous history of high BP or its treatment, the use of birth control pills or other hormones, cardiac or renal disease, stroke, and other cardiovascular risk factors, including diabetes, cigarette smoking, a high salt intake, lipid abnormalities, or family history or high BP or its complications. A history of weakness, muscle cramps, and polyuria suggests further screening for aldosteronism. A history of headaches, palpitations, or excessive sweating suggests further study for pheochromocytoma.

2. Physical evaluation

In addition to two or more BP measurements (one standing), the pretreatment physical examination includes the items listed below:

  a. Height and weight

  b. Funduscopic examination of the eyes for hemorrhages, exudates, and papilledema; especially

Recommended Action for Initial BP Measurement

Systolic/Diastolic	Recommended Action
	All adults
Diastolic 120 or higher	Prompt evaluation and treatment
	All adults
150/95 or higher	Confirm BP elevation within 1 month
	Under age 50
140/90 to 160/95	BP check within 2-3 months
	Age 50 or older
140/90 to 160/95	Check within 6-9 months

Follow-up Recommendations for Referral to Treatment

Average Diastolic Blood Pressure	Recommended Action
120 or higher	Immediate evaluation and treatment indicated
105-119	Treatment indicated
90-104	Individualize treatment
Under 90	Remeasure BP at yearly intervals

important in persons with diastolic BPs of 110 mm Hg or higher

   c. Examination of the neck for thyroid enlargement, bruits, and distended veins

   d. Auscultation of the lungs

   e. Examination of the heart for increased rate, size, precordial heave, murmurs, arrhythmias, and gallops

   f. Examination of the abdomen for bruits, large kidneys, or dilation of the aorta

   g. Examination of the extremities for edema, peripheral pulses, and neurologic deficits associated with stroke

3. Basic laboratory tests

Baseline laboratory tests listed below are obtained before initiating therapy:

   a. Hematocrit

   b. Urinalysis for protein, blood, and glucose (dipstick)

   c. Creatinine and/or blood urea nitrogen

   d. Serum potassium

   e. Electrocardiogram

Other tests that may be helpful include a chest x-ray, blood sugar, serum cholesterol, HDL, LDL, cholesterol/HDL ratio, serum uric acid, microscopic urinalysis, and blood count. (Ordering automated blood chemistries reduces the cost to the patient.) Clinical judgment or abnormal findings obtained during the routine evaluation may suggest other tests such as a intravenous urogram and urinary catecholamines.

4. Explanation of findings to the patient and treatment plans

The patient must be given adequate information to under-stand the disease and what actions he or she must take, and the opportunity to ask questions or discuss points of concern. It is crucial to high BP control that the patient understand the following:

   a. The seriousness and lifelong nature of high BP and the possible consequences of not treating it—there is *no* cure; however, hypertension can be controlled

   b. The importance of taking medication as directed to maintain BP control. BP medications are now available for treatment all forms of high BP.

   c. The importance of adhering to other methods recommended to control BP such as weight loss, reduced intake of animal fats and food high in sodium or salt, not smoking, reduced intake of alcohol (not more than $1^1/_2$ to 2 drinks per day is the recommendation), and mild-to-moderate exercise programs as prescribed by the physician; frequently the physician recommends some combination of the above methods for controlling high BP

   d. The asymptomatic nature of the disease—how the patient feels may not reflect the level of BP or the need to continue taking medication

   e. The importance of keeping follow-up appointments

   f. That treatment of any form of high BP markedly reduces the risk of stroke, heart attack, heart failure, kidney failure, and blindness

Patients not requiring further study or treatment should be reassured, but the importance of an annual BP measurement must be strongly emphasized.

Long-Term Maintenance

Management of high BP must be considered a lifelong endeavor; BP treatment is considered effective if levels are controlled. Patients must be periodically monitored to ensure control and to make certain that they continue therapy. After control has been demonstrated and the patient's BP is stable, remeasurement every 3 to 6 months should be adequate for most patients. Physicians order laboratory and baseline tests according to each patient's age, the initial severity of BP, and the target organ damage.

After normal levels are achieved, it may be possible to reduce drug therapy; however, the patient must understand that it is normally impossible to discontinue treatment. BP may be measured at home when appropriate or when frequent monitoring is deemed necessary.

Most patients with uncomplicated essential hypertension have few, if any, symptoms related to their hypertension; however, they should be warned about drug therapy that may produce unwanted effects. Every effort should be made to adjust drugs and their dosages to eliminate or minimize such unpleasant effects and, at the same time, to gain patient acceptance of any that remain. Those responsible for monitoring antihypertensive regimens should also be aware of pharmacologic interactions and adverse effects of antihypertensive agents and should be alert to discover and/or prevent them.

Numerous reports over the past 20 years show that control of BP can reduce the occurrence of stroke by as much as 40% and the occurrence of heart attacks by 15% in patients with even mild forms of high BP. In patients with severe forms of high BP, treatment can reduce these risks by as much as 70%.

High-Blood Pressure Myth

The *major myth* about high BP is that people can feel when their BP is elevated. It is *very rare* that a person can tell when the BP is elevated unless it is very high. Studies have shown that the signs and symptoms that are frequently associated with hypertension (that is, headache, dizziness, fatigue, shortness of breath, and nosebleeds) are much more common in people with normal BP than they are in patients with hypertension. Therefore, it is recommended that everyone has his or her BP measured to determine the reading. If it is within normal ranges, it should be rechecked every 1 to 2 years.

Instruments for Measuring Blood Pressure

BP is measured with two instruments, a *sphygmomanometer* (sfig-mo-mah-nom' e-ter) and a *stethoscope* (steth'o-skop). Various models of each and combination kits are available (Figure 2-15).

Sphygmomanometers. Two common types of sphygmomanometers (*sphygmo*, pulse; *manos*, slight; *meter*, to measure) are available for general use: the mercury manometer, which uses a column of mercury to measure the BP, and the aneroid (*a*, not; *neroid*, liquid) manometer, which uses compressed air. Acoustic sphygmomanometers are also available.

Each type has advantages and disadvantages. The mercury manometer offers total reliability because, once calibrated at the factory, accuracy is ensured. But it can only be used when the column of mercury is in a vertical position, and it is more fragile and larger than the aneroid type. The aneroid manometer, on the other hand, must be adjusted periodically and calibrated against a mercury manometer. But it is smaller, thus

---

Figure 2-15 *Various types of sphygmomanometers.* **A,** *Wall mercury sphygmomanometer;* **B,** *portable sphygmomanometer;* **C,** *Critikon Vital Signs Monitor.*
(Courtesy Welch-Allyn, Inc.)

A
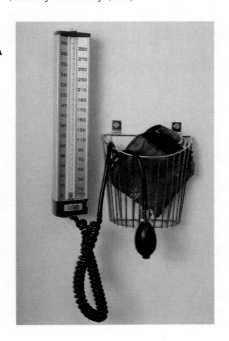

B
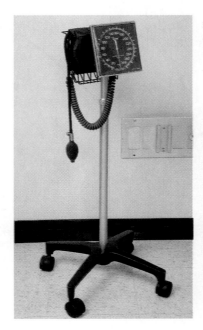

C
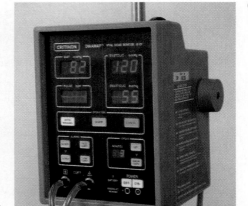

offering more convenience and easier portability. Each manometer has four basic parts (Figure 2-16).

1. *Pressure Indicators.* Pressure indicators are the scales used to read the BP. The mercury manometer has a glass tube with numbers on the side to indicate the height of the column of mercury in millimeters. When the cuff is inflated, mercury is forced up into the tube; as the cuff is deflated, the column of mercury falls. At certain points the level of the column of mercury is noted to provide the BP reading. In the aneroid manometer an internal gear rotates in response to inflation and deflation of the cuff, which in turn moves a needle across a calibrated dial to provide the BP reading.

2. *Cuff.* The compression cuff is a rectangular, inflatable rubber bag covered with a nonstretch material. This is wrapped around the patient's arm and secured with Velcro material or with clasps. On older models, the end of the cuff is tucked under one of the turns wrapped around the arm. Various sizes of cuffs are available to ensure a proper fit. Small cuffs are used on children or very thin people; larger cuffs are used on obese people or when taking a pressure reading on the leg (Table 2-2).

3. *Inflation bulb.* This bulb is used to pump air into the cuff through a rubber tube.

4. *Pressure control valve.* A valve on the inflation bulb is regulated with a thumbscrew to allow the air in the cuff to escape at different rates as it is opened and closed.

Stethoscopes. The second instrument used to measure BP is the *stethoscope,* a basic diagnostic instrument that amplifies sounds produced by the BP, the heart, and other internal body sounds. The key parts of the stethoscope are shown in Figure 2-17.

Measuring Blood Pressure

Auscultation method. Auscultation (aws"kul-ta'shun) is the process of listening for sounds representing the pressure inside the arteries. The artery most frequently used is the

Figure 2-17 *Key parts of the stethoscope.*

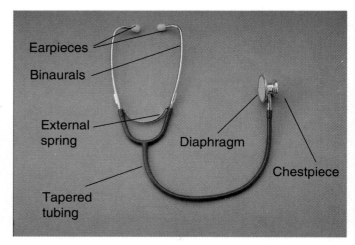

Figure 2-16 *Four basic parts of a sphygmomanometer.*

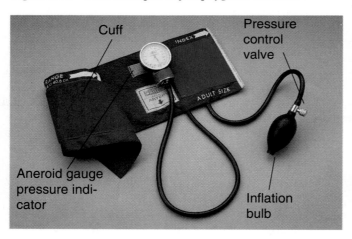

TABLE 2-2	
Recommended Widths of Compression Cuffs	
Age	Width of inflatable bladder
Newborn infants	2.5 cm (1 in.)
Children (1-4 yr)	6 cm (2.3 in.)
Children (4-8 yr)	9 cm (3.5 in.)
Adults	13 cm (5.1 in.)
Obese adults	20 cm (8 in.)

VOCABULARY

Binaurals—Rigid metal tubes that connect the tubing to the earpieces.

Chestpiece—Has one, two, or three "heads" consisting of bell-shaped or various diaphragm-type sensors that "pick up" body sounds.

Diaphragm—A waferlike sound sensor; its shape and the pressure applied to it determine which sound frequencies, low to high, are picked up.

Earpieces—Tips of the stethoscope to be positioned in the examiner's ear.

Spring—The external spring that holds the binaural so that the earpiece is firmly positioned in the ear.

Tubing—Tapered, flexible rubber or plastic tubing through which sound travels from the chestpiece to the binaurals.

brachial artery at the antecubital space opposite the elbow. Other locations that may be used are the popliteal artery behind the knee or, less commonly, the pedal artery on the foot.

When measuring BP you listen for a series of sounds called *Korotkoff sounds.* These sounds are produced by the blood as it flows through the artery. You hear these sounds through the stethoscope placed over the artery as you are deflating the BP cuff. Particular phases of these sounds are what determines the systolic and the diastolic BP readings.

1. *Phase I.* This is the first in a series of faint but clear tapping sounds. These sounds gradually increase in intensity. The first two consecutive sounds represent the systolic pressure.
2. *Phase II.* As the cuff is further deflated, the sounds change to a swishing or murmur. Occasionally these sounds disappear and reappear as the cuff is further deflated by 10 to 40 mm Hg. The period of silence is called the auscultory gap. This is present especially in patients who have hypertension (high BP). Failure to notice this gap may cause serious errors in obtaining a BP reading.
3. *Phase III.* The sounds become crisp and loud. The blood is flowing through an increasingly open artery.
4. *Phase IV.* As the cuff is further deflated, the sounds become dull and muffled. This change of sound is the first diastolic sound.
5. *Phase V.* This is the point at which all sound disappears. This is the second diastolic sound.

Sometimes two figures are used to record the diastolic pressure. The first one used is the number observed when the sound changes in Phase IV. The second figure used is the number observed at the point when all sound disappears. An example of this type of recording: BP 124/82/0. If all of the sounds disappeared when the first diastolic sound was heard, the BP would be recorded as 124/82/82.

Taking a blood pressure reading on the leg
1. The procedure is the same as outlined in the box on page 42, except that the arterial locations differ and the patient should be lying down. A leg pressure may be taken by either of the following methods:
   a. Placing a cuff around the thigh and the bell or diaphragm of the stethoscope over the popliteal artery behind the knee (see Figure 2-13).
   b. Placing the cuff around the calf of the leg and the bell or diaphragm of the stethoscope over the pedal (dorsalis pedis) artery on the foot (see Figure 2-13). This is not a commonly used procedure.

These locations can be used when the brachial artery is inaccessible because of a cast or dressing, or when an arteriovenous shunt for hemodialysis is present in the arm.

Palpation method for measuring blood pressure. This
is an alternative method for measuring blood pressure. When the blood pressure is inaudible by stethoscope, you may use this method, but only when the physician directs you to use it, because it is generally thought to be inaccurate.

The procedure is similar to the auscultation method, except that you use your fingers rather than a stethoscope.
1. Place your fingers over the patient's brachial artery.
2. Pump cuff to at least 20 to 30 mm Hg after pulsation in the artery has ceased.
3. Release the air valve slowly.
4. Read the *systolic pressure* the moment you feel the first pulsation in the artery.
5. The pulse increases in force and tension and then gradually becomes softer; at this point of change, record the *diastolic pressure* if you can feel it. (*Some believe that this reading is not accurate because it is difficult to obtain; therefore they do not obtain a diastolic reading for BP taken by the palpation method.*)
6. Chart and indicate that the BP was obtained by palpation on the brachial artery.

Orthostatic blood pressure. When a patient is on antihypertensive drug therapy, dehydrated, or suffering from hemorrhagic shock, it may take longer than normal for the BP to stabilize when the patient is changed from a lying position to a sitting or standing position. The BP readings taken after this change are known as orthostatic readings.

PHYSICAL MEASUREMENTS OF HEIGHT AND WEIGHT

The two other important physical or clinical measurements to obtain are the height and weight of the patient. It is common practice to take these measurements as part of a physical examination for the following reasons:
1. Because they may provide relevant information for diagnosing, treating, preventing, or evaluating a condition
2. To determine a child's growth pattern (see Unit Four)
3. The patient's weight is used as a guide for determining the dosage to be administered for certain drugs
4. The patient's weight must be known before a magnetic resonance imaging (MRI) examination (see Unit Fourteen) because the machine used must be adjusted to the patient's weight

Recommended standards have been set for the average weight that individuals should be for their height, but these are only ranges, not absolute standards; differences in body types must be considered.

Being overweight or underweight can cause serious health complications. Frequent complications of overweight include hypertension (high BP), heart disease, and diabetes mellitus. Being underweight may indicate malnourishment or metabolic disorders. Either may be the result of psychologic problems.

Many patients are very self-conscious about their weight; therefore it is advisable to have the scales located in an area that ensures privacy. Also to reduce embarrassment, you may

Text continues on page 47.

TAKING BLOOD PRESSURE READING ON THE ARM

Equipment

Sphygmomanometer
Stethoscope
70% Isopropyl alcohol
Cotton balls or alcohol sponges
Paper and pencil

General Instructions

1. Before taking the patient's BP, ask if he or she has been or is currently under treatment for high BP. Anyone under treatment should be encouraged to continue, especially if BP is normal at the time of screening, and should be urged to report an elevated BP to the physician. The potential dangers of discontinuing antihypertensive treatment and the desirability of controlling BP must be strongly emphasized.
2. Ensure as much confidentiality as possible during the recording of the BP.
3. Be sure the patient is relaxed and in a comfortable position. Depending on the physician's orders, the patient may be sitting, standing, or lying.
4. If possible, take all subsequent observations with the patient in the same position and using the same arm.
5. Do not leave the cuff inflated any longer than necessary because prolonged pressure affects the accuracy of the readings and is unpleasant for the patient.

6. On all new patients, BP should be taken on both arms. If a discrepancy exists, the arm with the higher pressure is used in future recordings. This discrepancy is to be recorded on the chart.
7. BP is taken routinely on the following patients, the frequency being determined by their condition:
   a. Patients receiving a complete physical examination
   b. Children before entering school
   c. Patients on hypertensive drugs
   d. Patients with a history of heart, kidney, or hypertensive disease
   e. New admissions to the hospital
   f. Pregnant patients
   g. Postpartum patients
   h. Preoperative patients
   i. Postoperative patients
   j. Patients in shock or those who are hemorrhaging
   k. All patients with neurologic disorders
   l. *All* patients as a preventive health measure
8. Check the sphygmomanometer regularly for loss of mercury and for leaks in the tubing, compression bag, and bulb.
9. Before and after each use of the stethoscope, clean the earpieces and the bell or diaphragm with a cotton ball soaked in alcohol or with an alcohol sponge.
10. Handle these instruments gently; misuse adversely affects their proper functioning.

PROCEDURE

1. Wash hands and obtain equipment. **Use appropriate personal protective equipment (PPE) as indicated by facility.**

2. Identify patient and explain the procedure.

3. Help the patient assume a comfortable position with the arm extended and supported.

4. Place a mercury sphygmomanometer on a level surface, in a position in which the scale can be easily read.

5. Expose the patient's arm well above the elbow.

6. Apply the cuff of the sphygmomanometer over the brachial artery (see Figure 2-13) 1 to 2 inches above the antecubital space, and wrap the remainder of the cuff around the arm so that each turn covers the previous one (Figure 2-18). On older model cuffs, tuck the end under one of the turns; some cuffs have clasps or hooks to fasten, and the newer models with Velcro closures adhere to the last turn on the cuff.

RATIONALE

Explanations help gain the patient's confidence and relaxation.

The patient may be sitting, standing, or lying down, depending on the physician's orders.

Having a mercury manometer at your eye level enables you to take a more accurate reading.

Clothing should be adjusted to avoid constriction and to prevent rustling of garments.

You should apply the cuff snugly and neatly. The arm may be flexed slightly after the cuff is applied. Use a child's or infant's cuff for small children or on extremely thin patients and the larger cuff on obese patients to obtain an accurate reading (see Table 2-2).

TAKING BLOOD PRESSURE READING ON THE ARM—cont'd

PROCEDURE	RATIONALE
7. Locate the strongest pulsation of the brachial artery in the antecubital space by palpating with your fingers at the bend of the elbow (Figure 2-19).	
8. Adjust the earpieces of the stethoscope in your ears, place the bell or diaphragm of the stethoscope over the artery pulsation, and hold in place (Figure 2-20).	*The bell or diaphragm should always be placed below, not under, the cuff and directly over the strongest pulsation of the brachial artery that is felt.*
9. With your dominant hand, close the air valve on the hand bulb by turning the thumbscrew in a clockwise direction. Pump air into the cuff of the manometer rapidly until the level of mercury is about 20 to 30 mm Hg above the palpated or previously measured systolic pressure (the procedure for taking BP by palpation is explained on page 41).	*Blood is cut off when the cuff is inflated. To identify the true systolic pressure, air must be pumped into the cuff rapidly, and then the cuff deflated slowly. Inflating the cuff slowly or sending the mercury to a higher level than necessary is very uncomfortable for the patient. To avoid missing the true systolic reading, pressure can initially be taken by the palpation method and then 15 to 30 seconds later the pressure reading can be taken by the auscultation method.*
10. Turn the thumbscrew counterclockwise to open the air valve slowly. Allow for a slow release of air to the cuff so that the pressure falls only 2 to 3 mm Hg at a time (Figure 2-21).	*Rapid deflation of the cuff causes you to miss the exact reading.*
11. Listen carefully and read the exact point on the mercury column (or spring gauge if using an aneroid manometer) at which the first distinct sound is heard. Keep this number in mind; this represents the systolic pressure.	*This sound is caused by the initial spurt of blood into the collapsed artery as deflation of the cuff occurs.* *This is Phase I of the Korotkoff sounds.*
12. Continue to allow the air to escape, thereby letting the cuff deflate slowly. The sounds get louder and then become like a murmur, then crisp, then dull and soft, then fade away (Figure 2-22).	*This is a continuation of Phases I, II, III, and into Phase IV of the Korotkoff sounds.*
13. Read the scale when the sound becomes dull or muffled. Keep this number in mind; it represents the diastolic pressure.	*The level of mercury at the point where the sound changes from loud to dull or muffled is the diastolic pressure, representing the pressure in the arteries during diastole of the heart.* *This is Phase IV of the Korotkoff sounds.*
14. Continue to deflate the cuff until the sound disappears. This is Phase V of the Korotkoff sounds. Remember this number because many physicians request that both numbers be reported for diastolic readings.	*This is Phase V of the Korotkoff sounds.*
15. Open the valve completely to release all the air from the cuff.	*The blood in the veins in the lower arm is not able to return to the heart if all the air in the cuff is not released.*
16. If there is any doubt of an accurate reading, wait 15 seconds, then repeat steps 7 through 15. Do not repeat more than twice on the same arm, because the reading will be inaccurate because of blood stasis (blood trapped in the arm).	*Between readings, the cuff must be completely deflated. Failure to do so produces erroneously high readings.*
17. Write the BP down on paper as a mathematic fraction. If your employer doesn't mind, you may inform the patient of the numeric value of the BP.	*Do not trust it to memory. Record systolic reading over diastolic reading as a mathematical fraction. (For example, 120/80 or 120/80-60 (60 indicating where the sounds disappear).*
18. Remove the cuff from the patient's arm.	
19. See that the patient is comfortable.	

TAKING BLOOD PRESSURE READING ON THE ARM—cont'd

PROCEDURE

20. Return the equipment to the designated area and prepare it for storage according to the type of apparatus used. Cleanse the earpiece and diaphragm of the stethoscope with alcohol sponge.

21. Record the BP on the patient's chart.

22. Notify the physician if you have obtained a relatively higher or lower reading than previously recorded.

RATIONALE

Charting example:
    October 1, 19__, 2 p.m.
      BP 118/86 rt arm
        or
    118/86-70
    Ann Banks, CMA

Further evaluation or only periodic measurement may be needed. Because an initial high reading may reflect only a transient increase, which could be due to anxiety or excitement, the BP should be measured on different days and after the patient has been able to relax for a time.

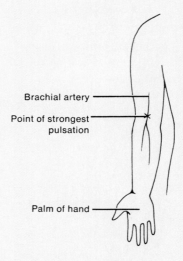

Brachial artery —

Point of strongest pulsation —

Palm of hand —

Figure 2-19 *Location of strongest pulsation in the antecubital space.*

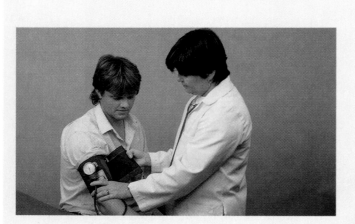

Figure 2-18 *Applying the cuff of the sphygmomanometer above the antecubital space of the right arm. Wrap cuff around the arm in the usual way. Make sure microphone is over brachial artery. With cuff in place, raise pressure to approximately 30 mm Hg beyond expected systolic pressure. Watch digital countdown as pressure automatically releases. Systolic pressure is displayed first, followed by diastolic pressure as the sphygmomanometer responds to appropriate sounds. When both systolic and diastolic readings are displayed, the touch of a button also lets you read pulse rate.*

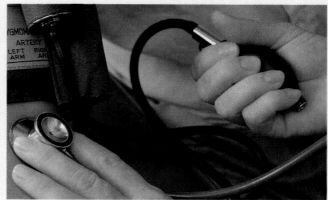

Figure 2-20 *Adjusting the stethoscope for taking BP.*

TAKING BLOOD PRESSURE READING ON THE ARM—cont'd

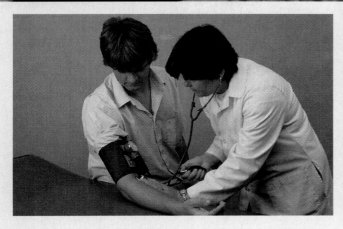

Figure 2-21 *Technique for taking BP using aneroid sphygmomanometer.*

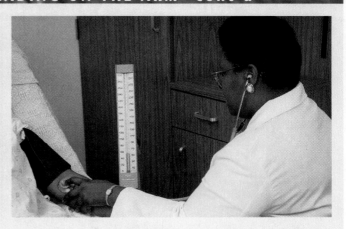

Figure 2-22 *Mercury column descending as air is released from the cuff.*

MEASURING ORTHOSTATIC BLOOD PRESSURE

Equipment

Sphygmomanometer
Stethoscope

PROCEDURE	RATIONALE
1. Identify the patient and explain the procedure.	*Explanations help gain the patient's confidence and relaxation.*
2. Have the patient assume a recumbent position for 5 minutes, and then take the BP and apical pulse.	
3. Instruct the patient to sit up at a 90-degree angle. Take the BP and apical pulse immediately. Ask how the patient feels.	*The patient may feel dizzy.*
4. Have the patient stand up at the side of the examining table. Take the BP and apical pulse immediately. Question the patient concerning a change in equilibrium.	*The patient may need to rest between the sitting and standing measurements. Standing pressure may be omitted, depending on the physician's order and/or the patient's condition.*
5. Chart the BPs and apical pulses on the patient's medical record. Indicate which readings were taken when the patient was lying down, sitting, and standing.	*Charting example:* *120/80—lying* *110/80—sitting* *90/70—standing* *August 22, 19____, 8 a.m.* *T. O'Connell, CMA*

6. Report the following to the physician:
   a. Any systolic change greater than 10 mm Hg in lying/sitting or lying/standing positions
   b. Any diastolic change greater than 20 mm Hg in lying/sitting or lying/standing positions
   c. Any apical pulse change greater than 20 beats per minute in a lying/sitting or lying/standing position	

MEASURING HEIGHT AND WEIGHT

Equipment

A weight scale with height measuring bar

PROCEDURE	RATIONALE
1. Wash your hands—**Use appropriate personal protective equipment (PPE) as indicated by facility.**	
2. Identify the patient and explain the procedure.	
3. Place a clean paper town on the scale foot stand.	*This is just one form of expected clean technique. Use a clean towel for each patient.*
4. Balance the scale. Ensure that both weights are on zero and that the balance bar hangs free before the patient steps onto the scale.	*Unbalanced scales result in an inaccurate weight measurement.*
5. Have the patient remove shoes and any jacket or heavy outer sweater. In some offices or agencies, the patient may be weighed in a patient gown.	*The removal of heavy outer clothing provides a more accurate reading.*
6. Direct and/or assist the patient onto the scale. NOTE: You may raise the height bar above the patient's estimated weight and have it in position before the patient steps onto the scale to avoid moving and manipulating it later.	
7. Ask the patients his or her usual weight, and then move the 50-pound weight to the 50-, 100-, 150-, 200-, or 250-pound mark, ensuring that the weight is resting securely in the weight indicator groove (Figure 2-23). Metric scales are marked using 10-kg increments.	*Unless the weight is secured correctly in the groove provided, the patient's weight measurement will be off by many pounds.*
8. Gradually move the upper weight across the individual pound register until the arm at the right end of the balance bar rests in a position in the center of the metal frame, not touching either edge of this frame.	*The weight is read when the balance bar is in the middle.*
9. Read the weight accurately to the nearest quarter of a pound *or* the nearest 0.1 kg. NOTE: Pediatric scales measure weights in pounds and ounces or grams and kilograms.	
10. Return the weights to zero.	

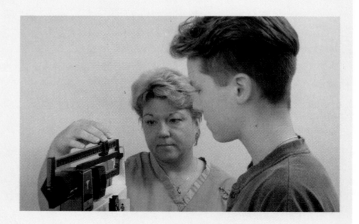

Figure 2-23   *Weighing the patient.*

MEASURING HEIGHT AND WEIGHT—cont'd

PROCEDURE	RATIONALE
11. Record the weight on the patient's chart.	*When charting, you must indicate if the patient was wearing street clothes or a patient gown.*
12. To measure height, either have the patient remain on the scale, standing erect and looking straight ahead, *or* have the patient face away from the scale.	*The patient must be standing very straight to obtain the correct height measurement.*
13. If the height bar was not raised previously (see step 6), raise it over the patient's head and extend the hinged arm.	
14. Carefully lower the height bar until it touches the top of the patient's head lightly (Figure 2-24).	
15. Read the height measurement.	*The number (in inches) indicating the patient's height is the last digit or fraction visible at the point where the movable part of the bar enters its stationary holder.*
16. Assist the patient off the scale if necessary and return the height bar to the resting position.	
17. Record the height accurately in feet and inches. Use accepted abbreviations. Some height bars use the metric scale. The height is then recorded in centimeters (cm).	*Charting example:* *October 27, 19___, 4 p.m.* *Ht. 5′ 2″* *Wt. 112 lb in street clothes, s [without] shoes.* *Annie Fox, CMA*

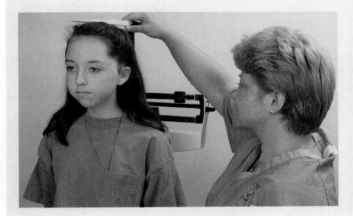

Figure 2-24 *Measuring the patient's height.*

have the patient stand with the back to the numbers on the scale. It is important in this procedure, as in all procedures, that you maintain a neutral facial expression to avoid communicating your impressions to the patient.

Be alert, and note any unusual weight gains or losses in established patients and comments regarding changes by new patients, either of which may be an important diagnostic aid.

Some scales are calibrated in kilograms, and others in pounds. To convert a weight, use the following formulas:

To convert kilograms to pounds (kg to lb):

1 kg = 2.2 pounds

Multiply the number of kilograms by 2.2
EXAMPLE: If a patient weighs 60 kg, multiply 60 × 2.2

60 × 2.2 = 132 pounds

To convert pounds to kilograms (lb to kg):
Divide the number of pounds by 2.2
EXAMPLE: If a patient weighs 132 pounds, divide 132 by 2.2

132 ÷ 2.2 = 60 kg

See Table 2-3 for the conversion of pounds to kilograms and Table 2-4 for the average heights and weights for adults.

For convenience, post a conversion chart near the area

TABLE 2-3

Conversion Table: Pounds to Kilograms*

Pounds	Kilograms	Pounds	Kilograms	Pounds	Kilograms
1	0.45	100	45.36	205	92.99
2.2	1.00	105	47.63	210	95.26
5	2.27	110	49.90	215	97.52
10	4.54	115	52.12	220	99.79
15	6.80	120	54.43	225	102.06
20	9.07	125	56.70	230	104.33
25	11.34	130	58.91	235	106.60
30	13.61	135	61.24	240	108.86
35	15.88	140	63.50	245	111.13
40	18.14	145	65.77	250	113.40
45	20.41	150	68.04	255	115.67
50	22.68	155	70.31	260	117.94
55	24.95	160	72.58	265	120.20
60	27.22	165	74.84	270	122.47
65	29.48	170	77.11	275	124.74
70	31.75	175	79.38	280	127.01
75	34.02	180	81.65	285	129.28
80	36.29	185	83.92	290	131.54
85	38.56	190	86.18	295	133.81
90	40.82	195	88.45	300	136.08
95	43.09	200	90.72		

*To convert:
Pounds to kilograms: multiply number of pounds by 0.45 (0.4536).
Kilograms to pounds: multiply number of kilogram by 2.2 (2.204).

CONCLUSION

You have now completed the unit on Physical Measurements, the most basic clinical procedures that you may be required to perform. When you have practiced these procedures and feel competent in performing them, arrange with your instructor to take the Performance Test.

You will be expected to demonstrate accurately your ability to prepare for and take the vital signs and height and weight measurements on individuals assigned to you by your instructor.

TABLE 2-4

Desirable Weights-ages 25 to 59 Based on Lowest Mortality*

	Men					Women†		
Height (in shoes with 1-inch heels)					Height (in shoes with 1-inch heels)			
Feet	Inches	Small frame	Medium frame	Large frame	Feet	Inches	Small frame	Medium frame	Large frame

Feet	Inches	Small frame	Medium frame	Large frame	Feet	Inches	Small frame	Medium frame	Large frame
5	2	128-134	131-141	138-150	4	10	102-111	109-121	118-131
5	3	130-136	133-143	140-153	4	11	103-113	111-123	120-134
5	4	132-138	135-145	142-156	5	0	104-115	113-126	122-137
5	5	134-140	137-148	144-160	5	1	106-118	115-129	125-140
5	6	136-142	139-151	146-164	5	2	108-121	118-132	128-143
5	7	138-145	142-154	149-168	5	3	111-124	121-135	131-147
5	8	140-148	145-157	152-172	5	4	114-127	124-138	134-151
5	9	142-151	148-160	155-176	5	5	117-130	127-141	137-155
5	10	144-154	151-163	158-180	5	6	120-133	130-144	140-159
5	11	146-157	154-166	161-184	5	7	123-136	133-147	143-163
6	0	149-160	157-170	164-188	5	8	126-139	136-150	146-167
6	1	152-164	160-174	168-192	5	9	129-142	139-153	149-170
6	2	155-168	164-178	172-197	5	10	132-145	142-156	152-173
6	3	158-172	167-182	176-202	5	11	135-148	145-159	155-176
6	4	162-176	171-187	181-207	6	0	138-151	148-162	158-179

Courtesy Metropolitan Life Insurance Co., New York, NY.
*Weights in pounds according to frame (in indoor clothing weighing 5 pounds for men and 3 pounds for women).
†For women between 18 and 25, subtract 1 pound for each year under 25.

REVIEW OF VOCABULARY

This is a sample of how a physician may write up part of a patient's case history. In the following sentences, words that have been defined for you in the unit are used. Read this and define the italicized terms.

PHYSICIAN'S STATEMENT OF A PATIENT'S *VITAL SIGNS* This 40-year-old patient was first seen with the chief complaint of frequent *dyspnea* and *orthopnea* at night. On examination of the chest, *rales* were heard, and *respirations* were *accelerated* to 30 per minute.
Patient stated that he often *hyperventilated*, especially in stressful situations.
Patient had a fever of 103° F, which remained *constant* over the first 24 hours after being seen in my office. The *onset* of this *fever* was apparently 2 days before this examination.
Bigeminal pulse rate, arrhythmia, and *pulse deficit* of at least eight beats—*apical pulse rate* was 130; *radial pulse rate* was 122, approximately. Venous pulse in the external jugulars was palpable and also very *irregular.*
BP—systolic, 164; *diastolic,* 128.
Pulse pressure 36. Height 5′ 6 ″; weight, 142 lbs.
Family history revealed that this patient's father has *hypertension,* mother has *hypotension,* and sister was diagnosed as having *malignant hypertension* at the age of 29.
For more information on this patient's history, please refer to past notes in the previous chart.
Y. Short, MD

CONSULTATION LETTER TO REFERRING PHYSICIAN

December 15, 19____

Dr. Y. Short
666 South W Street
Anytown, USA

Dear Dr. Short:

Mrs. Alice Price was seen initially on 9/27/93 at your request because of her progressing nocturnal choking sensations during the past year.

It was of interest to learn that I had seen her sometime before 1979 for a respiratory allergy syndrome that was attributed to dust and other inhalants following some testing procedures.

She indicates that she has been living in the same residence for the past 14 years and has had the same pet, a chihuahua, for the past 12 years. There has been some sputum production without blood with the present illness but no chest pain or peripheral edema. She had retired from her employment as a janitress with the City and County of Anytown 2 years ago.

Past history shows T & A [tonsillectomy and adenoidectomy] age 27, appendectomy and hysterectomy proximate to that date, and a whiplash 3 years ago.

The weight is in the 168-lb range, and she indicates an allergy to pork and fish, which she believes may precipitate her nocturnal dyspneic events. She has had nocturia three times nightly for the past year; she drinks two cups of coffee and tea per day, uses no cigarettes, and her alcohol intake is moderate. Her medications are limited to the Tri-Pro-Hist prescribed by you for her asthma.

The various laboratory data of 9/10/93 were not remarkable, except for liver enzyme elevation, and it was noted the PME equaled 2% on the differential. Chest x-ray film in 1986 was reportedly negative, and was noted the PME equaled 2% on the differential. Chest x-ray film in 1986 was reportedly negative, and no changes were seen on the 9/27/93 repeat film. Physical signs showed height 66 inches, weight 169 lbs; the general findings were normal except for BP 160/109.

Vital capacity was 3.0 liters (90% normal) with mild FEV$_1$ [full expiration volume 1] delay, and EKG showed an intermediate heart with changes suggesting hypocarbia.

It was my belief that Mrs. Alice Price has the following conditions:
1. Arterial hypertension, mild
2. Exogenous obesity, approximately 30 lbs
3. Paroxysmal nocturnal dyspnea, atopic, possibly associated with food and/or inhalants
4. Hepatic insufficiency, metabolic origin

I advised her of these several entities, prescribed Aldactazide one daily for antihypertensive effect, and suggested that she continue on the antihistamine prescribed by you. When reviewed on 10/3/93, she had had significant diuretic effect, fewer nocturnal events, and BP was 150/92.

I therefore advised her to remain on the Aldactazide daily and supplement the antihistamine with Elixophyllin 0.2 on a prn basis for dyspnea.

She will report back in 1 month, and if there are any unusual circumstances, I shall promptly advise you.

Sincerely yours

R. G. Lewis, MD

CASE STUDY

The following examples contain variations from normal vital signs. Read each and be able to discuss the italicized terminology.

1. A patient telephones the office to advise of a *constant oral* temperature higher than 100° F for 18 hours. This is the third episode of *pyrexia* of undetermined origin in 2 months.
2. A patient has a *B/P* of 140 and the doctor has recommended immediate evaluation and treatment, including daily monitoring of BP at home because of suspected *arrhythmias*.

3. In reviewing the *TPR* on the chart of an 82-year-old female, a *thready pulse* was indicated following an episode of syncope.
4. While cleansing the *diaphragm* of the *sphygmomanometer* and *stethoscope* with *isopropyl alcohol*, the medical assistant noticed the *binaurals* were bent and inserted a new set.

REVIEW QUESTIONS

1. List three purposes for taking a patient's vital signs.
2. For the following situations, indicate if you would normally see an increase or a decrease in each of the following: temperature, pulse rate, respiratory rate, and BP:
   a. A patient who faints
   b. A patient who has a severe infection in her
   c. A patient who is hemorrhaging
   d. A patient who has just jogged for 2 miles
   e. A patient who has a brain stem injury
   f. A patient who becomes extremely excited or upset
   g. A patient who is sleeping
   h. A child as compared with an adult
3. List the normal average readings for the following:
   a. Oral temperature in adults
   b. Axillary temperature in adults
   c. Rectal temperature in adults
   d. Pulse rate in adults
   e. Respiratory rate in adults
   f. BP in adults
4. Convert the following temperatures to centigrade degrees:
   a. 98.6° F
   b. 97.8° F
   c. 100.4° F
   d. 99.6° F
5. Convert the following temperatures to Fahrenheit degrees:
   a. 39.5°C
   b. 36° C
   c. 38.2° C
   d. 37.2° C
6. List four benefits of tympanic thermometry over glass mercury thermometers.
7. Why is the tympanic membrane an accurate indicator of body temperature?

8. List and describe the location of the seven most common arteries where a pulse may be felt.
9. If a patient has an extremely sore mouth, how would you take the temperature?
10. What is meant by the pulse rate? The respiratory rate?
11. What is meant by the rhythm of the pulse rate? The rhythm of the respiratory rate?
12. You have just taken a patient's respiratory rate and found it to be 10 respirations per minute. Would you consider this a normal and adequate rate or a throat?
13. What action is taking place in the heart during systole? During diastole?
14. Why does BP usually increase in the elderly?
15. If a patient had plaster casts on both arms, where and how would you take the BP?
16. A patient's BP is 130/92. What is the pulse pressure? Is this pulse pressure in the normal range?
17. What medical condition is commonly referred to as the "silent killer?" Explain why.
18. List four conditions that may be prevented if hypertension is treated successfully.
19. List four methods that may be used to control high BP.
20. Convert the following body weights to measurements in pounds:
    a. 52 kg
    b. 68.5 kg and how would you take the BP?
    c. 47 kg
    d. 56 kg
21. Convert the following body weights to measurements in kilograms:
    a. 112 lb
    b. 174 lb
    c. 136 lb
    d. 155 lb

PERFORMANCE TEST

In a skills laboratory, a simulation of a joblike environment, the medical assistant student must demonstrate knowledge and skill in performing the following procedures without reference to source materials. For these activities the student needs a watch with a second hand, rectal and oral thermometers, a stethoscope, a sphygmomanometer, alcohol sponges, containers for used thermometers, a scale with height measuring bar, various individuals to play the role of a patient, and patient chart. The instructor assigns time limits and the number of patients to be tested for each procedure.

Given an ambulatory patient and the appropriate equipment and supplies, obtain and record accurately:

- Oral temperature
- Axillary temperature
- Rectal temperature (a model may be used for this procedure)
- Pulse rate
- Respiratory rate
- BP taken on the brachial artery
- BP taken on the popliteal artery
- Apical heartbeat
- Orthostatic BP
- Height and weight

Grading

Grading systems are flexible in order to meet each instructor's preference. The instructor may wish to use a satisfactory/unsatisfactory grading system, a pass/fail system, or a point-value system for each step on the checklist. It is recommended that each procedure be assigned a time limit by the instructor.

Performance Tests, Checklists, and Evaluation Charts for the instructor's use when evaluating the student's performance of a skill are provided in the Instructor's Manual.

The student is expected to perform the above procedures with 100% accuracy.

*Results obtained for the pulse rates and the respiratory rates are acceptable if within two beats or respirations as determined and recorded by the instructor. Results for BP readings are acceptable if within 2 to 4 mm Hg, as determined and recorded by the instructor. The student is expected to become proficient in these procedures before progressing to others in this book.

Health History and Physical Examinations

COGNITIVE OBJECTIVES

On completion of Unit Two, the medical assistant student should be able to:

1. Define and pronounce the vocabulary terms and define the medical abbreviations listed.
2. List the eight major components of a patient's medical history/record, and describe the information that is recorded in each.
3. List and define the six parts of the patient's medical history.
4. List eight reasons why information gathered during a history and physical examination is valuable to the physician.
5. List and describe six methods of examination used by the physician when performing a physical examination on a patient, giving an example of when or how each is used.
6. List the essential parts of a physical examination.
7. Differentiate between information obtained in the review of systems and that obtained during the physical examination.
8. Discuss the steps taken by a physician when making a diagnosis.
9. List five forms of treatment.
10. List three reasons for diagnostic studies.
11. Discuss the purpose of the patient's medical record.
12. Discuss the importance of correct documentation and confidentiality of the patient's medical record.
13. State who owns the patient's medical record.
14. State reasons for and the technique used to make corrections in a patient's medical record.
15. Discuss options for retaining medical records.

TERMINAL PERFORMANCE OBJECTIVE

On completion of Unit Three, the medical assistant student should be able to:

1. Help obtain and record a brief medical history or statement of the patient's chief complaint.

The student is expected to perform these objectives with 100% accuracy 90% of the time (9 out of 10 times).

The consistent use of universal precautions is required by all health care professionals in all health care settings as a method of infection control. It is assumed that these precautions are used in all of the following procedures. Review Unit One if you have any question on methods to use as the methods/techniques will not be repeated in detail in each procedure presented in the unit.

Be sure to consult the latest guidelines issued by the Centers for Disease Control and Prevention and consult with infection control practitioners when needed to identify specific precautions that pertain to your particular work situation.

THE MEDICAL RECORD

To provide a basis for decision making and planning for the care of a patient, different kinds of information must be gathered, compiled, and maintained in an orderly and confidential manner. Lack of needed information and confidentiality may jeopardize appropriate patient care. The patient's confidential medical record is a compilation of information concerning the patient, the care provided, the progress, and the results obtained. The medical record is a *legal document belonging to the physician or clinical agency.* Because the patient records are legal documents, use only blue or black ink. Do not erase information or use other corrective solutions.

When a physician sees the patient for the first time, identifying information (such as name and address) and all the information necessary for diagnosing the case, prescribing treatment, and planning future care are obtained. Every diagnostic workup has six major components: the history, the physical examination, the summary of positive findings, the interpretation of completed diagnostic studies, the examiner's impression based on all the information gathered, and the care plans, including suggested further study.

On subsequent visits the progress or status of the patient's condition is recorded as progress notes. Eventually, when the patient is discharged or the condition has been resolved, the date of discharge and status of the patient at that time are recorded as the discharge summary.

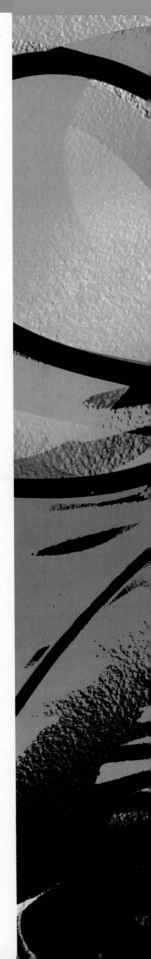

VOCABULARY

Health—The state of mental, physical, and social well-being of an individual; not merely the absence of disease.

Negative findings—*No* evidence of disease or body dysfunction.

Positive findings—Evidence of disease or body dysfunction.

Prodrome—An early symptom indicating the onset of a disease, such as an achy feeling before having the flu.

Prognosis—A statement made by the physician indicating the probable or anticipated outcome of the disease process in a patient; usually stated simply as *good, fair, poor,* or *guarded.*

Sign—Sometimes called a *physical sign*; any objective evidence (apparent to the observer) representing disease or body dysfunction. Signs may be observed by others or revealed when the physician performs a physical examination; examples include swollen ankles, a distended rigid abdomen, elevated blood pressure, and decreased sensation.

Symmetry—Conformity in form, size, and arrangement of parts on opposite sides of the body.

Symptom—Sometimes called a subjective symptom; any subjective evidence of disease or body dysfunction; a change in the physical or mental state of the body that is perceptible or apparent only to the individual experiencing the change; examples include anorexia, nausea, headache, pain, itching, and dizziness.

Syndrome—A combination of symptoms resulting from one cause or commonly occurring together to present a distinct clinical picture; an example is the dumping syndrome, which consists of nausea, weakness, varying degrees of syncope, sweating, palpitation, and sometimes diarrhea and a feeling of warmth. This may occur immediately after eating in patients who have had a partial gastrectomy.

This compilation of information is kept together and called the patient's medical record. These confidential records and reports are arranged in a file folder, binder, or other special type of folder, which is generally referred to as the patient's chart or file.

The medical assistant plays a very important role in obtaining and maintaining data on patients. This responsibility varies with the preference and specialty of the physician. In some instances the medical assistant is expected to relieve the physician of much of the data collection. In these cases, the medical assistant obtains identifying information from the patient; measures the patient's height, weight, temperature, pulse rate, respiration rate, and blood pressure; and takes the medical history. In other situations, the medical assistant may be required to obtain only the identifying information. In addition to recording data, the medical assistant is responsible for preparing the examination room for the examination of the patient, preparing the equipment and supplies needed, preparing the patient both physically and mentally, assisting the patient and the physician, collecting specimens as requested, and organizing the results of diagnostic studies in the patient's record (see also Unit Ten).

Some hospitals have now computerized many parts of their medical records. Physicians have their own secret signature code or password to call up information on their patients. With the appropriate hardware in the office or clinic, physicians can call up certain reports and information about their patients in the hospital to keep them abreast of ongoing care. They can also obtain the discharge summary with a current laboratory summary and recent vital signs for patients leaving the hospital. These reports are then put into the patient's med-

ical record in the office to help the physician provide continuity of care in the clinic or office. Hospital laboratory reports can also be obtained for clinic or office patients.

This unit discusses the components and related information of a patient's medical record, related vocabulary, medical abbreviations, and the problem-oriented medical record. Unit Four presents vocabulary, procedures, and techniques used when preparing for and assisting with various types of physical examinations.

Actual medical reports are cited at the end of the unit in the Review of Vocabulary to help the medical assistant student correlate the contents of this unit with the ways physicians record information about the patient.

HISTORY AND PHYSICAL EXAMINATION

The history and general physical examination are extremely valuable diagnostic tools used by a physician to gather information about the physiologic and sometimes psychologic condition of a patient. Many people now recognize the value of a regular physical examination in preventing disease or treating in the early stages. Most medical authorities recommend that everyone have at least one a year.

Information gathered from a history and general or special physical examination can be used by the physician to determine the following:

- The individual's level of health
- The body's level of physiological functioning
- A tentative diagnosis of a condition or disease
- A confirmed diagnosis of a condition or disease

- The need for additional special examinations or testing
- The type of treatment to be prescribed
- An evaluation of the effectiveness of the prescribed treatment
- Preventive measures to be used

Preventive techniques include educating patients about healthful living habits, administering vaccinations to prevent communicable diseases, using screening procedures such as blood pressure checks and Pap smears, and treating conditions in the early stages to avoid more serious diseases.

The order followed by physicians when taking a history and performing a physical examination may vary somewhat, but the end result is the same, since the same basic areas are covered. One of two types of forms may be used to record the information obtained: a preprinted outline form (Figure 3-1) or a blank sheet of standard-size paper on which the physician writes out all the information gathered. The preprinted form serves as a reminder so that essential factors not overlooked, and it minimizes writing.

HISTORY

The history is a record of the information provided by the patient and/or family or from the patient's health record. It is the systematic account of past medical and psychologic occurrences in a patient's life and other factors that may have an effect on the patient's health. It includes a series of questions and answers regarding the patient.

History taking reveals information about the patient's general health status and physical or emotional problem areas, including both current and potential problems that call for preventive care and advice. Focus is also on the patient's behaviors and feelings about the illness.

History is composed of the following:

1. *Chief Complaint (CC)*. The chief complaint is a brief statement made by the patient describing the nature of the illness and duration of symptoms that led the patient to consult the physician. Chief complaint is abbreviated CC.
2. *History of Present Illness (HPI or PI)*. The history of present illness includes the present illness discussed in detail, the health status of the patient until the onset of the present illness, the onset of symptoms, the character and duration of each, and any other pertinent facts or relation to other events, such as shortness of breath after exertion.
3. *Past History (PH)*. The past history is a summary of all prior illnesses, allergies, drug sensitivities, childhood diseases, surgical procedures, hospital admissions, and serious injuries and disabilities, including the date of each. For women, the number of pregnancies, live births, and abortions, if any, are also recorded. Past history is abbreviated PH.
4. *Family History (FH)*. The family history is the health status and age of immediate relatives; if deceased, the date, age at death, and cause are noted. Diseases among relatives that are thought to have a hereditary or familial tendency or cases in which contact may play a role are also recorded. Examples would be cardiovascular, renal, endocrine, metabolic, mental, or infectious diseases, neoplasms or carcinoma, and allergies.
5. *Social and Occupational History*. The social and occupational history (may also be referred to as personal history and patient profile) includes information relating to where the patient has lived, occupation(s), and environment. This includes statements about the patient's lifestyle and habits, any of which may have a bearing on the development of disease, and the patient's general health status and perception of his/her health. These factors may include the following:
   - Use of tobacco, alcohol, drugs, coffee, tea
   - Diet, sleep, exercise, hobbies, and interests
   - Marital history, children, home life; religious convictions; occupation and employment
   - Sexual preferences, problems, and attitudes
   - Causes, levels of, and ways of reacting to stress
   - Defense mechanisms
   - Resources for support and assistance
   - Cultural, educational, and environmental factors that may be related to health status
6. *Review of Systems (ROS)*. Review of systems is the last category in the history. The purpose of this systematic review is to reveal subjective symptoms that either the patient forgot to discuss or at the time seemed relatively unimportant to the patient. An analysis of the subjective findings, as related by the patient when questioned by the physician, generally gives a clue to the diagnosis and indicates the nature and extent of the physical examination required.

The following are the major headings in the order in which they appear in the patient's ROS and the items that are usually reviewed by the physician. The physician questions the patient as to the usual or unusual presence or condition and/or occurrence of any of these.

The physician asks if there has been or is a history of the following conditions and whether, as well as what, kinds of medications are currently being used for any of the following:*

- General—Chills, fever, sweats, weight gain or loss, fatigue, weakness, nightmares, insomnia, nervousness, loss of memory
- Head—Headaches, trauma, sinus pain, fainting
- Eyes—Vision, pain, burning, eyestrain, redness, photophobia, diplopia, blurred vision, excessive tearing, discharge, any eye diseases, prescription glasses, date of last eye examination
- Ears—Hearing loss, pain, discharge, tinnitus, dizziness, mastoiditis, trauma, noise exposure, vertigo
- Nose—Smell, head colds, discharge, postnasal drip, epistaxis, pain, obstruction, trauma, allergies
- Mouth—Taste, dryness or excessive salivation, condition of lips, tongue, gums, teeth, dentures

*See Appendix A for definitions and pronunciation keys for many of the terms listed.

Figure 3-1 *Preprinted forms used for patient history and physical examination.* **A,** *Front;*
Courtesy Histacount Corp., Melville, N.Y.

GENERAL PRACTICE—cont'd

A

CASE NO.

PATIENT'S NAME

ADDRESS _____ INSURANCE _____ DATE _____

TEL NO _____ REFERRED BY _____ OCCUPATION _____ AGE ___ SEX ___ S.M.W.D.

CASE NO.

FAMILY HISTORY: FATHER _____ MOTHER _____

BROTHERS _____ SISTERS _____

CANCER _____ TUBERCULOSIS _____ INSANITY _____ DIABETES _____ HEART DISEASE _____ RHEUMATISM _____

GOUT _____ GOITER _____ OBESITY _____ NEPHRITIS _____ EPILEPSY _____ OTHER _____

PAST HISTORY: DIPHTHERIA _____ MEASLES _____ MUMPS _____ CHICKEN-POX _____ SCARLET FEVER _____ SMALL POX _____

INFANTILE PARALYSIS _____ TYPHOID _____ MALARIA _____ PNEUMONIA _____ DYSENTERY _____ JAUNDICE _____ BOILS _____

RHEUMATIC FEVER _____ TUBERCULOSIS _____ ASTHMA _____ HEART DISEASE _____ HYPERTENSION _____ DIABETES _____

INFECTIONS _____ GONORRHEA _____ SYPHILIS _____ TONSILLITIS _____ NEPHRITIS _____ OPERATIONS _____

MENSTRUAL: ONSET _____ PERIODICITY _____ TYPE _____ DURATION _____ PAIN _____ L M P _____

MARITAL: MISCARRIAGES _____ ABORTIONS _____ CHILDREN _____ STERILITY _____

HABITS: ALCOHOL _____ TOBACCO _____ DRUGS _____ COFFEE _____ TEA _____ MEALS _____ WATER _____

SLEEP _____ BOWEL MOVEMENTS _____ EXERCISE _____ AMUSEMENTS _____

PRESENT AILMENT: _____

PHYSICAL EXAMINATION: TEMP ___ PULSE ___ RESP ___ B P ___ HT ___ WT ___

GENERAL APPEARANCE _____

SKIN _____ MUCOUS MEMBRANE _____

EYES VISION _____ PUPIL _____ FUNDUS _____

EARS _____

NOSE _____

THROAT _____ PHARYNX _____ TONSILS _____

CHEST _____ BREASTS _____

HEART _____

LUNGS _____

ABDOMEN _____

GENITALIA _____

RECTUM _____

VAGINA _____

EXTREMITIES _____

LYMPH NODES: NECK _____ AXILLA _____ INGUINAL _____ ABDOMINAL _____

REFLEXES _____

REMARKS: _____

LABORATORY FINDINGS:

(Urine · Blood · Sputum · Smears · Exudates Transudates · Feces · Gastric Contents · Wassermann Kahn · Chemistry · Pregnancy Tests · X-Ray Fluoroscopy · Schick · Dick · Etc.)

Date	

PATIENT'S NAME

DIAGNOSIS _____

TREATMENT _____

SYMBOLS: √ NORMAL, ___ ABNORMAL (UNDERLINE WORD)
DEGREE OF ABNORMALITY: X   XX   XXX

Figure 3-1 cont'd B, *back.*

GENERAL PRACTICE

| CASE No. | PATIENT'S NAME | | | B |

DATE			SUBSEQUENT VISITS AND FINDINGS	ACCOUNT RECORD		
MO.	DAY	YR.		CHARGE	PAID	BALANCE

- Throat—Redness, sore throat, tonsillitis, hoarseness, laryngitis, voice changes, speech defects, dysphagia
- Neck—Pain, tenderness, swelling, limitation of motion, trauma
- Respiratory—Chest pain, cough, expectoration, hemoptysis, asthma, wheezing, dyspnea, orthopnea, hyperventilation, night sweats, recurrent respiratory tract infections
- Cardiovascular (CV)—Chest pain, hypertension, palpitation, tachycardia, bradycardia, peripheral edema, varicosities, cyanosis, dizziness, syncope
- Gastrointestinal (GI)—Appetite, anorexia, bulimia, abdominal pain, nausea, vomiting, hematemesis, food intolerance, indigestion, dysphagia, diarrhea, constipation, laxatives, color and form of stools, melena, jaundice, distention, flatus, colic, hemorrhoids, rectal pain, presence of blood, pus, or mucus, pruritus ani, hernia or masses
- Genitourinary (GU)—Dysuria, oliguria, polyuria, frequency, hesitancy, nocturia, incontinence, enuresis, urgency, retention, hematuria, pyuria, glycosuria, abnormal color or odor, pain, renal colic, stones, pruritus, discharge, sexually transmitted disease(s), sexual habits, potency, prostate disease, testicular masses, history of urinary tract infections
- Female reproductive—Leukorrhea, discharge, itching, pain, dyspareunia, date and results of last Pap smear, breast self-examination routine

  Menses (menstrual periods)—Age at onset, regularity, amount, duration, date of last menstrual period, premenstrual tension, dysmenorrhea, amenorrhea, irregular bleeding, spotting, menopause (age of onset), postmenopausal bleeding, menopausal symptoms

  Obstetric—Number of pregnancies, live births, and living children; complications during pregnancy and labor; abortions if any

  Birth Control—Method if used
- Metabolic—Change in weight and appetite
- Endocrine—Excessive thirst, goiter, hair distribution, falling hair, change in skin texture or color, temperature intolerance, speech, voice, growth changes, sexual vigor and abnormalities, symptoms of diabetes, hormone therapy
- Blood—Bruising or bleeding tendencies, blood disorders
- Skin—Allergies, rash, pruritus, moles, sores or ulcers, color change (redness, jaundice, cyanosis, pallor), infections, dryness, sweating, alopecia, past dermatitis
- Musculoskeletal (MS)—Muscle or joint pain, swelling, stiffness, limitation of movement, spasm, tetany, weakness, numbness, coldness, deformities, atrophy, dislocations, fractures, discoloration, varicosities, cramping, edema, thrombophlebitis
- Neurologic—Headaches, vertigo, fainting, sense of balance, nervousness, sleeping irregularities, tremor, convulsions, loss of consciousness, memory, paralysis, paresthesia, pain
- Psychiatric—Personality type, emotional stability, previous mental illness

Assisting with the Patient History/Interview

At times, you may be responsible for obtaining some of the information for the patient history. The interview is often the first step in developing a relationship with the patient, with the patient's well-being established as the mutual concern. A positive relationship opens the door to providing opportunities for health education and possibly counseling now or at a later time. You will be collecting data on the various dimensions of the patient's health. To help guide you in this responsibility, keep the following guidelines in mind:

1. Make sure that the environment is as quiet and private as possible. This helps put the patient at ease and also enhances your own concentration.
2. Introduce yourself and explain to the patient what you will be doing and *why* you are doing this interview before the patient sees the physician.
3. Call the patient by name. Express friendliness and concern without losing professional mannerisms or perspective.
4. Speak slowly, clearly, and distinctly.
5. Listen to the patient attentively.
6. Use eye contact appropriately, observing the patient's body language and facial expressions while doing so. *Do not* stare at the patient or at your outline.
7. Treat the patient the way you would want to be treated. Successful interviewing begins with your attitude toward the patient. Think of the interview as a conversation rather than a task of filling out a preprinted form. By doing this, the quality of information that you get from the patient will be improved. Avoid interrogation (that is, asking a series of blunt questions). Create an atmosphere of mutual respect and trust by showing genuine interest, concern, and empathy. Be calm. A conversation is a two-way communication. Allow the patient time to complete sentences, even if he/she starts to ramble. You can redirect your questioning as necessary.
8. Encourage the patient to give specific information. This enables both you and the physician to care for the patient's needs. Besides medical information, personal information about the patient, such as stressors at home or work, can help to identify factors that may be affecting the patient's health. It is a well-documented fact that stress can lead to a number of physical and emotional problems.
9. Use direct and open-ended questions to ask the patient the reason for the visit to the physician, and when applicable, to describe the chief complaint and symptoms or problems that have been experienced. You may start simply by asking, "How are you feeling?" Most patients will then focus on their chief complaint. The responses given to these questions help the physician determine the nature and extent of the physical examination required.

When you ask the patient about symptoms, you must get specific information but be careful not to influence the patient's answer. You must ask questions that will answer *"what," "where,"* and *"when."* For example, if the patient is complaining of pain (the *"what"*), ask the patient to describe the type of pain experienced. Do not ask "Is it a sharp or dull pain?" Ask *where* the pain is and have the patient show you where he or she feels the pain. Watch the patient's facial expression and other body language as the pain area is pointed out. Ask *when* the pain first occurred and if there are any special times that it occurs; ask whether anything seems to bring on the pain and how long it lasts. If the patient can't remember when the pain first started, try to pinpoint the time by asking questions such as, "Did you have pain on the July 4th holiday?" or similar questions. Be aware that some patients may prefer to use another word rather than pain (for example, a pediatric patient may associate better with the word "hurt.") (See also "Vocabulary to Describe Pain" on page 66.)

10. Listen carefully to the patient and pay attention to the sound of his or her voice. The patient may be anxious or upset, or maybe the pain is so intense that the patient is about to cry. Listen for offhand comments such as, "I probably have this pain because I'm under so much stress. I really shouldn't be here at all." You must reassure the patient that the right decision was made by coming to see the doctor and encourage the patient to discuss any problems with the physician. Alert the physician to these types of comments. The physician can then ask the patient what is really bothering him or her. It may be that the patient does not wish to disclose an intimate problem to you but may be more willing to discuss it if the physician appears to be receptive and willing to inquire and listen.

11. Accept what the patient states. Often saying "um-hm" or giving a nod will encourage the patient to go on.

12. Summarize the information that you have gathered. Ask the patient if there is anything else that he or she would like to add or if there is anything that you may have left out.

13. Be willing and prepared to answer questions that the patient may have. Respond with interest. If you cannot answer the question, refer it to the physician. Explain that the physician will discuss the answer to the patient's question(s).

PHYSICAL EXAMINATION

After the history is completed, the physician proceeds with the physical examination, often referred to as a physical or a PE. This differs from the history in that it involves a thorough examination of the patient from head to toe for anatomic and physiologic functioning.

The key to a physical examination is systematic thoroughness. Generally a physician formulates a logical, methodic approach by examining each body system or part, beginning with the head and working down. The information obtained in the history or the chief complaint as stated by the patient helps determine the extent of the examination to be performed. Sometimes either a limited or a specific examination of one body part or system may be indicated.

The physician uses various methods of physical examination. The standard methods follow (Figure 3-2).

Inspection. Inspection is the visual observation of the body as a whole and of its individual parts. The physician observes the patient's general appearance, the color of the skin, and the size and shape of the body as a whole and of the individual parts. The physician also notes any rashes, scars, trauma, deformities, swelling, injuries, and nervousness.

In the detailed examination, the physician use the otoscope to look into the ears and the ophthalmoscope to inspect the eyes. A tongue blade is helpful when inspecting the mouth and throat.

Palpation. Palpation is performed by applying the tips of the fingers, the whole hand, or both hands to the body part. Pressure may be slight or forcible, continuous or intermittent. The physician feels, touches, and sometimes manipulates the external surface of the various parts of the body to determine the physical characteristics of tissues or organs and also to note if pain or tenderness is present.

Also involved are the physician's senses of temperature, vibration, position, and kinesthesia (the sense used to perceive movement, position, and weight) as the examination is in progress. Some of the organs and parts of the body examined by this method are the breast, chest, abdomen, liver, kidney, bladder, and lymph nodes. In conjunction with external palpation, internal palpation may be done on the uterus, ovaries, rectum, and prostate. Palpation is used to determine the size, position, and location of pelvic and abdominal organs, and if any abnormalities or masses are present.

Percussion. In medical diagnosis, percussion is done by tapping the body lightly but sharply with the fingers. The physician places one or two fingers of one hand on the part of the body to be examined and then strikes those fingers with the index or middle finger of the other hand.

The purpose of percussion is to determine the density, size, and position of the underlying organs and also to determine the presence of pus or fluid in a cavity. The differing densities of the various parts of the body give off different sounds when struck by the examiner's fingers. The more hollow the part struck, the more drumlike the sound. The sounds that are emitted help the physician make a diagnosis. A solid mass in a hollow organ can be noted because of a change from the normal density. Also, the border of certain organs such as the heart can be mapped out by comparing the density in the organ with surrounding tissues. Percussion is most commonly used on the chest and back for examination of the heart and lungs, but may also be done on the abdomen, bladder, or bones.

A physician may also use an instrument, the percussion hammer, to check a patient's reflexes by striking the tendon just below the knee and also at the elbow or ankle with this instrument. Failure of the desired reflex gives the physician more information for a diagnosis.

Figure 3-2 *Methods of physical examinations.* **A,** *Inspection,* **B,** *Palpation,* **C,** *Percussion,* **D,** *Auscultation.*

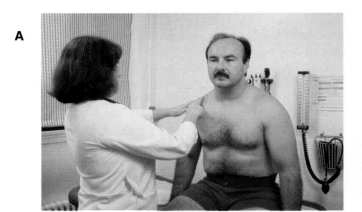

A

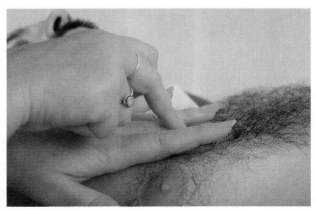

C

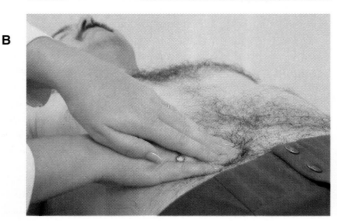

B

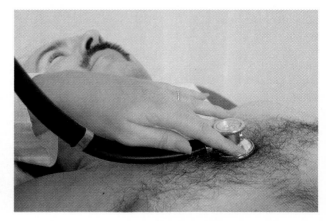

D

Auscultation. Auscultation is the process of listening to sounds produced in some of the body cavities as the organs perform their functions. A stethoscope is usually used, but it can also be done by placing an ear directly over a bared or thinly covered body surface. It is used chiefly on the chest to listen to the heart and lungs and also on the abdomen to diagnose an abdominal aneurysm or listen to fetal heart sounds or peristaltic waves. Listening to the sounds produced in these body cavities helps determine the physical condition of the organs.

Mensuration. Mensuration is the process of measuring. Clinical measurements include weight, height, temperature, pulse, respirations, and blood pressure. Head circumference is also measured in young children. When recorded and compared with previous measurements, these are extremely important guides for some diagnoses. The chest may also be measured to ascertain the amount of expansion and retraction on each side that accompanies inspiration and expiration. This is important when diagnosing or treating chest conditions such as emphysema, in which there is often a loss of elasticity of the lungs. Circumference of the extremities may be measured, especially when determining neuromuscular problems.

Smell. Smell is a much less frequently used method but it is still a relevant method for detecting a disease process. Odors from the breath, sputum, urine, feces, vomitus, or pus can

provide valuable information to help the physician make a diagnosis.

Essentials of a Thorough Physical Examination

The physician observes, tests, and measures each of the following for normal or abnormal structure and function and records his findings.

- General inspection—General appearance, nutritional status, apparent age, color, sex, height, weight, attitude, communication
- Vital signs—Temperature, pulse, respiration, blood pressure
- Skin—Color, texture, turgor, warmth, hair distribution, pigmentation, rashes, scars, lesions, moles, warts
- Head—Position, proportion to rest of body, distribution of hair, masses, evidence of trauma
- Face—Symmetry, size, appearance, facial expression, tenderness
- Eyes—Visual fields, visual acuity, eyeball movement, conjunctiva, sclera, cornea, iris, pupils, eyelids, ptosis, tearing, discharges
- Ears—Hearing, ear canals, tympanic membranes, cerumen, discharge
- Nose—Size, shape, color, deformity, septum, airways, mucosa, discharge, bleeding

- Mouth—Breath, lips, gums, teeth, tongue, mucosa
- Throat—Tonsils, pharynx, larynx
- Neck—Suppleness, thyroid gland, lymph nodes, vessels, carotid pulses, position of trachea, tenderness, stiffness, masses
- Breasts—Size, contour, symmetry, nipples, masses, discharge, tenderness
- Chest—Shape, symmetry, expansion, lesions
- Lungs—Rate and quality of respiration, breath sounds, cough, sputum, friction rubs, resonance, fremitus
- Heart—Rate, rhythm, point of maximum impulse (PMI), sounds, murmurs, dullness, thrills, gallop
- Arteries—Pulses, vessel walls, bruits
- Veins—Pulsation, dilation, filling
- Lymph nodes—Enlargement
- Abdomen—Contour; appearance; liver, kidneys, and spleen (KS); bladder; scars, peristalsis; tenderness; rigidity; spasm; masses; fluid; hernia
- Female genitalia—External appearance, Bartholin and Skene glands, discharge, masses; vaginal—bimanual examination of uterus and adnexa, tenderness, masses, Pap smear if required
- Male genitalia—Penis, scrotum, scars, lesions, discharge, tenderness, masses, atrophy, enlargement
- Rectum—Spincter tone, prostate gland, seminal vesicles, fissure, fistula, hemorrhoids, masses, discharge, feces
- Back and spine—Posture, curvature, balance, mobility, gait, tenderness, masses, costovertebral tenderness
- Extremities—Proportion to trunk, range of motion, color, pulses, edema, swelling, deformity, tenderness, ulcers, varicosities
- Fingernails—Contour, color
- Neurologic status—Consciousness, cranial nerves, reflexes, coordination, gait, balance, muscle tone and strength, tactile, pain (deep and superficial), discriminatory sensation
- Mental status—Orientation to time, place, and person; appearance, behavior; mood and thought content

Other tests that a physician may have performed as part of the physical examination include a routine urinalysis (UA), a complete blood count (CBC), a chest x-ray film, and electrocardiogram (ECG or EKG). Physical examination varies according to the needs or complaints of a patient. Frequently a patient may have a complaint or situation that can be handled in a few minutes or that requires a special type of examination such as a sigmoidoscopy. Other patients may require a complete physical examination, in this case, all of the preceding information is obtained.

Special Examinations

Certain types of examinations are more specific and restricted. These are local or special examinations, which are confined to specific parts and organs or special functions of the body. They are extensive and detailed and performed to establish complete information of a complex

nature. Frequently they are done to examine the interior of body cavities and passages. Some of the local or special examinations are vaginal and obstetric examinations, proctoscopy, sigmoidoscopy, cystoscopy, bronchoscopy, and skin tests. Other specialized examinations include ultrasound, roentgenologic, neurologic, ophthalmologic, and cardiac studies.

SUMMARY OF POSITIVE FINDINGS

On the basis of the subjective findings related by the patient and the objective findings of the physician during the physical examination, the physician sometimes briefly summarizes all of the positive findings of the case.

DIAGNOSTIC DATA

Diagnostic studies are performed—
- To determine (diagnose) the condition from which the patient is suffering so that treatment may be started if feasible.
- To discover disease in its early stage before the patient has any signs or symptoms. This is called screening. Screening often makes it possible to cure or delay the progression of a disease such as cancer or hypertension because treatment can be started in the early stages.
- To evaluate past or ongoing treatment received by the patient.

As the field of medical science continues to expand, newer, more accurate, and more sophisticated techniques are made available to help physicians diagnose disease processes. Diagnostic procedures and studies include but are not limited to physical examinations, surgical intervention, and laboratory studies. Laboratory data may include a set of routine laboratory examinations that were performed at the time of the patient's physical examination, with the results recorded if the tests have been completed. Other procedures used in diagnosing and treating disease processes may involve the specialized areas of radiology (roentgenology), nuclear medicine, special skin tests, physical medicine, physiotherapy, and electrocardiography. These areas of health care and treatment are elaborated on in later units of this book.

IMPRESSION

Once all of this information have been gathered, the physician gives an impression of the patient's condition that may include any or all of the following:
- Diagnosis
  Primary diagnosis—A statement that indicates the cause of the patient's current, most important problem/condition
  Secondary diagnosis—A statement that indicates a problem/condition that is less important or urgent than the patient's primary diagnosis
- Tentative or provisional diagnosis—A probable diagnosis that reflects the physician's impression of the patient's con-

dition, but it is made before any further tests have been completed and a final diagnosis has been reached

- Differential diagnosis—A possible diagnosis that is based on comparison of the signs and symptoms of two or more similar diseases to determine, by a process of elimination, the disease from which the patient is suffering
- Rule out (R/O)—A statement that indicates the conditions that the physician believes might be causing the patient's problem. Each condition is investigated thoroughly and ruled out as a diagnosis, if and when negative testing results are obtained. Again, by a process of elimination, a diagnosis may be reached. (Currently the term *rule out* is being replaced by the term *possible diagnosis*, which some believe to be a better description of the process.)
- Problem list—This is used in the most recent system of recording called the Problem-Oriented System (POS). A problem is any situation, disease, or condition for which the patient needs help or any question that requires a solution. In the problem list, each problem drawn from the data base is numbered, dated, and listed in order of occurrence. (Data base refers to all of the preceding parts of the medical record as discussed.) Problems may be stated in terms of the following:

    Diagnosis
    Symptom of physical findings
    Physiologic findings
    Abnormal laboratory results
    Social or personal problems
    Environmental problems
    Behavior factors
    Patient education
- Additional explanations of the problem-oriented system and the problem-oriented record will be discussed at the end of this unit.
- Prognosis—a statement of the probable or anticipated outcome of the patient's condition.

CARE PLANS AND SUGGESTED FURTHER STUDY

The next part of the medical record details the physician's specific plans, which may include one or a combination of the following forms of treatment: drug therapy, physical therapy, diet therapy, surgery, and psychotherapy. Treatments prescribed and medications ordered are entered on the record in detail. If hospitalization is required, this is noted. Patient education should be included.

Suggested further studies list the laboratory tests, x-ray film studies, or any other special tests that the physician deems necessary for the treatment and care of the patient. Instructions for follow-up visits are stated. There may be a statement that the patient has been referred to another physician for consultation or treatment when this is advisable.

After special tests or consultations are completed, a report is made, which is then incorporated into the patient's medical record.

PROGRESS NOTES

After each future visit, the physician's observations, the status of the patient's condition, and the patient's own report, it if is relevant, are added to the medical record. This is called the progress report or progress note, and each entry must be dated and signed. In a hospital, other health care providers (for example, physical therapists) write progress notes.

DISCHARGE SUMMARY

If the patient is discharged, the date and final statement about the patient's health and condition at that time are recorded on the medical record. These may be written at the end of the progress notes or on a separate form.

If the patient death, a statement describing the cause of death is recorded, and the history is marked *"deceased."*

Hospital discharge summaries contain more detailed information, including:
- Admission date, discharge date
- Admitting diagnosis, final diagnosis
- Summary of the history—sex, age, chief complaint, brief history of present illness, pertinent past history
- Pertinent physical findings
- Pertinent laboratory and x-ray film findings
- Treatment (for example, surgery, drugs, x-ray films, and diet)
- Hospital course (uneventful or list of any complications)
- Condition on discharge
- Prognosis (good, fair, poor, guarded)
- Recommendations on discharge (for example, special orders, follow-up care, and medications)
- Date, hour, and physician's signature

A copy of the patient's hospital discharge summary should be obtained from the hospital for the patient's permanent office record. The summary is helpful to the physician for providing continuity of care to the patient on return visits to the office or clinic. It is also used for research, statistical, insurance, billing, and legal purposes.

PROBLEM-ORIENTED MEDICAL RECORD

Over the years, the problem-oriented medical record (POMR) has gained great momentum and support from health care providers in a variety of settings. Pioneered by Lawrence L. Weed, MD, of the University of Vermont College of Medicine, the POMR provides a systematic way of recording data pertinent to patient care. Its purpose is to obtain and record in an organized manner all the facts needed to accurately diagnose, treat, and provide complete follow-up care for a patient's condition/disease or situation. It consists of four basic parts.

1. Data base
2. Problem list
3. Plans
4. Progress notes

The *data base* provides the essential data necessary to identify and solve the problem(s). It consists of the patient's medical history, the physical examination, and known laboratory data, all of which were described previously.

The *problem list* results from the information obtained in the data base. All the problems identified are titled, numbered, and dated in order of occurrence. This information is usually placed on the front page of the patient's chart to provide a quick diagnostic profile of the patient. The problems may be stated in various terms as outlined in the following paragraphs.

At subsequent visits any new problems are noted as they arise, dated, and numbered consecutively. As problems are resolved, the fact is noted with the date it occurred. The number of a resolved problem is not used again for another problem.

The problem list can be adapted in various ways to accommodate short-term or temporary problems that are seen frequently in the physician's office or clinic. One recommendation is the use of two problem lists: one for short-term or temporary problems, the other for long-term or permanent problems. When a short-term problem persists beyond a reasonable time or when it recurs frequently, it is removed from the short-term list and added to the long-term or permanent list.

Another recommendation is to use only one problem list, but not to record quickly resolved temporary problems on it. Temporary problems are simply indicated as such in the progress notes and are not numbered.

Plans state what will be done to start to solve the problem(s). They are made for each titled and numbered problem. A plan for a problem may be classified as follows:
- *Diagnostic* (that is, evaluative studies such as laboratory tests and x-ray films, consultations requested, and interviews with the patient's family), all of which help acquire additional information
- *Therapeutic* (that is, medical, surgical diet, psychologic, and/or physical treatment used to meet the goals of the physician when providing health care)
- *Educative,* (that is, what the patient is told about the therapy and condition, what instructional material, if any, the patient received, and what the patient is expected to do as a partner in the care and treatment of pain)

The *progress notes* are added to the record as the plan(s) are carried out. Each progress note is dated and titled and numbered according to the corresponding problem number. Each problem is evaluated for current status, with a notation of new findings or thoughts, changes in treatment plans, and resolution of the problem.

Each progress note should contain four parts and should be recorded according to the following format:

Number and title of the problem

S   *Subjective findings*—Statements made by the patient; how the patient feels; other information from the patient's family.

O   *Objective findings*—What the examiner observes or measures; specific things done for/to the patient; results of laboratory, x-ray, and other diagnostic reports.

A   *Assessment*—Evaluation and interpretation of the patient's status (S plus O). Assessment may be what the examiner thinks is happening, reasons for changing management of the problem, or significance of the findings; it may be expressed as an impression or as a diagnosis.

P   *Plan*—Diagnostic, therapeutic, and/or educative methods that will be used.

After the data base has been completed and evaluated, the POMR may appear as follows:

Problem list

Nov. 4, 19__

    Problem No. 1: Hypertension, essential arterial

    Problem No. 2: Obesity, exogenous

    Problem No. 3: Upper abdominal pain—Resolved ll/7/__

Plan

Nov. 4, 19__

    Problem No. 1: Aldactazide 50 mg, 1 tab bid; recheck patient in 1 week

    Problem No. 2: 1200-calorie diet; multivitamin X1 daily: suggested to patient to join a weight reducing group

    Problem No. 3: UGI series; oral cholecystogram

Progress notes

Nov. 4, 19__

    Problem No. 1: Hypertension, essential arterial

      S—patient states that fatigue and headaches decreasing somewhat

      O—BP ↓ 20 points to 160/84

      A—positive effects from the medication

      P—continue medication for 2 weeks; then to be checked

    Problem No. 2: Obesity

      S—patient has joined a weight reducing group, but states that she hates dieting

      O—wt. down to 4 lb to 176

      A—dieting effective

      P—continue 1200-calorie diet and multivitamin X1 daily

    Problem No. 3: Upper abdominal pain

      S—patient states that the abdominal pain is less severe but persists

      O—UGI and GB series negative; no abdominal distention

      A—deferred until all results complete

      P—abdominal ultrasound

Nov. 11, 19__

    Problem No. 1: Hypertension

      S—patient states that headaches have stopped, but she still remains fatigued

      O—BP 140/84

A—medication effective
P—reduce Aldactazide to 1 tab daily
Problem No. 2: Obesity
S—patient states is now adjusting to the diet much better
O—wt. ↓ 2 lbs to 174
A—weight loss will benefit problem No. 1
P—continue 1200-calorie diet
Problem No. 3: Upper abdominal pain
S—patient states pain has subsided 11/7/__
O—x-ray results and ultrasound reports negative
A—temporary condition, resolved 11/7/__
P—patient to report if pain recurs and advised that x-ray film studies and ultrasound were negative

As you can see, the POMR is an orderly method of providing a chronologic profile of a patient that helps the physician and other health care providers conduct total patient care. This system provides a quick current reference of the patient's medical record, including problem management. It greatly reduces the possibility of an oversight, especially for patients receiving long-term care or those with multiple problems.

RECORDS MANAGEMENT

RECORDS AND DOCUMENTATION

The medical record is the most important tangible element in legal medicine. The patient's record provides the information necessary to determine if medical services were given in accordance with the standards of care recognized by law, and it should include the patient's acceptance or refusal of medical advice. The record should clearly indicate the patient's failure to comply with treatment plans or keep necessary appointments for follow-up care and the physician's attempts to inform the patient of the necessity of care.

The physician and any other personnel responsible for making contributions to the patient's record should be careful to avoid unprofessional comments such as slang or colloquial terms; criticisms of patient's lifestyle, previous physicians, or medical care; or terms such as *error, mistake,* and *inadvertently.*

Although the *medical record* is considered the *property of the physician* because he or she acquired, compiled, and interpreted the information, other persons have legal access to it. Patients or their attorneys may acquire copies for review. If a lawsuit is filed, the patient's records become available to the legal representatives of the plaintiff and defendant and to the court. They are also available to federal or state agencies responsible for payment of the medical care or private (health, life, or disability) insurance companies with the written consent of the patient.

It is in the patient's and the physician's best interests if the records are accurate, complete, and legible. If these three criteria are met, the physician has an important tool in the prevention of or defense against professional liability claims.

Confidentiality

Properly maintaining and storing patients' medical records ensures the confidentiality of the information contained in them. You should think of the record as the person and provide the same privacy for the record as you would provide for the patient. This creates an atmosphere in which the patient can feel confident in being totally frank with the physician.

Permanent Protection

A medical record is a permanent proof of care and is credible, regardless of the time elapsed since an entry was made. Since a lawsuit may be filed years after an event, the record is considered more reliable than the physician's memory. For the record to provide protection, it must be carefully prepared and maintained.

Entries

Unalterable entries. The entries in a medical record are unalterable. In other words, notes written in a patient's medical record cannot be changed or removed. Should an error be recognized, a specific technique should be used to correct it. If records are handwritten, all notations should be made in a neat and legible manner.

Authorized personnel. Because of the importance of the medical record, office policy should be established that indicates which personnel are authorized to make entries in a patient's record. As a professional medical assistant, you will undoubtedly be responsible for medical records, including entry making. You must always keep in mind the importance of the medical record for patient care and for legal purposes.

Entries to be avoided. A thoughtless comment in a patient's chart could give the impression that the physician is uninterested in the care or prejudiced in his or her opinion of the patient. This impression can influence the credibility of the physician and the quality of care provided. Humorous or sarcastic remarks should never be written in a patient's record. Physicians and assistants should also take care not to attempt to describe another physician's findings or treatments. Information provided by the patient can be enclosed in quotation marks to indicate the source. If more information is required, the patient can sign a records release so that the other physician's records can be acquired.

Corrections

Reasons for corrections. Occasionally it is necessary to make a correction in the progress notes of a patient's record. This occurs when incorrect data are recorded in the patient's record or when an entry is made in the wrong chart. For example, as you record a patient's weight as 103 pounds, you note that it was recorded as 156 pounds on a previous visit. One of the notations must be incorrect. The fact should be rechecked, and the entry corrected. If you have several charts in your hands at one time, you could inadvertently make an entry intended for the chart of one patient in the progress notes of another. Again, a correction is in order.

Correction technique. Any information noted in the chart, whether factual or not, becomes part of the permanent record. You must *never* attempt to obliterate a chart entry. If an error in charting is discovered, you should:

1. Strike a single line through the error.
2. Date and initial the strikeout.
3. If the data are incorrect, enter the correct information directly below the strikeout. Date and initial the entry.
4. If the entry is made in the wrong chart, follow Step 1 and note "Recorded in chart by error. Information transferred to chart of John C. Adams."
5. Date and sign the strikeout and explanation.

Step four is vital for legal purposes, because the information can be verified and moving the information from one file to another is not considered a breach of confidentiality.

Statistical Information

Physicians may wish to gather and evaluate data on the effectiveness of a treatment plan or follow the course of several patients with the same diagnosis. Medical records can provide this information, which can be abstracted and maintained in a separate file. The increasing use of computers to store records and abstract data is a great help with statistical information. You should remember, however, that this information, whether abstracted by you or a computer, is still confidential and must be protected.

RETENTION OF MEDICAL RECORDS
Period of Retention

Debates are ongoing concerning the amount of time that records should be retained after certain events such as treatment of a minor, closure of a case, death of a patient, retirement of the physician, and death of the physician. Opinions vary from one state to another and according to whether they belong to an attorney, a medical association, or a management consultant.

When care involves a minor, the record should always be kept at least until the child becomes an adult and thereafter until the local statute of limitations runs out.

Closure of a case (for example, the care of a specialist) may warrant destroying a chart after a given period of time. Most agree that the chart should be retained for at least 10 years.

If the death of a patient is uncomplicated, some suggest that the chart be retained through the statute of limitations and then destroyed.

If a physician retires, the charts of deceased patients may be destroyed after a specified period of time following the death. Following appropriate notification, the records of living patients may be transferred to the physician who continues the practice or to a physician of the patient's choice on receipt of a written authorization.

When a physician dies, the patient's records are put under the care of a custodian of records, often the physician's spouse or a former employee who is willing to perform the duties involved. The disposition of the record is similar to that for a physician's retirement.

General Advice

Because of the increasing frequency of professional liability suits and the variations in statutes, many authorities are beginning to agree that the only safe option is to retain medical records forever. If the physician retires or dies, records that are requested should be forwarded, and the others retained by the physician or his or her heir.

Storage Sites

Inactive records may be stored in specifically designed file storage boxes in a storage area on the office premises, with a professional storage company, or on microfilm. For an ongoing practice, storing the records on the premises is ideal because inactive records may be needed from time to time. Professional storage facilities are appropriate if the physician has retired or dies. Microfilm is an ideal option from the perspective of saving space, but it is relatively expensive.

SPECIAL VOCABULARY

VOCABULARY USED TO DESCRIBE PAIN

In performing the complete history and physical examination, the examiner must deal with a variety of terms relating to pain. The following are some of these particular terms, along with an explanation of each term.

Pain is a very subjective symptom, usually having both a physical and a mental component. The experience and related feelings vary greatly among people. How a person expresses, does not express, or tolerates pain is also subjective. Some people don't express pain, but that doesn't mean they are not experiencing it; often they adapt to it. Adaptation can be dangerous because pain may be a warning signal, and becoming used to it and ignoring it can result in damage to the body. On the other hand, people who have pain for long periods often have a decreased tolerance to pain. All pain is real and must be acknowledged. Recognition and proper management of pain is an important part of total patient care.

VOCABULARY USED WHEN RECORDING PHYSICAL FINDINGS

The following vocabulary lists *some* of the terms that the examiner may use when recording the *objective* findings of the physical examination of a patient. Each term is presented under the body part or system for which it is used when reporting the findings of the physical examination. If you have completed studies in medical terminology, these terms should be familiar; if not, by referring to Appendix A, you should be able to define, pronounce, and become familiar with each term.

Skin

Abrasion	Laceration
Avulsion	Petechiae
Contusion	Purpura
Cyanosis	Turgor
Ecchymosis	Urticaria
Erythema	Ulcer
Jaundice	

Eyes

Acuity	Nystagmus
Adnexa	Papilledema
Arcus senilis	Ptosis
Fundus of the eye	

Ears

Tympanic membranes	Cerumen

Nose

Nares	Nasal septal defect

Neck

Supple	Range of motion
Carotid pulse	

Cardiovascular system (CVS)

Bruit	Ischemia
Congestion	Murmur
Ecchymosis	Petechiae
Engorgement	Purpura
Erythema	Resuscitation
Gallop	Rub
Infarction	Thrill

Respiratory system

Fremitus	Rhonchi
Friction rub	Sputum
Rales	Stridor
Resonance	

Abdomen

Ascites	Hernia
Contour	Protuberant
Distention	Rigidity
Flaccid	Scaphoid

Gastrointestinal (GI) system

Caries	Fistula
Distention	Hemorrhoid
Fissure	Peristalsis

Reproductive system

Adnexa	Introitus
Atrophy	Involution
Gravida	Parous

Genitourinary system (GU)

Introitus	Discharge

Musculoskeletal system (MS)—neurological and extremities examination

Claudication	Lordosis
Clubbing	Passive congestion
Crepitation	Protuberance

Edema	Rigidity
Exostosis	Scoliosis
Flaccid	Supple
Gait Ulcer	
Kyphosis	Varicosity

General

Cachexia	Fingerbreadth
Diaphoresis	Lethargic
Dehydration	Patulous *or* distended
Emaciation	Tenderness

MEDICAL ABBREVIATIONS

In a patient's medical case history, physical examination report, and notes on the chart, you will encounter a variety of abbreviations. The following list includes some of the more common abbreviations. They are grouped together according

PAIN

Colicky—Acute intermittent abdominal pain usually caused by spasmodic contractions.

Excruciating—Torturing extreme pain, often intractable.

Exquisite—Immense pain to which an individual is extremely sensitive.

Guarding—A reflex usually related to abdominal pain; the action of tensing muscles, drawing up knees, and/or placing a hand over a part to prevent examination and/or protect against increasing pain.

Intractable—Unmanageable; not controllable with conventional means such as rest, heat, or medication.

Radiating—Diverting from a common central point (for example, gallbladder pain begins in the right upper quadrant of the abdomen, and it is diverted from that central point to the right flank and right scapular area).

Rebound tenderness—A sensation of pain felt when pressure applied on a body part is released.

Stabbing—Deep, sharp, intermittent pain

Threshold—The level that must be exceeded for an effect to be produced; the level of pain that an individual can tolerate without external intervention. Threshold is unique to each individual, and the overall physio-psychologic makeup of an individual must be considered when evaluating pain.

Transient—Fleeting, brief, passing, coming and going.

Types of pain

- Superficial or cutaneous
- Deep pain—From muscles, tendons, joints
- Visceral pain—From the visceral (any large interior organ in any great body cavity, especially those in the abdomen)

to general usage. You should know some of these; others are new. Pay special attention to when capital letters are and are not used. Prescription abbreviations are given in Unit Seven. Others are given in the appropriate units.*

Body systems
HEENT—head, eyes, ears, nose, and throat
ENT—ear, nose, and throat
CR—cardiovascular system
GI—gastrointestinal
GU—genitourinary
CNS—central nervous system
MS—musculoskeletal
NS—nervous system
NM—Neuromuscular

Patient's history
CC—chief complaint
PI *or* HPI—present illness or history of present illness
PH—past history
LMD—local medical doctor
UCHD *or* UCD—usual childhood diseases
FH—family history
a & w *or* A & W—alive and well
ROS—review of systems
PTA—prior to admission
c/o—complains of

Physical examination (PE)
wd—well-developed
wn—Well-nourished
IPPA—inspection, percussion, palpation, and auscultation
P & A—percussion and auscultation
BP—blood pressure
TPR—temperature, pulse, and respirations
WNL—within normal limits
wt—weight
ht—height

Diagnosis
Diag *or* Dx—diagnosis
R/O—rule out
POS—problem-oriented system

Ears
TM—tympanic membrane(s)

Eyes
REM—rapid eye movement
L & A—light and accommodation
PERLA—pupils equal and reacting to light and accommodation
EOM—extraocular movement
RRE—round, regular, and equal

OS—left eye
OD—right eye
OU—both eyes

Chest (heart and lungs)
P & A—percussion and auscultation
PND—paroxysmal nocturnal dyspnea
SOB—shortness of breath
PMI—point of maximal intensity (or impulse)
MCL—midclavicular line
ICS—intercostal space
NSR—normal sinus rhythm
RSR—regular sinus rhythm
ASHD—arteriosclerotic heart disease
MI—myocardial infarction
EKG *or* ECG—electrocardiogram
AV—arteriovenous, atrioventricular
CHF—congestive heart failure
RHD—rheumatic heart disease
URI—upper respiratory infection
CPR—cardiopulmonary resuscitation
PVC—premature ventricular contraction
COPD—chronic obstructive pulmonary disease
CHD—coronary heart disease

Abdomen and GI
LKS—liver, kidney, spleen *or* LKKS—liver, kidneys, and spleen
GB—gallbladder
BM—bowel movement

Female reproductive system
BUS—Bartholin, urethral, and Skene glands
LMP—last menstrual period
OB—obstetrics
PID—pelvic inflammatory disease
GYN—gynecology
EDC—expected date of confinement
FHT—fetal heart tones
FHR—fetal heart rate
L & D—labor and delivery
PP—postpartum
IUD-intrauterine device
SAB—spontaneous abortion (miscarriage)

Musculoskeletal system
EMG—electromyogram
MS—multiple sclerosis
LOM—loss of movement or motion
cva—costovertebral angle
DTR—deep tendon reflexes
Li, La, etc.—first lumbar vertebra, second lumbar vertebra, etc.
Ti, Ta, etc.—first thoracic vertebra, second thoracic vertebra, etc.

Central nervous system (CNS)
CSF—cerebrospinal fluid
CVA—cerebrovascular accident
EEG—electroencephalogram
DTR—deep tendon reflexes

*According to the style of the American Medical Association, medical and pharmaceutical abbreviations are to be written *without* the use of periods (for example, rather than writing a.c. as was done in the past, you will now write ac).

Laboratory
CBC—complete blood count
UA—urinalysis
O_2—carbon dioxide
CO_2—carbon dioxide
CSF—cerebrospinal fluid
SMA—sequential multiple analysis
HGB *or* HG *or* hb—hemoglobin
Hct—hematocrit
WBC—white blood count
RBC—red blood count
Diff—differential (blood count)
Protime or PT—prothrombin time
PTT—partial thromboplastin time
pH—hydrogen ion concentration, referring to the degree of acidity or alkalinity of a solution
BUN—blood urea nitrogen
Sedrate—sedimentation rate
Rh—Rhesus blood factor
PKU—phenylketonuria
FBS—fasting blood sugar
GTT—glucose tolerance test
PBI—protein-bound iodine
PCV—packed cell volume
RhA—rheumatoid arthritis
STS—serologic test for syphilis
VDRL—Venereal Disease Research Laboratory (blood test for syphilis)
C & S—culture and sensitivity
CPK—creatine phosphokinase
LDH—lactic dehydrogenase
SGOT—serum glutamic oxaloacetic transaminase (now known as AST)
AFB—acid-fast bacillus
O & P—ova and parasites
Chol—cholesterol
HDL—high-density lipoproteins
LDL—low-density liproproteins
HGH—human growth hormone
EMIT—enzyme immunoassay for drug screening
staph—staphylococcus
strep—streptococcus
2 hr pc—2 hours post cibal (2 hours after a meal)
2 hr pp—2 hours post prandial (2 hours after a meal)
T3, T4 — thyroid tests
X-ray film studies
A-P and Lat—anterior-posterior, and lateral
IVP—intravenous pyelogram
GBS—gallbladder series
CT—computed tomography
MRI—magnetic resonance imaging
BE—barium
KUB—kidneys, ureter, bladder
UGI—upper gastrointestinal series
Surgical Studies

T & A—tonsillectomy and adenoidectomy
D & C—dilation and curettage
I & D—incision and drainage
TUR—transurethral resection
TURP—transurethral resection of the prostate
Hospital departments
ICU—intensive care unit
CCU—coronary care unit
ER—emergency room
OR—operating room
RR *or* PAR—recovery room or postanesthetic room
Lab—laboratory
Path—pathology
OPD—outpatient department
Peds—pediatrics
RT—respiratory therapy
PT—physical therapy
OT—occupational therapy
General
Ca *or* CA—cancer or carcinoma
D/c *or* D/C—discontinue
DOA—dead on arrival
OD—overdose
cm—centimeter
lb—pound
kg or kilos—kilograms
ac—before meals
pc—after meals
stat—immediately
prn—whenever necessary
ad lib—as desired
ASAP—as soon as possible
BR—bed rest
BP—blood pressure
I & O—intake and output
IM—Intramuscular
IV—intravenous
sc or SubQ—subcutaneous
LP—lumbar puncture
NPO—nothing by mouth
D/W—dextrose in water
S/W—saline in water
DOB—date of birth
FUO—fever of unknown (or undetermined) origin
CDC—Centers for Disease Control and Prevention
DPT—diphtheria, pertussis, tetanus (immunizations)
Dx—diagnosis
Rx—prescription
STD—sexually transmitted disease (the newer term replacing VD for venereal disease)
TB—tuberculosis
LLQ—left lower quadrant (of the abdomen)
LUQ—left upper quadrant (of the abdomen)
RLQ—right lower quadrant (of the abdomen)
RUQ-right upper quadrant (of the abdomen)

WF, BF—white female, black female
WM, BM—white male, black male
y/o—years old
GC—gonococcus or gonorrhea
K—potassium
LE—lupus erythematosus
NYD—not yet diagnosed
PM—postmortem
O_2—oxygen
CO_2-carbon dioxide
pt—patient
TLC—tender loving care
Symbols
>—greater than
<—less than
♂—male
♀—female

↑—above, increase
↓—below, decrease
×—times (multiply by)
%—percentage
#—number *or* pound
=—equals
+ —plus *or* positive
− —minus *or* negative
ō — none
c̄—with
s̄ —without
ā —before
p̄ —after

Additional abbreviations frequently used for medications are given in Unit Eight.

CONCLUSION

You have now completed the unit on Health History and Physical Examinations. You will be expected to discuss the parts a patient's health history and its importance, together with other components that make up a medical record. In addition you should be able to describe the methods used by a physician when performing a physical examination. When you are familiar with the contents of this unit, arrange with your instructor to take a performance test.

REVIEW OF VOCABULARY

The following are samples of a patient's medical history and physical examination. A consultation letter and a hospital discharge summary as dictated by a physician are also included. These are to help familiarize you with the format and contents of medical reports. Read these and be prepared to discuss the contents and define all the medical terms that are used. You should recognize some of the terms; others are new, and you may have to refer to Appendix A or to a medical dictionary for the definitions.

HISTORY AND PHYSICAL EXAMINATION

PATIENT: Patrick Nelson

PHYSICIAN: S. Kennedy, MD

DATE: November 12, 19__

CHIEF COMPLAINT: None

HISTORICAL DATA: This 27-year-old white male enters for a physical evaluation. Actually he has no complaints but thinks that it is wise to have a general physical evaluation.

PAST MEDICAL HISTORY: The patient states that he had the usual childhood diseases. He had the flu in 1984, moderately severe. The patient received all of his immunizations.

Operations: Tonsillectomy as a child.

Injuries: Broken bones and unconsciousness, none.

PERSONAL HISTORY: The patient is single and works with his father.

FAMILY HISTORY: His father and mother are both living, middle-aged, and well. He has an older sister and a younger brother, both in good health.

HABITS: The patient smokes a package to a package and a half of cigarettes per day. Alcoholic intake, about 4 oz per week.

MEDICATIONS: None.

SYSTEM REVIEW

Head and neck

Eyes: The patient is myopic and wears glasses all the time. He denies headaches or visual disturbances.

Ears. nose, and throat: Not remarkable.

Cardiorespiratory: The patient denies all symptoms in this system, except for being soft. He states that he gets no regular exercise and when he does sudden exercise, he becomes short of breath.

Gastrointestinal: His appetite is excellent. His weight is stable at approximately 160 pounds. Digestion is good. Bowels are regular with use of laxatives. He states that he had some minor hemorrhoid problems in the past.

Genitourniary: The patient denies nocturia. He urinates several times daily without difficulty. There is no history of kidney stones, bladder infections, or bleeding.

Neuromuscular osseous: The patient recently had a backache from which he has made a satisfactory recovery. Orthopedic consultation at that time was negative.

PHYSICAL EXAMINATION

Height: 72 inches.

Weight: 167 pounds.

Blood pressure: 144/80.

Pulse: 76 and regular.

Respiration: 16 per minute.

The general impression is that of a well-developed, well-nourished white male, who appears to be in no acute distress. He is slightly obese, pleasant, and cooperative.

Head and neck

Eyes: Patient has a positive cover test, with a latent exophoria. He is highly myopic. Funduscopic examination is otherwise not remarkable.

Ear, nose, and throat: Normal. The neck is supple. The trachea is in the midline. The thyroid is not palpable. The neck veins are collapsed.

Chest: Clear to percussion and auscultation. There is good diaphragmatic descent bilaterally. Breath tones are normal. No adventitious sounds are heard.

Heart: The left border of cardiac tonus is 6 cm from the midsternal line, with the point of maximum impulse at the fourth intercostal space. The rhythm is regular. No murmurs or adventitious sounds are heard.

Abdomen: Slightly rotund. The liver, spleen, and kidneys are not palpable. There are no masses or tenderness.

Genitalia: There is a normal male escutcheon. The penis is circumcised. Testes are in the scrotum. The inguinal rings are intact.

Rectal: Examination discloses good sphincter tone. The prostate is small, smooth, and symmetric. The ampulla is filled with soft, brown stool.

Extremities: There is no evidence of edema, cyanosis, or jaundice. Peripheral pulses are adequate. Most notable is the finding of several small glomus tumors on the fingers. Some of these are painful; others are not.

Neurologic: Intact.

Skin: Negative.

Lymphatics: Negative.

IMPRESSIONS

1. Normal, healthy male.
2. Glomus tumors.
3. Latent exophoria.

RECOMMENDATIONS

1. Routine urine and CBC.
2. Chest x-ray film.
3. Lose 10 pounds of weight.
4. Return as needed.

S. Kennedy, MD

DISCHARGE SUMMARY

HISTORY: The patient is a 36-year-old, juvenile-onset male with diabetes, with multiple problems involving the gastrointestinal, genitourinary, and musculoskeletal systems.

PROBLEM NO. 1: Diabetes mellitus: onset at age 15 years, with two episodes of diabetic ketoacidosis at ages 15 and 20, with multiple admissions for hypoglycemic and hyperglycemic symptoms. The patient states he has taken 55 units of Lente in the morning and 15 units of Lente in the evening for 20 years, with slight increases in these periodically, covering himself with regular, 15 units in the a.m. and 10 units in the p.m. The patient is presently on 45 units of Lente and 15 units of regular in the morning, and 15 Lente and 10 regular in the PM, with urines running negative to 2+, with no ketones. The patient states he has not changed his dose or altered his eating habits or skipped a dose in the past 48 hours.

Twelve hours before admission, the patient noted the onset on mild nausea and vomiting, with abdominal distention, bloating, and intermittent diarrhea (brown). The patient denies bright red blood per rectum or per mouth, or melena. He denies loss of consciousness or lethargy, fever, chills, night sweats, cough, dysuria, pyuria, but does admit to polydipsia on a chronic basis. Complications from the diabetes include retinopathy, which was first noted in 1986 and treated with lasers; he denies any renal or neurologic complications (impotence, bladder, bowel). The patient has also had numerous abscesses in the perianal area and urinary tract infections, including pyelonephritis times one.

PROBLEM NO. 2: Gastrointestinal complaints: The patient has a greater than 15-year history of peptic ulcer disease, with a history of hematemesis and melena in 1984, for which he had an upper GI series that showed a suggestion of a swollen duodenal bulb and an endoscopy that read out as a normal examination. The patient also had acid studies done, which showed a basal secretion of 7.86 mEq per hour, going to a post-Histalog stimulation level of 35.7 mEq per hour. The findings were consistent with an ulcerogenic picture. It was elected not to do surgery at that time, because of the lack of anything treatable. The patient was noted to have decreased gastric emptying, which was thought to be caused by an inadvertent vagotomy during his hiatal hernia repair in 1985.

The patient presently complains of epigastric pain, worse on lying, with heartburn, relieved by eating and taking antacids. The patient gives a history of melena for 3 days and hematemesis, two episodes in the past 2 months, without recurrence. The patient also takes aspirin for back pain. The patient has a past history of infectious hepatitis, treated in 1980, without recurrence.

PROBLEM NO. 3: Back pain, chronic: In 1985 the patient suffered trauma to his back, secondary to lifting a heavy object, which resulted in marked decrease in the strength in his lower extremities. The patient was evaluated at that time with an electromyogram (EMG), which was normal, and a myelogram, which showed protrusion of the nucleus pulposus in the L4-5 area. The patient was taken to surgery, where partial hemilaminectomy was done in December 1985. The patient states that he has had no cessation or relief of his back pain secondary to the operation. The patient denies any paresthesia, weakness, or asymmetry in motor sensory involvement in his lower extremities.

PROBLEM NO. 4: Chest pain, hypertension: The patient has a history of cardiac "attacks" in 1984 and 1985 times two and in 1986, requiring hospitalization. The patient was told each time that there was no heart damage. The patient describes the pain as substernal, radiating to the neck and back, without associated shortness of breath, palpitations, diaphoresis, but does state that it is precipitated by exercise on occasion or emotional stress. The patient has never had any EKG changes consistent with ischemia and/or infarct. The patient's history of high blood pressure runs in the 140/90 range and has been treated for 1 1/2 years in the past, but he has presently been off medications. The patient states that episodes of chest pain come approximately one to two times per month and only last for seconds. The patient has been treated in the past with nitroglycerin in 1986, but no longer takes the medication.

PROBLEM NO. 5: Kidney problems: At the age of 10 years, the patient had pyelonephritis and subsequent recurrent urinary tract infections, which may or may not have included flank pain, fever, and chills. The patient has been treated in the past with antibiotics for his urinary tract infections, the most recent being 7 years ago. The patient has a past history of renal stones in 1986, left-sided, with a normal intravenous pyelogram. The patient was evaluated for calcium, phosphate, and oxalate in his urine, which were all within the normal range. The patient's creatinine in the past has run around 1, with a BUN around 18 in 1986.

PAST MEDICAL HISTORY: Allergies: None. Illness: As above. Surgery: Note above. Habits: 25 years of smoking a pack a day; no alcohol. Medications: Note history of present illness.

SOCIAL HISTORY: The patient lives in Anytown, California, works as a chef, and presently is living with a girlfriend. The patient has been married three times and has one child, who is 14 years old, by his first wife.

FAMILY HISTORY: The family history is positive for diabetes in a maternal uncle and maternal great-grandmother. There is no history of myocardial infarction, high blood pressure, cerebrovascular accident, tuberculosis, rheumatic heart disease, endocrinopathies, or cancer.

REVIEW OF SYSTEMS: This is significant for head, eyes,

ears, nose, and throat. He did have a headache in 1986, which was evaluated with an EEG and skull films, all of which were within normal limits; presently without complaint of headache. Lungs: He has been without pneumonia; negative PPD within the last year and half. Neurologic: The patient has a questionable history of psychiatric disease in the past with "rage attacks." The patient has not been evaluated further.

PHYSICAL EXAMINATION: Blood pressure was 140/96 lying, with a pulse of 92, going to 140/100 standing up, with a pulse of 116. Respirations were 20, temperature was 37{{ring}}C. Generally , a well-developed male, appearing in no acute distress.

Skin: The skin had a abdominal scar and an abscess scar on the left medical buttock area. There were ingrown hairs on his anterior and posterior thoracic walls. There was no diaphoresis.

Head, eyes, ears, nose, and throat: Atraumatic; extraocular movements were positive; pupils were equal, round, and reactive to light, without nystagmus. The fundi were remarkable for increased tortuosity of his vessels, with hemorrhages and exudates present in both retinae; his discs were flat. Tympanic membranes showed old scarring, but normal light reflexes. Oropharynx was clear and edentulous.

Neck: Supple, without increase, decrease, or asymmetric thyroid enlargement; there were no bruits.

Node: No cervical, supraclavicular, axillary, or epitrochlear nodes. He did have positive occipital and inguinal nodes, old.

Lungs: Decreased respiratory movements; there was a slight increase in his AP diameter; positive end-inspiratory wheezing, with inspiration: expiration ratio of 1:1.2. The patient was without rales; he did have scattered rhonchi. There was no E to A change; no increased or decreased vocal or tactile fremitus was noted.

Cardiovascular examination: The cardiovascular examination showed a point of maximal impulse in the fifth intercostal space, midclavicular line; no heave, thrill, or thrust; no S-3, S-4, or murmur. Pulses were + 2 and equal throughout, without bruits. The carotids were good and up bilaterally, without bruits.

Abdomen: The liver was 12 cm by percussion; no spleen, kidney, or bladder palpable; bowel sounds were active, without distention.

Rectal examination: The rectal examination was guaiac-negative; prostate was symmetrically enlarged, without nodularity or mass.

Extremities: There was full range of motion, without cyanosis, clubbing, or edema.

Neurologic examination: Oriented times three. Abstract thought and short- and long-term memory were intact.

There was no sensory, motor, or cerebellar abnormality in his lower or upper extremities. Cranial nerves II through XII were within normal limits. His reflexes were + 1 and equal throughout, except for absent ankle jerks, with down-going toes. Negative straight-leg raising. No root, grasp, or suck reflexes were noted.

LABORATORY DATA: He had a pH of 7.38, pO2 of 40 on room air, with a bicarbonate of 24. His glucose was 855. His urinalysis showed PLUS 4 glucose, negative ketones. Chest x-ray film was without cardiopulmonary disease, and there was no air under the diaphragm. KUB showed no abnormalities. Sodium was 122, potassium 3.6, bicarbonate 28; BUN was 21 and creatinine was 1.6. His EKG showed normal sinus rhythm, without acute changes.

HOSPITAL COURSE: The patient's hospital course was one of treatment with intravenous insulin and normal saline to correct the abnormalities noted from the hyperosmolar effect of the increased glucose load intravascularly. The patient responded well to rehydration and to IV insulin, receiving 10 units of IV insulin over a 4- to 6-hour period, with a blood glucose drop from 855 to 328. The patient at no time showed any evidence of ketoacidosis, with urines running in the 3 to 4 PLUS range, with negative ketones, and bicarbonate staying in the 28 to 30 range. By morning, the glucose was 106, with negative-negative urine and a bicarbonate of 30. The patient was treated as an outpatient and started on a normal regimen, with 45 units of Lente and 15 units of regular in the morning, and 15 units of Lente and 10 units of regular in the evening. The patient responded well to therapy and is being discharged today for follow-up in my clinic.

The patient continued to be guaiac-negative in the hospital for the 2 days. The patient's epigastric complaints will be followed on an outpatient basis and worked up accordingly.

CHEST PAINS: The patient did have one episode of chest pain while in the hospital, with EKG during chest pain showing no abnormalities. The pain lasted for seconds and went away without medication.

The patient is being discharged with the following medications: Lente and regular insulin—45 units of Lente and 15 units of regular in the a.m., and 15 units of Lente and 5 units of regular in the p.m.. Tylenol and codeine, one po q4h prm for low back pain.

DISCHARGE DIAGNOSIS
Diabetes, out of control, secondary to noncompliance
Epigastric pain
Low back pain
Chest pain
N.J. Hopew, MD

REVIEW OF VOCABULARY—cont'd

CONSULTATION LETTER TO REFERRING PHYSICIAN

October 1, 19__

W.F. Mayhan, MD
124 Medical Drive
San Francisco, CA 94119

Dear Doctor Mayan:

Ms. Catherine Holmes was seen for neurologic evaluation on September 28, 19__.

She is a 21-year-old, white, right-handed, single supermarket checker who complains of headaches.

The patient stated that on the evening of September 27, 19__, she fell and struck the back of her head against an upholstered arm of a couch. She was not rendered unconscious but did have a headache afterwards. Nevertheless, the remainder of the evening passed uneventfully, and she went to bed. The following morning she woke up and went to work. However, at approximately 10 o'clock she had the onset of a relatively severe headache with a feeling that her ears were popping and her eyes were glassy. In addition, she felt very tired. She complained of some nausea but did not vomit. She took aspirin, which has given her some degree of relief.

At the time of her examination, the patient was continuing to complain of a mild headache, but one that was not severe. She did feel extremely tired and wanted to rest at home. Approximately 1 year ago the patient had a concussion; however, she was not hospitalized and suffered no long-term adverse effects. She denies any history of other neurologic or general medical problems. She did have eye surgery a number of years ago for an extraocular muscle imbalance. She denied any history of surgery, fractures, or allergies. She smokes approximately a package of cigarettes per day and occasionally partakes of wine. Currently she is taking birth control medication, but no other agents.

Family history reveals her father to be suffering from hypertension. Her mother died approximately a year ago at the age of 46 from a cerebral hemorrhage, which, from her description, may have been a ruptured aneurysm. While speaking of her mother, the patient did become quite tearful.

EXAMINATION: The examination revealed a well-developed, well-nourished, white female. She was in no acute distress. She was alert, oriented, and cooperative.

Cranial nerve examination was normal. Deep tendon reflexes were active and symmetric. Plantar responses were downgoing.

Motor testing showed no upper extremity drift. No other evidence of gross of focal motor weakness was noted.

Sensory testing was intact to pinprick, as well as vibratory, sensation. Romberg test was negative.

Cerebellar testing showed no incoordination or decomposition of movements.

The patient's gait was normal for all modalities, including heel, toe, and tandem. No cranial or carotid bruits were heard. There was a full range of motion to her head and neck. Blood pressure was 100/60, right arm sitting.

IMPRESSION: Status 1 day after head injury.

DISCUSSION: This patient's neurologic examination is unremarkable. She does complain of a residual headache that is the result of the blow she received to her head the evening before this examination. Currently she is feeling better with very minimal symptomatic treatment, and it is quite possible that this will resolve without any further aggressive management. I have given her a prescription for Darvocet-N 50 mg in the event her headache recurs or becomes more severe. In addition, I have indicated to her that if further difficulties arise, she should again contact us.

Thank you for giving me the opportunity to meet this very nice patient.

With best personal regards,

E. Schroeder, MD

CASE STUDY

The following are brief medical histories. Read and discuss the italicized terminology.

1. The patient is a 76-year-old lady seen because of difficulty walking and taking care of herself. Her husband had a *CVA* in March and has recently been transferred to a *rehabilitation* hospital for further care. She has been living alone in a two-story house, has been able to *ascend* and *descend* the stairs, and until recently has been able to manage her own affairs. Apparently during the past month, she has been eating poorly, her hands have begun shaking, and she "has had trouble picking up her heels."

2. The patient is a 73-year-old right hand-n-*dominant* white male with a *positive finding* of old right *AKA* who presents *signs and symptoms* of *acute* left *hemiparesis* and *dysarthria.* He was well until yesterday, when he noted the acute onset of these symptoms not associated with any loss of *consciousness, vertigo,* headache, or nausea. There is no history of previous *cerebrovascular accident. Prognosis* is guarded.

3. Physical examination
   a. General: Patient *denies* chills, fever, change in weight, or sleep disorder.
   b. Head: There is *symmetry* of facial features. Large *verruca* noted on right *supraorbital* ridge; one episode of *syncope* 2 months ago.
   c. Eyes: Vision *corrected* to 20/20 with contact lenses.
   d. Ears: Denies earache, discharge, *tinnitus.*
   e. Nose: Seasonal stuffiness and watery discharge. No *rhinorrhea.*
   f. Throat: No pain, hoarseness, or *dysphagia.*
   g. Neck: No masses or tenderness *elicited.*
   h. Respiratory: Lungs clear to *percussion* and *auscultation.*
   i. Cardiovascular: See present illness.
   j. Gastrointestinal: Right lower *quadrant* pain and a mass *palpated* on physical examination.
   k. *Genitourinary:* Complains of increasing *hesitancy* but denies *dysuria, urgency,* or *nocturia.*
   l. *Hemopoietic: Unremarkable.*
   m. *Lymphatic:* Unremarkable.
   n. *Musculoskeletal:* Morning stiffness in major joints.

REVIEW QUESTIONS

1. Information gathered on a history and physical examination is used for various purposes. List four of these purposes.
2. List and define the six parts of a patient's history.
3. The following information has been obtained from the physician's notes. For each statement, indicate where on the patient's record this information is recorded. Choose your answers from the following headings: chief complaint, history of present illness, past history, family history, social or occupation history, review of systems, physical examination, and impression.
   a. The patient is a 25-year-old white, obese female who was in good health until approximately 10 p.m. last evening.
   b. There is no history of past operations.
   c. Neck: Thyroid is not enlarged.
   d. Head: there is no history of headaches, sinus pain, or trauma.
   e. The arteries are full, soft, and readily compressible.
   f. "I have a lump in my left breast."
   g. Patient had measles and chickenpox when she was a child.
   h. R/O diabetes.
   i. Muscle tone is decreased in all four extremities.
   j. Patient's father has a history of hypertension for 5 years.
   k. GU system: There is no history of dysuria, hematuria, frequency, or nocturia.
   l. The patient denies the use of alcohol, tobacco, and drugs of any kind.

4. Define the following methods of examination, and state one body part or system that is examined in each method.
   a. Inspection
   b. Percussion
   c. Palpation
   d. Auscultation
   e. Mensruation
5. Describe the difference between the ROS and the PE.
6. List five forms of treatment that may be used for the care of a patient.
7. List three reasons why diagnostic studies are important for patient care.
8. State the purpose of the problem-oriented medical record.
9. List and explain the four parts of the problem-oriented medical record.

PERFORMANCE TEST

In a skills laboratory, a simulation of a joblike environment, the medical assistant student is to demonstrate knowledge and skill in obtaining identifying information and the medical history from a patient. The student may use a preprinted history form or make a list of questions that should be asked of the patient from the information presented in this unit. For these activities the student needs a person to play the role of the patient and the necessary supplies. Time limits for the performance of this procedure are to be assigned by the instructor. (See also "GRADING" on page 52 in Unit Two).

The student is to perform the above procedures with 100% accuracy 90% of the time (9 out of 10 times.)

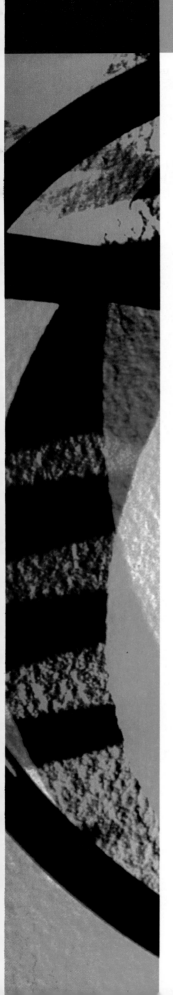

Preparing for and Assisting with Routine and Special Physical Examinations

COGNITIVE OBJECTIVES

On completion of Unit Four, the medical assistant student should be able to:

1. Define and pronounce the vocabulary terms.
2. State in summary form the medical assistant's responsibilities when assisting the physician during the examination of a patient.
3. List, identify, and state the function of each instrument commonly used during a complete physical examination, including rectal and vaginal examinations; a proctosigmoidoscopy; a neurologic examination; an ear examination; an eye examination.
4. State two purposes for positioning a patient and three purposes for gowning and draping a patient for physical examinations.
5. State the purpose of and discuss the following special examinations: neurologic, ear, eye, gynecologic, obstetric, 6 weeks' postpartum visit, breast self-examination, and pediatric.
6. Discuss the special instructions that must be given to the patient before a Papanicolaou (Pap) smear is taken.
7. Discuss the five classifications that are used to report the results of a Pap smear.
8. List the information that should be included on a laboratory requisition when sending a specimen for a cytologic examination.
9. Discuss the American Cancer Society's guidelines for examinations for the early detection of cancer in people without symptoms.
10. List seven warning signals of cancer.
11. Differentiate between cancer that is localized and cancer that has metastasized.
12. Briefly discuss major cancer sites with reference to:
    a. Risk factors
    b. Risk reduction
    c. Examinations used for early detection
    d. Warning signs
    e. Treatment
    f. Special information listed
13. State the purpose for the Snellen Big E eye chart and when it is used.
14. Differentiate between an alpha-fetoprotein blood test, an amniocentesis, and a chorionic villi sampling test. State the purpose(s) of each test.
15. State the two broad classifications of pediatric patient physician office visits. State the purpose of each type of visit.
16. Discuss the guidelines for health supervision for a child's care.
17. Discuss general points that should be considered for a physical examination and office visit of a pediatric patient.
18. Discuss the reasons why keeping growth charts for infants and children is important. List the measurements that are recorded on these charts.
19. Discuss the disease *phenylketonuria (PKU)* and the recommended treatment. List the tests performed to diagnose this condition and state when each is usually performed.
20. Discuss the recommended schedule for an immunization program for an infant and child.
21. List six common immunizations given to children. State how each is administered.

TERMINAL PERFORMANCE OBJECTIVES

On completion of Unit Four, the medical assistant should be able to:

1. Prepare a patient for a physical examination by providing clear, simple instructions and explanations that are easy to understand.
2. Position and drape a patient in the positions outlined in this unit.
3. Select, identify, and prepare for use equipment and supplies required for:
    a. A complete physical examination, which is to include a rectal examination and a pelvic examination with Pap smear.
    b. A proctosigmoidoscopy.
4. Demonstrate correct assisting techniques during physical examinations.

5. Assist the patient before, during, and after the examination.

6. Record the procedures and results (when applicable) of physical examinations.

7. Perform a breast self-examination. Discuss this method of examination with a female patient.

8. Measure a preschooler's and an adult's distance visual acuity using the Snellen eye charts.

9. Measure a patient's near visual acuity.

10. Measure color vision in a patient.

11. Assist a parent/caregiver in completing an initial health history form for a pediatric patient.

12. Demonstrate how to carry an infant in the cradle, upright, and football positions.

13. Take the following measurements on a child and record the results in the medical record and on the growth chart:
    a. Length/stature
    b. Weight
    c. Head circumference
    d. Chest circumference
    e. Vital signs

14. Demonstrate the method used to obtain a urine specimen from a child that is not toilet trained.

15. Obtain a blood specimen from an infant for a screening test for PKU.

16. Demonstrate the procedures used for performing a urine test to screen an infant for PKU.

17. Locate the sites and demonstrate the procedure used to give an intramuscular injection to a child.

18. Record the required information on a child's medical record after a vaccination has been administered.

The student is to perform these skills with 100% accuracy 90% of the time (9 out of 10 times).

The consistent use of universal precautions is required by all health care professionals in all health care settings as a method of infection control. It is assumed that these precautions are used in all of the following procedures. Review Unit One if you have any question on methods to use, as the methods/techniques will not be repeated in detail in each procedure presented in the unit.

Be sure to consult the latest guidelines issued by the Centers for Disease Control and Prevention and consult with infection control practitioners when needed to identify specific precautions that pertain to your particular work situation.

PREPARING FOR AND ASSISTING WITH PHYSICAL EXAMINATIONS

The physical examination is done in an examination or treatment room, whereas frequently the history is obtained from the patient in the physician's private office.

This unit covers gowning, positioning, and draping the patient for an examination and preparing for and assisting with the common examinations performed by a physician—*one* method of conducting examinations and *one* group of instruments and equipment are included for each. The physician(s) or agency for whom you work may use other methods and equipment; you must be able and willing to adapt to individual needs as required.

General instructions to be followed and responsibilities to be assumed by medical assistants when assisting with every procedure and examination are listed in the next section. Keep them in mind as you prepare for all examinations, since they are not repeated in each individual procedure.

Frequently, during any of the examinations that are outlined in this unit, various types of specimens may be obtained. Detailed information for collecting and labeling specimens is covered in Unit Seven.

Cleansing and sterilization techniques to be used in the care of used, nondisposable equipment is discussed in Unit Five. Refer to these units for more specific information.

The instruments used for a physical examination are described in Figure 4-1.

VOCABULARY

ACS—American Cancer Society

Bimanual (bi-man'u-al)—With both hands, as bimanual palpation.

Bronchoscopy (bron-kos' ko-pi)—Internal inspection of the tracheobronchial tree with the use of a bronchoscope; used for diagnostic or treatment purposes. For diagnosis, the physician inspects the interior of the bronchi and may obtain a sample of secretions or a biopsy of tissue; for treatment, foreign bodies or mucus plugs that may be causing an obstruction to the air passages can be located and removed.

Cystoscopy (sis-tos'kop-i)—Internal examination of the bladder with a cystoscope. Samples of urine for diagnostic purposes can be obtained by passing a catheter through the cystoscope into the bladder or beyond, up into the ureters and kidneys. Also, radiopaque dyes may be injected through the cystoscope into the bladder or up into the ureters when taking x-ray films of the urinary tract.

Digital (dij' it-al)—The use of a finger to insert into a body cavity such as the rectum for palpating the tissue.

Endoscopy (en-dos' ko-pi)—Visual examination of internal cavities of the body with an endoscope (for example, a proctoscope, bronchoscope, cystoscope, gastroscope, and laryngoscope).

Gastroscopy (gas' tros' ko-pi)—Internal inspection of the stomach with a gastroscope.

Oral examination—Examination pertaining to the mouth.

Papanicolaou (Pap) smear or test (pap"ah-nik"o-la′oo)—A smear examined microscopically to detect cancer cells from body excretions (urine and feces), secretions (vaginal fluids, sputum, or prostatic fluid), or tissue scrapings (as obtained from the stomach or uterus); most commonly done on a cervical scraping to detect abnormal or cancerous cells in the mucus of the uterus and cervix.

Pelvic examination—Examination of the external and internal female reproductive organs.

Prodrome—An early symptom indicating the onset of a disease (for example, an achy feeling before having the flu).

Roentgenologic (rent-gen-ol′oj-i-cal)—Pertaining to an examination with the use of x-ray film (radiographs).

Sign (physical sign)—Any objective evidence (apparent to the observer) of disease or body dysfunction. Signs may be observed by others or revealed when a physician performs a physical examination (for example, swollen ankles, a distended rigid abdomen, elevated blood pressure, or decreased sensation).

Symptom—Any subjective evidence of disease or body dysfunction; a change in the physical or mental state of the body that is perceptible or apparent only to the individual (for example, anorexia, nausea, headache, pain, or itching).

Syndrome—A combination of symptoms having one cause or commonly occurring together to present a distinct clinical picture; an example is the dumping syndrome, which consists of nausea, weakness, varying degrees of syncope, sweating, palpitation, and sometimes diarrhea and a feeling of warmth. This may occur immediately after eating in patients who have had a partial gastrectomy.

Subjective symptom—Symptom of internal origin that is apparent or perceptible only to the patient (for example, pain or dizziness [vertigo]).

Symmetry (sim′et-ri)—Conformity in form, size, and arrangement of parts on opposite sides of the body.

Figure 4-1   Instruments used for physical examinations. **A,** *Laryngoscope;* **B,** *Hirschman anoscope.*
B, Courtesy Miltex Instrument Co., Division of Miltenberg, Inc., Lake Success, NY.

A

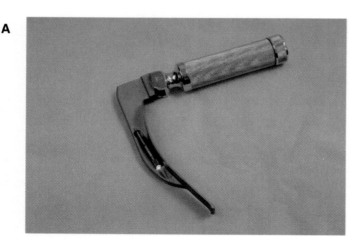

Larnygoscope

B

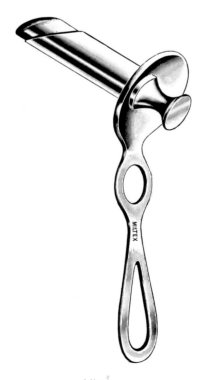

Hirshman anoscope

Figure 4-1—cont'd *Instruments used for physical examinations.* **C,** *Tuning forks;* **D,** *otoscope;* **E,** *Boucheron and Toynbee ear specula to be used with an otoscope;* **F,** *Miltex fiberglass tape measure;* **G,** *Tischler cervical biopsy punch forceps.*
C and E through G, Courtesy Miltex Instrument Co., Division of Miltenberg, Inc., Lake Success, NY.

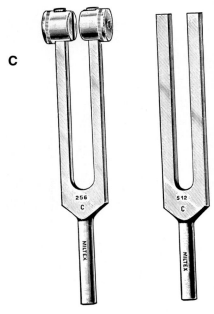

C

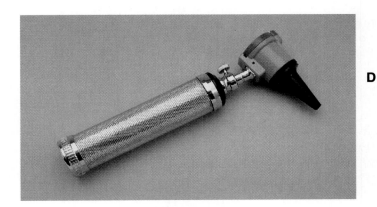

Otoscope

D

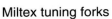

Miltex tuning forks

E

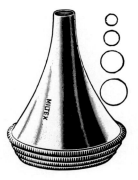

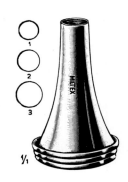

Boucheron and Toynbee ear specula to be used
with an otoscope

F

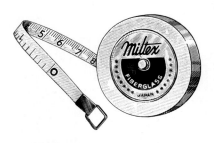

Miltex fiberglass tape measure

G

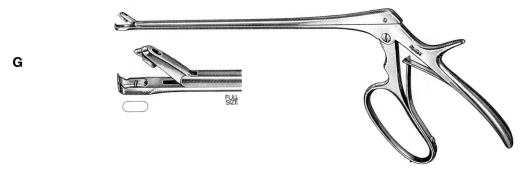

Tischler cervical biopsy punch forceps

Figure 4-1—cont'd *Instruments used for physical examinations.* **H,** *Frankel head band and mirror set;* **I,** *Wartenberg neurologic pinwheel;* **J,** *Laryngeal mirror;* **K,** *insufflator;* **L,** *percussion hammer;* **M,** *Graves vaginal speculum.*
H through J, L, and M Courtesy Miltex Instrument Co., Division of Miltenberg, Inc., Lake Success, NY.

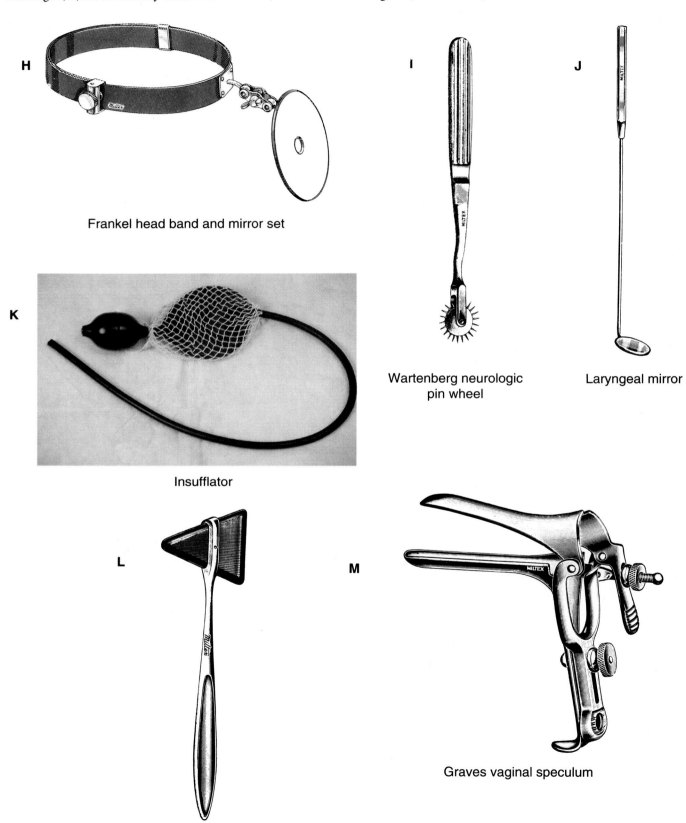

Frankel head band and mirror set

Wartenberg neurologic
pin wheel

Laryngeal mirror

Insufflator

Taylor percussion hammer

Graves vaginal speculum

Figure 4-1—cont'd *Instruments used for physical examinations.* **N,** *Ophthalmoscope;* **O,** *Kelly proctoscope;* **P,** *Sonnenschein nasal speculum;* **Q,** *Tonometers* **(2).**
O through Q Courtesy Miltex Instrument Co., Division of Miltenberg, Inc., Lake Success, NY.

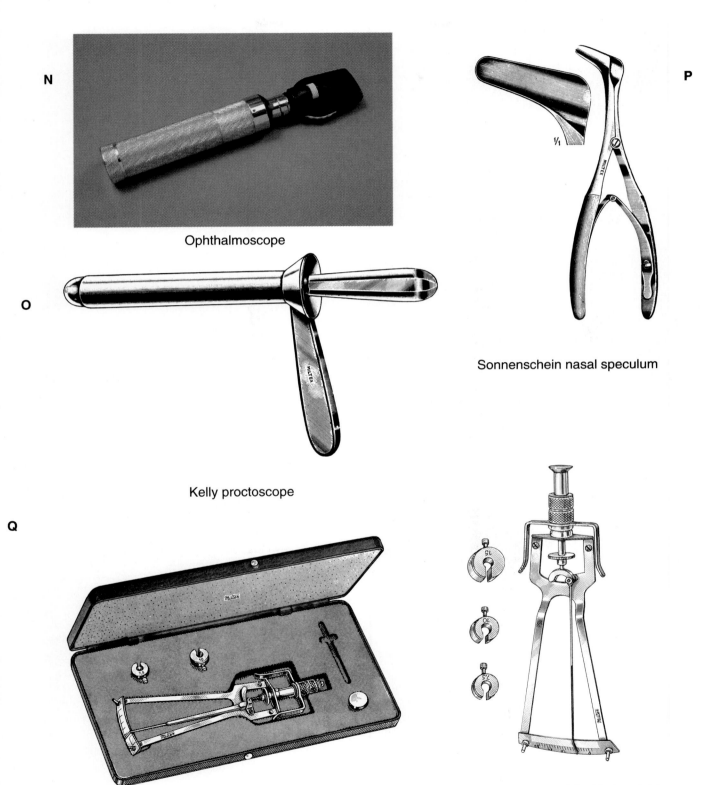

Ophthalmoscope

Sonnenschein nasal speculum

Kelly proctoscope

Original model with 3 weights (5,5,7,5, and 10g) plunger, flootplate, and test block

Improved model with 4 weights (5,5,7,5,10, and 15g) mirror insert on scale reduces error or parallax

Figure 4-1—cont'd *Instruments used for physical examinations.* **R**, *Yeoman biopsy forceps;* **S**, *60 cm fiberoptic flexible sigmoidoscope (1) and metal 25- to 30-cm sigmoidoscope (2).*

R Courtesy Miltex Instrument Co., Division of Miltenberg, Inc., Lake Success, NY.

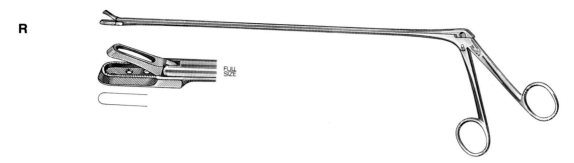

Yeoman biopsy forceps

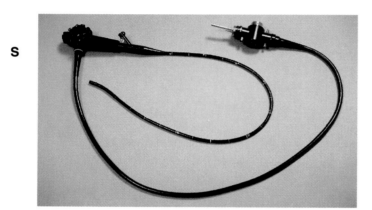
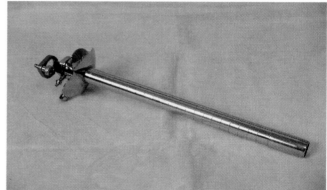

Fiberoptic flexible colonoscope and metal sigmoidoscope

V O C A B U L A R Y

anoscope (an' no-skop)—A speculum or endoscope inserted into the anal canal for direct visual examination.

Applicator—A slender rod of wood with a pledget of cotton on one end used to apply medicine or to take a culture from the body.

Biopsy (bi' op-se) **forceps**—Two-pronged instruments of varying sizes and shapes used to remove tissue from the body for examination.

Bronchoscope (brong' ko-skop)—An endoscope designed specifically for passage through the trachea to allow visual examination of the interior of the tracheobronchial tree.

Cystoscope (sist' o-skop)—A hollow metal tube (endoscope) designed specifically for passing through the urethra into the urinary bladder to permit internal inspection. The bladder interior is illuminated by an electric bulb at the end of the cystoscope. Special lenses and mirrors allow the bladder mucosa to be examined for calculi (stones), inflammation, or tumors.

Endoscope (en' do-skop)—A specially designed instrument made of metal or rubber (rigid or flexible) that is used for direct visual examination of hollow organs or body cavities. All endoscopes have similar working elements, even though the design varies according to its specific use. The viewing part (scope) is a hollow tube fitted with a lens system that allows viewing in a variety of directions. Each endoscope has a light source, power cord, and power source; examples include bronchoscope, cystoscope, proctoscope, and sigmoidoscope.

Insufflator (in' suf ' fla-tor)—An instrument, device, or bag used for blowing air, powder, or gas into a cavity.

Laryngeal (lar-in' je-al) **mirror**—An instrument used to view the pharynx and larynx, consisting of a small, rounded mirror attached to the end of a slender (metal or chrome plate) handle.

Laryngoscope (lar-in'go-skop)—An endoscope used to examine the larynx. It is equipped with mirrors and a light for illumination of the larynx.

Nasal speculum (na′ zl spek′ u-lum)—A short, funnellike instrument used to examine the nasal cavity.

Ophthalmoscope (of ′ thal′ mo-skop)—An instrument used for examining the interior parts of the eye. It contains a perforated mirror and lens. When the ophthalmoscope is turned on and brought close to the eye, it sends a narrow, bright beam of light through the lens of the eye. By looking through the lens of the instrument, the physician is then able to examine the interior parts of the eye, including the lens, anterior chamber, retinal structures, and blood vessels, to detect any possible disorders. Many ophthalmoscopes come with an interchangeable otoscope, throat illuminator head, or nasal illuminator head.

Otoscope (o′to-skop)—An instrument used to examine the external ear canal and eardrum.

Percussion (pur-kush′ un) **hammer**—A small hammer with a triangular-shaped rubber head used for percussion.

Proctoscope (prok ′ to-skop)—A specially designed tubular endoscope that is passed through the anus to permit internal inspection of the lower part of the large intestine.

Sigmoidoscope (sig-moy ′ do-skop)—A tubular endoscope used to examine the interior of the sigmoid colon.

Speculum (spek ′ u-lum)—An instrument used for distending or opening a body cavity or orifice to allow visual inspection; a bivalve speculum is one having two parts or valves.

Sims vaginal speculum—A form of bivalve speculum used in the examination of the vagina and cervix. Vaginal specula come in three sizes: small, medium, and large. They are made of metal or disposable plastic.

Stethoscope—An instrument used in auscultation to amplify the sounds produced by the lungs, heart, intestines, and other internal organs; also used when taking a blood pressure reading (see page 39).

Tongue blade—A flat, thin, smooth piece of wood or metal with rounded ends approximately 6 inches long; also called a tongue depressor. It is used for pressing tissue down to permit a better view when examining the mouth and throat. In addition, it may be used for application of ointments to the skin.

Tonometer (to-nom ′ e-ter)—An instrument used to measure tension or pressure, especially intraocular pressure.

Tuning fork—A steel, two-pronged, forklike instrument used for testing hearing; the prongs give off a musical note when struck.

GENERAL INSTRUCTIONS AND RESPONSIBILITIES FOR THE MEDICAL ASSISTANT

1. Always wash your hands thoroughly before setting up the required equipment for an examination and assisting the physician.
2. Prepare the patient, the examination room, and the equipment and instruments required by the physician for the examination according to office or agency policy.
3. Make certain that electrical and battery-operated equipment and all lights are in working condition.
4. Place the equipment for the examination so that it is conveniently located for the physician's use.
5. Make sure that the examination room is comfortably warm, well aired, and spotlessly clean.
6. Cover the examination table with a clean cover, either a cotton or muslin sheet, crepe paper, or a covered rubber sheet on the lower part of the table. A towel may be placed over a pillow at the end of the table.
7. Always have the patient empty his or her bladder before an examination begins. If a urine specimen is needed, collect it at this time.
8. Assist the patient as required. Have a sturdy stepstool for the patient to use when getting on and off the examining table. Offer support; guard against falling. Never leave a confused patient or a child alone on the examining table because of the danger of falling.

9. Assist the physician as required. You must learn the physician's methods and preferences for each examination.
10. *Never* expose the patient unnecessarily. Only those parts of the body being examined are to be exposed.
11. A female assistant should remain in the room if the patient is female and the physician is male. Your presence may not only help the anxious patient to feel more relaxed, but it also protects the physician from unwarranted lawsuits. There can be no false allegations if you witness the entire examination.
12. Observe the patient for various types of reactions. A change in facial expression may indicate that the patient is apprehensive or experiencing pain. Note any unusual weakness, change in breathing pattern, change in skin color, or fainting. Your observations may provide the physician with important information that will help make a diagnosis and provide treatment for the patient.
13. Inform the patient of any special instructions. When the physician has completed the examination, inform the patient that he or she is free to leave after getting dressed, or if required, to check at the front desk to schedule a future appointment or a laboratory or x-ray film examination. Often the physician requests that certain tests be run or specimens be gathered. Some offices and agencies have a printed sheet on which the physician can check each test that is to be performed on the patient. The medical assistant makes the proper arrange-

ments, notifies the technologist, or collects the specimens requested before the patient leaves.

14. Handle specimens obtained according to office or agency policy.

15. On completion of the examination, carry out your responsibilities for the disposal, cleansing, disinfecting, or sterilizing of the used equipment and the treatment room to prevent the spread of microorganisms.

16. Record findings from the examination accurately and completely. Use correct medical abbreviations, when applicable, in recording all information. Most physicians record all the necessary information on the patient's chart; thus frequently this is not one of the medical assistant's responsibilities. The policy regarding this varies and is established by the physician or agency for whom you work. If it is your responsibility, the following items are usually to be included:

a. Date, time, and type of examination and the findings/results, when applicable

b. Name of the examiner

c. If specimens were obtained, the type, how they were handled, snf the test(s) to be performed

d. Any pertinent observations that you have made that will describe the patient's general condition; be specific in the type of information you record (for example, "patient complained of slight nausea and a transient pain in the right lower abdominal quadrant")

e. Future directions given to the patient

f. Your signature

GOWNING, POSITIONING, AND DRAPING THE PATIENT FOR PHYSICAL EXAMINATIONS

A physical examination is facilitated by the use of an examining table and proper gowning, positioning, and draping of the patient. The purposes of positioning a patient are:

• To allow for better visibility and accessibility for the physician during the examination of the patient.

• To provide support for the patient when being examined.

The purposes of gowning and draping the patient are:

• To avoid unnecessary exposure of the patient's body during an examination, thereby protecting the patient's modesty.

• To contribute to the patient's feeling of being cared for, which helps the patient relax.

• To provide some comfort and warmth and to avoid chilling.

The principle of gowning and draping is that only the part of the body that is being examined should be exposed, other than the head, arms and sometimes the legs, and only when the physician is about to begin the examination.

There are different positions used for various types of examinations. In all positions the patient must be well supported, since most positions are uncomfortable and difficult to maintain for any length of time. The position chosen depends on the type of examination or procedure to be performed and on the patient's age, sex, and physical and emotional condition. The various positions used most frequently in a general or special physical examination are presented along with the instructions for gowning, positioning, and draping the patient.

Text continues on page 90.

DORSAL-RECUMBENT AND LITHOTOMY POSITIONS

Equipment

Examination table
Patient gown, either cotton or disposable paper
Paper or sheet to cover the table
Small towel, cloth or paper
Small pillow
Drape sheet; two drape sheets are needed for the jackknife and Trendelenburg positions
Stirrups on the examining table for the lithotomy position
A binder to support the patient on the table when placed in the Trendelenburg position

In the lithotomy position the patient's feet normally are placed in stirrups that are raised approximately 12 inches from table level, although the stirrups on some examining tables cannot be elevated. These positions are used almost exclusively for pelvic, bladder, and rectal examinations (Figures 4-2 and 4-3).

• The patient lies on the back with the legs separated and flexed.

• The feet are supported in stirrups, or the soles of the feet are flat on the table.

• The buttocks are brought to the edge of the examining table.

• The arms are placed either at the side or crossed over the chest or under the head.

DORSAL-RECUMBENT AND LITHOTOMY POSITIONS—cont'd

PROCEDURE	RATIONALE
1. Place clean paper or sheet on the examination table.	
2. Identify the patient and explain the procedure.	*The medical assistant must explain what is required and why it is necessary in order to gain full cooperation from the patient. Clear explanations also help reassure the patient.*
3. Have the patient disrobe and put on the patient gown.	*For a pelvic examination the patient should disrobe from the waist down. For a pelvic and breast examination, the patient should disrobe completely and put the gown on with the opening in the front.*
4. Have the patient lie down on the table; place a small pillow under the head.	*Help make the patient as comfortable as possible.*
5. Cover the patient with a drape sheet, placing it in a rectangular arrangement. One point of the sheet faces the patient's neck and covers the chest; the opposite corner is placed between the legs or feet. The other corners extend over the sides of the patient.	
6. Have the patient move buttocks down to the extreme edge of the table with knees flexed and the feet firmly on the table, or at table level in stirrups.	
7. Place a small towel under the buttocks.	*This catches discharge that may be excreted from the patient's body.*
8. Have the patient cross arms under the head or over the chest, or place along the sides of the body.	
9. Take the lateral corners of the sheet and wrap them around the feet in a spiral fashion.	
10. When the examination begins, the corner of the sheet that covers the perineum is pulled back and upward toward the abdomen to expose the perineal area. Place this part of the sheet neatly over the patient's abdomen.	*Avoid letting the sheet fall over the perineum, as it would obstruct the physician's examination.*
11. If you are to position the patient in the lithotomy position, the same procedure is followed, except that the patient's legs are elevated in the stirrups. In this position the lateral corners of the sheet are wrapped around the legs and feet that are supported in the stirrups. The stirrups are generally raised at least 1 foot above the table level and positioned to the sides of the table.	*The knees are placed sufficiently apart to allow exposure of the perineum.*

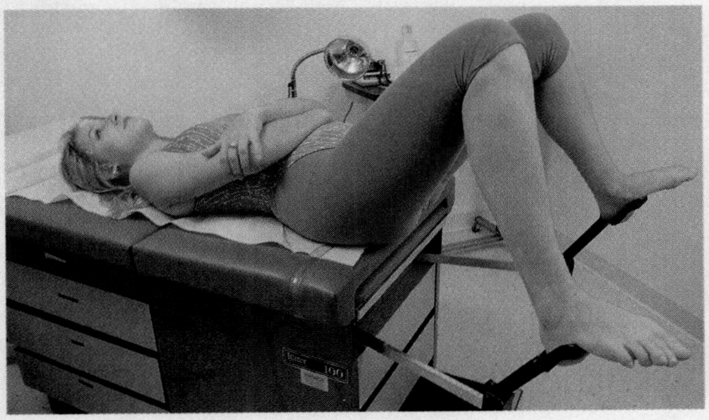

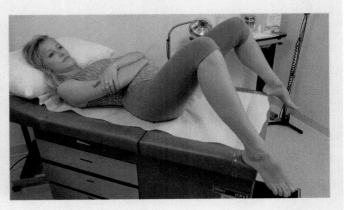

Figure 4-2 *Dorsal-recumbent position.*

Figure 4-3 *Lithotomy position.*

JACKKNIFE OR PROCTOLOGIC POSITION

Equipment

Examination table
Patient gown, either cotton or disposable paper
Paper or sheet to cover the table
Small towel, cloth or paper
Small pillow
Drape sheet; two drape sheets are needed for the jackknife and Trendelenburg positions
Stirrups on the examining table for the lithotomy position
A binder to support the patient on the table when placed in the Trendelenburg position

General Instructions

The patient lies on the abdomen with both the head and legs lowered, so that the buttocks are elevated. Arms are placed along the side of the head.

This position is used for rectal examinations and occasionally for surgery. A special examining table that can be adjusted to facilitate this position is required.

PROCEDURE

1. Place clean paper or sheet on table and a small towel over the area of the table where it will be split.

2. Identify the patient and explain the procedure.

3. Have the patient disrobe completely and put on a patient gown with the opening in the back.

4. Have the patient lie on the table and roll over onto the abdomen.

5. The table is split so that the patient's head and legs are lowered, and the buttocks are elevated. Arms may be placed under the head or stretched out in front of the head.

6. Place a small pillow under the patient's head.

7. Cover the patient's body with one sheet, and put another sheet over the legs.

8. When the examination begins, the lower part of the sheet covering the patient's body is drawn back and folded over the lumbar region.

RATIONALE

The towel helps soak up any discharge that may be excreted from the patient during the examination and can be removed or folded over before the patient gets up.

This helps to put the patient at ease and cooperate.

If only a rectal examination is to be done, a female does not have to remove her bra.

The patient's legs are braced against the lowered part of the table. Good support is required, as this position is difficult to maintain.

Make the patient as comfortable as possible.

Do not bind the legs together, as frequently it is necessary for them to be separated for proper examination.

This exposes only the rectal region, which is being examined, and maintains the patient's modesty as well as can be expected.

KNEE-CHEST POSITION

Equipment

Examination table
Patient gown, either cotton or disposable paper
Paper or sheet to cover the table
Small towel, cloth or paper
Small pillow
Drape sheet; two drape sheets are needed for the jackknife and Trendelenburg positions
Stirrups on the examining table for the lithotomy position
A binder to support the patient on the table when placed in the Trendelenburg position

Figure 4-4 *Knee-chest position.*

General Instructions

The patient rests on the knees and chest, with the head turned to one side. Arms may be placed under the head to partially help support the patient. Buttocks extend up in the air, and back is straight.

This position is used for the rectal examination and sometimes for vaginal and prostatic examinations (Figure 4-4).

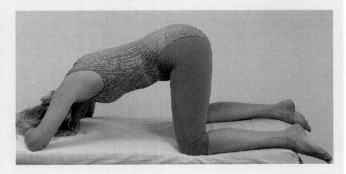

PROCEDURE

1. Place clean paper or sheet on the table.

2. Identify the patient and explain the procedure.

3. Have the patient disrobe and put on the patient gown. The opening of the gown should be in the back.

4. Have the patient kneel on the table, keeping the buttocks elevated and back straight.

5. Have the patient turn the head to one side.

6. The arms should be flexed at the elbow and extended, placing them under or near the side of the head.

7. Cover the patient's body with a drape sheet, and place a smaller drape sheet over the legs.

8. When the examination begins, the drape sheet is pulled back and folded over the top of the buttocks.

RATIONALE

This helps reassure the patient and helps the patient understand what to expect and the reason for assuming this position.

The patient is resting on the chest in this position. A small pillow may be placed under the chest for support and comfort.

This helps support the patient.

The patient should be fully draped.

This exposes only the rectal and vaginal areas, which are to be examined.

SIM'S OR LEFT LATERAL POSITION

Equipment

Examination table
Patient gown, either cotton or disposable paper
Paper or sheet to cover the table
Small towel, cloth or paper
Small pillow
Drape sheet; two drape sheets are needed for the jackknife and Trendelenburg positions
Stirrups on the examining table for the lithotomy position
A binder to support the patient on the table when placed in the Trendelenburg position

General Instructions

The patient lies on the left side and chest, with the left leg slightly flexed and the right leg sharply flexed on the abdomen.
The left arm is drawn behind the body with the body inclining forward.
The right arm is positioned forward according to the patient's comfort.
The buttocks are brought up to the long edge of the table.

This position is used frequently for rectal examinations and when giving enemas. The vagina and abdomen can also be examined in this position, and it may be used for older women when the lithotomy position is too difficult to maintain (Figure 4-5).

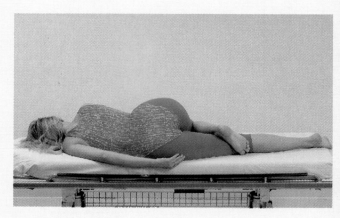

Figure 4-5 *Sim's or left lateral position.*

PROCEDURE

1. Place clean paper or sheet over table.

2. Identify the patient and explain the procedure.

3. Have the patient disrobe completely and put on the patient gown. The opening of the patient gown should be in the back.

   You may help the patient assume this position properly by placing your hand along the long side of the table, so that the patient's buttocks touch your hand when they are over to the side far enough.

4. Instruct the patient to lie down on the table and then to roll over onto the left side and chest, moving the buttocks up to the long edge of the table.

5. The left arm is drawn behind the body with the body inclining forward. The right arm is positioned in front of the body, where it provides support and is most comfortable for the patient

6. Place a small pillow under the patient's head. One may also be placed under or near the chest.

RATIONALE

This provides the patient with some understanding of why this position is to be assumed, thus enabling the patient to cooperate.

Provide comfort and support for the patient.

SIM'S OR LEFT LATERAL—cont'd

PROCEDURE	RATIONALE
7. Instruct the patient to flex the right leg sharply over the abdomen and to flex the left leg slightly.	*This position provides good access to the anal canal, rectum, and sigmoid colon.*
8. Place a small towel under the buttocks.	*The towel catches discharge and can be removed before the patient gets up.*
9. Cover the patient with the drape sheet.	
10. When the examination begins, fold back the drape sheet so that only the anal and vaginal areas are exposed.	

TRENDELENBURG POSITION

Equipment

Examination table
Patient gown, either cotton or disposable paper
Paper or sheet to cover the table
Small towel, cloth or paper
Small pillow
Drape sheet; two drape sheets are needed for the jackknife and Trendelenburg positions
Stirrups on the examining table for the lithotomy position
A binder to support the patient on the table when placed in the Trendelenburg position

General Instructions

In the Trendelenburg (tren-del´ en-burg) position, the patient lies on the back with the head lower than the rest of the body. The body is elevated at an angle of about 45 degrees, and the knees are flexed over the lower section of the examining table, which is lowered. The patient should be well supported to prevent slipping.

This position is not used routinely for an office examination, but often it is used in the operating and x-ray rooms. It displaces the intestines into the upper abdomen.

An alternate form of the Trendelenburg position is one in which the patient's body is placed on an incline with the feet elevated at an angle of 45 degrees and the head lowered. This position is used to prevent shock or when the patient is in a state of shock or has low blood pressure. It is also used for some abdominal surgery. Some physicians have the patient positioned in the Sims position, along with this form of the Trendelenburg position, for rectal examinations (Figure 4-6).

A

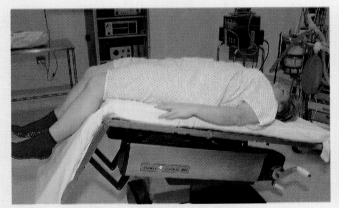

B

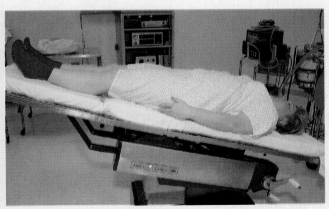

Figure 4-6 **A** *and* **B,** *Trendelenburg positions.*

TRENDELENBURG POSITION—cont'd

PROCEDURE

1. Place clean paper or sheet on the examining or x-ray table.

2. Identify the patient and explain the procedure.

3. Have the patient disrobe and put on the patient gown. Have the opening of the gown in the front.

4. Assist the patient onto the table and instruct the patient to assume a supine position. Place a small pillow under the head.

5. Instruct the patient to cross arms over the chest region or place alongside the body.

6. Cover the patient from the shoulders to the feet with a drape sheet.

7. Support the patient with a binder to prevent slipping. This is placed over the abdominal region and secured to both sides of the table.

8. Adjust the examining table. The body is on an inclined plane with the head slightly lowered. In the operating room the knees will be flexed over the lower end of the table. In the x-ray room, the table is raised so that the head is lowered and the feet are elevated. Feet and legs are straight.

RATIONALE

This enables the patient to understand the need for this position and what to expect. Your caring attitude will also help reassure the patient.

Make the patient as comfortable as possible.

SUPINE POSITION

The patient lies flat on the back, arms placed at the side, and head elevated slightly on a pillow. This position is used for examinations of the abdomen and breasts, for some surgical and x-ray film procedures, and on occasion for examination of the chest (Figure 4-7).

PRONE POSITION

The patient lies flat on the abdomen, arms flexed under the head, which is turned to one side. This position may be used in examinations of the back in musculoskeletal and neurologic examinations and for some surgical procedures (Figure 4-8).

FOWLER'S POSITION

The patient is sitting up. This position is used for examining the head, ears, eyes, nose and throat, neck, chest, and breasts (Figure 4-9).

SEMI-FOWLER'S POSITION

The patient is lying in a supine position, with the head of the table or bed raised 18 to 20 inches above the level of the feet. This may be used rather than the supine or Fowler position when the comfort and physical condition of the patient require it (for example, for a patient with dyspnea [Figure 4-10]).

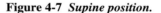

Figure 4-7 *Supine position.*

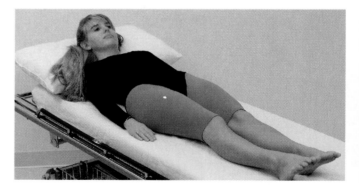

Figure 4-8 *Prone position.*

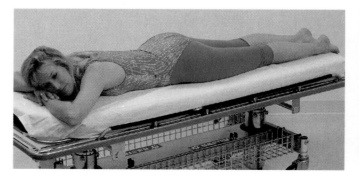

Figure 4-9 *Fowler's (sitting) position.*

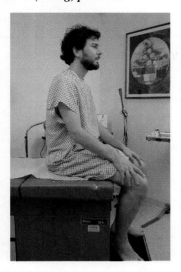

Figure 4-10 *Semi-Fowler's position.*

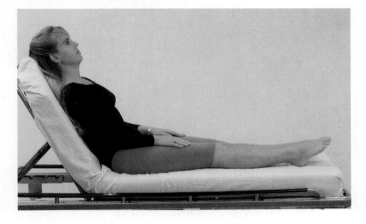

ERECT OR STANDING POSITION

The patient stands erect with arms at the sides, feet facing forward. This position is used for part of a neurologic and musculoskeletal examination and also during some x-ray film procedures (Figure 4-11).

The following instructions apply to positioning and draping the patient in the supine, prone, Fowler's and semi-Fowler's positions.

1. Provide the patient with a gown. Depending on the examination to be performed, the patient should be instructed to disrobe completely; at times the patient may leave underpants on. If the chest is to be examined, it is advisable to instruct the patient to put the gown on with the opening in the front because this provides for comfort and easier accessibility to this region during the examination.

2. Instruct and assist the patient in assuming the correct position as required.

3. Place a drape sheet over the midtrunk and legs.

Figure 4-11 *Standing position.*

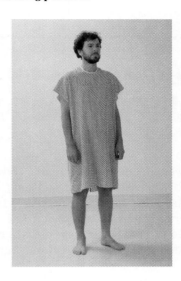

4. When the examination begins, the drape sheet may be folded back to expose the area on the body that is being examined.

GYNECOLOGIC EXAMINATION

Gynecology is the branch of medicine that deals with maintaining the health of the female reproductive tract and with the diseases and conditions that affect it. The medical specialist in this branch of medicine is called a *gynecologist.*

A *gynecologic examination* may be included as part of a complete physical examination of a female as discussed in the previous procedure or it may be performed as a separate examination. When performed by itself, a gynecologic examination generally included the following.

* A breast examination performed by the physician and instructions to the patient on how to perform a breast self-examination (BSE) (Figure 4-12)
* A pelvic examination
* A Pap smear
* Individual cultures and smears for suspected vaginal infections (for example, trichomoniasis vaginitis, candidiasis, gonorrhea, chlamydia, herpes simplex viruses (HSV), and the human papillomavirus ([HPV or genital warts]). These infections and the cultures and smears that are used to diagnose them are discussed in Unit Eleven (also see Table 11-2).

BREAST SELF-EXAMINATION

Generally the physician examines the patient's breasts at each physical examination. Between examinations, women should examine their own breasts to detect any abnormality, which can be brought to the physician's attention immediately. The following information is supplied to the public for their general information by the American Cancer Society.

Figure 4-12 *Breast self-examination: a new approach.*
Courtesy American Cancer Society, San Francisco, Calif.

Breast Self-Examination:
A NEW APPROACH

All women over 20 should practice monthly breast self-examination (BSE). Regular and complete BSE can help you find changes in your breasts that occur between clinical breast examinations (by a health professional) and mammograms.

Women should examine their breasts when they are least tender, usually seven days after the start of the menstrual period. Women who have entered menopause, are pregnant or breast feeding, and women who have silicone implants, should continue to examine their breasts once a month. Breast feeding mothers should examine their breasts when all milk has been expressed.

If a woman discovers a lump or detects any changes, she should seek medical attention. Nine out of ten women will not develop breast cancer and most breast changes are *not* cancerous.

Remember the seven P's for a complete BSE:

1 **Positions**
2 **Perimeter**
3 **Palpation**
4 **Pressure**
5 **Pattern**
6 **Practice with Feedback**
7 **Plan of Action**

1 Positions
Visual Inspection: Standing

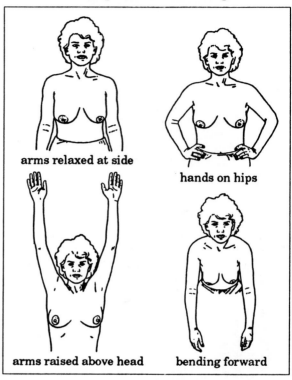

arms relaxed at side

hands on hips

arms raised above head

bending forward

In each position, look for changes in contour and shape of the breasts, color and texture of the skin and nipple, and evidence of discharge from the nipples.

Palpation: Side-lying & Flat
Use your left hand to palpate the right breast, while holding your right arm at a right angle to the rib cage, with the elbow bent. Repeat the procedure on the other side. The side-lying position allows a woman, especially one with large breasts, to most effectively examine the outer half of the breast. A woman with small breasts may need only the flat position.

Side-lying Position:
Lie on the opposite side of the breast to be examined. Rotate the shoulder (on the same side as the breast to be examined) back to the flat surface.

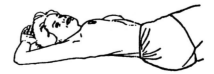

Figure 4-12—cont'd *Breast self-examination: a new approach.*

Flat Position:

Lie flat on your back with a pillow or folded towel under the shoulder of the breast to be examined.

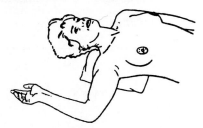

2 Perimeter

The examination area is bounded by a line which extends down from the middle of the armpit to just beneath the breast, continues across along the underside of the breast to the middle of the breast bone, then moves up to and along the collar bone and back to the middle of the armpit. Most breast cancers occur in the upper outer area of the breast (shaded area below).

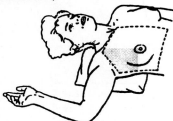

3 Palpation With Pads of the Fingers

Use the pads of three or four fingers to examine every inch of your breast tissue. Move your fingers in circles about the size of a dime.

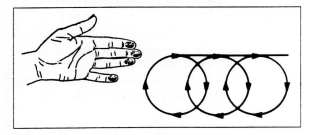

Do not lift your fingers from your breast between palpations. You can use powder or lotion to help your fingers glide from one spot to the next.

4 Pressure

Use varying levels of pressure for *each palpation*, from light to deep, to examine the full thickness of your breast tissue. Using pressure will not injure the breast.

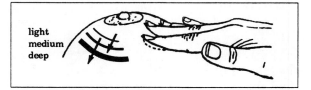

5 Pattern of Search

Use one of the following search patterns to examine all of your breast tissue. Palpate carefully beneath the nipple. Any incision should also be carefully examined from end to end. Women who have had any breast surgery should still examine the entire area and the incision.

Vertical Strip:

Start in the armpit, proceed downward to the lower boundary. Move a finger's width toward the middle and continue palpating upward until you reach the collarbone. Repeat this until you have covered all breast tissue. Make at least six strips before the nipple and four strips after the nipple. You may need between 10 and 16 strips.

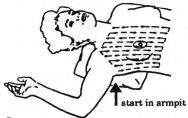

Wedge:

Imagine your breast divided like the spokes of a wheel. Examine each separate segment, moving from the outside boundary toward the nipple. Slide fingers back to the boundary, move over a finger's width and repeat this procedure until you have covered all breast tissue. You may need between 10 and 16 segments.

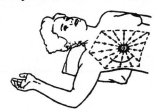

Figure 4-12—cont'd *Breast self-examination: a new approach.*

Circle:

Imagine your breast as the face of a clock. Start at 12 o'clock and palpate along the boundary of each circle until you return to your starting point. Then move down a finger's width and continue palpating in ever smaller circles until you reach the nipple. Depending on the size of your breast, you may need eight to ten circles.

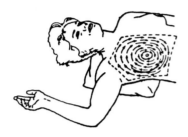

Nipple Discharge:

Squeeze your nipples to check for discharge. Many women have a normal discharge.

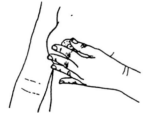

Axillary Examination:

Examine the breast tissue that extends into your armpit while your arm is relaxed at your side.

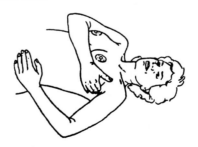

6 Practice With Feedback

It is important that you perform BSE while your instructor watches to be sure you are doing it correctly. Practice your skills under supervision until you feel comfortable and confident.

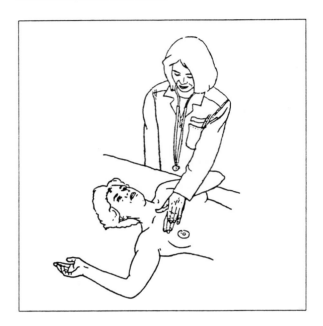

7 Plan of Action

Every woman should have a personal breast health plan of action:

✔ Discuss the American Cancer Society breast cancer detection guidelines with your health care professional.

✔ Schedule your clinical breast examination and mammogram as appropriate.

✔ Do monthly BSE. Ask your health professional for feedback on your BSE skills.

✔ Report any changes to your health care professional.

COMPLETE PHYSICAL EXAMINATION

Equipment

The exact amount and type of equipment to be assembled for a physical examination depends on the following:

> Purpose of the examination
> Type and extent of the examination
> Preferences of the physician
> Condition of the patient

In some physician's offices and agencies, the equipment required for examination is kept on a special tray ready for use and in a central location. In others it may be necessary for you to assemble all the equipment that will be needed. Although there are differences among physicians and agencies, the following list includes items that are commonly used, and should be available, ready for use (Figure 4-13).

> Examination table covered with a clean sheet
> Patient gown, either cloth or paper
> Draping material, drape sheet, small towel
> Watch with a sweep second had
> Stethoscope
> Thermometer
> Sphygmomanometer
> Scale with height measure rod
> Tape measure
> Tuning fork
> Percussion or reflex hammer
> Tongue blades
> Laryngeal mirror
> Head mirror
> Flashlight and/or gooseneck lamp
> Otoscope
> Ophthalmoscope
> Nasal speculum
> Safety pin
> Tissues

> Cotton balls
> Alcohol or prepackaged alcohol swabs
> Urine specimen bottle
> Laboratory request form
> X-ray film request form
> Emesis basin or waste container used for soiled equipment and/or waste

Additional equipment is required for a visual acuity test, vaginal, and rectal examinations. This varies with the purpose of the examination, the condition of the patient, and the physician's preference.

Visual acuity test
> A Snellen eye chart is used most frequently to measure distance visual acuity.

Vaginal examination
> Vaginal speculum
> Disposable single-use exam gloves
> Water-soluble lubricant such as K-Y jelly
> Uterine sponge or uterine dressing forceps
> Sponges
> Two glass slides for smears; or one glass slide and one sterile culture tube with applicator
> Cotton-tipped applicators or wooden cervical spatulas
> Fixative spray or cytology jar with solution
> Plastic container for slides if using the fixative spray
> Laboratory require form

Rectal examination
> Rectal glove or sterile rubber gloves or rubber finger cot
> Lubricant, such as K-Y jelly
> Rectal speculum, proctoscope, or anoscope (depending on the extent of the examination)
> Tissues
> Sponge forceps
> Sponges
> Cotton-tipped applicators

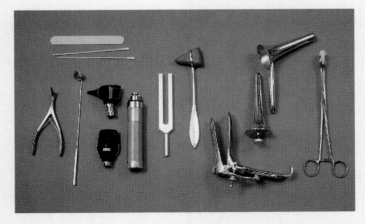

Figure 4-13 *Instruments and supplies commonly used for a physical examination.* **Left to right,** *Nasal speculum, laryngeal mirror, otoscope (top) and ophthalmoscope (bottom) attachments with battery-operated handle, tuning fork, percussion hammer, vaginal speculum, anoscope, and sponge stick (forceps) with sponge;* **Top left corner,** *Tongue blade, cotton-tipped applicators.*

COMPLETE PHYSICAL EXAMINATION—cont'd

PROCEDURE	RATIONALE
1. Wash your hands. **Use appropriate personal protective equipment (PPE) as indicated by facility.**	
2. Assemble and prepare the necessary equipment for the physician. Equipment is to be arranged on a table or tray covered with a clean towel.	
3. Identify the patient and explain the procedure.	*An explanation helps the patient to understand the procedure (that is, what will occur, how it may feel, and how she or he can help in the examination). It also helps to reassure for the patient.*
4. Have the patient void to empty the bladder. Instruct the patient how to collect a urine specimen if one is required (see Unit Eleven).	*When the bladder is full, it is difficult for the physician to palpate the abdomen adequately. It is also very uncomfortable for the patient to have a full bladder while being examined.*
5. Take the following physical measurements and record accurately: TPR BP Height Weight This varies with your job requirements. At times the physician may wish to do these tests rather than have you do them. Height and weight should be taken after the patient removes shoes and heavy outer clothing.	
6. Instruct the patient to disrobe completely and put on a patient gown with the opening in the front.	*Gown donned with opening in the front permits access to the chest for examination while the shoulders and back are still covered.*
7. Have the patient sit on the edge of the examining table with a towel under the buttocks. Place a drape sheet over the patient's lap.	
8. Call the doctor when the patient is ready and when you have completed all the necessary recordings and assembled the equipment. Give the patient's chart to the physician before the examination begins. A female assistant should remain in the room if the patient is female and the physician male and/or if the physician requires your assistance when performing the examination (see page 83).	
9. Assist the physician as required. Depending on the physician's preference, you may have to be ready to hand the instruments as needed. The physician proceeds with the examination from head to toe, examining the body systems and parts as described previously under the physical examination in Unit Three.	
10. While the patient is in a sitting position, the physician examines the head, ears, eyes, nose, mouth, and throat; the neck and axillae; the chest, breasts, and heart; and the neuromuscular reflexes and sensations such as the pinprick. He or she generally observes skin and body symmetry.	**Equipment**

Equipment

Tuning fork	*Flashlight*
Otoscope	*Head mirror*
Ophthalmoscope	*Laryngeal mirror*
Nasal speculum	*Stethoscope*
Tongue blade	*Safety pin*
	Percussion hammer

COMPLETE PHYSICAL EXAMINATION—cont'd

PROCEDURE	RATIONALE
11. If handing used equipment and/or specimens, don gloves. When handing or accepting a tongue blade from the physician, hold it in the center. Without touching the end used, discard in the emesis basin or waste container.	*By handling the tongue blade this way you avoid contamination to the patient and also to yourself.*
12. Warm the laryngeal mirror by placing the mirrored end under warm running water or in a glass of warm water. Be sure to dry it before it is used.	*It must be warmed to prevent fogging.*
13. After Step 10 is completed, the patient is to assume a supine position. Help the patient attain this position if necessary. Give reassurance and support as needed.	*Often just placing your hand on the patient's shoulder or arm gives the patient a feeling of support and of being cared for.*
14. Place the drape sheet to cover the patient from shoulders to feet. Move it down when the physician is ready to examine the breasts and abdomen. When the physician examines the breasts, fold the sheet down to the patient's waist and open the patient's gown. When the patient is in this position, the physician palpates breasts, liver, spleen, and other abdominal organs. The groin is checked for a possible hernia.	
When the abdomen is being examined, the patient's gown can be used to cover the breasts; fold the drape sheet down to the pubic hair line. The physician may use a stethoscope to listen to abdominal sounds as part of the examination of the abdomen.	
15. For a vaginal and rectal examination, help the patient assume the correct position. Assist the physician as required. Positions and procedures for these examinations are discussed next. Vaginal and rectal examinations are included in the complete physical examination of a female patient. For the male patient, the physician examines the genitals, the rectum, and prostate gland.	
16. Observe the patient for any unusual reactions such as a feeling of weakness or pain, facial grimace, change in color.	
17. When the examination has been completed, the patient may sit up. It may be advisable to allow the patient to remain in the supine position for a few minutes before getting up.	
18. Ask if patient has any questions.	*Frequently a patient may have questions, but does not feel free to ask or may feel that there isn't time to do so.*
19. Inform the patient of any special instructions.	*(Also see rationale for No. 13). Frequently patients are left in the room after the examination, not knowing if they are to talk further to the physician or are free to leave. Do not let this happen.*
20. If necessary, help the patient dress; otherwise leave the room so that the patient may have some privacy.	

COMPLETE PHYSICAL EXAMINATION—cont'd

PROCEDURE	RATIONALE
21. On returning to the examining room, assemble all used equipment and supplies to be disposed of properly. Remove all linens and place in the soiled laundry. Place disposable equipment in a covered waste container. Take instruments to your cleanup area. You may rinse some instruments with cool water or wash or soak them in soap and water until you are ready to prepare them for sterilization or disinfection (see Unit Five). Others (for example, the tuning fork) you may wipe off and replace them in the usual storage area. 22. Resupply clean equipment as needed. 23. Clean the examination table and put on a fresh cover. 24. If smears or cultures were obtained, send them to the laboratory or place them in a refrigerator or a cool dark place until you can transfer them to the laboratory. Make sure that specimens are properly labeled and that you have completely filled out the appropriate laboratory request form. 25. Remove gloves if worn. Wash your hands. 26. Do any recording required of you completely and accurately (see No. 16, page 84). Use accepted medical abbreviations when recording.	*Charting example:* *Jan. 27, 19__, 1 p.m.* *Complete physical examination done by Dr. Short. Patient referred to lab for a CBC (complete) and UA (urinalysis) and to the x-ray department for a chest x-ray film. Patient to return in 1 week to discuss the results of these tests with the doctor.* *Ann O'Reilly, CMA*

Reasons for monthly BSE. Most breast cancers are first discovered by women themselves. Since breast cancers found early and treated promptly have excellent chances for cure, learning how to examine your breasts properly can help save your life. Use the sample six-step BSE procedure shown in Figure 4-12.

Best time to perform BSE. Follow the same procedure once a month about a week after your period, when breasts are usually not tender or swollen. After menopause, check breasts on the first day of each month. After hysterectomy, check with your doctor or clinic for an appropriate time of the month. A monthly BSE coupled with an annual physical examination reassures you there is nothing wrong.

What to do if you find a lump or thickening. If a lump or dimple or discharge is discovered during BSE, it is important to see your doctor as soon as possible. Don't be frightened. Most breast lumps or changes are not cancer, but only your doctor can make the diagnosis.

The medical assistant should see that the office or clinic has literature for women on this subject. (See also "Mammography" in Unit Thirteen.)

PELVIC EXAMINATION AND A PAP SMEAR

Pelvic (vaginal) examinations and Pap smears are essential for the adult female. Most general practitioners and internists, as well as gynecologists and obstetricians, perform them routinely. These examinations, done for diagnostic purposes of the female reproductive system, include inspection of the vulva, vagina, and cervix for any abnormalities and a bimanual palpation of the uterus, fallopian tubes, and ovaries. The physician notes the size, shape, position, and consistency of the uterus and whether any masses are present in the uterus, fallopian tubes, or ovaries. Developed by Dr. George Papanicolaou in the 1940s, the *purpose* of the Pap smear is to detect precancerous conditions or any unusual cell growth and to detect cancer of the cervix or uterus. The value of the test is that it can detect potential problems early so that they can be treated. It is recommended that all women have a pelvic examination every 3 years and that all women who are or have been sexually active or have reached age 18 have an annual Pap smear and pelvic examination. After three or more consecutive normal examinations, the Pap test may be performed less frequently at the discretion of the woman's physician.

Special instructions must be given to the patient before they have a Pap smear taken. It is often the responsibility of the medical assistant to provide the patient with the following information.

1. Do not douche or put any vaginal medications, creams or foams, lubricants or contraceptive products such as spermicides in the vagina for 24 hours (some suggest 48 to 72 hours) before having a Pap smear taken. These products interfere with the specimen obtained and make the test invalid.

2. Abstain from sexual intercourse for 1 to 2 days before the test.

3. Try to schedule the Pap smear so that it takes place between the twelfth and sixteenth days of the menstrual cycle. A Pap smear must not be taken during the patient's menstrual period because the red blood cells interfere with obtaining accurate findings.

The federal government and several states have passed legislation to regulate the laboratories that evaluate Pap smears. These relatively new laws establish training requirements and proficiency testing for technologists and place a limit on the number of slides that they can review in 1 day. The smear should be examined in a certified laboratory by a pathologist or qualified technologist who reports the findings as one of five classifications that follow.

- Class I—Normal. Only normal cells are seen.
- Class II—Possibly abnormal. Some atypical cells are seen. These may be the result of inflammation of the vagina or cervix. Occasional dysplasia.
- Class III—Abnormal. Mild to moderate dysplasia. Suspicious, some precancerous cells. Another Pap smear and/or biopsy would be suggested.
- Class IV—Abnormal. Severe dysplasia, suspicious cells. High probability of cancer. Biopsy should be done to confirm findings.
- Class V—Abnormal. Carcinoma cells are seen.

When the Pap smear is abnormal, it doesn't mean that the patient has cancer, except if the findings were in Class V. Abnormal findings indicate the need for further diagnostic studies. Frequently a physician first does a colposcopy. In this examination an instrument called a colposcope magnifies and focuses an intense light on the cervix. This allows the physician to observe the cervical anatomy in greater detail. If the colposcopy reveals an inflammatory process, a vaginal cream may be all that is needed for treatment. If the colposcopy reveals areas of abnormal tissues, the physician may use one or more diagnostic and therapeutic procedures, including a biopsy, cryosurgery, endocervical curettage, possibly a cone biopsy using either traditional surgery, laser surgery, or more extensive surgery (also see Table 4-3).

NEW USES FOR THE PAP SMEAR

Technologic advances combined with the traditional techniques and better sampling and interpretation guidelines are making the Pap smear more effective than ever in detecting early disease. The PAPNET, a computerized method for analyzing Pap smears, is being used to retest Pap smears that have been interpreted by technologists. The PAPNET computer duplicates the process that the human eye and mind use to identify abnormal cells. It is hoped that this method will eventually replace many of the examinations now done by hand.

Another test, the *ViraPap*, was approved by the FDA in 1989. It is used to screen for the presence of HPV or genital warts in Pap smear samples. HPV is linked to the incidence of cervical cancer, and this test could detect the disease before cancer develops.

RECTAL EXAMINATION

The rectal examination is used to detect polyps, early cancer, lesions, inflammatory conditions, and hemorrhoids. In addition, examination of the rectum can show how far the uterus is displaced and if there are any masses in the rectum or pelvic region in a female; and the size, any enlargement, and texture of the prostate gland in a male.

The prostate is a gland just below the bladder in the male genital tract. It has the second highest incidence of cancer in men 55 years of age and older. Recommendations for prostate cancer screening for men over age 50 include a digital rectal examination and a blood test, the prostate specific antigen (PSA). The PSA is a very sensitive test used to screen for prostate disease, but it is not specific for cancer. Some elevated PSA tests are discovered that are not related to cancer and some cancer patients have normal PSAs. However, the digital and PSA test together are an excellent screen for prostate cancer. One without the other is thought to be inadequate by many physicians.

The American Cancer Society recommends that after age 40 an annual health checkup for everyone include a digital rectal examination. A more extensive examination of the interior surfaces of the rectum is done by a proctoscopy.

ENDOSCOPIC EXAMINATION: PROCTOSCOPY AND SIGMOIDOSCOPY

The purpose of a proctoscopy (prok-tos′ ko-pi) and sigmoidoscopy (sig″moi-dos′ ko-pi) is to examine the rectum and lower sigmoid colon for possible lesions, tumors, ulcers, polyps, inflammatory conditions, strictures, varicosities, and hemorrhages. Carcinoma may appear as a nodular, often cauliflower-like growth with superficial ulceration. Polyps are recognized easily by their pedicle. In doubtful cases, a biopsy of the growth is done.

Text continues on page 108.

PELVIC EXAMINATION AND PAP SMEAR

Equipment (Figure 4-14)

Examination table (stirrups if available) covered with a clean sheet or paper
Patient gown
Drape sheet
Small towel
Small pillow
Gooseneck lamp
Vaginal speculum (metal or disposable plastic)
Water-soluble lubricant, such as K-Y jelly
Disposable single-use exam gloves
Uterine sponge or uterine dressing forceps
Sponges or cotton balls
Two glass slides for smears or one glass slide and one sterile culture tube with applicator

Two cotton-tipped applicators or wooden cervical spatulas
Fixative spray such as Cyto-Fix or Spray-cyte or cytology jar with solution (for example, 95% isopropyl alcohol solution is preferred, although formalin 10% may be used)
Plastic container for slides when using the fixative spray
Tissues
Laboratory request form

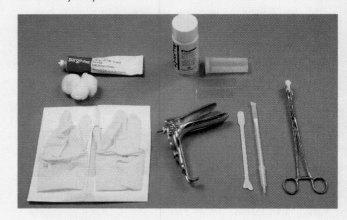

Figure 4-14 *Equipment for pelvic examination and Pap smear.*

PROCEDURE

1. Wash your hands. **Use appropriate personal protective equipment (PPE) as indicated by facility.**

2. Assemble and prepare the necessary instruments and equipment. Prepare the room. Make sure the lamp is working and that there is a clean paper or sheet on the table.

3. Identify the patient. Explain the procedure, and reassure the patient.

4. Have the patient empty her bladder. Explain to the patient how to collect a specimen if a urinalysis is to be done.

5. You may be required to take the patient's pulse and blood pressure.

6. Provide a patient gown and have the patient remove all clothing from the waist down. Shoes may be left on if the heels fit into the stirrups.

7. Position the patient on the table in a dorsal-recumbent or lithotomy position and drape as explained previously.
   a. Place the stirrups far enough out so the knees are apart.
   b. Avoid exposing the patient unnecessarily.
   c. Make sure there is a small towel under the buttocks.

RATIONALE

An explanation helps the patient understand the need for the examination and what to expect (that is, what will occur and how it may feel).

This is usually done if the woman is taking birth control pills and often routinely in many offices as a screening process for high blood pressure.

This varies with the physician's preference and the patient's condition. The Sims position may also be used for a vaginal examination of an elderly woman.

PELVIC EXAMINATION AND PAP SMEAR—cont'd

PROCEDURE

8. Call the physician. NOTE: You may call the physician into the room and then have the patient assume the required position. Remain in the room (refer to No. 11, page 83).

9. Assist the physician as required.
   a. Lower the foot of the examining table (if it is a table that splits), or push the foot piece in on newer-model tables.
   b. Pull back the drape sheet, exposing *only* the perineal region.
   If you do not have to assist the physician with the instruments and materials, give your attention to the patient. You may stand by the patient on one side and offer support and reassurance. Frequently support can be given just by having your hand placed gently on the patient's arm or shoulder.

10. Be prepared to hand the physician the various instruments and materials that he may need. Some physicians request that you put some water-soluble lubricant such as K-Y jelly out on a gauze sponge; others squeeze it out when they are ready to lubricate the disposable single-use exam gloves and vaginal speculum. Direct the light on the area being examined. The vaginal speculum may be warmed by running warm water over it. Alternatives used in some offices and agencies are to keep the instruments on a heating pad or in a warming pan. Other agencies use plastic, disposable specula; it is not necessary to warm them.

11. If a smear is to be obtained, mark the patient's name on the slides and the cytology jar *or* on the container where they will be placed after using a fixative spray. Label the slides No. 1 and No. 2. Attach paper clips to the ends of the slides.

12. You may instruct the patient to breathe deeply through the mouth.

13. The *physician* begins the examination. If a Pap smear is to be obtained, the physician:
    a. Inserts a dry speculum into the vagina (Figure 4-15).
    b. Opens the speculum so that he or she can see the cervix clearly.
    c. Inserts a cotton-tipped applicator or wooden vaginal spatula and draws it across the cervix to obtain a specimen, which is then smeared evenly and moderately thinly across the No. 1 glass slide (Figure 4-16).

RATIONALE

Attaching paper clips to the ends of the slides prevents them from sticking together if they are to be placed in a cytology jar with the isopropyl alcohol or formalin solution.

This helps relax muscles.

NOTE: *If a smear is not to be obtained, the speculum is lubricated for easier insertion into the vagina. Steps (c) through (e) would then be omitted.*

PELVIC EXAMINATION AND PAP SMEAR—cont'd

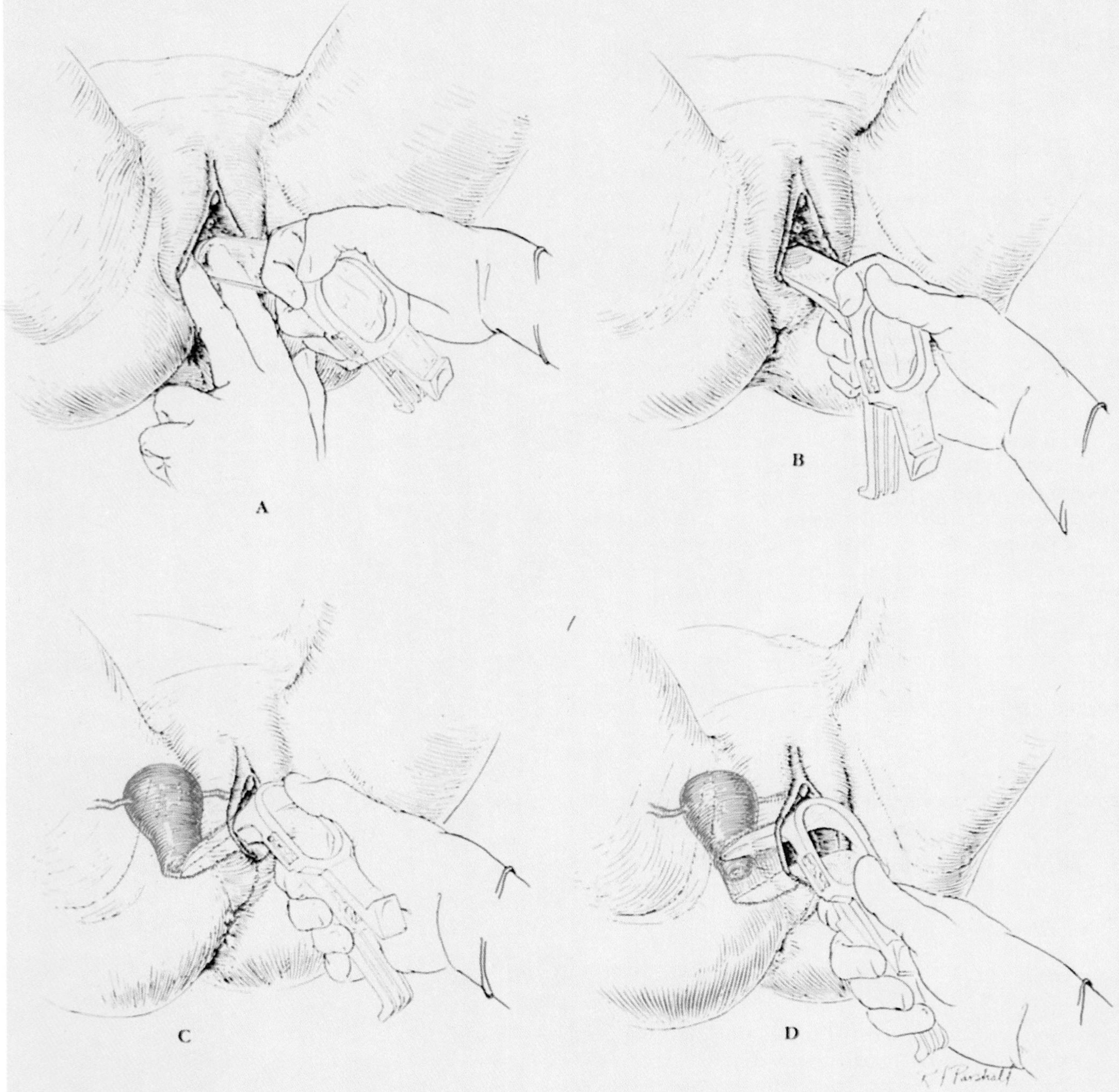

Figure 4-15 ***Procedure for vaginal examination.* A, *Opening of the introitus;* B, *oblique insertion of the speculum;* C, *final insertion of the speculum; and* D, *opening of the speculum blades.***

From Malasanos L, et al: *Health assessment*, ed 4, St. Louis, 1990, Mosby.

PELVIC EXAMINATION AND PAP SMEAR—cont'd

PROCEDURE

d. Inserts another applicator or spatula and draws it across the posterior fornices or pools of the vaginal canal to obtain a second specimen, which is then smeared evenly and moderately across the No. 2 glass slide. If the material is spread too thickly, it is difficult for the laboratory worker to visualize individual cells.

e. Places these two slides immediately (within 4 seconds to prevent drying and death of cells) into the cytology jar with solution, or sprays them thoroughly with the cytologic fixative spray and places them in the designated container after the fixative has dried thoroughly (drying takes about 5 to 10 minutes). NOTE: The *medical assistant* may be required to hold the slide while the physician smears the specimen on the slide and then to spray the slide with the cytologic fixative spray. Don disposable single-use exam gloves if you will be handling the slides. (See also Unit One and the CDC guidelines for handling specimens.) When spraying the slides, hold the nozzle of the can at least 5 to 6 inches away from the slide and spray lightly from left to right and then from right to left (Figure 4-18). Allow the slides to dry thoroughly before placing them in the designated container for transport to an outside laboratory (Figure 4-19).

NOTE: Send these slides with a properly labeled cytology laboratory request form to the laboratory for cytologic examination. Enter the following on the request form:
• Date
• Physician's name and address
• Patient's name and age
• Source of specimen
• Test(s) requested

Also enter all of the following that apply:
• Date of last menstrual period (LMP)
• Hormone treatment (which includes birth control pills)
• Postmenopausal
• Postpartum
• Pregnant
• Previous surgery
• X-ray film treatment
• Previous normal
• Previous abnormal and date

NOTE: Rather than making two smears, many agencies and physicians obtain one endocervical smear for cytology studies and one culture for gonorrhea screening. This is done more frequently now because often an infection is present without any signs or symptoms. This has been found to be a very beneficial screening process that enables early treatment when an asymptomatic infection is present. *Other specimens* may be obtained at this time for *any* suspected vaginal infection(s).

RATIONALE

NOTE: *Frequently an endocervical smear is more desirable than one obtained from the posterior vaginal pool. In this case, the physician inserts an applicator into the cervical os, rotating it completely around the os until the cotton is saturated. A smear is then prepared with this specimen (Figure 4-17).*

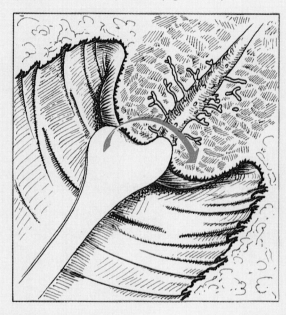

Figure 4-16 *Cervical smear.*
From Malasanos L, et al: Health assessment, ed 4, St. Louis, 1990, Mosby.

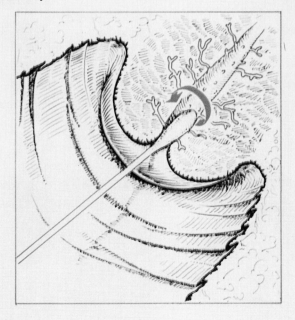

Figure 4-17 *Endocervical smear.*
From Malasanos L, et al: Health assessment, ed 4, St. Louis, 1990, Mosby.

PELVIC EXAMINATION AND PAP SMEAR—cont'd

PROCEDURE

f. Remove the speculum and place it in an area designated for used equipment.

g. Apply water-soluble lubricant to the gloved index finger of the dominant hand.

h. Insert the gloved, lubricated finger into the vagina to palpate internally for any abnormalities such as displacement or growths of the uterus, cervix, ovaries, and fallopian tubes. Place the other hand on the patient's abdomen and apply pressure so that the movable abdominal organs may be felt more easily during this bimanual examination (Figure 4-20).

14. When the physician has completed the examination, wipe off the excess lubricant or discharge from the patient's perineal region. You may use tissues or the small towel that was placed under the patient's buttocks.

15. Remove small towel from under the patient's buttocks.

16. Raise or pull out the foot of the examining table.

17. Help the patient remove her feet from the stirrups and place her legs down on the table.

18. The patient may now slide up toward the head of the table and then sit up. Frequently it is desirable or advisable to allow the patient to rest for a few minutes before getting up.

19. Remove drape sheet.

20. If necessary, help the patient get up and get dressed. Provide extra tissue and a sanitary pad and belt if required.

21. Inform the patient of any special instructions, if she is free to leave after she is dressed, or if the physician wishes to speak to her further. Ask the patient if she has any questions (see No. 13, page 83). Provide accurate and complete information, or refer the patient's questions to the physician if you cannot answer them.

RATIONALE

This varies with the type of examining table used.

If you are helping the patient lower her legs, lift and move both legs together to avoid any undue strain to the pelvic area.

Always provide for the patient's safety, comfort, and well-being.

Part of patient care includes patient education and providing information and answers as necessary.

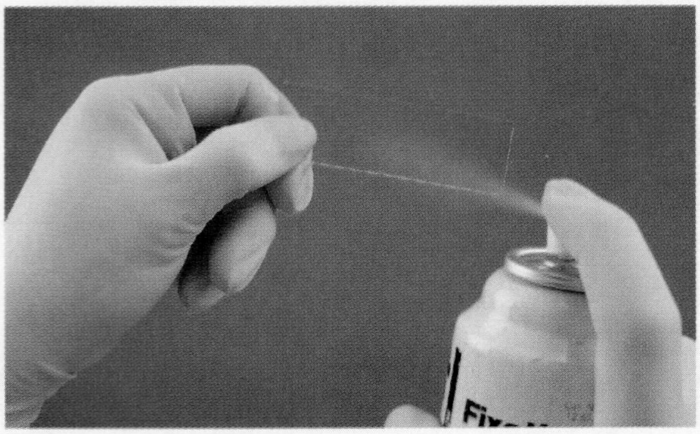

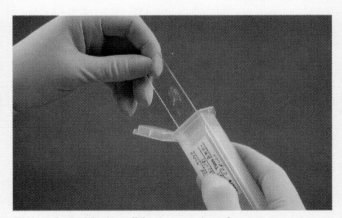

Figure 4-18 *Spraying smear with a cytological fixative spray.*

Figure 4-19 *Placing slides in container for transport to a laboratory.*

PELVIC EXAMINATION AND PAP SMEAR—cont'd

PROCEDURE

22. Leave the patient to dress in privacy if your assistance is not required.

23. Don gloves and return to the examining room to assemble all used equipment and supplies to be disposed of properly.

    Remove any linens and place them in the soiled laundry. Place disposable equipment in a covered waste container.

    Take instruments to your cleanup area. Rinse the instruments with cool water. They can be soaked in soap and water until you are ready to prepare them for sterilization (see Unit Five).

24. Resupply clean equipment as needed.

25. Clean the examination table and put on a fresh cover.

26. If smears or cultures were taken, send them to the laboratory with request form; or place in a cool, dark place until you can transfer them to the laboratory. It is important that all the required information appears on the cytology lab request, including notation of cervical and vaginal smears (see NOTE to No. 13e of this procedure).

27. Remove gloves.

28. Wash your hands.

29. Do any recording required of you completely and accurately (see No. 16, page 84).

RATIONALE

Charting example:
  January 27, 19____, 2 p.m.
    Pelvic exam done by Dr. Short. Pap smear sent to laboratory for cytology studies. Patient had no specific complaints and left office in good spirits.
      Sandi Wilcox, CMA

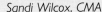

A

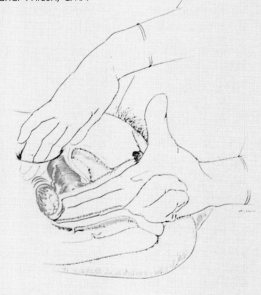

B

Figure 4-20 A, *Bimanual palpation of the uterus;* **B,** *Bimanual palpation of the adnexa.*
From Malasanos L, et al: Health assessment, ed 4, St. Louis, 1990, Mosby.

RECTAL EXAMINATION

Equipment (Figure 4-21)

Examination table
Sheet or paper to cover the table
Patient gown
Drape sheet
Small pillow
Small towel
Tissues
Disposable single-use exam gloves
Water-soluble lubricant (example, K-Y jelly)
Sponge forceps
Sponges
Rectal speculum and/or anoscope
Cotton-tipped applicators

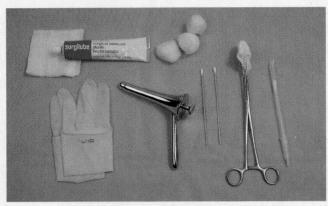

Figure 4-21 *Equipment for rectal examination including a Culturette (on the far right) to obtain a culture.*

PROCEDURE

1. Wash your hands. **Use appropriate personal protective equipment (PPE) as indicated by facility.**

2. Identify the patient and explain the procedure.

3. Have the patient empty the bladder. Explain to the patient how to collect a specimen if a urinalysis is to be done (See Unit Seven).

4. Provide a patient gown; have the patient remove all clothing from the waist down and put the gown on with the opening in the back.

5. Assemble the necessary instruments and equipment.

6. Position the patient on the examination table in a Sims, jackknife, or knee-chest position.

7. Drape the patient. Refer to pages 84 to 91 for positioning and draping techniques.

8. Call the physician.

9. When the examination is ready to begin, pull the drape sheet back, exposing only the rectal area.

10. Assist the physician as required. A female assistant should remain in the room if the patient is female and the physician is male, even if she does not have to assist during the examination (see. No. 11, page 83).

11. Be prepared to hand the physician the various instruments and equipment. Some physicians request that you put some water-soluble K-Y jelly out on a piece of gauze; others get it themselves to lubricate the gloved finger and anoscope if used. If a light is used, direct it on the part to be examined (the rectal region).

RATIONALE

An explanation helps the patient understand the need for the examination and provides some reassurance.

This varies somewhat, depending on the extent of the examination to be done and the physician's preference. Frequently only the glove and lubricant are necessary.

This varies according to the physician's preference.

NOTE: You may call the physician and then position the patient. By doing this, you prevent the patient from having to be in an uncomfortable position for an excessive period of time.

Avoid exposing the patient unnecessarily.

RECTAL EXAMINATION—cont'd

PROCEDURE

12. If you do not have to assist the physician, give your attention to the patient. Provide support and observe for any unusual reaction such as a feeling of weakness, a change in skin color, or facial grimace, which may be an indication of pain.

13. The *physician* begins the examination by inserting a gloved, lubricated finger into the rectum, then palpating the rectum internally to determine if there are any hemorrhoids, polyps or other observations, growths, or enlargements. This is done gently because it is often painful for the patient. If the anoscope is used it is lubricated; then the physician inserts it into the anal canal gently and removes the obturator. If there is any bleeding or discharge, the physician may insert the sponge forceps and sponge through the anoscope to swab the area dry. This allows better viewing of the internal surfaces. A good light is needed so that the physician can view the internal lining of the anal canal. If a culture is to be taken, the physician puts a cotton-tipped applicator through the anoscope and swabs the area. The cotton-tipped applicator is then placed in a sterile culture tube, often one that has a special broth solution in it, so that the culture does not dry out.

14. When the physician has completed the examination, wipe the patient's anal region for any excess lubricant or discharge. You may use tissues, or the small towel under the patient's buttocks, which is then removed.

15. Help the patient, if required, assume a supine position. Frequently it is desirable to allow the patient to remain lying down for a few minutes.

16. Remove the drape sheet.

17. If required, assist the patient to a standing position and in getting dressed. Provide extra tissues to the patient, if required, for additional cleansing of the anal region.

18. Tell the patient of any special instructions, if the patient is free to leave after getting dressed, or if the physician wishes to speak further to the patient in the office. Inquire if the patient has any questions. (see No. 13, page 13). Always provide complete and accurate information. Refer the patient's questions to the physician if you cannot answer them completely and accurately. Never leave a patient in the examining room wondering if the office visit and examination are completed.

19. If your assistance is not required, leave the patient to dress in private.

RATIONALE

Always provide for the comfort and welfare of the patient at the conclusion of an examination.

RECTAL EXAMINATION—cont'd

PROCEDURE	RATIONALE
20. On returning to the examining room, assemble all used equipment and supplies to be disposed of properly. Don disposable gloves and remove any linens and place in soiled laundry. Place disposable equipment in a covered waste container. Take instruments to your cleanup area; rinse with cool water. These may be soaked in soap and water until you are ready to prepare them for sterilization (see Unit Five). Follow Universal Precautions for cleanup activities (see Unit One).	
21. Resupply clean equipment as needed.	
22. Clean the examination table and put on a fresh cover.	
23. If smears or cultures were obtained, send them to the laboratory or place them in a refrigerator or a cool, dark place until you can transfer them to the laboratory. See Unit Eleven for the technique for obtaining a stool specimen. Make sure that specimens are properly labeled and that you have completely filled out the appropriate laboratory request form.	Proper care and labeling of specimens is essential.
24. Wash your hands.	

25. Do any recording required of you completely and accurately (see No. 16, page 84).	Charting example:
	Jan. 27, 19 ___ 3 p.m.
	   Rectal exam done by Dr. Short. No specimens were obtained. Patient complained of a sharp, continuous pain in the anal region when leaving the office and will call the doctor if it continues.
	   Betty Fox, CMA

If found early and treated properly, 75% to 80% of all cases of cancer of the rectum and lower bowel can be cured. Most cases occur in individuals 55 to 75 years of age. Bowel cancers tend to grow slowly and are possible to detect at the most curable stage, before symptoms appear. Anyone with a personal or family history of rectal or colon cancer, of polyps in the rectum or colon, or of ulcerative colitis should be examined carefully. If cancer is found, surgery, sometimes combined with radiation therapy, is the most effective method of treatment. Recently chemotherapy has shown to be beneficial when given to patients after surgery in certain early colon cancer cases.

The American Cancer Society recommends that individuals have the following (Figure 4-22):

- An annual digital rectal examination after age 40
- An annual stool test for occult (hidden) blood after age 50 (see Unit Eleven)
- A proctosigmoidoscopy examination every 3 to 5 years after age 50 (*following* two initial negative annual examinations that were performed 1 year apart)

These guidelines apply only to people without symptoms. If a person has a change in bowel habits or has rectal bleeding, they should see a physician immediately.

Figure 4-22 *Examinations of the rectum and colon. 1, Anus; 2, rectum; 3, limit of digital-rectal examination; 4, colon; 5, limit of rigid procto examination; 6, limit of flexible sigmoidoscope (35 cm) examination; 7, limit of flexible sigmoidoscope (60 cm) examination; 8, limit of stool blood test.*

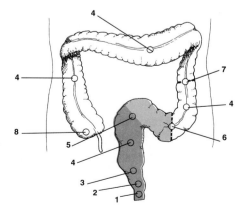

Some people are at higher risk for cancer and may need tests earlier and more often. Check with your physician to see what's right for you.

Text continues on page 118.

PROCTOSCOPY AND SIGMOIDOSCOPY

Equipment

Examination table covered with a clean sheet

Patient gown

Drape towel

Drape sheet

Small towel

Small pillow

Place and assemble the following equipment from the contents of the rectal diagnostic set on a clean drape towel (Figure 4-23):

Sigmoidoscope with obturator (depending on the physician's request, either a 30- to 65-cm, flexible fiberoptic sigmoidoscope or a rigid, 30-cm sigmoidoscope; with the flexible fiberoptic sigmoidoscope the physician can view a greater portion of the intestinal tract)

A rigid 15-cm proctoscope with obturator (depending on the physician's request)

Transilluminators (light source)

Rheostat

Extension cord

Insufflator with bulb attachment

Suction tip for suction machine

Biopsy forceps (sterile)

Metal sponge holder or 12-inch long sponge sticks

When the above have been assembled, add:

Disposable single-use exam gloves

Doctor's fluid-resistant gown

Rectal dressing forceps

Cotton-ball sponges

4 × 4-inch gauze

Tissues

Water-soluble lubricant (such as K-Y jelly)

Specimen bottle with preservative if biopsy is to be taken

Laboratory request form

Kidney basin

Suction machine

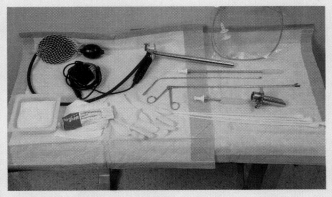

Figure 4-23 *Equipment for sigmoidoscopy.*

PROCEDURE

1. Wash your hands. **Use appropriate personal protective equipment (PPE) as indicated by facility.**

2. Assemble and prepare the necessary equipment and supplies on a clean drape towel. Disposable scopes may be used instead of the metal ones.

3. Test the suction apparatus and the light on the scopes.

4. Identify the patient and explain the procedure carefully.

5. Have the patient empty the bladder. Explain to the patient how to collect a specimen if a urinalysis is to be done. (Refer to Unit Seven for specimen collection procedure.)

6. Have the patient remove all clothing from the waist down and put on the patient gown.

7. Position the patient.
   a. Knee-chest position: Many examining rooms have a special proctoscopic table that is tilted in a way that supports the patient in the knee-chest position (see Figures 4-4 and 4-5). Draping remains the same.

   b. Sims or left lateral position: Position of the patient may vary with the physician's preference.

RATIONALE

Make sure they are working properly.

This helps the patient understand the need for the examination and what to expect (that is, what will occur and how it may feel). It also enables the patient to cooperate more readily and to feel somewhat reassured.

This is often preferred as it allows the abdominal contents to fall away from the pelvis, making it easier and less painful for the patient to be examined.

NOTE: *This is an uncomfortable position and usually cannot be tolerated for a long period.*

This may be more comfortable for the patient, depending on age, weight, and condition.

PROCTOSCOPY AND SIGMOIDOSCOPY—cont'd

PROCEDURE	RATIONALE
8. Drape the patient completely. Refer to draping procedures on page 84.	
9. Call the physician into the room.	NOTE: You may call the physician into the room and then position the patient, as this would avoid the necessity of having the patient in an uncomfortable position for an excessive period of time.
10. When the physician is ready to begin the examination, pull the drape sheet back to expose only the anal area.	Avoid exposing the patient unnecessarily.
11. Assist the physician as required. Be prepared to hand the physician the various instruments and equipment. A female assistant should always remain in the room if the patient is female and the physician is male (see No. 11, page 83). If you do not have to assist the physician, give your full attention to the patient. Provide support and reassurance. Observe the patient for any unusual reaction	
12. The physician begins the examination.	***Method of examination:***
a. Put a generous amount of water-soluble lubricant on 4 × 4-inch gauze square, and place on the towel with the equipment. Use this for lubricating the instruments and the physician's gloved finger when the examination begins.	The physician first does a manual rectal examination. A liberal amount of lubricant is applied to the gloved index finger for easier insertion into the anal canal.
b. Warm the metal scopes by placing them in warm water or by rubbing them with your hand. Avoid additional discomfort for the patient that a cold instrument would cause.	This varies with office or agency preference. Disposable scopes do not need to be warmed.
c. Hand the physician the scope. Attach the inflation bulb to the scope.	The physician or you then lubricates the distal end of the scope with the obturator in place.
d. To help the patient relax the anal sphincter for easier insertion of the scope, instruct the patient to bear down slightly, as though having a bowel movement, at the same time the physician inserts the scope. Also, instruct the patient to take deep breaths through the mouth because this also helps relax the anus and rectum..	If right-handed, the physician separates the buttocks with the left hand and then slowly and gently inserts the scope about 3 to 4 cm. Force is never used when inserting the scope, because it could cause injury to the bowel. The obturator is removed and can be placed in the kidney basin
e. Attach the light source to the scope and adjust the light to the proper intensity. Note: You may turn off the lights in the room when the physician begins the visual examination through the scope. This allows for better inspection.	The physician visually inspects the bowel thoroughly as he or she advances the scope to its full length.
f. Observe the patient throughout the procedure for fatigue, weakness, or fainting.	Next, the physician pumps the inflator bulb attachment slowly to inject a small amount of air into the bowel. Although this is quite painful for the patient, it is necessary for proper inspection of the bowel. NOTE: This step is omitted in cases of ulcerative colitis or diverticulitis, because of fragility of the bowel.
g. Turn on the suction machine if it is to be used.	When there is bleeding or loose discharge in the bowel, the physician may place a long metal sponge holder with a sponge through the scope to swab the area clean, or the suction tip may be used.
h. You may hand the biopsy forceps to the physician. A biopsy forcep is placed through the scope if a biopsy is required.	

PROCTOSCOPY AND SIGMOIDOSCOPY—cont'd

PROCEDURE

i. Have ready a labeled specimen jar.

j. Continue to offer reassurance and support to the patient. Frequently, just placing your hand on the patient's shoulder, arm, or hand gives the patient a feeling of being cared for as an individual.

13. At the completion of the examination, take tissues and wipe the anal area for any lubricant and/or body discharge.

14. Help the patient assume a supine position. Frequently, it is desirable to allow the patient to rest for a few minutes before getting up, as he or she may feel faint.

15. Remove the drape sheet.

16. When required, help the patient get up and get dressed. Provide the patient with extra tissues to cleanse the anal region more completely.

17. Inform the patient of any special instructions. Inquire if the patient has any questions (see No. 13, page 83). Provide complete and accurate information. Never leave a patient alone in a room after an examination without an understanding of what is to be done after getting dressed.

18. If your assistance is not required, leave the patient to dress in privacy.

19. If specimens were obtained, send them to the laboratory. Be sure that all specimens are properly labeled and sent to the laboratory with the correct requisition form.

20. Don disposable single-use exam gloves and return to the examining room to assemble all used equipment and supplies. Remove linens and place in soiled laundry. Take the instruments to your cleanup area. Following Universal Precautions (see Unit One), rinse thoroughly with running water. You may then soak the instruments in soap and water until you are ready to prepare them for sterilization (Unit Five).
   NOTE: Do not soak the light attachment for the scope; cleanse it thoroughly with an alcohol sponge. Disposable equipment should be removed and placed in a covered waste container.

21. Wash the examination table with a disinfection solution and cover with a clean sheet or paper.

22. Resupply clean equipment as needed.

23. Wash your hands.

24. Do any recording required of you completely and accurately (see No. 16, page 84).

RATIONALE

When a specimen is obtained, it should be placed immediately into the labeled specimen jar.
On completing the examination, the physician removes the scope slowly, which may then be placed in the kidney basin.

Provide for the patient's comfort.

Always provide for the safety and comfort of the patient.

This prepares the examination room for the next patient.

Charting example:
   Jan. 29, 19___, 1:15 p.m.
      Sigmoidoscopy done by Dr. Short. Tissue biopsy sent with requisition to laboratory.
      Gary Greaves, CMA

Cancer Facts

How Cancer Works*

Normally the cells that make up the body reproduce in an orderly manner so that worn-out tissues are replaced, injuries are repaired, and growth of the body proceeds.

Occasionally certain cells undergo an abnormal change and thus begin a process of uncontrolled growth and spread. These cells may grow into masses of tissue called tumors. Some tumors are benign, and others are malignant (cancerous).

The danger of cancer is that it invades and destroys normal tissue. In the beginning, cancer cells usually remain at their original site, and the cancer is said to be localized. Later, cancer cells may metastasize (that is, they invade distant or neighboring organs or tissues). This occurs either by direct extension of growth or by cells becoming detached and carried through the lymph or blood systems to other parts of the body.

Metastasis may be regional—confined to one region of the body—when cells are trapped by lymph nodes. If left untreated, however, the cancer is likely to spread throughout the body. That condition is known as advanced cancer and usually results in death. Because cancer becomes more serious with each stage, it is important to detect it as early as possible. Aids to early detection include the Seven Warning Signals and the Cancer Risk Factors. (Tables 4-1 to 4-3)

Courtesy American Cancer Society, San Francisco, Calif.

TABLE 4-1

Five Most Common Cancer Sites By Age and Sex—1988

Age:	0-14	15-34	35-44	45-54	55-64	65-72	75+
Rank			Males				
1	Leukemia	Kaposi's Sarcoma	Kaposi's Sarcoma	Lung	Lung	Prostate	Prostate
2	Brain	Testis	Non-Hodgkin's Lymphoma	Colorectal	Prostate	Lung	Lung
3	Non-Hodgkin's	Non-Hodgkin's	Melanoma	Non-Hodgkin's	Colorectal	Colorectal	Colorectal
4	Hodgkin's Disease	Melanoma	Lung	Melanoma	Bladder	Bladder	Bladder
5	Bone/Soft Tissue	Hodgkin's	Testis	Oral	Oral	Oral	Stomach

Age:	0-14	15-34	35-44	45-54	55-64	65-74	75+
Rank			Females				
1	Leukemia	Breast	Breast	Breast	Breast	Breast	Breast
2	Brain	Thyroid	Cervix	Lung	Lung	Lung	Colorectal
3	Kidney	Cervix	Melanoma	Colorectal	Colorectal	Colorectal	Lung
4	Soft Tissue	Melanoma	Thyroid	Corpus	Corpus	Corpus	Corpus
5	Non-Hodgkin's Hodgkin's Lymphoma	Ovary	Ovary	Ovary	Ovary	Ovary	Non-Lymphoma

Courtesy American Cancer Society, San Francisco, Calif.

TABLE 4-2

Summary of American Cancer Society Recommendations for the Early Detection of Cancer in Asymptomatic People

Test or Procedure	Sex	Population Age	Frequency
Sigmoidoscopy preferably flexible	M & F	50 & over	Every 3-5 years
Fecal Occult Blood Test	M & F	50 and over	Every year
Digital Rectal Examination	M & F	40 and over	Every year
Prostate Exam*	M	50 and over	Every year
Pap Test	F	All women who are or who have been sexually active, or have reached age 18, should have an annual Pap test and pelvic examination. After a woman has had three or more consecutive satisfactory normal annual examinations, the Pap test may be performed less frequently at the discretion of her physician.	
Pelvic Examination	F	18-40 Over 40	Every 1-3 years with Pap test Every year
Endometrial Tissue Sample	F	All menopause, if at high risk†	At menopause and thereafter at the discretion of the physician
Breast Self-examination	F	20 and over	Every month
Breast Clinical Examination	F	20-40 Over 40	Every 3 years Every year
Mammography‡	F	40-49 50 and over	Every 1-2 years Every year
Health Counseling and Cancer Checkup§	M & F M & F	Over 20 Over 40	Every 3 years Every year

*   *Annual digital rectal examination and prostate-specific antigen should be performed on men age 50 and older. If either is abnormal, further evaluation should be considered.*
†   *History of infertility, obesity, failure to ovulate, abnormal uterine bleeding, or unopposed estrogen or tamnoxifen therapy.*
‡   *Screening mammography should being by age 40.*
§   *To include examination of cancers of the thyroid, testicles, ovaries, lymph nodes, oral region, and skin.*

Nutrition guidelines
1. Maintain a desirable body weight.
2. Cut down on total fat intake.
3. Include a variety of both vegetables and fruits in the daily diet.
4. Eat more high-fiber foods such as whole grain cereals, legumes, vegetables and fruits.
5. Limit consumption of alcoholic beverages, if you drink at all.
6. Limit consumption of salt cured, smoked, and nitrate-preserved foods.
7. Eat a varied diet.

Cancer's seven warning signals
1. Change in bowel or bladder habits
2. A sore that does not heal
3. Unusual bleeding or discharge
4. Thickening or lump in breast or elsewhere
5. Indigestion or difficulty in swallowing
6. Obvious change in wart or mole
7. Nagging cough or hoarseness

If you have a warning signal, see your doctor.

Courtesy American Cancer Society, San Francisco, Calif.

Major Cancer Sites

	Cancer Risk Factors	Risk Reduction	Early Detection (Asymptomatic Persons)
Bladder	Tobacco use; higher in African American than whites; aniline dye used in textile, rubber and cable industries; personal history of bladder cancer.	Avoid use of tobacco products; use work place safety precautions if working in high-risk industry.	Health-related check-ups may identify early signs or symptoms.
Brain	Increasing among older persons; second leading cause of death in children.	None known.	Health-related check-ups may identify early signs or symptoms.
Breast	Age; family history in mother or sisters; precancerous condition on breast biopsy; first child born after age 30; obesity; never had children	Follow ACS's nutrition guidelines to increase fiber intake and lower fat consumed; maintain normal weight.	Mammography; breast self-examinations annual breast examinations.
Cervix	Early age at first intercourse; multiple sexual partners; smoking; Papilloma virus infections; low-socioeconomic status; poor compliance to screening programs or never had screening.	Have safe sex; avoid use of tobacco products.	Pap smear and pelvic examination.
Colorectal Cancer	Personal or family history of colorectal cancer, colorectal polyps; diets high in fat and low in fiber; inflammatory bowel disease.	Removal of polyps. Follow the ACS's nutrition guidelines for diets high in fiber and low in fats.	Stool blood test; digital rectal examination; sigmoidoscopy.
Endometrium	Infertility; obesity; use of unopposed postmenopausal estrogens; hypertension; diabetes.	Follow ACS's nutrition guidelines to maintain normal weight. When considering estrogen replacement therapy, benefits and risks must be considered by woman and her physician to decide on best action for the woman.	Pelvic exam endometrial tissue sampling at menopause if high risk.
Hodgkin's Disease	Viral causes have been suggested but not proved.	None known.	Health-related check-ups may identify early signs and symptoms.
Non-Hodgkin's Lymphoma	AIDS in some cases; transplantation and immunosuppression therapy; viral causes have been suggested in some types; increased risk in certain genetic diseases.	Use measures to avoid AIDS in high-risk populations.	Health-related check-ups may identify early signs and symptoms.

Courtesy American Cancer Society, San Francisco, Calif.

Table 4-3—cont'd
Major Cancer Sites

Warning Signs	Treatment	Special Information
Blood in urine.	In-situ state-surgery and possible installation of drugs. Later stages-surgery at times with radiation therapy or chemotherapy. Metastatic disease-radiation therapy and chemotherapy.	Modifications of surgical techniques to preserve bladder continence are under study.
Headaches, convulsions, personality changes, visual problems, unexplained vomiting.	In adults-surgery, chemotherapy and radiation. In children-surgery, radiation therapy, chemotherapy.	Metatases to brain occur with many other cancers. Symptoms may be reduced by using cortisone-like drugs and radiation therapy.
Breast lump or a thickening; bleeding from nipple; skin irritation; retraction.	Early stage-mastectomy or local removal with radiation therapy. Adjuvant therapy-hormones and/or combination chemotherapy. Later stage-combination chemotherapy or hormones and radiation therapy for selected clinical problems.	Bone marrow transplantation is being tested in women with advanced disease. Breast reconstruction after mastectomy has had good cosmetic results. ACS has special Reach to Recovery programs to help women.
Abnormal vaginal bleeding.	Percursor lesions-cryotherapy (kills cells by cold), electro-coagulation (kills cells by heat from an electrical current), surgery. Localized-surgery or radiation therapy. Invasive-surgery or radiation therapy. Metastatic-chemotherapy and radiation therapy.	The use of the Pap test has greatly reduced the death rate from cervical cancer. The Pap test must be made available to women who have never had the test or who have had infrequent screening. Mature and underserved women may not have the test available. Such women should be prime targets for screening programs.
Rectal bleeding, change in bowel habits, blood in the stools.	Surgery at times combined with radiation therapy or chemotherapy. Chemotherapy in advanced cases is under study.	Colostomy is seldom necessary now for colon cancer and is infrequently needed for rectal cancer patients. New helpful adjuvant treatments have been reported recently.
Abnormal vaginal bleeding in menopause.	For uterine hyperplasia, progestins may be used. Surgery sometimes with radiation therapy. Advanced metastases-progestins/chemotherapy.	The cure rate for endometrial cancer is high because tumors tend to be well-differentiated and localized.
Night sweats, itching, unexplained fever, lymph node enlargement.	Early stages-radiation sometimes with chemotherapy. Advanced stages-combination chemotherapy.	There has been dramatic improvement in the outcome of this cancer. Most patients are cured.
Lymph node enlargement, fever.	Usually disseminated at time of diagnosis; chemotherapy is used. At times autologous bone marrow transplantation may be used.	Surgery may be useful when lymphoma is found in the gastrointestinal tract and to remove the spleen when it is overactive.

Table 4-3—cont'd

Major Cancer Sites

	Cancer Risk Factors	Risk Reduction	Early Detection (Asymptomatic Persons)
Leukemia	Persons with genetic abnormalities like Down's Syndrome; ionizing radiation; exposure to certain chemicals; certain forms are related to retro-virus, HTLV-1.	Reduce exposure to radiation and hazardous chemicals.	Health-related check-ups may identify early signs and symptoms.
Lung	Tobacco use; voluntary and involuntary smoking; occupational exposure such as asbestos.	Avoid tobacco products in all forms; stop smoking; follow workplace safety practices; avoid second-hand smoke.	Chest x-rays for high-risk persons.
Melanoma	Fair skin; sun exposure; severe sunburn in childhood; familial conditions like dysplastic nevus syndrome; large congenital moles.	Protect against sun exposure, especially in childhood; use protective clothing and sunscreens when exposed to the sun.	Annual skin examinations by an experienced physician; monthly self-exams.
Oral	Tobacco use; excessive use of alcohol; poor dentition.	Avoid tobacco products in all forms and if you must drink alcohol, do so in moderation.	Regular oral exams.
Ovary	Increases with age. Possible dietary factors. Older women who have never had children are at a risk. History of breast, endometrial or colon cancer. Family history.	Following ACS's nutrition guidelines may be helpful.	Health-related check-ups may identify early signs or symptoms.
Pancreas	Increases after age 50, with most cases between age 65 and 79. More common in smokers. Occurs more frequently in African Americans. May be associated with pancreatitis, diabetes, and diet.	Following ACS's nutrition guidelines may be helpful.	Health-realted check-ups may identify early signs or symptoms.
Prostate	Age is the most important risk factor. Eighty percent of all prostate cancer occurs in men over age 65. Dietary fat may play a role. High in African Americans.	While not certain, prudent action would be to follow ACS's nutrition guidelines.	Digital rectal examination. Prostate ultrasound and a blood test for prostate-specific antigen are under study.
Stomach	Occurs in those 50-70 years old; pernicious anemia; certain types of pastritis; possible gastric ulcers; dietary factors.	Avoid food high in nitrates.	Health-related check-ups may identify early signs or symptoms.
Testes	Undescended testes.	Correction of undescended testes.	Testicular self-examination in young males has been suggested.

Table 4-3—cont'd

Major Cancer Sites

Warning Signs	Treatment	Special Information
Fatigue, pallor, repeated infection, easy bruising, nose bleeds.	Combination chemotherapy; bone marrow transplantation may be used in some cases.	There has been dramatic improvement in the outcome of acute childhood leukemia. The majority of children are cured and live into adulthood leading normal lives.
Nagging cough, coughing up blood, unresolved pneumonia.	Surgery, radiation and chemotherapy depending on type. In small-cell lung cancer, chemotherapy alone or combined with radiation may be the first choice.	Lung cancer rates in men have begun to decrease, but the rates in women continue to increase.
A change in a mole or a sore that does not heal.	Early-surgery Advanced cases-surgery, radiation, chemotherapy, immunotherapy.	Melanoma is increasing due to environmental and lifestyle changes. For early detection follow ABCD rule: A-Asymmetry of mole (one side does not match the other); B-Border irregularity (edges are irregular); C-Color (color is not uniform); D-Diameter (the size is greater than 6 millimeters).
Sore in mouth that does not heal; color change in mouth.	Radiation and surgery; chemotherapy is being studied. Surgery, radiation and chemotherapy.	This cancer is significantly affected by alcohol and tobacco use.
Often "silent"; abdominal enlargement may occur.	Surgery, radiation therapy and chemotherapy may be used. Disease is often advanced at the time of diagnosis.	The use of chemotherapy has improved the outcome of this cancer. Markers such as CA125 are being studied.
Vague abdominal symptoms, pain.	Early stage-surgery or sometimes radiation therapy. Later stages-radiation therapy, hormone treatments or anti-cancer drugs. Radiation therapy can ease painful areas in the bones.	Two percent of pancreatic cancers occur in the insulin-producing cells. Thirty percent of these patients live 3 years or more after diagnosis.
Difficulty passing urine; blood in urine. These symptoms can be due to benign (noncancer) conditions.	Surgery; combination chemotherapy may be helpful.	New operations that save nerves and blood supply can preserve potency. New hormonal treatments are being tested.
Indigestion.	Early stage-surgery at times with radiation therapy.	Decreasing in the U.S., but an important cancer in Japan, Chile, Iceland, and other countries.
Testicular mass or enlargement.	Advanced-chemotherapy.	This is a cancer in which there has been a dramatic improvement in survival due to therapy. Many patients are cured of disease.

Many physicians also recommend that a sigmoidoscopy be included as part of the annual physical examination for men over age 40 because of the relatively high incidence of cancer of the rectum and sigmoid colon in this age group.

A proctosigmoidoscopy takes approximately 10 to 15 minutes and requires special preparation of the patient beforehand.

Check with your physician or agency for specific instructions. It is the medical assistant's responsibility to check that the patient is prepared before the examination begins. Generally the preparation includes a laxative the evening before (type and amount as prescribed by the physician), only liquids for breakfast, and tap water or saline enemas until the return is clear, usually 1 hour before the examination. NOTE: Enemas are usually avoided for patients who have colitis, bleeding from the rectum, or Crohn's disease.

An alternate preparation is the *Golytely prep*, is a commonly used prescription drug (cathartic or purgative) used to promote defecation and bowel evacuation. Golytely is supplied in powder form in a plastic one-gallon (4-liter) container. Water is to be mixed with the powder as directed. Many suggest that the mixture tastes better if it is premixed and refrigerated for a few hours before being ingested. No solid foods are to be eaten 3 to 4 hours before drinking the Golytely mixture. Clear fluids are allowed until the patient starts to drink the mixture at intervals as directed.

Depending on the physician's orders and the time of the examination, the patient may drink the Golytely the night before *or* 2 hours before the examination begins. The patient must have clear liquid bowel movements at least 1 hour before the examination begins.

The *Colyte prep* is very similar to the Golytely prep described in the preceding paragraphs, but it has the advantage of being supplied in a pineapple flavor, which is appealing to some patients.

Cancer risk varies considerably by age with fewer than 1% of all cancers occurring after the age of 65. In fact, 50% of all cancers occur between the ages of 55 to 74, and more cancers occur after age 85 than between birth and age 35.

Cancers occurring before the age of 15 are typically nonepithelial in origin, with the most common types being leukemias, tumors of the brain and nervous system, and lymphomas. Five-year survival rates for childhood cancers vary considerably, depending on the type of cancer, but in general survival is excellent.

Within California, cancer patterns in young adult males differ somewhat from patterns in other geographic areas in that the most common cancer among males between the ages 15 and 44 is Kaposi's sarcoma. Melanoma is an important cancer among young adults of both sexes. Breast cancer is the most common cancer among all ages of adult women. After age 35, lung cancer is among the top three cancers for both men and women. Cancer patterns change relatively little after age 65, with the four most common cancers remaining the same within each sex group.

NEUROLOGIC EXAMINATION

The neurologic examination tests for adequate functioning of the cranial nerves, the motor or sensory systems, and the superficial and deep tendon reflexes.

Equipment and Supplies

- Pins and cotton to test the senses of touch, sensation, and pain on the external surfaces of the body (Figure 4-24)
- Tuning fork to test hearing
- Ophthalmoscope to examine the interior of the eye
- Flashlight to test pupil reactions and equality
- Tongue depressor to test the gag and corneal reflexes, and also pharyngeal sensation
- Percussion hammer to test superficial and deep tendon reflexes (Figure 4-25).
- Test tubes with hot and cold water to test the skin for heat and cold sensation
- Bottles of sweet, bitter, salty, and sour solutions to test the sense of taste
- Bottles of substances that have common familiar odors to test the sense of smell

The physician also observes the patient's level of consciousness, behavior, and the higher functions of speech and writing. Coordination, balance, gait, muscle tone, and strength are noted for adequate functioning of the motor system. The sense of touch, pain (deep and superficial), temperature, and discriminatory sensations are noted in the examination of the sensory system.

Figure 4-24 *Alternate use of the dull end of the pin for evaluation of sensation and pain.*

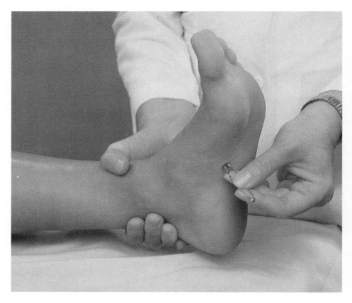

Figure 4-25 *Elicitation of the patella reflex. A tap with the percussion hammer is applied directly inferior to the patella. A, With the patient sitting and legs hanging over the examining table; B, with the patient in a supine position. The normal response is the leg kicking out or extension of the leg.*

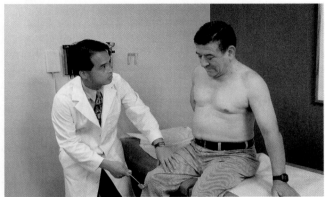

A

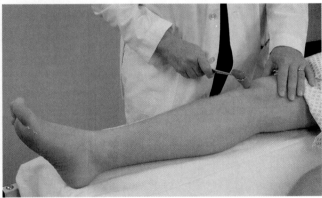

B

Figure 4-26 *Examination of the ear with an otoscope. A, The patient's head is tipped toward the opposite shoulder; B, The audiometer is used to measure the patient's acuity of hearing bilaterally. Patient dons earphones and responds to various frequencies of sound waves by hand signalling.*

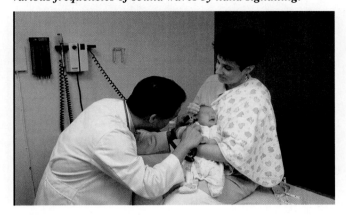

A

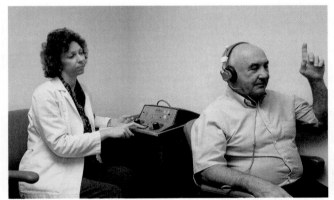

B

HEARING EXAMINATION

To detect impaired hearing, the physician uses an otoscope to inspect the external ear canal and eardrum (Figure 4-26, *A* and *B*) and a tuning fork to test for hearing acuity.

The tuning fork is used to determine the distance at which the patient can hear a certain sound (air conduction test) and for bone conduction tests. In the bone conduction test, the vibrating end of the tuning fork is placed on the patient's skull. This test is valuable in distinguishing between perceptive and transmission deafness (Figure 4-27, *A* and *B*).

A more accurate test to gauge and record the hearing sense is done with the use of an audiometer, a delicate instrument consisting of complex parts. For audiometry the patient is placed in a soundproof room and puts on earphones. Timing circuits, sound wave generators, and other complex pieces of equipment are used to measure the patient's acuity of hearing for the various frequencies of sound waves. Results are plotted on a graph called an audiogram. No special preparation of the patient is required for this test. Physicians, audiometric technicians, or other specially trained individuals perform this test.

Figure 4-27 *Hearing examination. A, Air conduction test.*

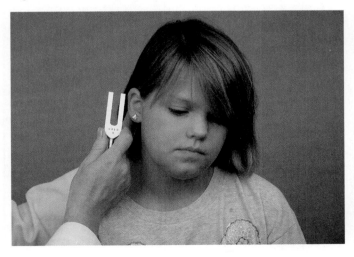

A

Figure 4-27—cont'd *Hearing examination.*
B, *Bone conduction test.*

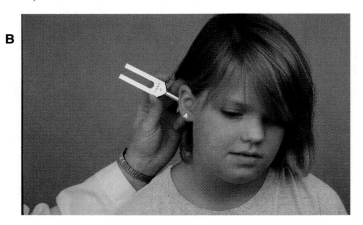

B

EYE EXAMINATION

EXTERNAL EYE EXAMINATIONS
Distance Visual Acuity

Visual acuity means acuteness or clarity of vision. Visual acuity may be measured on patients having complete physical examinations; but more specifically it is measured because patients have a specific visual complaint, because of employment requirements, or to meet requirements of the Department of Motor Vehicles to drivers' licenses. The visual acuity test is also performed in schools and on preschool-aged children as a means of vision screening.

Imperfect refractive powers of the eye include conditions known as *myopia* (nearsightedness), *hyperopia* (farsightedness), and *astigmatism* (another refractive error of the eye resulting from irregularities in the curvature of the cornea and/or surfaces of the lens of the eye).

Myopia occurs when the lens of the eye is too thick or the eyeball is too long. Correction is made by using a concave lens to help the light rays come to a focus on the retina. Within the last 5 years technologic advances have ushered in a new era for treatment for myopia using a surgical procedure called radial keratotomy (RK). This is of special interest to people who do not want to depend on glasses or contact lens for corrected vision.

Hyperopia occurs when the lens of the eye is too thin or the eyeball is too short. Here the eye focuses on an image at a hypothetic distance behind the retina. With hyperopia a person finds it difficult to view objects at an average reading distance. Correction is made by using a convex lens to help light rays focus on the retina. As people age, another type of farsightedness, called *presbyopia*, frequently develops. It results from a loss of elasticity of the lens of the eye.

In an astigmatism light rays cannot be focused clearly in a point on the retina because there is uneven curvature of the cornea or lens. Vision is blurred, and using the eyes causes discomfort. Correction is made by using contact lenses or eye glasses ground to neutralize the defect.

These conditions can be detected by using the *Snellen eye chart* to measure distance visual acuity. The *Snellen eye chart* (Figure 4-28) consists of varied-sized block letters arranged in rows in gradually decreasing sizes. Another chart used for preschoolers, individuals unable to speak English, slow learners, and those unable to read is the *E chart*, which consists of the letter "E" arranged in different directions in decreasing sizes. Charts with pictures of common objects such as a house and truck are

Figure 4-28 **A,** *Snellen eye chart consisting of varied-sized letters arranged in rows in gradually decreasing sizes;* **B,** *Snellen Big E eye chart consisting of the letter "E" arranged in different directions in decreasing sizes. These charts are used to measure distance visual acuity;* **C,** *objects Chart for non-English speaking people.*

A
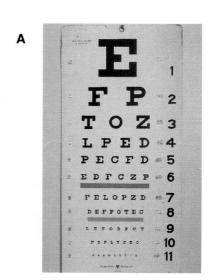

B
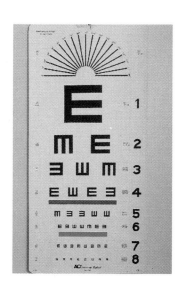

C
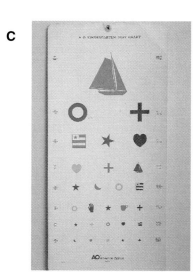

available to use when testing preschoolers, although some children are unable to identify the objects because of lack of knowledge rather than a defect in visual acuity.

On the *Snellen* chart there are two standardized numbers on the side of each row of letters; these numbers, shown one on top of the other, indicate the degree of visual acuity measured from a distance of 20 feet, the standard testing distance. The top number is 20, indicating the number of feet between the chart and the person taking the test; the bottom number indicates the distance in feet from which the normal eye can read the row of letters. The large letter on the top of the chart can be read by the normal eye at a distance of 200 feet. This is indicated as 20/200. In each of the succeeding rows, from top to bottom, the size of the letters decreases to the point at which the normal eye can read the row of letters at distances of 100, 70, 50, 40, 30, 25, 20, 15, 13, and 10 feet. The row marked 20/20 indicates normal visual acuity and is expressed as 20/20 vision. A measurement of visual acuity of less than 20/20 vision is an indication of a refractive error or some other eye disorder (for example, when the letters on the row marked 20/50 are read, the person is said to have 20/50 vision). This means that the person can read at only 20 feet what the normal eye can read at 50 feet. The larger the bottom number of the row that can be read, the poorer the vision. A reading of 20/15 indicates above-average distance vision (see Figure 4-28, *A* and *B*).

This test is to be given in a well-lit room, with the person taking the test standing or sitting 20 feet away from the chart and the chart placed at eye level to the person. Each eye is to be tested separately, with and without glasses or contact lenses. However, reading glasses should not be worn during the test because they tend to blur distant vision. The results must be recorded indicating the reading for each eye without and with glasses or contact lenses. Usually, each eye is tested separately because the stronger eye usually compensates for the weaker eye. Patients who are unable to see even the largest numbers on the Snellen chart (top line 20/200) are given additional tests to determine if they can see enough to count fingers (this is recorded as C.F.), perceive hand movements (H.M.), perceive light (L.P.), or perceive light with projection (L.P.cP.). N.L.P. is used to record "no light projection." An ophthalmologist considers patients to be blind when they cannot even perceive light. **Legal blindness** is defined as vision of 20/200 or less in both eyes when wearing correction glasses.

For office space that does not have a 20-foot hallway or space, charts are available that can be used at a distance of 10 feet; or the patient can stand or sit 10 feet away from the standard Snellen chart, and the results recorded would indicate that the test was performed at a distance of 10 feet (for example, if the patient's distance visual acuity were measured using the standard eye chart at a distance of 10 feet, the results would be recorded as "20/20 at 10 feet"). The physician then converts the results. This test is not as reliable as the test recorded at 20 feet because at a distance of 10 feet the eye has to focus, whereas at a distance of 20 feet the eye does not have to focus.

Electric Vision Testing Devices

Electric testing devices such as the Titmus II Vision Tester, which is the product of advances in computer-designed optics I (see Figure 4-32), are also on the market. This one compact instrument, using eight test slides, can screen patients of all ages (preschool through adults) for *all* common vision problems—problems that the standard wall chart misses. *The Titmus II Vision Tester measures acuity (both far and near), hyperopia, binocularity, muscle balance, color perception, depth perception, and, with the optional equipment, peripheral vision and intermediate vision, all within 5 minutes.* The standard wall chart measures only distance vision. The fiber optics perimeter system determines if peripheral vision is adequate, a basic requirement for employees who operate machinery and mobile equipment. The intermediate distance feature tests the intermediate distance (20 to 40 inches) viewing capabilities important to machine workers and to the increasing number of video display terminal operators. Because of its extremely compact and lightweight design, the Titmus II Vision Tester can be used virtually anywhere. It is especially convenient when performing vision screening tests on large groups or in small areas where space is less than 20 feet. Only 5 square feet of space is required for using this instrument. Patients of all ages and statures can be easily screened because of the unit's balanced height adjustment. The face mask of the unit eliminates outside light and is designed to accommodate all sizes and types of eyeglasses. A training manual complete with an instructional cassette supplied as standard equipment provides correct testing techniques that are easy to learn. The Titmus II Vision Tester is a complete system for all vision screening in each individual office situation (Figure 4-29).

Figure 4-29 *Titmus II Vision Tester.*
Courtesy Titmus Optical, Inc., Petersburg, Va.

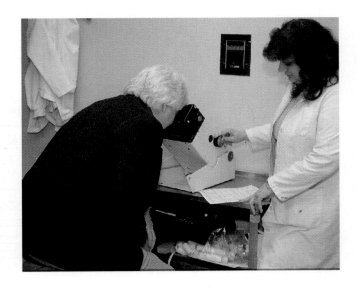

MEASURING DISTANCE VISUAL ACUITY (SNELLEN CHART)

Equipment

Snellen eye chart (see Figure 4-28, A and B)
Opaque card or eye cover or occluder

Pen
Paper

PROCEDURE	RATIONALE
1. Wash your hands. **Use appropriate personal protective equipment (PPE) as indicated by facility.**	
2. Prepare the room; determine location of 20 feet from where the chart will be posted to where the patient will be positioned. When this test is used frequently, this distance can be permanently marked to save time.	
3. Assemble the supplies and equipment.	
4. Identify the patient and explain the procedure. Do not allow time for the patient to study and memorize the chart before the examination begins.	*Explanations help the patient to feel comfortable and more relaxed, in addition to gaining the patient's confidence as you proceed with the examination.*
5. Position the patient comfortably, either standing or sitting, 20 feet from the location of the chart.	*Twenty feet is the standard testing distance.*
6. Position the center of the Snellen eye chart at eye level to the patient.	*To position the chart correctly, the patient must first be positioned.*
7. Provide the patient with the opaque card or eye cover or occluder. Instruct the patient to cover the left eye with the card, keep the left eye open at all times, and not to put pressure on the eye with the card or occluder.	*The right eye (OD) is traditionally tested first. The hand or fingers are not to be used to cover the eye not being tested. The covered eye is to be kept open because closing one eye often causes the other to squint inadvertently.*
8. Instruct the patient to use the right eye and to verbally identify the letters as you point to each row. Start at row 20/70 (or a row several rows above the 20/20 row) (Figure 4-30). The patient is to read as many letters as possible in the rows as you point to them.	*Starting with row 20/70, which has larger letters than those on row 20/20, allows the patient to gain confidence in identifying the letters.*
9. As the patient identifies the letters in the first row that you point to, proceed down the chart until the patient has identified as many rows of letters as possible. Proceed until three out of four symbols *or* three out of five symbols *or* four out of six symbols cannot be read. If the patient is unable to identify row 20/70, proceed up the chart, having the patient identify the rows of letters until the smallest row of letters is identified.	
10. Provide instructions to the patient during the test, such as what line to read and not to squint. Observe the patient for any unusual reactions, such as tearing of the eyes, blinking, squinting, or leaning forward to read the chart.	*These reactions may indicate the patient is experiencing difficulty with the test and must be recorded.*
11. Continue testing until the smallest line of letters that the patient can read is reached or until a letter is misread.	

MEASURING DISTANCE VISUAL ACUITY (SNELLEN CHART)—cont'd

PROCEDURE

12. Record the results of visual acuity of the right eye on a piece of paper. It is important to write the result down when it is determined to avoid errors when charting the results on the patient's record. When testing the covered eye, please allow time for the eye to adjust to the room's lighting before starting the test.

13. Instruct the patient to cover the right eye with the opaque card or eye cover and keep the eye open (see Figure 4-30).

14. Measure the visual acuity of the left eye (OS), using the method described in steps 8 through 12.

15. Give further instructions to the patient as required.

16. Replace equipment and leave the room neat and clean.

17. Record the results for each eye on the patient's chart, using proper medical abbreviations. When one or two letters are missed or misread in a row, the results are recorded with a minus sign. The number of letters missed or misread is recorded next to the bottom number (for example, if the patient identified the rows of letters down to row 20/25 and could not read two letters in this row, you would record this result as 20/25-2). Record as s̄ correction (without correction) when the patient isn't wearing glasses or contact lenses, and c̄ correction (with correction) when the patient is wearing glasses or contact lenses.

RATIONALE

Charting example:
October 31, 19____, 5 p.m.
   Snellen chart eye test given. Results without glasses:
   OD 20/20 sc
   OS 20/14-2 sc
      H. McMullen CMA

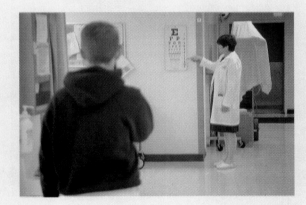

Figure 4-30 *Using the Snellen chart for distance visual acuity testing.*

Measuring Distance Visual Acuity in Preschoolers

For testing distance visual acuity in preschoolers (*and also for testing non-English speaking or illiterate people*), the Snellen Big E eye chart can be used (Figure 4-31, *B*). This chart uses the capital letter E pointing in four directions. This test is very similar to the preceding procedure using the Snellen eye chart. Children and others "read" the chart by showing the direction of the letter E or use a large duplicate E to match the E that you are pointing to on the chart. Before beginning the test, use a practice E card and have the child practice identifying which direction the "legs of the E" are pointing (Figure 4-31, *A*). Teach the child how to use the eye cover to cover one eye

while the other eye is being tested (Figure 4-31, *B*). Instruct the child to keep both eyes open during the test. Position the child comfortably, either standing or sitting, 20 feet away from the chart.

If the child wears glasses, test only with the glasses on. First test both eyes together, then the right eye, and then the left eye. Begin with the 40- or 30-foot line and proceed. If the child is thought to have very poor vision, begin the test using the 200-foot line and proceed until three out of four or four out of six symbols cannot be read. Use a pointer to point to one symbol at a time. Observe the child's eyes during the test and record any evidence of excessive blinking, tearing, squinting, or redness and any head tilting or thrusting the head forward. Record the results of the test accurately.

Figure 4-31 A, *Have a child point to the direction in which "the legs of the E" are pointing;* **B,** *teach a child how to cover one eye with an eye cover/occluder while the other eye is being tested.*

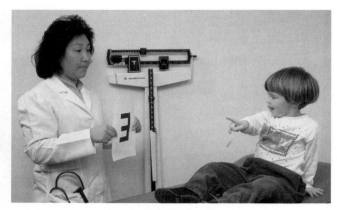

A

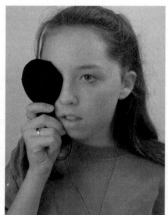

B

Measuring Near Visual Acuity

The tests for near vision are used to determine if the patient can read average-sized type at a normal reading distance of 14 inches. A sample of newspaper printing or a specially designed chart such as the Rosenbaum or Jaegar charts can be used. The Rosenbaum chart consists of a series of numbers, Es positioned in different ways, Xs, and Ox, all in varying sizes. Each eye should be tested separately, traditionally beginning with the right eye. The eye not being tested should be kept covered with an eye occluder or an opaque card. If the patient wears reading glasses, they should be worn during the test. This must be recorded along with the results. In a well-lit area, have the patient assumed a comfortable position, hold the chart 14 inches away from the eye, and read the smallest line possible. The test results are recorded as either distant equivalents such as 20/25 or 20/30 or Jaegar equivalents such as J-1 or J-2. Both of these measurements are given on the chart. J-2 indicates normal near visual acuity. If you give the patient a newspaper to read for this test, he or she should be able to read it without difficulty when it is held at least 14 inches away from the eyes (Figure 4-32). State the distance tested when recording the results.

Figure 4-32 *Rosenbaum chart for testing near vision.*
From Seidel H, et al: Mosby's guide to physical examinations, ed 2, St. Louis, 1991, Mosby.

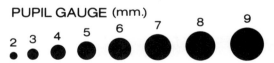

Card is held in good light 14 inches from eye. Record vision for each eye separately with and without glasses. Presbyopic patients should read thru bifocal segment. Check myopes with glasses only.

DESIGN COURTESY J. G. ROSENBAUM, M.D.

Visual Fields

The patient is asked to look directly at a central point; then the extent of peripheral and side vision is spot checked with an instrument called a perimeter. A target screen method may also be used. The patient is asked to focus on a small target that is moved to different points on a screen. The patient has a visual field defect in the areas where the target cannot be seen.

Color Vision

Color vision should be tested when a defect is suspected or when employment requires a person to be able to differentiate colors such as is required in certain vehicle operation and industrial jobs. Deficiency in color perception is inherited in approximately 7% of men and 0.5% of women. Visual acuity is normal, but perceptions of color are depressed to varying degrees. Diseases of the optic nerve and the fovea centralis (an area at the center of the retina of the eye where cone cells are concentrated and there are no rod cells), some nutritional disturbances, and ingestion of toxic drugs can all interfere with color vision. Testing color vision should include testing with color plates. The plates have numbers outlined in one color surrounded by confusion colors that are similar in color or intensity. The tests vary in degree of difficulty. The patient is asked to identify colored numbers on various color plates from a standardized distance, usually 75 cm (30 inches). The color-deficient person is unable to see the numbers on color plates, numbers that are easily recognizable to the person with normal color vision.

Commonly used color plates for color vision screening are the Ishihara plates. This series provides quick and easy assessment of total color blindness or a red-green deficiency, both of congenital origin. The Ishihara book contains 24 test plates. The first 17 plates consist of primary colored dots arranged to form different numbers against a background of dots in contrasting colors. The patient is asked to identify the number on each of these plates within 3 seconds. The first plate is designed to be read correctly by everyone so that it can be used to explain the method of the test to the patient. Plates 18 through 24 are used for patients who cannot read numbers such as non-English speaking or illiterate patients and preschoolers. The patient is asked to trace with a brush winding colored lines between two X's. Each tracing should be completed within 10 seconds. The plates should be held 75 cm (30 inches) away from and at right angles to the patient's line of vision (Figure 4-33).

It is not necessary to use the whole series of plates for every screening. Omit plates 16 and 17 if you are testing primarily to determine a color defect versus normal color appreciation. The test may also be simplified to an examination of only six plates. For this you would use:

- Plate No. 1
- One of plates Nos. 2, 3
- One of Nos. 4, 5, 6, 7
- One of Nos. 8, 9
- One of Nos. 10, 11, 12, 13, and
- One of Nos. 14, 15

Explanation of the plates and how the test is interpreted is provided with the plates. An assessment of the results obtained from the reading of plates 1 to 15 determines if color vision is normal or defective. Color vision is regarded as normal if 13 or more plates are read normally. Color vision is regarded as deficient if 9 or less plates are read normally. It is rare to find a person whose recording of normal answers is between 14 and 16 plates. For the shorter version of the test when only six plates are used, a normal recording of all plates indicates normal color vision. The test is to be given in a room well lit by natural daylight. Unnatural light can lead to inaccurate results because it may cause a change in the appearance of the shades of color. When not in use, the book of test plates should be kept closed to help prevent fading of the colors on the plates.

Refraction. A physician instills atropine drops (or any mydriatic, a drug used to dilate the eyes) into the eye. With the use of these drops, the lens of the eye is unable to accommodate, thus allowing the physician to determine eye function when the lens is at rest.

INTERNAL EYE EXAMINATIONS
Ophthalmoscopic Examination

With the use of the ophthalmoscope, the physician examines the anterior chamber, the lens, the vitreous body, and the retina of the eye. When using the ophthalmoscope, the physician may want the room darkened because this causes the pupils to dilate and thus aids the examination. Visualization of the retina with the ophthalmoscope is known as a funduscopic examination (Figure 4-34).

Figure 4-33 *Testing color vision. Hold the color plate 75 cm (30 inches) away from and at right angles to the patient's line of vision.*

Figure 4-34 *The physician is using the ophthalmoscope to examine the lens and vitreous body of the eye from a distance of about 12 inches.*

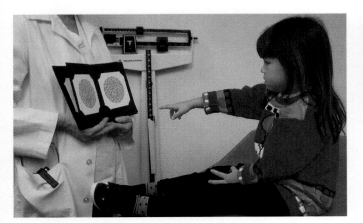

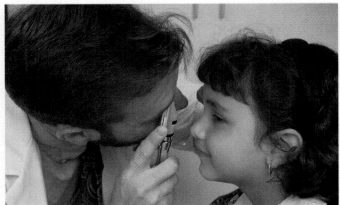

Tonometry

After instillation of a local anesthetic into the eye, a tonometer is gently rested on the eyeball, or other special equipment is used to touch the eyeball to measure the tension of the eyeball and intraocular pressure. This method is referred to as *applanation tonometry* and is the most accurate method. *"Puff" tonometry* is a type of non-contact tonometry (NCT). This method does not require an anesthetic. Puff tonometry uses a special piece of equipment to determine intraocular pressure.

Tonometry is an important test to determine the presence of an eye condition termed *glaucoma*, in which the pressure within the eyeball is increased.

Most glaucoma is a chronic condition in which the fluid pressure in the eye is abnormally high. If left untreated, the buildup of this pressure damages the sensitive visual structures in the back of the eye and results in a gradual loss of vision. Left untreated, glaucoma can cause total blindness. It is the second most common cause of new blindness in the United States.

Special eyedrops are the most common form of treatment for glaucoma. Other treatment choices include ointments and pills. However, when none of these treatments work, traditional ocular surgery or a new infrared laser surgery using a highly concentrated beam of light is necessary to relieve the pressure. Since glaucoma seldom causes symptoms until it is very advanced, ophthalmologists recommend that every adult over the age of 40 get regular eye pressure checks. Normal tonometry reading is 11 to 22 mm Hg. A reading of 24 to 32 mm Hg suggests glaucoma.

OBSTETRIC EXAMINATIONS AND RECORD

Obstetrics is the branch of medicine that deals with the care of the mother and fetus during pregnancy, labor and delivery, and the immediate postpartum period, which is called the puerperium. Pregnancy lasts approximately 280 days or 40 weeks from the day of fertilization. The puerperium lasts about 6 weeks after delivery. It is during that time that the mother's body, which has undergone many anatomic and physiologic changes during pregnancy, returns to a normal prepregnancy state and the mother adjusts to the new responsibilities of motherhood. When a woman suspects that she may be pregnant after missing her regular menstrual period, she may call the physician's office or clinic for an appointment to be tested for pregnancy. To test for pregnancy, most laboratories now do a blood test, called the human chorionic gonadotropin (HCG) beta subunit test, commonly referred to as the serum pregnancy test. This test can be done 10 to 14 days after the woman thinks she may have conceived. Other laboratories prefer to do the blood test 6 weeks after the date of the first day of the woman's last menstrual period, or 1 to 2 weeks after the first missed menstrual period. The results of this test are reported as either + (positive) or − (negative). Results of 100 mIU of HCG per milliliter or greater are

positive. In special circumstances an HCG quantitative serum pregnancy test or a radioimmunoassay (RIA) test may be ordered to rule out the possibility of an ectopic pregnancy or a spontaneous abortion (SAB). The results of this test are reported as a number. Any number less than 5 mIU/ml HCG indicates a negative result (Figure 4-35). In the medical office, urine pregnancy tests are often used because they provide immediate results and are easy to perform (see Unit Twelve, page 410).

After pregnancy has been confirmed, monitoring both the physical well-being of mother and fetus and the progress of the pregnancy is highly recommended and considered vital by some. Prevention of health problems or early detection, diagnosis, and treatment of health problems is accomplished by close supervision of the mother throughout the entire pregnancy. The mother should be seen by the physician at regular intervals. After the initial visit, the expectant mother should see the physician once a month for the first 6 months, every 2 weeks during the seventh and eighth months, and then once a week until the baby is born. For patients with medical problems such as diabetes, these prenatal visits are often scheduled every week throughout the pregnancy.

Six weeks after the baby is born, the mother should return to the office or clinic for a postpartum physical examination to have her general physical condition evaluated.

HEALTH CARE DURING PREGNANCY

To provide the best care and supervision of the expectant mother during her pregnancy, the physician must know the patient as an individual and as a member of her family. On the basis of her health status, the physician can determine what, how much, and when care is required. The initial assessment is made on the basis of the mother's medical history and the results of a physical examination. The data gathered initiates the prenatal or antepartum record (Figure 4-36, A to C). This record contains much of the same information as the health history and physical examination discussed in Unit Three. The data collected are also essential in identifying high-risk patients. Follow-up visits and examinations monitor the progress of the pregnancy.

Patient History

This includes the patient's past medical history and also an obstetric history if this is not the first pregnancy; the family history, which also includes information on the father's health and family history; the social and occupational history; the review of systems, including the history of the patient's menstrual cycles—the age at onset, regularity, amount, duration, and the date of the last menstrual period (LMP) (see page 131 and Figure 4-36). Particular attention is given to habits, and conditions, or diseases that could influence the health of the mother and fetus during the pregnancy. The physician plans to watch and give more care during and after the pregnancy if the patient has a present or past history of one or more of the following:

Figure 4-35   *Laboratory request form to order a pregnancy test.*

CODE	TEST	NORMAL	RESULTS
3150	T₃ AND T₄ COMBINATION (includes free thyroxine index)		
3151	T₃ UPTAKE	30-40%	%
3153	T₄	4.5-11.5 ug%	ug%
	FREE THYROXINE INDEX	0.5-1.7	
3163	FERRITIN	25-125 ng/ml	ng/ml
3579	HB$_s$AG	NEG.	
3165	SERUM PREGNANCY		
6268	SERUM ESTRIOL		
3384	TSH	0.8-5.0 mIu/ml	
3167	HCG QUANT		

RIA GL 4063 | ST | BD

ROUTINE REQUEST DRAWN AT: ___ TIME ___ DATE

IF REQUEST IS OTHER THAN ROUTINE, PLACE STICKER WITH APPROPRIATE INSTRUCTIONS IN THIS SPACE

RIA — PLEASE PRINT — PRESS HARD

TIME IN   TECHNOLOGIST   TIME TELEPHONED OR TELETYPED   TIME OUT

MEDICAL RECORD

- Age under 17 or over 35 years
- Problematic pregnancies, which may include repeated spontaneous abortions, premature deliveries, stillbirths, eclampsia, or toxemia
- Previous cesarean section(s)
- An infectious disease such as a sexually transmitted disease or a urinary tract infection
- Medical conditions such as kidney, cardiovascular, or respiratory diseases; hypertension; obesity; and nutritional deficiencies
- A metabolic disorder such as hyperthyroidism or diabetes
- A family history of genetic diseases
- Rh negative blood when the father has Rh positive blood
- Use of alcohol, tobacco, and/or drugs (which includes over-the-counter, prescription, or street drugs)

In addition, with domestic violence seen as "epidemic," the Surgeon General of the United States is asking all health care providers to take an active role in addressing this public health concern. Assessment for abuse during pregnancy must be standard care for all pregnant women.

Personal History of the Present Pregnancy

The personal history of the pregnancy includes the date of the first day of the LMP, symptoms of pregnancy, warning signs, and the expected date of confinement (EDC).

The patient is asked to explain what, if any, early symptoms of pregnancy she has experienced. These symptoms may include fatigue, nausea and vomiting (morning sickness), frequent urination, and breast changes such as a tingling sensation in the breasts, tenderness, enlargement of the nipples, and darkening of the areolae.

The patient is also asked if she has experienced any warning signs. The physician must explain what these warning signs are and stress that the patient must notify the physician if and when any of the following appear:

- Sudden increase in vaginal discharge
- Bleeding from the vagina—especially if it is heavy or coupled with abdominal or back pain. Bleeding and cramping early in pregnancy may signal a miscarriage.
- Sudden continuous or intermittent abdominal pain or cramping
- Continuous or severe nausea and vomiting
- Blurred vision or seeing spots before her eyes

Figure 4-36 A *to* **C,** *Prenatal records.*

<u>OBSTETRICS AND GYNECOLOGY CLINIC</u>

A

PROBLEM LIST	ONSET	COMMENTS	PLAN
1.			
2.			
3.			
4.			
5.			
6.			
7.			

DATING SHEET

LNMP _____ ⟶ EDC _____   LMP _____ ⟶ EDC _____

FIRST SYMPTOMS OF PREGNANCY (date) _____

(+)   PREGNANCY TEST   a. URINE (date) _____ at _____ wks

b. SERUM (date) _____ at _____ wks

FIRST EXAM (date) _____ SIZE _____ at _____ wks GA

QUICKENING (date) _____ at _____ wks GA

20 WK STETH FHT (date) _____ at _____ wks GA

Utx at umbilicus? _____

SIZE = DATES?

SONO #1 (date) _____ (findings) _____ ⟶ SONO EDC

SONO #2 (date) _____ (findings) _____ ⟶ SONO EDC

BEST ESTIMATE OF EDC

Figure 4-36—cont'd *Prenatal records.*

B

ANTEPARTUM RECORD

☐ IDENTIFIED HIGH RISK

LAST NAME		FIRST NAME
ADDRESS		
BIRTHDATE	AGE	SEX	CLASS
PHYSICIAN		

PEDIATRICIAN

DATE	PHONE

PATIENT (LAST NAME - FIRST NAME)	MAIDEN NAME	REFERRED BY

PATIENT'S ADDRESS (STREET, CITY, STATE, ZIP CODE)	HOME PHONE	BUSINESS PHONE

AGE	BIRTHDATE	BIRTHPLACE	RELIGION	HEIGHT FT. IN.	AVER. WT. LB.	OCCUPATION	MAY WORK UNTIL (DATE)

MARRIED YES ☐ NO ☐	FATHER'S NAME	AGE	HEIGHT	WEIGHT LB.	BLOOD TYPE	OCCUPATION

FATHER'S HEALTH HISTORY	FATHER'S FAMILY HISTORY

HISTORY

CTA ONSET DATE	INTERVAL (DAYS)	DURATION (DAYS)	AMOUNT	DYSMENORRHEA	LMP	EDC	

PRESENT PREGNANCY HISTORY

	QUICKENING DATE	MOTHER TO NURSE? ☐ YES ☐ NO	ANESTHETIC

PREVIOUS PREGNANCIES – PARITY

YEAR	DURATION	LABOR	ANESTHESIA	SEX	WEIGHT	RHOGAM	✱ PREMATURITY	✱ FETAL LOSS

✱ RECORD REASON

FAMILY

DIABETES	HYPERTENSION	TWINS	CONGENITAL DEFECTS

PERSONAL

RH. FEV.	DIABETES	HEPATITIS	RUBELLA	ANEMIA	CARDIAC	THYROID	ALLERGIES

DRUGS	TRANSFUSIONS	URINARY TRACT	CONVULSIONS	PHLEBITIS	VARICOSITIES

SERIOUS ILLNESS, SURGERY, HOSPITALIZED:

INITIAL PHYSICAL EXAMINATION

BLOOD PRES.	PULSE	ENT	TEETH	HEART	LUNGS	EXTREMITIES

ABDOMEN	BREASTS

PELVIMETRY	PELVIC
D.C.	OUTLET
BIS	VAGINA
SPINES	CERVIX
S.S. LIG.	CORPUS
ARCH.	ADNEXA
SACRAL HOLLOW	RECTUM
FORE PELVIS	
DATE	SIGNATURE

INITIAL LABORATORY WORK

PCV.	HGB.	SEROLOGY	BLOOD TYPE	RH.	ALBUMIN	SUGAR	ATYPICAL ANTIBODIES	Rh TITRE	CYTOLOGY

COPY TO HOSPITAL IN APPROXIMATELY 30 WEEKS

PHYSICIAN

Figure 4-36—cont'd ***Prenatal records.***

C

ANTEPARTUM RECORD
(CONTINUATION)

NAME

LAST NAME FIRST NAME
ADDRESS
BIRTHDATE AGE SEX CLASS
PHYSICIAN
DATE PHONE

SUBSEQUENT VISITS

DATE	WEIGHT	BLOOD PRESSURE	HEIGHT OF FUNDUS	POSITION AND PRESENTATION	FETAL HEART	URINE: ALBUMIN	URINE: SUGAR	HEMOGLOBIN	SYMPTOMS: HEADACHE	SYMPTOMS: DIZZINESS	SYMPTOMS: EDEMA	SYMPTOMS: NAUSEA & VOMITING	SYMPTOMS: BLEEDING		INITIALS

DATE	PROGRESS NOTES	TEST	DATE	FINDINGS
		Rh TITRE		
		AMNIO-CENTESIS		
		ULTRA-SONOGRAM		
		X-RAY		
		OTHER		

QUICKENING DATE	MOTHER TO NURSE? ☐ YES ☐ NO	ANESTHETIC	PEDIATRICIAN

SEND COPY TO HOSPITAL AT APPROXIMATELY 38 WEEKS.

______________________ M.D.
SIGNATURE

PHYSICIAN

- Chills and/or fever
- Severe pain in the lower abdomen, frequently beginning on one side, during early pregnancy. This is the classic indication of an ectopic pregnancy.

Later in the pregnancy additional warning signs to watch for and report include the following:

- Pelvic pressure
- Sudden gush of water from the vagina with subsequent leakage, indicating that the amniotic sac has ruptured
- Fainting spells or loss of consciousness
- Swelling or puffiness of the hands or face and/or marked swelling of the ankles and feet
- Rapid weight gain in a short period of time
- Pain or a burning sensation on urination
- Painless contractions
- Low, dull backache
- Rashes or lesions

By using Nägele's rule and the date of the first day of the LMP, you or the physician determine the EDC. This is determined by adding 7 days to the date of the first day of the LMP, subtracting 3 months, and adding 1 year.

EXAMPLE:

EDC = date of first day of LMP
   + 7 days − 3 months + 1 year
EDC = April 4, 19___ plus 7 days
         =April 11, 19___
 − (minus) 3 months
         =January 11, 19___
 + (plus) 1 year
         = January 11 of the following year

Thus the baby will be delivered on approximately January 11 of the following year, or more commonly within 1 week before or 1 week after the EDC (see also Table 4-4).

Initial Prenatal Physical Examination and Diagnostic Tests

The initial prenatal examination includes a physical examination as described on pages 95 to 98. Among other findings, the patient's *blood pressure* and *weight* are recorded at this and all subsequent visits. By keeping a continuous record of the blood pressure and weight, the physician can determine any excessive elevation of the BP or a sudden and rapid weight gain from one visit to the next. Such elevations may be early warning signs of a serious problems such as preeclampsia and require further follow-up. Weight measurements are also helpful in determining the stages of fetal growth. The American College of Obstetrics and Gynecology recommends a weight gain of 22 to 26 pounds during pregnancy. Just as important as total weight gain is the rate of the gain. The mother's weight should increase only slightly in the first 3 months—about 1 pound per month. Then she should begin a steady rate of gain of $1/2$ to 1 pound per week until the birth of the baby. It is critical that the added weight gain be from increased consumption of the necessary food groups, not simply overloading on calories.

Of particular importance during the physical examination are the *breast, abdomen,* and *pelvic examinations.* In addition to the routine examinations of these areas of the body, the breasts are observed for any breast changes that accompany pregnancy as described previously. During the abdominal examination the initial measurement of the height of the fundus of the uterus is recorded. This is the distance in centimeters between the superior aspect of the symphysis pubis and the top of the fundus of the uterus (Figure 4-37). This provides a baseline for future measurements. During the pelvic examination a *Pap smear* and a *culture for gonorrhea and chlamydia* are usually taken. By feeling the uterus, the physician can learn about its position, shape, and size and how long the patient has been pregnant. As estimation of pelvic measurements is also made to determine a difficult delivery in cases of cephalopelvic disproportions. The *vaginal examination* is done to check the birth canal for any abnormalities and obtain further pelvic measurements.

Samples of urine and blood are collected for the following tests. (At times the patient may be sent to an outside laboratory to have these specimens collected.) On the first visit a *complete urinalysis* is performed; then on subsequent visits the urine is checked for *albumin and sugar.* The presence of albumin in the urine can be an early warning sign of toxemia. The presence of sugar in the urine can be a warning sign of a prediabetic state or diabetes. Both of these conditions require careful medical supervision and treatment. Blood tests to be performed include a complete blood count to assess the general health status of the expectant mother. Of special importance are the hemoglobin and hematocrit results, which determine if the mother is anemic. If anemia is present, special treatment is given, and further hemoglobin and hematocrit evaluations are done. Other blood tests include the Rh factor and blood typing of the ABO blood groups, a Venereal Disease Research Laboratory (VDRL) or a rapid plasma reagin (RPR) test for syphilis, and a rubella titer to determine if the patient has immunity to rubella (German measles) (see also Units Twelve and Thirteen).

For other high-risk patients, a blood test that screens for hepatitis B may also be performed. This is a blood serum test that tests for the presence of the hepatitis B surface antigen (HbsAG). If the results are positive, a liver function test may then be performed.

Some physicians may order a *Tine or Mantoux test* to screen the patient for tuberculosis (see also Unit Nine). The physician usually only orders a chest x-ray film to screen for tuberculosis if the patient has had a positive Tine or Mantoux test in the past, when the mother has been exposed to tuberculosis, or if other family members have tuberculosis.

After the examination has been completed, the physician discusses with the patient *general health care during pregnancy;* care of the teeth; proper diet; the need for rest and relaxation; types of exercise and work that can be continued; weight gain; the use of tobacco, alcohol, and drugs; and the need for follow-up prenatal visits. Pamphlets containing simi-

TABLE 4-4

Pregnancy Table for Expected Date of Delivery

Find the date of the last menstrual period in the top line (light-face type) of the pair of lines. The dark number (bold-face type) in the line below will be the expected day of delivery.

	1	2	3	4	5	6	7	8	9	10	11	12	13	14	15	16	17	18	19	20	21	22	23	24	25	26	27	28	29	30	31	
Jan.	1	2	3	4	5	6	7	8	9	10	11	12	13	14	15	16	17	18	19	20	21	22	23	24	25	26	27	28	29	30	31	
Oct.	**8**	**9**	**10**	**11**	**12**	**13**	**14**	**15**	**16**	**17**	**18**	**19**	**20**	**21**	**22**	**23**	**24**	**25**	**26**	**27**	**28**	**29**	**30**	**31**	**(1**	**2**	**3**	**4**	**5**	**6**	**7**	**Nov.**
Feb.	1	2	3	4	5	6	7	8	9	10	11	12	13	14	15	16	17	18	19	20	21	22	23	24	25	26	27	28				
Nov.	**8**	**9**	**10**	**11**	**12**	**13**	**14**	**15**	**16**	**17**	**18**	**19**	**20**	**21**	**22**	**23**	**24**	**25**	**26**	**27**	**28**	**29**	**30**	**(1**	**2**	**3**	**4**	**5**				**Dec.**
Mar.	1	2	3	4	5	6	7	8	9	10	11	12	13	14	15	16	17	18	19	20	21	22	23	24	25	26	27	28	29	30	31	
Dec.	**6**	**7**	**8**	**9**	**10**	**11**	**12**	**13**	**14**	**15**	**16**	**17**	**18**	**19**	**20**	**21**	**22**	**23**	**24**	**25**	**26**	**27**	**28**	**29**	**30**	**31**	**(1**	**2**	**3**	**4**	**5**	**Jan.**
April	1	2	3	4	5	6	7	8	9	10	11	12	13	14	15	16	17	18	19	20	21	22	23	24	25	26	27	28	29	30		
Jan.	**6**	**7**	**8**	**9**	**10**	**11**	**12**	**13**	**14**	**15**	**16**	**17**	**18**	**19**	**20**	**21**	**22**	**23**	**24**	**25**	**26**	**27**	**28**	**29**	**30**	**31**	**(1**	**2**	**3**	**4**		**Feb.**
May	1	2	3	4	5	6	7	8	9	10	11	12	13	14	15	16	17	18	19	20	21	22	23	24	25	26	27	28	29	30	31	
Feb.	**5**	**6**	**7**	**8**	**9**	**10**	**11**	**12**	**13**	**14**	**15**	**16**	**17**	**18**	**19**	**20**	**21**	**22**	**23**	**24**	**25**	**26**	**27**	**28**	**(1**	**2**	**3**	**4**	**5**	**6**	**7**	**Mar.**
June	1	2	3	4	5	6	7	8	9	10	11	12	13	14	15	16	17	18	19	20	21	22	23	24	25	26	27	28	29	30		
Mar.	**8**	**9**	**10**	**11**	**12**	**13**	**14**	**15**	**16**	**17**	**18**	**19**	**20**	**21**	**22**	**23**	**24**	**25**	**26**	**27**	**28**	**29**	**30**	**31**	**(1**	**2**	**3**	**4**	**5**	**6**		**April**
July	1	2	3	4	5	6	7	8	9	10	11	12	13	14	15	16	17	18	19	20	21	22	23	24	25	26	27	28	29	30	31	
April	**7**	**8**	**9**	**10**	**11**	**12**	**13**	**14**	**15**	**16**	**17**	**18**	**19**	**20**	**21**	**22**	**23**	**24**	**25**	**26**	**27**	**28**	**29**	**30**	**(1**	**2**	**3**	**4**	**5**	**6**	**7**	**May**
Aug.	1	2	3	4	5	6	7	8	9	10	11	12	13	14	15	16	17	18	19	20	21	22	23	24	25	26	27	28	29	30	31	
May	**8**	**9**	**10**	**11**	**12**	**13**	**14**	**15**	**16**	**17**	**18**	**19**	**20**	**21**	**22**	**23**	**24**	**25**	**26**	**27**	**28**	**29**	**30**	**31**	**(1**	**2**	**3**	**4**	**5**	**6**	**7**	**June**
Sept.	1	2	3	4	5	6	7	8	9	10	11	12	13	14	15	16	17	18	19	20	21	22	23	24	25	26	27	28	29	30		
June	**8**	**9**	**10**	**11**	**12**	**13**	**14**	**15**	**16**	**17**	**18**	**19**	**20**	**21**	**22**	**23**	**24**	**25**	**26**	**27**	**28**	**29**	**30**	**(1**	**2**	**3**	**4**	**5**	**6**	**7**		**July**
Oct.	1	2	3	4	5	6	7	8	9	10	11	12	13	14	15	16	17	18	19	20	21	22	23	24	25	26	27	28	29	30	31	
July	**8**	**9**	**10**	**11**	**12**	**13**	**14**	**15**	**16**	**17**	**18**	**19**	**20**	**21**	**22**	**23**	**24**	**25**	**26**	**27**	**28**	**29**	**30**	**31**	**(1**	**2**	**3**	**4**	**5**	**6**	**7**	**Aug.**
Nov.	1	2	3	4	5	6	7	8	9	10	11	12	13	14	15	16	17	18	19	20	21	22	23	24	25	26	27	28	29	30		
Aug.	**8**	**9**	**10**	**11**	**12**	**13**	**14**	**15**	**16**	**17**	**18**	**19**	**20**	**21**	**22**	**23**	**24**	**25**	**26**	**27**	**28**	**29**	**30**	**31**	**(1**	**2**	**3**	**4**	**5**	**6**		**Sept.**
Dec.	1	2	3	4	5	6	7	8	9	10	11	12	13	14	15	16	17	18	19	20	21	22	23	24	25	26	27	28	29	30	31	
Sept.	**7**	**8**	**9**	**10**	**11**	**12**	**13**	**14**	**15**	**16**	**17**	**18**	**19**	**20**	**21**	**22**	**23**	**24**	**25**	**26**	**27**	**28**	**29**	**30**	**(1**	**2**	**3**	**4**	**5**	**6**	**7**	**Oct.**

lar information may be given to the patient to use as a reference. Many obstetric offices also have videotapes on pregnancy for the patient to watch and learn from.

Follow-Up Prenatal Visits

The antepartum record also includes essential data obtained during the follow-up prenatal visits (see Figure 4-31). Data measured and recorded include the patient's weight, blood pressure, height of the uterine fundus, position and presentation of the fetus, the fetal heart rate after the fourth month (Figure 4-38), urine tests for albumin and sugar, blood tests for hemoglobin and a hematocrit or a complete blood count if deemed necessary, any symptoms or early warning signs experienced by the patient, and any concerns or questions that the patient may have. A vaginal examination is done only periodically and usually 2 to 3 weeks before the EDC. All this information aids the physician in determining and evaluating the progress of the pregnancy and in planning good patient care.

All visits should also include educating the mother in healthful living habits and various aspects of her pregnancy, since education is an integral part of antepartum care. The follow-up visits provide the perfect opportunity to reinforce healthful living habits to the mother and to provide explanations of the physical and emotional changes that she is experiencing and explanations about the growth pattern of the fetus. Information on the LaMaze method of childbirth may be given later in the pregnancy. You may be responsible for scheduling the LaMaze childbirth classes and possibly classes on the fundamentals of newborn care for the mother and father.

Other topics to be discussed and reviewed include exercise, rest, diet, sexual intercourse, partner support, labor (the signs of labor, how long it will last, anesthetics), delivery of the baby, postpartum care, and, possibly, family planning.

Other Prenatal Tests

In California and a few other states, it is now a state law that the *alpha fetoprotein (AFP)* blood test be offered to the mother around the sixteenth week of pregnancy. The mother is at liberty to accept or deny this test. AFP is produced in the fetus' liver and gastrointestinal tract and is normally found in the mother's blood. The AFP test is nondefinitive and is used *only* as a screening test. It may be used to help rule out conditions such as neural tube defects, abdominal wall defects, chromosome problems, Down syndrome, fetal demise, and also twins. If the results of this test are positive, *further testing is required.* First an ultrasound examination is performed to check for the exact gestational time, since AFP levels vary at different times during pregnancy. This may be followed by a repeat serum test and/or amniocentesis and possibly another ultrasound examination. Counseling and patient education are vital during all of this testing.

Recent research studies found a correlation between high levels of AFP in a mother's blood and late miscarriage, usually in the third trimester. This is an important development in terms of defining high-risk pregnancies, which is a serious problem in obstetrics. The AFP test is different from other prenatal tests available for early diagnosis of genetic and biochemical disorders in a fetus (for example, the *chorionic villi sampling* (CVS) and *amniocentesis*). The latter tests are currently recommended only for certain pregnant women:

- Women age 35 years or older
- Women who have previously borne a child with chromosomal abnormalities
- Women who are likely to bear a child with other genetic abnormalities because they are known carriers of a detectable genetic disorder, including sickle cell anemia, Tay Sachs disease, and thalassemia.

The primary advantage of CVS over amniocentesis is earlier prenatal diagnosis of disorders. This procedure is performed between the eighth to the tenth week of pregnancy. A small amount of tissue surrounding the fetus, the chorionic villi, is suctioned out for laboratory analysis. Results are reported in less than a week. Some controversy still exists over CVS because of isolated cases of fetal damage or the potential for such damage and the increased risk of spontaneous abortion after this test is performed—especially in women who have a history of spontaneous abortion, who have spotting or bleeding during pregnancy, or whose placenta is located on either side of the uterus or in the area of

Figure 4-37 *Measuring the height of the uterine fundus.*

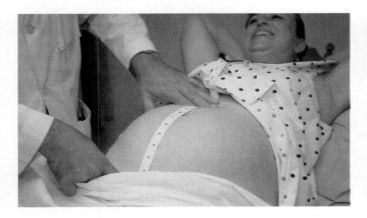

Figure 4-38 *Listening to the fetal heart rate.*

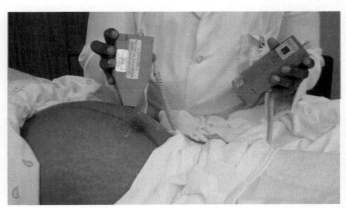

the uterus farthest from the cervix. Amniocentesis is performed around the fourteenth to the sixteenth week of pregnancy. A small amount of amniotic fluid is removed for laboratory study. Results are reported in 2 to 3 weeks.

Another prenatal screening test, *ultrasound,* uses high-frequency sound waves to produce an image of the fetus on a video screen and on a photographic picture. Ultrasound may be used to confirm the presence of twins, to check fetal age, and to identify defects in the structure of the fetus.

Counseling and patient education are vital before, during, and after any of these tests.

Six-Weeks' Postpartum Visit

Six weeks after a vaginal delivery, the patient is advised to return to the physician's office for a visit so that her general condition can be evaluated. If the patient had a cesarean section, she should return for a checkup 2 weeks after delivery and then 4 to 6 weeks postpartum. Procedures that are performed at this visit include the following:

- Vital signs (TPR and BP)—Any unusual elevation must be noted, since it could indicate potential problems.
- Weight—The patient's weight loss after delivery is noted. Nutritional counseling may be necessary if the mother is having difficulty losing the weight that she gained during pregnancy.
- Breast examination—The breasts are checked for any unusual lumps or masses. Any tenderness should be noted. The nipples are examined for cracks, soreness, and redness in mothers who are breast feeding.
- Abdominal and pelvic examination—The physician determines if the uterus has returned to its normal size and state, if the cervix has healed, and if the abdominal wall and pelvic floor have regained muscle tone. The vagina is checked for any abnormal discharge. Some physicians do a Pap smear at this time; others wait until 3 months after delivery before doing a Pap smear.
- Rectal examination—To examine for the presence of hemorrhoids.
- Blood tests—Hemoglobin and hematocrit levels are done to screen for anemia, which may have resulted from blood loss during delivery.

The physician also discusses breast feeding, any problems the patient may be having with it (if doing so), sexuality, birth control, diet, exercise, and any other concerns that the patient may have. It is an opportune time for patient education and to reinforce healthful living habits.

MEDICAL ASSISTANT'S RESPONSIBILITIES

In addition to the general instructions and responsibilities for the medical assistant listed on pages 83 and 84 and the procedures for assisting with a physical examination as outlined on pages 95 to 98, the medical assistant's responsibilities include the following:

- Acquire some of the information to be recorded on the antepartum record (see Figure 4-36). The amount of information collected by the medical assistant varies

according to the physician's preference. Some physicians may obtain all of the history and have the medical assistant obtain only the vital signs and height and weight measurements.

- Assemble additional equipment that is be required for prenatal examinations. This would include:
    A flexible centimeter tape measure used to measure the height of the fundus of the uterus.
    A pelvimeter used for taking pelvic measurements.
    A fetoscope or Doppler fetal pulse detector and an ultrasound coupling agent used to listen to the fetal heart ones
- Develop a good rapport with the patient so that she feels comfortable and confident enough to ask questions of you and the physician; help the patient to relax and gain confidence in your abilities and functions.
- Schedule the follow-up prenatal visits.
- Make certain that the patient understands all of the instructions that were given to her.
- Reinforce the need for healthful living habits.
- Take part in patient education as discussed previously.
- Remind the patient to call the physician immediately if she experiences any of the early warning signs of problems during the pregnancy.
- Remind the patient to call the office with any questions she may have about the pregnancy and her care.

PEDIATRIC EXAMINATIONS

Pediatrics is the branch of medicine that deals with the care and development of neonates (the first 28 days of life), infants, children, and adolescents and with the diseases and treatment affecting them. The physician specialist in pediatrics is called a pediatrician.

There are two broad classifications of pediatric-patient physician office visits. They are the well-child visit and the sick-child visit. In an effort to accommodate working parents, pediatric practices often have extended office hours. It is not unusual for a pediatrician's office to be open evenings as late as 9 p.m. and at least part of the day on Saturday. During both types of visits health teaching and anticipatory guidance can and should be provided. Family interrelationships can be observed, and progress of any chronic problem(s) can be assessed. Parents (and patients) are often ready and motivated to learn when they are seeking help for a medical problem. All information given, observed, or obtained should be recorded on the patient's chart. In this way proper treatment and referrals can be made.

During both the well-child and the sick-child visit, the medical assistant may perform or assist with many of the procedures already discussed in this unit or in other units (for example, measuring and recording temperature, pulse, respiration, and blood pressure; assisting with different types of examinations; and measuring distance visual acuity). Procedures and techniques that are specifically related to the pediatric patient are presented here.

WELL-CHILD VISITS

A schedule of well-child visits should be planned for each child to assess growth and development (i.e., physical, mental, and emotional maturation), provide immunizations, detect deviations, and provide health teaching and anticipatory guidance. Assessing the child's growth and development is best accomplished by monitoring and comparing each child's growth and development with that of other children within the same age group using established norms and expectations (Figure 4-39; also see Figure 4-45). Guidelines for health supervision for a child's care are outlined in Table 4-5. Table 4-6 contains general trends in physical growth during childhood. The guidelines in Table 4-5 are for children who have no apparent health problem and who are growing and developing satisfactorily. When any variation from the normal standards are detected, additional visits and care may become necessary. Table 4-7 contains more current recommendations for immunizations, and Appendix D contains expanded information on the most current immunization recommendations. In addition, in December 1992 the American Medical Association (AMA) established new Guidelines for Adolescent Preventive Services (GAPS), which call for physicians to make preventive services a greater part of their clinical practice. The main issues of the new recommendations of the GAPS plan suggest that all adolescents ages 11 to 21 years "should have an annual preventive services visit that addresses both the biomedical and psychosocial aspects of health." A physical examination and health guidance for the patients and their adult caregivers/parents should be provided in three of these visits—one each during early, middle, and late adolescence. Annually, physicians should screen and ask adolescents about each of the following:

- Eating and other emotional disorders
- High blood pressure and other heart disease risks such as obesity, a sedentary lifestyle, diabetes, stress, family history of heart attacks, high blood cholesterol
- Alcohol, tobacco, or drug use or abuse
- Sexual behavior that could lead to sexually transmitted diseases (STDs) or unwanted pregnancy

The specialists who developed the guidelines for health supervision emphasize the great importance of continuity of care. Prenatal visits, as discussed under "Obstetric Examinations" in this unit, for anticipatory guidance are strongly recommended. Health supervision for the newborn should begin in the hospital at the time of birth. The medical assistant should emphasize to the parent(s) or caregiver the need for well-child visits. When the parent(s) or caregiver(s) do not follow the recommendations for physician visits, follow-up should be provided. This can be accomplished by special reminders mailed to the parents/caregivers and/or by a phone call suggesting a date and time for the visit. A brief explanation of what the visit will include should also be provided so that the parent/caregiver hopefully understands the need for completing the recommended schedule of visits.

A sample of a health history that the parent may fill out before the physician examines the child is shown in Figure 4-40. The medical assistant may have to explain parts of this form to the parent and/or help the parent to complete the form.

Today's well-child checkups are designed to prevent, detect, and stop health problems early. By monitoring a child's growth and such things as dietary habits through routine visits, situations such as a tendency toward obesity and heart disease can be detected early, and steps can be taken to avoid these conditions. The checkups cover routine health tests, immunizations, behavior problems, and diet and exercise programs. Home safety is a topic that should be discussed at every checkup, since most parents do not realize that accident, not disease, are the number one cause of death among children. By the time the child is 2 years old, some doctors start making recommendations for a low-fat diet. Because of today's busy lifestyles, the physician must also help the families come up with a plan that includes the right foods and plenty of exercise (rather than the frequent use of fast-food items that commonly are high in fat and salt). Cultural, ethnic, and socioeconomic factors should be included in the plan of action for review and follow-up care because they may influence the assessment of growth and development of the child.

General Points for Pediatric Visits

Any physical examination is approached on the basis of the child's age, development, level or wellness or illness, and past experience with the health care system. The examiner and attendants take into consideration physical, mental, and emotional developmental milestones to reduce or eliminate anxiety that many children experience during a physical examination. The examiners should begin to observe from the time the child and parent/caregiver enter the physician's office. Everyone involved in the process must work together to make the visit and examination a positive experience for the child, the parent/caregiver, and the medical personnel. It is very important that a feeling of trust and confidence be developed between the child, the parent, and the health care workers. A special rapport should be established to solicit cooperation between the child and medical personnel. Interacting with children requires special skills and practice. Knowledge of normal growth and development patterns and how to approach children of different ages is particularly helpful. It is suggested that you refer to a pediatric textbook and other books and pamphlets to review the stages and changes for growing and developing children, since it is not within the limits of this text to describe growth and development in detail. It is important to note that it is quite normal for a sick child to regress to an earlier stage of expected behavior.

Explanations are of the utmost importance. Always explain a procedure to children who are capable of understanding and to the parent. Both need reassurance. Be honest when you are describing a procedure. If the procedure will hurt, *never* tell children that it will not hurt. Tell them that it will hurt but just for a short time; then offer praise after the procedure, telling them how brave they were, because this will help them feel a

Text continues on page 138.

Figure 4-39 *Guideposts in motor development, emphasizing the average child.*
From Cole G: *Basic nursing skills and concepts,* ed 1, St. Louis, 1991, Mosby.

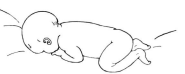

Birth
Keeps his legs tucked up under him and bears his weight
on his knees, abdomen, chest, and head.

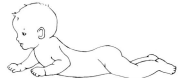

2-3 months
Extends his legs and lifts his chest and
head to look around.

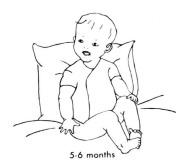

5-6 months
Can sit up with support, hold his head up,
and is alert to surroundings.

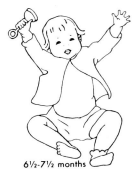

6½-7½ months
Sits up alone and steadily without support.
Legs are bowed to help balance.

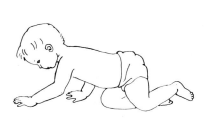

8-9 months
Creeping; the trunk is carried free from floor. With practice,
rhythm appears and only one limb moves at a time.

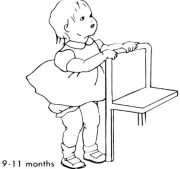

9-11 months
Pulls himself up and stands holding onto furniture. Feet
far apart, head and upper trunk carried forward.

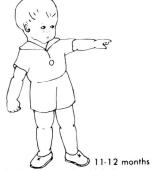

11-12 months
Stands alone, can walk with help.

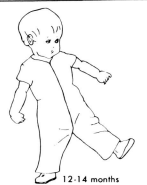

12-14 months
Walks alone on wide base with legs far apart.

TABLE 4-5

AAP Guidelines for Health Supervision

	Infancy							Early Childhood				Late Childhood				Adolescence[1]			
Age[2]	by 1 mo.	2 mos.	4 mos.	6 mos.	9 mos.	12 mos.	15 mos.	18 mos.	24 mos.	3 yrs.	4 yrs.	5 yrs.	6 yrs.	8 yrs.	10 yrs.	12 yrs.	14 yrs.	16 yrs.	18 yrs.	20+ yrs.
History Initial/interval	•	•	•	•	•	•	•	•	•	•	•	•	•	•	•	•	•	•	•	•
Measurements Height and Weight	•	•	•	•	•	•	•	•	•	•	•	•	•	•	•	•	•	•	•	•
Head Circumference	•	•	•	•																
Blood Pressure										•	•		•	•	•	•	•	•	•	•
Sensory Screening Vision	S	S	S	S	S	S	S	S	S	S	o	o	o	o	S	o	o	S	o	o
Hearing	S	S	S	S	S	S	S	S	S	S	o	o	S[3]	S[3]	S[3]	o	S	S	o	S
Devel./Behav.[4] Assessment	•	•	•	•	•	•	•	•	•	•	•	•	•	•	•	•	•	•	•	•
Physical Examination[5] Procedures[6]	•	•	•	•	•	•	•	•	•	•	•	•	•	•	•	•	•	•	•	•
Hered./metabolic[7] Screening	•																			
Immunization[8]		•	•	•			•	•	•		•						•			
Tuberculin Test[9]	←———•———→							←———•———→									←———•———→			
Hematocrit or Hemoglobin[10]	←———•———→							←———•———→				←——•——→					←——•——→			
Urinalysis[11]																				
Anticipatory[12] Guidance	•	•	•	•	•	•	•	•	•	•	•	•	•	•	•	•	•	•	•	•
Initial Dental[13] Referral																				

1. Adolescent related issues (e.g., psychosocial, emotional, substance usage, and reproductive health) may necessitate more frequent health supervision.
2. If a child comes under care for the first time at any point on the schedule, or if any items are not accomplished at the suggested age, the schedule should be brought up to date at the earliest possible time.
3. At these points, history may suffice: if problem suggested, a standard testing method should be employed.
4. By history and appropriate physical examination: if suspicious, by specific objective developmental testing.
5. At each visit, a complete physical examination is essential, with infant totally unclothed, older child undressed and suitably draped.
6. These may be modified, depending upon entry point into schedule and individual need.
7. Metabolic screening (e.g., thyroid, PKU, galactosemia) should be done according to state law.
8. Schedule(s) per Report of Committee on Infectious Disease, 1986, Red Book.
9. For low risk groups, the Committee on Infectious Diseases recommends the following options: (1) No routine testing or (2) testing at three times–infancy, preschool, and adolescence. For high-risk groups, annual TB skin testing is recommended.
10. Present medical evidence suggests the need for reevaluation of the frequency and timing of hemoglobin or hematocrit tests. One determination is therefore suggested during each time period. Performance of additional tests is left to the individual practice experience.
11. Present medical evidence suggests the need for reevaluation of the frequency and time of urinalysis. One determination is therefore suggested during each time period. Performance of additional tests is left to the individual practice experience.
12. Appropriate discussion and counselling should be an integral part of each visit for care.
13. Subsequent examinations as prescribed by dentist.
N.B: **Special chemical, immunologic, and endocrine testing** are usually carried out upon specific indications. Testing other than newborn (e.g., inborn errors of metabolism, sickle disease, lead) are discretionary with the physician.
Key: •, To be performed; S, subjective, by history; o, objective, by a standard testing method.
From American Academy of Pediatrics: Guidelines for Health Supervision II, Elk Grove Village, IL, 1988, American Academy of Pediatrics.

TABLE 4-6

General Trends in Physical Growth During Childhood

Age	Weight*	Height*
Infants Birth-6 months	Weekly gain: 140-200 g (5-7 ounces) Birth weight doubles by end of first 6 months†	Monthly gain: 2.5 cm (1 inch)
6-12 months	Weekly gain: 85-140 g (3-5 ounces) Birth weight triples by end of first year	Monthly gain: 1.25 cm (0.5 inch) Birth length increases by approximately 50% by end of first year
Toddlers	Birth weight quadruples by age 2-1/2 years Yearly gain: 2-3 kg (4.4-6.6 pounds)	Height at 2 years is approximately 50% of eventual adult height Gain during second year: about 12 cm (4.8 inches) Gain during third year: about 6-8 cm (2.4-3.2 inches)
Preschoolers	Yearly gain: 2-3 kg (4.4-6.6 pounds) Yearly gain: 6-8 cm (2.4-3.2 inches)	Birth length doubles by 4 years of age
School-age children(2 inches)	Yearly gain: 2-3 kg (4.4-6.6 pounds)	Yearly gain after 6 years: 5 cm Birth length triples by about 13 years of age
Pubertal growth spurt Females—between 10 and 14 years	Weight gain: 7-25 kg (15-55 pounds) Mean: 17.5 kg (38.1 pounds)	Height gain: 5-25 cm (2-10 inches); 95% of mature height achieved by onset of menarche or skeletal age of 13 years Mean: 20.5 cm (8.2 inches)
Males—between 12 and 16 years	Weight gain: 7-30 kg (15-65 pounds) Mean: 23/7 kg (52.1 pounds)	Height gain: 10-30 cm (4-12 inches); approximately 95% of mature height achieved by skeletal age of 15 years Mean: 27.5 cm (11 inches)

Reproduced with permission from Wong: Essentials of pediatric nursing, ed 4, Mosby, 1993, St. Louis.
*Yearly height and weight gains for each age group represent averaged estimates from a variety of sources.
†A study has shown the mean doubling time for birth weight to be 4.7 months and mean tripling time to be 14.7 months (Jung E, Czaijka-Narins DM: Birth weight doubling and tripling times: an updated look at the effects of birth weight, sex, race, and type of feeding, Am J Clin Nutr *42:182-189, 1985.).*

little better and accept what has occurred in a more positive way. Children between the ages of 2 and 3 have short attention spans. They often respond well if you make the procedure a game or get them to assist you. You may let them listen to your heartbeat with the stethoscope and then to their own heartbeat before you attempt to take their apical heart rate or blood pressure (Figure 4-41, *A*). Compliment children during and after the procedure, and ask them questions (for example, what is your favorite game). Be friendly—talk to children during a procedure. You can also use actions to demonstrate what you want to convey to children. Use hand gestures or point to the item while you are talking. Be sensitive to children. Note their psychologic attitude (for example, are they happy, sad, depressed, anxious, irritable, or withdrawn). When asking children to describe how they feel, whether they are happy, or how much pain (hurt) they feel, you may want to use the Wong-Baker Faces Pain Rating

Scale (Figure 4-41, *A* to *C*) and let them identify their feelings from the diagrams.

Infants under 2 years of age have not yet associated pain and discomfort with the physician's office; thus they are often very agreeable to being weighed and measured or to other procedures, although some may cry when being undressed. In this case have parent undress the child. Often these children don't cry before an immunization and can be comforted quickly after the injection by you, the parent, or a toy.

Toddlers and preschool-age children may be more disagreeable and reluctant to be examined and treated. By this age children have learned to associate pain with visits to the physician and may be fearful of all equipment that they see, even the scale or thermometer. They can associate past pain with this visit. Here you may let the child hold the thermometer before you use it. Often when children become familiar with an instrument, they are more apt to let you use it on

TABLE 4-7

Recommended Schedule for Immunization of Healthy Infants and Children in the United States[a]

Recommended Age[b]	Immunizations[c]	Comments
2 months	DTP, HbCV[d], OPV	DTP and OPV can be initiated as early as 4 weeks after birth in areas of high endemicity or during epidemics
4 months	DTP, HbCV[d], OPV	2-month interval (minimum of 6 weeks) desired for OPV to avoid interference from previous dose
6 months	DTP, HbCV[d]	Third dose of OPV is not indicated in the United States but is desirable in other geographic areas where polio is endemic
15 months	MMR[e], HbCV[f]	Tuberculin testing may be done at the same visit
15-18 months	DTP[g,h], OPV[i]	(See footnotes)
4-6 years	DTP[i], OPV	At or before school entry
1-12 years	MMR	At entry to middle school or junior high school unless second dose previously given
14-16 years	Td	Repeat every 10 years throughout life

Modified from American Academy of Pediatrics: Report of the Committee on Infectious Diseases, ed 22, Elk Grove Village, Ill, 1991, The Academy.
Reproduced with permission from Wong D: Essentials of pediatric nursing, ed 4, St. Louis, 1993, Mosby.
[a]*For all products used, consult manufacturer's package insert for instructions for storage, handling, dosage, and administration.*
[b]*These recommended ages should not be construed as absolute. For example, 2 months can be 6 to 10 weeks. However, MMR usually should not be given to children younger than 12 months. (If measles vaccination is indicated, monovalent measles vaccine is recommended, and MMR should be given subsequently, at 15 months.)*
[c]*DTP, Diphtheria and tetanus toxoids with pertussis vaccine; HbCV, Haemophilus b conjugate vaccine; OPV, oral poliovirus vaccine containing attenuated poliovirus types 1, 2, and 3; MMR, live measles, mumps, and rubella viruses in a combined vaccine; Td, adult tetanus toxoid (full does) and diphtheria toxoid (reduced dose) for adult use.*
[d]*Two HbCVs are approved for use in children younger than 15 months.*
[e]*May be given at 12 months of age in areas with recurrent measles transmission.*
[f]*Any licensed Haemophilus b conjugate vaccine may be given.*
[g]*Should be given 6 to 12 months after the third dose.*
[h]*May be given simultaneously with MMR and HbCV at 15 months or at any time between 12 and 24 months; priority should be given to administering MMR at the recommended age.*
[i]*Can be given up to the seventh birthday.*

them. This age group frequently reacts to a situation or injury by crying and kicking in anticipation of the effects.

School-age children often approach the examination room with apprehension. Many 10- to 12-year-olds prefer to see the physician without their parent present in the examination room. Check with the physician as to how he or she prefers to handle these situations.

Use any opportunity that arises to inform and teach the patient and parent about health and prevention of illness or about the form of treatment that the patient will be receiving. Tell them to write all of their questions down so they won't forget to ask the physician. This also is a form of reassurance; you are letting them know that you are interested in them and in their treatment. You may also refer parents to classes on child development that are being offered in your community. It is good to keep a list of these classes readily available. Let the parent be as involved with caring for the child as is possible during the visit (for example, the mother may hold the baby or child on her lap while the physician is doing part of the examination, or the mother may help in restraining the child during a procedure or part of the examination). Ask the parent if the child knows why she or he is seeing the physician. The child deserves to be told the truth. When the parent and child are ready to leave the office, always check to see if either one still has questions. Reconfirm the information that the parent and patient have received, check if they both understand it, and check if the physician explained things to their satisfaction. Follow that by setting up the next appointment if one is needed.

When scheduling appointments, avoid having a lot of children in the reception room at the same time. When possible schedule well-child visits at certain hours of the day and sick-child visits at other times. In this way you can avoid exposing well children to sick children who may have an infectious disease that could be readily transmitted.

Growth Patterns

Assessing growth and development of a child requires measuring and comparing the child's growth and development with that of other children within the same age group. *Length/stature* and *weight* should be measured and plotted on a standardized chart (Figure 4-42) at least five times during the first year of life and then yearly through adolescence at

Fig 4-40 *Pediatric patient history.*

PEDIATRIC PATIENT HISTORY

Name: _____ Birthdate: _____ Age: _____
     last   first

Phone number: home (H) _____ work (W) _____

Informant: (indicate relationship to child) _____
Previous pediatrician _____ Location _____

_____

Present concerns (if "none", please state):

Past medical history
Birth history: Birthplace (indicate hospital) _____

HISTORY OF PREGNANCY

1. Illness	No	Yes
2. Drugs/medicine	No	Yes
3. Prematurity	No	Yes
4. Hospitalized	No	Yes
5. Bleeding	No	Yes
6. Smoking	No	Yes
7. Drinking	No	Yes
8. Other	_____	

Comments on "Yes" responses

LABOR AND DELIVERY

9. Caesarean section	No	Yes
10. Prolonged	No	Yes
11. Complications	No	Yes

Newborn History birth weight _____

12. Prolonged stay	No	Yes
13. Yellow jaundice	No	Yes
14. Other		

CHILD'S HISTORY (AS APPLICABLE)

1. Allergies to		
a. medications	No	Yes
b. others	No	Yes
2. Childhood illnesses		
a. ear infections	No	Yes
b. chickenpox	No	Yes
c. strep throat	No	Yes
d. other	No	Yes

3. Dental problems	No	Yes
4. Injuries/poisonings	No	Yes
5. Emergency room visits	No	Yes
6. Vaccination reactions	No	Yes
7. Hospitalizations	No	Yes
8. Surgeries	No	Yes
9. Blood transfusions	No	Yes
10. Current medications	No	Yes

Comments on "Yes" responses:

Fig 4-40—cont'd *Pediatric patient history.*

GROWTH AND DEVELOPMENT (AS APPLICABLE)

Nutrition

Breastfed	No	Yes	
if yes, how long? _____			
problems with?	No	Yes	
feeding	No	Yes	
weight	No	Yes	
anemia	No	Yes	
other _____			
Sleeping difficulties	No	Yes	

Bowel/bladder habits

Bedwetting	No	Yes
Constipation/soiling	No	Yes
Diarrhea	No	Yes
Toilet-trained	No	Yes

Behavioral problems

At home	No	Yes
At school	No	Yes
With peers	No	Yes

Development

Do you have specific concerns about your child's physical, language, or social development?   No   Yes

Comments on "Yes" responses:

Education (if applicable):

Name and location of child's day care or school:

Grade level:

Is your child's performance thought to be satisfactory?:

Family history

Any immediate family members who have a special medical problem or who
are on special medications?   No   Yes _____

Any immediate family members who have died of medical reasons under the
age of 50?   No   Yes _____

Any immediate family members with the following conditions?

Allergies (asthma, eczema)	No	Yes
High cholesterol, triglycerides	No	Yes
Tuberculosis or positive skin test	No	Yes
Anemia, blood disorder or bleeding	No	Yes
Diabetes	No	Yes
Visual or hearing problems	No	Yes
Speech or learning problems	No	Yes
High blood pressure	No	Yes
Heart disease	No	Yes
Cancer	No	Yes
Seizure disorder (fits)	No	Yes
Alcoholism/drug dependency	No	Yes
Birth defects	No	Yes
Mental disorder	No	Yes
Liver or liver problems	No	Yes
Sudden infant death (crib death)	No	Yes

Fig 4-40—cont'd *Pediatric patient history.*

Family environment

Are there any special circumstances the could potentially have
an impact on the health of your child?   No   Yes

Family Unit

Persons living at home (indicate age and relation to patient)

       Usual language(s) spoken at home:
       Usual caretaker(s) of child:

Family resources

Occupation of family members

Father	Place of work	WK No.
Mother	Place of work	WK No.
	Place of work	WK No.
	Place of work	WK No.

Family pedigree (to be completed by physician):

Signature_____   Reviewed by_____M.D.
                                   Date_____
      (relationship to child)

Additional comments:

each physical examination. Length and weight should be obtained on a newborn to use as a baseline. The average length for a newborn is 18 to 20 inches. The average weight of a newborn ranges from 7 to 7 1/2 pounds. Male infants on the average are usually longer and heavier than the female infant.

The growth charts show the growth pattern of the child over time. They can give the physician an indication as to whether the child is maintaining his/her own growth pattern as compared to the accepted ranges. Any child who is plotted on the chart and is found to be in the fifth percentile or lower or in the 95th percentile or higher requires a careful evaluation. The most common causes of a child's growth deviation from the accepted norm on the chart are related to the genetic influences of both parents and grandparents and to nourishment (see Table 4-6).

Another measurement that is routinely measured and plotted on the chart is the *head circumference*. When comparing the head circumference with the *chest circumference,* height, and weight, the physician can determine if the head is growing normally or if a pathologic condition may exist. Head circumference is usually measured in children under 36 months of age or in any child whose head size appears abnormal. At birth the infant's head circumference exceeds the chest circumference by 1 inch (2 to 3 cm). At age 1 to 2 years, the head circumference equals the chest circumference, and during childhood, the chest circumference will exceed the head circumference by about 2 to 3 inches (5 to 7 cm).

Recording growth patterns The medical assistant may be responsible for taking these measurements and plotting the results on the growth carts (see Figure 4-42).

1. To record the results on the growth charts, follow the following procedure.
   a. In the vertical column locate the length or stature or weight of the child. (Record recumbent length on 0 to 36-month chart and status on 2- to 18-year chart.)
   b. In the horizontal column locate the child's age.
   c. Using imaginary lines extending from these values, locate the point at which the two lines would cross on the graph.
   d. Place an "X" at this location on the chart.
2. To determine the percentile in which the child is compared to that of other children, proceed as follows.
   a. From the marked "X," follow the percentile line or the area between the two percentile lines upward to the right side of the chart.
   b. Read the percentile value located on the right side of the chart.

Vital Signs

Temperature. Many now recommend that the temperature be take by the axilla method in children up to the age of 5 to 6 years and then orally. In the past, for most children under the age of 5 years, the temperature was taken rectally. The rectal method is used less frequently now because of the possibility of causing trauma to the rectal area and because there have been cultural complaints from the parents about penetrating the child's body with a thermometer. If there is any doubt as to the accuracy of the axilla or oral temperature, the rectal method should be used. Also, when the child is very sick or septic, a rectal temperature is still the method of choice. In many facilities the use of tympanic thermometry is becoming more common. See Unit Two for the procedures for all of the methods listed.

Pulse. The pulse rate in children is usually obtained apically or radially. Take an apical pulse in children under 2 years of age. In a child the pulse rate should be counted for a full minute since, frequently there are some normal irregularities. See Unit Two for the procedure for taking a pulse rate.

Respiration rate. Count the respiration rate for a full minute. Note the rate, rhythm, and any retractions. See Unit Two for the procedure for taking the respiratory rate.

Text continues on page 153.

Figure 4-41 **A,** *Make a game of the procedure;* **B,** *Let the child listen to his or her own heartbeat;* **C,** *Wong-Baker Faces Pain Rating Scale.*

A
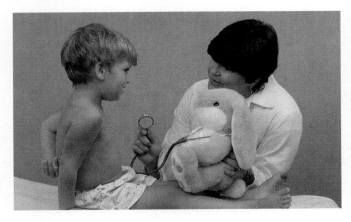

B
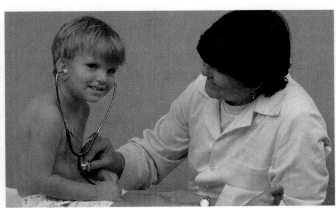

Figure 4-41—cont'd   C, *Wong-Baker Faces Pain Rating Scale.*

From Wong D, Whaley L: *Clinical manual of pediatric nursing,* ed 4, St. Louis, 1993, Mosby.

C

Pain scale	Instructions	Comments
Faces Scale* (Wong and Baker, 1988)	Explain to child that each face is for a person who feels happy because there is no pain (hurt) or sad because there is some or a lot of pain. Face 0 is very happy because there is no hurt. Face 1 hurts just a little bit. Face 2 hurts a little more. Face 3 hurts even more. Face 4 hurts a whole lot, but Face 5 hurts as much as you can imagine, although you don't have to be crying to feel this bad. Ask child to choose face that best describes how the pain feels.	Can be used with children as young as 3 years.

| 0 | 1 | 2 | 3 | 4 | 5 |

Pain scale	Instructions	Comments
Poker Chip (Hester, 1979, 1989)	Use four red plastic (poker) chips. Explain to child that these are "pieces of hurt." One piece is a "little bit of hurt," and four pieces is the "most hurt." Ask child to choose number of pieces that describes the pain. If child replies "no pain," record a 0.	Recommended for children as young as 4½ years.
Color Tool (Eland, 1985)	Ask child to identify things that have hurt in the past and what has hurt the worst. Give child 8 crayons or markers (yellow, orange, red, green, blue, purple, brown, and black) in a random order. Ask child which color is like the worst pain experienced. Place that crayon or marker aside and ask child to identify crayon that is like a hurt not quite as bad as the worst hurt. Place that crayon aside and ask which other crayon is like something that hurts just a little. Place that crayon with the others and ask child which crayon is like no hurt at all. Show four crayon choices to child in order from worst hurt color to no hurt color. Ask child to show on body outline where it hurts using crayon of color that most nearly is like the pain feeling. When colors are ranked, assign them a numeric value of 0 to 3.	Recommended for children as young as 4 years provided children know their colors and are not color blind.
Oucher† (Beyer, 1988)	Consists of six photographs of child's face representing "no hurt" to "biggest hurt you could ever have." Child chooses face that most nearly describes the pain. Also includes a vertical scale with numbers from 0 to 100. Child chooses number that best describes the pain.	Photographic scale may be appropriate for children as young as 3 years; use numeric scale for children who can count to 100 by ones.
Numeric Scale	Explain to child that at one end of the line is a 0, which means that a person feels no pain (hurt). At the other end is a 10, which means the person feels the worst pain imaginable. The numbers 1 to 9 are for a very little pain to a whole lot of pain. Ask child to choose the number that best describes how the pain feels.	May be appropriate for children as young as 5 years, although children who cannot count may have difficulty with scale.

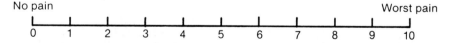

No pain ───────────────────────────── Worst pain

0   1   2   3   4   5   6   7   8   9   10

Pain scale	Instructions	Comments
Simple Descriptive Scale	Explain to child that at one end of line is *no pain* because person feels no hurt. At the other end is *worst pain* because person feels the worst pain imaginable. The words in between are *mild* for just a little pain, *moderate* for a little more, *quite a lot* for even more, and *very bad* for a whole lot of pain. Ask child to choose word that best describes how the pain feels.	May be appropriate for children as young as 5 years, although words may need explanation.

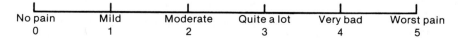

No pain   Mild   Moderate   Quite a lot   Very bad   Worst pain
0   1   2   3   4   5

*Available from Purdue Frederick Company, 100 Connecticut Avenue, Norwalk, CT 06856 (1-800-243-5667, ext 4010).

†Available from Judith E. Beyer, PhD, RN, School of Nursing, University of Colorado Health Sciences Center, Campus Box C-288, 4200 E 9th Avenue, Denver, CO 80262 (303) 270-4317.

(Figures may be photocopied for clinical use.)

Figure 4-42 *Growth charts.*

Reprinted with permission of Ross Laboratories, Columbus, Ohio.

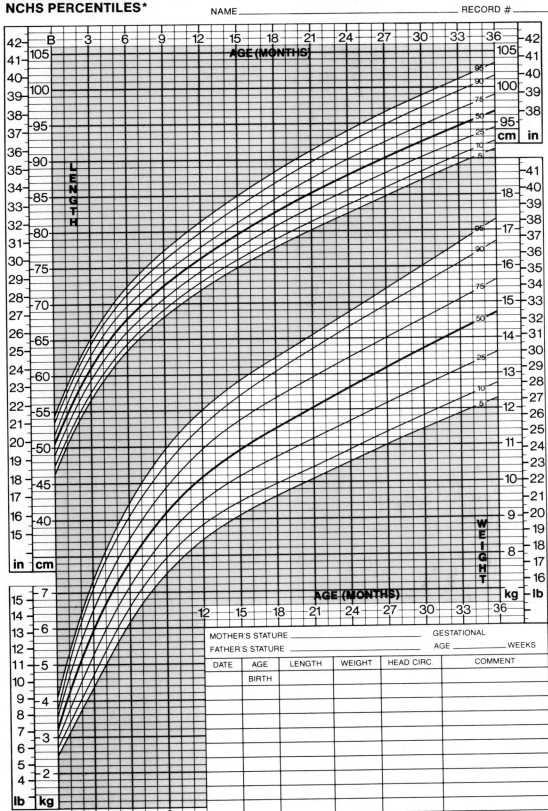

BOYS: BIRTH TO 36 MONTHS
PHYSICAL GROWTH
NCHS PERCENTILES*

Figure 4-42—cont'd *Growth charts.*
Reprinted with permission of Ross Laboratories, Columbus, Ohio.

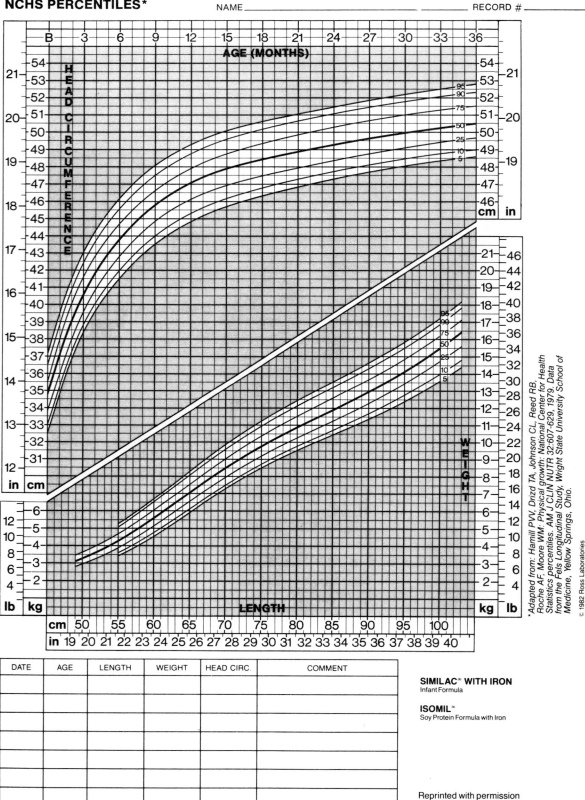

BOYS: BIRTH TO 36 MONTHS
PHYSICAL GROWTH
NCHS PERCENTILES*

NAME _____ RECORD # _____

DATE	AGE	LENGTH	WEIGHT	HEAD CIRC.	COMMENT

*Adapted from: Hamill PVV, Drizd TA, Johnson CL, Reed RB, Roche AF, Moore WM: Physical growth: National Center for Health Statistics percentiles. AM J CLIN NUTR 32:607-629, 1979. Data from the Fels Longitudinal Study, Wright State University School of Medicine, Yellow Springs, Ohio.

© 1982 Ross Laboratories

SIMILAC® WITH IRON
Infant Formula

ISOMIL®
Soy Protein Formula with Iron

Reprinted with permission
of Ross Laboratories

Figure 4-42—cont'd *Growth charts.*
Reprinted with permission of Ross Laboratories, Columbus, Ohio.

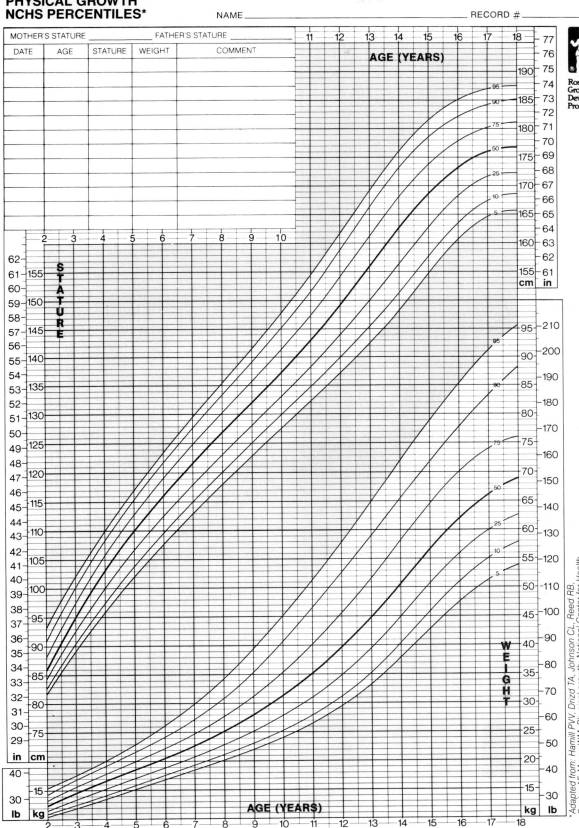

Figure 4-42—cont'd *Growth charts.*
Reprinted with permission of Ross Laboratories, Columbus, Ohio.

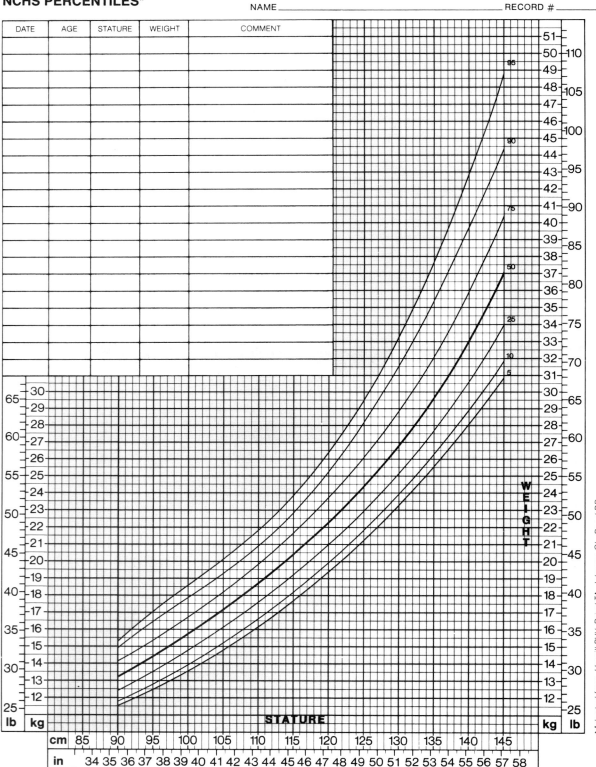

Figure 4-42—cont'd *Growth charts.*
Reprinted with permission of Ross Laboratories, Columbus, Ohio.

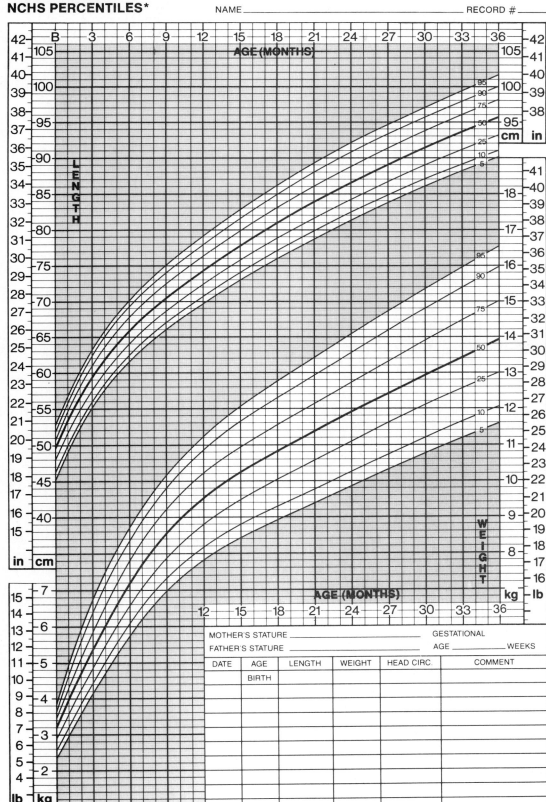

GIRLS: BIRTH TO 36 MONTHS
PHYSICAL GROWTH
NCHS PERCENTILES*

Figure 4-42—cont'd *Growth charts.*

Reprinted with permission of Ross Laboratories, Columbus, Ohio.

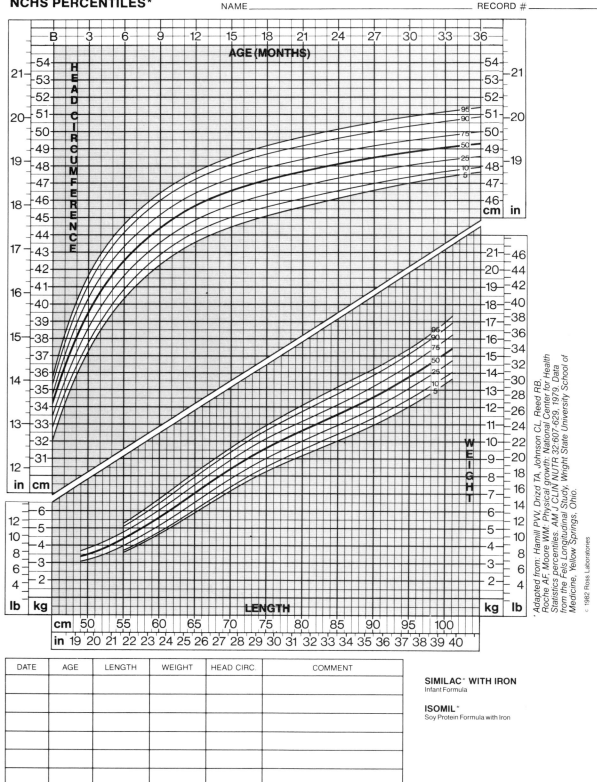

GIRLS: BIRTH TO 36 MONTHS
PHYSICAL GROWTH
NCHS PERCENTILES*

NAME _____ RECORD # _____

* Adapted from: Hamill PVV, Drizd TA, Johnson CL, Reed RB, Roche AF, Moore WM: Physical growth: National Center for Health Statistics percentiles. AM J CLIN NUTR 32:607-629, 1979. Data from the Fels Longitudinal Study, Wright State University School of Medicine, Yellow Springs, Ohio.

© 1982 Ross Laboratories

DATE	AGE	LENGTH	WEIGHT	HEAD CIRC.	COMMENT

SIMILAC® WITH IRON
Infant Formula

ISOMIL®
Soy Protein Formula with Iron

Reprinted with permission
of Ross Laboratories

Figure 4-42—cont'd *Growth charts.*

Reprinted with permission of Ross Laboratories, Columbus, Ohio.

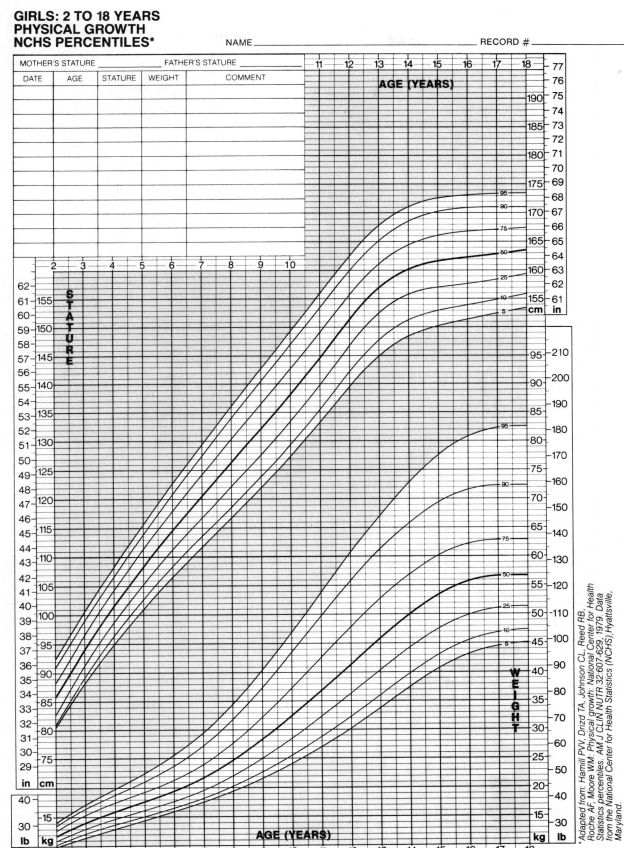

GIRLS: 2 TO 18 YEARS PHYSICAL GROWTH NCHS PERCENTILES*

Figure 4-42—cont'd *Growth charts.*

Reprinted with permission of Ross Laboratories, Columbus, Ohio.

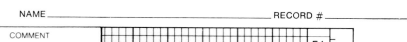

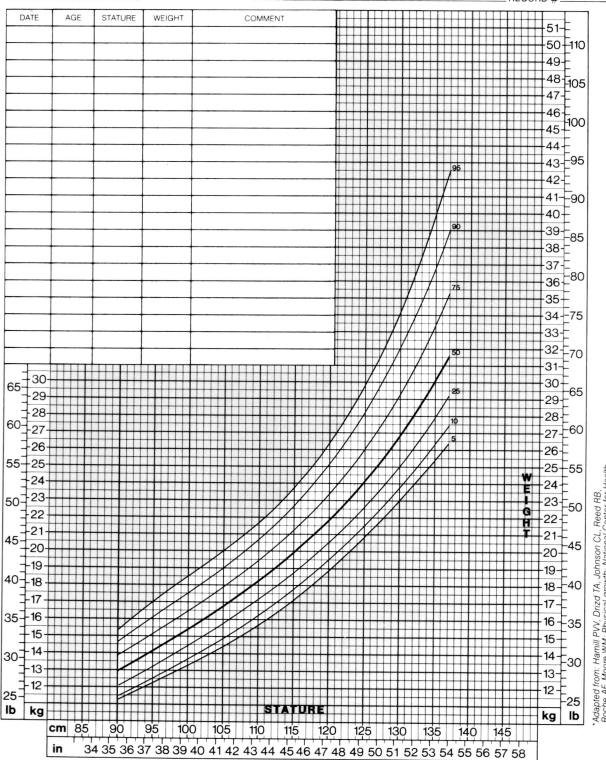

GIRLS: PREPUBESCENT
PHYSICAL GROWTH
NCHS PERCENTILES*

*Adapted from: Hamill PVV, Drizd TA, Johnson CL, Reed RB, Roche AF, Moore WM: Physical growth: National Center for Health Statistics percentiles. AM J CLIN NUTR 32:607-629, 1979. Data from the National Center for Health Statistics (NCHS) Hyattsville, Maryland.

SIMILAC® WITH IRON
Infant Formula

ISOMIL®
Soy Protein Formula with Iron

Reprinted with permission
of Ross Laboratories

Blood pressure. Take the blood pressure before the child becomes excited. Blood pressure in a child can be measured by either the auscultation or the palpation method. The size of the cuff is important for both of these methods. See Unit Two for the procedures for taking a blood pressure and the recommended size of cuff to use. In many facilities automatic blood pressure monitors are used. One such monitor is the Dinamap adult/pediatric monitor. The machine is set according to the manufacturer's directions, the cuff is placed on the patient's arm, the machine is turned on, and the results are displayed on the monitor within seconds.

Blood pressure should be measured once a year in children 3 years of age through adolescence, in children with a tendency toward hypertension, and in high-risk infants.

Techniques for Carrying an Infant

When lifting or carrying an infant, you must provide for his or her safety and comfort. You must always provide support for the infant's head and neck because the muscles in these areas are not as strong at this age as they will be in the future years. Three basic carrying and lifting techniques follow.

Cradle position. When you carry the infant in the cradle position, you support the head, buttocks, and back adequately by your arms (Figure 4-43).
*   Slide your left arm under the infant's head and back and gently grasp the infant's upper arm with your hand.
*   Slide your right arm up and under the infants buttocks. Let your hand provide support for the infant's back.
*   The infant is cradled in your arms with his/her body resting against your chest.

Upright position. With fingers spread apart, put your right hand against the infant's head and neck. Always support the head and neck until the infant can do so for himself or herself (Figure 4-44).
*   Put your left forearm under the infant's buttocks. This supports the weight of the infant.
*   Allow the infant to rest against your chest with the cheek on your shoulder. The infant's head should not come in contact with your face.

Football position. In the football position you support the infant's head with your hand and the neck and back with your forearm, and you maintain a firm hold by supporting the infant's buttocks between your hip and elbow (Figure 4-45).
*   With fingers spread, place your left hand under the infant's head and neck.
*   The infant's back rests on your forearm.
*   Maintain security by gently pressing the infant's buttocks between your hip and elbow.

This position is very useful when you need your other hand free for another activity.

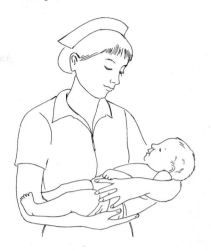

Figure 4-43 *Cradle position.*

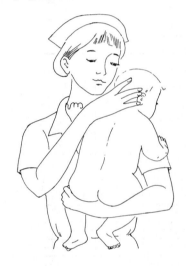

Figure 4-44 *Upright position.*

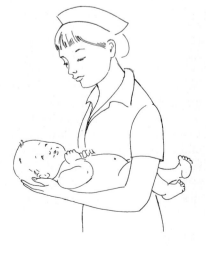

Figure 4-45 *Football position.*

Measuring the Weight of an Infant

It is important to weigh an infant accurately because the weight reflects the status of the infant and is used for determining nutritional needs and medication dosages when administered. A baby scale or pediatric scale is used for children up to 14 months of age. This is a basket-type scale (Figure 4-46). When the child can stand alone, a regular scale is used (see Unit Two), or the parent may hold the child on a regular scale, in which case the parent's weight is subtracted from the total weight of parent and child together. The procedure for using a pediatric scale follows.

1. Wash your hands. **Use appropriate personal protective equipment (PPE) as indicated by facility.**
2. Identify the infant.
3. Explain the procedure to the parent/caregiver.
4. Place a clean, impervious paper on the scale basket. Do not use linen to drape the scale because fluids such as urine may seep through the material and contaminate the scale. The paper drape on the scale *must* be changed between each infant. The use of a drape on the scale makes the surface warmer for the infant and also prevents the indirect spread of infection.
5. Ensure that the scale is balanced after the drape has been placed on it.
6. Undress the infant *or* have the parent undress the infant.
7. Gently place the infant in the basket of the scale, face facing up.
8. Place your hand over the infant to protect him or her from falling. Do not touch the infant (see Figure 4-46).
9. Adjust the weight on the scale. Adjust the pound weight and then the ounce weight. Read the results in pounds and ounces.
10. Return the weights to zero.
11. Remove the infant from the sale. You may have the parent hold the infant while you record the weight or you may proceed to measure the infant.
12. Record the infant's weight in the chart. Give the time, date, and infant's age. Sign your name.
13. Remove and discard the drape.

NOTE: Weigh older children in their underwear (no shoes) standing on an upright scale (see the weighing procedure in Unit Two). When recording the weight, indicate what the child was wearing when weighed.

The procedure for weighing an adolescent is the same as the procedure for weighing an adult (see Unit Two).

Measuring the Length of an Infant

To determine the length of a child up to 24 to 36 months, you measure the recumbent length (Figure 4-47). This is the measurement from the top of the head to the heels of the feet when the child is lying flat and straight with toes pointing upward. Older children can be measured in a standing position on a scale with a height bar as described in Unit Two or by having the child stand erect with back to the wall (with shoes removed) against a measuring scale. Standing height is

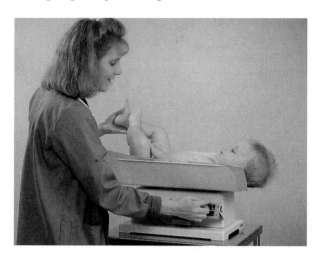

Figure 4-46 A, *Weighing an infant lying on a scale;* B, *weighing an infant sitting on a scale.*

A

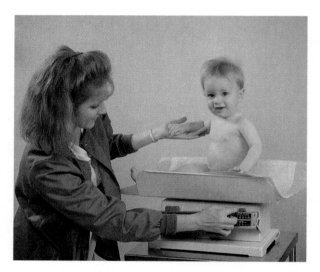

B

also referred to as stature. Note this on the growth charts in Figure 4-42. The procedure for measuring length follows.

1. Wash your hands. **Use appropriate personal protective equipment (PPE) as indicated by facility.**
2. Identify the infant.
3. Explain the procedure to the parent/caregiver. You may wish to ask the parent for help in supporting the infant while you take the measurement.
4. Have a clean disposable drape on the examining table.
5. Place the infant on the back of the disposable drape.
6. Place the vertex (top) of the head at the beginning of the measuring tape.
7. Grasp the knees and gently push them toward the table so that the infant's legs are fully extended. While you are extending the infant's legs, the parent can be holding and supporting the infant's head in position.

Figure 4-47 *Measuring the length of an infant.*

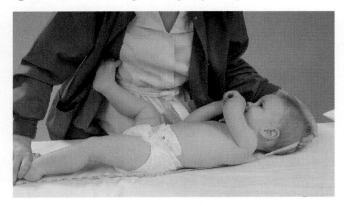

Figure 4-48 *Measuring the head circumference of an infant.*

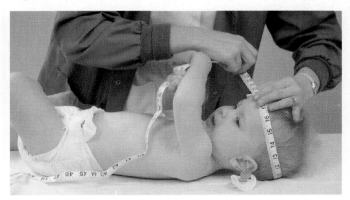

8. Take the measurements from the top of the infant's head to the heels of the feet with the toes pointing upward.

9. If you are doing this procedure alone, position the infant's head and draw a pencil mark on the disposable drape at the tip of the head. Then grasp and straighten the knees and draw another pencil mark on the disposable drape where the heels of the feet are. Remove the infant from the table and provide for his or her safety. With a tape measure, measure the distance between the head and feet marks. This gives you the length of the infant.

10. Record the measurement on the infant's chart. If required, record the measurement on the infant's growth chart. Give the date, time, and infant's age and sign your name to the record.

Measuring Head Circumference

To measure the infant's head circumference place the infant in a supine position or have the parent hold the him or her. Place a measuring tape around the greatest circumference of the head (that is, from slightly above the eyebrows and top point of the earlobes to the occipital prominence of the skull in the back of the head) (Figure 4-48).

Measuring Chest Circumference

Place the infant in a supine position. Place a measuring tape around the chest and across the nipple line. Ideally, take a measurement during inspiration and a measurement during expiration. Take the average of these two measurements as the chest circumference.

Obtaining a Urine Specimen from a Child Who is not Toilet Trained

A plastic disposable urine collector can be affixed to the perineal area of an infant to obtain a urine specimen. Wearing gloves, clean the perineal area of the infant with soap and water or other cleansing agent. Dry the skin thoroughly. Peel off the gummed backing on the urine collector; spread the infant's legs apart and place the adhesive portion of the bag firmly against the infant's perineal region (Figure 4-49, *A* and *B*). The adhesive adheres to the skin. To aid the flow of urine by gravity, you can place the infant in a sitting position. Check the bag frequently until the desired amount of urine is obtained. When the desired amount of urine is voided, remove the bag. Hold it against the child's skin at the bottom and gently peel the adhesive from the skin from top to bottom. Transfer the urine to a specimen bottle. The specimen is now ready to be tested in the office, you should prepare it to be sent to the laboratory for testing (see Unit Eleven).

SICK-CHILD VISITS

Any sign or symptom of illness or disease should be evaluated by the physician to ensure proper and adequate diagnosis and treatment. Follow-up visits or phone calls to note the patient's progress are also very important.

Today it is possible for children to be treated in the physician's office for illnesses that once required hospitalization. For example, children suffering from a variety of childhood infections can receive injectable antibiotics in the office. Also, many outpatient treatments for children with asthma or those who need potent antibiotics are available, and some of these can even be administered in the home. The physician discusses the diagnosis, treatment, and home care for the specific illness with the parent and the patient if he/she is old enough to understand. Both parent and patient must understand medication directions and any other directions.

Phenylketonuria

Phenylketonuria (PKU) is an inherited disease that must be diagnosed early to avoid serious brain damage and mental retardation. Although it is not a common condition, it is thought to affect one in every 10,000 births. This disease is characterized by a deficiency in the liver enzyme, phenylalanine hydroxylase, which is essential for converting phenylalanine to tyrosine. Phenylalanine is an essential amino acid that is necessary for growth. Any excess of phenylalanine in the body should be converted to tyrosine. However, a newborn with PKU is unable to convert any excess.

Figure 4-49 **A** *and* **B,** *Obtaining a urine specimen from a child who is not toilet trained.*
Boy sketch from Sorrentino S: *Mosby's textbook for nursing assistants*, ed 3, St. Louis, 1992, Mosby.

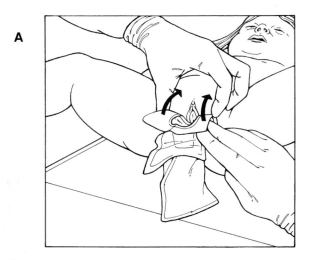

A

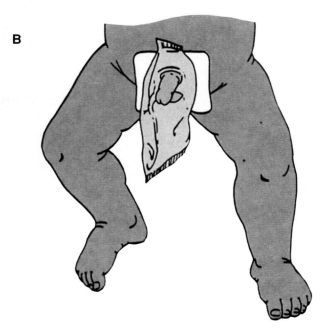

B

Phenylalanine and its metabolites then accumulate in the body and can lead to severe developmental delays and other neurologic problems. Eventually the phenylalanine spills over into the urine. If the condition is not treated, severe mental retardation and brain damage can result. Dietary control is used to help regulate the amount of phenylalanine present in the body. This therapy must begin early because, if the amount of phenylalanine is not restricted, mental retardation progresses.

Blood and urine tests are available to diagnose PKU. The most common blood test is the Guthrie test. The Guthrie blood test is required in all states in an effort to screen new-

borns for PKU. This test is normally done before the newborn is discharged from the hospital. If it is not done in the hospital, arrangements should be made to have it done as soon as possible after discharge. Proper timing for this test is important. The newborn must have ingested an ample amount of phenylalanine, which is a constituent of both human and cow's milk. Therefore it is recommended that this test not be performed before the infant has had breast feedings or formula for 2 to 3 days.

A urine test (either the diaper test or the Phenistix test) is usually done 6 weeks after birth and frequently at the infant's first checkup. If the first test was negative, this follow-up test is usually done to ensure that the first test was not a false-negative as a result of inadequate ingestion of milk. It is also done to ensure identification of all those with the deficiency so that special dietary protocols can be begun. When the urine PKU test is positive, a blood phenylalanine test should be performed to confirm the findings.

Before any of the tests are performed:
- Explain to the parent(s) the purpose of the test and the procedure.
- Assess the infant's eating patterns. The test must be done 2 to 3 days after milk feedings. Inadequate amounts of ingested protein before the test can cause false-negative results.
- Check the infant's age. Urine tests are recommended for infants who are at least 6 weeks of age.
- Complete the information section on the test card.

Diaper test. This urine test to screen for PKU is *not* to be used until the infant is at least 6 weeks old. The diaper test is frequently performed at the infant's first checkup after discharge from the hospital.

Drop 10% ferric chloride on a diaper that contains fresh urine. A green spot on the diaper is considered to be a positive result. This test indicates the *possibility* of PKU.

Phenistix test. This urine test to screen for PKU is not to be used until the infant is at least 6 weeks old. The Phenistix test is frequently performed at the infant's first checkup after discharge from the hospital or 6 weeks after delivery. It is not accurate unless the infant is at least 6 weeks old.

Press a Phenistix test reagent strip against a diaper containing urine *OR* dip a Phenistix reagent strip into a urine specimen. Compare color changes on the reagent strip with the color chart on the reagent strip bottle. A green color reaction indicates probable PKU.

Positive test results. When all tests are positive, the infant is put on a formula low in phenylalanine such as Lofenalac. Since phenylalanine is necessary for growth, it must be included in the diet. Severe neurologic impairment can be prevented if the patient remains on a diet low in phenylalanine. There is disagreement as to how long this special diet must be followed. Some believe that it should be maintained

GUTHRIE TEST

Equipment

PKU Guthrie test card (filter paper) (Figure 4-50)
Mailing envelope for the test card
Sterile lancet

Alcohol sponge
Cotton balls
Disposable single-use exam gloves

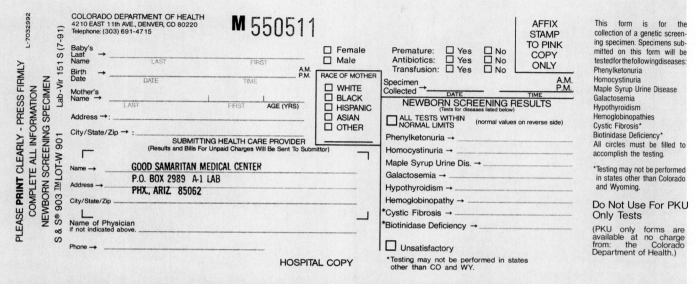

Figure 4-50 *PKU Test Card. Fill in the requested information before obtaining the specimen.*

PROCEDURE

1. Wash your hands, assemble equipment, and don disposable single-use exam gloves. **Use appropriate personal protective equipment (PPE) as indicated by facility.**

2. Place the infant prone on a flat surface. Make the heel accessible.

3. Grasp the infant's heel and cleanse with the alcohol sponge. Allow the alcohol to dry.

4. Grasp the infant's heel. With the sterile lancet, puncture the side of the heal at a right angle (Figure 4-51). The puncture should be at right angles to the lines on the skin and approximately 2 to 3 mm deep.

5. Wipe away the first drop of blood.

6. Collect the next drops of blood in the circles on the special test filter paper (Figure 4-52). Press the filter paper against the infant's heel and exert enough gentle pressure to obtain an adequate sample.

7. Fill each of the circles on the test card with blood. The blood must soak through the filter paper from one side to the other.

8. Apply pressure with a cotton ball to the puncture site.

9. Observe the infant after collecting the specimen.

10. Remove your gloves and wash your hands.

RATIONALE

This position lessens the opportunity for the infant to kick at you.

The first drop of blood may be diluted with tissue fluid.

An adequate sample is required for testing. The test would have to be repeated if the blood sample was not adequate.

This aids in controlling bleeding from the puncture site.

Ensure that clotting takes place and bleeding is prevented.

GUTHRIE TEST—cont'd

PROCEDURE

11. Allow the test card to dry on a nonabsorbent surface. Do not stack cards on top of one another. Drying takes approximately 2 hours.

12. Record the procedure in the patient's chart.
Record on the lab slip the infant's date and time of birth and the number of days taking milk, in addition to the usual identifying information requested.

13. Place the dry test card in the protective envelope supplied with the test card and send it to the laboratory within 48 hours for testing.

RATIONALE

A wet specimen cannot be sent in the protective envelope. This would cause contamination plus invalidate the test.

Charting Example:
Oct. 10, 19___, 2 p.m.
Rt heel puncture for PKU testing. Specimen on filter paper sent to laboratory at 4 p.m. Small amount of bleeding after heel puncture. Mother instructed about the test and gave permission. She expressed interest in the results.
J.A. Lee, SMA

The laboratory should receive the test within 48 hours to ensure accurate testing.

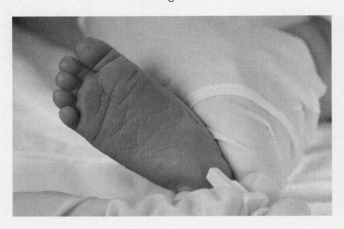

Figure 4-51 *Grasp the infant's heel. Using a sterile lancet puncture the side of the heel at a right angle to obtain a blood sample.*

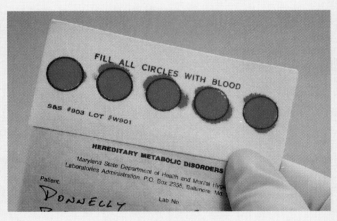

Figure 4-52 *Collect drops of blood in the circles on the special PKU test filter paper. Fill each of the circles with blood.*

for life; others suggest that it should continue through the sixth year of life when maximum brain development occurs. Therefore close supervision and long-term follow-up, especially nutritional counseling, is very important. Explanation, counseling, and support must be provided for the parents of the infant. The dietary treatment is monitored by urine and blood testing.

A woman who has PKU and wants to become pregnant should be instructed to begin a low-phenylalanine diet before conception and continue it throughout the pregnancy (assuming that she has not been following this type of diet for some time). If the woman continues on a general diet, the risk of having a mentally retarded infant is very high.

Intramuscular, Subcutaneous, and Intradermal Injections

The technique for administering injections in a child are the same as those used for an adult. See Unit Eight and Figure 4-53. The child may need to be restrained before the injection is given. Another person should help you with this. Even the parent can hold and restrain the child while you are administering the medication. Tell the child that the medicine will help him orher to feel better and that it will hurt a little bit but only for a very short time. Praise the child after the injection is given, telling the child how brave he or she was. You or the parent can give an infant a hug. Give the child something to play with after the injection is given. This helps to distract the child and allows him or her to associate something pleasant with the experience other than discomfort. You can also place an adhesive strip with a happy face decoration over the puncture mark. This can be comforting to the child and provides a distraction.

Immunizations

Immunization is the process of rendering a person immune (protected from or not susceptible to a disease) or of becoming immune. It is frequently called vaccination or inoculation. Immunization is a process by which a person is artificially prepared to resist infection by a specific pathogen. Immunity, the antigen-antibody reaction, and the different types of immunity are discussed in Unit Five.

Several vaccines are available for routine use to protect children from many communicable diseases. They should be administered according to a standardized schedule during well-child visits. Common vaccines available include the following:

- Diphtheria and tetanus toxoid combined with tetanus vaccine (DPT). This is given intramuscularly.
- Diphtheria, tetanus toxoid (Td or DT). This is given intramuscularly.
- Trivalent oral polio vaccine (OPV). This is given by mouth.
- Measles (rubeola), mumps (parotitis), and rubella (German measles [MMR]). This is given subcutaneously.
- *Haemophilus* b polysaccharide vaccine (HBPV) (also called hemophilus influenza type b vaccine). This is given intramuscularly.
- Hepatitis B vaccine (in late 1992 specialists started to recommend hepatitis B vaccine for all children under 6 years of age). This is given intramuscularly.

Medical assistants should be familiar with the different types of vaccinations given, the use of each, the contraindications, the possible side effects, the dosage, the route of administration, and the methods of storage and handling. Package inserts are provided with each vaccine with valuable information. Drug reference books can also be used for obtaining the necessary information. Also see Table 4-7, Appendix D, and Figure 4-54.

Before a child receives a vaccination, information must be provided to the parent/caregiver both verbally and in writing. Forms containing information for each immunization must be given to the parent so that he or she understands the importance of the immunization and the possible side effects. After reading this form, the parents must sign a consent form if he or she agrees to have the infant or child immunized (Figure 4-54). Once immunized, an immunization card should be given to the parents for their permanent home records. This record may also be needed for school and/or travel purposes.

The National Childhood Vaccine Injury Act of 1988 requires the following information to be recorded in the child's permanent medical record for all childhood mandated vaccinations.

1. Type, manufacturer, and lot number of the vaccine.
2. Date of administration.
3. Name, address, and title of the person administering the vaccine.

Other information that is suggested to be recorded includes:

1. The site and route of administration.
2. The expiration date of the vaccine.

Figure 4-53 *Intramuscular injection sites in children. A, Vastus lateralis; B, ventrogluteal; C, dorsogluteal; D, deltoid.*
From Wong D, Whaley L: *Clinical manual of pediatric nursing*, ed 4, St. Louis, 1993, Mosby.

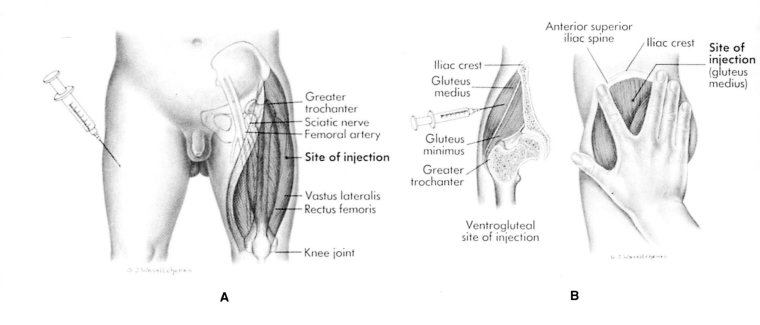

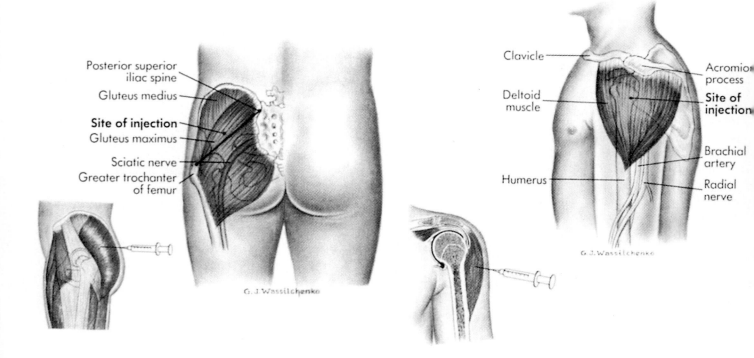

Figure 4-54 *A to C, Immunization consent forms.*

Reproduced with permission from Kaiser Permanente, The Permanente Medical Group, Inc., 1993.

KAISER PERMANENTE
Kaiser Foundation Hospitals
The Permanente Medical Group, Inc.

☐ Antioch	☐ Hayward	☐ Oakland	☐ Richmond	☐ San Rafael	☐ Stockton
☐ Davis	☐ Martinez	☐ Park Shadelands	☐ Roseville	☐ Santa Clara	☐ Vallejo
☐ Fairfield	☐ Milpitas	☐ Petaluma	☐ Sacramento	☐ Santa Rosa	☐ Walnut Crk
☐ Fremont	☐ Mt. View	☐ Pleasanton	☐ San Francisco	☐ Santa Teresa	
☐ Fresno	☐ Napa	☐ Rncho Crdva	☐ S F (French)	☐ So. Sacto.	
☐ Gilroy	☐ Novato	☐ Rdwd Cty	☐ San Jose	☐ So. S.F.	

ROUTINE CHILDHOOD IMMUNIZATIONS:
INFORMATION AND CONSENT

IMPRINT AREA

In the United States today, immunization is routinely recommended for all healthy children and adolescents for the following diseases: diphtheria, tetanus, pertussis (commonly abbreviated as DTP), poliomyelitis, measles, mumps, and rubella. Furthermore, vaccination against Haemophilus influenzae type B (HIB) is recommended for all children 5 years of age and under, and against hepatitis B virus (HBV) for all infants and certain people at increased risk (your physician will review these risks with you).

The following table gives the recommended schedule for the administration of those vaccines:

Birth – 2 months	Hepatitis B vaccine (HBV) #1
2 to 4 months	Hepatitis B vaccine #2
2 months	DTP #1; Polio #1; HIB #1
4 months	DTP #2; Polio #2; HIB #2
6 months	DTP #3; HIB #3
6 – 18 months	HBV #3
15 months	Measles-Mumps-Rubella (MMR) #1
15 – 24 months	DTP #4; Polio #3; HIB #4
4 – 6 years	DTP #5; Polio #4; Measles or MMR #2
14 – 16 years	Tetanus-Diphtheria (Td), repeat every 10 years

By signing below, the legal representative of the child, _____ (his/her parent or legal guardian) acknowledges the following:

1. I have received written documents explaining the severity of the above diseases and the risks and benefits of the vaccines. It is emphasized that most experts agree that the known benefits of immunization far outweigh the possible side effects of the vaccines.

2. I have been given appropriate information on how to evaluate and report any possible adverse effects of the vaccines. Any vaccine side effects should be reported to your child's physician or advice center, or to the federal government at 1-800-822-7967.

3. All of my questions have been adequately answered prior to my child receiving the vaccines.

4. I request that my child receives the routine immunizations as recommended above. Should any circumstances arise where I or my child's physician decide that any of the above vaccines may be contraindicated or no longer wanted, I will be able to revoke the consent for that/those particular vaccine(s), after discussion with my child's physician.

DATE	NAME OF CHILD	MEDICAL RECORD #
NAME OF LEGAL GUARDIAN	WITNESS	
SIGNATURE OF LEGAL GUARDIAN		

95804 (4-92)

Figure 4-54—cont'd *A to C, Immunization consent forms.*

Reproduced with permission from Kaiser Permanente, The Permanente Medical Group, Inc., 1993.

B

KAISER PERMANENTE
Kaiser Foundation Hospitals
The Permanente Medical Group, Inc.

☐ Antioch ☐ Hayward ☐ Oakland ☐ Richmond ☐ San Rafael ☐ Stockton
☐ Davis ☐ Martinez ☐ Park Shadelands ☐ Roseville ☐ Santa Clara ☐ Vallejo
☐ Fairfield ☐ Milpitas ☐ Petaluma ☐ Sacramento ☐ Santa Rosa ☐ Walnut Crk
☐ Fremont ☐ Mt. View ☐ Pleasanton ☐ San Francisco ☐ Santa Teresa
☐ Fresno ☐ Napa ☐ Rncho Crdva ☐ S F (French) ☐ So. Sacto.
☐ Gilroy ☐ Novato ☐ Rdwd Cty ☐ San Jose ☐ So. S.F.

INFORMATION ABOUT HEPATITIS B VACCINE FOR CHILDREN AND ADOLESCENTS

IMPRINT AREA

THE DISEASE:

Hepatitis B is a viral infection caused by hepatitis B virus (HBV) and affects 200,000 to 300,000 individuals in the US each year. It causes inflammation of the liver, jaundice, abdominal pains and loss of appetite. Most people recover completely, but 1-2% of infected individuals die from the acute infection, and 5-10% become chronic carriers of the virus. Carriers have no symptoms, but can transmit the virus to others, and may develop chronic liver disease, including cirrhosis and liver cancer. The virus is highly contagious through exposure to blood, blood stained secretions and other infected body fluids, through sexual contact, and from infected mothers to infants primarily at the time of birth.

THE VACCINE:

Hepatitis B vaccine is a non-infectious unit viral vaccine manufactured in a purified form by recombinant DNA technology using yeast cells. It is not a blood product. More than 95% of healthy individuals who receive 3 doses demonstrate evidence of protective antibodies (anti-HBs). Full immunization requires 3 doses. Persons who have already been infected with HBV will not benefit from immunization. The duration of immunity is unknown at this time, and the need for booster doses is not yet defined. The vaccine is contraindicated in patients with yeast hypersensitivity. This HBV vaccine is not protective against other causes of hepatitis.

POSSIBLE VACCINE SIDE EFFECTS

The vaccine does not cause hepatitis B infection. The incidence of side effects is very low, consisting primarily of soreness at the injection site. Low grade fever may occur. Rash, nausea, joint pain and mild fatigue have been reported. These side effects can be treated with analgesics. Any more severe reaction should be reported to your physician, the advice center, or to the federal government at 1-800-822-7967.

WHO SHOULD GET THE HEPATITIS B VACCINE?

1. All infants. The first dose is recommended between birth to 2 months of age, the 2nd dose at 2 to 4 months, and the 3rd dose between 6-18 months.
2. All adolescents in communities where there is a high risk of exposure to hepatitis B.
3. Other groups: all health care workers with patient contact, adults with new sexual partners, household contacts of patients with hepatitis B, and other individuals at risk for hepatitis B as advised by their physicians.

If you have any questions about hepatitis B or hepatitis B vaccine, please ask your doctor or our advice center.

CONSENT: I request the hepatitis B vaccine to be administered to my child or to me:

NAME OF VACCINE RECIPIENT	MEDICAL RECORD #
SIGNATURE/NAME OF VACCINE RECIPIENT OR LEGAL GUARDIAN	DATE

DECLINATION:

I have read the above statement and have had all my questions answered to my satisfaction.

☐ I decline to receive the hepatitis B vaccine.

☐ I decline to have the hepatitis B vaccine given to my child _____
NAME OF CHILD

WITNESS	DATE	SIGNATURE OF VACCINE RECIPIENT OR LEGAL GUARDIAN

95802 (4-92)

Figure 4-54—cont'd *A to C, Immunization consent forms.*

Reproduced with permission from Kaiser Permanente, The Permanente Medical Group, Inc., 1993.

KAISER PERMANENTE
Kaiser Foundation Hospitals
The Permanente Medical Group, Inc.

☐ Antioch	☐ Hayward	☐ Oakland	☐ Richmond	☐ San Rafael	☐ Stockton
☐ Davis	☐ Martinez	☐ Park Shadelands	☐ Roseville	☐ Santa Clara	☐ Vallejo
☐ Fairfield	☐ Milpitas	☐ Petaluma	☐ Sacramento	☐ Santa Rosa	☐ Walnut Crk
☐ Fremont	☐ Mt. View	☐ Pleasanton	☐ San Francisco	☐ Santa Teresa	
☐ Fresno	☐ Napa	☐ Rncho Crdva	☐ S F (French)	☐ So. Sacto.	
☐ Gilroy	☐ Novato	☐ Rdwd Cty	☐ San Jose	☐ So. S.F.	

IMMUNIZATION AGAINST HAEMOPHILUS INFLUENZAE TYPE B INFECTIONS

IMPRINT AREA

BACKGROUND:

Haemophilus influenzae type B (HIB) is the most common cause of bacterial meningitis in infants and young children. About 2 to 5% of infected infants die from this disease, and 10 to 45% of survivors may be left with neurological disorders including hearing defects, learning disabilities and motor function abnormalities.

This bacterium can also cause pneumonia, bone and joint infections, soft tissue infections (cellulitis), epiglottitis (a severe life threatening throat infection), and blood infections (sepsis).

Prior to the availability of the vaccine, 1 in 500 children less than 5 years of age acquired severe infection from HIB.

THE VACCINE:

A safe and effective vaccine made of a purified piece of the bacterial sugar-protein envelope of the HIB bacteria has been used for over a decade. The present vaccine has an efficacy rate of greater than 98%. It is given in a series of 3 or 4 doses given at 2, 4, and 6 months of age, with a booster dose at 15 months. Older children may need fewer doses.

Side effects are very rare and usually mild. Soreness and redness at the injection site and fever occur in less than 2% of children. These side effects can be treated with analgesics. Any more severe reactions should be reported to your child's physician, the advice center, or to the federal government (1-800-822-7967).

CONSENT:

After reviewing the above information and having all my questions answered, I request the HIB vaccine series to be administered to my child.

DATE _____   NAME OF CHILD _____

SIGNATURE OF LEGAL GUARDIAN _____

DECLINATION:

After reviewing the above information and despite my child's physician's recommendations, I decline the HIB vaccine

for my child _____ .
NAME OF CHILD

DATE _____   SIGNATURE OF LEGAL GUARDIAN _____

WITNESS _____

95803 (4-92)

CONCLUSION

You have now completed the unit on Preparing for and Assisting with Routine and Specialty Physical Examinations. After you have practiced the procedures and are ready to demonstrate your skills and knowledge attained, arrange with your instructor to take a performance test. You will be expected to accurately demon-

strate your ability in preparing for and assisting with procedures and examinations discussed in this unit and to measure a patient's distance and near visual acuity. In addition, when questioned by your instructor, you will be expected to identify by name the equipment and instruments used for each examination.

REVIEW OF VOCABULARY

The following are samples of a patient's admission note and a hospital discharge note as dictated by a physician. These are to help familiarize you with the format and contents of medical reports. Read these and be prepared to discuss the contents and define all the medical terms that are used. You should recognize some of the terms; others are new, and you may have to refer to Appendix A or a medical dictionary for the definitions.

Medical Center
PHYSICIAN'S REPORT
PATIENT: ☒ ADMISSION NOTE
  McFerrin, Sandra ☐ CONSULTATION
PHYSICIAN:
  Robert Scott, MD ☐ DISCHARGE SUMMARY
  9/13/___ Admitted
  _____ Discharged

CHIEF COMPLAINT: Abdominal pain.
PRESENT ILLNESS: The patient is a 19-year-old woman who, for the first 5 days, has had progressively severe abdominal pain. There has been no nausea until the day of admission, when she became nauseated driving over to the hospital. There has been no vomiting, chills or fever. The patient has not been bothered by constipation or diarrhea. She had a normal bowel movement the day before admission. The patient's menstrual period started the day before admission and the previous one approximately a month ago was normal.
The patient was seen in my office the day before admission, and epigastric tenderness was noted. Donnatal and Maalox were prescribed, but this afforded little if any relief. The pain became more acute, more severe, and awoke the patient from sleep and prompted her present admission.

PAST HISTORY: The patient's past health has been quite good, except for an automobile accident approximately a year and half ago in which her pelvis and bladder were fractured and lacerated respectively. No sequelae followed. Approximately 7 to 8 years ago, patient was treated prophylactically with INH for a year for exposure to tuberculosis.
FAMILY HISTORY: There is no family history of diabetes, cancer, or premature cardiac disease. The patient's sister had pulmonary tuberculosis when the patient was young, and the patient received a year's course of prophylactic INH. The patient's skin test was positive.
REVIEW OF SYSTEMS: There are no symptoms of respiratory, cardiac, or genitourinary disease.
PHYSICAL EXAMINATION: Blood pressure 130/80, pulse 90, temperature 36.6° C.
General appearance: The patient is a young, well-developed woman who is lying in bed crying because of abdominal pain. *Skin:* no rash. *Eyes:* Sclera clear. The pupils are found, regular and equal. *ENT:* The tongue and mucous membrane are somewhat dry. *Neck:* Supple. *Breasts:* Clear. *Heart:* Normal sinus rhythm, no murmurs. *Lungs:* clear. *Abdomen:* Flat, the bowel sounds are hypoactive. There is marked epigastric and left upper quadrant tenderness. There is no guarding or rigidity. There is no rebound tenderness. There is no adnexal tenderness. Rectal examination negative. Extremities negative.
IMPRESSION: Acute abdominal pain, etiology to be determined.
RS:vy
D:9/13/___
T:9/13/_____
Robert Scott, MD

REVIEW OF VOCABULARY—cont'd

DISCHARGE NOTE
PATIENT: Marion Dale
PHYSICIAN: Scott Douglas, MD
DATE: April 15, 19___

The patient is a 45-year-old, premenopausal white woman presenting a history of a recent dark vaginal discharge with a negative Pap test in April of last, but a recent Pap test showed dyskeratotic cells and atypical class III cells. Biopsy the next month was positive for epidermoid carcinoma with lymphatic permeating present.

Pelvic examination revealed a lacerated eroded cervical canal, and, under anesthesia, pelvic examination showed uterine enlargement to approximately twice the normal size with a freely mobile uterus; however, no evidence of parametrial induration or other pelvic pathology was present.

Following endometrial curettage, a tandem and colpostat radium-containing applicator were inserted, with the applicator carrying a total of 90 mg homogenous distribution in a circular e.5 cm colpostat, 20 mg radium in the base and 20 mg in the tip of the tandem with $1/2$ mm plantinum intrinsic filtration and 1.5 mm Monel extrinsic-filtration, representing total equivalent of 1 mm plantinum filtration.

The applicator was inserted to be removed after 72 hours for a total dosage of 6480 mg hours. Following the course of radium, a complete pelvic cycle with external irradiation is recommended. Intravenous pyelogram showed no obstructive nephropathy or ureteral constriction or displacement. Portable AP and lateral views of the pelvis confirming the position of the applicator in situ are to be obtained. Three rolls of iodoform packing in the vaginal canal firmly secured the applicator in contact with the cervical lips, and a loose ligature affixed the colpostat to the anterior cervical lip during the surgical procedure.

Scott Douglas, MD

CASE STUDY

Positioning patients for various examinations and giving emotional as well as physical support is a vital part of the medical assistant's responsibility. Read the following excerpts from office progress notes and discuss ways to alleviate any physical and emotional discomfort resulting from positioning and examination. Discuss the italicized terminology.

1. An 18-year-old female experiencing left *lower quadrant pain* and severe cramping during *menstruation* presents for her first *pelvic examination* and *Pap smear*. Discuss the positioning of a patient for *gynecologic* examination, including *Papanicolaou smear* and suggestions for emotional support for this patient's initial pelvic examination. What instruments and equipment are used in addition to the *vaginal speculum*? Explain the use of these instruments to the patient, as well as *inspection and digital and bimanual examination of the cervix and rectum.*

2. An elderly 89-year-old gentlemen presents with symptoms of severe *diarrhea* accompanied by *nausea* and *rectal* pain for the past 5 days. He exhibits signs of *dehydration, pallor,* and weakness. The doctor directs you to prepare the patient for a *proctologic* examination. Discuss positioning the patient in the *jackknife* position and emotional support for this *debilitated* patient. What instruments and equipment are required?

3. The gentleman in the above example returns to the office for an *endoscopy* of the *sigmoid*. Discuss positioning and emotional support for this patient. Keep in mind his continued *debilitated* condition and need for additional comfort.

1. List and summarize the medical assistant's general responsibilities when assisting the physician with a complete physical examination.
2. Indicate what body part or system is examined with the following instruments:
   a. Otoscope
   b. Laryngeal mirror
   c. Ophthalmoscope
   d. Anoscope
   e. Tuning fork
   f. Bronchoscope
   g. Cystoscope
   h. Percussion hammer
   i. Stethoscope
3. In what position is the patient placed for:
   a. A vaginal or pelvic exam?
   b. A rectal examination and proctosigmoidoscopy?
   c. A chest examination?
   d. An examination of the ears and eyes?
4. List the purpose(s) and the common instruments required for the following examinations:
   a. General physical examination
   b. Vaginal examination
   c. Pap smear or test
   d. Rectal examination
   e. Proctosigmoidoscopy
5. If a physician suspects a growth in the sigmoid colon that is considered doubtful as to being benign or malignant, what procedure does he or she usually perform?

6. You have a 50-year-old obese patient who cannot tolerate the jackknife position for a sigmoidscopy. Name an alternate position that may be used for this examination.
7. Explain why it is important for a female assistant to remain in the room when a female patient is being examined by a male physician.
8. List some of the common unusual reactions for which you observe a patient during an examination.
9. Explain why it is important that you check battery-operated and electrical equipment before an examination.
10. List the instruments and equipment that are used for a neurologic examination.
11. What is a Snellen chart and how is it used?
12. When increased pressure is present in the eyeball, what common condition is suspected?
13. Albumin in the urine during a pregnancy is thought to be a serious sign of what condition?
14. List seven warning signals of cancer.
15. Explain how a woman can perform a breast self-examination.
16. Why should every woman examine her breasts monthly?
17. When is the best time of the month for a woman to examine her breasts for any unusual lump or thickening?
18. List two types of pediatric visits.

PERFORMANCE TEST

In a skills laboratory, a simulation of a joblike environment, the medical assistant student is to demonstrate knowledge and skill in performing the following procedures without reference to source materials. For these activities, the student needs a person to play the role of a patient and the necessary equipment and supplies. Time limits for the performance of each procedure are to be assigned by the instructor (see also page 52).

1. Given an ambulatory patient, the student is to position and drape the patient in the following positions, and state when each is used:
   a. Dorsal-recumbent
   b. Lithotomy
   c. Sims
   d. Knee-chest
   e. Supine
   f. Prone
   g. Trendelenburg

2. Given an ambulatory patient, the student is to prepare for and assist with the following:
   a. A complete physical examination that is to include a vaginal and rectal examination
   b. A proctosigmoidoscopy, including a description of the patient preparation that is to be completed before the examination
   c. A pelvic examination and a Papanicolaou smear
   d. An obstetric examination
   e. Pediatric examinations

3. Given an ambulatory patient, the student is to prepare for and measure:
   a. Distance visual acuity using the Snellen eye chart
   b. Near visual acuity
   c. Color vision

4. Demonstrate how to obtain the following measurements on an infant:
   a. Length/height
   b. Weight
   c. Head circumference
   d. Chest circumference

5. Demonstrate the procedures used for performing a urine test to screen an infant for phenylketonuria.

6. Demonstrate the method used to obtain a blood specimen from an infant to perform a test to screen for phenylketonuria.

7. Given an ambulatory patient, the student is to instruct and assist the patient with the performance of a breast-self examination.

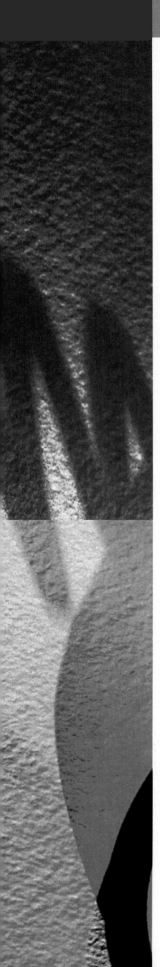

Infection Control: Practices of Medical Asepsis and Sterilization

COGNITIVE OBJECTIVES

On completion of Unit Four, the medical assistant student should be able to:

1. Define and pronounce the terms presented in the vocabulary and throughout the unit.
2. List the five classifications of microorganisms that are capable of causing a disease process, giving examples of diseases caused by each.
3. List the six factors that are essential for the development of an infectious process, discussing briefly components in each.
4. Differentiate between the types of human reservoirs—overt cases, subclinical cases, and human carriers.
5. Compare direct transmission with indirect transmission of a disease process.
6. List and describe the body's natural defense mechanisms used to control or prevent disease and infection.
7. State the function of the immune system.
8. List and briefly discuss the four critical phases of each immune response.
9. Discuss and compare the various types of immunity.
10. List the classic signs and symptoms of inflammation and briefly describe the inflammatory process.
11. List five diagnostic tests that may be used to diagnose an infectious process.
12. Differentiate between medical and surgical asepsis; list and describe procedures used to accomplish each and medical situations in which each is used.
13. Differentiate between sanitization, disinfection, and sterilization; describe the procedures used with these methods when working with contaminated instruments, syringes and needles, rubber goods, and other equipment and select the most effective method for controlling microscopic agents.
14. Explain the importance of sterilizing instruments and supplies before using them for medical procedures.
15. List and briefly describe five methods used for sterilizing equipment and two methods used for disinfecting equipment.
16. Describe how items are to be wrapped, positioned, and removed from a sterilizer for sterilization to be effective, and how items are to be positioned and removed from a boiler.
17. List three critical factors in steam sterilization.
18. State the recommended exposure times for sterilizing and disinfecting the various types of equipment and supplies that are used in the physician's office.
19. Describe types of and state the reason for using sterilization indicators.
20. Discuss problems encountered in sterilization techniques and causes of insufficient sterilization.
21. Discuss how, where, and the how long sterile supplies should be stored.

TERMINAL PERFORMANCE OBJECTIVES

On completion of Unit Five, the medical assistant should be able to:

1. Demonstrate how to wash hands, wrists, and forearms, explaining the reasons for the actions taken.
2. Given various items assumed to be contaminated, demonstrate how to sanitize, disinfect, and sterilize each, using the methods discussed in this unit.
3. Demonstrate how to inspect instruments before they are sterilized. State the reason for the actions taken.
4. Given packs that have been removed from an autoclave, determine if sterilization has been effective and then store each for use at a later date.
5. Given items to be sterilized, demonstrate how each should be wrapped before placing it in the sterilizer.

The student is to perform these objectives with 100% accuracy 90% of the time (9 out of 10 times).

The consistent use of universal precautions is required by all health care professionals in all health care settings as a method of infection control. It is assumed that these precautions are used in all of the following procedures. Review Unit One if you have any question on methods to use as the methods/techniques will not be repeated in detail in each procedure presented in the unit.

Be sure to consult the latest guidelines issued by the Centers for Disease Control and Prevention and consult with infection control practitioners when needed to identify specific precautions that pertain to your particular work situation.

BASIC CONCEPTS AND GOALS

Since the early days of civilization, there has been concern with the control of disease and the spread of infection. The history of medicine documents the wealth of knowledge attained by numerous individuals about the anatomy and physiology of the human body, certain diseases, and many therapeutic agents. However, not until the last half of the nineteenth century was a connection between disease and pathogenic microorganisms established through the work of Louis Pasteur and Robert Koch. Among the findings documented, Pasteur discovered important properties of bacteria, and Koch was credited with establishing the germ theory of disease. Koch's theory states that to prove an organism is actually the specific pathogen causing the disease, one must establish a causal relationship between the microbe and the disease.

Microorganisms (microbes) are defined as minute living creatures that are too small to be seen by the naked eye. The classifications or divisions of microscopic life include viruses, rickettsiae, bacteria, fungi, and parasites. Microorganisms in each of these divisions that cause disease are termed *pathogens*. It is important to keep in mind that many members of these microscopic divisions are either beneficial or harmless to humans or animals. The term *medical microbiology* implies the study of pathogens, which involves identification and development of effective methods of control or elimination.

Pathogenic microorganisms are everywhere around us. They are easily spread directly from person to person, or indirectly by animate and inanimate vehicles to humans. Disease or infection occurs when pathogens invade a susceptible host. Although antibiotics are available for use in the treatment of many infectious processes, the best means of controlling infection is to prevent the spread of disease-producing microorganisms. It is the responsibility of health professionals to take an active, conscientious role in the process of infection control. Lack of knowledge about how pathogens spread or how to control the process is frequently the cause of major outbreaks of infection or disease. The goals of infection control are to prevent the spread of pathogenic microorganisms, to attain a state of asepsis (absence of pathogens), and to edu-

cate the public in the ways that they too can help. Asepsis, or aseptic technique, is divided into two categories: medical asepsis and surgical asepsis. It is important to distinguish between these two methods.

The rest of this unit discusses disease-producing organisms, how they are spread, the body's own defense mechanisms, the immune system, infection control precautions, and medical and surgical asepsis with techniques and sterilization procedures used to prevent transmission of pathogens. Surgical asepsis (aseptic technique) is discussed in greater length in Unit Six. Universal Precautions for blood and body substance are presented in Unit One.

INFECTIOUS PROCESS AND CAUSATIVE AGENTS

The mere presence of a pathogenic microorganism is not enough to promote infection. For the infectious process to develop, there must be a sequential connection between the following factors (Figure 5-1):

1. A cause or an etiologic (e-ti-o-loj′ ik) agent (pathogen)
2. A source or a reservoir of the etiologic agent
3. A means of escape of the etiologic agent from the reservoir (portal of exit)
4. A means of transmission of the etiologic agent from the reservoir to the new host
5. A means of entry of the etiologic agent into the new susceptible host (portal of entry)
6. A susceptible host

Figure 5-1 *The chain of the infectious process. To prevent the spread of disease this sequential connection must be broken.*

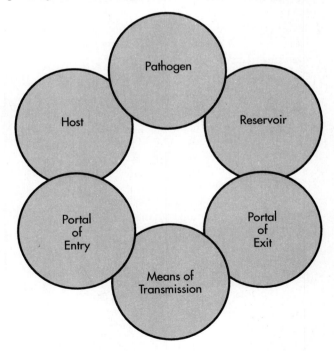

VOCABULARY

Antiseptic (an' ti-sep' tik)—A substance capable of inhibiting the growth or action of microorganisms, without necessarily killing them; generally safe for use on body tissues.

Asepsis (a-sep' sis)—The absence of all microorganisms causing disease; absence of contaminated matter.

Bactericide (bak-ter' i-sid)—A substance capable of destroying bacteria but not spores.

Bacteriostatic (bak-te"'Pre-o-stat' ik)—A substance that inhibits the growth of bacteria.

Contaminated, contamination (kon-tam" i-na'shun)—The act of making unclean, soiling, or staining, especially the introduction of disease germs or infectious material into or on normally sterile of objects.

Disinfectant (dis"in-fek' tant)—A substance capable of destroying pathogens, but usually not spores; generally not intended for use on body tissue because it is too strong.

Disinfection—A process that destroys most harmful microorganisms but rarely kills spores.

Fungicide (fun' ji-sid)—A substance that destroys fungi.

Germicide (jer' mi-sid)—A substance that is capable of destroying pathogens.

Immunization (im"u-ni-za' shun)—The process of rendering a person immune (protected from or not susceptible to a disease) or of becoming immune; frequently called vaccination or inoculation. A process by which a person is artificially prepared to resist infection by a specific pathogen.

Incubation (in"ku-ba' shun) period—The interval of time between the invasion of a pathogen into the body and the appearance of the first symptoms of disease.

Infection (in-fek' shun)—A condition caused by the multiplication of pathogenic microorganisms that have invaded the body of a susceptible host.

   Acute—Rapid onset, severe symptoms, and usually subsides within a relatively short period of time.

   Chronic—Develops slowly, milder symptoms, and lasts for a long period of time.

   Latent—Dormant or concealed; pathogen is ever-present in the host, but symptoms are present only intermittently, often in response to a stimulus. At other times the pathogen is dormant.

   Localized—Restricted to a certain area.

   Generalized—Systemic; involving the whole body.

Medical microbiology—The study and identification of pathogens, and the development of effective methods for their control or elimination.

Necrosis (ne-kro' -sis)—The death of a cell or a group of cells because of injury or disease.

Normal flora—Microorganisms that normally reside in various body locations such as the vagina, intestine, urethra, upper respiratory tract, and skin. These microorganisms are nonpathogenic and do not cause harm (although they may become pathogenic and cause harm if they are introduced into a body area in which they do not normally reside).

Pathogenic (path"o-jen'ik)—Productive of disease. *P. microorganism*—one that produces disease in the body.

Reservoir (rez'er-vwar)—The source in which pathogenic microorganisms grow and from which they leave to spread and cause disease.

Resistance (re-zis' tans)—The ability of the body to resist disease or infection because of its own defense mechanisms.

Sepsis(sep' sis)—A morbid state or condition resulting from the presence of pathogenic microorganisms.

Spore (spor)—A reproductive cell, usually unicellular, produced by plants and some protozoa, and possessing thick walls to withstand unfavorable environmental conditions. Bacterial spores are resistant to heat and must undergo a prolonged exposure to extremely high temperatures to be destroyed.

Sterile (ster' il)—Free from all microorganisms.

Toxin (tok' sin)—A poisonous substance produced by pathogenic bacteria and some animals and plants. The toxins produced by bacteria include toxic enzymes, exotoxins, and endotoxins. Toxins in the body cause antitoxins to form, which provide a means for establishing immunity to certain diseases.

Vaccination (vak"si-na' shun)—The introduction of weakened or dead microorganisms (inoculation) into the body to stimulate the production of antibodies and immunity to a specific disease.

Virulence (vir' u-lens)—The degree of ability of a pathogen to produce disease.

CAUSE OR ETIOLOGIC AGENT

Infection begins with the invasion of the body by a pathogen that is the causative agent of the disease in question. The pathogenic organisms must be present in a sufficiently high concentration and be adequately capable of causing disease. Examples of causative agents or pathogens are viruses, rickettsiae, and bacteria.

Viruses

Viruses (vi´ rus) are the smallest pathogens and require susceptible host cells for multiplication and activity. To observe viruses, an electron microscope must be used. A phenomenon that characterizes viral infections as the most insidious is the fact that viruses, as intracellular parasites, can only multiply inside a living cell. Viruses attach themselves to a living cell, inject a compound of protein and nucleic acid, either deoxyribonucleic acid (DNA) or ribonucleic acid (RNA), and take over the normal cellular metabolism. The cell proceeds to make new cells in addition to new viruses, then bursts, dies, and releases numerous viruses that can then invade other cells. Chemotherapy for viral diseases is extremely difficult, because the viruses surviving an initial dose of a drug have the ability to change their characteristics so that they rapidly become resistant to the drug.

Viruses are also more resistant to chemical disinfection than bacteria, but they can be destroyed by heat, as is done when sterilizing equipment in an autoclave.

There is a greater variety of viruses than of any other category of microbial agents of disease. Viruses are the causative agents of influenza, poliomyelitis, colds, mumps, measles, rabies, smallpox, chickenpox, as well as hepatitis A, hepatitis B, and herpes simplex I, and herpes simplex II.

Rickettsiae

Rickettsiae (rik-et´ si-a) like viruses, are obligate intracellular parasites. This means that they can only survive within the host organism. They differ from viruses in that they are visible under a conventional microscope by special staining techniques and are also susceptible to antibiotic suppression of replication.

Rickettsiae are the causative organisms for the various "spotted fevers" such as Rocky Mountain spotted fever, and also typhus, Q fever, and trench fever. They are generally tick-borne and therefore are not common in sanitary urban areas.

Bacteria

Bacteria (bak-te´ re-ah) can readily multiply outside of living cells. Bacteria are single-celled microorganisms that can be cultivated on artificial media and, with appropriate staining techniques, can be readily visible under a microscope. These characteristics make bacteria much simpler to identify than viruses and rickettsiae. There are many varieties, only some of which cause disease; most are nonpathogenic, and many are useful. Bacteria are classified in three groups according to their shape and appearance (morphology) (Figure 5-2):

1. Cocci (kok´v si) are spheric bacteria; among the cocci are the following three types:
   a. Staphylococci (staf"il-o´kok´si)—Forming grapelike clusters of cells, these are the most common pus-producing organisms known to humans. They are readily found in pimples, boils, suture abscesses, and osteomyelitis.
   b. Streptococci (strep"to-kok´si)—Forming chains of cells, these are the cause of strep throat, rheumatic heart disease (RHD), scarlet fever, and septicemia (infection in the bloodstream)
   c. Diplococci (dip-lo-kok´si)—Forming pairs of cells, different types of diplococci are the causative organisms for gonorrhea, pneumonia, and meningitis.
2. Bacilli (bah-sil´i) are rod-shaped bacteria; these organisms cause tuberculosis (TB), typhoid and paratyphoid fever, tetanus (lockjaw), gas gangrene, bacillary dysentery, and diphtheria.
3. Spirilla (spi-ril´ah) are spiral organisms; these organisms cause cholera, syphilis, and relapsing fever.

Fungi

Fungi (fun´ ji) are the lowest form of infectious agents that bridge the gap between free-living and host-dependent parasites.

Fungi are unicellular or multicellular. They can be grown on artificial media and then identified under the microscope. Fungi appear in the form of molds and mushrooms, as well as in microscopic growth. Disease-producing fungi are seen as the causative agent in some infections of the skin such as athlete's foot and ringworm.

The fungus *Candida albicans* (Monilia) is responsible for the disease known as thrush (an infection of the mouth and throat) and also some vaginal infections.

Parasites

Parasites (par´´ ah-sit) are organisms that live in or on another organism from which they gain their nourishment. Parasites include single-celled and multicelled animals, fungi, and bacteria. Viruses are sometimes considered to be parasitic. Examples include the following:

Figure 5-2 *Classification of bacteria according to their morphology.*

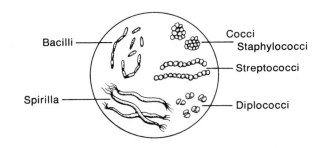

1. Protozoa (pro″to-zo′ah) are single-celled microscopic organisms. Some can be cultivated, fixed, and stained for viewing under a microscope. The most well-known protozoa cause malaria, amoebic dysentery, and trichomonas infections of the vagina.
2. Metazoal (met″ah-zo′al) parasites are multicellular organisms, causing conditions such as pinworms, hookworms, tapeworms, and trichinosis in pork.
3. Ectoparasites (ek″to-par′ah-sit) can superficially affect the host (for example, lice and scabies mite) or can invade the integument (for example, the larvae of dipterous flies).

SOURCE OR RESERVOIR OF ETIOLOGIC AGENT

Areas where organisms grow and reproduce are called reservoirs and are found mainly in human beings and animals. Organisms can also exist in soil, water, and equipment.

Human reservoirs include:
- Overt carriers: people who are obviously ill with the disease
- Subclinical carriers: abortive (undeveloped) and ambulatory (walking) cases of the disease (for example, "walking" pneumonia). Infection goes unnoticed because of lack of symptoms.
- Human carriers: people unaware of their condition who circulate freely in their communities until detected and diagnosed (for example, the "Typhoid Marys," or people who are in the convalescent stage of an infection).

Animal reservoirs include mainly domestic animals and rodents. Zoonosis (zo-on′asis) is the term given to an animal disease that is transmissible to humans. In this case, the infection is usually derived from the animal and is not further transmitted from human to human. An example is rabies.

MEANS OF ESCAPE OF ETIOLOGIC AGENT FROM RESERVOIR

Pathogens commonly exit from their reservoir through one or more of the following *(portals of exit)*:
- Respiratory tract in secretions from the nose, nasal sinuses, nasopharynx, larynx, trachea, bronchial tree, and lungs
- Intestinal tract through discharge with the feces
- Urinary tract through discharge or in the urine
- Skin or mucous membranes, or open lesions or discharges on the surface of the body
- Reproductive tract through discharges
- Blood
- Across the placenta

MEANS OF TRANSMISSION OF ETIOLOGIC AGENT

The means of transmission is the method by which the pathogen is transmitted from the portal of exit in the reservoir to the portal of entry in the new host. After an infecting organism has escaped from its reservoir, it can cause a new infection only if it finds its way to a new susceptible host. Transmission may occur by either of the following:
- *Direct transmission:* The organism passes from one person to another through inhalation, by actual physical contact such as sexual contact or kissing, or by direct contact with an open lesion. The organism goes from one host to another without the aid of intermediate objects. Also called person-to-person transmission.
- *Indirect transmission:* The organism is capable of survival for a period of time outside the body and is transferred to the new host by a vehicle, which is either animate or inanimate. Animate vehicles are people who touch contaminated material, don't wash their hands, and then carry the microorganism on their hands to a susceptible host. Other animate vehicles are called vectors and include the various insects that spread infection. Inanimate vehicles, called fomites, are nonliving objects or substances and include water, milk, foods, soil, air, excreta, clothing, bedding, towels, instruments, syringes and needles, toiletries, or any contaminated article.

MEANS OF ENTRY OF ETIOLOGIC AGENT

The infecting organism enters a new host through a part of the body, which is called the portal of entry. The main portals of entry are:
- Respiratory tract—Organisms may be inhaled
- Gastrointestinal tract—Organisms may be ingested
- Skin or mucous membranes—Organisms may be introduced via cuts, abrasions, or open wounds
- Urinary tract—Organisms may be introduced through external body orifices
- Reproductive tract—Organisms may be introduced through external body orifices
- Blood
- Across the placenta

Although avenues of escape or portals of exit correspond to the portals of entry, the pathogen can escape from one site in the reservoir and enter the new host in another site. An example of this is when the pathogen leaves from the respiratory tract in the reservoir (as through sputum or water droplets) and enters the new host through the skin (as through an open wound when a dressing is being changed).

SUSCEPTIBLE HOST

For the infectious process to be completed, the pathogenic organism must enter a host whose resistance is so low that it cannot fight off the invading organism. Even though a pathogen gains entry to the body, disease or infection may not develop, since the body possesses certain defense mechanisms to protect itself. These mechanisms may also help destroy invading pathogens. Such defense mechanisms are called resistance, and, if they are great enough, they constitute immunity (i-mu′ni-te).

Table 5-1 outlines the six essential factors of the infectious process for two diseases. All infectious diseases can be outlined in this manner.

STAGES OF AN INFECTIOUS PROCESS

The stages of an infectious process generally include the following:

1. The invasion and multiplication of the pathogen in the body
2. The incubation period, which may vary from a few days to months or years
3. The prodromal period when the first mild signs and symptoms appear; the person is highly contagious during this period
4. The acute period when signs and symptoms are at the most severe stage
5. The recovery and convalescent period when signs and symptoms begin to subside and the body heals itself, returning to state of health.

THE BODY'S DEFENSES AGAINST DISEASE AND INFECTION

The body's resistance level to undesirable microorganisms is influenced by the general health status of the individual and other related circumstances:

- Amount of rest, sufficient or insufficient
- Dietary intake of nutritional foods, adequate or inadequate
- How one copes with stress
- Age of the individual (the young and aged are most susceptible to infection because of the immaturity of the immune system in the young and the decline of this system in the aged)
- Presence of other disease processes in the body
- Condition of the external environment such as poor living conditions
- Influence of genetic traits (for example, people with diabetes mellitus and sickle cell anemia are more prone to some infections than are other individuals)

PHYSICAL AND CHEMICAL BARRIERS

The body has natural defense mechanisms, either physical or chemical, that act as barriers to the invasion of pathogenic organisms.

Skin. This tissue is the largest barrier against infection. As long as it remains intact, the skin is a physical barrier to a tremendous number of microorganisms. Chemical barriers of the skin include the acid pH of the skin (which inhibits bacterial infection), sweat, and lysozyme (which functions as an antibacterial enzyme in the skin).

Mucous membrane. This tissue holds in check many microorganisms because of the repelling forces in the secretions that bathe these membranes. The cilia of some mucous membranes serve to keep their surfaces swept clean.

Respiratory tract. The muscosal lining of this tract is very sensitive and thus readily stimulated by foreign matter. Certain reflexes such as coughing or sneezing help remove foreign matter, including microorganisms. The hairs lining the nostrils, along with the moist membranes, serve as a physical barrier. The cilia lining the bronchi beat upward to carry mucus and small, interfering foreign materials such as dust, bacteria, and soot to the throat. The bending passageway from the mouth to the lungs also serves as a barrier.

TABLE 5-1

Factors of Infectious Process

Disease	Cause/Agent	Reservoir/Source	Means of Escape from the Reservoir	Means of Transmission from Reservoir to New Host	Means of Entry into New Host	Susceptible Host
German measles (rubella)	Virus	Humans	Mouth, nasopharynx	Water droplets	Mouth	Humans
Pneumonia	Bacteria	Humans	Mouth, nasopharynx	Droplets	Mouth, sputum Fomites, such as a pencil (indirect transmission)	Humans respiratory mucosa

Gastrointestinal tract. Hydrochloric acid in the stomach has an important bactericidal action, destroying many disease-producing agents. Bile in the small intestine is thought to have a germicidal effect.

Blood and lymphoid tissue. These tissues contain and produce cells and antibodies that can exert a tremendous influence in protecting the body against disease. White blood cells (leukocytes) are particularly active when pathogenic microorganisms invade the body. In the inflammatory process, some leukocytes surround, engulf, and digest the pathogens. This process is known as phagocytosis (fag´ o-si-to´sis), which is basically the ingestion of the pathogen or "cell-eating." Lymphoid tissue produces antibodies, which are protein compounds that help combat infection.

ANTIGEN-ANTIBODY REACTION

Another internal defense mechanism that the body gradually develops against invasion by foreign substances (antigens) is the formation of antibodies. Antibodies are protein substances produced mainly in the lymph nodes, spleen, bone marrow, and lymphoid tissue in response to invasion by an antigen. Different types of antibodies are produced in response to different antigens, with each antibody being effective only against the specific antigen that stimulates its production. The antibodies can either neutralize the antigens, render them harmless, rupture their cell membrane, or prepare the antigen so that they are more susceptible to destruction by phagocytes (cells that ingest and destroy microorganisms, cells, and cell debris).

The antigen-antibody reaction is this reaction of the body to the invasion of antigens. When antibodies are produced in sufficient quantities, the body becomes immune. Since the body is capable of continuing to produce antibodies for weeks to several years, it is possible for immunity to last for months or years.

IMMUNE SYSTEM

The immune system is a complex system that defends us against microorganisms and cancer cells. Its general function is to produce immunity, that is, resistance to disease. The structures of the immune system are not organs. It is made up of trillions of separate cells and molecules performing many different functions. It includes the white blood cells (especially the neutrophils and lymphocytes), the connective tissue cells or macrophages, and protein molecules or antibodies. The effects and functions of immune system cells are not yet completely understood, but because of recent research our understanding of this system is increasing by leaps and bounds. To fully grasp the complexities of the immune system requires a thorough knowledge of human biology, which is beyond the scope of this book. However, a general view of the immune response is provided in Figure 5-3.

The four critical phases to each immune response are:

1. *Recognition of the enemy:* When a pathogen enters the body the immune system must recognize that a foreign agent has invaded the body.

2. *Amplification of defenses:* To be effective, defense mechanisms that fight the recognized pathogen must be produced in large numbers.

3. *Attack:* The T and B cells (the specific cells of the immune system) and the antibodies (produced by the B cells) seek out and destroy infected cells and disable free-floating pathogens.

4. *Slowdown:* After the pathogen has been contained and/or eliminated, the suppressor T cells halt the entire range of immune responses, preventing them from getting out of control and depleting the system.

A properly functioning immune system is needed to help prevent or conquer disease once it has invaded the body. Without a normal functioning immune system, the body becomes a victim to serious and potentially life-threatening disease(s).

Immunity

Immunity, the resistance of the body to pathogenic microorganisms and their toxins occurs as a result of the antigen-antibody reaction. Specific types of immunity follow:

- Active immunity develops when antigens are introduced into the body.
- Passive immunity develops when ready-made antibodies are introduced into the body.
- Natural immunity is an inborn resistance to a disease as a result of antibodies that are normally present in the blood.
- Acquired or induced immunity results from antibodies that are not normally present in the blood.
- Active and passive immunity can be either natural or acquired.

Natural immunity. Natural immunity can be active or passive. *Inherited (active) immunity* is acquired by being a member of a race or species. Some races are more or less susceptible to certain diseases. The longer a race has been exposed to a certain disease, the less susceptible its members become. Humans do not contract many diseases common to lower species of animals, and lower species of animals do not contract most human diseases.

Congenital (passive) immunity is the immunity possessed at birth; antibodies are passed from the mother through the placenta to the fetus. The duration of this immunity can last from 5 to 6 months.

Acquired immunity. Acquired immunity can be active or passive. *Natural active immunity* results from being a carrier, recovering from or having a disease, or having an atypical or subclinical case of the disease.

Artificial active immunity is acquired through vaccinations with inactivated (dead) or attenuated (weakened) organisms. Inactivated or dead vaccines include the typhoid, whooping cough, and influenza vaccines, as well as the Salk vaccine for polio. Attenuated vaccines include vaccines for polio (the Sabin vaccine), smallpox, measles (rubeola), mumps, and German measles (rubella). Toxoids are exotoxins that have

Figure 5-3 *The four phases of the immune system and how they function.*
Courtesy The National Geographic Society.

CELL WARS

About one trillion strong, our white blood cells constitute a highly specialized army of defenders, the most important of which are depicted here in a typical battle against a formidable enemy.

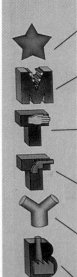

VIRUS
Needing help to spring to life, a virus is little more than a package of genetic information that must commandeer the machinery of a host cell to permit its own replication.

MACROPHAGE
Housekeeper and frontline defender, this cell engulfs and digests debris that washes into the bloodstream. Encountering a foreign organism, it summons helper T cells to the scene.

HELPER T CELL
As a commander in chief of the immune system, it identifies the enemy and rushes to the spleen and lymph nodes, where it stimulates the production of other cells to fight the infection.

KILLER T CELL
Recruited and activated by helper T cells, it specializes in killing cells of the body that have been invaded by foreign organisms, as well as cells that have turned cancerous.

B CELL
Biologic arms factory, it resides in the spleen or the lymph nodes, where it is induced to replicate by helper T cells and then to produce potent chemical weapons called antibodies.

ANTIBODY
Engineered to target a specific invader, the Y-shaped protein molecule is rushed to the infection site, where it either neutralizes the enemy or tags it for attack by other cells or chemicals.

SUPPRESSOR T CELLS
A third type of T cell, it is able to slow down ro stop the activities of B cells and other T cells, playing a vital role in calling off the attack after an infection has been conquered.

MEMORY CELL
Generated during an initial infection, this defense cell may circulate in the blood or lymph for years, enabling the body to respond more quickly to subsequent infections.

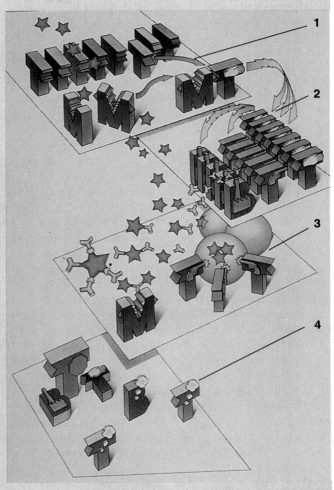

A miracle of evolution, the human immune system is not controlled by any central organ, such as the brain. Rather it has developed to function as a kind of biologic democracy, wherein the individual members achieve their ends through an information network of awesome scope. Accounting for one percent of the body's 100 trillion cells, these defender white cells arise in the bone marrow. They fall into three groups: the phagocytes, or "cell eaters," of which the stalwart macrophage is one, and two kinds of lymphocytes, called T and B cells. All share one common objective: to identify and destroy all substances, living and inert, that are not part of the human body, that are "not self." These include human cells, which have turned from self to nonself, friend to foe.

There are four critical phases to each immune response: recognition of the enemy, aplification of defenses, attack, and slowdown. Each immune response is a unique local sequence of events, shaped by the nature of the enemies. Chemical toxins and a multitude of inert environmental substances, such as asbestos and smoke particles, are normally attacked only by phagocytes. Organic invaders inlist the full range of immune responses. Besides viruses, these include single-celled bacteria, protozoa, and fungi, as well as a host of multicelled worms called helminths. Many of these enemies have evolved devious methods to escape detection. The viruses that cause influenza and the common cold, for example, constantly mutate, changing their fingerprints. The AIDS virus, most insidious of all, employs a range of strategies, including hiding out in healthy cells. What makes it fatal is its ability to invade and kill helper T cells, thereby short-circuiting the entire immune response.

1. **THE BATTLE BEGINS**
As viruses begin to invade the body, a few are consumed by macrophages, which seize their antigens and display them on their own surfaces. Among millions of helper T cells circulating the bloodstream, a select few are programmed to "read' that antigen. Binding to the macrophage, the T cell becomes activated.

2. **THE FORCES MULTIPLY**
Once activated, helper T cells begin to multiply. They then stimulate the multiplication of those few killer T cells and B cells that are sensitive to the invading viruses. As the number of B cells increases, helper T cells signal them to start producing antibodies.

3. **CONQUERING THE INFECTION**
Meanwhile, some of the viruses have entered cells of the body—the only place they are able to replicate. Killer T cells will sacrifice these cells by chemically puncturing their membranes, letting the contents spill out, thus disrupting the viral replication cycle. Antibodies then neutralize the viruses by binding directly to their surfaces, preventing them from attacking other cells. Additionally, they precipitate chemical reactions that actually destroy infected cells.

4. **CALLING A TRUCE**
As the infection is contained, suppressor T cells halt the entire range of immune responses, preventing them from spiraling out of control. Memory T and B cells are left in the blood and lymphatic system, ready to move quickly should the same virus once again invade the body.

been modified to reduce the toxicity (for example, diphtheria and tetanus toxoids).

Artificial passive immunity is obtained by injecting various products that are usually prepared commercially, to produce a high level of antibodies immediately. These products are used to modify, treat, or prevent disease; they include gamma globulin and antitoxins.

Gamma globulin, obtained from the blood, is sometimes used for treatment, but is more frequently used for the prevention of viral hepatitis and measles. Antitoxins include the following:

- Diphtheria antitoxin, produced by vaccinating horses and then extracting the gamma globulin fraction of the blood, is used for the immediate prevention and treatment of diphtheria.
- Tetanus antitoxin, obtained by extracting the gamma globulin fraction from the blood of people recently vaccinated with the tetanus toxoid, is used for the immediate prevention and treatment of tetanus.
- Immune sera, either bacterial or viral in origin, are obtained from the gamma globulin fraction of blood from an artificially immunized animal. The rabies immune sera and the pertussis (whooping cough) immune sera are the most commonly used products.

Table 5-2 provides a guide to common vaccines and toxoids.

Vaccination records should be kept current. Parents must understand the purposes and possible risk factors when a child is immunized. As of August 1992, federal law states that a parent or guardian must be informed and sign a consent form allowing the child to be immunized (see also Pediatric Examinations in Unit Four). At times people must be vaccinated against particular diseases for travel purposes. A special certificate booklet must be completed verifying the required vaccination(s). These booklets can be obtained from your local U.S. Government Printing Office or from the Superintendent of Documents, U.S. Government Printing Office, Washington, D.C. 20402 (Figure 5-4).

INFLAMMATORY PROCESS

The inflammatory process is a nonspecific defense response of the body to an irritating, invasive, or injurious foreign substance. In other words, it is a process by which the body responds to injury. Acute inflammation is stimulated by necrosis and degeneration of tissue (injuries), invading microorganisms (infection), and antigen-antibody reactions (allergies). The inflammatory process includes dilation of the blood vessels because of increased blood flow, oozing of watery fluids and protein into tissue spaces (exudation) from the dilated blood vessels because of their increased permeability, and infiltration of neutrophils and monocytes (white blood cells) from the blood into the tissue of the injured area to phagocytize (ingest) necrotic tissue and bacteria, if present.

After phagocytosis is complete, the liquefied remains diffuse back into the blood vessels or are carried away by the lymphatic vessels that drain into regional lymph nodes. Here the contents are filtered to prevent the spread of foreign substances

or bacteria to other parts of the body. By now the process of repair has started at the original site of inflammation.

Signs and Symptoms

Classic signs and symptoms of inflammation include both local signs and symptoms, which are a result of the changes seen in the blood vessels and the effect on the surrounding tissues, and systemic signs and symptoms.

Local
  Redness
  Heat or warmth
  Swelling
  Pain or tenderness
  Limitation of function in the area
Systemic
  Leukocytosis (increased number of white blood cells in the blood)
  Fever
  Increased pulse rate
  Increased respiration rate

INFECTION
Signs and Symptoms

Common signs and symptoms of infection follow. The patient may have only a few of the signs and symptoms listed for each type of infection. At other times all of the listed signs and symptoms may be present. Common sexually transmitted diseases are discussed in Unit Eleven (see pages 363 to 370 and Table 11-1).

Localized infections
  Edema, redness of the area
  Exudate or drainage that is clear, cloudy, serous, purulent, or bloody
  Itching (in some infections)
  Pain
  Redness
  Swelling
  Tenderness
  Warmth
Generalized infections
  Altered mental status
  Confusion
  Congestion
  Convulsions
  Decreased appetite
  Fatigue
  Fever
  Headache
  Hypotension
  Increased pulse rate
  Jaundice (in some infections)
  Joint pain
  Light-headedness
  Malaise
  Muscle aches
  Possible elevation of white blood cell count

Shock
Gastrointestinal infections
  Abnormal bowel sounds
  Chest pain
  Congestion
  Cough
  Elevated white blood cell count
  Fever
  Increased pulse rate
  Positive sputum culture
  Positive throat culture
  Positive x-ray film findings
  Productive cough (sputum)
  Rhinitis
  Shortness of breath
  Sore throat
Genitourinary Infections
  Dysuria
  Elevated white blood cell count
  Fever
  Flank or pelvic pain
  Frequency
  Hematuria
  Positive urine culture
  Purulent or foul discharge
  Urgency

DIAGNOSTIC DATA

None of the local or systemic signs and symptoms of the inflammatory process are diagnostic in themselves. Many of these signs and symptoms are seen in disease processes other than the infectious process. However, they do provide clues that aid in the diagnosis of a suspected infection. Diagnostic tests in conjunction with an evaluation of the patient's general health status are required to confirm a diagnosis and initiate therapeutic decisions. Examples of diagnostic tests used to obtain data follow. Each of these tests is discussed in detail in its respective unit in this book.

* Microbiologic tests—bacterial, viral, and fungal cultures and the Gram stain; cultures are commonly obtained from blood, sputum, urine, spinal fluid, aspirates of body fluids, and body discharges at any possible site of infection
* Blood counts
* Urinalysis
* Skin tests
* Radiologic examinations
* Ultrasound examinations
* Gallium scans
* CT scans

The techniques for collecting and handling laboratory specimens must be correct to ensure accurate results (see Unit Eleven for the methods of properly handling and collecting specimens.) Inaccurate results lead to a false diagnosis and an inappropriate form of therapy for the patient. Knowledge of the infectious disease process, of the signs and symptoms of an infectious process, and of prevention and control measures are vital to control and prevent all infectious disease processes.

INFECTION CONTROL

To control and prevent the infectious process, the sequential connection between the six factors involved in this process must be broken at the weakest point. Various medical and surgical aseptic practices can break this cycle so that microorganisms cannot spread to and invade a susceptible host (see Figure 5-1).

MEDICAL ASEPSIS

Medical asepsis refers to the destruction of microorganisms after they leave the body. Techniques used to accomplish this include practices that help reduce the number and transfer of pathogens. We observe many of these practices in everyday living (for example, washing one's hands after using the bathroom or before handling food; covering one's nose and mouth when sneezing or coughing; and using one's own hair comb, toothbrush, and eating utensils).

Common medical aseptic practices to follow to break the cycle of the infectious process when working with patients include the following:

* Wash your hands before and after handling supplies and equipment, and before and after assisting with each patient. The handwashing procedure is discussed in detail in this unit.
* Handle all specimens as though they contain pathogens.
* Use disposable equipment when available, and dispose of it properly according to office policy. All equipment is considered contaminated after patient use.
* Clean nondisposable equipment before and after patient use.
* Use gloves to protect yourself (See Universal Precautions in Unit One).
* Avoid contact of used supplies with your uniform to prevent the transfer of pathogens to yourself and other patients.
* Place damp or wet dressings, bandages, and cottonballs in a waterproof bag when discarding them to prevent the possible spread of infection to individuals who handle the garbage.
* Cover any break in your skin as a protective measure against self-infection.
* Discard items that fall on the floor or clean before using, because all floors are contaminated.
* Use damp cloths for dusting or cleaning to avoid raising dust, which carries airborne microorganisms.

If you are unsure whether supplies are clean or sterile, clean or sterilize them before use.

These practices are used during "clean" procedures, which involve parts of the body that are not normally sterile. Specific examples include aseptic procedures used when tak-

Text continues on page 184.

Guide for Use of Selected Vaccines and Toxoids

This guide is intended to serve as a quick reference for commonly employed immunization procedures. It is based on recommendations made by the Public Health Service Advisory Committee on Immunization Practices (ACIP) and the Report of the Committee on Infectious Diseases 1982 (RED BOOK) of the American Academy of Pediatrics. Reference should be made to the complete published reports of these two committees for more detailed information on general considerations and specific applications of accepted immunization practices.

IMPORTANT: Avoid immunizing persons ill or febrile in preceding 24 hours. Carefully read the product description and directions supplied with each immunizing agent as potency (dosage) may vary with the manufacturer. In addition, agents may contain substances to which patients may be sensitive such as

Disease	Immunizing Agent	Age Range	Administration	Immunization Interval(s)	Booster Doses	Comments
Diphtheria, tetanus, and pertussis	Toxoids of diphtheria and tetanus, alum precipitated or adsorbed, combined with pertussis antigen (DTP)	For infants and children ages 6 weeks through 6 years	Three doses: 0.5 ml each IM Fourth dose: 0.5 ml IM	4-8 weeks 6-12 months	At age 4-6 years, preferably at time of school entrance. Dose: 0.5 ml IM	Do not use after 7th birthday.
Tetanus and diphtheria (for adults)	Toxoids of tetanus and diphtheria, alum precipitated or adsorbed, combined (contains 1-2 Lf units diphtheria toxoid) (Td)	7 years through adult	Two doses: 0.5 ml each IM Third dose: 0.5 ml IM	4-8 weeks 6-12 months	Every 10 years for life	For severe wounds, it is unnecessary to use booster doses if the patient has completed a primary series and has had a booster dose within the preceding 5 years (within 10 years for clean minor wounds)
Influenza	Inactivated (killed) polyvalent, bivalent or monovalent influenza virus vaccine (grown in chick embryo tissue)	All ages, from 6 months. Seasonally for high risk groups such as the elderly and those with chronic illness	May change from year to year. See instructions on manufacturer's package insert	4 weeks or more, if 2 doses are needed	Seasonally for high risk groups	Does not protect after exposure. "Split", or "subunit" vaccine generally recommended for children
Poliomyelitis	Inactivated (killed) trivalent, poliovirus vaccine (IPV) Types 1, 2, 3 combined	All ages. Begin: 6 weeks	Three doses: 1.0 ml each IM Fourth dose: 1.0 ml IM	4-8 weeks 6-12 months	Booster dose every 5 years through age 17	To be used in persons with altered immune states and in their households

Vaccine	Age	Dose	Number of doses / spacing	Recommended recall	Comment
Attenuated (live) trivalent oral poliovirus vaccine (TOPV). Types 1, 2, 3 combined	Begin: 6 weeks Routine use in persons age 18 and over in the United States is not needed	Three oral doses	Between doses: 1 and 2: 6-8 weeks; 2 and 3: 6-12 months	Preschool age (4-6 years) and when traveling to endemic areas. Repeated "booster" doses are not needed	Can be given to pregnant women in outbreak situations. Avoid in persons with altered immune states
Measles (rubeola)* Attenuated (live) measles virus vaccine	Age 15 months or older	One dose: 0.5 ml sc One dose: 0.5 ml sc	One dose only. However, measles vaccine should be given again if there is a history of receiving a) killed measles vaccine only, or live vaccine within 2 years of receiving killed vaccine; b) vaccine before the first birthday; c) live *further* attenuated vaccine with immune serum globulin (ISG) or measles immune globulin (MIG).		Contraindications: Altered immune states such as leukemia, lymphoma, antimetabolite and radiation therapy, and generalized malignancy. As with any live virus vaccine, avoid during pregnancy
Mumps* Attenuated (live) mumps virus vaccine	Age 12 months or older*	One dose: 0.5 ml sc	One dose only		As with any live virus vaccine, avoid during pregnancy and in persons with altered immune states.
Rubella* Attenuated (live) rubella virus vaccine	Susceptibles age 12 months or older*	One dose: 0.5 ml sc	One dose only		SHOULD NOT BE GIVEN DURING PREGNANCY. Women of childbearing age may be considered for immunization if advised of necessity to avoid pregnancy for three months following vaccine administration. Avoid in persons with altered immune states
Smallpox	As of 1980 there is no medical indication for smallpox vaccination in any part of the world except for persons handling variola/vaccinia-group viruses in research laboratories.				

Courtesy State of California, Department of Health Services, Infectious Disease Section, revised April 1983.
IM, Intramuscular; sc, subcutaneous.
**Combined live attenuated vaccines are available for these viruses (measles-mumps-rubella; measles-rubella; and mumps-rubella). If combined vaccine including measles vaccine is used, give at age 15 months or older.*

Figure 5-4 *International certificates of vaccination. Administration of vaccinations needed for international travel must be documented in this booklet and carried as the person travels. (Courtesy U.S. Department of Health, Education and Welfare)*

INTERNATIONAL CERTIFICATES OF VACCINATION

AS APPROVED BY
THE WORLD HEALTH ORGANIZATION
(EXCEPT FOR ADDRESS OF VACCINATOR)

CERTIFICATS INTERNATIONAUX DE VACCINATION

APPROUV'ES PAR
L' ORGANISATION MONDIALE DE LA SANT'E

(SAUF L'ADRESSE DU VACCINATEUR)

TRAVELER'S NAME-NOM DU VOUYAGEUR

ADDRESS-ADRESSE   (Number- Nem'ero)   (Sttreet-Rue)

(City-Ville)

(County-Departement)   (State-Etat)

U.S. DEPARTMENT OF
HEALTH, EDUCATION, AND WELFARE

PUBLIC HEALTH SERVICE

PHS-731 (REV. 1-74)
===

Figure 5-4—cont'd *International certificates of vaccination.*

INSTRUCTIONS TO TRAVELERS

International Certificates of Vaccination or Revaccination are official statements verifying that proper procedures have been followed to immunize you against a disease which could be a threat to the United States and other countries. The Certificates are second in importance only to your passport in permitting uninterrupted international travel. THEY MUST BE COMPLETE AND ACCURATE IN EVERY DETAIL, or you may be detained at ports of entry.

When your itinerary is complete, you may obtain information on immunizations required or recommended for foreign travel from your local or State Health Department.

How to Complete Your International Certificates of Vaccination
1. Enter your name and address on the cover of the booklet before presenting it to your physician.

2. On the Certificates required for your travel, print your name on the first line; sign your name on the second line; indicate you sex; and indicate your date of birth in the following sequence: day, month, year. Example: 5 June 1940.

3. Vaccination against smallpox and cholera may be given by any licensed physician in the United States. After the physician completes his part of the Certificate, take it to your local health department to be validated. Yellow fever immunization may be obtained only at a designated Yellow Fever Vaccination Center. The Certificate must be stamped with the official stamp of the Yellow Fever Vaccination Center.

4. It is your responsibility to have the Certificates validated with an "approved stamp." THE CERTIFICATES ARE NOT VALID WITHOUT AN "APPROVED STAMP."

INSTRUCTIONS TO PHYSICIAN

INFORMATION REQUESTED ON EACH CERTIFICATE MUST BE COMPLETE FOR THE CERTIFICATE TO BE VALID.

1. The space for primary vaccination against smallpox is to be used only when a person receives his vaccination for the first time. If unsuccessful, and new Certificate must be used for a repeat primary vaccination.

2. The dates on each Certificate are to be written with the day in arabic numerals, followed by the month in letters and the year in arabic numerals. Example: 1Jan. 1971.

3. Vaccinations may be given by nurses and medical practitioner. The WRITTEN signature of the physician or other person authorized by him must appear on the Certiticate. A signature stamp is not acceptable.

4. If smallpox vaccination is contraindicated on medical grounds, you should provide the patient with a written statment, on your letterhead, signed and dated, indicating the nature on the contraindication.

5. Information concerning officail immunization requirements for international travel and the location of Yellow Fever Vaccination Centers in your area may be obtained from your local or State Health Department.

DO NOT THROW THIS BOOKLET AWAY. YOU MAY HAVE OCCASION TO USE THE CERTIFICATES FOR FUTURE TRAVEL AND AS A RECORD OF YOUR VACCINATION HISTORY.

Figure 5-4—cont'd *International certificates of vaccination.*

PERSONAL HEALTH HISTORY

The information which follows is a record of other immunizations which the traveler has obtained as an additional health protection for international travel. These immunizations are NOT usually required for entrance by any country. Space is also provided for a personal health record in case of illness or accident while traveling abroad.

OTHER IMMUNIZATIONS (Typhus, Typhoid, Plague, Poliomyelitis, Tetanus, etc.)

Date	Vaccine	Dose	Physician's Signature

Figure 5-4—cont'd *International certificates of vaccination.*

REMARKS CONCERNING VACCINATIONS-REMARQUES CONCERNANT LES VACCINATIONS

Date	Notes	Physician's signature and address Signature et adresse du me'decin

This information is to assist any physician called upon to treat an ill traveler.
Cette information est pour aider le me'decin qui peut etre appel'e pour traiter un voyageur malade.

Date	Rh type Type Rh	Blood group Groupe sanguin	Name and address of physician-Signature et adresse du medecin

Name and address of person to
notify in case of emergency.

Nom et adresse de la personne
a aviser en cas d'urgence.

REMARKS concerning state of health, medical treatments, or known sensitivities:
REMARQUES concernant I'etat de sante, traitements medicaux, ou sensibilites connues:

OPHTHALMIC INFORMATION (Prescription Glasses)

	Sphere	Cylinder	Axis	Prism	Base
(OD) Ocular Dexter					
(OS) Ocular Sinister					

Add _____   Base Curve _____
Other _____

ing a temperature; obtaining urine, stool, or sputum specimens; obtaining smears or cultures from the throat or vagina; administering oral medications; removing and discarding used supplies; and cleaning a treatment room after use. See Universal Precautions in Unit One .

Handwashing

To prevent the spread of microorganisms, handwashing is one of the first procedures that all health personnel must learn. *Correct handwashing is the foundation of aseptic technique.* Hands that are not properly cleansed frequently spread infection because the hands are in constant use when working with or around patients.

This procedure must become an automatic part of your work. Its importance *cannot* be overemphasized, and your conscientiousness *cannot* be overstressed. The time involved to wash the hands, wrists, and forearms well should be 1 to 2 minutes (2 to 4 minutes if they are highly contaminated).

The use of bar soap is being discouraged because of the possibility of cross-contamination between people using it. In addition, a wet bar of soap is a good reservoir for microorganisms. Liquid soap or soap granules are preferred and recommended, especially in areas where many people use the same facilities. When liquid soap is used, the dispenser should be replaced or cleaned and filled with fresh product when empty; liquids should not be added to a partially full dispenser.

The following handwashing procedure includes information on using a bar of soap *ONLY when it is the only form of soap available. Remember, liquid soap is preferred and* **MUST** **be used when available.**

The Centers for Disease Control and Prevention (CDC) recommends the following guidelines:
- Wash your hands for 2 minutes before beginning to work with patients. This provides effective protection.
- Wash your hands for 30 seconds after each patient contact. This ensures minimal spread of infection.
- Wash your hands for 1 minute immediately after handling contaminated equipment, supplies, or organic material.

Also see Barrier Precautions and Handwashing in Unit One.

SURGICAL ASEPSIS

Surgical asepsis refers to the destruction of all microorganisms, pathogenic as well as nonpathogenic, before they enter the body. The goal of surgical asepsis is to prevent infection or the introduction of microorganisms into the body.

Practices of surgical asepsis are usually referred to as sterile techniques and are used when an area and supplies in that area must be made and kept sterile. These techniques are used in all procedures in which entry into normally sterile body parts occurs (for example, when administering injections, when changing dressings on a wound, and during all surgical procedures).

HANDWASHING

Equipment

Clean paper towels
Sink with running water

Soap—liquid preferred
Orangewood stick or nail brush

PROCEDURE	RATIONALE
1. Remove jewelry, except plain wedding band. Remove watch or move it up. Provide complete access to area to be washed.	*Jewelry may harbor microorganisms.*
2. Stand in front of the sink, making sure that your clothing does not touch the sink.	*Sinks are always contaminated.*
3. Turn water on; adjust it to a lukewarm temperature and a moderate flow to avoid splashing.	*Warm water makes better suds than cold water; hot water may burn or dry the skin.*
4. Wet hands and apply soap. When using bar soap, keep the bar in your hands throughout the whole procedure. For liquid soap use approximately 1 teaspoon. Apply enough soap to develop a good lather. If you drop the bar of soap, you must repeat the procedure.	*Only the inside of a bar of soap is clean when in use; all other objects are considered contaminated.*

HANDWASHING—cont'd

PROCEDURE

5. Wash hands (palm, sides, and back), fingers, knuckles, and between each finger, using a vigorous rubbing and circular motion (Figure 5-5, page 186). If wearing a wedding band, slide it down the finger a bit and scrub skin underneath it. You must wash *all* areas on the hands. Interlace fingers and scrub between each finger (Figure 5-5).

6. During the procedure, keep the hands and forearms at elbow level or below and hands pointed down.

7. Rinse hands well under running water.

8. Wash wrists and forearms as high as contamination is likely.

9. If soap bar was used, rinse it off and drop it on a rack in the dish without touching the dish. Bar soap should ONLY be used when liquid soap or soap granules are not available.

10. Rinse hands, wrists, and forearms under running water (Figure 5-6, page 186).

11. Clean nails with orangewood stick or nail brush at least once a day when starting work and each time hands are highly contaminated; then rinse well under running water (Figure 5-7, page 186).

12. Repeat steps 3 through 10 when the hands are highly contaminated.

13. Thoroughly dry hands, wrists, and forearms with paper towels. Use a dry towel for each hand.

14. Use another dry paper towel to turn water faucet off (Figure 5-8, page 186).

15. Use hand lotion as necessary.

RATIONALE

Friction caused by vigorous rubbing mechanically removes dirt and organisms.

This prevents water from running down to the elbows, which are areas of less contamination than the hands.

Washing the wrists and forearms after the hands prevents the spread of microorganisms from the hands to these areas.

Soap bars are excellent media for the growth of bacteria; therefore they must be rinsed after use. The soap dish is considered contaminated and therefore must not be touched. Bar soap should be kept on racks that allow drainage of water so that the soap can dry.

Running water rinses away the dirt and organisms that have been loosened during the washing process.

Microorganisms collect and can remain under the nails unless cleansed away.

A second washing is necessary when the hands are heavily contaminated to ensure that all the microorganisms have been removed.

Drying the skin completely prevents chapping.

The faucet is contaminated; using a paper towel allows the hands to remain clean.

Lotion helps replace the skin's natural oils and prevents chapping. Chapping skin is more difficult to keep clean and more likely to crack. Once the skin is broken, microorganisms can easily enter and cause an infection.

HANDWASHING—cont'd

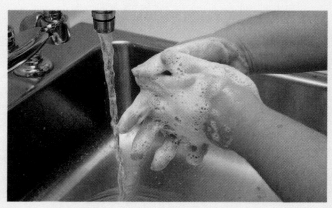

Figure 5-5 *Handwashing technique. Interlace the fingers to wash between them. Create a lather with the soap. Keep hands pointed down.*

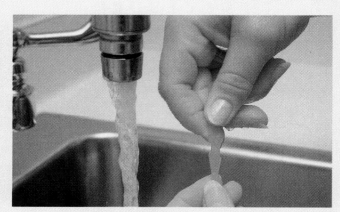

Figure 5-7 *Use the blunt edge of an orangewood stick to clean under the fingernails.*

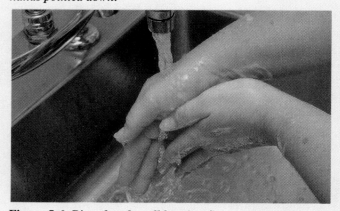

Figure 5-6 *Rinse hands well keeping fingers pointed down.*

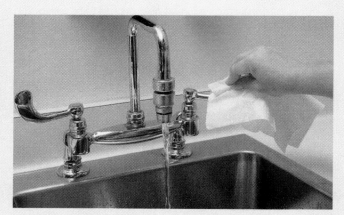

Figure 5-8 *After drying your hands, turn water faucet off, using a dry paper towel.*

Measures used to obtain and provide surgical asepsis include absolute sterilization of all instruments and supplies that come in contact with normally sterile body parts and open wounds, thorough handwashing with a detergent or surgical soap, and wearing sterile gloves during sterile procedures, other than when administering injections. During surgical procedures, the physician and those directly involved with the procedure also wear a sterile gown, a cap, and a mask to help prevent contamination.

Methods of sterilization and disinfection are discussed in this unit. The use of other surgical aseptic or sterile techniques and practices is discussed in Unit Six.

METHODS TO CONTROL MICROSCOPIC AGENTS

Sanitization, disinfection, and sterilization are the three principal methods used for inhibiting the growth of and destroying microscopic life. Each represents a different level of decontamination, and though often used jointly, one must not be confused or substituted for the other.

Sanitization, the first step that must always be done before items can be reliably disinfected or sterilized, is a process of cleansing and scrubbing items with agents such as water and detergents, or chemicals. Ultrasonic cleaners are also used (see Figure 5-19).

Disinfection involves methods that destroy "most" infectious microorganisms. However, some resistant and spore-forming bacteria and some viruses such as the hepatitis B virus are not adequately destroyed by these methods. Agents used to disinfect items include various types of chemical germicides and boiling water or flowing steam.

Sterilization is a precise scientific term with a single, exact meaning when applied to medical supplies and instruments. Sterilization is defined as the processes or methods that completely destroy all forms of microscopic life.

Using specific procedures, sterilization is accomplished by subjecting the object(s) to chemical or physical agents that are capable of killing the microorganisms. It must be emphasized that there are no degrees of sterility—*objects are either sterile or unsterile.*

SANITIZING INSTRUMENTS

PROCEDURE

1. Bulk rinse the instruments in water containing a blood solvent, a low-sudsing detergent, or any *approved* germicide solution.

2. Rinse the instruments in another sink or pan of fresh water.

3. Scrub each instrument thoroughly with a brush and a warm nonionizing detergent solution (such as Tide or Joy). Keep the instrument under a flow of water or in water when scrubbing with the brush (Figure 5-9). Pay special attention to serrated edges and other areas where blood, oil, or grease may collect.

4. Using hot water, thoroughly rinse all detergent off the instruments.

5. Remove the excess moisture from the instruments by rolling them in a towel.

6. Check all instruments for working condition, and check to see that they are thoroughly cleaned. Never oil instruments, even if they are stiff when using them.

7. Wrap the instruments for sterilization.

8. When instruments cannot be cleaned immediately after use, soak them in a solution of water and an effective blood solvent. Never soak an instrument in saline.

RATIONALE

This first step is to clean all debris, oil, blood, and grease off the instruments.

Any detergent residue on an instrument prevents dininfection.

Drying instruments helps to prevent rusting.

Oil on an instrument may keep a contaminated area from a sterilizing agent.

Soaking prevents blood or other organic matter from drying or hardening on the instrument (which would be more difficult to remove later). Saline causes corrosion to the instrument.

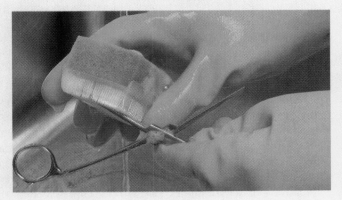

Figure 5-9 *When scrubbing, wear heavy rubber gloves over disposable gloves.*

Sterilization plays a vital role in protecting the health and life of patients who seek treatment in both physicians' offices and hospitals. The use of presterilized disposable equipment has greatly helped reduce the spread of microorganisms and the need for sterilization procedures. Almost all equipment used in a physician's office or clinic is now available in disposable materials. Nonetheless, certain nondisposable items and equipment such as a stethoscope are used repeatedly on many patients. Therefore the microorganisms that contaminate nondisposable supplies must be destroyed by appropriate measures.

Methods used to accomplish sterilization include:

- Dry heat
- Moderately heated chemical gas mixtures
- Chemical agents
- Steam under pressure (autoclaves)
- Unsaturated chemical vapor (Chemiclaves)

The first three methods are limited to certain applications and require longer exposure periods to sterilize items; therefore they are not often used. The autoclave, the most commonly used sterilizing method, and the Chemiclave are considered the most efficient, reliable, and practical answers to meet the sterilizing needs in the physician's office or clinic.

STERILIZATION

Preparation of materials. The initial step when sterilizing or disinfecting contaminated items is to remove them from the treatment room to the work area designated for dirty equipment. Take care to avoid contamination to yourself or injury from any sharp instrument, and to prevent dulling any sharp blade or scissors while you are handling instruments. When you handle contaminated items or if you have any break in your skin, wear heavy rubber gloves with long cuffs over disposable gloves, a plastic apron or gown, and safety glasses, goggles, or personal glasses with added solid side shields or a chin length face shield when sanitizing supplies.

After you clean supplies, your hands are contaminated. Wash them as described previously (see also Barrier Precautions in Unit One.)

Inspection of instruments. The purpose of checking instruments is to ensure that they are in proper working order and in alignment before they are needed for use in a procedure. Check instruments in a well-lit clean area. Instruments should be dry before you check them.

1. Check that the serrations of each instrument meet evenly.
2. Check that the ratchets close easily and that they do not spring open.
3. Check that the instruments open and close easily.
4. Check that all parts are present (for example, that the screws of a speculum are intact).
5. Coat instruments with a water-soluble lubricant such as instrument milk* to protect from corrosion and to provide lubrication for the hinges.
6. Air-dry for 20 minutes.
7. If imperfections are found, separate out and follow agency policy for dealing with broken equipment.
8. The instruments are now ready to be wrapped for sterilization.

Wrapping instruments and related supplies for sterilization. The next step before sterilizing items that are to be stored for future use is to wrap them in protective coverings such as clean muslin or special disposable paper bags. These materials are used because they can be permeated by steam or the chemical vapor from the sterilizer, but not by airborne or surface contaminants during handling and storage.

Items that will be used immediately or those that do not have to be sterile when used (for example, supplies used for "clean" procedures) can be sterilized by placing them in the sterilizer tray with muslin or other material designated by the manufacturer under and over them. When you have completed the sterilizing process, remove the items with sterile transfer forceps and then either use or place them in the proper storage area.

Wrap the items that are to be kept sterile for future use. Wrap together materials and instruments that will be used together. Leave hinged instruments such as hemostats open

*Preplube Solution recommends 1:10. Review and follow the manufacturer's directions.

when they are being sterilized for immediate or future use. Sterilize containers with lids on their sides with the lid off; place the lid at the side or bottom of the container, with the inner surface facing outwards.

The method for wrapping instruments and other supplies such as dressings is the same. Figure 5-10 explains and illustrates the method to be used for wrapping these items. Study and practice this procedure of preparation. Keep packs small. Wrap loosely but firm enough for handling.

Another aid to sterilization has been the introduction of disposable packaging materials, including paper, pouches and tubing of paper and plastic. They are convenient for sterilizing and storing syringes, tubing, and special purpose items.

ATI Steriline bags are made of a special heavy-duty, wet-strength, surgical grade paper that allows rapid steam penetration during sterilization. They also act as a barrier against airborne bacteria during storage.

Each Steriline bag is printed with a temperature and steam-sensitive indicator consisting of an indicator line that changes color during sterilization to show that an item has been processed through the sterilizer (Figure 5-11, *A*).

ATI pouches and tubing offer a clearly labeled package that can be used either for steam or ethylene oxide gas sterilization. They offer advantages similar to those of Steriline bags, plus the benefits of content visibility and an easy, peel-open feature. Their use minimizes the risk of damaging expensive items by using the wrong sterilizing method. The steam indicator changes color from blue to grey/black during processing in either a gravity displacement or pre-vacuum, high-temperature steam sterilizer. The gas indicator changes color from yellow to rust/red during processing in an ethylene oxide gas sterilizer (Figure 5-11, *B*).

ATI Instrument Protectors are convenient, disposable holders for delicate surgical instruments. They protect instrument tips from being cracked or broken and help prevent the instrument from penetrating the pouch or package in which it is placed. Chemical indicators on each protector verify steam or ethylene oxide (EO) gas processing. To use these holders, first insert the instrument through the slots of the protector until the tip is completely covered by the plastic flap. Open hinged instruments such as scissors, and fold the antilock flap forward between the handles. For added protection and holding ability, tuck the antilock flap into the top slot. Slide the loaded instrument protector into a sterilization pouch, with the instrument facing the film side. Seal the pouch in the normal manner and sterilize (Figure 5-11, *A* to *C*).

Wrapping reusable syringes and needles. Syringes are best wrapped in special disposable paper bags or peel pouches that are available for sterilization (see Figure 5-11).

AUTOCLAVE—STEAM STERILIZATION

Any appreciation of infection control must include an understanding of the basic principles and procedures of sterilization. Although different methods of sterilization are available, steam sterilization still remains one of the most effective, economical, and safe procedures and is considered the method of choice whenever applicable.

Figure 5-10 *Wrapping technique.*

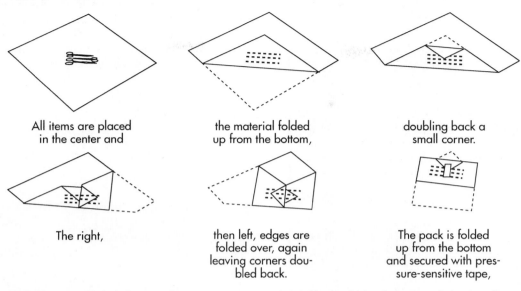

All items are placed in the center and

the material folded up from the bottom,

doubling back a small corner.

The right,

then left, edges are folded over, again leaving corners doubled back.

The pack is folded up from the bottom and secured with pressure-sensitive tape,

then dated and labeled according to its contents. The pack should be firm enough for handling, but loose enough to permit proper circulation of steam. The materials included in each pack can be varied to suit the needs of each office, but the same wrapping pattern should be followed for all packs.

The *purpose* of sterilization is to completely destroy all living microorganisms, including spores and viruses that may be present in the item being sterilized. The process must destroy or kill *all* microorganisms , including those that cause infection or disease (pathogens). There is no such thing as an object being "almost sterile" or "partially sterile."

Bacterial Life Cycle

The reason why sterilization must be an absolute process is based on our knowledge of the bacterium and its life cycle. Bacteria have a very high rate of reproduction and can multiply rapidly into millions within hours. If only a few of these bacteria enter an operative wound from a supposedly sterile item, their multiplication may delay or inhibit recovery. Some may even cause the death of a patient. Bacteria in their vegetative form are easily destroyed by correct sterilization methods; but their spores are far more resistant. Spore forming is a protective mechanism by which the bacteria are able to remain dormant for extended periods of time, even years. In this state, they can survive conditions that would quickly kill their active or vegetative form. However, when these spores are again placed in a favorable condition for development, they become active bacteria capable of causing infection and death. Surgically critical microorganisms such as anthrax and clostridium can pose a real threat to the human body if not completely destroyed. Thus sterilization must be absolute and destroy both active bacteria and their spores.

Critical Factors in Steam Sterilization

Heat and moisture. Since microorganism destruction must be absolute, a knowledge of the factors controlling steam sterilization is essential. The killing power of saturated steam depends on three main factors: *heat, moisture,* and *time*. Heat by itself can readily kill bacteria. This is accomplished by disrupting the cell's life functions through coagulation of cell protein. However, spores are more resistant to dry heat but are readily destroyed by sufficient moist heat. Saturated steam is a gas and is therefore able to circulate by convection. This process allows it to penetrate porous objects in the steam sterilizer.

Time. At any given temperature, exposure must be for a specific period of time in order to completely disrupt and destroy all the microorganisms. Steam sterilization may be adequately accomplished at any temperature above 212° F (100° C), provided the related time period of exposure is used. You should always adhere to the required time period; otherwise unsterile supplies may result.

Research recommends a minimum of 12 minutes of direct exposure to saturated steam at 250° F (121° C) for surgical sterilization. In practice, it usually takes longer for direct exposure to take place throughout the pack (see Exposure Times).

When the temperature is increased, the length of time needed for sterilization decreases. Conversely, if the temperature is lowered, more time is needed to ensure sterilization. This time-temperature ratio can vary from 0.9 minutes at 275° F (135° C) to 834 minutes at 212° F (100° C).

Temperature/pressure. Since saturated steam is a gas, it is subject to the physical laws of gasses. Although a detailed discussion of the subject is not possible here, two physical relationships between temperature and pressure should be mentioned. First, saturated steam cannot undergo a

A

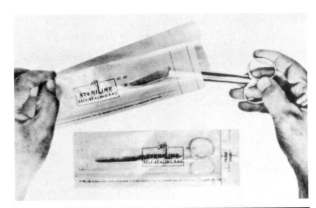

Figure 5-11 A to C, *ATI Instrument Protectors are thick, disposable paper holders designed to protect delicate surgical instruments during sterilization. They hold instruments snugly in place and help prevent the instrument from penetrating the pouch in which they are placed. Each Instrument Protector has steam and EO gas indicators to verify processing in a sterilizer.*
Courtesy ATI, a division of PyMaH Corp, Somerville, NJ.

B

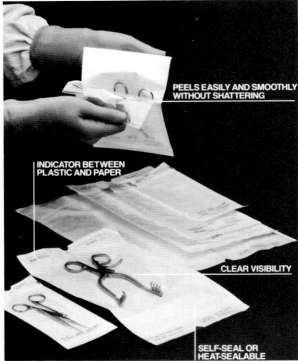

PEELS EASILY AND SMOOTHLY
WITHOUT SHATTERING

INDICATOR BETWEEN
PLASTIC AND PAPER

CLEAR VISIBILITY

SELF-SEAL OR
HEAT-SEALABLE

C

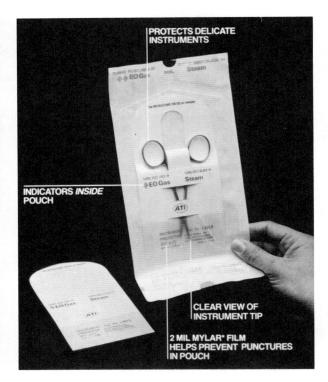

PROTECTS DELICATE
INSTRUMENTS

INDICATORS *INSIDE*
POUCH

CLEAR VIEW OF
INSTRUMENT TIP

2 MIL MYLAR* FILM
HELPS PREVENT PUNCTURES
IN POUCH

reduction in temperature without a corresponding lowering of pressure (the opposite is also true). Second, in high-altitude regions, it is necessary to use greater steam pressure to reach the minimum temperature range for sterilization. This is because atmospheric pressure decreasing with an elevation in altitude.

Steam quality. It should be briefly noted that steam can exist in various physical states, all of which have an effect on sterilizer performance. The three most common forms are:

1. *Saturated steam:* Steam containing pure gaseous water holding as much water as possible for its temperature and pressure. It is the most effective form of steam for sterilization.

2. *Wet steam:* This is usually formed when water from the boiler or condensate from the pipes carrying the steam is injected into the sterilizer. The result is an excess of water that can cause items in the sterilizer to become wet.

3. *Superheated steam:* Steam formed from saturated steam that is further subjected to higher temperatures. The steam becomes "dried out" and lacks sufficient water vapor, resulting in the loss of essential moisture necessary for sterilization.

General Procedures

Correct sterilization technique is essential for the destruction of microorganisms and their spores. Remember that steam is lighter than air and that air must be eliminated from the sterilizer.

The following is an abbreviated discussion of recommended procedures.

Positioning loads in an autoclave. Proper positioning of all instruments and materials is extremely important because of the pattern that steam follows as it circulates through the autoclave.

WRAPPING REUSABLE SYRINGES AND NEEDLES

PROCEDURE

1. Write the size of the syringe and the date on the outside of the bag.

2. Wrap barrel and plunger of the syringe separately in gauze.

3. Place matching separated syringe barrel and plunger inside the bag (or peel pouch) with the top of both facing the same direction.

4. Fold the top of the bag and seal securely.

5. When the needle is to be sterilized with the syringe, place the needle in a disposable paper form.

6. Label the bag with the size of syringe and needle and the date.

7. Place the needle in the bag with the syringe and plunger; fold the top of the bag and seal.

8. When the needle is to be sterilized individually, place it in a plastic pouch as described in Figure 5-12, A and B.

RATIONALE

Size must be indicated for identification. Date must be indicated, because if not used within 21 to 30 days (varies with office or agency preference), it must be rewrapped and resterilized.

The paper form protects the point of the needle, allows steam penetration, provides a means for sterile handling when putting the needle on the syringe tip for use, and also prevents the needle from piercing the bag.

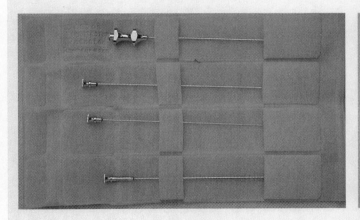
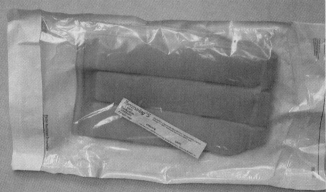

B

Figure 5-12   A *and* **B,** *Needles in packets ready for autoclaving. Some surgical needles are reusable, but the sterilization process is handled by central sterilization supplies in hospitals. Sterilization of needles generally is not handled in offices.*

A direction booklet, which must be read carefully, is supplied with every sterilizer. Usually, when the sterilizing cycle begins, steam builds up at the top of the inside chamber and moves downward from the point of admission. Dry, cool air is forced downward and out an exhaust drain at the bottom front part of the chamber. You must place all materials so that steam can flow between the packs and penetrate them. To avoid the formation of air pockets, you must place containers, tubes, cups, and similar items on their sides so that cool air can drain out in a downward direction and be replaced by

steam. If they are placed upright, air becomes trapped in the item, which in turn prevents steam from contacting all surfaces, resulting in incomplete sterilization.

Place syringes wrapped in disposable paper bags horizontally (on their sides) in the sterilizer tray so steam can circulate inside the syringe barrel. Place constriction or test tubes with needles horizontally so that steam can circulate inside the tube. Place linen and dressing packs in a vertical position.

When sterilizing linen packs and hard items in the same load, place the linen packs on top and the hard items on the bottom to prevent water condensation from dripping down on the linen packs. Items should not rest against plastic utensils to allow plastics to retain their shape even though exposed to very high temperatures.

Above all, *do not* overload the sterilizer chamber, regardless of the number of items being sterilized. Place the articles as loosely as possible inside the chamber. Leave a 1- to 3-inch space between all articles and the surrounding walls in the chamber. Correct positioning and spacing of all materials allows effective sterilization to occur when the proper *temperature, pressure,* and *time* requirements are also met (Figure 5-13, *A,* and *B*).

NOTE: Do not try to open the door of the sterilizer for any reason once the sterilizing cycle has begun. If you do open the door while the cycle is in progress, the steam under pressure may cause severe injury to you. At that time it may be impossible to re-close the door because of the presssure remaining inside the sterilizer. If the door is opened before the exhaust phase has been completed, the sterlizing process will be ineffective.

Exposure times. All loads placed in a sterilizer must be timed carefully after the sterilizer has attained the proper temperature. The length of sterilization time varies with the items and whether a wrapper, paper, or fabric is used. Suppliers of such materials supply correct exposure data to ensure observance of adequate exposure periods.

The *high temperature* attained is the *sterilizing influence* that destroys the microorganisms. The amount of pressure used only makes it possible to develop the high temperature. An accurate thermometer on the autoclave should be used to provide a positive indication that sterilizing conditions have been met in the chamber. Thus the three variables in the sterilizing cycle of an autoclave are *time, temperature,* and *pressure.* Altering any one of these means that you must alter the others.

In the autoclave, when steam is in contact with all surfaces of the items, 30 to 45 minutes and 15 to 17 pounds of pressure

at 250° F (121° C) is adequate time to kill all known microorganisms. However, in practice, longer periods are necessary to achieve this exposure. Recommended exposure times for items placed in an autoclave at 250° F (121° C) follow.

Wrapped surgical instruments	30 minutes
Wrapped syringes and needles	30 minutes
Wrapped rubber good (excessive exposure causes heat damage to the rubber)	20 minutes
Wrapped dressings	30 minutes
Wrapped suture materials	30 minutes
Wrapped treatment trays	30 minutes
Unwrapped utensils, glassware, and similar items, when inverted or placed on edge	15 minutes
Unwrapped instruments covered with muslin	20 minutes

Again, you must scrupulously watch methods of wrapping, time of exposure, and temperature, since the purpose of autoclaving is to sterilize every article completely. Each manufacturer's direction booklet must be read and followed carefully to achieve adequate sterilization.

Care and cleaning of the autoclave. It is essential to follow the manufacturer's instructions for cleaning and maintenance. Follow the spore check schedule for maintaining the autoclave.

Chemical sterilization indicators. Numerous commercial devices are used to indicate the effectiveness of the sterilization process. Used correctly, these devices, known as chemical sterilization indicators, are adequate assurances that the parameters of the sterilization process are met. These indicators work on the principle that specifically prepared dyes will change color when exposed to the high temperature and saturated steam in the autoclave for a specific time. Individual disposable indicators for which color changes are to be observed after sterilization include the Sterilometer-

Figure 5-13 **A,** *Instruments in autoclave for sterilization must be well spaced, and hinged handles left open.* **B,** *Linen packs spaced correctly in an autoclave.*

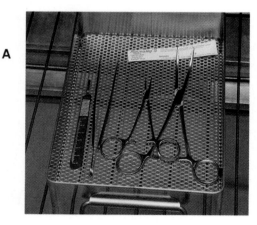

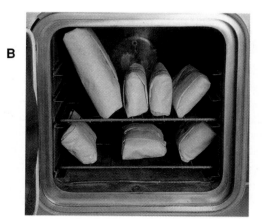

REMOVING LOADS FROM THE STERILIZER

PROCEDURE	RATIONALE
1. Exhaust steam pressure from the chamber. Read and follow precisely the manufacturer's directions for exhausting steam.	
2. When the pressure has reached 0 and the temperature has decreased to 212° F, open the door of the autoclave *slightly* (Figure 5-14). Only *"crack"* open the door.	*Stand back from the door to avoid steam burns to the face and hands. An open sterilizer door allows condensation from outside cool air; this results in wet packs.*
3. Allow the contents to dry for approximately 15 minutes before removing them. Some modern autoclaves automatically provide a sterilization cycle that includes drying, thus eliminating the need for these steps.	*Packs must not be removed wet or damp. If wet or damp packs are touched, they will be contaminated. Also, if a pack is hot and placed on a cool surface, moisture condenses and contaminates the pack.*
4. Regardless of the type of sterilizer you use, all dry, wrapped items and unwrapped items that do not have to remain sterile can then be removed with your clean, dry hands. Do not remove unwrapped metal objects too soon with bare hands.	*Metal retains heat, and you could get burned.*
5. Remove unwrapped items that are to remain sterile for immediate use with sterile transfer forcep; place items to be used later in sterile storage containers.	

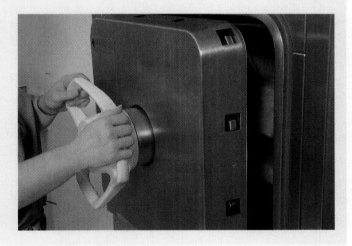

Figure 5-14 *When the sterilization cycle is finished, "crack" open the door* slightly *and allow the contents to dry for 15 minutes before removing them.*

Plus and Sterilo-meters (Figure 5-15, *A* and *B*). Sterilometer-Plus represents one of the most precise, complete chemical indicators available. It consists of two indicator bars covered by a clear plastic overlay. The indicator bars contain a special reactive pigment that changes color from purple to green only in the presence of steam and not in the presence of heat alone (the water molecules in the steam actually are part of the color-change reaction, so that the reaction cannot take place without steam present). The clear plastic overlay prevents the indicator areas from coming into contact with items being sterilized.

When the indicator is exposed to steam in a sterilizer, the steam begins to work on the indicator inks. The heat energy and water content of the steam react with the purple pigment in the ink and cause it to turn green. The ink contains other chemicals that carefully control the amount of time necessary for the ink to completely change color, so that the indicator changes only when the conditions necessary for complete sterilization have been met.

The Sterilo-meter is a disposable tag that is placed in the center of a pack with the nonindicator end extended outside the wrapper. This enables the indicator to be removed without touching the contents of the pack. Sterilization conditions of adequate steam, temperature, and time are ensured if the wide bar at the opposite end has changed completely from white to black. If these color change standards do not result, the pack must be reprocessed and resterilized.

Also, specific areas or markings on the outside of commercially prepared packages and on special disposable bags that are available for wrapping instruments, syringes, and needles change color if sterilization standards have been met (see Figure 5-15). These preceding indicators are superior to the frequently used autoclave tape indicators, because the dark diagonal lines that appear on the tape at the end of the sterilization cycle merely indicate that the pack has been exposed to steam and the autoclaving process (Figure 5-16). There are many other indicators available for various types of sterilization processes. Figure 5-17 illustrates the dry heat steriliza-

Figure 5-15 A, *Sterilometer-Plus sterilization indicators. Color changes from purple to green on the indicator bars, pointing out when the conditions necessary for sterilization have been met.* **B,** *Sterilometer sterilization indicators. Sterilization conditions are ensured if the wide bar at one end has changed completely from white to black.*
Sterilometer-Plus and Sterilometer are registered trademarks of PyMah Corp., Somerville, NJ.

A
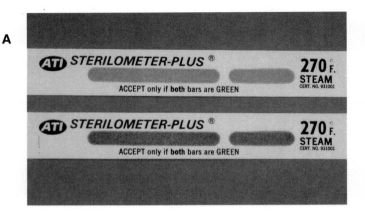

B

Figure 5-16 *Autoclave indicator tape used to seal and label packages before sterilization.*

Figure 5-17 *Dry heat sterilization indicator labels.*

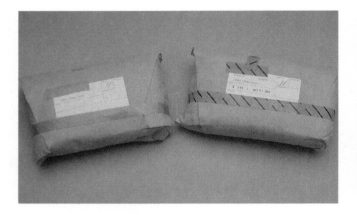

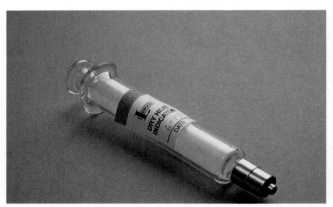

tion indicator on a pressure-sensitive label, which changes from tan to black when exposed for 5 minutes.

Evidence of sterility of equipment can *only* be obtained if a culture is taken from the equipment after it has been processed in the sterilizer. This means that the pack would have to be opened, and once opened it would be contaminated by the air. *Biologic indicators and monitors* in test packs placed in the sterilizer can provide definitive biologic verification that conditions to kill spores were met in the sterilizer. An example of biologic monitors are small strips of specially impregnated paper to which a precise number of live, nonpathogenic resistant spores have been applied. They are designed to validate both the actual sterilizer "kill" function and the operator's wrapping and processing technique. The biologic strips are placed in hard-to-reach parts of the sterilizer, cycled with a normal load of instruments and then cultured (provided with nutrition and incubation) and tested 24 and 48 hours later. If the spores grow, sterilization has not been achieved. A biologic monitor should be used daily in each sterilizer or according to

agency policy. This helps to ensure that the sterilization process is effective and safe.

Causes of Insufficient Sterilization

Failure of the indicators to change colors completely indicates a serious lack of steam penetration into the pack. This is a warning that there may be a sterilizer malfunction or an error in the sterilization technique. *Never neglect this warning.* Causes of sterilization failure are numerous, elusive, and often difficult to locate. The problem may require minute examination of every part of the sterilizer and/or a complete reexamination of your preparation, wrapping, and loading techniques. Some of the most common problems are:
1. Faulty preparation of materials
2. Improper loading of the sterilizer
3. Faulty sterilizer
4. Air in the sterilizer
5. Wet steam

Sanitize all materials completely beforehand, and wrap and secure them properly as described previously. You must position the load correctly in the sterilizer and not overload the chamber. Timing for adequate exposure times must begin *after* the sterilizer has attained the proper temperature. If all of these conditions have been met satisfactorily and sterilization has not taken place, you must have the equipment checked for a defect and repaired as necessary (Table 5-3).

Storing sterile supplies. Special storage places for each type of supply should be maintained away from areas where contaminated materials are handled. Storage places must be clean, dry, and dustproof. Sterile items wrapped in cloth or special sterilization paper can safely be stored for 21 to 30 days. Wrapped items that are placed in sterile plastic duster covers can be stored for 6 months, and items wrapped in plas-

tic teel-packs (special envelopes with one side of transparent plastic and the other side of paper) for 3 months. When these time periods are elapsed, all packs should be reprocessed and resterilized before use. Create a system for storing supplies (for example, load sterilizer or new items on the right side of the shelf and remove them for use from the left side). If supplies are stored in longer, narrower shelves, put the oldest supplies in the front and the new in the back. With these systems, the oldest supplies are always stored on the left side of the designated shelf so that they will be used first. Set a time once a month, to review the examination rooms and all cupboards and shelves to ascertain adequate inventory levels, expired dates, and defective or contaminated packages. Remove any defective or outdated supplies and reprocess them for sterilization.

TABLE 5-3

Problems Encountered in Sterilizing Technique

Probable Causes	Corrections
Damp or wet loads	
Clogged strainer in exhaust line; clogged steam trap	Remove strainer; free openings of lint and sediment daily; use trisodium phosphate solution weekly
Placing warm sterilized packs on cold surfaces	Allow packs to cool before removing from sterilizer, or place on surfaces covered with several layers of towels or drapes
Sterilized goods removed too soon from sterilizer following completion of cycle	Allow goods to remain in sterilizer at completion of cycle an additional 15 minutes—door slightly opened 1/2 inch
Improper loading; tightly loaded packs	Leave space between items; arrange items to present least possible resistance to passage of air and steam through layers of load; position load so water does not collect in utensils; place packs on edge
Pools of water on floor of chamber	Bottom of sterilizer must lean toward exhaust port so condensation can drain
Wet steam	Contact manufacturer in charge of maintenance
Deposits on interior	Weekly cleaning of sterilizer
Corroded instruments	
Poor cleaning; residual organic debris (for example, blood)	Improve cleaning; do not allow protein to dry on instruments; use correct cleaning solution for each instrument
Improper use of instrument milk, or other water-soluble lubricant	Follow procedures for instrument milk or other instrument lubricant used
Moisture—not dried properly	Check sterilizer for drying efficiency; packs should air dry in sterilizer; store packs in dry area
Exposure to harsh chemicals	Do not expose instruments to harsh chemicals and abrasives such as steel wool and powder cleaner
Metallic deposits resulting from reaction with sterilizer components	Keep sterilizer free of deposits on chamber walls, shelves, and trays

Instruments sterilized unwrapped are to be used immediately and are not to be stored if they are to be sterile when used.

In summary, remember the following points when sterilizing items in an autoclave (steam sterilization). Treat all items as follows:

- Sanitize (clean) properly before sterilization.
- Correctly wrap, seal, and label (for identification) or cover to prevent recontamination; when using cloth or paper wrapper, include a chemical sterilization indicator in and on the pack.
- Position correctly in the sterilizer so steam contacts all surfaces.
- Load only items able to fit easily into the chamber — *do not overload.*
- Expose to saturated steam at 250° F (121° C) for 15 to 30 minutes (varies with the items).
- Allow to dry before removal from the sterilizer.
- Store in specific clean, dry, and dustproof places.
- Check at intervals to determine if the period (date) of sterility has been exhausted.
- Reprocess and resterilize when they are no longer sterile because of wrap damage or date expiration.
- Replace the wrapper and all chemical indicators (inside and outside of the pack) of all items that need to be reprocessed; rewash any fabric items in the package and the wrapper; discard and replace nonwoven wrappers and gauze sponges.

UNSATURATED CHEMICAL VAPOR STERILIZATION

A practical, efficient, and reliable method of sterilization, the unsaturated chemical vapor sterilizer (now known as the MDT/Harvey Chemiclave, Figure 5-18, *A* and *B*) depends on pressure, heat, and a specific solution, the Vapo-Sterile Solution, a formulation of proven effective liquid bactericidal chemicals and minimal water. When it is heated and pressurized to 270° F (132° C) and at least 20 pounds per square inch pressure, all living microorganisms are consistently killed within 20 minutes.

First clean all items to be sterilized. To avoid hand scrubbing of instruments and the possibility of transmitting pathogenic microorganisms among patients and medical personnel, use an ultrasonic cleaning device such as the Vibraclean 100, 200, or 300 (Figure 5-19). When the instruments are clean, thoroughly rinse them in cold running water to remove any residue or ultrasonic solution or detergent that would inhibit sterilization or damage the sterilizer, and towel dry them before placing them in the sterilizer. Dip small, hard-to-dry items in a shallow tray of Vapo-Steril solution in lieu of drying. Place the items in an instrument tray lined with a Harvey chemically pure, hard-surface tray liner. If storage of sterile instruments is desired, sterilize them in Harvey Sterilization Indicator bags. These bags permit penetration by the chemical vapor but preclude contamination by air-borne bacteria.

The Chemiclave (the unsaturated chemical vapor sterilizer) uses mechanical principles substantially different from those of other systems. The sterilizer is preheated before the initial use and remains at 270° F (132° C) for immediate use. No further preheating is necessary. Unlike the steam autoclave, in

Figure 5-18 A, *Ultrasonic cleaning and sterilization. The MDT Decacheck System for instrument recycling and sterilization;* **B,** *MDT/Harvey Chemiclave 8000.*
Poster on wall in A courtesy MDT Corporation, Torrance, Calif.

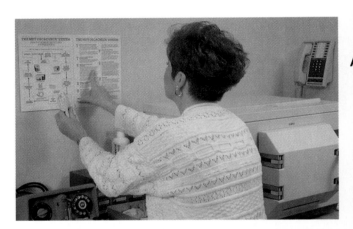

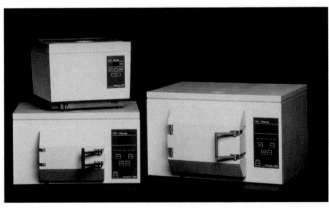

Figure 5-19 *Harvey 300-Vibraclean, an ultrasonic cleaner.*

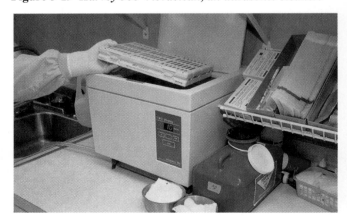

which an unmeasured amount of water is recirculated over the heating element, the unsaturated vapor sterilizer valving system measures a precise amount of solution into the closed, preheated chamber. This solution condenses on the cooler objects in the chamber to begin bactericidal activity. As the objects heat, vaporization of the solution occurs, and unsaturated chemical vapor acts to complete the sterilization cycle. Temperature monitoring is unnecessary because this sterilizer provides both audible and visual signaling on completion of the cycle. A thermostatically controlled heating unit maintains the chamber temperature, and a temperature indicator light registers that the heating element is functioning properly. Any failure in the system is immediately evident, since the pressure

in the chamber will not be attained and, unless all operating criteria are met, the pressure switch will not activate the cycle timer.

Cutting edges, even those of carbon steel, and surgical instruments, handpieces, forceps, and similar items vulnerable to dulling, corroding, rusting, or loss of temper in autoclaves or dry heat units are safely and effectively sterilized in a Chemiclave. Many "soft" items can also be safely sterilized in this unit; and since sterilization is achieved in a water-unsaturated environment, materials such as gauze and cotton are dry and ready for immediate use when the cycle is completed. Only low-grade plastic and rubber items, liquids, agars, and items damaged at 270° F (132° C) *should not* be

PROCEDURE FOR CHEMICAL STERILIZATION

PROCEDURE

1. Sanitize items as discussed for autoclaving.

2. Pour chemical solution into a designated container with an airtight cover (Figure 5-20). Follow the directions for each chemical accurately.

3. Completely immerse the item into the solution and close the cover.

4. Leave for required time, which varies with the chemical and strength used. Exposure time may be from 20 minutes to 3 hours or more. Items must soak for 1 to 4 hours in Cidex, 1 hour in Metricide, and up to 10 hours in glutaraldehyde.

5. Before using, lift tray out of container and rinse items in pan of sterile distilled water. Wear gloves when handling supplies.

6. Using sterile transfer forceps, remove items from the tray for use.

7. Change the solution in the container every 7 to 14 days or as recommended by the manufacturer.

RATIONALE

Some chemicals must be diluted before use, but if diluted too much, the solution loses its effectiveness.

Correct exposure time is extremely important to ensure sterilization.

Often the solutions used are toxic; therefore items must be thoroughly rinsed before being used on patients.

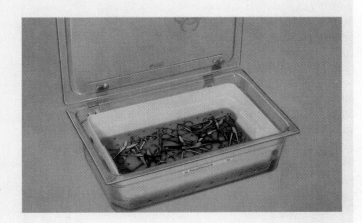

Figure 5-20 *Instrument container with cover used for chemical disinfection and sterilization.*

placed in the Chemiclave. As with all sterilizers, the directions for operation from the manufacturer must be followed explicitly to obtain maximum results.

You must adhere to regulations made by the Environmental Protection Agency (EPA) and the Occupational Safety and Health Administration (OSHA) when using this equipment. In addition, individual states may set additional regulations that you must followed when using this equipment.

DRY HEAT STERILIZATION

To sterilize items with dry heat, a special, combined autoclave-dry heat sterilizer or an individual dry heat sterilizer is required. In essence they are like an oven.

Thoroughly clean all items before sterilizing them. Place instruments and glass items such as syringes placed on the tray or wrap them in aluminum foil. Place sharp items on gauze in racks or wrap them in aluminum foil. Disperse rubber goods and dressings in a container or wrap them in aluminum foil. As for all methods of sterilization, consider both exposure time and temperature. Dry heat sterilizers require longer exposure periods and higher temperatures than do the autoclave (steam under pressure). The exposure time for dry heat is at least 1 hour at 320° F (160° C). If the items being sterilized cannot tolerate this temperature, reduce the temperature and extend the time proportionately. This method is suggested for instruments that corrode easily, sharp cutting instruments, and glass syringes because moist heat dulls the cutting edges and the ground-glass portion of the syringe. Needles, powders, oils, ointments, lensed instruments, dressings, rubber goods, and polyethylene tubing can also be sterilized by this method.

GAS STERILIZATION

Gas sterilizers that use moderately heated mixtures of ethylene oxide gas are useful for sterilizing heat and moisture-sensitive items, including rubber and plastic goods, delicate items such as lensed instruments, glass, ophthalmologic surgical instruments, catheters, telescopic instruments (for example, endoscopes, opthalmoscopes, otoscopes, sigmoidoscopes, and arthroscopes), and anesthesia equipment. Clean, wrap, and position items to be sterilized in the gas chamber using the same steps that were discussed for autoclaving. The temperature in a gas sterilizer is lower (140° F or 50° C); thus the exposure time is extended to suit the temperature, moisture, and gas concentration being used. Time required is 2 to 6 hours, with additional time required for aeration, which can be as long as 5 to 7 days for certain porous materials. Specific instruments for the times and temperatures required are supplied by the manufacturer and must be followed explicitly. Adhere to EPA and OSHA regulations when this method is used. Physician's offices may contract with outside agencies to process equipment in this manner.

CHEMICAL STERILIZATION

Many studies have shown that chemical sterilization (cold sterilization) is difficult to accomplish. Therefore this method generally is limited to items that are heat-sensitive such as delicate cutting instruments and nonboilable sutures, or it is used when heat sterilization methods are not available. Chemical solutions are more commonly used for disinfection rather than for sterilization. Nonetheless, a variety of chemical solutions are on the market. Classifications include germicidal, bactericidal, disinfectants, and antiseptics.

Three chemical solutions that have been recognized as reliable for both sterilization and disinfection procedures are *Cidex, Metricide,* and *glutaraldehyde.* These solutions are capable of destroying bacteria (including spore-forming types) and viruses and are safe to use on instruments, rubber, and plastic goods. Reliable manufacturers always indicate which microorganisms can be expected to be killed by the chemical solution, which items the solution can and cannot be used on, and specific directions for use, including the amount of time that the item must soak in the solution.

ULTRASONIC CLEANING AND STERILIZATION PROCEDURES

To avoid cleaning instruments by hand and risking the possibility of contamination, many health care clinics and offices are now using ultrasonic cleaners for sanitizing instruments before they are sterilized. See Figure 5-18 for processing instruments using an ultrasonic cleaner and preparing instruments to be sterilized and stored.

DISINFECTION PROCEDURES
Chemical Disinfection

Many medical procedures are termed "clean" procedures; therefore they do not require the use of strict aseptic (sterile) technique. Instruments and equipment used in clean procedures are in contact only with the patient's skin or shallow body orifices. Since they do not bypass the body's natural defenses, they can be used safely after being disinfected. Examples of such supplies are thermometers, percussion hammers, laryngeal mirrors, blunt instruments not used on open skin surfaces or on sterile materials (for example, dressings that will touch an open wound), and stainless steel goods such as kidney basins.

When disinfecting such items, thoroughly wash, rinse, and dry as for sterilization. Then apply a disinfectant or antiseptic solution to the surface of the item or immerse it completely in such a solution (refer to the procedure under chemical sterilization).

Certain items such as sphygmomanometers, stethoscopes, and opthalmoscopes may be ruined if washed and immersed in any solution. Disinfect these items only by wiping them off with gauze or cloth moistened with a disinfectant (Figure 5-21). Chemical solutions suggested for use include *Cidex, Solucide, 70% to 90% isopropyl alcohol, Deo-Fect, iodophor solutions, Chlorophenyl,* and *Metricide.*

SUMMARY

When instruments and other equipment are used, the spread of numerous pathogens can be prevented only by the proper sterilization of reusable items or by the use of presterilized disposable items, in addition to meticulous aseptic technique.

Because few procedures more directly affect the continued health of the patient, the physician, and yourself, you must pay conscientious attention to sterilizing all items at all times. Periodically reexamine the techniques used to check their adequacy.

The use of disposable equipment is highly recommended to help control infectious processes and has been found to be most economical in the long run.

Figure 5-21   *Disinfecting a stethoscope. Both earpieces and diaphragm should be disinfected after each use.*

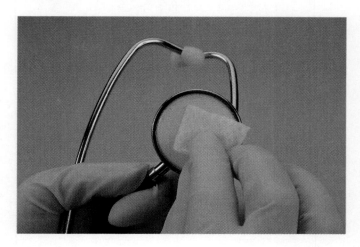

CONCLUSION

You have now completed the unit on Infection Control. After you have practiced the procedures and are ready to demonstrate your skills and knowledge attained, arrange with your instructor to take a performance test. You will be expected to demonstrate accurately your skill in preparing for and performing all of the procedures outlined in this unit. In addition, you should be prepared to discuss briefly the infectious process and the methods used for infection control.

REVIEW OF VOCABULARY

Read the following and define the italicized terms.

When *chemically disinfecting* supplies after use, you may use a variety of preparations that are on the market. These are designated as being a *bactericide* or *bacteriostatic, a germicide,* or a *disinfectant.* When making your choice for use, keep in mind that most of these solutions do not destroy *spores* and that the most effective method for decontaminating items is by using the process of *sterilization.* Remember also to keep *contaminated* supplies away from your clean working area.

Sterile or *aseptic technique* is a very important factor in *infection control* and is to be used in numerous medical procedures. A common example of a time when these techniques are used to prevent *infection* from developing is the administration of injections—the syringe and needle used must be *sterile,* and the patient's skin must be cleansed with an *antiseptic* before the injection is administered.

When a *pathogenic organism* leaves its *reservoir,* it may invade a new *susceptible host,* and, depending on its *virulence* and the *resistance* of the new host, it may cause *infection, sepsis,* and even *necrosis* to the tissues involved.

Immunizations (vaccinations) are given to build up *resistance* to various infectious diseases such as diphtheria, which has an *incubation period* of 2 to 5 days.

CASE STUDY

An employee from another practice calls you today for information about processing instruments. Be prepared to discuss the italicized terminology in the following paragraph.

Contrast the difference between *disinfection* and *sterilization.* Define *physical disinfectants, bactericide, pathogenic microorganisms,* and *antisepsis;* discuss *biologic testing* for the effectiveness of sterilization techniques to kill *spores.*

Suggest methods, products, and techniques for both. She has been using a chemical for cold processing of instruments, along with an anti-rusting tablet. She relates that the manufacture of the anti-rusting tablet has been discontinued and asks for a suggested replacement or technique. She has also been soaking the instruments before processing and rinsing them afterward in a saline bath. What affect would the saline have on the instruments? Discuss *sterile water* versus *saline.* What application would naval jelly have on the rusting problem?

REVIEW QUESTIONS

1. State three goals of infection control, and explain how you and the general public can play an active role in this.
2. Differentiate between a local and generalized infection.
3. Differentiate between artificial passive and active immunity.
4. List five diagnostic tests that may be used to help diagnose an infection.
5. Describe the inflammatory process, listing five local and four systemic signs and symptoms of inflammation.
6. You are given three pieces of equipment: one to sanitize, one to disinfect, and the other to sterilize. Explain the differences among these three processes, and list methods used to accomplish each effectively.
7. At your place of employment you have an autoclave, a Chemiclave, a dry-heat sterilizer, a gas sterilizer, and chemical solutions. List a least three items that you would sterilize in each of these.
8. If you are busy and cannot clean soiled instruments immediately after use, what should you do?
9. When an instrument is to be boiled for 20 minutes, when do you start to time the exposure period?
10. On checking your storage area of sterile supplies, you find a pack that has been there for 1 ½ months. What should your next action be regarding this pack?
11. When removing a dry pack from the autoclave, you observe that the sterilization indicator has not changed color. What would you do?

PERFORMANCE TEST

In a skills laboratory, a simulation of a joblike environment, the medical assistant student is to demonstrate skill in performing the following procedures without reference to source materials. Time limits for the performance of each procedure are to be assigned by the instructor (see also page 52).

1. Given soap, perform a medical aseptic handwash.
2. Given reusable syringes and needles and instruments, sanitize these items and then wrap them for sterilization.
3. Given wrapped supplies for sterilization, position these correctly in the chamber of the sterilizer.
4. Given various types of sterilizers and the manufacturer's instructions, sterilize wrapped and unwrapped items, correctly remove them from the sterilizer on completion of the sterilizing cycle, and determine if sterilization has been effective.
5. Given thermometers, a percussion hammer, and a variety of blunt instruments, correctly disinfect these items using chemicals; disinfect blunt instruments using boiling water.

Surgical Asepsis and Minor Surgery

COGNITIVE OBJECTIVES

On completion of Unit Six, the medical assistant student should be able to:

1. Define and pronounce the vocabulary terms.
2. State at least 15 principles and practices of surgical aseptic technique.
3. Describe how to handle sterile supplies to avoid contamination—that is, how to open sterile peel-down and envelope-wrapped packages, how to pour sterile solutions into sterile containers, and how to don sterile gloves.
4. List at least six minor surgical procedures that may be performed in a physician's office, and list three responsibilities of the medical assistant during each procedure.
5. List and differentiate between three types of local anesthesia.
6. State the information that must be obtained from a patient before administering a local anesthetic, and explain why this is important.
7. State the purpose of suture materials, differentiate between absorbable and nonabsorbable suture material, give an example of each and state when each may be used.
8. Given the numeric sizes of suture material, identify which is the thickest, and arrange in order down to the thinnest; state a procedure in which each size may be used.
9. Discuss and differentiate between the different types of suture needles available.
10. Discuss the meaning and purpose of "informed consent."
11. Discuss the preparation of the patient for minor surgery.
12. List the equipment and supplies that are (1) basic to all minor surgical procedures, (2) required for preparing the patient's skin, (3) required for the administration of a local anesthetic, and (4) required for the minor surgical procedures as outlined in this unit.
13. Differentiate between an open wound and a closed wound. Give one example of a closed wound and five examples of open wounds.
14. Describe briefly the healing process of wounds.
15. List two goals of wound care.
16. Differentiate between dressings and bandages and know the types and purposes of each. List eight purposes of dressings and four purposes of bandages.
17. Explain the criteria for acceptable bandaging techniques.
18. Describe the five basic turns used to apply roller bandages, and explain when each is most appropriately used.
19. State the purposes of casts. Discuss instructions for the patient on the care of a cast.

TERMINAL PERFORMANCE OBJECTIVES

On completion of Unit Six, the medical assistant student should be able to:

1. Open and handle sterile supplies and equipment in a manner that prevents contamination.
2. Don sterile gloves in a manner that prevents contamination.
3. Prepare the patient physically and mentally for a minor surgical procedure.
4. Select, assemble, and prepare sterile and nonsterile supplies and equipment needed for a minor surgical procedure using aseptic technique.
5. Assist the patient and the physician during a minor surgical procedure.
6. Prepare the patient's skin for a minor surgical procedure.
7. Remove sutures as directed by the physician.
8. Assist the physician with the application of a cast.
9. Change the patient's dressing, and obtain a wound culture.
10. Identify by name, and explain the use and care of the instruments and supplies used in minor surgical procedures.
11. Apply roller, triangular, and Tubegauz bandages.

The student is to perform these objectives with 100% accuracy 90% of the time (9 out of 10 times).

The consistent use of universal precautions is required by all health care professionals in all health care settings as a method of infection control. It is assumed that these precautions are used in all of the following procedures. Review Unit One if you have any question on methods to use as the methods/techniques will not be repeated in detail in each procedure presented in the unit.

Be sure to consult the latest guidelines issued by the Centers for Disease Control and Prevention and consult with infection control practitioners when needed to identify specific precautions that pertain to your particular work situation.

This unit discusses the common practices of, and some procedures requiring, surgical asepsis (sterile technique). To control the sources and spread of infection when one is performing and assisting with certain medical procedures, knowledge of and adherence to the correct performance of aseptic practices are essential.

It is helpful to review Unit Five, which discussed concepts of infection control, medical and surgical asepsis, practices of medical asepsis, and the disinfection and sterilization of supplies.

BACKGROUND OF STERILE TECHNIQUE

Sterile techniques as we know them today have gradually evolved since the turn of the century. The history of medicine shows evidence of some understanding of asepsis as early as the time of Hippocrates, the father of medicine, in 460 BC. It was Hippocrates who started to use boiled water when irrigating wounds; later Galen (131-210 AD) boiled instruments before using them when caring for wounds. Throughout the centuries up to the present, numerous individuals, too many to mention here, played vital roles in describing diseases and their causes, theories for contagious diseases, the spread of infection by improperly washed hands, the role of bacteria in causing disease, the inhibition of the growth of microorganisms by heat, and the germ theory for the causes of disease.

It was Joseph Lister (1827-1912) who introduced the use of chemicals to destroy microorganisms in the infected wounds (antisepsis) and later procedures to exclude bacteria from surgical fields (asepsis). Surgery as we know it today was essentially Lister's gift to humanity.

In the later years of the 19th century, the concept of vaccinations against disease were introduced. Edward Jenner discovered the value of vaccination against smallpox. This was a discovery that led to further advances, such as Louis Pasteur's principle of inoculation by means of vaccines against viral and bacterial diseases.

Sterilization of items by boiling began around 1880, and the principles and practices of autoclaving (steam under pressure)

began around 1886. Rubber gloves were first used to protect the hands from harsh antiseptics. Eventually they were accepted and used as a protective measure to prevent contamination to the patient. Thus sterile technique or aseptic practices, as we know them, evolved.

PRINCIPLES AND PRACTICES OF SURGICAL ASEPSIS

Surgical asepsis, more commonly referred to as *sterile technique* or *aseptic technique,* is the practice used when an area and supplies in that area are to be made and kept sterile. The goal of surgical asepsis is to prevent infection or the introduction of microorganisms into the body. These techniques are used in all procedures in which entry is made into normally sterile body parts, such as when administering an injection, when making a surgical incision, or when caring for any break in the skin such as open wounds or skin ulcers. Strict sterile or surgical aseptic technique is required at all times in such procedures, because body tissues can easily become infected. Breaks in technique may lead to infections that the body cannot combat. Even mild infections delay recovery and are costly—mentally, physically, and financially—to the patient. It is the responsibility of the medical assistant and the physician to adhere to the following principles and practices at all times when assisting with or performing a sterile procedure.

1. Sterilize all supplies used for sterile procedures either previously or at the time for immediate use.
2. When in doubt about the sterility of anything, consider it nonsterile.
3. When putting sterile gloves on, do not touch the outside of the gloves with bare hands.
4. People who are wearing sterile gloves must touch only sterile articles; people who are not gloved must touch only nonsterile articles, except when using sterile transfer forceps to move sterile items.
5. During a sterile procedure, if a glove is punctured by a needle or instrument, remove the damaged glove, wash your hands, and put on a new glove as promptly as patient safety permits. Remove the needle or instrument from the sterile field.
6. The outer wrappings and the edges of packs that contain sterile items are not sterile and thus are handled and opened by the person who is not wearing sterile gloves.
7. Open sterile packages with the edges of the wrapper directed away from your body to avoid touching your uniform or reaching over a sterile field.
8. Touch only the outside of a sterile wrapper.
9. Once a sterile pack has been opened, use it; if it is not used, replace any fabric items, sponges, and dressing materials and rewrap and resterilize the pack.

VOCABULARY

Abscess (ab˝ses)—A cavity containing pus and surrounded by inflamed tissue. An abscess is usually caused by specific microorganisms (characteristically staphylococci) that invade tissues often by way of small breaks or wounds in the skin. Healing usually occurs when an abscess drains or is incised.

Anesthesia (an˝es-the´ze-ah)—The loss of sensation or feeling.

Asepsis (a-sep´sis)—The state of being free from infection or infectious matter. The absence of all microorganisms causing disease; absence of contaminated matter.

Biopsy (bi´op-se)—Removal of tissue from the body for examination.

Incisional biopsy—Incision into and removal of part of a lesion.

Excisional biopsy—Removal of an entire small lesion.

Aspiration/needle biopsy—Removal of matter from an internal organ by means of a hollow needle inserted through the body wall and into the affected tissue.

Fine-needle aspiration (FNA) biopsy—Insertion of a thin needle into a lump from which a cell specimen is taken and evaluated for cancer. FNA has been used to diagnose lesions and lumps of the breast, thyroid, lymph nodes, soft tissue, prostate, abdomen, lung, salivary glands, liver, and brain.

Punch biopsy—Biopsy in which tissue is obtained by a punch (a type of instrument).

Cautery (kaw´ter-e)—A closed capsule or sac containing fluid or a semi-solid substance.

Sebaceous cyst (se-ba´shus)—A benign cyst of a sebaceous gland containing the fatty secretion of the gland; also called a wen. They are most common on the back, scrotum, and scalp.

Don—To put an article on, such as gloves or a gown.

Ligate (li´gat)—To apply a ligature.

Ligature (lig´ah-tur)—A suture; material used to tie off blood vessels to prevent bleeding, or to constrict tissues.

Mayo (ma´o) **stand**—A stand with a flat metal tray used to hold sterile supplies during an aseptic procedure.

Postoperative (post-op´er-ah-tiv)—Pertaining to the period of time following surgery.

Preoperative (pre-op´er-ah-tiv)—Pertaining to the time preceding surgery.

Sterile field—A work area prepared with sterile drapes (coverings) to hold sterile supplies during a sterile procedure.

Sterile setup—Specific sterile supplies used in a specific sterile procedure.

Suture (soo´cher)—Various types and sizes of absorbable and nonabsorbable materials used to close a wound with stitches.

Transfer forceps—A type of instrument (forcep) that is kept in a chemical disinfectant or germicide and used for transferring or handling sterile supplies and equipment.

10. Avoid sneezing, coughing, or talking directly over a sterile field or object.
11. Do not reach across or above a sterile field or wound. Your clothes and skin are not sterile. If you touch the sterile field or drop debris onto it or into the wound, contamination results. Movements around the area should be kept to a minimum.
12. Avoid spilling solutions on a sterile setup. Any moisture that soaks through a sterile area to a nonsterile one produces a means of transporting bacteria to a sterile area. Thus the wet areas are considered contaminated and must either be covered with sterile towels or drapes until the top surface is dry or be removed and redraped.
13. Hold sterile objects and gloved hands above waist level or level to the sterile field. Anything below this level is considered unsterile. Keeping objects or hands in sight helps avoid contamination.
14. Since skin cannot be sterilized, any object that touches it is considered contaminated.
15. Have a special receptacle or plastic bag to receive contaminated materials.
16. A sterile field should be away from drafts, fans, and windows. Microorganisms can be carried in air currents to the patient or the sterile field.

17. Store sterile packages in dry areas. If they become wet, they must be repacked and resterilized or discarded.
18. Hands are the greatest source of contamination; therefore wash frequently, using correct technique.
19. Be constantly aware of the need for very clean surroundings.

In summary, remember these five basic rules:
- Know what is sterile.
- Know what is not sterile.
- Keep sterile items separate from nonsterile items.
- Prevent contamination.
- Remedy a contaminated situation immediately.

HANDLING STERILE SUPPLIES

OPENING STERILE PACKAGES

Many commercially prepared sterile packages have instructions for opening printed on them. Read these directions carefully before opening the package to avoid contamination of the contents. To open peel-down packages, such as those in which syringes and dressing materials are supplied, use the following procedure.

OPENING PEEL-DOWN PACKAGES

PROCEDURE

1. Wash your hands. **Use appropriate personal protective equipment (PPE) as dictated by facility.**

2. Using both hands, grasp both sides of the extended edges provided.

3. Pull evenly along the sealed edges (Figure 6-1, A).

4. Do not touch the inside of the wrapper; place on a flat surface.

    or

   Using sterile forceps, remove the contents from the wrapper and transfer to a sterile field, or use immediately in a sterile procedure such as a dressing change (Figure 6-1, B).

    or

   Holding the bottom of the package with the edges folded back, allow a person wearing sterile gloves to take the contents (Figure 6-1, B).

    or

   If the item is a syringe to be used by you, grasp the plunger end of the syringe with one hand while holding onto the package with your other hand.

RATIONALE

Pull evenly in a downward motion to avoid tearing.

The inside of the wrapper is sterile and can be used as a sterile field until using the contents.

Keep your fingers away from the contents to avoid contamination.

The bottom part of the plunger does not have to remain sterile, because this is how you take hold of the syringe to remove it from the sterile package, provided you are going to use it immediately and not place it on a sterile field.

A
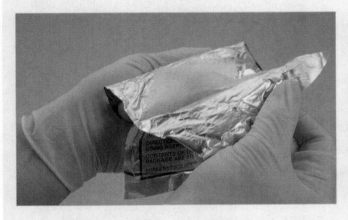
B
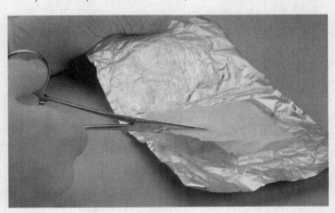

Figure 6-1 A, *Technique for opening peel-down package with sterile contents.* **B,** *Technique for removing a sterile dressing from package.*

OPENING AN ENVELOPE WRAP

PROCEDURE

1. Wash your hands. **Use appropriate personal protective equipment (PPE) as dictated by facility.**

2. Place package on a flat surface so that the folded edges are on top.

RATIONALE

PROCEDURE

3. Remove tape or string fastener, and discard in waste container. At this time you should also check the date and sterilization indicator.

4. Pull out the corner that is tucked under, if present, and unfold this top flap away from you (Figure 6-2). Avoid touching the pack with your uniform or person.

5. Using both hands, grasp the second layer of folded corners, and open these flaps to the sides of the package (Figure 6-3), or open first one side and then the other. The contents of the package are still covered with the last layer of the wrapper.

6. Without reaching over any of the uncovered area, grasp the last fold or fourth corner, and open toward your body (Figure 6-4). Lift this corner up and toward you, dropping it on the surface holding the package. Do not touch the inside of the package or the contents with bare hands.

RATIONALE

Check to make sure that the contents are safe for use.

Unfolding away from you avoids the necessity of reaching over the sterile field later and causing contamination.

Touching would contaminate everything.

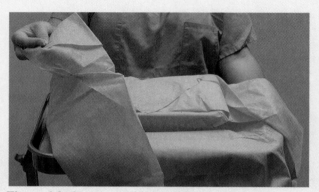

Figure 6-3 *Open second layer of flaps to each side.*

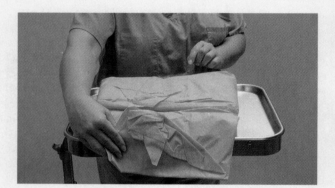

Figure 6-2 *Unfold top flap away from you.*

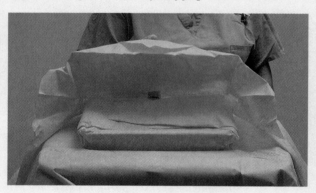

Figure 6-4 *Open last flap toward your body.*

You now have a sterile field that can be used as a sterile work area. Additional sterile items that may be needed for the procedure may be added to this sterile field. To organize the items contained in the package you just opened, use individually wrapped sterilized hemostats or don sterile gloves (Figure 6-5). Small packages can be held in the hand and unwrapped in the same fashion. Have someone who is wearing sterile gloves take the item from the opened wrap, or remove it with sterile transfer forceps, or carefully place the item on a sterile field, avoiding contamination to the item and field. Be sure that the wrapper corners do not touch the sterile field.

Treat the edges of a sterile field on a flat surface as if they were contaminated. Some recommend that the outside 1-inch border of the field be considered contaminated. Parts of the wrap that fall over the side of the surface are considered to be contaminated.

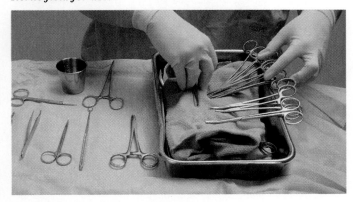

Figure 6-5 *Using sterile gloves, arrange sterile supplies on sterile field for use.*

POURING STERILE SOLUTIONS

When required to pour a sterile solution, you must use aseptic technique to avoid contamination to the solution.

DONNING AND REMOVING STERILE GLOVES

Sterile gloves are worn to protect the patient from infection caused by microorganisms that may be on your hands and to provide a means of safely handling sterile supplies and equipment without contaminating these items. Gloves are also worn to protect the health care worker from possible contamination or infection (see also Unit One).

MINOR SURGERY

Minor surgery is sometimes performed in the physician's office, although frequently even these procedures are done in the emergency room or outpatient department of a hospital or in a clinic.

Minor surgical procedures include those that can be done with or without the use of a local anesthetic such as the suturing of a laceration; the incision and drainage of an abscess or cyst; incision and removal of foreign bodies in subcutaneous tissues; removal of small growths such as warts, moles, and skin tags; various types of biopsies; cauterization of tissue (such as cauterization of the uterine cervix or of a wart, mole, or skin tag); and insertion of an intrauterine device (IUD). After minor surgery performed in the office or at the hospital, the patient may come to the physician's office for dressing changes and for the removal of sutures as part of the postoperative care. The wound is also inspected that time to determine the amount of healing that has occurred and to ensure the absence of a developing infectious process.

As the physician's assistant, you may be called upon to assist with the surgical procedures or to change a dressing for a patient. Assisting in any surgical procedure is a highly responsible job, and you must always use strict surgical aseptic technique. The nature of the surgery or postoperative care governs the duties and responsibilities of the medical assistant.

ANESTHESIA

For minor surgery and extremely painful treatments, some type of local anesthetic is usually required. *Local anesthesia* refers to the absence of feeling or sensation and pain in a limited area of the body without the loss of consciousness. The extent and severity of the procedure determines the type and amount of anesthetic used, which can be administered by injection or by topical application. Local anesthetics produce their effects in 5 to 15 minutes. These effects may last from 1 to 3 hours, depending on the type and dose administered.

Types of Local Anesthesia

* Infiltration—The anesthetic solution is injected under the skin to anesthetize the nerve endings and nerve fibers at the site of the procedure. The sensory nerves become insensitive and remain so for several hours, depending on the amount of drug administered. (Rules for the administration of medications and injections described in Unit Seven apply here.) Examples of infiltration anesthetics include procaine (Novocain) 1% to 2% and lidocaine (Xylocaine) 1% to 2%.
* Nerve block or block anesthesia—The anesthetic solution is injected into or adjacent to accessible main nerves, thus desensitizing all the adjacent tissue. Examples of nerve block anesthesia include procain (Novocaine) 1% to 2% and lidocaine (Xylocaine) 1% to 2%.
* Topical or surface anesthesia—The anesthetic solution is painted or sprayed directly onto the skin or mucous membrane involved to deaden sensation and relieve pain. Examples of topical anesthetics include lidocaine 4% solution for accessible mucous membranes of oral and nasal cavities and ethyl chloride spray for external topical use, because it is too harsh for use on mucous membranes. Before a topical anesthetic is applied, the patient's skin must be washed and dried well.

Allergic reactions. Before the administration of a local anesthetic, you must ask every patient if he or she is allergic to any drug, if he or she has any cardiac or respiratory problems, and if he or she has had any type of anesthetic before. This information is most important because some local anesthetics can cause anaphylactic shock or violent allergic reactions. Frequently skin tests are made beforehand when deemed necessary. An *emergency tray* with sterile syringes and needles, sterile alcohol sponges, and ampules of a stimulant such as epinephrine (Adrenalin) must be kept in reach when an anesthetic is to be administered, in case an emergency does arise. (See also Unit Seven, "Emergency Tray," page 261).

SUTURE MATERIALS AND NEEDLES

The purpose of sutures is to hold the edges of a wound together until healing occurs. When suture materials are needed for a procedure, they can be added to your sterile field. The most frequently used are the sterile prepackaged sutures with or without an attached suture needle

POURING STERILE SOLUTIONS

PROCEDURE

1. Wash your hands. **Use appropriate personal protective equipment (PPE) as dictated by facility.**

2. Obtain the solution and check the label.

3. Obtain sterile container to be used for the solution, and unwrap. Follow procedure for unwrapping as described previously.

   NOTE: When using prepackaged sterile trays, a container for the solution may be included in the pack.

4. Remove bottle cap; place on a level surface with the top of the cap resting on the surface, or hold it in your hand with the top facing downward (Figure 6-6).

5. Check the label again. Hold the bottle with the label in the palm of your hand about 6 inches above the container (or less, when pouring very small amounts of solution), and pour the solution (Figure 6-7). Pour a small amount of solution into a waste container to cleanse the side of the bottle, and then pour from the same area.

6. When pouring a solution on a sponge, pick up the sponge with forceps and pour the solution over the sponge. The excess solution will drip into the basin or discard container (see Figure 6-7).

7. Pick the cap up by the sides and replace it on the bottle securely.

8. Check the label of the bottle and replace it in the correct storage area.

RATIONALE

Solutions are drugs. All drug labels must be checked three times before using or administering:
- When removing from storage area
- Before pouring
- When replacing container in the storage area

The inner part of the cap is considered sterile. If you place the cap with top facing up, you have contaminated the inner surface, which then cannot be replaced on the container until it has been resterilized.

Holding the bottle this way prevents damage to the label if the solution runs or spills; you also avoid undue splashing.

Do not contaminate the inside of the cap, because it is considered sterile and must cover the sterile solution in the bottle.

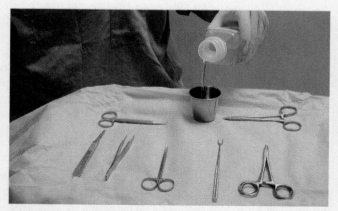

Figure 6-6 *Pouring soluton into container on sterile field. Hold top of container in your hand with top facing downward.*

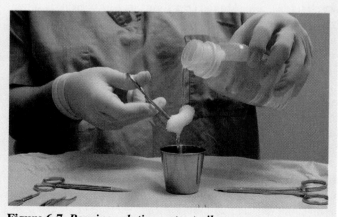

Figure 6-7 *Pouring solution onto sterile sponge.*

DONNING AND REMOVING STERILE GLOVES

PROCEDURE

1. Wash your hands. **Use appropriate personal protective equipment (PPE) as dictated by facility.**

2. Place wrapped gloves on a clean, dry, flat surface with the cuff end toward you.

3. Open the outside and inside wrapper by handling only the outside of the packages.

4. Using your left hand, pick up the right-hand glove by grasping the folded edge of the cuff, and lift up and away from the wrapper (Figure 6-8). The folded edge of the cuff will be against your skin and is contaminated as soon as you touch it. *Do not* touch the outside of the glove with your ungloved hand.

5. Pulling on the edge of the cuff, pull the right glove on. Keep your fingers away from the rest of the glove.

6. Place fingers of the right gloved hand under the cuff of the left-hand glove (Figure 6-9). Be sure that your gloved fingers do not touch your skin.

7. Lift the glove up and away from the wrapper, and pull it onto your left hand. Be sure that the left thumb does not stray up and touch the right glove. Keep the right gloved fingers under the cuff and straight; keep the right gloved thumb back.

8. Continue pulling the left glove up over your wrist

9. With the gloved left hand, place fingers under the cuff of the right glove and pull the cuff up over your right wrist (Figure 6-10).

10. Adjust the fingers of the gloves as necessary. If, when putting on either glove, the fingers get into the wrong space, you must proceed with the rest of the gloving procedure, and then adjust the gloves with gloved hands.

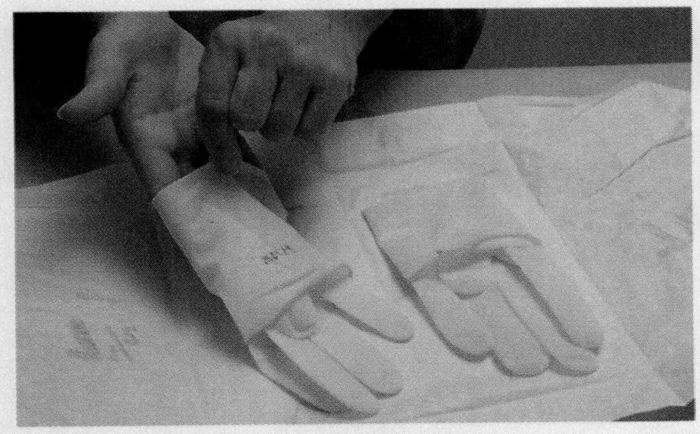

RATIONALE

The inside part of the wrappers is sterile.

The area inside the folded cuff is considered sterile.

Avoid touching skin.

The area inside the folded cuff is considered sterile.

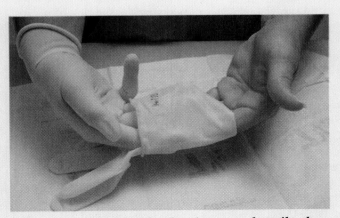

Figure 6-8 *Technique for donning first sterile glove. Grasp folded edge of cuff, lift up and away from wrapper and pull onto right hand.*

Figure 6-9 *Technique for donning second sterile glove. Place fingers of gloved hand under cuff of other glove and pull onto left hand.*

DONNING AND REMOVING STERILE GLOVES—cont'd

PROCEDURE

11. If either glove tears during the procedure, remove and discard. Begin the procedure again with a new pair of gloves.

12. To remove gloves:
    a. Grasp the cuff of the right-hand glove with your left hand.
    b. Pull the glove down over the hand.
    c. Discard in appropriate place.
    d. Repeat, using the right hand to remove left glove. Grasp the inside and top of the left-hand glove with your right hand, pull the glove down over the hand, and discard. Reusable gloves must be washed and resterilized; disposable gloves are discarded in the appropriate waste container. Do not touch the outside of the glove.

RATIONALE

Glove touches glove. You do not touch your skin, thus avoiding contamination of your skin.

The glove turns inside out as it comes off.
The glove is considered contaminated after use. Skin touches skin.

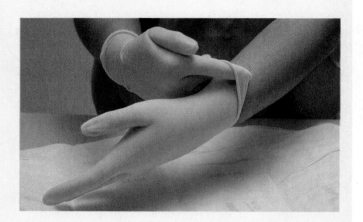

Figure 6-10 *Technique for donning sterile glove. Adjust cuffs on gloves avoiding contamination.*

(Figure 6-11). The label on these packages indicates the type, length, and size of the suture and the type and size of the needle enclosed. Sutures are prepared from materials that are either absorbable or nonabsorbable. *Absorbable sutures* do not have to be removed when used because they are absorbed or digested by the body fluids and tissues during and after the healing process, usually 5 to 20 days after insertion, varying with the type used. An example of absorbable suture material is surgical gut (catgut), which is made from the submucosa of the intestine of sheep. Absorbable suture material is generally used in surgical procedures involving the suturing of internal organs and subcutaneous tissue, and when ligating vessels.

Nonabsorbable sutures used on outer skin surfaces are removed after the wound has healed because body fluids and cells do not absorb or digest them (for example, cotton, silk, nylon, and stainless steel and metal clips or staples). When used internally, they are not removed and remain as foreign bodies; usually they become encysted and cause no trouble. The most commonly used nonabsorbable suture material is black surgical silk. The silk is dyed black so that it can readily be seen in the tissue in which it is used. The size, or gauge, of most sutures is labeled in terms of 0s (for example, 0, which is the thickest, followed by 00, 000, each decreasing in size up to 10-0, which is the thinnest). Sizes 2-0 up to 6-0 are used most frequently; 4-0 black silk may be used to suture a laceration on the arm. 5-0 and 6-0 are frequently used for repair in delicate tissues such as the tissues on the face and neck. The

finer the suture, the less scar formation; therefore fine sutures are most desirable when cosmetic results are important. 10-0 silk, which is extremely fine, is used for ophthalmologic and vascular procedures. A few types of sutures are designated as 1, 2, 3, 4, and 5 (the thickest); others are designated simply as fine, medium, and coarse. The size and type of the suture used is determined by the area and the purpose for which it is being used and the physician's preference. Thicker sutures are used when closing large wounds, medium ones are used

Figure 6-11 *Prepackaged sterile suture materials. Cover of package indicates type, length, and size of suture material. The curved line under the suture label represents the type and size of needle included.*

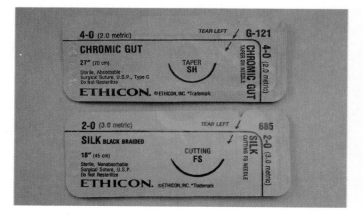

on lacerations, and very fine sutures are used on more delicate tissues, such as the eye or facial tissues.

Sutures must remain in place until the incision or break in the tissue has healed. The physician decides when to remove sutures. Generally sutures in the skin on the neck or head are removed in 3 to 5 days; sutures in the skin of the hand, arms, legs, and other areas are removed in 7 to 10 days.

Suture needles are either straight or curved and have either a sharp, cutting point or a round, noncutting point. They are supplied in individual packages or in packages with suture materials (see Figure 6-11). Some needles have an eye through which you thread the suture material. Other needles come attached to the suture material as one unit. These are called *swaged needles* (Figure 6-12). Packages containing these will be labeled as to the type and size of the needle and the type, size, and length of the suture material.

Sharp cutting needles are used on stable tissues such as the skin, where the sharp point is useful in getting the needle through the tissue. Round, noncutting needles are used on less firm tissues, such as subcutaneous tissues and on the internal organs of body cavities. Curved needles are held in a needle holder (see Figure 6-12, *D*) when used so as to be able to get in and out of the tissue, as when suturing small skin incisions. Straight needles are used by hand as they are pushed through adjoining tissues as when suturing large skin incisions. The size and type of suture needle used is determined by the area and the purpose for which it will be used.

An *alternative* to the use of sutures for holding the edges of tissue together is the use of adhesive skin closures. These are sterile nonallergic tapes that are supplied in a variety of lengths and widths. An example of a commercial adhesive

Figure 6-12 *Types of suture needles:* **A,** *Straight;* **B,** *swaged needle positioned for use in needle holder;* **C,** *curved with sharp point;* **D,** *swaged.*
A, B and C courtesy of Miltex Instrument Co., Lake Success, N.Y.

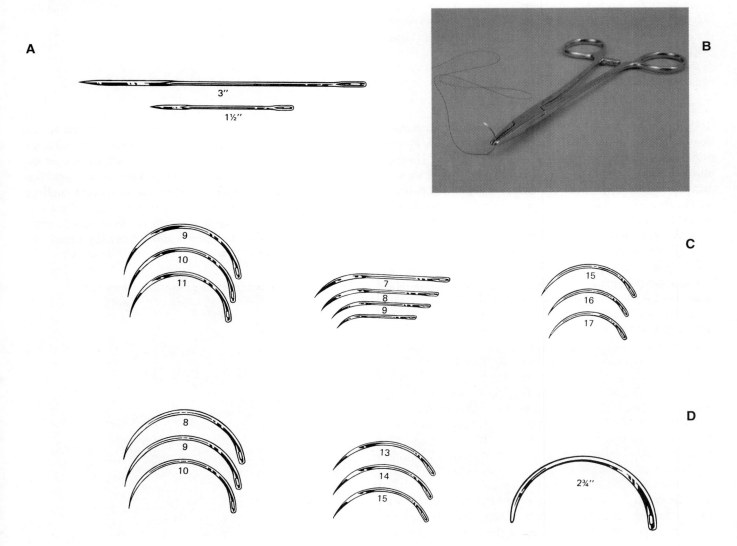

skin closure is the Steri-Strip. The edges of the tissue are held together, and the Steri-Strips are applied transversely across this area and left in place until the wound has healed.

The medical assistant may be responsible for setting up the supplies needed by the physician for suturing tissue. The physician will tell you what size and type of suture material and needle are required. The materials required for suturing tissue are given on page 220.

INSTRUMENTS USED FOR MINOR SURGERY

Surgical instruments are tools or devices designed to perform a specific function such as cutting, grasping, retracting, or suturing (Figure 6-13). They are usually made of steel and are treated so that they are durable, rust-resistant, heat-resistant, and stain-proof. Proper care of all surgical instruments is essential. You must see that they are used correctly, handled carefully, inspected for any defects, and sterilized and stored correctly. As a medical assistant, you should be able to identify a variety of surgical instruments; know how they are used, sterilized, and stored; and be able to select the correct instruments for a variety of minor surgical procedures that may be performed in the physician's office or clinic. Some of the more common surgical instruments are discussed. Figure 6-13 illustrates many of these instruments. Additional figures in this unit illustrate tray set-ups for specific procedures with some of these instruments.

Scalpels

Scalpels (skal´ pel) are used to make incisions into tissues. They are small surgical knives that usually have a convex (rounded, somewhat elevated) edge. Scalpel blades are supplied in various sizes and shapes that are designed for making different types of incisions in various tissues. Scalpels are now disposable, and some are supplied with a disposable handle. The No. 3 and No. 7 handles are the most commonly used, the No. 7 handle being thinner.

Scissors

Surgical scissors are used to cut or dissect tissues and to cut sutures. Other are used to cut bandages when they are to be removed. These instruments consist of two opposing cutting blades, which may be straight or curved. The tips on the blades vary. On some scissors both tips are sharp; on others both tips are blunt; others have one sharp tip and one blunt tip. *Bandage scissors* have one blunt tip and one tip that has a flat blunt probe. These are used to remove bandages and dressings without puncturing the tissues. *Suture scissors,* used to remove sutures, have one blunt tip and a hook on the second tip. When removing sutures, the hook goes under the suture. The blunt tip prevents puncture to the tissue. Short, straight Iris scissors with two sharp tips are also used to remove sutures. Common *dissecting scissors* are the straight or curved Mayo scissors; the short, curved Metzenbaum scissors, which are used on superficial, delicate tissue; and the long, blunt, curved Metzenbaum, which are used on deep, delicate tissue. The tips of dissecting scissors are blunt so that tissue is not inadvertently punctured. *Operating scissors* have straight blades and may have any of the combination types of blades (sharp/sharp, blunt/blunt, or sharp/blunt). The type of scissors used in a procedure varies, depending on its intended function and physician's preference.

Forceps

Forceps are instruments of varied sizes and shapes used for grasping, compressing, or holding tissue or objects. They are two-pronged instruments with either a spring handle or a ring handle with a ratchet closure. The ratchet is a toothed clasp that allows for different degrees of tightness to be applied to the tissue or object on which the instrument is used. The inner surfaces of some forceps have sawlike teeth that are called serrations (Figure 6-14). Serrations prevent tissue from slipping out of the forceps jaw. The tips may be either straight or curved and plain-tipped or toothed-tipped. Plain-tipped forceps are used to pick up tissue, dressings, or other sterile objects. A toothed-tipped forcep is especially useful for

Figure 6-13 *Instruments used for minor surgery.* **A(1),** *Korvorkian curette;* **A(2),** *uterine tenaculum,* **A(3),** *endometrial suction curette;* **A(4),** *Kovorkian biopsy forceps;* **B,** *cryosurgery unit and probe.*

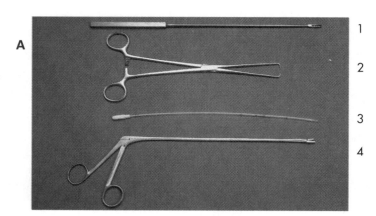

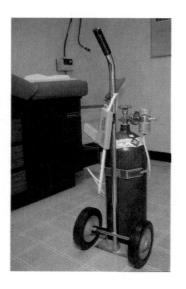

Figure 6-14 **LEFT,** *Serrated tip on forceps;* **RIGHT,** *serrated tip with groove in the middle as seen on some needle holders.*

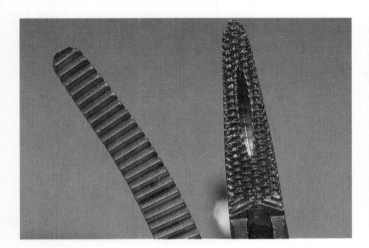

grasping tissue. The teeth prevent the tissue from slipping out of the grasp of the instrument.

Examples of forceps with a *spring handle* are the thumb, tissue, splinter, and dressing forceps. Examples of forceps with a *ring handle* and ratchet closure are Allis tissue forceps, Foerster sponge forceps, Backhaus towel clamps, and straight or curved hemostatic forceps or hemostats. Hemostats include Halsted mosquito hemostatic forceps, Kelly hemostatic forceps, Rochester-Pean hemostatic forceps, and Ochsner-Kocher hemostatic forceps.

Forceps with a *toothed-tip* include standard tissue forceps, Allis tissue forceps, and Ochsner-Kocher hemostatic forceps. *Plain-tipped* forceps include standard thumb forceps, plain splinter forceps (these have sharp points), Adson dressing forceps, and the Halsted mosquito, Kelly, and Rochester-Pean hemostatic forceps.

Sponge forceps are used for holding sponges and have serrated ringlike tips. *Towel clamps* have two sharp points and are used to hold the edges of sterile drapes or towels together. *Hemostats* are used to compress, hold, or grasp a blood vessel. They are also used by some people to apply or remove a dressing.

Needle Holders

Needle holders have a ring handle, a ratchet closure, and serrated tips. Some needle holders have a groove in the middle of the serrations (see Figure 6-14). These instruments are designed to hold a curved needle used for suturing tissues.

Retractors

Retractors are instruments used to hold back the edges of tissues or organs to maintain exposure of the operative area. Examples include a double-ended Richardson retractor and a Volkmann rake retractor.

Probes

Probes are slender, long instruments used for exploring wounds or body cavities or passages. The end of a probe may be straight or curved. The body area being explored determines the type of probe to be used.

Biopsy Instruments

Biopsy instruments are used to obtain a small piece of tissue from the body for examination. There are various sizes and shapes of biopsy forceps. Three common ones that you may see in the office or clinic are the rectal biopsy punch, the cervical biopsy forceps, and a 6-mm biopsy punch used to obtain a small sample of skin.

Instrument Care

Keep in mind the following points for the care of instruments:

1. Use the instrument *only* for the intended purpose and in the correct manner. "Handle with care."
2. Rinse or soak and then sanitize and sterilize instruments as described in Unit Five as soon as possible after use.
3. Inspect each instrument for proper working condition and for any defect.
4. Never toss instruments around or pile them on top of each other; damage could result.
5. Keep sharp and lensed instruments separate from other instruments to prevent damage.
6. Keep ratchet handles open when not in use. This prolongs the usefulness of the instrument.

PREPARING THE PATIENT FOR MINOR SURGERY

When a patient is to have minor or major surgery or other major forms of therapy, the physician must explain the nature and risks of the procedure and the alternatives available. This allows the patient to give *informed consent* for the procedure. Informed consent is a *right*, not merely a privilege. By law, the patient's consent is required for these types of treatment. A consent form (Figure 6-15) giving the physician permission to perform the procedure must be signed by the patient before the procedure is started. The patient *must* understand what he or she is signing. If this is not done, numerous legal complications may result. Although the explanation is the physician's responsibility, frequently the medical assistant must briefly explain the procedure once again on the day of the surgery while preparing the patient and be ready to answer numerous questions that the patient may have. Remember, any surgical procedure is an invasion into body parts; and although the surgical procedure may be minor, it often does not appear minor to the patient. Many patients are anxious, nervous, or concerned about what is going to happen. You can and must help the patient relax and allay any fears or apprehensions. Prepare supplies and equipment required for the procedure in advance. Have everything ready when the patient arrives. Make sure that the room is spotlessly clean, well lighted, and at a comfortable temperature. Do not have instruments exposed for the patient's view because seeing them may make some patients more apprehensive.

When the patient arrives in the office, greet and usher him or her into the treatment room. Have the consent form ready to sign. Provide a patient gown and give directions for the removal of clothing. Attend to the patient's needs for comfort and communication, and give emotional support and reassurance. Once again, a simple explanation of the procedure may be needed. Be willing to answer any questions that the patient may have. Always maintain a calm and confident manner as you are preparing the patient. This in itself can help to reassure and relax the patient.

The best of care can be enhanced by evaluating every patient and situation individually. In this way you can pro-

Figure 6-15 *Sample consent form required for surgical procedures and other medical procedures.*

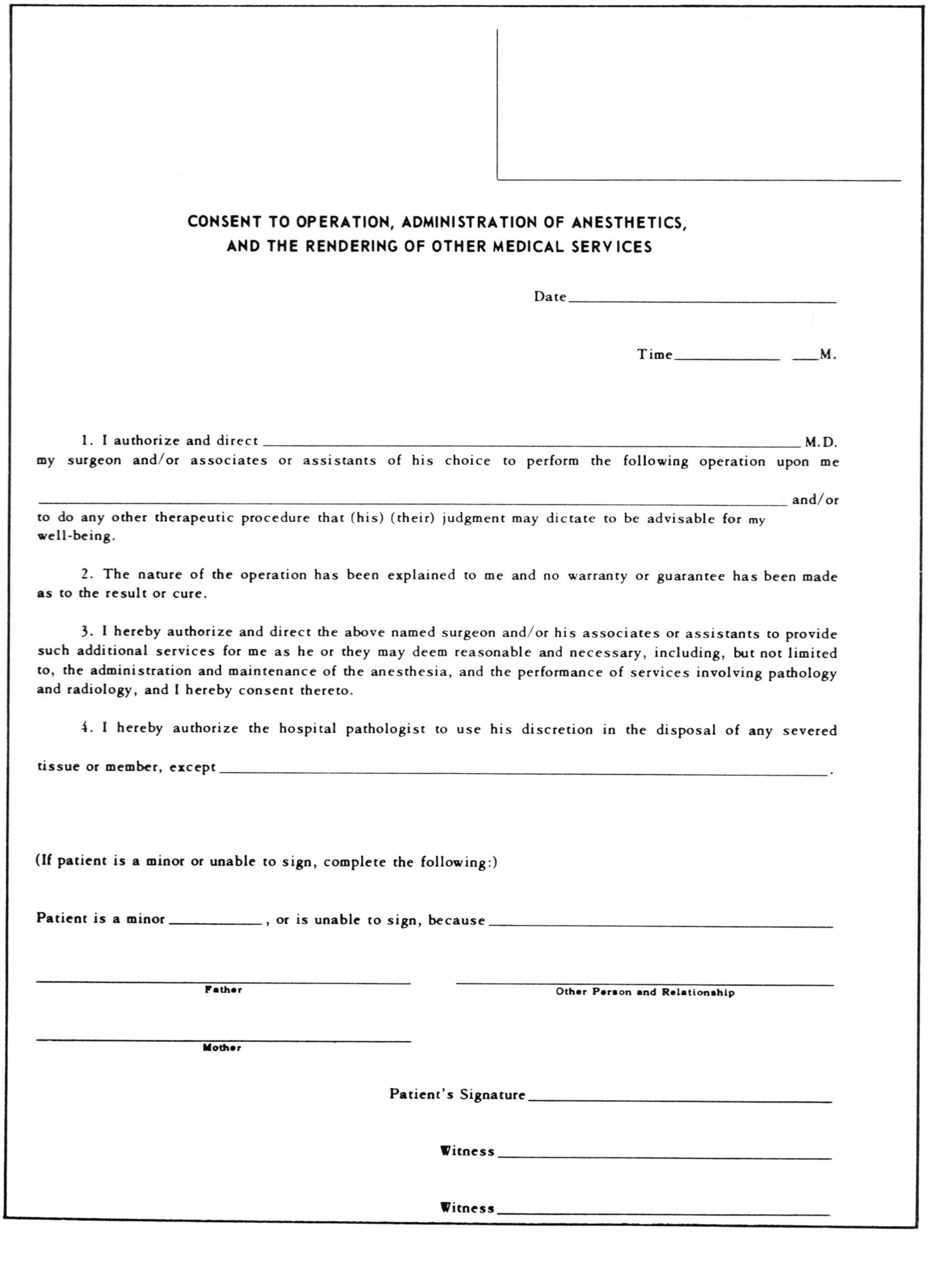

CONSENT TO OPERATION, ADMINISTRATION OF ANESTHETICS, AND THE RENDERING OF OTHER MEDICAL SERVICES

Date _____

Time _____ ___M.

1. I authorize and direct _____ M.D. my surgeon and/or associates or assistants of his choice to perform the following operation upon me

_____ and/or to do any other therapeutic procedure that (his) (their) judgment may dictate to be advisable for my well-being.

2. The nature of the operation has been explained to me and no warranty or guarantee has been made as to the result or cure.

3. I hereby authorize and direct the above named surgeon and/or his associates or assistants to provide such additional services for me as he or they may deem reasonable and necessary, including, but not limited to, the administration and maintenance of the anesthesia, and the performance of services involving pathology and radiology, and I hereby consent thereto.

4. I hereby authorize the hospital pathologist to use his discretion in the disposal of any severed tissue or member, except _____ .

(If patient is a minor or unable to sign, complete the following:)

Patient is a minor _____ , or is unable to sign, because _____

_____   _____
Father   Other Person and Relationship

_____
Mother

Patient's Signature _____

Witness _____

Witness _____

vide the most suitable environment for each individual. Also, when deemed necessary, ascertain that the patient has arranged to have someone accompany her or him to the office or clinic and provide transportation home.

ASSISTING WITH MINOR SURGERY

Careful preparation and adherence to aseptic technique are required when preparing for office or clinic surgery. The responsibilities of the medical assistant during minor surgery include preparing the room and supplies; preparing the patient, both physically and mentally; and assisting the physician as needed. An efficient assistant can make the procedure easier for the patient and the physician by giving attention to both. Similar preparatory steps and equipment are used in most minor surgical procedures, although they may vary according to the physician's preferences. A general procedure for assisting with minor surgery is presented, followed by sample lists of materials needed for the most common surgical procedures performed in a physician's office or clinic.

ASSISTING WITH MINOR SURGERY

PROCEDURE

1. Check that the room is spotless clean, well ventilated, and well lighted.

2. Wash your hands. **Use appropriate personal protective equipment (PPE) as dictated by facility.**

3. If electrical or battery-run equipment is to be used, check it for working order.

4. Assemble and prepare supplies and equipment.
   a. Open and place a sterile drape towel on a clean and dry tray or Mayo stand. This will be used as a sterile field.
   b. Place the required supplies and instruments on this sterile field. Sterile supplies are to be handled with sterile transfer forceps or sterile hands (refer to the section on handling sterile supplies).
   When the required instruments come wrapped in the same package or in a commercially prepared package, open the wrapper and use it for the sterile field. Then, with individually-wrapped sterilized hemostats or gloved hands, organize the instruments for use (Figure 6-16, A). Refer to the previous section on opening sterile packages.

5. Cover this sterile setup with a sterile towel until ready to use (Figure 6-16, B).

RATIONALE

Avoid contamination to the sterile setup.

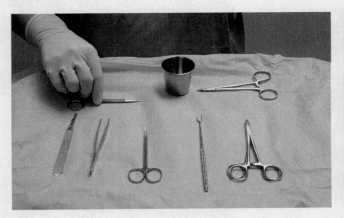

A

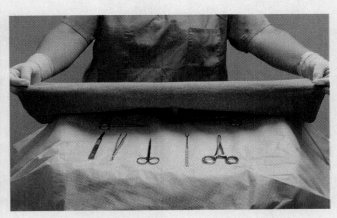

B

Figure 6-16 A, *Using sterile gloves to organize instruments for minor surgery.* **B,** *Cover sterile setup with a sterile towel until ready to use.*

<table>
<tr><td>

PROCEDURE

</td><td>

RATIONALE

</td></tr>
<tr><td>

6. Obtain any medications or solutions that will be required during the procedure.

7. Open outer wrap of the sterile glove pack for the physician.

8. Prepare the patient. Refer to the preceding discussion on preparing the patient for minor surgery.
   a. Explain the procedure. Have the necessary consent forms ready for the patient to sign.
   b. Provide a gown, and instruct what clothing must be removed.
   c. Have the patient void if necessary.
   d. Position the patient according to the type and location of surgery that is to be performed. The patient must be made comfortable, whether sitting or in a prone or supine position
   e. If required, wash the operative site with soap and water and shave the area. (Materials for preparing the skin are listed on page 220.)

SKIN PREPARATION
   a. Pull skin taut to shave (Figure 6-17).
   b. Rinse and dry the shaved area.
   c. Wash area with an antiseptic soap, using a firm, circular motion. Start at the center and move outward (Figure 6-18). Do not return to the washed area.
   d. Rinse and blot dry with sterile gauze.

9. Summon the physician. The physician dons gloves, injects the local anesthetic (when one is required), paints the skin with an antiseptic solution such as povidone iodine, and drapes the operative area with sterile drapes.

</td><td>

Avoid any undue tension or movement during the operation.

The skin cannot be sterilized. Washing helps to reduce the risk of contamination. Microorganisms can also grow on hair; therefore the physician may request that you shave the operative area and surrounding skin.

These drapes provide a sterile area around the operative area, thus helping to reduce contamination to the surgical wound.

</td></tr>
</table>

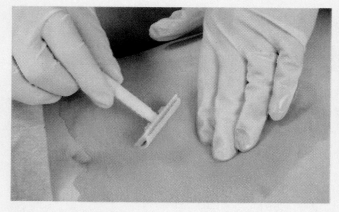

Figure 6-17 When shaving the skin in preparation for minor surgery, pull the skin taut and be careful not to cut it.

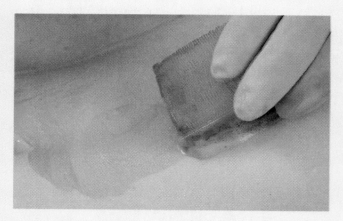

Figure 6-18 Using an antiseptic soap, wash operative area with a firm circular motion. Start at the center and move outward.

ASSISTING WITH MINOR SURGERY—cont'd

PROCEDURE	RATIONALE
10. When the physician has donned the sterile gloves, remove the sterile towel that is covering the tray of instruments. Standing behind or to the side of the instrument tray, carefully grasp the two distal corners of the towel. Slowly lift the towel off by lifting it toward you. You must not touch anything but the two distal ends of the towel.	*If you touch anything, you may contaminate the sterile setup.*
11. Assist the physician as requested. If additional supplies are needed, you must use surgical aseptic technique when handing them to the physician or placing them on the sterile field. Refer to the previous section on Handling Sterile Supplies.	
12. Offer the patient physical and emotional support. It may be necessary for you to steady the patient's arm, hand, leg, head, or any body part so that moving or jerking is avoided while the physician is operating. Casually and calmly talk to the patient.	*Casual and calm conversation may help to direct attention from any pain or discomfort being experienced and may help the patient relax.*
13. Do not stand between the patient and the physician, between the physician and the light source, or too near the sterile setup.	*The operative area must not be obstructed. Sterile supplies must not be contaminated.*
14. If you actually help the physician and handle the sterile supplies during the procedure, you must again scrub your hands thoroughly before the procedure begins, don sterile gloves, and sometimes also don a sterile gown. During the procedure, you are expected to hand the instruments to the physician and to receive them after use. When directly assisting the physician with the instruments, you must anticipate the physician's needs (that is, you must know when the physician will need an instrument or other supplies). You must hand an instrument over so that, when the physician grasps it, it is ready to use without need for adjustments.	
15. Hold containers for collecting specimens, drainage, or discharge near the work area when needed (Figure 6-19). Wear disposable single-use exam gloves when you think that there is any chance that you will have direct contact with a specimen or drainage.	*Wear gloves for your protection.*
16. Place soiled instruments in a basin or container, out of the patient's view, when they are no longer needed. Avoid contaminating the remaining sterile supplies.	
17. Place soiled sponges and dressings in a plastic bag. Do not allow wet items to sit on a sterile field.	*Contamination will result.*
18. When a biopsy is obtained, immediately place it into the designated jar containing a preservative solution (see Figure 6-19). Hold the lid of the container so that the underside of the lid is facing down.	*Do not touch the inside of a specimen jar because it is sterile. Holding the lid in this position helps to prevent contamination of the underside of the sterile lid by microorganisms in air currents or by objects touching it.*
19. Label the specimen jar with the patient's name, the date, and the source of the specimen. Ensure that the lid of the jar is closed securely.	

ASSISTING WITH MINOR SURGERY—cont'd

PROCEDURE	RATIONALE

20. After the surgery, it is often advisable to allow the patient to rest for a short while. When sedation has been administered, never leave the patient alone on the examining table unless it has guard rails.

21. Help the patient prepare to leave the office. Do not allow the patient to leave the office without the physician's knowledge. Check with the physician regarding future treatments, medications, and appointments. Frequently the physician gives the patient instructions regarding postoperative care to be performed at home by the patient.

22. Provide clear and concise postoperative instructions to the patient, when necessary. When indicated, make sure that the patient knows and understands about
    a. Compresses
    b. Elevation of the affected part(s)
    c. Presence of a drain
    d. Changing dressing—how often, how it should be down, what to look for (drainage, healing, and so on), and how long to continue
    e. The possibility of pain and the use of medications ordered for this

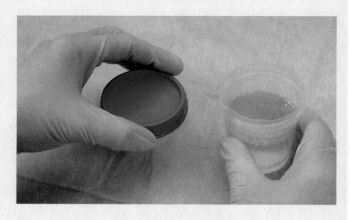

Figure 6-19 *Hold container for receiving specimens or discards near the work area.*

23. Send any specimen(s) collected to the laboratory along with a properly completed laboratory requisition. See Unit Eleven, "Collecting and Handling Specimens." Record in the patient's chart the date and time that the specimen was sent to the laboratory.

This provides documentation that the specimen was properly attended to.

24. When the patient has left, attend to sanitization of the reusable instruments and supplies, discard disposables properly, and clean and prepare the room for the next patient. When time permits, clean all instruments for sterilization, sterilize, and return them to the proper storage area, following the procedures presented in Unit Five.

25. Wash your hands.

MATERIALS FOR OFFICE SURGERIES

The following are sample lists of equipment used for minor office surgeries that may vary with the individual physicians' preferences and the case. Supplies and instruments can be added or deleted to meet the requirements of the particular situation. Once you learn the physician's preferences, you can prepare lists for each procedure and use them as a reference when preparing for minor surgery. Figure 6-20 shows standard instruments used for medical-surgical purposes, Figure 6-21 shows supplies and instruments used for procedures involving incisions *without* suture closure, and Figure 6-22 shows supplies and instruments used for procedures involving an excision of tissue and closure *with* sutures. Figure 6-23 shows a setup for major surgery.

Materials basic to all procedures
- Individually wrapped sterile forceps
- Sterile gloves for the assistant when directly assisting with the procedure

NOTE: When using instruments for the following setups that have been soaking in a chemical solution, rinse them in sterile water before using.

Figure 6-20 *Instruments used for medical-surgical purposes.* **A,** *Types of scissors.* **Left to right,** *Straight iris scissors, curved iris scissors, suture scissors, curved Metzenbaum blunt blade scissors, disposable suture scissors, bandage scissors with the flat blunt tip to prevent puncturing skin when cutting away bandage;* **B, Top (left to right),** *punch biopsy forceps, No. 11 scalpel blade and handle.* **Bottom (left to right),** *Straight mosquito forceps, curved mosquito forceps, straight Kelly forceps, curved Kelly forceps, tissue forceps plain tip, tissue forceps toothed tip, Allis clamp, needle holder.*

A
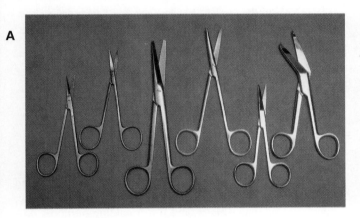

B
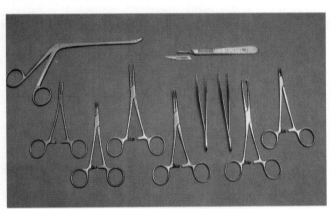

Figure 6-21 *Supplies and instruments used for minor surgery involving incision* without *suture closure. Materials for preparing the skin: container with sponges in surgical detergent and razor with blade. Materials for local anesthesia: vial of local anesthetic medication , 3-cc syringe with needle, alcohol sponge (other antiseptic solutions could be used rather than alcohol sponge). Other supplies and instruments: sterile gloves for the surgeon, 4 × 4 inch and 2 × 2 inch sponges and instruments, (left to right) - No. 3 scalpel blade and handle, scalpel blades (top to bottom, No. 11, No. 10, No. 15), curved iris scissors, straight mosquito forceps, tissue forceps (plain tip).*

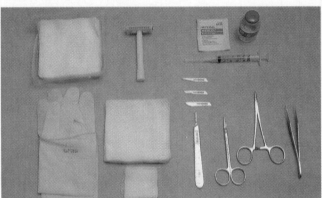

Figure 6-22 Supplies and instruments used for minor surgery when excising tissue and closing the skin with suture materials. Left side of illustration and along the top includes materials for preparing the skin, administering local anesthesia, sponges, and sterile gloves for the surgeon. Additional supplies and instruments from left to right include: No. 3 scalpel blade handle, No. 10, (top) and No. 15, scalpel blades, toothed tissue forceps, curved iris scissors, curved and straight mosquito forceps, straight and curved Kelly forceps, suture scissors, needle holder with mounted curved atraumatic needle with suture materials, and container for specimen with preservative solution.

Materials for preparing the skin area

- Surgical detergent for washing the skin
- Sterile sponges (cotton balls and gauze—2 × 2 inch and 4 × 4 inch)
- Sterile forceps
- Antiseptic solution such as povidone-iodine for disinfecting the skin
- Razor and blade (if skin is to be shaved)
- Draping materials

Materials for administering local anesthesia

- Sterile antiseptic in sterile container such as povidone-iodine solution
- Applicators or cotton balls and a forceps to use when painting the skin; prepackaged sterile povidone ioxide applicators are available and may be used instead.

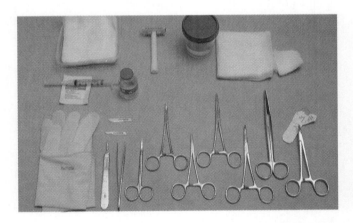

- Sterile syringe (3 cc or 5 cc)
- Sterile needles: 25-gauge, 1/2 inch, and 23- or 24- gauge, 1 1/2 inch (size and gauge vary with site to be infiltrated)
- Local anesthetic: ampules or vials of lidocaine 1% or 2% or procaine hydrochloride 1% or 2%. For a topical spray anesthetic, ethyl chloride may be used

Figure 6-23 *Setup for major surgery. Note the difference in the instrument setup required for major surgery versus that presented in Figures 6-21 and 6-22 for minor surgery.*

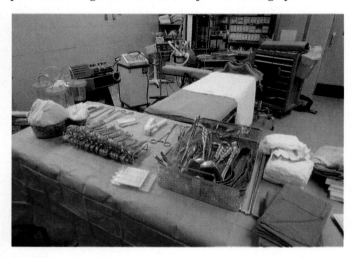

- Alcohol sponge to cleanse the vial top
- Sterile gloves (depending on physician's preference and procedure to be performed)

This setup may be prepared individually or added to the sterile setup used for the procedure.

Materials for suturing lacerations

- Materials for preparing the skin
- Local anesthetic setup
- Sterile gloves
- Toothed tissue forceps
- Hemostat
- Needle holder
- Suture scissors
- Suture material with suture needle
- Sterile gauze 2 × 2 inch and 4 × 4 inch (for sponging and dressing wound; larger dressings are needed for lacerations larger than 3 inches)
- Adhesive or, preferably, hypoallergenic tape and bandage scissors to cut it
- Container for used instruments and sponges

NOTE: If the wound is infected or abscesses are to be incised, suture material is not needed because infected wounds are usually not sutured.

Materials for incision and drainage (I&D) of an abscess or cyst (see Figure 6-21)

- Materials for preparing the skin
- Local anesthetic setup
- Sterile gloves
- No. 3 scalpel handle and blade; usually a No. 11 blade—or a No. 15 blade for finer and smaller incisions
- Iris (small) sharp scissors to dissect and cut with; sometimes larger blunt scissors are also needed

- Tissue forceps
- Hemostat
- Rubber drain to be inserted to provide for drainage during healing, when indicated. (Size varies with the size of the incision and area drained. If the drain is sutured to the skin for support, suture material, suture needle, and needle holder are needed)
- Sterile gauze for sponging and dressing the wound (2 × 2 inch and 4 × 4 inch)
- Adhesive or, preferably, hypoallergenic tape and bandage scissors to cut it
- Container for used instruments and gauze sponges

Materials for removing foreign bodies in subcutaneous tissues, small growths, and tissue biopsy specimens (see Figure 6-22)

- Materials for preparing the skin
- Local anesthetic setup
- Sterile gloves
- Mosquito forceps, straight and curved
- Kelly forceps, straight and curved
- No. 3 scalpel handle and blade (No. 10 or No. 15 blade) and the electrocautery unit, including a lubricated lead plate, that is placed under the patient for grounding purposes; this plate is not needed when the table is grounded; some tables are supplied with an electrical system that is grounded to an electrical wall outlet
- Iris scissors (small sharp scissors)
- Toothed tissue forceps
- Suture scissors
- Suture material and needle
- Needle holder
- Sterile gauze for sponging and dressing the wound (2 × 2 inch and 4 × 4 inch)
- Adhesive or, preferably, hypoallergenic tape and bandage scissors to cut it
- Container for used instruments and sponges
- Specimen bottle containing a preservative solution for a tissue biopsy specimen; Zenker's solution or formalin 10% are the preferred solutions used to preserve small tissues, warts, and moles
- Biopsy forceps are also needed for obtaining a biopsy from certain body sites such as the uterine cervix; in this case, dressing materials or tampons are needed to pack the area after the biopsy has been obtained, in addition to instruments used in pelvic examination (see Unit Four)
- Laboratory requisition

Materials for a cervical biopsy

- Materials for preparing the skin—skin antiseptic solution
- Sterile gloves
- Vaginal speculum
- Uterine dressing forceps
- Cervical biopsy punch
- Coagulant gel or foam
- Sponges

- Uterine tenaculum
- Vaginal packing or tampon
- Specimen bottle with preservative solution such as 10% Formalin
- Laboratory requisition

Colposcopy

A colposcopy is an examination of the vagina and cervix done with a colposcope. A colposcope is a lighted instrument with lenses that magnify and focus an intense light on the tissues of the vagina and cervix. This allows the physician to observe the anatomy of these tissues in greater detail. Through the colposcope the physician can see areas of abnormal tissue that can be removed by biopsy or cryosurgery. A colposcopy is performed to assess patients with cervical lesions that were observed during a pelvic examination, to assess the cervical cells and tissues when the results of a Pap smear fall within abnormal ranges, to visualize abnormalities, to assess patients who were exposed to diethylstilbestrol in utero, to obtain a biopsy specimen, and at times to substitute for a cone biopsy when the physician is evaluating the cause of abnormal cervical cytologic findings.

If biopsy specimens were taken, the patient may have some vaginal bleeding. Provide a perineal pad for the patient. Inform her that she may have a coffee-colored granular discharge for about 3 days. Also instruct her to call the physician if she has excessive bleeding or discharge. (See also Pelvic Examination and Papanicolaou Smear in Unit Four.)

Endocervical Curettage

Depending on the findings from a colposcopy and to further examine for precancerous conditions, the physician may perform an endocervical curettage (ECC) and/or cryosurgery. In an ECC cells are scraped from inside the cervical canal. This is necessary when the physician cannot see this area during a colposcopy. The ECC can help the physician determine a more precise diagnosis and plan treatment accordingly.

Cryosurgery

When the endocervical curettage shows that the cervical canal has no dysplasia (an alteration in the shape, size, and organization of cells or an abnormal development of cells), cryosurgery may be performed. Cryosurgery (also known as cryotherapy) in this area of the body is commonly used to treat any type of cervical erosion or chronic cervicitis. Freezing temperatures ($-40°$ to $-80°$ C) are used in this treatment method. The physician uses the colposcopy to magnify the surface of the cervix. Then a low-temperature probe is applied to the affected area, freezing and destroying the involved cells. The patient may experience some cramping resembling menstrual cramps and may be given a mild analgesic such as Anaprox or Advil before the procedure and a prescription for the same after the procedure. It is important that she use sanitary pads and not tampons because she would not want to irritate the tissues that had been treated. Explain to the patient that she will most likely have a clear, watery discharge for

about the next 4 weeks, to report any foul odor or unusual discharge to the physician, to abstain from sexual intercourse for 4 weeks, to douche with a dilute vinegar and water solution, and to schedule a return visit in 6 weeks so that the physician can determine if the cervix is healing properly. The new cells that grow during healing are usually normal.

Endometrial Biopsy (EMB)

An endometrial biopsy is done for the following reasons.

- To detect endometrial carcinoma and precancerous conditions
- To monitor the effects of hormonal therapy on the uterine endometrium, including the effects of estrogen in patients with suspected ovarian dysfunction, or to determine adequate levels of circulating progesterone
- To routinely screen selected patients for early detection of endometrial carcinoma; the American Cancer Society recommends that women at high risk have this done at menopause; a woman is considered to be at high risk if she has a history of infertility, obesity, failure to ovulate, or abnormal bleeding or if she is undergoing estrogen therapy
- To determine if ovulation has occurred
- To detect inflammatory conditions or polyps
- To assess abnormal uterine bleeding

As for the previous gynecologic procedures, the patient is placed in a lithotomy position (see Unit Four) and the physician performs a bimanual pelvic examination by placing one hand on the woman's abdomen and one or two gloved fingers of the other hand in the woman's vagina to determine the position of the uterus (see Figure 4-20). The physician then administers the local anesthetic. After the anesthetic has taken effect, the physician inserts the uterine sound and then the Knovak suction tube curette into the uterus to obtain the specimens, *or* the physician may use an endometrial suction curette that has centimeter markings on it so that uterine sounding can be done with the same instrument. Specimens are obtained and placed in the specimen bottles containing 10% formalin and sent to the laboratory for histologic examination. After the procedure, provide the patient with a sanitary pad. Inform her that some vaginal bleeding is to be expected but, if excessive bleeding occurs, she must inform the physician. Also tell her that she should not douche or have sexual intercourse for the next 72 hours. A mild analgesic may be prescribed for any discomfort.

Materials for a colposcopy

- Sterile gloves
- Vaginal speculum
- Sterile gauze 4 × 4 inch
- Long (8-inch) sterile cotton-tipped applicators
- 3% Acetic acid (some physicians may use Lygol's solution instead of or in addition to acetic acid)
- Kevorkian biopsy forceps (for a cervical biopsy)
- Endocervical curette (for an endocervix tissue sample)
- Two specimen bottles with 10% formalin preservative. Label bottle No. *cervical* and bottle No. 2 *endocervical*

- Coagulating agents (Monsel's solution or silver nitrate applicators may be used after a biopsy has been taken)
- Perineal pad
- Laboratory requisition

Materials for a vulvar biopsy

- Sterile gloves
- Materials for preparing the skin area
- Sterile needle: 30 gauge, 1 inch
- Sterile syringe: 3 cc or 5 cc
- 1% lidocaine
- Cervical punch biopsy forceps
- Coagulating agents (Monsel's solution on a 6-inch applicator or silver nitrate applicators)
- Perineal pad
- Laboratory requisition

Materials for an endocervical curettage (ECC)

- Sterile gloves
- Povidone-iodine
- Long cotton-tipped applicators
- Cotton balls
- 4 × 4 sterile gauze
- Two specimen bottles with 10% formalin (one is used and labeled for the ECC and the second bottle is used and labeled for the EMB)
- Sanitary pad
- Vaginal speculum
- Kovorkian curette
- Uterine tenaculum
- Laboratory requisitions

Materials for an endometrial biopsy (EMB)

In addition to the materials needed for the endocervical curettage add the following:

- 1% lidocaine
- 22-gauge spinal needle
- 10-cc syringe
- Uterine sound
- Knovak suction curette with a 10-cc 3-ring syringe, *or an* endometrial suction curette such as the Z endometrial sampler or Pipelle
- Kidney stone or straight packing forceps

Materials for cryosurgery

- Sterile gloves
- Vaginal speculum
- 3% acetic acid solution
- Long cotton-tipped applicators
- Cryosurgery unit
- Sanitary pad

Materials for a 6-mm skin biopsy

- Materials for preparing the skin—skin antiseptic solution or an alcohol sponge
- Local anesthetic setup—sterile needle: 25-gauge, $5/_8$-inch or 30-gauge, $1/_2$ inch; 3-cc syringe; 1% lidocaine

- Sterile gloves
- No. 3 scalpel handle and a No. 15 blade
- 6-mm biopsy punch
- Suture set with straight sharp scissors (scissors used to remove the top two layers of skin)
- Suture material: 5-0 black silk and curved needle
- Needle holder
- Sterile gauze—2 × 2 inch and 4 × 4 inch
- Specimen bottle with 10% formalin
- Adhesive bandage (used for the dressing over surgical site)
- Laboratory requisition

Materials for an aspiration (needle) biopsy of the breast

- Materials for preparing the skin
- Sterile gloves
- Topical spray anesthetic (ethyl chloride is frequently used)
- 12-cc syringe, No. 18 needle, and a sterile culture tube to receive the specimen; most laboratories prefer to receive the specimen in the culture tube because each laboratory may use different procedures for fixing, staining, and examining the specimen
- An adhesive bandage is usually sufficient for the dressing
- Laboratory requisition when a specimen is sent for cytologic or histologic examination

For a fine-needle aspiration (FNA), many use a No. 20 gauge $2^1/_2$-inch needle with a 20-cc syringe.

For a core biopsy, add:

- Biopsy syringe gun
- No. 14- or No. 16-gauge needle
- 2 or 3 microscopic slides
- Container with preservative and label for the slides

Materials for electrocauterization (Figure 6-24)

- Materials for skin preparation
- Local anesthetic setup, depending on extent and site of area to be cauterized; at times this may not be required
- Sterile gloves
- Electrocautery unit
- Extension electrode for the cautery and instruments used for a pelvic examination (see page 100) for cauterization of the uterine cervix
- Container for used instruments, sponges
- Dressing materials: size and type determined by size and type of area cauterized; an adhesive bandage may be applied to a small area to protect it from irritants; frequently dressings are not applied to small, superficial areas

INSERTION OF AN INTRAUTERINE DEVICE

An intrauterine device (IUD) is inserted into the uterus for the purpose of contraception. Only two types of IUDs are available in the United States: the Progestasert (a T-shaped IUD containing progesterone) and the Copper-T 380A (a T-shaped IUD wrapped with copper wire). The Progestasert IUD must be replaced every year, whereas the Cooper-T 380A can remain in place for up to 4 years. The physician insert the IUD usually on the third day of the patient's menstrual period because at this time the cervix may be dilated some and it is assumed that the patient is not pregnant. Before the insertion of an IUD, the patient should have had a Pap smear. On occasion, the physician may choose to insert an IUD 5 to 10 days after the patient's menstrual period. The patient is positioned and draped as for a pelvic examination. A consent form must be signed before an IUD is inserted (Figure 6-25).

Figure 6-24 *Supplies and instruments for electrocauterization.*

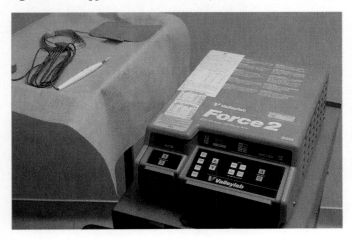

Figure 6-25 *Consent form for insertion of an IUD.*

OB/GYN CLINIC
IUD CONSENT FORM

I have been informed by my physician of alternative methods of birth control and have chosen to use the IUD. I have received literature explaining the use of the IUD. I have read the literature and I understand it. I also understand the risks of insertion and use of an IUD. Some serious complications which may occur are an increased chance of infection, rarely leading to sterility, and possible uterine perforation. I understand that there is still a possibility of pregnancy with an increased risk of miscarriage or, rarely, a tubal pregnancy.

Signed_____
patient
Date_____

Date of insertion_____

Lot number of IUD_____

Name of IUD_____

Date to be changed_____

VOCABULARY

Types of open wounds

Abrasion (ab-ra-zhun)—A scrape on the surface of the skin or on a mucous membrane (for example, a skinned knee).

Avulsion (a-vul´shun)—A piece of soft tissue torn loose or left hanging as a flap.

Incision—A straight cut caused by a cutting instrument such as a scalpel (surgical knife) for surgical purposes.

Laceration (las´e-ra´shun)—A tear or jagged-edged wound of body tissues.

Puncture—A small, external opening in the skin made by a sharp, pointed object such as a needle or nail.

Pathogenic organisms that can cause wounds

Staphylococci (staf-il-o-kok´si)—Bacteria that occur in grapelike clusters; gram-positive cocci. Pathogenic species cause suppurative (pus-producing) conditions

Streptococci (strep´´to-kok-si)—A type of bacteria occurring in chains; gram-positive cocci

Colon bacillus (*Escherichia coli* or *E. coli*)—A type of bacteria; a normal inhabitant of the intestinal tract; gram-negative bacteria. Pathogenic *E. coli* are responsible for many infections of the urinary tract and for many epidemic diarrheal diseases, especially in infants.

Gas bacillus (*Clostridium perfringens*)—A type of bacteria; gram-positive bacteria; anaerobic; the most common cause of gas gangrene. (Gas gangrene is a condition often resulting from dirty lacerated wounds in which the muscles and subcutaneous tissue become filled with gas and serosanguineous exudate. It is caused by the species of *Clostridium* that breaks down tissue by gas production and toxins. An exudate is material that has escaped from blood vessels and has been deposited in a body cavity, in tissues, or on the surface of tissues, usually as a result of inflammation).

Tetanus bacillus (*Clostridium tetani*)—A type of bacteria; gram-positive bacteria; anaerobic; spore-forming rods; the causative organism of tetanus or lockjaw. This organism enters the body through a break in the skin, especially through puncture wounds. In this case infection is often obvious. Tetanus and gas bacilli are common in puncture wounds because they are anaerobic (that is, they grow in the absence of oxygen).

Terms that describe drainage

Serous—Consisting of serum (clear, straw-colored liquid)

Sanguineous—Consisting of blood or blood in abundance

Serosanguineous—Consisting of blood and serum

Purulent—Consisting of or containing pus (a pale, yellow, creamy, yellow-green sticky fluid exudate)

INSERTING AN IUD

Equipment (Figure 6-26)

Surgical soap and water
Alcohol or povidone-iodine
Sterile sponges
Vaginal speculum
Sterile gloves
Sterile single-toothed tenaculum
Sterile uterine sound
Sterile sponge stick
Sterile suture scissors
IUD and inserter

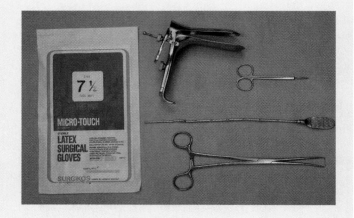

Figure 6-26 *Equipment for the insertion of an intrauterine device. Left to right, Sterile gloves, (top) suture scissors, uterine sound, single-toothed tenaculum, sponge stick.*

PROCEDURE

The physician will:

1. Introduce the vaginal speculum into the vagina.

2. Perform a pelvic examination.

3. Prepare the cervix with surgical soap and water and then with alcohol or povidone-iodine.

4. Grasp the cervix with the single-toothed tenaculum.

5. Introduce the uterine sound into the uterus to check for depth.

6. Prepare and insert the IUD.

7. Withdraw the IUD inserter.

8. Cut the string attached to the IUD with suture scissors.

9. Perform a digital examination.

PROCEDURE

The medical assistant should now:

10. Wash hands and assemble the equipment. **Use appropriate personal protective equipment (PPE) as dictated by facility.** (Step 10 should be completed before patient's arrival.

11. Help the patient assume a supine position for 5 to 10 minutes to prevent the state of shock.

12. Elevate the patient's head 45 degrees to 50 degrees for 5 minutes.

13. Have the patient sit up with legs over the side of the table and maintain this position for a few minutes to ensure that the patient's condition is stable.

14. Give the patient further instructions:
    a. If bleeding, fever, or pain occurs, notify the physician.
    b. Check for the presence of the IUD string in the vagina once a month after her menstrual period. (If she cannot find the string, she should make an appointment to see the physician.)
    c. A yearly checkup with the physician is necessary.
    d. The Progestasert IUD must be changed every year because effectiveness decreases after that time span.
    e. Once dressed, she is free to leave.

15. Ask the patient if she has any questions; answer them adequately, or refer the patient to the physician.

SUTURE REMOVAL

After the physician has inspected a wound and suture line, the medical assistant may be directed to remove the sutures. (Agency policy and state law will determine who can remove sutures.) The condition of the suture line and the progress of healing will determine when suture materials can be removed. Depending on the location of the sutures and the progress of healing, sutures are generally removed from the third to the tenth or twelfth day postoperatively. Sutures that are left in place longer than necessary may be a source of infection.

WOUNDS

A wound is a break in the continuity of external or internal soft body parts, caused by physical trauma to the tissues. An *open wound* is one in which the skin and mucous membranes

REMOVING SUTURES

Equipment (Figure 6-27)

Sterile gloves
Suture removal kit that includes suture scissors, plain-tipped tissue forceps, sterile gauze 4 × 4 inch
Antiseptic solution in container (or disposable povidone-iodine applicators)
Sterile applicators or gauze or cotton balls
Container for removed sutures, used instruments, and sponges

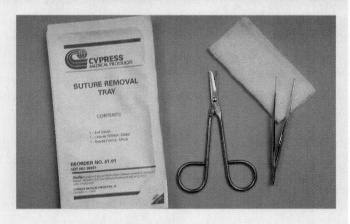

Figure 6-27 *Sterile disposable suture removal kits.*

PROCEDURE	RATIONALE
1. Wash your hands and assemble the equipment. **Use appropriate personal protective equipment (PPE) as dictated by facility.**	
2. Identify the patient and explain the procedure. Explain that the patient will feel a slight pulling sensation as the suture is removed.	*Explanations provide reassurance and help the patient to relax.*
3. Don sterile gloves.	*Maintain surgical asepsis.*
4. Cleanse the suture line with an antiseptic (for example, povidone-iodine). Start from the incision line and work outwards. One stroke per cotton ball or applicator.	*Remove bacteria from the incision line.*
5. Using plain-tipped tissue forceps, grasp the knot of the suture and gently pull it away from the skin.	
6. Using suture scissors cut the suture below the knot (the part that is closest to the skin).	
7. To remove the suture, pull it straight up from the skin and place it in the container. Pull gently to keep pain and tissue damage to a minimum.	*Using a smooth continuous motion to remove the suture reduces tension on the suture line and patient discomfort. Cutting the suture as close as possible to the skin prevents pulling previously exposed contaminated suture through the skin.*
8. Continue to remove all sutures in this manner.	
9. Count the number of sutures that you removed.	*Ensures that all sutures were removed.*
10. Note the condition of the suture line.	
11. Cleanse the suture line with an antiseptic.	
12. Apply a sterile dressing or leave open to the air as applicable.	*A dressing would protect the wound site. Dressing may not be needed unless the patient's clothing would irritate the wound site.*
13. Give the patient any instructions as needed.	
14. Dispose of supplies properly.	
15. Remove your gloves and wash your hands.	

16. Record the procedure. Note the date, time, how many sutures were removed, the location of the wound, the condition of the wound site, and any directions given to the patient. Sign your name.	*Charting Example:*
	Sept. 23, 19____, 4 p.m.
	  6 sutures removed from palm of right hand. Suture line is dry and appears to be healing well.
	    E.M. Day, CMA

are broken; in a *closed wound,* the skin is not broken, but there is a contusion (bruise) or a hematoma (hem-a-to´ ma), a tumorlike mass of blood.

Types of open wounds include the following (Figure 6-28): abrasions, avulsions, incisions, lacerations, and punctures.

Microorganisms can invade both open and closed wounds, and an infection can result. Signs and symptoms that indicate the presence of an infection include redness, heat, pain, swelling, and at times, the presence of pus and a throbbing sensation at the wound site. Fever often accompanies infection. As the temperature rises, pulse and respiration rates also rise. An indication that an infection is spreading from a wound caused by needle pricks, splinters, or small cuts is the presence of a red streak running up the extremity from the wound site.

Wounds that are most susceptible to infection are those in which there is not a free flow of blood, those in which there is a crushing of the tissues, and those in which the break in the skin closes or falls back in place, thus preventing entrance of air, as seen in puncture wounds.

Common pathogenic organisms causing a wound infection include the following:

staphylococci, streptococci, colon bacillus, gas bacillus, and tetanus bacillus.

One of the body's natural defense mechanisms against infection or trauma is the inflammatory process. It works to limit damage to the tissue, remove injured cells, and repair injured tissues (see also page 177).

THE HEALING PROCESS

Wounds heal by first intention or by second intention, depending on damage or loss of tissue. When the edges of wounds can be brought together, as in sutured surgical incisions, or when there is a minimal amount of tissue loss or damage, as in a relatively clean and small cut, they heal by first intention. There will be little inflammation and minimal scarring, if any.

When the wound edges cannot be approximated because of extensive tissue loss or damage, healing by second intention occurs. This is seen in open and infected trauma or surgical wounds such as after the incision and drainage of abscesses or in major lacerations. Since large amounts of granulation tissue form to fill the gap between the wound edges and to allow epithelial cells to migrate across the wound surfaces from the edges, this healing process is also known as healing by granulation or indirect healing. This is a slower process than healing by first intention; thus it involves a greater risk of infection and usually produces greater scarring.

The healing process normally occurs in three stages.

1. Lag phase: Blood serum and cells form a fibrin network in the wound. A clot is formed that fills the wound and begins to knot the edges together with shreds of fibrin. Dried proteins then form a scab.
2. Fibroplasia: Granulation tissue (fragile, pinkish red tissue) forms as the fibrin network absorbs and epithelial cells start forming from the edges to form a scar.
3. Contraction phase: Small blood vessels are absorbed, fibroblasts (cells from which connective tissue develops) contract, and the scar begins to shrink and changes in color from red to white.

The body's ability to heal after any trauma is affected by the general health status of the individual. Good health helps the body deal successfully with injuries and infections.

Figure 6-28 *Types of wounds.*

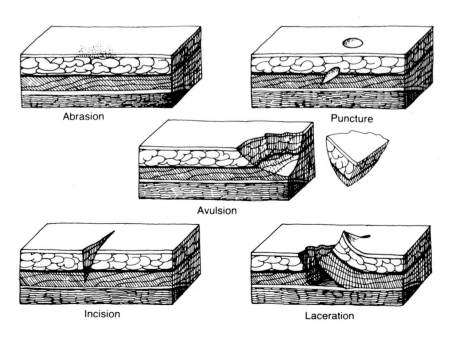

CARE OF WOUNDS

The goals of wound care are to promote healing and prevent additional injury. There are two schools of thought regarding the care of a wound: some prefer to leave the wound undressed, and others prefer to dress a wound.

Most closed wounds are left undressed, as well as some wounds that have sealed and can be protected from additional injury, irritation, and contamination. Exposure to the air helps keep the wound dry and can promote healing. Open wounds covered with a dressing provide a warm, dark, moist area that is suitable for growth of microorganisms. Dressings applied incorrectly can interfere with adequate circulation to the area, which will interfere with the healing process; also, if a dressing does not stay in place, it can cause further irritation to the wound and possibly cross-contamination.

Regardless of the method used (dressed or undressed), a wound must be kept clean, have dead tissue removed, and then be allowed to drain freely.

When a dressing is changed, it and the wound must be inspected for the amount and character of drainage, if present. The amount is best described as scant, moderate, or large; the character refers to the color, odor, and consistency of the drainage. Common terms that describe drainage are as follows: serous. sanguineous, serosanguineous, and purulent.

The condition of the wound, the degree of healing, and the integrity of sutures and drains must also be observed during a dressing change.

DRESSINGS AND BANDAGES

Techniques of applying dressing and bandages vary according to the extent and location of wounds, injuries, or burns; the materials to be used; and the purpose for which they are applied.

DRESSINGS

Dressings are materials of various types placed directly over wounds, open lesions, and burns as the immediate protective covering. When used correctly, dressings serve eight purposes.

1. To protect wounds from additional trauma
2. To help prevent contamination of the wound
3. To absorb drainage
4. To provide pressure for controlling hemorrhage, promoting drainage, and reducing edema
5. To immobilize and support the wound site
6. To ease pain
7. To provide a means for applying and keeping medications on the wound
8. To provide psychologic benefits for the patient by concealing, protecting, and giving support to the wound.

To prevent contamination and the possibility of an infection developing, sterile technique and sterile dressing materials must be used when applying or changing a dressing. The only exception is in emergency situations when the patient has serious bleeding. On those rare occasions, it is more important to stop the bleeding than to worry about contaminating the wound with unsterile materials.

Dressing Materials

Various types and sizes of commercial sterile dressings are available (Figure 6-29). Many are made of gauze, such as folded gauze sponges* available in various sizes (for example, 2 × 2 inch, 4 × 4 inch, and 3 × 4 inch) and gauze fluffs, which are loosely folded, large gauze squares used to absorb large amounts of drainage or to pack an opening. Some dressings are made from viscose rayon and cellulose materials such as folded Topper* sponges supplied in 3 × 3-inch, 4 × 3-inch, and 4 × 4- inch sizes; still others are made from a unique, nonwoven binderless soft fabric called Sofwik,* (for example, Sof-wik dressing sponges, available in 4 × 4-inch and 2 × 2-inch sizes). Larger absorbent gauze and dressings made from similar materials are available for dressing large wounds, major burns, or major surgical wounds (for example, Surgipad Combine Dressing* supplied in 5 × 9-inch, 8 × ½-inch, and 8× 10-inch sizes) and ABDs.

Other dressing materials have a special covering over the gauze to prevent them from sticking to an open or draining skin area. These are called nonadhering dressings. Examples of these include the Band-Aid Surgical Dressing* which is a complete dressing in a single package, consisting of a nonadherent facing, enclosing an absorbent filler, and backed by Dermicel* tape, available with 4 × 6-inch tape and 4 × 3-inch pad; or 8 × 6-inch tape and 8 × 3-inch pad. Telfa† is a gauze dressing with a plasticlike covering on the side that is to be placed over the wound; it is also available in various sizes. Steripak is another complete dressing, made of layers of absorbent cellulose and covered with a nonadhering, perforated plastic material that is secured to a vented adhesive

*Johnson & Johnson, New Brunswick, N.J.
†Kendall Co., Greenwich, Conn.

Text continues on page 232.

Figure 6-29 *Dressing matrials representing a system of wound management products for use in the care of lacerations and abrasions, multiple trauma, and burns.*

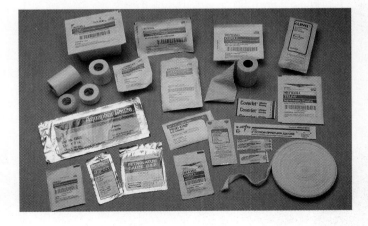

DRESSING CHANGE WITH A WOUND CULTURE

Equipment (Figure 6-30)

To obtain the culture

Sterile applicator(s) in a sterile culture tube(s) or a Culturette.* The type of culture tube varies, depending on the specific organism that is suspected. Check with your laboratory to ensure accuracy. Most laboratories request that an anaerobic Culturette* be used for wound cultures. Always check the expiration date on the outside wrapper before using to assure stability of the culture medium at the time of use. See Unit Eleven for additional information on cultures and materials used.

To change the dressing

Sterile dressing or a prepackage sterile dressing set containing:

Tissue forceps

Hemostat

Scissors

Gauze sponges 2 × 2-inch, or cotton balls, or antiseptic swabs

Dry dressings (for example, 4 × 4-inch gauze, Topper sponges, Sof-wik sponges)

Small container for antiseptic solution

Antiseptic solution

*Marion Scientific Corp.

Additional equipment

Antiseptic solution, if not supplied in the prepackaged dressing set, such as povidone-iodine, hydrogen peroxide, alcohol 70%

Tape, preferably hypoallergenic

Plastic bag for soiled dressing and disposable equipment

Disposable single-use exam gloves

Draping materials, as needed

Laboratory requisition

Optional equipment

Acetone or benzine or commercial tape remover to moisten tape on old dressing for easier removal

Sterile saline to moisten a dressing that has stuck to a wound to allow for easier removal

Sterile towels

Additional dressing supplies appropriate to the condition of the wound site (for example, Telfa, adhesive bandages, Steripak, Surgipads, Adaptic dressing, roller gauze bandage, Kling elastic gauze bandage)

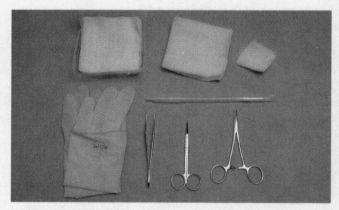

Figure 6-30 *Supplies and instruments for dressing change with wound culture.*

PROCEDURE

1. Wash your hands. **Use appropriate personal protective equipment (PPE) as dictated by facility.**

2. Assemble your equipment. Place the supplies on a flat, clean surface, convenient for use.

3. Identify the patient and explain the procedure. Explain that you will remove the soiled dressing, obtain a culture of the discharge from the wound, and apply a sterile dressing. The culture will then be sent to the laboratory for study. When the physician receives the laboratory report, the appropriate medication to eliminate the causative organism(s) of the infection may then be prescribed.

RATIONALE

Provide reassurance, and gain the patient's cooperation.

DRESSING CHANGE WITH A WOUND CULTURE—cont'd

PROCEDURE	RATIONALE

PROCEDURE

4. Have the patient put on a patient gown, if necessary. Position the patient, providing for comfort and relaxation. Drape if and as needed, exposing the area where the wound is located. When the wound is on the arm or leg, place a towel under the area to be dressed. Remind the patient not to touch the open wound once the dressing has been removed and not to talk over it because microorganisms can spread into the wound. Gowning, positioning, and draping vary with the location of the wound.

5. a. Open the dressing set. Using sterile gloves, arrange supplies in their order of use.
   b. Open plastic bag. Place the bag in a convenient place to receive the soiled dressing and used disposable supplies. Use surgical aseptic technique at all times. The wrapper on the dressing set is used for the sterile field.
   c. Pour the antiseptic solution into the sterile container located on the sterile field.

   NOTE: When the antiseptic solution is supplied in the dressing tray set, do not pour the solution until after you have donned sterile gloves.

   d. Cut pieces of tape that will be used to secure the clean sterile dressing when applied. These may be tagged onto the side of your dressing tray.

6. Loosen tape on the present dressing (Figure 6-31). Loosen and pull tape gently, pulling toward the wound so you don't tear newly formed tissue. When the tape doesn't pull away easily, moisten it with a sponge soaked with acetone, benzine, baby oil, or a commercial tape remover.

7. Loosen and remove the soiled dressing with a (Figure 6-32) gloved hand. Do not pull on the dressing. A dressing can also be removed by placing your hand inside a plastic bag. Then grasp and lift the dressing off, inspect for drainage, and invert bag over the dressing. Handle all dressings as if they are contaminated. Use forceps for this step only; then set aside or, if disposable, discard in the bag with the soiled dressing. If a dressing is difficult to remove, a sterile saline may be applied to help loosen it.

8. Inspect the dressing and discard it in the plastic bag. Observe the amount and type of drainage on the dressing.

9. Observe the wound. Note the location, type, and amount of drainage coming from the wound and the presence of pus, necrosis, and/or a putrid odor. Note the degree of healing and, when sutures are present, if they are intact.

RATIONALE

The important thing to remember is that the part of the body from which the culture is to be obtained and the dressing changed must be well supported and exposed. In addition, the patient's modesty must be protected.

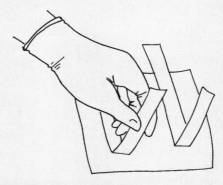

Figure 6-31 *Technique for loosening tape on dressing.*

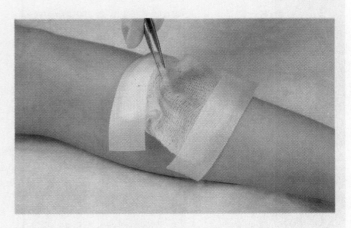

Figure 6-32 *Remove soiled dressing with a forceps.*

DRESSING CHANGE WITH A WOUND CULTURE—cont'd

PROCEDURE

RATIONALE

10. Remove the sterile applicator from the sterile culture tube or Culturette.* Swab the drainage area of the wound once to obtain a specimen. If you need more of the drainage for culturing, you must use another applicator. Swab only the draining area of the wound. Do not spread the infection to a clean area on the wound. Swab the wound only once in one direction. Never go back and forth over the area.

11. Place the applicator(s) in the culture tube(s) and set aside. Secure the lid tightly to prevent air from getting into the tube.

Air causes the specimen to dry, thus destroying the microorganisms.

12. Remove disposable single-use exam gloves. Dispose of them in the plastic bag.

13. Don sterile gloves as described previously to complete the dressing change.

Gloves are donned to prevent any microorganisms that may be on your hands from entering the wound and also to keep your hands clean.

14. Pick up gauze sponge with forceps or hemostat (whichever is most comfortable for you to use).

15. Dip the sponge into the antiseptic cleansing solution to wet through. Do not oversaturate the sponge. Keep sponge and forceps facing downward.

16. Gently, but thoroughly, cleanse the wound using single strokes over and parallel to the incision, one sponge per stroke. Starting at the center of the wound, stroke toward the ends. Cleanse the side farthest from you, working outward from the incision, and then repeat on the side closest to you (Figure 6-33).

Bacterial count is usually lowest at the center of the incision and greatest at the edges. Always work from the least contaminated areas to most contaminated areas to avoid contaminating uncontaminated sites.

17. Discard each sponge in the plastic bag for waste after use. Do not touch the bag with the forceps.

18. Repeat the process directly over the wound until it is cleansed to your satisfaction. Use a clean sponge for each single stroke.

19. When cleansing a drain site or a very small wound, move the antiseptic sponge in a circle around the site (Figure 6-34). Cleanse around and away from the wound in an ever-widening circle. Do not go back over a clean area.

20. Discard the sponge, and repeat.

21. Apply the sterile dressing. Center it over the wound area. Gloved hands are used to apply the dressing. Additional layers of dressings are added as indicated by the type of wound and amount of drainage (when present).

22. Discard disposable forceps and gloves in plastic waste bag. Close the plastic bag by tying a knot in the top. Put gloves to the side of the sterile field or in a container for used supplies. Remove gloves by pulling on the cuff and turning inside out.

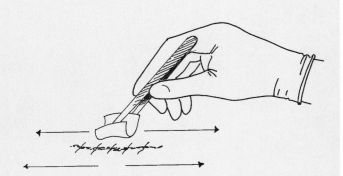

Figure 6-33 *Cleanse wound, starting at center going toward the end. Use one sponge per stroke.*

*Marion Scientific Corp.

DRESSING CHANGE WITH A WOUND CULTURE—cont'd

PROCEDURE

23. Secure the dressing with tape applied so that it conforms to body contours and movement. Ensure that it is adequately spaced; do not cover the entire dressing with tape (Figure 6-35). Place each strip of tape over the middle of the dressing and press down gently on both sides, working toward the ends. Hypoallergenic tape is preferred. Have equal lengths of tape on both sides of the dressing—not too short or too long. Tape should not cover the entire dressing. Distribute tension away from the incision. Do not tape too snugly.

24. Attend to the patient's comfort; you may reposition patient if necessary. Observe patient for any undue reaction. Provide further instructions as indicated or as ordered by physician. Check if the patient has any questions. Inform the patient if he or she is free to leave. Help the patient dress when necessary.

25. Label culture tube(s) or Culturette(s)* completely and accurately. Complete and attach the appropriate laboratory requisition. The label should include the following:
    Patient's name
    Physician's name
    Date
    Time
    Source of specimen
    Test requested

26. Take or send the culture to the laboratory. Avoid delay.

27. Remove used items from the treatment room; dispose of correctly. Discard soiled items and disposable equipment in a covered container according to agency policy. Wearing disposable single-use exam gloves, rinse reusable instruments under running water and then soak in detergent and water until you are ready to prepare them for sterilization (see Unit Five).

28. Wash your hands.

29. Replace supplies as needed. Leave the treatment room clean and neat.

30. Record the procedure and observations on the patient's chart, using correct medical abbreviations.

RATIONALE

If tape covers the entire dressing, it interferes with air circulation; if tape is too snug, it may constrict blood flow to the wound and interfere with the healing process.

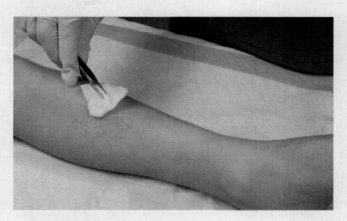

Figure 6-34 *Cleanse small wound or drain site using circular strokes, working from center to outside portion of wound site.*

Delay could cause drying of the specimen.

Charting example:
    March 4, 19___, 1 p.m.
        Rt. forearm dressing changed.
        Moderate amount of thick, yellow, purulent drainage on lower end of laceration.
        Culture taken and sent to label for C & S [culture and sensitivity].
        Wound cleansed and dry sterile dressing applied.
            Ann Michaelson, CMA

*Marion Scientific Corp.

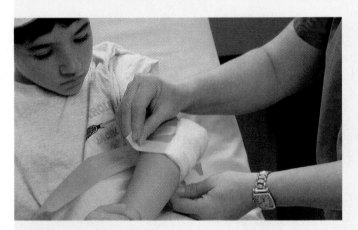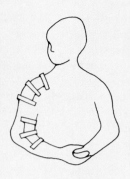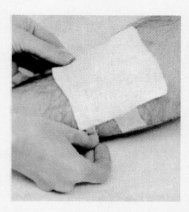

Figure 6-35 *Correct method of securing a dressing to conform to body contour and movement.*

tape. Steripak is available in 4 × 8-inch, 4 × 4-inch, and 2 × 4$^1/_2$-inch sizes. The Adaptic* nonadhering single-layer dressing, made of a highly porous weave, is used as the immediate covering over a wound under an absorbent secondary dressing; it is available in a foil envelope in 3 × 3-inch, 3 × 8-inch, 3 × 16-inch sizes and in a bottle in dimensions of $^1/_2$ inch × 4 yards for a packing strip. Vaseline* petrolatum gauze, a fine-mesh, absorbent gauze impregnated with white petrolatum, is a nonadhering dressing that clings and conforms to the wound. It is used over open or draining wounds to prevent the top dressing from sticking to the wound or disrupting newly formed tissue.

A third type of dressing materials is kept moist in a package; some are premedicated. These are used for debriding tissue, for treating open or ulcerated wounds, and sometimes for dermatologic conditions.

There are also spray-on dressing materials that, when sprayed over the wound, form a transparent, protective film. These are nontoxic and somewhat bacteriostatic and allow for close observation of an incision or wound site. Fluff cotton or cotton balls are never to be used for dressings because the fibers may get embedded in the wound and are difficult to remove if they do.

To hold dressings in place securely, various types and sizes of tape are available. The types of tape include hypoallergenic cloth tape, hypoallergenic paper tape, transparent tape, elastic cloth tape, and adhesive tape; sizes range from $^1/_2$ inch to 3 inches.

When changing or applying an initial dressing, select the dressing materials according to the purposes to be accomplished; in other words, know why the wound is to be dressed. This enables you to select the proper types and amounts of dressing materials. Any dressing must be large enough to cover the wound completely and extend at least an inch or more beyond.

*Chesebrough Pond's Inc., Greenwich, Conn.

In addition to patients who have had minor surgery in the office, patients who have had surgery in the hospital may come to the physician's office for a dressing change or wound culture when necessary. You may assist the physician with these procedures or perform them alone.

Dressing Change with a Wound Culture

When infection is suspected, a wound culture is taken to determine the presence and type of microscopic organism that is causing the infection. Cultures can be obtained from wounds on any part of the body. Soiled dressings are removed and replaced by a sterile dressing.

BANDAGES

Bandages are strips of soft, pliable materials used to wrap or cover a body part. When used correctly, bandages serve four basic purposes:
1. To hold dressings or splints in place
2. To immobilize or support body parts
3. To protect an injured body part
4. To apply pressure over an area

Bandaging materials should be clean, but not necessary sterile, because they should never come into direct contact with an open wound, as do dressings.

Bandaging Materials

There are several types of bandages prepared commercially.

Adhesive and elastic tape. Adhesive and elastic tape are supplied in rolls of various widths. When tape is used for a bandage, it is applied directly to the skin. When wrapping a body part with tape, be careful not to cut off circulation by wrapping too tightly. Elastoplast is an example of an elastic adhesive bandage.

Roller bandages. Roller bandages are available in various widths and materials. *Gauze,* a porous, light-weight, nonstretch material, has little absorbency, does not self-adhere, and does not conform readily to body contours. However, it is relatively inexpensive.

A preferred type of gauze bandage is the *elastic gauze bandage,* such as Kling. Kling conforms to all body contours, stretches, adheres to itself, and is absorbent; it does not slip with movement and therefore eliminates frequent rebandaging. It is nonocclusive, allowing for wound aeration; thus it does not interfere with wound healing.

Elastic bandages. Elastic bandages, made of women cotton with elastic fibers, are particularly useful for bandaging areas that require firm support, immobilization, or the application of pressure. Frequently used are the Ace bandage or the Peg bandage, which is self-adhering. Once wrapped around a body part, nonadhering elastic bandages are secured with bandage clips or tape. (See Figure 6-38, which illustrates the application of a Peg bandage).

Triangular bandages. Triangular bandages are large pieces of cloth, usually cotton, in the shape of a triangle. These bandages are usually used for slings on an injured arm, but can be adapted for use on almost any part of the body (Figure 6-36). A cravat bandage can be made by folding the point of a triangular bandage to the midpoint of the base and continuing to fold it lengthwise until the desired width is

Figure 6-36 **A,** *Triangular bandage;* **B,** *triangular bandage used for arm sling.*

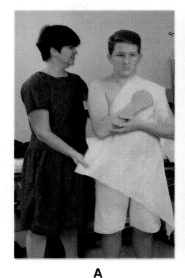
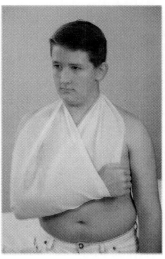

A   **B**

obtained (Figure 6-37). A cravat bandage can be used to hold a dressing in place, to help support an injured joint, to hold a splint in place, and if necessary, as a tourniquet.

Figure 6-37 **A to D,** *Cravat bandage.*

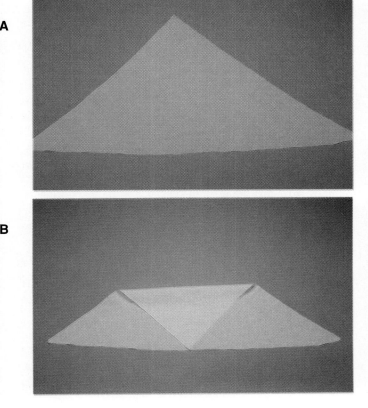

A

B

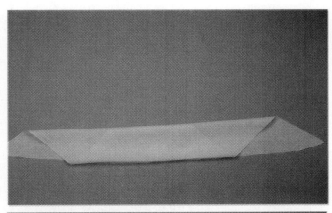
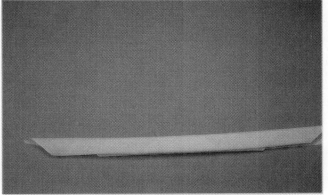

C

D

Tubegauz. Tubegauz, a seamless, tubular-knitted, cotton bandage, is adaptable and conformable to all body areas. Because Tubegauz is tubular, it stays in place with little or no adhesive tape. A finger or cage-type appliance is used to apply Tubegauz to provide a neat and strong bandage (see Figure 6-40 for instructions on applying Tubegauz bandages.)

Tubegauz is supplied in various sizes from $5/8$ inch to 7 inches. The size of the bandage to be used is determined by the size of the body part to which it will be applied (for example, a $5/8$ bandage can be used on small fingers and a toe of either infants or adults; 1-inch Tubegauz can be used on larger fingers and toes of adults and also on the hands and feet of infants; $1^{1}/_{2}$-inch Tubegauz may be used on the arms and legs of infants and on the arms and feet of children; $2^{5}/_{8}$ inches may be used on the arms and lower legs of adults or the legs and thighs of children; 3 $5/8$-inch Tubegauz may be used on the heads, arms, shoulders, legs, and thighs of adults and possibly on the trunks of infants; 5-inch Tubegauz is used on the heads and small trunks of adults, and the 7-inch Tubegauz can be used on the trunk of an adult).

Application of Bandages

Important criteria for acceptable bandaging techniques are that the bandage perform its function and that it not cause additional problems or pain. The following measures promote safety and comfort when applying bandages.

- Observe the principles and practices of medical asepsis when applying a bandage.
- Select a bandage of appropriate size for the area to be bandaged.
- Apply bandages to areas that are clean and dry. When an open wound is present, apply a bandage over a dressing.
- Do not have two skin surfaces touching each other under a bandage. Use absorbent material between touching skin surfaces (for example, when bandaging two fingers together, place a padding between them to prevent the skin from rubbing together). Other areas that need similar techniques include the axillary areas (an individual's perspiration provides a moist environment that is conducive to the growth of microorganisms), the areas under the breasts, areas in the groin or folds of the abdomen, and areas between the toes.
- Pad bony prominences and joints over which a bandage must be placed to prevent skin irritation, to provide comfort, and to maintain equal pressure on body parts.
- Apply bandages on a body part while in its normal functioning position and when placed in a resting position (1) so that deformities will not result, and (2) to avoid muscle strain. Joints should be slightly flexed rather than extended or hyperextended.
- Apply bandages with sufficient pressure to attain the intended function (that is, pressure, support, or immobilization), but do not apply the bandage too tightly because this interferes with circulation to the area. Ask the patient if the bandage feels comfortable.
- Wrap the bandage from the end of a limb toward the center of the body to avoid congestion and circulatory interferences in the distal part of the extremity.

- When possible, leave a small portion of an extremity such as a finger or toe exposed so that any change in circulation can be observed. Signs that indicate that the bandage is too tight include coldness and numbness to the part, pain, swelling, cyanosis, and pallor. If any of these signs occur, the bandage must be loosened immediately.
- Apply bandages so that they are secure and do not move about over the area, causing irritation or the need for rebandaging frequently.
- Apply chest bandages so that they do not interfere with breathing.
- Avoid unnecessary layers of bandages; too many layers are comfortable. Use only the amount of bandage material needed to accomplish its purpose.
- Place securing materials such as clips, pins, or knots well away from the wound or inflamed area and off pressure points and bony prominences to avoid undue pressure and irritation to the area.
- Check (or inform the patient to check) the bandage at regular intervals to note the circulation to the part and to see if the bandage needs to be reapplied (for example, when it has slipped out of place or loosened to the point at which it is no longer accomplishing its purpose). Also, it is very important to check bandages frequently on injuries or burns involving swelling to ensure that they are not becoming too tight.
- Replace bandages as required. Many bandages can be washed or autoclaved and then reused. Gauze should be discarded and replaced with clean gauze.

Basic wrapping techniques. There are five basic turns used alone or in combination when applying a roller bandage. The type of turn used depends on the purpose and the area being bandaged (Figure 6-38).

When beginning a wrap with a roller bandage, you may anchor it by placing the outer portion on a bias next to the patient's skin; the bandage is circled around the body part, allowing the corner edge to protrude; the protruding edge is then folded down over the first turn and covered with the second encircling turn of the bandage.

The circular turn encircles the part, with each layer of bandage overlapping the previous one. This turn is used most frequently for anchoring a bandage at the start and at the end and on body parts that are even in size such as the hand, fingers, toes, and circumference of the head.

The spiral turn is applied by angling the turns of the bandage in a spiral fashion with each turn overlapping the previous one by one-third to one-half the width of the bandage. This turn is used on body parts that increase in size where circular turns are difficult to make and on cylindric parts such as the forearm, fingers, legs, chest, and abdomen.

The figure-eight turn consists of diagonal turns that ascend and descend alternately around a part, making a figure eight. This turn is used over joint areas such as the wrist, ankle, elbow, or knee to support the joint, support a dressing, or to apply a pressure bandage.

Figure 6-38 *Bandage-wrapping techniques illustrating the circular, spiral, and figure-eight turns. The Peg Self-Adhering elastic bandage is used in these illustrations.*
Courtesy Becton-Dickinson, Division Becton, Dickenson and Co., Rutherford, N.J.

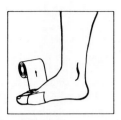

Foot and ankle Use 3-inch width. Hold foot at right angle to leg. Start bandage on ridge of foot just back of the toes.

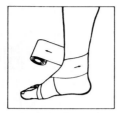

Pass bandage around foot from inside to outside. After two or three complete turns around foot, ascending toward the ankle on each turn, make a figure eight turn by bringing bandage up over

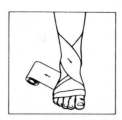

the arch—to the inside of the ankle—around the ankle—down over the arch—and under the foot

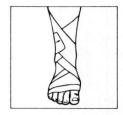

Repeat the figure eight wrapping two to three times. Fasten end by pressing the last 4 to 6 inches of unstretched bandage to the preceding layer.

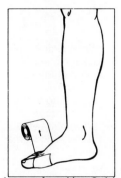

Lower leg: Use 3-4-inch width depending on the size of the leg. A leg wrap requires two rolls of bandage. Hold foot at right angle to leg. Start bandage on ridge of foot just back of the toes.

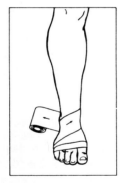

Pass bandage around foot from inside to outside. After two complete turns around foot, make a figure eight turn by bringing bandage up over the arch—to the inside of the ankle—around the ankle—

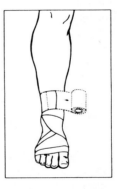

down over the arch—and under the foot. Start circular bandaging, making the first turn around the ankle. To begin the second roll of bandage, simply overlap the unstretched ends by 4 to 6 inches, press firmly, and continue wrapping.

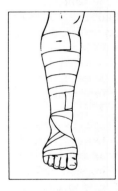

Wrap bandage in spiral turns to just below the kneecap. Fasten end by pressing the last 4 to 6 inches of unstretched bandage to the preceding layer.

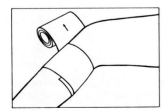

Knee Use 4-inch width. Bend knee slightly. Start with one complete circular turn around the leg just below the knee.

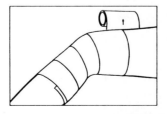

Start circular bandaging, applying only comfortable tension. Cover kneecap completely.

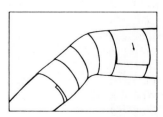

Continue wrapping to thigh just above the knee. Fasten end by pressing the last 4 to 6 inches of unstretched bandage to the preceding layer.

Figure 6-38—cont'd *Bandage-wrapping techniques illustrating the circular, spiral, and figure-eight turns.*

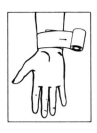 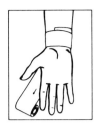 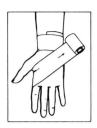 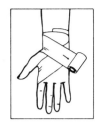 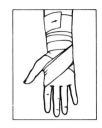

Wrist Use 2-or 3-inch width. Anchor bandage loosely at the wrist with one complete circular turn.

Carry the bandage across the back of the hand, through the web space between the thumb and index finger

and across palm to the wrist. Make a circular turn around the

wrist and once more carry the bandage through the web space and back to the wrist.

Start circular bandaging, ascending the wrist. Fasten end by pressing the last 4 to 6 inches of unstretched bandage to the preceding layer.

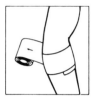 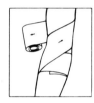 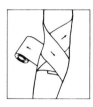 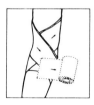 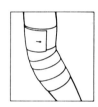

Elbow Use 3- or 4-inch width, depending on the size of the arm. Two rolls of bandage are required to complete the wrap. Start with a complete circular turn just below the elbow.

Wrap bandage in loose figure eights

to form a protective bridge across the front of the elbow joint.

Fasten end by pressing 4 to 6 inches of unstretched bandage to preceding layer. Start second bandage with a circular turn below the elbow

over the first wrap. Continue spiral bandaging over the elbow, ascending to the lower portion of the upper arm. Fasten end with a circular turn.

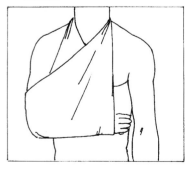 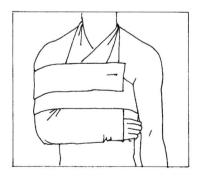 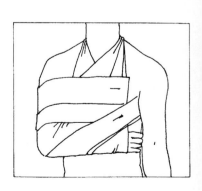

Shoulder A shoulder wrap is used to provide additional support for an arm in a sling. Use 4- or 6-inch width. One or two rolls of bandage may be used. Start under the free arm.

Carry the bandage across the back, over the arm in the sling, across the chest and back under the free arm in complete circular, overlapping turns. Fasten the end by pressing 4 to 6 inches of unstretched bandage to underlying bandage.

Additional support can be obtained with a second bandage. Start at the back just behind the flexed elbow in the sling. Carry the bandage under the elbow, up over the forearm, around the chest and back, and repeat. Fasten end.

Figure 6-38 illustrates the circular, spiral, and figure-eight turns, along with wrapping techniques for the Peg self-adhering, elastic bandage.

The *spiral-reverse turn* is a spiral turn in which reverses are made halfway through each turn; the bandage is directed downward and folded on itself, wrapped around the part so that, when it circles around, it is parallel to the lower edge of the previous turn. Each turn overlaps the previous one by two thirds the width of the bandage. Spiral-reverse turns allow for a neater fit because they take up the slack on the lower ends of the bandage applied to cone-shaped parts or parts that vary in width such as the leg, thigh, or forearm.

The *recurrent turn* is a series of back-and-forth turns anchored by circular or spiral turns. After the bandage has been anchored, it is folded at right angles and passed across and back over the center of the part. Each subsequent fold is slightly angled and overlaps the previous fold by two thirds the width of the bandage, first on one side and then on the other side of the centerfold. To finish the bandage, a circular turn is made around the part and secured with tape, clips, pins, or a knot. The recurrent turn is used to bandage the head, fingers, toes, or the stump of an amputated limb (Figure 6-39).

Application of Tubegauz bandages. When a Tubegauz bandage is applied, there is one basic method used for application to any body part being bandaged. Figure 6-40 illustrates areas where the Tubegauz may be applied, basic instructions for all Tubegauz applications, and a simple arm or leg bandage.

Figure 6-39 *Bandage wrapping technique: recurrent turn used for head bandage.*

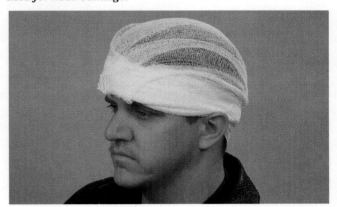

Figure 6-40 *Tubegauz bandage applications.*

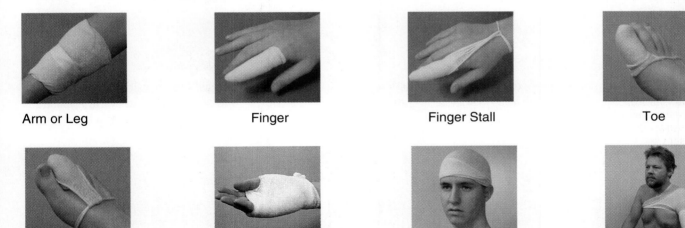

Arm or Leg · Finger · Finger Stall · Toe

Toe Splint · Palm of Hand · Head · Shoulder

TUBEGAUZ

Tubegauz is a seamless, tubular-knitted cotton bandage designed as an improved method of bandaging.
Tubegauz is:
- Quick and easy to apply
- Efficient and neatly conformable
- Produced from quality cotton yarns
- Adaptable to all body areas
- Economical to use
- Strong yet soft in texture

Figure 6-40—cont'd *Tubegauz bandage applications.*

BASIC INSTRUCTIONS FOR ALL TUBEGAUZ APPLICATIONS

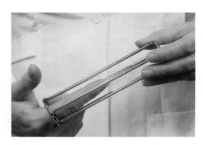

1 To apply any Tubegauz, first select a cage-type applicator that fits comfortably over the area to be bandaged.

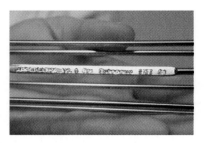

2 Next, select the size Tubegauz as printed on the cage-type applicator. For example, see Tubegauz size 01 for applicator No. 1.

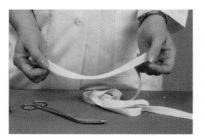

3 To load the Tubegauz onto the applicator, place the "channeled end" of the applicator of a flat surface and pull several feet of Tubegauz from the dispenser box.

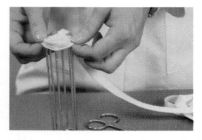

4 While spreading open the end of the tubular knit, slip the Tubegauz over the "smooth end" of the applicator.

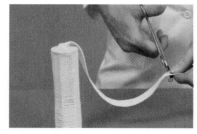

5 Complete loading by gathering sufficient Tubeqauz to complete the bandage, onto the applicator and cut off near the dispenser box opening.

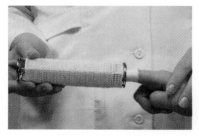

6 With the applicator loaded, pass the channeled end of the applicator over the limb to the middle of the dressing.

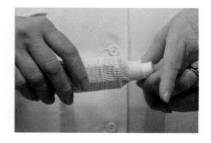

7 Pull the Tubegauz over the channeled end of the applicator, holding it lightly in place around the dressing.

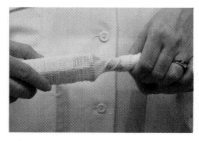

8 Continue to secure the dressing and Tubegauz end with one hand while slightly rotating clockwise to anchor as you withdraw the applicator over the limb.

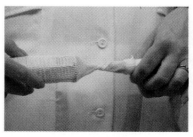

9 Withdraw the applicator several inches below the dressing or to the extremity, then rotate one full clockwise turn to anchor or close.

Figure 6-40—cont'd *Tubegauz bandage applications.*

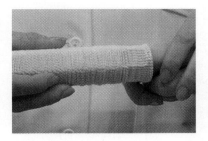

10 Move the applicator forward past the starting point and anchor with slight rotation several inches above the dressing.

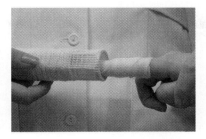

11 Continue this "back and forth" action until the desired layers of Tubegauz have been applied. Complete the last layer by stopping at the end of the bandage nearest the mesial plane.

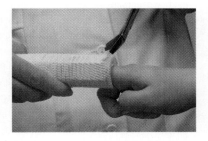

12 To finish, snip a small hole in the channeled rim, and continue cutting the Tubegauz from the applicator using the channeled rim as a cutting guide. If necessary, adhesive tape may be used to secure either end.

Remember....

Tubegauz is often applied over a sterile dressing that covers broken skin. Tubegauz is not sterile, but can be autoclaved on or off a metal applicator if desired.

Always load sufficient Tubegauz onto the applicator. It is difficult to complete a neat bandage when you have run out of Tubegauz in the middle of a procedure.

SIMPLE ARM OF LEG BANDAGE

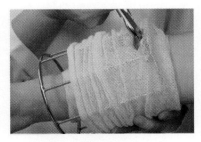

1 With applicator loaded as directed, bring the Tubegauz over the channeled end over sterile dressing.

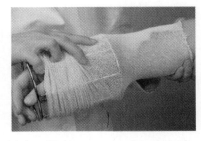

2 Hold the Tubegauz on the dressing with one hand and withdraw the applicator with the other hand letting the Tubegauz roll off the applicator to cover the desired area (usually just below the sterile dressing.)

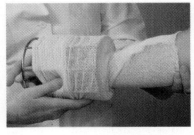

3 Rotate clockwise about 1/2 to 3/4 turn to anchor slightly and proceed in opposite direction to above dressing.

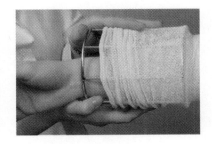

4 Rotate again in the same direction and return to base of bandage.

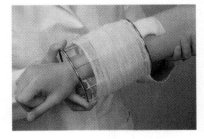

5 Cut Tubegauz off in channeled rim.

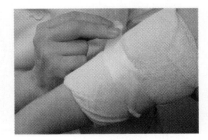

6 Secure with adhesive or slit and tie.

Adhesive tape may be applied at center of bandage by allowing a little more Tubegauz so that, after anchoring at base, the raw edge finishes in the center.

CASTS

Casts are a type of bandage made of either plaster-of-Paris or synthetic materials such as fiberglass, polyester, plastic, or other materials. The synthetic casts are stronger, lighter, and more resistant to water. However, they are more expensive and have a rough exterior. Casts are used to immobilize broken bones, injuries, joint disorders, or congenital disorders such as a dislocated hip or club foot. They are also used to protect the affected area and to reduce pain. Immobilization of a fractured bone holds bone fragments in place until healing takes place. Immobilization usually includes the joints immediately proximal and distal to the fractured bone. The healing time for a fracture depends on the type of fracture, the kind of bone affected, and the age of the person (see also Fractures in Unit Seventeen and Figure 17-13). A child's bones generally heal much faster than those of an adult. Patients with simple fractures are frequently treated in the physician's office or clinic. The patient with a cast can generally carry on with most activities of daily living without causing any further damage to the injured site. However, a plaster-of-Paris cast may restrict some activities because of its weight and inflexibility. If a cast is not applied correctly or cared for properly, it can *cause* physical injury. Patients must be provided with instructions on the proper care of a cast and on what signs to watch for that may indicate problems and/or complications. You may be required to assist the physician when a cast is applied or removed and to give the patient important information and instructions.

PLASTER OF PARIS CAST APPLICATION

Equipment

Plaster-of-Paris bandages (appropriate width)—Various widths from 5 to 20 cm or 2, 3, 4, and 6 inches.

Webril sheet wadding—A thick, nonabsorbent cotton web covered with starch to hold it together. Used as padding for casts. Available in widths of 5 inches by 6 yards.

Felt or sponge rubber pads—Used over bony prominences to protect them from pressure if needed.

Tubular stockinette (appropriate width)—A seamless rib knit material of natural color. It is available in widths of 3, 6, 10, and 12 inches or 5 to 45 cm; used as a lining or thin padding for the cast.

Bandage scissors

Rubber gloves and rubber or plastic protective apron for the physician

Cast knife—Used for trimming the ends of the cast that may be rough after the cast has hardened.

Bucket of water lined with a cloth or plastic to catch waste plaster. The water should be warm—70° to 75° F (21° to 24° C).

After x-ray films have been taken to determine the extent of the injury, the physician reduces the fracture (returns the bone fragments to their normal position) and then applies the cast.

PROCEDURE

1. Wash your hands and assist with the procedure as required. **Use appropriate personal protective equipment (PPE) as dictated by facility.**

2. Place sheet wadding over the affected area.

3. Place felt or sponge rubber over bony prominences.

4. Apply tubular stockinette over the padding. Apply it so that it extends over the edge to cover the round edges of the plaster.

5. When the physician is ready to apply the cast, you should:
   a. Place the bandage in the bucket of warm water for 5 seconds. Place only a few bandages in the water at a time.
   b. Carefully remove the bandage from the water. Hold it horizontally with an end in the palm of each hand and gently compress it to remove excess water (Figure 6-41). Remove it carefully so that none of the plaster is lost. *DO NOT* wring the cast material. Squeeze it at the ends, pushing toward the center.

RATIONALE

Sheet wadding helps to protect the skin.

This protects these areas from pressure.

The stockinette serves as a lining for the cast.

PLASTER OF PARIS CAST APPLICATION—cont'd

PROCEDURE

c. Quickly hand the bandage to the physician so that it can be applied before it begins to set (Figure 6-42).

d. Continue to prepare as many bandages as needed. At the end, you usually fold the excess stockinette and sheet wadding back over the cast and bind them down with a final roll of plaster (see No. 5 of this procedure). Use the knife to trim any sharp or rough edges.

e. When the procedure is completed, remove and discard the cloth or plastic liner from the bucket (Figure 6-43). Any waste plaster will have collected in the liner of the bucket. Discard it in the regular garbage can.

f. Discard water down sink. Check that there is no plaster in the water.

g. Attend to the patient's safety and comfort. Provide the patient with any further instructions if directed to do so by the physician. Explain that the cast will feel warm immediately after it is applied because the plaster was dipped in warm water to make it moldable to the limb. A chemical reaction between the plaster and water causes the cast to feel warm.

h. Clean the work area.

i. Wash your hands.

j. Do any recording required of you. The physician usually records this procedure, along with other recordings regarding the fracture and the patient's condition.

RATIONALE

Plaster bandages start to harden within 3 to 7 minutes.

Plaster in the water could clog the drain in the sink.

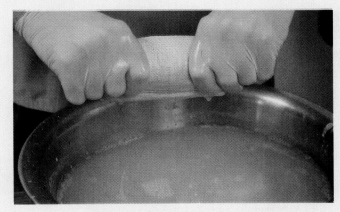

Figure 6-41 *Remove plaster bandage from the water; hold it horizontally, using both hands, and gently compress it to remove excess water. Quickly hand this to the physician so it can be applied before it dries.*

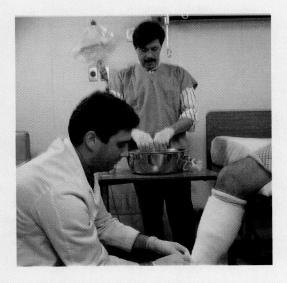

Figure 6-42 *Physician applying cast to patient's leg.*

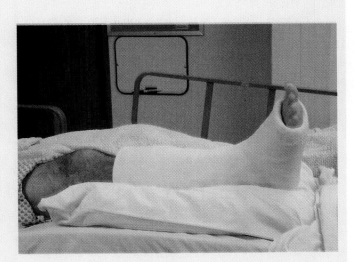

Figure 6-43 *Plaster-of-Paris cast on the leg.*

FIBERGLASS CAST APPLICATION

Equipment

Fiberglass bandages
Webril (sheet wadding)
Felt or sponge rubber pads
Tubular stockinette

Bandage scissors
Rubber gloves and rubber or plastic protective apron for the
  physician
Cast knife
Bucket and cold water

PROCEDURE

1. Follow steps 1 through 4 as outlined for application of a plaster cast.

2. When the physician is ready to apply the cast, you should:

   a. Place the bandage in a vertical position in the bucket of cold water. The water should be at least 1/4 inch above the bandage. Only a few bandages should be placed in the water at a time.
   b. Carefully remove the bandage from the water when the water stops "bubbling." Shake water out of the bandage.
   c. Continue to prepare and hand the physician as many bandages as needed.
   d. When all the bandages are applied, the physician rubs the bandages a number of times to make sure that all the bandages adhere and that the bandage is smooth. It is vital that the cast be set correctly to maintain the correct support and body alignment required for proper healing of the bone(s).

3. Attend to the patient as required.

4. Clean the work area and discard any waste.

RATIONALE

DO NOT squeeze water out of the bandage because fiberglass hardens very quickly and the physician needs enough time to apply the cast before it starts to harden.

NOTE: A fiberglass cast frequently dries within 1 hour. A fan or air gun may be used to hasten the drying process. NEVER use a heat blower or heat lamp to dry a fiberglass cast because the fiberglass material becomes hot and could burn the patient's skin under the cast material.

If a fiberglass cast becomes wet, it will swell. If swelling is excessive, it could compress tissue and cause problems. Therefore you must emphasize to the patient to keep the cast dry. You should also caution the patient against using a blow dryer on the cast (should it become wet) to prevent burning the skin beneath the cast.

CARE OF CASTS

Plaster casts dry on their own. Thin casts may dry completely in several hours. Thick casts dry completely in 2 to 3 days, releasing heat and moisture. During this time, casts must be handled with care. Instruct the patient to lift or move the cast with the palms of the hands, not the fingers, and to support the entire length of the cast on a pillow to reduce the chance of denting. A dent on the outside of the cast causes a bump on the inside, which causes pressure on the skin. It is best to lie still until the cast dries to prevent misshaping the new cast. Instruct the patient to avoid resting the cast on hard or sharp surfaces because dents can cause sores; to expose the cast to air to promote drying; to keep it uncovered, even at night, because it is still drying and needs air flow; and not to stand on a walking cast until it is completely dry. The cast is completely dry when it no longer feels damp or slightly soft to touch.

Ongoing Care: Instructions for the Patient

- Keep the cast dry. Cover it with a waterproof cover whenever you are going to come in contact with water or while bathing (Figure 6-44). Wrap plastic around the edges of the cast before you wash the surrounding skin. Plaster casts become soft and heavy when wet. Synthetic casts may cause skin softening if exposed to moisture frequently.
- Avoid excessive activity and hot rooms because heat causing perspiration can make the cast very uncomfortable.
- Whenever possible, elevate the limb in the cast to help prevent swelling.
- Avoid tight clothing that could restrict circulation.

Figure 6-44 *ShowerSafe waterproof cast and bandage cover. This is a durable, reusable, and pliable plastic covering used to keep casts, wounds, and bandages dry during showering or bathing. ShowerSafe reduces the risk of infection and preserves the integrity of a cast or bandage.* **A,** *Arm;* **B,** *elbow;* **C,** *knee; and* **D,** *foot and ankle.*
ShowerSafe cast and bandage protectors courtesy Trademark Corp., Fenton, Mo.

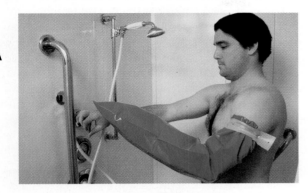

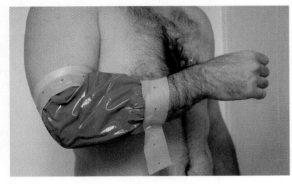

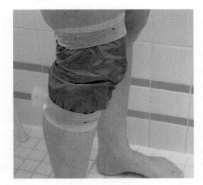

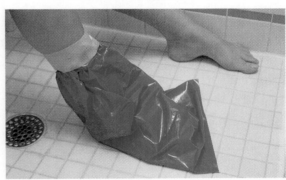

- Do not put anything down a cast such as a ruler or a knitting needle. An itching sensation under the cast is normal. If it persists or becomes troublesome, consult the physician.
- Do not cut or trim the cast. See the physician if it causes discomfort. You can use masking tape to cover sharp edges.
- Never use powders or creams under a cast. You may use rubbing alcohol on the skin around the cast to protect and toughen the skin.
- If you have a cast on the leg, keep a sock or knit cap over the toes to keep them warm.

Contact the physician immediately if you notice any of the following:
- Broken, cracked, soft, or loose places on the cast.
- Skin irritation caused by the cast rubbing the skin.
- Raw or red skin under the edges of the cast.
- A bad odor coming from the cast.
- The cast feels too tight.
- Prolonged swelling.
- Fingers or toes below the cast become numb, difficult to move, discolored, or cold. Casts are applied snugly but are fit to allow adequate circulation necessary for proper healing.
- General discomfort because of constant or severe pain.
- A burning sensation, especially over a bony prominence.
- Bleeding or a red-pink discoloration on the cast.

CAST REMOVAL

Before the cast is removed, more x-ray films are usually taken to be sure that the bones have healed sufficiently to allow safe removal. A special tool, the manual or electric plaster cutter, or cast cutter, is used to cut the cast. The blade of the cast cutter vibrates instead of spinning. It can only cut hard surfaces such as casts and not soft things, like the skin. The patient needs to be reassured that the cast cutter will not cut his or her skin. Some pressure or vibration and heat will be felt, but it will not be painful. The cast is bivalved (opened or split) at a site away from an incision line or surgical area. The padding and stockinette are cut off with scissors. The skin under the cast is usually dry and scaly. You can instruct the patient to wash the skin with a mild soap and water and to use skin lotion and/or bath oil to help it return to normal. There is usually some stiffness in the joints; thus the limb should be moved gently. Exercises are usually prescribed for the joint and the extremity. When a leg cast has been removed, elastic bandages may also be prescribed to help prevent dependent edema. Always remind patients to check with the physician if, at a later time, they have any questions or problems about the body part from which the cast was removed.

CONCLUSION

trict aseptic technique is needed at all times when handling sterile supplies and assisting with sterile or surgical procedures. Never be reluctant to admit a possible break in technique.

Be honest and admit contamination of sterile equipment, even if you are the only one who realizes that the equipment is not sterile. It is no disgrace to contaminate sterile equipment. The only disgrace is to use if after you know it is contaminated, because you would then subject the patient to the great danger of infection.

Learn the principles and practice the sterile techniques to be used when handling sterile supplies and equipment and when assisting with sterile procedures. Practice handing instruments so that the physician can grasp them in the way most convenient to use during a procedure. Be prepared to select and arrange the supplies and equipment required for the minor surgeries listed in this unit.

When ready to accurately demonstrate your skills, arrange with your instructor to take the performance test.

REVIEW OF VOCABULARY

The following is a sample of a minor surgery report using terms that have been defined for you. Read it and be able to define or explain the terms that are italicized.

OPERATIVE REPORT
DIAGNOSIS: Lipomas in right buttock and posterior thigh (Rt); large mole, right posterior thigh.
POSTOPERATIVE DIAGNOSIS: Same.
OPERATION: Excision of lipomas; *cauterization* of mole.
ANESTHESIA: Local infiltration—Lidocaine 1%
SURGEON: A. Joseph, MD
PROCEDURE: *Sterile field* and *setup* prepared. *Sterile gloves donned.* With the patient in a prone position, the usual *skin preparation* was performed, and then *sterile drapes* were applied. The *local anesthetic* was administered. The tumors were excised without any difficulty, and two *biopsy* specimens were sent to the laboratory for cytology studies. The tissues were approximated with *000 black silk.*
The *cautery* unit was then used to remove a questionable mole on the right posterior thigh.
Dry dressings were applied to the surgical sites.
POSTOPERATIVE STATUS: The patient left the office with minor complaints of discomfort in the surgical areas.
Patient to return in 1 week for removal of sutures and for follow-up care.
Andrew Joseph, MD

PATHOLOGY REPORTS
The following minor surgery pathology reports were received in a physician's office. After reading these, you should be able to discuss the contents of these reports with your instructor. Reference sources may be used to obtain definitions of terms with which you are not familiar.

Patient No. 1

CLINICAL DATA: 63-year-old black male with sebaceous cyst of the left axilla and skin tag of the right arm.
CLINICAL DIAGNOSIS: Epidermoid inclusion cyst, left axilla, and right arm skin tag.
MATERIAL FROM: Excision of the above.
GROSS DESCRIPTION: The specimen is received in formalin in two parts:
Part 1, labeled "left axilla," consists of a soft, round lesion with an opaque, glistening serosal surface, measuring $1.5 \times 1.3 \times 0.7$ cm. Sectioning reveals a cystic character of the lesion with brown, friable contents. Representative sections are submitted.
Part 2, labeled "right upper arm," consists of a brown piece of tissue covered with skin and measuring $0.7 \times 0.3 \times 0.2$ cm. Sectioning reveals a pale, pinkish tan, fibrous core. Representative sections are submitted.
MICROSCOPIC: Sections show features listed in the diagnosis.
DIAGNOSIS
1. Epidermal inclusion cyst (excision biopsy, left axilla).
2. Fibroepithelial skin tag with hyperkeratosis (excision biopsy, right upper arm).
J. D. Wynn, MD

Patient No. 2

CLINICAL DATA: 29-year-old white female with a recent onset of a right breast mass with nipple retraction.

CLINICAL DIAGNOSIS: Right breast mass.

MATERIAL FROM: Breast biopsy.

GROSS DESCRIPTION: Received fresh, labeled "breast mass," are two pieces of fibrofatty tissue measuring 1.8 × 1.3 × 1.3 cm and 1.7 × 1.7 × 0.6 cm, weighing 2.1 and 1 g, respectively. Serial sections reveal homogeneous fibrofatty tissue. The specimen is submitted in its entirety.

MICROSCOPIC: Sections show features listed in the diagnosis.

DIAGNOSIS: Focally acute and chronically inflamed breast tissue with fat necrosis and fibrosis; see note (right breast biopsy).

NOTE: The peripheral nature of this inflammatory process suggests that it may represent the wall of an abscess.

J.D. Wynn, MD

Patient No. 3

CLINICAL DATA: 34-year-old white female with a lump in the upper outer left breast.

CLINICAL DIAGNOSIS: Same as above.

MATERIAL FROM: Left breast biopsy.

GROSS DESCRIPTION: Received in formalin are three pieces of pale tan, firm, fibrous tissue with attached yellow fat measuring 2.2 × 1.4 × 0.5 cm, 1.1 × 1.0 × 0.3 cm, and 0.4 × 0.2 × 0.1 cm. Serial sectioning reveals similar homogenous, white, fibrous tissue. Representative sections are submitted.

MICROSCOPIC: Sections show features listed in the diagnosis.

DIAGNOSIS: Mammary dysplasia characterized by cyst, adenosis, and apocrine metaplasia (left breast biopsy).

J.D. Wynn, MD

CASE STUDY

Read the following explanation of local anesthesia and be able to differentiate among the various types. Define the underlined terminology.

Local infiltration is an *intracutaneous or subcutaneous* injection of an *anesthetic agent* into the tissues at the *incisional site* to block *peripheral nerve stimuli* at their origin. It may be used in suturing *superficial lacerations* or the *excision* of minor *lesions*.

Regional application is the injection of the anesthetic agent in or around a specific nerve or group of nerves to depress the entire *sensory nervous system* of a limited, *localized* area of the body. The injection is at a distance from the operative site. The anesthetized area is wider and deeper than simple local infiltration. An example includes *nerve block*, which is performed to interrupt sensory, motor, or *sympathetic transmission*.

Example: The patient was seen and treated with a series of three *epidural steroid injections*. The patient was experiencing lower back pain and left-sided *radicular* symptoms that responded well to this series of three injections. She reports that she did well until shortly after a *D&C* was performed. Presumably secondary to the stress of the *lithotomy* position, the patient noticed immediate lower *lumbar* pain.

I reviewed all the presently available *therapeutic* options, including: bed rest, *traction*, *NSAID*, oral *steroids*, *physical therapy*, *epidural* steroids, and surgery. The procedure of epidural steroids was discussed in detail, along with the attendant risks, including: back pain, *subdural puncture* and subsequent headache, infection, *epidural hematoma*, and nerve injury.

The patient was placed in the seated position. After sterile *prep and drape* in the usual fashion, 1% *Xylocaine* for *local anesthesia* with an *18-gauge Touhy needle* was used at the *L4-5 interspace*. After confirming proper placement of the needle through *negative aspiration of blood or CSE*, 80 mg. of *Depo-Medrol* diluted into a total volume of *10 cc.* with *preservative free normal saline* was slowly injected into the epidural space. The patient tolerated the procedure well.

REVIEW QUESTIONS

1. Having opened a sterile suture removal kit for use, the physician then decides not to remove the patient's sutures. What would you now do with these instruments?
2. When pouring a solution into a sterile container on a sterile field, you accidentally spill some of the solution on the sterile field. What would you do to remedy this contamination?
3. While directly assisting with a minor surgical procedure, you accidentally puncture your sterile glove with a needle. What should be your next actions?
4. Differentiate between a sterile field and a sterile setup.
5. When assisting with minor surgery, the physician asks for the thinnest black silk suture material. What size (number) would you provide?
6. Surgical asepsis is commonly referred to as sterile technique or surgical aseptic technique. Explain what is meant by these terms.
7. List 15 of the principles and practices of surgical aseptic (sterile) technique.
8. Why do you open envelope-wrapped sterile packages with the top flap going away from your body?
9. Before pouring a sterile solution for use, why do you first pour a small amount into a waste container?
10. List two reasons for wearing sterile gloves during a procedure.
11. Name and describe three methods used to administer a local anesthetic for a minor surgical procedure.
12. List the supplies and equipment that you would assemble and prepare when the physician is to:
    a. Incise and drain an abscess
    b. Remove sutures
    c. Repair a laceration by suturing
    d. Obtain an aspiration (needle) biopsy of breast tissue
    e. Remove a wart on the patient's left hand
    f. Insert an IUD
13. Describe how to prepare a patient for minor surgery.
14. State the purpose of an IUD.
15. List and explain four terms that describe the character of drainage from a wound.
16. Describe the five types of open wounds, and explain the healing process.
17. List eight purposes of dressings and four purposes of bandages.
18. List and explain the five basic turns used to apply roller bandages, indicating when each may be most appropriately used.
19. List and briefly describe four types of dressing materials and four types of bandage materials.
20. State the purpose of the casts.

PERFORMANCE TEST

In a skills laboratory, a simulation of a joblike environment, the medical assistant student will demonstrate skill and knowledge when performing the following activities without reference to source materials. Time limits for the performance of each procedure are to be assigned by the instructor (see also page 52).

1. Given a pair of sterile gloves, don them, avoiding contamination, and then remove.
2. Given the choice of a variety of sterile instruments and prepackaged instrument sets, select, identify by name, and prepare for use those that will be used for:
    a. Preparing the patient's skin for minor surgery
    b. Administering a local anesthetic
    c. Suturing a laceration
    d. Incision and drainage of an abscess or cyst
    e. Removal of a foreign body in subcutaneous tissue, a wart and a mole, and a tissue biopsy from the skin surface
    f. Cervical biopsy
    g. Aspiration (needle) biopsy of breast tissue
    h. Insertion of an IUD
    i. Vulvar biopsy
    j. Endocervical curettage
    k. Endometrial biopsy
    l. Cryosurgery
    m. Colposcopy
    n. A 6 mm skin biopsy
    o. Suture removal
    p. Dressing change with a wound culture
    q. Application of a plaster-of-Paris cast
3. Given a sterile hemostat, while gloved, hand it to the physician in the way most convenient for immediate use.
4. Demonstrate and proper procedures for:
    a. Preparing the skin for a minor surgical procedure
    b. Removing sutures
    c. Assisting with the application of a plaster-of-Paris cast
5. Demonstrate the proper procedure for changing a dressing and obtaining a wound culture.
6. Demonstrate the application of a roller, triangular, and Tubegauz bandage.
7. At the completion of the preceding activities, be able to discuss with the instructor at least ten of the principles of surgical aseptic technique, how to prepare a patient physically and mentally for minor surgery, and how to assist the physician during a minor surgical procedure.

The student must be able to perform the above activities with 100% accuracy 90% of the time. If the student contaminates any item during the performance of these skills, the correct actions to remedy the contaminated site must be employed 100% of the time.

Principles of Pharmacology and Drug Administration

COGNITIVE OBJECTIVES

On completion of Unit Seven, the medical assistant student should be able to:

1. Define and pronounce the terms listed in the vocabulary.
2. List and briefly describe the uses, sources, names, classification, and types of drugs.
3. Select and name official and other reference books on drugs.
4. Differentiate between a controlled substance, a prescription drug, and a nonprescription drug.
5. Define "prescription"; list and explain the seven parts of a prescription.
6. Differentiate between administering, dispensing, and prescribing medications.
7. Interpret abbreviations and symbols commonly used when administering medications.
8. State and discuss drug standards and the laws governing drug usage.
9. State and describe the various types of pharmaceutical preparations.
10. Explain how drugs should be stored, handled, and labeled.
11. List examples of drugs that may be kept on an emergency tray.
12. List additional supplies that should be kept near the emergency tray for emergency situations.
13. List eight signs and symptoms of hypoxemia.
14. Describe the difference between an oxygen mask and a nasal cannula. Discuss how each should be placed on a patient when oxygen is to be administered.
15. State the usual amount of oxygen administered through an oxygen mask and through a nasal cannula.
16. State and discuss the legal requirements for controlled substances inventory and the prescriber's record.
17. List 12 routes by which medication may be administered, briefly describing each.
18. List at least 15 rules for administering medications and 15 specific rules for administering injections.

19. Calculate the correct dosage of a medication to be administered.
20. List the five rights for preparing and administering medications. State a sixth right that has been added by many medical authorities.
21. State the correct size needle and syringe for intramuscular and subcutaneous injections; list factors that influence these choices.
22. List at least eight factors that influence drug dosage and action.
23. Discuss aspects of patient education when drug therapy is initiated.
24. State six reasons why medication is administered by an injection.
25. List six to eight dangers involved when giving injections and the sites that are to be avoided.
26. List anatomic sites for administering an intramuscular injection, a subcutaneous injection, and an intradermal injection.
27. Describe how drugs are placed into a syringe from a vial, from an ampule, and from a prefilled sterile cartridge-needle unit.
28. Explain how the skin is prepared before an injection is administered.
29. Explain why the skin disinfectant should be allowed to dry before you give an injection.
30. Explain why it is recommended that the needle be inserted and removed quickly and the medication be injected slowly when giving an injection.
31. Discuss eight guidelines suggested for use to prevent needlesticks.
32. List four sites used for administering an insulin injection.
33. Discuss the concepts of rotating injection sites for insulin injections.
34. State four factors that influence the absorption of insulin.
35. State at least 10 points to consider for the administration of insulin.
36. Explain what to do with a syringe and needle after use.
37. List three reasons for the administration of solutions by an intradermal injection.

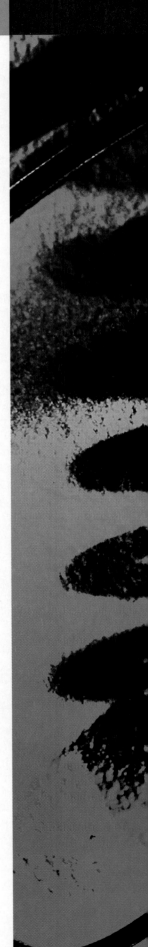

TERMINAL PERFORMANCE OBJECTIVES

On completion of Unit Seven, the medical assistant student should be able to:

1. Given medication orders, interpret these, and calculate the dosage of the drug to be administered.
2. Given a medication order, prepare and administer safely and efficiently a subcutaneous and an intramuscular injection using (a) a sterile disposable syringe and needle of the correct sizes, and (b) a reusable injector (for example, Tubex injector) with a prefilled sterile cartridge-needle unit.
3. Given a medication order, prepare and administer safely and efficiently an intramuscular injection using the Z-Track technique.
4. Demonstrate how to identify the correct sites for administering a subcutaneous and an intramuscular injection by palpating definite anatomic landmarks.
5. Demonstrate how to fill a syringe with a medication from a vial; from an ampule.
6. Demonstrate how to reconstitute a powdered drug for administration by injection.
7. Demonstrate how to administer insulin using the correct insulin syringe for the insulin preparation available.
8. Demonstrate how to place an oxygen mask and a nasal cannula on a patient for the administration of oxygen.
9. Given the PDR or other reference pharmacology book, obtain information on a variety of drugs.

The student is to perform these objectives with 100% accuracy.

The consistent use of universal precautions is required by all health care professionals in all health care settings as a method of infection control. It is assumed that these precautions are used in all of the following procedures. Review Unit One if you have any questions on methods to use as the methods/techniques will not be repeated in detail in each procedure presented in the unit.

Be sure to consult the latest guidelines issued by the Centers for Disease Control and Prevention and consult with infection control practitioners when needed to identify specific precautions that pertain to your particular work situation.

Of the many duties of a medical assistant, none is more important than administering medications responsibly. As a member of a professional team involved with the medical care of the public, the medical assistant must seek all possible knowledge of a drug—its use or abuse, correct dosage, methods and routes of administration, symptoms of overdose, and abnormal reactions that may occur when it is administered—before administering them to a patient. Although it is beyond the scope of this book to include a detailed presentation of pharmacology, general concepts, basic information on drugs, and procedures for the correct methods of administration are discussed. Reference sources for more detailed information on drugs are cited.

PHARMACOLOGY AND DRUGS

Pharmacon is Greek for drugs. Pharmacology is the science that deals with the study of drugs—their origin, properties, uses, and actions. Drugs are any medicinal substances or mixtures of substances that are used for therapeutic, prophylactic, or diagnostic purposes. Drugs are either medicinal, therefore therapeutic, or poisonous, depending on dosage and use. The therapeutic use of drugs includes the application of these substances to treat or cure a disease or condition, to relieve undesirable symptoms such as pain, and to provide substances that the body is not producing or not producing in sufficient amounts (for example, insulin, used for diabetes mellitus, and thyroid extract, used for hypothyroidism). Prophylactically, drugs are used to prevent diseases such as vaccinations given to prevent communicable diseases. Drugs can also help a physician diagnose an illness, as seen when a contrast medium is given to a patient in a diagnostic x-ray film procedure, or when antigens are used to detect skin allergies in a patient.

Pharmacology has undergone tremendous changes during the past few decades and continues to be dynamic. Through constant study and research, new drugs arrive on the market, and some old ones are withdrawn, either because newer ones are more effective, or because complications arising from the use of the older drugs prove to be too hazardous to the patient's health.

Drugs are derived from four main sources:

1. Plant sources—Obtained from plant parts or products. Seeds, stem, roots, leaves, resin, and other parts yield these drugs; examples include digitalis and opium.
2. Animal sources—Glandular products from animals such as insulin and thyroid.
3. Mineral sources—Some drugs are prepared from minerals (for example, potassium chloride and lithium carbonate [an antipsychotic]).
4. Synthetic sources—Laboratories duplicate natural processes. Frequently side effects can be eliminated and potency of the drug increased (for example, barbiturates, sulfonamides, and aspirin).

DRUG NAME: BRAND (TRADE), GENERIC, AND CHEMICAL

A typical drug may be known by as many as three names, as follows:

1. A brand or trade (proprietary) name
2. The generic name
3. The chemical name

When a drug is developed and marketed, it is assigned a specific name that is patented by the pharmaceutical company that has manufactured it. This is called the *trade* or *brand name* of the drug and is the exclusive property of the manufacturer. After a patent has expired (drug patents run 17 years), other companies may manufacture and sell the drug either under different brand names or under the drug's

VOCABULARY

Addiction (ah-dik′ shun)—An acquired physiologic and/or psychologic dependence on a drug with tendencies to increase its use.

AMA—American Medical Association.

Adulteration (ah-dul′ ter-a′ shun), adulterated—The addition of an impure, cheap, or unnecessary ingredient to a substance to cheapen, cheat, or falsify the preparation.

Anaphylactic (an″ah-fi-lak′ tuk) shock—An intense state of shock brought on by hypersensitivity to a drug, foreign toxin, or protein. Early symptoms resemble an allergic reaction; they increase in severity rapidly to dyspnea, cyanosis, and shock. It can be fatal if emergency measures are not taken immediately (see also First Aid for Allergic Reactions to Drugs in Unit Seventeen).

BNDD—Bureau of Narcotics and Dangerous Drugs (a federal government agency of the DEA).

Broad-spectrum—Adjective describing the ability of an agent to be effective against a wide range of microorganisms (for example, a broad-spectrum antibiotic such as tetracycline).

Chemotherapy (ke″mo-ther′ ah-pe)—The use of drugs (chemicals) to treat disease; a type of therapy used for cancer patients in which powerful drugs are used to interfere with the reproduction of the fast-multiplying cancer cells.

Contraindication (kon′tra-in″di-ka′shun)—Condition in which the use of certain drugs or treatments should be withheld or limited.

Crude drug—An unrefined drug.

Cumulative action of a drug—A drug accumulates in the body; it is eliminated more slowly than it is absorbed.

DEA—Drug Enforcement Administration. This is the federal law enforcement agency charged with the responsibility of combating drug diversion.

Dilute—To weaken the strength of a substance by adding something else.

Drug idiosyncrasy (id″e-o-sing′krah-se)—An unusual or abnormal response or susceptibility to a drug that is peculiar to the individual.

Drug tolerance—The decreased susceptibility to the effects of a drug after continued use. An increased dosage would be required to produce the desired effects because the initial dose is ineffective.

Cross-tolerance—Cross-tolerance can develop when tolerance to one drug increases the body's tolerance to drugs in the same category (for example, a tolerance to one depressant drug leads to a tolerance of other depressant drugs).

FDA—Food and Drug Administration (a federal government agency).

Habituation—Emotional dependence on a drug due to repeated use, but without tendencies to increase the amount of the drug.

HHS—Health and Human Services (a federal government agency).

Parenteral (pah-ren′ter-al)—Not through or in the digestive tract, e.g., intramuscular, subcutaneous, intravenous, or intradermal injection

Parenteral dosage—A drug given by injection; administering a drug by a route that bypasses the digestive tract.

PDR—Physician's Desk Reference, a book on drugs.

Placebo (plah-se′bo)—An inactive substance resembling and given in place of a medication for its psychologic effects to satisfy the patient's need for the drug; it hopefully will produce the same effect as the real medication through psychologic means. A placebo may be used experimentally.

Prophylaxis (pro″fi-lak′sis)—Prevention of disease.

Pure drug—A refined drug; one that has been processed to remove all impurities.

Side effect—A response in addition to that for which the drug was used, especially an undesirable result.

Untoward effect—An undesirable side effect.

Stock supply—A large supply of medications kept in the physician's office or pharmacy.

Toxicity (tok-sis′ i-te)—The nature of exerting harmful effects on a tissue or organism. The level at which a drug becomes toxic to the body. Minor or major damage may result.

Unit-dose—A system that supplies prepackaged, premeasured, prelabeled, individual portions of a medication for patient use.

USP-NF—*United States Pharmacopeia-National Formulary*, a drug book listing all official drugs authorized for use in the United States.

Generic Name	Brand or Trade Name	Pharmaceutical Company
hydrocodone bitartrate	Vicodin	Knoll
diazepam	Valium	Roche
naproxen	Naprosyn	Syntex

generic name. These exact copies of the original drug are often called generic drugs. Each drug has an official or non-proprietary name, which is also called the *generic name*. This name is often descriptive of the chemical composition or class of the drug and is assigned to the drug in the early stages of its development for general recognition purposes. Thus every drug has a generic name. Generic names are established by the U.S. Adopted Name Council (USAN). Except in the case of older drugs, the generic (USAN) name is identical to the USP (United State Pharmacopeia) or NF (National Formulary) name. A generic drug may be manufactured by any number of companies and placed on the market under a different brand or trade name. Examples follow. Brand names are prominently used in advertising a drug to the medical profession, although the generic name must appear in advertising and labeling in letters at least half as big as that of the brand name.

When prescribing a drug, the physician may use either the generic or the trade name. Currently the trend is to write more prescriptions using the generic name, if one is marketed (many trade names are still under patent protection and are not available from other manufacturers by the generic name), because it is generally less expensive for the patient to purchase. Sometimes the physician orders a specific trade name; but most states now have laws that state that the patient is entitled to ask the pharmacist for the medication under its generic name unless the physician has specifically directed otherwise, either orally or in handwriting. Also, the pharmacist filling the prescription order for a drug product prescribed by its trade or brand name may select another drug product of the same generic drug type (that is, the generic or chemical name of the drug that is considered to be therapeutically equivalent or "bioequivalent") unless the physician has specifically directed otherwise either orally or in handwriting, and only when the drug product selected costs the patient less than the prescribed drug product. Since both trade- and generic-named drugs represent the same chemical formula and must heed the same FDA standards, they can be used interchangeably according to most state laws. When the substitution is made, the use of the cost-saving drug product dispensed must be communicated to the patient, and the name of the dispensed drug product must be indicated on the prescription label, except when the pre-scriber orders otherwise.

The third name a drug may be assigned is the *chemical name*. This represents the drug's exact formula (that is, the chemical makeup or molecular structure). Generally this name is used only by the manufacturer and on occasion by the pharmacy when compounding a drug because for the chemical name of most drugs is long and complex.

REFERENCES AND OFFICIAL BOOKS ON DRUGS

Established standards and up-to-date information on drugs are published in various books; some of the more common ones follow.

United States Pharmacopeia (USP)-National Formulary (NF)

Once two individual books, the USP and NF are now published as a single volume. The National Formulary was acquired by the U.S. Pharmacopeial Convention, Inc., in 1975 and now publishes the USP-NF approximately every 5 years. This is an authoritative book establishing the standards for drugs. Only "official" drugs are listed in this book. All drugs sold under the name listed in the USP-NF must legally conform to the standards set forth. Detailed information on the description of drugs, standards for purity, strength and composition, storage, use, and dosage are given. Drugs that meet the standards set by the *Pharmacopeia* bear the initials USP on their labels. Some drugs listed in the USP section of the book are cross-referenced to the NF chapter. The NF chapter of the book deals primarily with the pharmaceutical ingredients of the drugs.

AMA Drug Evaluations

This book is published annually by the American Medical Association (AMA). New drugs that are not yet listed in the USP but that have been evaluated by the Council on Drugs of the AMA are presented.

Physician's Desk Reference (PDR)

Although not official, the PDR is a common reference book used by most medical personnel. It is published annually by Medical Economics, Inc., and is automatically distributed free of charge to medical offices, agencies, and hospitals. The *PDR* has seven sections that list the following:

1. Names, addresses, emergency telephone numbers, and a partial list of products available from the manufactur-ers who have provided information for the *PDR*
2. Products by brand name in alphabetic order
3. Products according to an appropriate drug category or classification
4. Products under generic or chemical name headings
5. Products shown in color and actual size under company headings
6. An alphabetic arrangement by manufacturer of over 2500 products; each is described as to composition, use and action, administration and dosage, precautions, contraindications, side effects, form in which each is supplied, and the common names and generic compositions or chemical names
7. An alphabetic arrangement by manufacturer of diagnostic products with descriptions for use
8. Name, address, and telephone numbers of Certified Poison Control Centers.
9. Key to Controlled Substances Categories
10. Information on Vaccine Adverse Event Reporting System

Supplements that provide new or revised product information developed after the *PDR* was published for the current year are published and distributed as necessary.

American Hospital Formulary Service (AHFS)

This book is published by the American Hospital Formulary Service. Subscribed to by all hospital pharmacists, it contains extensive, unbiased drug information kept current by periodic supplements. The *AHFS* arranges drugs into therapeutic or pharmacologic classes according to official (generic) names.

Medical assistants should be familiar with these publications and always keep one or more up-to-date copies in the physician's office as a reference source, for both the physician and themselves.

DRUG STANDARDS AND LAWS GOVERNING USE

When physicians or other qualified medical practitioners prescribe, administer, or dispense drugs, including narcotics, they must comply with federal and state laws that regulate such transactions. Comprehensive laws have been passed by the U.S. Congress and individual state legislatures to regulate the manufacture, sale, possession, administration, dispensing, and prescribing of a range of drugs.

To assist physicians in complying with the legal obligations required of them, medical assistants should know and understand the laws regulating drugs and narcotics in the state in which they are employed, because individual states may supplement federal legislation with their own laws.

All drugs available for legal use are controlled by the Federal Food, Drug and Cosmetic Act of 1938. This act contains detailed regulations to ensure the purity, strength, and composition of food, drugs, and cosmetics. The general purpose of this act, which is based on interstate commerce, is to control movement of impure and adulterated food and drugs. Amended periodically, the Federal Food, Drug and Cosmetic Act is enforced by the Food and Drug Administration (FDA), a department within the Department of Health and Human Services (HHS), formerly the Department of Health, Education and Welfare (HEW). There are also other federal and differing state laws that regulate the development, sale, and use of drugs.

LEGAL CLASSIFICATION OF DRUGS
Controlled Substances

Drugs having the potential for addiction and abuse, including narcotics, stimulants, and depressants, are termed controlled substances. Control of these drugs at all levels of manufacturing, distribution, and use is mandatory. Federal legislation that outlines these controls is the Controlled Substances Act of 1970 (the Comprehensive Drug Abuse Prevention and Control Act), which became effective May 1, 1971 and supersedes the Harrison Narcotic Act of 1914. This act is enforced by the Drug Enforcement Administration (DEA) in the U.S. Department of Justice. It is designed to improve the administration and regulation of the manufacturing, distribution, and dispensing of controlled substances by providing a "closed" system for legitimate handlers of these drugs. Such a closed system should help reduce the widespread diversion of these substances out of legitimate channels into the illicit market. Under this act, drugs that are under federal control are classified into one of five schedules. Each schedule (Schedule I through Schedule V) reflects decreasing levels of addiction and abuse potential, with Schedule I being the classification with highest potential for drug addiction and abuse. Complete listings of the drugs in each schedule are available from district DEA offices. Only a few examples are included here. All controlled substances listed in the *PDR* are indicated by the symbol C, with the Roman numeral II, III, IV, or V printed inside the C to designate the schedule in which the substance is classified.

- Schedule I—These drugs, having the highest potential for addiction and abuse, have not been accepted for medical use in the United States. Their use is limited to research purposes only after the research facility has obtained government approval and agreement to research protocol to test drugs for medical indications. Examples are heroin, marijuana, LSD, and mescaline.
- Schedule II—These drugs have a high potential for abuse and addiction, but are acceptable for medical use for treatment in the United States. Examples are amobarbital, amphetamine, cocaine, codeine, meperidine, methadone, methamphetamine, morphine, opium, and secobarbital.
- Schedule III—These drugs have less potential for abuse than the drugs in Schedules I or II and have a moderate or low addiction potential. They are acceptable for medical use for treatment in the United States. Examples are APC with codeine, butabarbital, methyprylon, nalorphine, and paregoric. Anabolic steroids became a Schedule III controlled substance in 1991. These drugs are synthetic preparations of the male hormone, testosterone. They have been used by some for a muscle-building effect.
- Schedule IV—These drugs have a lower potential for abuse and a more limited addiction liability than those in Schedule III. They are acceptable for medical use for treatment in the United States. Examples are chloral hydrate, diazepam, meprobamate, paraldehyde, and phenobarbital.
- Schedule V—These drugs have a low potential for abuse and a limited addiction liability relative to drugs in Schedule IV. They are acceptable for medical use for treatment in the United States. Examples are drugs of primarily low-strength codeine (less than those compounds included in Schedule III) combined with other medicinal ingredients, as well as preparations containing limited quantities of certain narcotic drugs generally used for antitussive (to suppress coughing) and antidiarrheal purposes.

For a complete listing of all the controlled substances, contact any office of the DEA.

Under federal law, every practitioner who administers, dispenses, or prescribes a controlled substance (with the exception of interns, residents, law enforcement officials, and civil defense personnel who meet special conditions outlined in the Federal Code of Regulations) must be registered with the Drug Enforcement Administration. Medical practitioners must also have a valid license to practice medicine in their chosen state. The practitioner's office location from which controlled substances are handled must be registered, and the certificate of registration must be kept at this location and available for official inspection. Applications for this registration can be obtained from any DEA regional office or from the DEA Section, PO Box 28083, Central Station, Washington, DC 20005. Registration must be renewed every 3 years.

Only DEA-registered practitioners can order and purchase controlled substances. Schedule II substances must be ordered with the Federal Triplicate Order Form (DEA0222). For example, the physician must fill out a Triplicate Order Form to obtain Demerol from the normal source of supply. Orders for Schedules III, IV, and V substances require only the practitioner's DEA registration number. In some states, when ordering Schedule II substances from out-of-state companies, a copy of the purchase agreement (*not* the Federal Triplicate Order Form) must be sent within 24 hours of placing the order to the office of the state attorney general.

Physicians who discontinue practice must return their Registration Certificate and any unused order forms to the nearest DEA office. It is suggested that the word "VOID" be written across the face of the order form before it is sent to the DEA. Physicians having controlled substances in their possession when they discontinue their practice should obtain information from the nearest field office of the DEA and from the responsible state agency on how to dispose of these drugs.

Some important duties of the medical assistant are to ensure that the physician is *currently* registered with the DEA, to obtain the correct federal forms for ordering and purchasing controlled substances, and to keep appropriate records of all transactions. Failure of the physician to comply with the laws regulating the use of controlled substances and other drugs can lead to considerable civil and criminal liability, in addition to the loss of the right to dispense or prescribe medications.

Prescription Drugs

These are drugs that may be obtained only when prescribed, administered, or dispensed by practitioners licensed by state law to prescribe drugs. The Federal Food, Drug and Cosmetic Act requires that these drugs bear on the label the legend "*Caution: Federal Law prohibits dispensing without prescription.*" Examples include digoxin and penicillin.

Nonprescription Drugs

Drugs easily accessible to the general public fall into this category. They are frequently referred to as "over-the-counter" (OTC) drugs because they can be obtained without a prescription (for example, vitamin tablets and aspirin).

CLASSIFICATION OF DRUGS

Drugs are classified in various ways, including the following:
- Drugs that have a principal action on the body (for example, analgesics and antidiarrheals)
- Drugs used to treat or prevent specific diseases or conditions (for example, hormones and vaccines)
- Drugs that act on specific organs or body systems (for example, cardiovascular drugs and gastrointestinal drugs)
- Forms of drug preparations (for example, solids or liquids)

You should be aware that frequently one drug may be used to treat different conditions either because it has multiple effects in addition to its primary effects or because it can affect different body systems by exerting its primary effect. For example, a broad-spectrum antibiotic can be used to treat various types of infectious processes, or a diuretic may be used to exert an effect on the cardiovascular system or on the urinary system.

Table 7-1 is a classification of drugs on the basis of their primary actions or effects on the body.

Table 7-2 lists 50 of the most frequently used prescription drugs.

PRESCRIPTIONS

A prescription is an order written by a licensed physician giving instructions to a pharmacist to supply a certain patient with a particular drug of specific quantity, prepared according to the physician's directions. It is a *legal document*. A prescription consists of the following seven parts (Figure 7-1):

1. Date, patient's name, and address (for children, age should be given)
2. Superscription, consisting of the symbol **R**, from the Latin *recipe*, meaning "take thou"
3. Inscription, specifying the ingredients and the quantities; the name of the drug, the dosage form, and the amount per dose

Text continues on page 256.

Figure 7-1 *Sample of a prescription.*

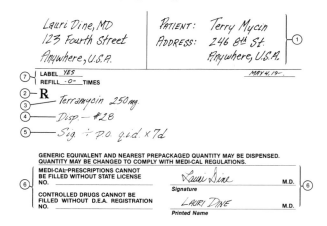

TABLE 7-1

Classification of Drugs Based on Actions or Effects on Body

Drug	Action	Examples
Amphetamine	Acts as stimulant on central nervous system: has temporary effect of increasing energy and mental alertness; sometimes used to depress the appetite	Amphetamine (Benzedrine), dextroamphetamine (Dexedrine)
Analgesic	Relieves pain	Aspirin, Empirin Compound with codeine, codeine, acetaminophen (Tylenol), phenacetin
Anesthetic	Produces generalized or local loss of feeling	Thiopental sodium (Pentothal Sodium), tetracaine hydrochloride (Pontocaine Hydrochloride), lidocaine hydrochloride (Xylocaine Hydrochloride)
Angiotensin-converting enzyme inhibitors	Used for hypertension	Capoten, Vasotec
Antacid	Counteracts acidity in stomach	Sodium bicarbonate, Maalox, Mylanta
Anthelminthics	Destructive to worms	Piperazine, mebendazole, Povan, mebendazole (Vermox)
Antianginal	Dilates coronary arteries or increases blood flow through collateral coronary vessels	Nitroglycerin (Nitrostat), isosorbide (Isordil), amyl nitrite, and drugs listed under calcium channel blockers and beta-adrenergic receptor antagonists
Antiarrythmic	Prevents harmful atrial and ventricular rhythms	Amiodarone hydrochloride (Cordarone), procainamide hydrochloride (Pronestyl), quinidine
Antibiotic	Inhibits growth and reproduction of or eliminates pathogenic bacterial microorganisms	Penicillin, ampicillin, tetracycline
Antidiabetic agents	Used to treat type I diabetes, insulin-dependent diabetes	Regular Insulin (Humulin R, Novolin R), Semilente Insulin, NPH Insulin, Lente Insulin, Ultralente Insulin
Antidiarrheal	Counteracts diarrhea	Lomotil, Kaopectate, codeine, paregoric, Imodium, tincture of opium
Anticoagulant	Inhibits blood-clotting mechanism	Heparin sodium, dicumarol warfarin sodium (Coumadin)
Anticonvulsant	Inhibits convulsions, as in epilepsy. Prevents or reduces the frequency or severity of seizures related to idiopathic epilepsy, as well as seizures secondary to drug reactions, hypoglycemia, eclampsia, alcohol withdrawal, or traumatic brain injury	Phenytoin (Dilantin), bromides, ethotoin, phenobarbital, primidone, trimethadione
Antidepressant	Relieves depression; often called mood elevator or modifier	*Tricyclic antidepressants*: Imipramine (Tofranil), Amitriptyline (Elavil), doxepin (Sinequan), desipramine (Norpramin) *Monoamine oxidase inhibitors (MAO)*: phenelzine sulfate (Nardil), tranylcypromine sulfate (Parnate) *Antimanic agents*: Lithium (Eskalith) *Miscellaneous*: Fluoxetine hydrochloride (Prozac)

Table 7-1—cont'd

Classifications of Drugs Based on Actions or Effects on Body

Drug	Action	Examples
Antidote	Neutralizes or acts as an antagonist to a poison or drug overdose	Lorfan, naloxone (Narcan) (narcotic antagonists)
Antiemetic	Counteracts nausea and vomiting	Dimenhydrinate (Dramamine), prochlorperazine (Compazine), triethobenzamide (Tigan)
Antifungal	Destroys or checks the growth of fungi; controls *Candida (Monilia)* infections in vagina	Mycostatin, nystatin
Antihistamine	Counteracts effect of histamine in the body; given to relieve symptoms of allergic reactions such as hay fever and also to relieve symptoms of common cold	Diphenhydramine (Benadryl), promethazine (Phenergan), chlorpheniramine (Chlortrimeton)
Antihypertensive (also referred to as hypotensive)	Reduces high blood pressure	Reserpine (Serpasil), guanethidine (Ismelin), hydrochlorothiazide (Esidrix)
Antiinflammatory agent	Reduces or relieves inflammation	*Nonsteroidal agents:* Indomethacin (Indocin), aspirin, naproxen (Naprosyn), piroxicam (Feldene) *Steroids:* triamcinolone (Kenacort), triamcinolone acetonide (kenalog), prednisone
Antiarthritic preparation	Acts against arthritic symptoms	Indomethacin (Indocin), phenylbutazone (Butazolidin), prednisone, piroxicam, naproxen
Antiseptic Skin antiseptic	Inhibits growth of microorganisms Urinary antiseptic to be taken internally	70% alcohol Nitrofurantoin (Macrodantin), nalidixic acid (NegGram)
Antineoplastic	Inhibits growth and spread of malignant cells	Chrlorambucil (Leukeran), busulfan (Myleran), melphalan (Alkeran), fluorouracil or 5-FU (Adrucil), megestrol acetate (Megace), tamoxifen citrate (Tamofen)
Antitussive	Inhibits cough reflex	Codeine, Benylin cough syrup, Benadryl, Sucrets Cough Control Lozenge
Astringent	Constricts tissue and arrests discharges or bleeding	Silver nitrate, alum, zinc oxide
Beta-adrenergic blockers	Used to treat angina, hypertension, cardiac arrhythmias, myocardial infarctions. Act as a shield against excessive stimulation to the sympathetic nerve endings in the heart tissue. Slow down the heartbeat besides making the heart less responsive to stimulations. Thus the heart performs more work with less oxygen demand and pain can be prevented	Inderal, Corgard, Lopressor, Tenormin, Visken (dieresis)
Bronchodilator	Causes dilation of bronchi, eases breathing	Aminophylline, Bronkotabs, isoproterenol (Isuprel), epinephrine (Adrenalin)
Calcium channel blockers	Used for hypertension, angina, and tachycardia	Diltiazem (Cardizem), nifedipine, nicardipine, verapamil (Isoptin)

Table 7-1—cont'd

Classifications of Drugs Based on Actions or Effects on Body

Drug	Action	Examples
Cardiogenic (heart stimulator)	Strengthens heart muscle action	Digoxin (Lanoxin)
Cathartic	Relieves constipation and promotes defecation; often classified according to the increased intensity of their action as laxatives, purgatives, and drastic purgatives	Cascara, mineral oil, castor oil, bisacodyl (Dulcolax)
Contraceptive	Prevents or diminishes likelihood of conception	Enovid, Ortho-Novum, Ovulen, Nordette, Norplant (an implant)
Cytotoxins	Toxic to certain cells. Used for treatment of cancer	*Cytoxan*, 6-mercaptopurine
Decongestant	Relieves swelling and congestion in upper respiratory tract	Actifed (combination decongestant and antihistamine); pseudoephedrine (Sudafed), phenylephrine (Neo-Synephrine)
Diuretic	Increases urinary output	Chlorothiazide (Diuril), furosemide (Lasix)
Emetic	Stimulates vomiting	Ipecac syrup
Estrogens	Used as oral contraceptives (see above); used in replacement therapy for conditions resulting from estrogen deficiency; also used to treat certain breast carcinomas and prostate cancer and some breast cancer in men	Estradiol (Estrace), conjugated estrogens (Premarin), estrone (Theelin and Femogen), ethinyl estradiol (Estinyl and Feminone)
Expectorant	Liquefies mucus in bronchi and aids in the expectoration of sputum, mucus, or phlegm	Terpin hydrate, potassium iodide, quaifenesen (Robitussin)
Hemostatic	Arrests flow of blood by helping coagulation	Vitamin K, thrombin
Hormone	Endocrine system produces hormones and secretes them directly into bloodstream; commercial preparations are available for patients whose own glands are malfunctioning	Cortisone, insulin, thyroxin
Hypnotic	Produces sleep	Glutethimide (Doriden), chloral hydrate
Immunosuppressive	Prevent rejection of transplanted organ	cyclosporine (Sandimmune), azathisprine (Imuran)
Laxative	Promotes movement of bowels	Mineral oil, senna (Senokot)
Miotic	Contracts pupils of eye	Pilacar ophthalmic solutions
Muscle relaxant	Relaxes muscles	Diazepam (Valium), carisoprodol (Soma) compound
Mydriatic	Dilates pupils of eye	Phenylephrine (neo-Synephrine) solution, atropine sulfate ointment
Narcotic	Produces sound sleep, stupor, and relief of pain	Drugs derived from opium; morphine, codeine; meperidine (Demerol) (a synthetic narcotic); Percodan, and Dilaudid (semisynthetics)
Psychedelic	Produces feelings of relaxation, freedom from anxiety, highly creative thought patterns, and perceptual changes; causes hallucinations, alters mental functions; highly controversial, potentially very dangerous, and used only under controlled supervision for experimental purposes	LSD, mescaline

Table 7-1—cont'd

Classifications of Drugs Based on Actions or Effects on Body

Drug	Action	Examples
Sedative	Quiets and relaxes patient without producing sleep	Phenobarbital
Stimulant	Increases activity of an organ or body system	Caffeine, amphetamine (Benzedrine)
Styptic	Checks bleeding by means of astringent quality	Styptic pencil
Sulfa preparations	Antibacterial	Sulfisoxazole (Gantrisin), Bactrim, Septra
Tranquilizers (also called ataractics)	Calms or quiets patients who are anxious or disturbed without causing drowsiness that a sedative would produce or the stimulation that antidepressants produce	*Antianxiety (anxiolytic)—minor tranquilizers* *Benzodiazepines* Librium, diazepam (Valium), Ativan, Serax, Halcion, Xanax, Dalmane *Nonbenzodiazepines* meprobamate (Equanil and Miltown) *Antipsychotic (neuroleptic)—major tranquilizers:* *Phenothiazines* chlorpromazine (Thorazine), Mellaril, prochlorperazine (Compazine), Haldol, Navane, Stelazine, Trilafon
Vaccine	Prevents infectious diseases	Salk polio vaccine, tetanus and typhoid vaccines, measles, mumps, and hepatitis B vaccines
Vasoconstrictor	Constricts blood vessels to increase force of heartbeat, relieve nasal congestion, raise blood pressure, or stop superficial hemorrhage	Epinephrine (Adrenalin), norepinephrine (Levophed), ephedrine sulfate
Vasaodilator	Dilates blood vessels and reduces blood pressure	Nitroglycerin, reserpine (Serpasil), amyl nitrite, nimodipine (Nimotop), Persantine
Vitamins	Organic substances found in foods that are necessary for body to grow and maintain health; commercial preparations of all these vitamins are available	Fat-soluble vitamins: A, D, E, K Water-soluble vitamins: B, C

4. Subscription, directing the pharmacist how to compound the drug(s). It generally designates the number of doses to be dispensed.
5. Signa (Sig), from Latin, meaning "mark," which gives instructions to the patient indicating when and how to take the drug and in what quantities
6. Physician's signature, address and phone number, registry number (this is the physician's license number), and, when prescribing controlled substances, the BNDD number (this is the same as the DEA number)
7. Number of times, if any, that the prescription may be refilled

Some state regulations require that the prescription form have a statement indicating that a generic equivalent may be dispensed. If this is not acceptable, the physician must write out "No substitutions" *or* "dispense as written" *or* initial a box that states "Do not substitute" or "Dispense as written." The pharmacist puts the name of the drug dispensed on the label of the container.

Current prescription writing has been greatly simplified, as pharmaceutical companies now prepare most drugs ready for administration. These preparations have largely eliminated the need for the pharmacist to compound or mix drugs and solutions.

When the physician writes a prescription, he or she gives it to the patient to take to a pharmacist, who dispenses the required medication. Once the prescription has been filled, the pharmacist must keep a record of that sale for 2 years (3 years in four states).

These records are subject to inspection and copying at any time by authorized employees of state and federal law enforcement and regulatory agencies. When a prescription is written for a Schedule II controlled substance (narcotic), a few states require the physician to use an official triplicate prescription blank. Where this is the case, one copy is kept for the physician's office files, and the original and other copy are given to the patient to take to the pharmacist. After filling the prescription, the pharmacist retains the original

TABLE 7-2

Top 50 Prescription Drugs

Rank	Drug	Classification
1	Amoxil*	Antibiotic
2	Premarin Oral	Hormone
3	Zantac	Antiulcer-histamine H_2 antagonist
4	Lanoxin	Cardiogenic (heart stimulator)
5	Xanax	Antianxiety - Benzodiazepine
6	Synthroid	Hormone
7	Ceclor	Antibiotic
8	Vasotec	Angiotens in converting enzyme inhibitor
9	Seldane	Antihistamine
10	Procardia XL	Calcium channel blocker
11	Tenormin	Beta-adrenergic blocker
12	Naprosyn	Antiarthritic preparation
13	Dyazide	Diuretic
14	Capoten	Angiotens in converting enzyme inhibitor
15	Tagamet	Antiulcer-Histamine H_2 antagonist
16	Calan SR	Calcium channel blocker
17	Cardizem	Calcium channel blocker
18	Augmentin	Antibiotic
19	Prozac	Antidepressant
20	Proventil Aerosol	Bronchodilator
21	Mevacor	Antihyperlipidemic (lowers cholesterol)
22	Ortho-Novum 7/7/7-28	Hormone
23	Lopressor	Beta-adrenergic blocker
24	Dilantin	Anticonvulsant
25	Ventolin Aerosol	Bronchodilator
26	Micronase	Antidiabetic
27	Cipro	Antibiotic
28	Provera	Hormone
29	Lasix Oral	Diuretic
30	Voltaren	Antiarthritic preparation
31	Trimox*	Antibiotic
32	Darvocet-N 100	Analgesic
33	Amoxicillin Trihydrate*	Antibiotic
34	Humulin N	Hormone (insulin)
35	Theo-Dur	Bronchodilator
36	Tylenol/Codeine	Analgesic
37	Coumadin Sodium	Anticoagulant
38	Halcion	Hypnotic
39	Lopid	Antihyperlipidemic (lowers cholesterol)
40	Triphasil-28	Hormone
41	Ibuprofen	Antiarthritic preparation
42	Cardizem SR	Calcium channel blocker
43	DiaBeta	Antidiabetic
44	Glucotrol	Antidiabetic
45	Feldene	Antiarthritic preparation
46	Polymox	Antibiotic
47	Hismanal	Antihistamine
48	Zestril	Angiotensin converting enzyme inhibitor
49	Pepcid	Antiulcer, Histamine H_2 antagonist
50	Duricef	Antibiotic

All are amoxicillin but manufactured by different companies.

and endorses the copy, which is forwarded to the Department of Justice at the end of the month in which the prescription was filled.

All prescriptions written for controlled substances in Schedule II must be wholly written in ink or indelible pencil or typewritten, and they must be signed by hand by the physician. A separate prescription blank must be used for each controlled substance ordered. These prescriptions must contain the following information:

- Name and address of the patient
- Date of prescription
- Name and quantity of controlled substance prescribed
- Directions for use
- Physician's DEA registration number (the BNDD number)
- Signature and address of physician

Prescriptions for controlled substances in Schedule II cannot be refilled, and some states require that they be filled within 7 days from the date written.

In a bonafide emergency, the physician may telephone a prescription order to a pharmacist for a Schedule II controlled substance. In these cases, the prescribed drug must be limited to the amount required to treat the patient during the emergency period. Within 72 hours the physician must furnish a written, signed prescription order to the pharmacy for the controlled substance prescribed. Pharmacies are required by law to notify the DEA if they have not received the written prescription order within the 72 hours. ("Emergency" means that the drug must be administered immediately for treatment, that there is no alternative treatment available, and that it is not possible for the physician to provide a written prescription form for the drug at that time.)

Prescriptions for controlled substances in Schedules III, IV, and V are written on the physician's standard prescription blank and need only to be signed by the prescriber. These prescriptions are limited to five refills within a 6-month period with proper authorization. A prescription for any controlled substance must be issued for a legitimate medical purpose by physicians acting in good faith in the course of their professional practice. Keep in mind that regulations for prescribing and dispensing controlled substances differ for each of the five schedules and may also be subject to stricter controls passed by many states. Therefore it is vital for you to learn what laws apply for your state.

Prescription pads should be kept in a safe place where they cannot be picked up easily by patients. Minimize the number of pads in use at one time. Use them only for writing prescriptions; *do not* use them for notes or memos. A drug abuser could easily erase the note and use the blank to forge a prescription. The DEA and the local police department are to be contacted if your office experiences any theft or loss of controlled substances or official order forms. Contact a local police department if you are aware of forged prescriptions.

Although medical assistants do not write prescriptions, a knowledge of prescription abbreviations and terms used is valuable and may be required to carry out the physician's orders, transcribe medical notes, take telephone messages,

answer questions for a patient regarding a prescription, verify information for a pharmacist, and understand instructions for the administration of medications. Table 7-3 is a list of the more common abbreviations and symbols used.

In addition to knowing prescription abbreviations, it is helpful for you to be familiar with general medical abbreviations. Table 7-4 includes some of the more common abbreviations. They are grouped together according to general usage. You should pay special attention to when capital letters are used and when they are not used. (A more detailed listing of these abbreviations can be found in Unit Three, pages 66 to 69.)

ADMINISTER, DISPENSE, PRESCRIBE

In the physician's office, medications may be handled in one of three ways: they may be administered, dispensed, or prescribed. A medication is administered when it is actually given to the patient to take by mouth or when it is injected, inserted, or given by any other method used for administering medications. It is dispensed when it is given to a patient by the physician or pharmacist at the pharmacy to be taken at a later time. It is prescribed when the physician gives the patient a written order, the prescription, to have filled by the pharmacist. Only the physician is licensed to prescribe medications. Depending on state law, various medical personnel may administer medications, and the physician and pharmacist dispense them. On occasion, under the physician's order and supervision, the medical assistant may also dispense stock medications to a patient in the physician's office or health agency.

PHARMACEUTICAL PREPARATIONS

Because of the various properties and uses of different drugs, there are different ways in which they are prepared for patient use. Drugs are supplies in either a solid or liquid state.

PROFESSIONAL RESPONSIBILITIES
STORAGE AND HANDLING OF DRUGS

If a physician keeps medications in the office, certain rules and precautions should be followed. Ideally, all medications should be stored in a separate room in a locked cabinet, and all *must* be kept in their original containers. Many medications must be stored in dark containers or dark areas or refrigerated. Some *must* also be in glass containers, because the chemical composition of the drug may react with plastic. Drugs that must be refrigerated are labeled as such. Because drugs deteriorate, it is necessary to have a review schedule so that outdated drugs can be discarded and replaced with a new supply. When discarding outdated, opened drugs, pour liquids down the sink; crush drugs that are in the solid form and flush them down the sink. You should also use this method if you have taken a drug out of its original container and then are unable to use it, since it is *never* to be replaced in the container once removed. This method of disposal of medications

TABLE 7-3

Common Prescription Abbreviations and Symbols*

Abbreviation or Symbol	Meaning	Abbreviation or Symbol	Meaning	Abbreviation or Symbol	Meaning
ā	before	L	liter	qam	every morning
āā	of each	liq	liquid	qd	every day
ac	before meals	m or min	minim	qh	every hour
ad lib	as desired	mcg	microgram	q2h or q2°	every 2 hours
amt	amount	mEq	millequivalent	(q3h or q3° and	every 3 hours
aq	aqueous	mEq/L	milliequivalents	so on)	
bid	twice a day		per liter	qhs	every night
c̄	with	mg	milligram	qid	four times a day
cap(s)	capsule(s)	ml	milliliter	qod	every other day
cc	cubic centimeter	mm	millimeter	qs	quantity sufficient
dil	dilute	npo (NPO)	nothing by mouth	℞	take thou
Dx or Diag	diagnosis	NS	normal saline	s̄	without
D/C or d/c	discontinue	noc(t)	night	sc or subq or	Subcutaneous
D/W	dextrose in water	od	daily or once a	SubQ	
dr	dram		day	Sig	directions
ʒ	dram	OD	right eye	sol	solution
ʒ₁	one dram	oint	ointment	ss or s̄s̄	one half
d	day	OS	left eye	subling	sublingual (under
Dr	doctor	OU	both eyes		the tongue)
fl or fld	fluid	oz	ounce	stat	immediately
gal	gallon	ʒ	ounce	S/W	saline in water
gm	gram	p̄	after, past	tid	three times a day
gr	grain	per	by or with	tinc or tr or	tincture
gt or gtt	drop(s)	pc	after meals	tinct	
H or hr	hour	po (or per os)	by mouth	tab	tablet
hs	hour of sleep or	prn	whenever neces	tsp	teaspoon
	bedtime		sary	Tbsp	tablespoon
IM	intramuscular	pt	pint (or patient)	ung or ungt	ointment
IU	international units	pulv	powder	U	units
IV	intravenous	q	every	wt	weight
kg	kilogram				

*According to the style of the American Medical Association, medical and pharmaceutical abbreviations are to be written without the use of periods. For example, rather than writing b.i.d. as was done in the past, you will now write.

eliminates the possible chance of drug abuse (that is, taking medications out of garbage containers and administering the drug to themselves or dispensing it to others). For unopened drug containers, consult pharmaceutical distributors for possible exchange policy. If no policy exists, dispose of unopened drugs in the same fashion as opened drugs.

To avoid medication errors, keep drugs for external use well separated from those to be used internally. Store disinfectants, cleansing preparations, and all drugs that are poisonous if taken internally in a location well separated from the other drugs. To facilitate easy access to the drugs, organize the central storage area. You may organize the drugs alphabetically or according to drug substance or classification (for

example, antibiotics, contraceptives, diuretics, hormones, vaccines). It is also recommended to label storage areas as external use only and internal use. You can further label areas such as drugs to be used for oral administration and those for parenteral administration.

In addition, federal law requires that all controlled substances be kept in a substantially constructed, separate, securely locked cabinet or safe. Some states require that these drugs be kept in a locked cupboard in a locked room. Extra security precautions must also be taken for the needles and syringes that are used for administering parenteral medications. Any loss or theft of controlled substances must be reported by the physician on discovery to the local police

VOCABULARY

Solid state (Figure 7-2)

Pills—Small, hard, molded objects of medication, either oval or round.

Tablets—Dried, powdered medications compressed into a round or disk-shaped object. Some are scored across the middle so that they can easily be broken in half.

Caplets—Tablets shaped like capsules with a special coating to make them easy to swallow. Like tablets, they are said to be virtually tamper proof.

Capsules—Liquid or powdered medications enclosed in a rod-shaped gelatin container.

Spansules—Granules of medication enclosed in a capsule that is prepared so that the medication will be released at various times after being ingested; a sustained-release capsule such as Dexamyl or Contac.

Powders—Medications or mixtures of medications ground into a powder.

Lozenges (also called troche [tro'ke])—A small, round, oval or oblong tablet that releases a drug while dissolving in the mouth. The lozenge contains a drug incorporated in a flavored, sweetened base made of sugar and mucilage or a fruit base.

Skin patch (transdermal patch)—An adhesive disK impregnated with a medication that is absorbed through the skin into the bloodstream over a period of time.

Thin, silicone-rubber capsules or rods (subdermal implants)—A thin capsule or rod of medication that is implanted under the skin. These are used for a slow release of a medication over an extended period of time.

Suppositories—Molded cone-shaped mixtures of medication dispersed in a firm base such as cocoa butter that dissolves and is absorbed when inserted into a body cavity such as the rectum or vagina.

Liquid State

Solutions—Liquid preparations consisting of one or more substances (solutes) that are dissolved or suspended in a substance (the solvent). The most frequently used solvents are distilled water, sterile water, normal saline, and alcohol. Solutes may be (1) a 100% full-strength or pure drug in a solid, liquid, or powder form; (2) tablets of a known specific amount of drug; or (3) stock solutions that are strong solutions of known strength used to prepare a weaker solution. To obtain a *true solution*, the solute must be completely dissolved in the solvent. If the solute is evenly dispersed throughout the solution but not dissolved, it is called a *suspension* or a *colloidal solution*. The difference between a true solution and a colloidal solution is determined by the molecular size of the particles of the solute; the colloidal solution contains very small particles. Drugs that are supplied in a suspension *must* be shaken before being administered; the label bears the instruction, "Shake well."

Diluent—A solution that is added to another to reduce the strength of the initial solution or mixture. Percentages or ratios are used to describe solutions. For example, a 15% solution means that 15 parts of the solute are mixed with 85 parts of the solvent. Some solutions come prepared for immediate use; others have to be mixed before they are suitable for use. When a solution must be prepared for use, it may be necessary to convert the apothecary system of weights and measures to the metric equivalents. Tables 7-7 and 7-8 on page 269 contain equivalents for these two systems and the preparation of solutions. Some solutions may be administered by injection, mouth, inhalation, irrigation, or lavage; others may be used topically on the skin, on dressings, or for cleansing purposes.

Emulsion—An oily substance suspended in a liquid with which it does not mix or in which it does not dissolve, such as fat globules in water with an emulsifying agent (for example, various ointments, Petrogalar (a laxative), and homogenized milk).

Tincture—An alcohol solution prepared from drugs or chemicals such as tincture of iodine, tincture of merthiolate, or tincture of Zephiran (benzalkonium).

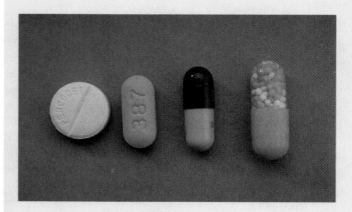

Figure 7-2 *Solid forms of drugs.*

Lotions—Aqueous preparations containing suspended particles used for local applications intended for soothing (for example, calamine lotion or Caladryl lotion).

Elixirs—Solutions containing water, alcohol, and sugar used frequently as flavoring agents or solvents (for example, terpin hydrate elixir or phenobarbital elixir).

Liniment—A liquid or soft mixture of drugs with soap, alcohol, oil, or water used for external application by rubbing it into the skin (for example, camphor liniment, or chloroform liniment).

Ointment—A mixture of drugs with a fatty substance used for external application (for example, A & D ointment, zinc oxide ointment, and various antibiotic ointments).

Aerosol—A suspension of a drug that is administered in a fine mist or spray. It can be inhaled for treatment of respiratory conditions; others are sprayed on topically. Examples include Alevaire, Bronkosol, and Mucomyst.

Spray—See aerosol.

Syrup—A thick, concentrated solution of a sugar in water or a watery liquid. A syrup can be used as a flavored vehicle for a medication.

Adrenalin (epinephrine)—A vasoconstrictor and antispasmodic; used to counteract anaphylactic shock, to relieve symptoms of allergic reactions, and as an emergency heart stimulant.

Albuter—A bronchodilator; an inhalant used to ease breathing, as for asthmatic patients.

Benadryl—An antihistamine; used to relieve symptoms of allergic reactions, itching, and anaphylactic shock.

Compazine—An antiemetic; used to counteract nausea and vomiting.

Dextrose 50%—Used for severe hypoglycemia.

Digoxin—A cardiac glycoside; used for congestive heart failure and certain cardiac arrhythmias.

Ipecac—An emetic; used to stimulate vomiting in some poisoning cases.

Lasix—A diuretic; used to promote the formation and excretion of urine.

Narcan—A narcotic antagonist; used in emergency situations for narcotic overdose.

Nitroglycerin—A vasodilator, used commonly for angina patients.

Pitocin—A hypothalmic hormone; stimulates uterine contractions to control postpartum bleeding in obstetric patients.

Steroids such as hydrocortisone, Solu-Cortef, or Solu-Medrol—Used for their antiinflammatory action.

Valium—A muscular relaxant and an antianxiety, minor tranquilizer; used to relax muscles or calm and quiet extremely anxious patients.

NOTE: Valium must be kept in a locked drawer or cabinet.

department and to the DEA field office in the area. The field office will provide information on what reports are required of the physician.

EMERGENCY TRAY

Keep a special container or tray with drugs needed for emergencies in a readily accessible location. Also keep sterile syringes, needles, alcohol sponges, diluents, and a tourniquet in this container. In most offices and clinics, the physician makes a checklist of the drugs and supplies to be kept in the emergency tray, varying with the need of the office and the physician's preference. You should be familiar with these specific drugs, knowing the use, usual dosage, and method of administration for each. Check this container or tray frequently to replace items that have been used and to discard outdated drugs or sterile supplies.

Listed in the box are examples of drugs that *may* be kept on the emergency tray. These vary according to the type of patient and possible emergency that you may encounter at your facility.

Additional supplies that may be kept near this tray for emergency situations include the following:
- Airway equipment (Ambu bag, laryngoscopes and airways of different sizes, and resuscitation masks of various sizes to fit adults, children and infants)
- Defibrillator
- Electrocardiogram machine
- Intubation equipment and other related materials
- Oxygen tank, mask, and/or nasal cannula with tubing
- IV sets
- Intravenous solutions (bottles or bags)
- Suction equipment

You should check the above equipment daily to make sure that it is in proper working order and to ascertain that there is sufficient oxygen in the tank.

LABELING

All drugs and solutions must be clearly labeled. Poisons should be clearly labeled as such and kept separate from other medications. Leave all drugs and solutions in the original labeled containers until they are administered or dispensed. Never use, but rather discard, medications or substances that are not clearly labeled or those in unlabeled containers. When pouring liquids from bottles, hold the bottle so that the label is facing the palm of your hand. Using this technique prevents soiling or obliterating the label if any of the liquid runs down the side of the bottle (see also page 265 and Figure 7-5, *A*). If a label becomes loose, soiled, or torn, type a new label with the exact information that was provided on the original. It is advisable to have someone else in the office check the new label for accuracy before you affix it to the container.

TABLE 7-4

Medical Abbreviatons

Body systems
HEENT—head, eyes, ears, nose, and throat
ENT—ear, nose, and throat
CR—cardiorespiratory
CVS—cardiovascular system
GI—gastrointestinal
GU—genitourinary
CNS—central nervous system
MS—musculoskeletal
NM—neuromuscular

Patient's history
CC—chief complaint
PI *or* HIP—present illness or history of present illness
PH—past history
LMD—local medical doctor
UCHD *or* UCD—usual childhood diseases
FH—family history
a & w *or* A & W—alive and well
ROS—review of systems
PTA—prior to admission
c/o—complains of

Physical examination (PE)
wd—well-developed
wn—well-nourished
IPPA—inspection, percussion, palpation, and auscultation
P & A—percussion and auscultation
BP—blood pressure
TPR—temperature, pulse, and respirations
WNL—within normal limits
wt—weight
ht—height

Diagnosis
Diag or DX—diagnosis
R/O—rule out
POS—problem-oriented system

Ears
TM—tympanic membrane(s)

Eyes
REM—rapid eye movements
L & A—light and accommodation
PERLA—pupils equal and reacting to light and accommodation
EOM—extraocular movements
RRE—round, regular, and equal
OS—left eye
OD—right eye
OU—both eyes

Chest (heart and lungs)
P & A—percussion and auscultation
PND—paroxysmal nocturnal dyspnea
SOB—shortness of breath
PMI—point of maximal intensity (or impulse)

MCL—midclavicular line
ICS—intercostal space
NSR—normal sinus rhythm
RSR—regular sinus rhythm
ASHD—arteriosclerotic heart disease
MI—myocardial infarction
EKG *or* ECG—electrocardiogram
AV—arteriovenous, atrioventricular
CHF—congestive heart failure
RHD—rheumatic heart disease
URI—upper respiratory infection
COPD—chronic obstructive pulmonary disease
CHD—coronary heart disease

Abdomen and GI
LKS—liver, kidney, spleen *or* LKKS—liver, kidneys, and spleen
GB—gallbladder
BM—bowel movement

Female reproductive system
BUS—Bartholin, urethral, and Skene glands
LMP—last menstrual period
OB—obstetrics
PID—pelvic inflammatory disease
GYN—gynecology
EDC—expected date of confinement
FHT—fetal heart tones
L & D—labor and delivery
PP—postpartum
IUD—intrauterine device
SAB—spontaneous abortion (miscarriage)

Musculoskeletal system
EMG—electromyogram
MS—multiple sclerosis
LOM—loss of movement or motion
cva—costovertebral angle
DTR—deep tendon reflexes
Fx—fracture
ROM—range of motion

Central nervous system
CSF—cerebrospinal fluid
CVA—cerebrovascular accident
EEG—electroencephalogram
DTR—deep tendon reflexes

Laboratory
CBC—complete blood count
UA—urinalysis
O_2—oxygen
CO_2—carbon dioxide
CSF—cerebrospinal fluid
SMA—sequential multiple analysis
HGB *or* HG *or* HB—hemoglobin
Hct—hematocrit

Table 7-4—cont'd

Medical Abbreviatons

WBC—white blood count
RBC—red blood count
Diff—differential (blood count)
Protime or PT—prothrombin time
pH—hydrogen ion concentration, referring to the degree
    of acidity or alkalinity of a solution
BUN—blood urea nitrogen
Sedrate—sedimentation rate
Rh—Rhesus blood factor
PKU—phenylketonuria
FBS—fasting blood sugar
PBI—protein-bound iodine
PCV—packed cell volume
RhA—rheumatoid arthritis
STS—serologic test for syphilis
VDRL—Venereal Disease Research Laboratory
C & S—culture and sensitivity
CPK—creatine phosphokinase
LDH—lactic dehydrogenase

X-ray film studies
A-P and Lat-anterior, posterior, and lateral
IVP—intravenous pyelogram
GBS—gallbladder series
CT—computed tomography
MRI—magnetic resonance imaging
BE—barium enema
KUB—kidneys, ureter, bladder
UGI—upper gastrointestinal series

Surgical terms
T & A—tonsillectomy and adenoidectomy
D & C—dilation and curettage
I & D—incision and drainage
TUR—transurethral resection
TURP—transurethral resection of the prostate

Hospital departments
ICU—intensive care unit
CCU—coronary care unit
ER—emergency room
OR—operating room
RR or PAR—recovery room or postanesthetic room
Lab—laboratory
Path—pathology
OPD—outpatient department
Peds—pediatrics
RT—respiratory therapy

General
Ca or CA—cancer or carcinoma
d/c or D/C—discontinue
DOA—dead on arrival
OD—overdose
cm—centimeter
lb—pounds

kg or kilos—kilograms
ac—before meals
pc—after meals
stat—immediately
prn—whenever necessary
ad lib—as desired
ASAP—as soon as possible
BR—bed rest
BP—blood pressure
I & O—intake and output
IM—intramuscular
IV—intravenous
sc or SubQ—subcutaneous
LP—lumbar puncture
NPO—nothing by mouth
D/W—dextrose in water
S/W—saline in water
DOB—date of birth
FUO—fever of unknown (or undetermined) origin
GC—gonococcus or gonorrhea
K—potassium
LE—lupus erythematosus
NYD—not yet diagnosed
PM—postmortem
TB—tuberculosis
O_2—oxygen
CO_2—carbon dioxide
pt—patient
TLC—tender loving care

Symbols
> —greater than
< —less than
♂—male
♀—female
↑—above, increase
↓—below, decrease
×—times (multiply by)
%—percentage
#—number
= —equals
+ —plus
− —minus
ō—none
c̄—with
s̄—without
ā—before
p̄—after

CONTROLLED SUBSTANCES INVENTORY AND PRESCRIBER'S RECORD

In addition to keeping a running inventory of all narcotics and controlled substances, a physician who dispenses or regularly engages in administering controlled substances is required to maintain a special record, either a card for each type or drug or a daily log book. All these records are to be kept for 2 years (3 years in some states), subject to inspection and copying by authorized employees of state and federal law enforcement and regulatory agencies.

Records kept on all Schedule II controlled substances dispensed, administered, or prescribed must show the date, name and address of the patient, character and quantity of the drug provided, and pathologic condition and purpose for which the drug was provided. *All records for controlled substances in Schedule II must be stored separately from other files.*

Records kept on all Schedule III, IV, and V controlled substances administered or dispensed from the office or medical bag must show the date, the name and address of the patient, and the quantity of the drug dispensed or administered. Schedule III, IV, and V records may be stored separately from other files or in such form that the information is readily retrievable from the practitioner's other business and professional records.

Medical assistants should play a major role in helping the physician keep all the appropriate records, guarding prescription pads, securing medication storage areas to prevent theft, ensuring the proper type of storage and correct labeling for all medications, and discarding and destroying outdated drugs.

OXYGEN ADMINISTRATION

Oxygen is commonly used as a drug for patients with hypoxia (oxygen deficiency) or hypoxemia (deficiency of oxygen in the blood). We cannot live without oxygen. Room air that we normally breathe is approximately 21% oxygen.

SIGNS AND SYMPTOMS OF HYPOXEMIA

- Anxiety or a feeling of impending doom
- Confusion
- Cyanosis
- Dyspnea
- Increased blood pressure
- Pale, cool extremities (caused by vasoconstriction)
- Restlessness
- Tachycardia

CONDITIONS FOR WHICH OXYGEN ADMINISTRATION MAY BE REQUIRED

- Apnea
- Carbon monoxide poisoning
- Congestive heart disease
- Chronic obstructive pulmonary disease (COPD)
- During surgical procedures
- Myocardial infarction
- Pulmonary edema
- Pneumonia
- Shock

METHODS OF OXYGEN ADMINISTRATION

Before oxygen is administered, the patient's respiratory condition must be assessed. This includes observing the respiratory rate and rhythm and the amount or nature of the difficulty in breathing that the patient is experiencing. When feasible, obtain and record baseline vital signs. Two methods used to administer oxygen in the physician's office or clinic are by using the face mask or the nasal cannula (Figure 7-3). Check the physician's order for the method and rate of oxygen administration.

Face Mask

This is a device that is shaped to fit snugly over the patient's mouth and nose. It can be secured in place with a strap that goes around the head, or it can be held with the hand. The mask has valves that allow oxygen to be inhaled or pumped

Figure 7-3 A, *Oxygen being administered through a nasal cannula;* **B,** *oxygen tank;* **C,** *mask, nasal cannula, and tubing.*

A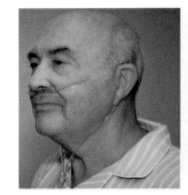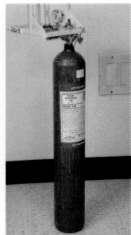

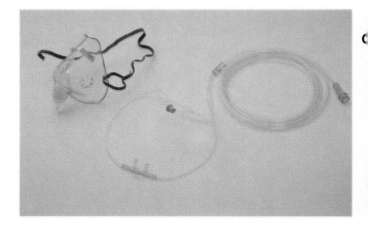

into the respiratory tract and carbon dioxide exhaled into the environment. Oxygen flows at a prescribed rate through a tubing to the mask. A flow rate of 8 to 15 liters per minute delivers 45% to 60% oxygen concentration.

Nasal cannula

This is a device that consists of two pronglike tubes that are placed into the nostrils to deliver oxygen. The nasal tubes should curve with the nasal passage to ensure delivery of the correct amount of oxygen. The patient must be instructed to breathe through the nose so that oxygen is not lost. Oxygen flows at a prescribed rate through a tubing to the nasal cannula. A flow rate of 2 liters per minute delivers 24% oxygen concentration. Flow rates higher than 5 liters per minute dry the nasal membranes if used for any length of time.

Keep the following points in mind when oxygen when administering oxygen:

- Do not use electrical appliances when oxygen is being administered. Do not connect or disconnect plugs when oxygen is in use.
- Do not use acetone and alcohol in the presence of oxygen.
- Do not use oil or grease on oxygen equipment. Your hands must also be free of grease when you are turning oxygen equipment on or off.
- Do not use oxygen tanks as a clothes rack.
- Keep all flammable substances away from the area where oxygen is in use.
- Post "No Smoking, Oxygen In Use" signs in areas where oxygen is being used.
- Patients *should not be allowed* to have cigarettes, lighters, or matches with them while oxygen is being used because they may forget that these items should not be used while oxygen is being administered and use them.
- When transporting an oxygen tank, fasten it to the platform of a carrier designed for that purpose.

ROUTES AND METHODS OF DRUG ADMINISTRATION

Drugs are supplied in various forms for different purposes (Table 7-5). Certain drugs can be administered in a variety of ways, and others must be administered in a specific way to be effective. Methods of administration are divided into two general categories: (1) drugs used for local effect, which are applied directly to the skin, tissue, or mucous membrane involved; and (2) drugs used for a systemic or general effect. A drug applied in this manner must be absorbed and circulate through the bloodstream to produce an effect on the body cells or tissues.

RULES FOR ADMINISTERING MEDICATION

There are certain rules to follow when preparing and administering medications. Additional guidelines and rules that apply specifically to medications given parenterally (by injection) are described later in this unit.

You must know and always adhere to the five rights of proper medication administration, which are as follows:
- *Right* drug
- *Right* dose
- *Right* route for administration
- *Right* time
- *Right* patient

It is the patient's *right* to expect the five *rights*.

A *sixth* right has been added by many medical authorities to the traditional five rights.
- *Right* documentation.

It is the patient's *right* to expect all six of the *rights*.

General Instructions

1. Wash your hands before preparing medications.
2. Give only medications and the correct dosage for which you have the physician's written order. A safe practice is to follow only *written* orders that are *complete*.
3. Prepare the medication in a well-lighted area away from distractions and interruptions. Give full attention to what you are doing.
4. **Read the label of the medication three times:**
   a. When removing from the storage area
   b. Before pouring the desired amount
   c. When replacing the container in the storage area
   Do not use unlabeled or illegibly labeled medications.
5. Know the drug that you are giving. Check the *PDR* or other reference books if you are unsure of the usual actions, uses, dosage, route of administration, and undesirable side effects.
6. Calculate a dosage accurately, when this is necessary. Consult another competent person for verification when you doubt your answer.
7. *Administration of liquid oral medications*—Shake well any medication that is in the form of an emulsion or suspension.
   a. Do not use medications that have changed color, turned cloudy, or have sediment at the bottom (except suspensions).
   b. Hold the bottle with the label in the palm of your hand to avoid damaging the label if the liquid runs or spills.
   c. Hold the medicine or graduate at eye level so that you can measure accurately as you pour the medication (Figure 7-5, *A*).
   d. Wipe the neck of the container before replacing the cap.
   e. Do not mix liquid medications unless specifically ordered to do so.
8. Administration of solid oral medications—Tablets, caplets, capsules, or spansules: Shake or drop the tablet or other preparation into the cap of the container; then drop it into a medicine cup. You must *not* handle the medication with your fingers (Figure 7-5, *B*).
9. Do not leave poured medications unattended.

TABLE 7-5

Routes and Methods Used for Administering Medications

Route of Administration	Method of Administration	Form of Drug
Oral	The patient is given the drug by mouth to swallow. This is the simplest method and the method most desirable to patients.	Pills, tablets, capsules, spansules, or solutions supplied in bulk form or as a unit dose.
Sublingual	The drug is placed under the patient's tongue and left to dissolve and be absorbed. It is not to be chewed or swallowed.	Tablets
Buccal	The drug is placed between the cheek and gum to dissolve and be absorbed.	Tablets
Inhalation	The drug is given via the respiratory tract. The patient inhales the drug using a nebulizer or a special mechanical apparatus.	Aerosols, sprays, mists, or steams medicated with drugs
Rectal	The drug is inserted into the rectum. This method is used when a patient cannot tolerate the drug orally; or if unconscious; or if the drug would be destroyed by digestive enzymes. Also may be administered by proctoclysis, a drip method.	Suppositories, enemas, or other solutions
Inunction	The drug is applied or rubbed into the skin. Disposable single-use exam gloves or tongue depressors should be used when applying drugs such as nitroglycerin, or those containing mercury to a patient. This prevents absorption of the drug into the system.	Ointments, lotions, sprays, solutions, powders, tinctures, liniments
Vaginal	The drug is inserted into or applied to the vagina.	Suppository; solution, as in a douche; or liquids or ointments to be applied for local effect on the cervix or vaginal canal; also contraceptive foams and creams
Instillation	The drug is applied in drops to a membrane, as into the eye or ear.	Solutions
Irrigation	The drug is flushed through a membrane or body cavity.	Solutions
Parenteral	The drug is given by injection through a needle. Types of injections include: • *Subcutaneous:* under the skin • *Intramuscular:* into a muscle • *Intradermal or intracutaneous:* into the upper layers of the skin. Used chiefly for skin reactions, as in allergy or tuberculosis testing • *Intraarticular:* into a joint for local effects • *Intraarterial:* into an artery; used in certain diagnostic procedures • *Lumbar puncture or intraspinal:* into the spinal canal between two vertebrae; used to administer drugs for diagnostic techniques or for spinal anesthetics • *Intravenous:* into a vein; used for immediate effect of a drug, for blood	A drug solution supplied in ampules for single use; in vials for single or multiple use; and in syringes or cartridges prefilled by the manufacturer. Drugs that deteriorate in solutions may be supplied in vials in powdered form to which a specified amount of diluent is to be added when prepared for use. Sterile hypodermic tablets that are to be dissolved before the drug is administered are also available. Larger amounts of solutions for intravenous use are supplied in bottles of 250 ml, 500 ml, or 1000 ml, such as dextrose in water and normal saline, to which other drugs may be added. Plasma and blood are also used for intravenous transfusions.

Table 7-5—cont'd

Routes and Methods Used for Administering Medications

Route of Administration	Method of Administration	Form of Drug
Transdermal patch (Figure 7-4)	The patch, an adhesive disk impregnated with medication, is applied to a clean dry skin area on the upper arms and legs, chest, and back (e.g., nitroglycerin—a vasodilator used for heart patients); or behind the ear (e.g., Transderm Scop used for motion sickness); or on the trunk of the body, including the abdomen and buttocks but not the breasts (e.g., Estraderm patch—a type of estrogen); or to a nonhairy site on the trunk or upper arm (e.g., Habitrol—a nicotine system used to help people stop smoking). The patches release a controlled amount of drug over a period of time. The drug is absorbed through the skin into the bloodstream.	Single-unit adhesive skin patch in a foil packet
Subdermal implant	A thin capsule or rod of medication is implanted under the skin commonly in the upper or lower arm. A local anesthetic is given before the implant is placed under the skin.	Thin silicone rubber capsules or rods

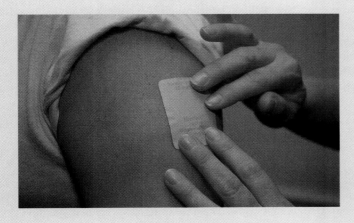

Figure 7-4   *Transdermal patch on patient's arm.*

10. Do not administer medications prepared by others. If an error is made, the person administering the medication is responsible.
11. Take both the drug and container to the physician for additional identification when you have prepared the medication to be administered by the physician.
12. Know your patient. You may ask the patient to state his or her name to ensure correct identification.
13. Make sure that the patient is not allergic to the medication before you administer it.
14. Stay with the patient until you are certain that an oral medication has been swallowed.
15. **Administration of rectal suppository**—Have the patient assume the Sim's position on the left side. Don gloves. Lubricate the suppository with a water-soluble lubricant, e.g., K-Y jelly. Spread the patient's buttocks and insert the suppository about 2 inches into the rectum. The anal canal of an adult is about 1 inch long. Inserting the suppository 2 inches into the rectum facilitates retention. The drug is absorbed through the mucous membrane when the suppository melts. It takes about 10 minutes for the suppository to melt.
16. Observe the patient for any unusual reactions to the drug administered.
17. Discard a medication that the patient refuses. Never replace a medication into the original container once it has been removed.
18. Report immediately to the physician if the patient refuses the medication or if an error was made so that appropriate action can be taken promptly or adjustments made for the patient's care.

Figure 7-5 **A,** *Hold the medicine or graduate at eye level so that you can measure accurately as you pour the medication;* **B,** *shake or drop tablet into cap of container.*

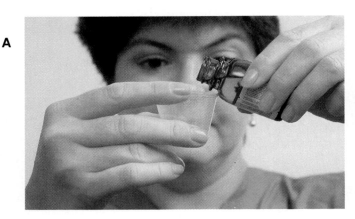

A

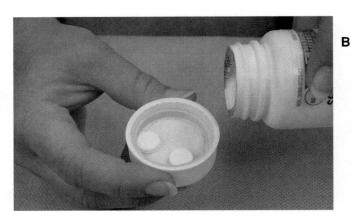

B

Follow any new orders that the physician may provide. Prompt corrective action is an important responsibility of the medical assistant if any error is made.

19. Record as soon as possible on the correct patient's chart the date, time, drug and amount given, route of administration, and your signature. *(Errors in administering drugs must also be recorded, describing the incident in full.)* Body locations must be recorded for drugs administered parenterally, by transdermal patch, or when implanted under the skin by the physician. In addition, if the medication administered was a narcotic or other controlled substance, you must record this information in the physician's controlled substances records.

DOSAGE: WEIGHTS, MEASUREMENTS, CALCULATIONS

A complete understanding of basic arithmetic is essential when preparing solutions or administering medications. A review of mathematic calculations is recommended at this time before you prepare to calculate dosages and administer medications.

The two primary systems of weights and measures used for describing dosages for medications are the apothecary system and the metric system. The *apothecary* system is our oldest system of measurement, the term being an ancient word meaning pharmacist or druggist. Today the trend is to use the *metric* system, the standard system of weights and measurements set up by the International Bureau of Weights and Measures, although it has not been completely adopted for use by everyone at this time. Therefore you must have an understanding of both systems.

The apothecary system units of fluid measurement are the minim, fluid dram, fluid ounce, pint, quart, and gallon. The units of solid measurement are the grain, dram, ounce, and pound. Roman numerals and fractions are used with this system (for example, HCI gtt X (hydrochloric acid drops ten); or nitroglycerin gr 1/150 (nitroglycerin grains one/one hundred fifty).

In the metric system, the units of fluid or volume measurements are the milliliter, cubic centimeter, and liter. Units of weight or solid measurements are the kilogram, milligram, and gram. Arabic numbers and the decimal system are used with this system. Example: $1/1000 = 0.001$, $1/100 = 0.01$, $1/10 = 0.1$ (for example, tetracycline 250 mg/ml or cc).

See Tables 7-6 through 7-9 for the equivalent values of apothecary and metric measurements for liquids and solids, and the equivalents of common household weights and measurements for these systems.

At times you may be required to calculate the dose of a medication that you are to administer. A simple formula to use is:

$$\frac{\text{Dose you want} \times \text{Quantity on hand}}{\text{Dose you have}} = \text{Quantity to administer}$$

Example: The physician has ordered 500 mg tetracycline, by mouth (po). The dose of tetracycline that you have on hand is labeled 250 mg/tablet.

Therefore:

$$\frac{\text{Dose you want (500 mg)} \times \text{Quantity (1 tablet)}}{\text{Dose you have (250 mg)}} = \text{Tablets to give (2)}$$

You would therefore give the patient two tablets of tetracycline 250 mg/tablet, so that the patient would receive 500 mg of tetracycline as was ordered.

The same formula can be used when preparing drugs supplied in a solution form.

Example: The physician has ordered 500 mg of tetracycline to be given intramuscularly (IM). The bottle you have on hand is labeled tetracycline 250 mg/ml. Therefore:

$$\frac{\text{Dose you want (500 mg)} \times \text{Quantity on hand (1 ml)}}{\text{Dose you have (250 mg.ml)}} = \text{dose in milliliters that you give (2 ml)}$$

TABLE 7-6

Metric System Equivalents

Dry weights

100 micro grams (μg)	= 1 milligram (mg)
1000 mg	= 1 gram (g)
1000 g	= 1 kilogram (kg)

Liquid volume

1000 milliliters (ml)	= 1 liter (L)
1000 cubic centimeters (cc)	= 1 L
1 ml	= 1 cc
1000 L	= 1 kiloliter

TABLE 7-7

Household System Equivalents

60 drops (gtt) = 1 teaspoon (tsp)
4 tsp = 1 tablespoon (Tbsp) = $^1/_2$ ounce (oz)
2 Tbsp = 1 fluid (fl) oz = 30 cc
8 fl oz = 1 cup (C) = 16 Tbsp
1 pint (pt) = 2 C = 16 oz = 480 cc (approximately)
1 quart (qt) = 4 C = 32 oz
1 gallon (gal) = 4 qt = 128 oz
16 oz = 1 pound (lb)

TABLE 7-8

Metric Doses with Approximate Apothecary Equivalents*

	Weights			Liquid Measures†	
Metric	Approximate Apothecary Equivalents	Metric	Approximate Apothecary Equivalents	Metric	Approximate Apothecary Equivalents
1 gram	= 15 grains	15 mg	= $^1/_4$ gr	1000 ml = 1	quart (qt)
2 grams (g)	= 30 grains (gr)	12 mg	= $^1/_5$ gr	750 ml = $1^1/_2$	pints
1.5 g	= 22 gr	10 mg	= $^1/_6$ gr	500 ml = 1	pint (pt)
1 g	= 15 gr	8 mg	= $^1/_8$ gr	250 ml = 8	fl ounces
1000 mg	= 15 gr	6 mg	= $^1/_{20}$ gr	200 ml = 7	fl ounces
0.75 g or 750 mg	= 12 gr	5 mg	= $^1/_{12}$ gr	100 ml = $3^1/_2$	fl ounces
0.6 g or 600 mg	= 10 gr	4 mg	= $^1/_{16}$ gr	50 ml = $1^3/_4$	fl ounces
0.5 g or 500 mg	= $7^1/_2$ gr	3 mg	= $^1/_{20}$ gr	30 ml = 1	fl ounces
450 mg	= 7 gr	1.5 mg	= $^1/_{40}$ gr	15 ml = $^1/_2$	fl ounce (4 fl drams)
300 mg	= 5 gr	1.2 mg	= $^1/_{50}$ gr	10 ml = $2^1/_2$	fl drmas
0.25 g or 250 mg	= 4 gr	1 mg	= $^1/_{60}$ gr	8 ml = 2	fl drams
200 mg	= 3 gr	0.8 mg	= $^1\backslash_{80}$ gr	5 ml = 75	minims ($1^1/_4$ drams)
0.15 g or 150 mg	= $2^1/_2$ gr	0.6 mg	= $^1/_{100}$ gr	4 ml = 1 fl	dram
120 mg	= 2 gr	0.5 mg	= $^1/_{200}$ gr	3 ml = 45	minims
0.1 g or 100 mg	= $1^1/_2$ gr	0.4 mg	= $^1/_{150}$ gr	2 ml = 30	minims
60 mg	= 1 gr	0.3 mg	= $^1/_{200}$ gr	1 ml = 15	minims
50 mg	= $^3/_4$ gr	0.25 mg	= $^1/_{250}$ gr	0.75 ml = 12	minims
40 mg	= $^2/_3$ gr	0.2 mg	= $^1/_{300}$ gr	0.6 ml = 10	minims
30 mg	= $^1/_2$ gr	0.15 mg	= $^1/_{400}$ gr	0.5 ml = 8	minims
25 mg	= $^3/_8$ gr	0.1 mg	= $^1/_{600}$ gr	0.3 ml = 5	minims
20 mg	= $^1/_3$ gr			0.25 ml = 4	minims
				0.25 ml = 4	minims
				0.2 ml = 4	minims
				0.2 ml = 3	minims
				0.1 ml = $1^1/_2$	minim
				0.06 ml = 1	minim

The approximate dose equivalents in this table represent the quantities that would be prescribed, under identical conditions, by physicians trained, respectively, in the metric or in the apothecary system of weights and measures.

†*A milliliter (ml) is the approximate equivalent of a cubic centimeter (cc).*

TABLE 7-9

Common Household Weights and Measurements with Metric and Apothecary Equivalents and Preparation

Household	Metric and Apothecary Equivalents	
	Metric	Apothecary
Liquid		
1 drop (gtts)		= 1 minim (m)
15 drops	= 1 milliliter (ml or cc)	= 15 minims
1 teaspoon (tsp) or (t)	= 4 ml	= 1 fluid dram (fl dr)
1 dessert spoon	= 8 ml	= 2 fl dr
6 teaspoons or 2 tablespoons (tbsp) or (T)	= 30 ml	= 1 fluid ounce
1 measuring cup	= 240 ml	= 8 fl ounces
2 measuring cups	= 500 ml	= 1 pint (pt) (16 fl oz)
4 measuring cups	= 1000 ml	= 1 quart (qt) or 2 pts or 32 oz
1 tbsp	= 15 ml	= 4 drams ($1/2$ oz)
Dry		
1/8 teaspoon	= 0.5 gram (g)	= $7^1/_2$ grains (gr)
1/4 teaspoon	= 1 g	= 15 gr
1 teaspoon	= 4 g	= 60 gr or 1 dram
1 tablespoon	= 15 g	= 4 drams
2 tablespoons	= 30 g	= 1 ounce

Preparation of Solutions		
Prescribed Strength	Amount of Full-strength Drug	Amount of Fluid
1:1000	1 teaspoonful	1 gallon (gal)
1:1000	15 drops	1 quart
$1/_{10}$ of 1%	15 drops	1 quart (qt)
1:500	2 teaspoonsful	1 gallon
1:500	30 drops	1 quart
1/5 of 1%	30 drops	1 quart
1:200	5 teaspoonsful	1 gallon
1:200	1-$1/4$ teaspoonsful	1 quart
$1/2$ of 1%	1 $1/4$ teaspoonsful	1 quart
1:100 (1%)	2 $1/4$ teaspoonsful	1 quart
1:50 (2%)	5 teaspoonsful	1 quart
1:25 (4%)	2 $1/2$ tablespoonsful	1 quart
1:20 (5%)	3 tablespoonsful	1 quart

When this formula is used, both the dose you want to give and the dose you have on hand must be expressed in the same measurements; that is, to give so many milligrams, the dose on hand must be in milligrams per milliliter for a solution, or in milligrams per tablet or capsule for drugs supplied in the solid form. If this is not the case, you have to convert one measurement into the equivalent value of the other. You should be familiar with the methods used for converting one system of measurements into the other. See Table 7-10 for conversion techniques for calculation of drug dosages.

It is recommended that you refer to some of the many books available with practice problems in the mathematics of drugs, solutions, and dosages to gain competence in this procedure. Use the tables of weights and measurements for a reference. When you doubt your calculations, always seek help from another competent person or the physician.

FACTORS INFLUENCING DOSAGE AND DRUG ACTION

Not all individuals respond to a given medication in the same manner. When prescribing a drug for a patient, the physician takes into account the following factors that influence the prescribed dosage and anticipated action.

TABLE 7-10

Conversion Techniques for Calculation of Drug Dosages

Metric measurements to apothecary measurements
1. *Grams to grains:* Multiply the number of grams by 15
2. *Milligrams to grains:* Divide the number of milligrams by 60
3. *Grams to ounces:* Divide the number of grams by 130
4. *Milliliters to fluid ounces:* Divide the number of milliliters by 30
5. *Milliliters to minims:* Multiply the number of milliliters by 15

Apothecary measurements to metric measurements
1. *Grains to grams:* Divide the number of grains by 15
2. *Grains to milligrams:* Multiply the number of grains by 60
3. *Ounces to grams:* Multiply the number of ounces by 30
4. *Fluid ounces to milliliters:* Multiply the number of fluid ounmces by 30
5. *Minims to milliliters:* Divide the number of minims by 15

Metric measurements to metric measurements
1. *Grams to milligrams:* Multiply grams by 1000
2. *Milligrams to grams:* Divide milligrams by 1000
3. *Liters to milliliters:* Multiply liters by 1000
4. *Milliliters to liters:* Divide milliliters by 1000

Pediatric dose calculation

The formula for calculating a pediatric dose is different. The calculation of a pediatric dose is based on the body weight of the child. The formula, called *Clark's Rule,* is as follows:

$$\frac{\text{Weight of child in points} \times \text{Usual adult dose}}{\text{divided by } 150} = \text{Safe dose for a child}$$

Example: The physician has ordered aspirin for a child that weighs 22.5 pounds. Knowing that the usual adult dose of aspirin is 10 grains, you would calculate as follows:

$$\frac{22.5 \text{ lb} \times 10 \text{ gr}}{150} = \frac{225}{150} = 1.5 \text{ grain}$$

You would therefore give the child 1.5 gr of aspirin, which is a safe dosage for a child.
For some drugs the pediatric dose is stated by the manufacturer in the literature accompanying the drug.

More examples and conversion problems are included in the Student Workbook that accompanies this textbook.

Age

Infants, young children, and the elderly usually require a smaller dosage of a medication.

Sex

The average woman is given a smaller dosage than the average man because of the difference in body structure and overall weight. Also, when a woman is pregnant, drugs and the dosage are monitored very closely to prevent harmful effects to the fetus.

Weight

The usual rule is the smaller or lighter the patient, the smaller the dosage of drug. Certain medication dosages are determined according to the weight of the patient.

Past Medical History and Drug Tolerance

If a patient has been taking a medication regularly for an extended period of time, a tolerance to the drug may have developed, and a larger dosage may be required to obtain the desired results. This is frequently seen with the use of narcotics, barbiturates, sedatives, and analgesics.

Physical or Emotional Condition of the Patient

A patient who has excruciating pain requires a larger dose of an analgesic than a patient who experiences intermittent pain. A severely depressed patient requires a larger dosage of an antidepressant than a patient suffering from mild depression.

Drug Idiosyncrasies or Allergies

At times the patient may experience an abnormal susceptibility or reaction to a drug. Alternate drugs with similar actions can then be prescribed.

Type of Action Desired or Produced

Drugs can produce local, systemic, selective, or cumulative actions. A *local action* occurs when the drug is absorbed and produces an effect at the site to which it was administered (for example, a local anesthetic administered to deaden sensation in the body area to be treated). A *systemic action* occurs when the drug is absorbed and circulates in the bloodstream to produce a general effect (for example, central nervous system stimulants and depressants). A *selective action* is a more specific effect of a drug on one special body area than on other areas (for example, bronchodilators). A *cumulative* action occurs when a drug accumulates in the body and exerts a greater effect than the initial dose; the drug accumulates in the body faster than it can be metabolized and excreted, such as alcohol does when a person drinks two or three drinks in 1 hour.

Route of Administration

Although there are exceptions, generally medications administered parenterally are given in smaller dosages than those given by mouth. Larger amounts of medications are used for topical application than for internal administration. Drugs administered parenterally produce their effects much more rapidly than drugs administered orally. When a systemic effect is desired from an irritating drug, it should be given intramuscularly rather than by other parenteral routes.

Time of Administration

For optimal effects, some drugs must be taken before meals; two, three, or four times a day; or after meals to avoid irritating the lining of the stomach. Drugs will be absorbed more quickly and have a more rapid effect if taken on an empty stomach.

Interactions of Drugs

Some drugs, when taken together, may enhance or counteract the effect of the other.

Interactions can be

- *Synergistic*: One drug augments the activity of the other drug; the action of the drugs is such that their combined effect is greater than the sum of their individual effects. For example, barbiturates taken with alcohol have up to four times the depressant effect that either drug would have if taken alone.
- *Potentiating*: A synergistic action in which one drug increases the effect of another drug when taken simultaneously, producing a combined effect that is greater than the sum of the effects of each drug taken separately.
- *Antagonistic*: One drug neutralizes or counteracts the action of the other drug when they are taken together.
- *Additive*: When the combined effect produced by the action of two or more drugs is equal to the sum of their separate effects.

Thus it is vital to know if the patient is taking any other medication and, in some cases, any alcoholic beverage, before a new medication is prescribed. It is also important to ask if the patient takes nonprescription drugs. Often patients do not consider drugs that they purchase over the counter to be medications; nonetheless, they are medications that may possibly interact adversely with a prescription drug.

SUMMARY

Drugs are potent substances that can provide individuals with extremely beneficial results when used properly and with care, but they are also capable of producing hazardous or fatal results when used indiscreetly. Toxic effects such as allergic reactions, adverse effects on the blood or blood-producing tissues, drug dependence, accidental poisoning, or drug overdose can be the result of careless or uninformed use of any drug on the market for legal use or from illegal drugs obtained in the streets. Always handle and administer drugs with extreme care because a life may depend on their proper use.

PATIENT EDUCATION

Patient education is a vital part of all medical care and treatment. When drug therapy is initiated, certain considerations and drug safety precautions must be brought to the patient's attention. The physician or medical assistant should instruct the patient to do the following:

- Inform the physician of all drugs, either prescription or over-the-counter drugs, that he or she is currently taking or take periodically. If the patient has more than one physician, tell each of them what drugs are being taken.
- Inform each physician of any reactions or allergies that he or she has to drugs.
- Know the name, dosage, and purpose of each medication that he or she is taking.
- Know how and for how long the drug is to be taken.

The patient should follow the instructions for taking the drug as prescribed. At times a drug should be taken with food, or before or after meals, or on an empty stomach. It is extremely important that these directions be followed precisely because there are sound medical reasons for these directions. Some drugs should be taken with food to avoid or minimize gastrointestinal irritation and reactions. Others should be taken on an empty stomach for proper metabolism and absorption. When drugs are to be taken three or four times a day, or every 6 hours, be sure that you understand the time schedule that must be followed. Again, there is a sound scientific reason for taking drugs on a specific schedule so that treatment will be maximized.

- If necessary, devise a calendar or diary as a reminder of what drug to take and when.
- Call the physician if there are any unusual reaction(s). (The patient should be informed of possible side effects).
- Don't stop taking the medication unless directed to do so by the physician. Some drugs such as antibiotics must be taken for 7 to 10 days to be effective; other drugs such as prednisone or synthroid should be tapered off slowly under the direction of the physician.

- Be aware that some drugs may lead to a dependency if misused or abused, and understand the dangers of dependency.
- Don't save old prescriptions. Look for the expiration date on all drugs being used. Old or outdated drugs should be flushed down the sink or toilet.
- *Never* give your medications to anyone else. They are only for *your* condition.
- Don't use alcohol when taking medications until the physician or pharmacist says it is safe.
- Avoid certain activities such as driving a motor vehicle when taking drugs that cause drowsiness.
- Check with the pharmacist where to store your medications. Some drugs need to be kept in a refrigerator. Others should be kept in a dry, cool atmosphere. Usually you should not keep medications in a hot, damp bathroom cabinet.
- Don't keep medications in a bedside stand. Take medications in a well-lit area so that he or she can read the label and be sure that the medication and dosage are correct.
- *Always* read the label of the container from which he or she removes the medication before taking it. Never assume that he or she is taking the right medication without reading the label on the container.
- If the patient has poor vision, ask the physician or pharmacist to print the name of the drug and the treatment schedule out clearly on a separate piece of paper or card.
- Keep all drugs out of the reach of children.
- Always ask or call the physician if he or she has any additional questions regarding the medication therapy.
- Be aware that all of the preceding directions are vital to a successful program of medical care.

INJECTIONS

Injections are an important means of administering chemotherapy treatment. Because two foreign objects, the medication and the needle, are being introduced into the patient's body, these procedures must be performed with extreme care and excellent technique. The effectiveness of the medication is influenced by the correct choice of injection site and the use of precise technique. Any injection administered into an inappropriate body site or with incorrect technique may interfere with the body's use of the medication and, more important, may cause irreparable damage. The practices of aseptic (sterile) technique (see Unit Six) must be observed when administering injections to minimize the danger of causing an infectious process.

REASONS PHYSICIANS ORDER INJECTIONS

1. To achieve a rapid response to the medication. When injected, a medication enters the bloodstream quickly and therefore is more effective.
2. To guarantee the accuracy of the amount of medication given.
3. To concentrate the medication in a specific area of the body such as into a joint cavity, fracture, or lumbar puncture.

4. To produce local anesthesia to a specific part of the body.
5. To administer the medication when it cannot be given by mouth or by other methods, either because of the physical or mental condition of the patient or the nature of the drug.
6. When the effect of the medication would be destroyed by the digestive tract or lost through vomiting, or when it would irritate the digestive system.

DANGERS AND COMPLICATIONS ASSOCIATED WITH INJECTIONS

1. Injury to superficial nerves or to a vessel
2. Introduction of infection resulting from the improper disinfection of the injection site and/or a contaminated needle or syringe, or from an operator with unclean hands
3. Breaking a needle in a tissue
4. Injecting a blood vessel rather than a muscle or subcutaneous tissue
5. Hitting a bone in a very thin patient
6. Allergic reactions that may be mild, severe, or even fatal
7. Toxic effects produced by the medication
8. Too much air entering the bloodstream in a venipuncture

BODY AREAS TO AVOID WHEN ADMINISTERING INJECTIONS

1. Burned areas
2. Scar tissue
3. Edematous areas
4. Cyanotic areas
5. Traumatized areas
6. Areas near large blood vessels, nerves, and bones
7. Areas where there have been a change in skin texture or pigmentation
8. Areas where there are other tissue growths such as a mole or wart

SUPPLIES AND EQUIPMENT FOR ADMINISTERING INJECTIONS
Syringes

Disposable plastic or glass and nondisposable glass syringes are available in several standard sizes and shapes. The most common sizes used in the physician's office are 2 cc, 3 cc, 5 cc, or 10 cc. The parts of the syringe are the barrel, the outside portion; the plunger, the portion that fits inside the barrel; and the tip, the point at which the needle will be attached, which is either a plain or a Luer-Lok tip (Figures 7-6 and 7-7). Other variations of syringes include the insulin syringe (Figure 7-8), tuberculin syringe (Figure 7-9), Tubex injector for use with a disposable needle-cartridge unit, and a disposable syringe unit-dose system.

There are a variety of systems available with a safety shield that is pulled up and over the needle after use. The purpose of the safety shield is to cover the needle without having to recap the needle after use. This provides protection for the user from a possible needlestick and/or contamination before the syringe is discarded (see Figure 7-6, *B*; Figures 7-10 to 7-12). Sterile disposable syringes come supplied in a paper wrapper or a rigid plastic container. Calibrations, usually in

Figure 7-6 A, *Parts of a syringe;* **B,** *SAFETY-LOK syringe.*

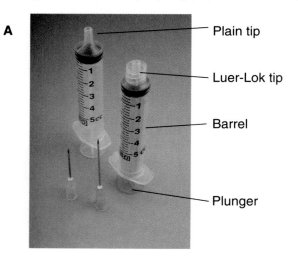

A

Plain tip

Luer-Lok tip

Barrel

Plunger

B

Precision glide needle
with X3 point

Safety shield

Bold scale

Crystal clear barrel
and shield

Large flanges

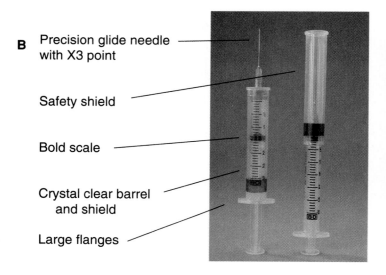

Figure 7-7 *Syringes, 5 cc and 10 cc, with needles attached. Calibrations are marked in cubic centimeters.*

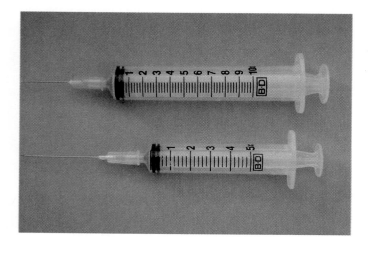

Figure 7-8 *Insulin syringes. Calibrations are marked in units per cubic centimeter.*

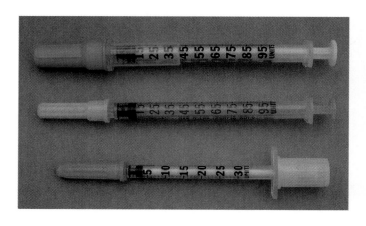

Figure 7-9 *Tuberculin syringe with fine calibrations up to 1 cc.*

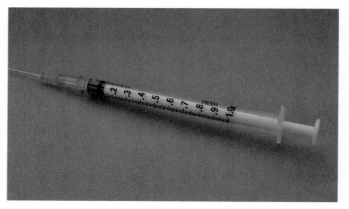

cubic centimeters (cc) and minims, are marked on the barrel of the syringe.

See Figure 7-10 for the procedure for using the Safety-Lok syringe and Figure 7-12 for a procedure for using the Monoject safety syringe.

Needles

Needles come in various lengths ranging from 1/4 inch to 6 inches, and with various gauges ranging from 13 to 30. The gauge of the needle and the length are indicated on the outside of the sterile protective cover or wrapper. Some manufacturers also color code the wrappers for quick and easy identification of the gauge. The parts of a needle are the point, the cannula or shaft, and the hub, which fits onto the tip of a syringe (Figure 7-13). The smaller the gauge of the needle, the larger the lumen or inside diameter. For example, an 18-gauge needle has a large lumen; a 26 gauge-needle has a small lumen. The size and length of a needle govern its use.

Today most practitioners use disposable needles and syringes to prevent all danger of cross-infection, although the reusable type is still available.

Figure 7-10 *Procedure for using the SAFETY-LOK syringe.*
Courtesy Becton-Dickinson, Division of Becton, Dickinson and Co., Rutherford, NJ.

Drawing the Medication

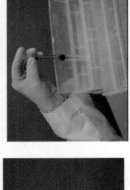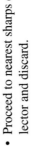

- Using your usual aseptic technique, prepare and draw up medication into the syringe.

- **Note:** The SAFETY-LOK Syringe requires no technique change for drawing medication.

Giving the Injection

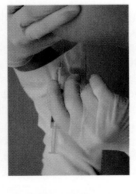

- Proceed to administer the injection following established technique.

- The SAFETY-LOK Syringe is primarily designed for IM and SUB-Q injections but can also be used for most IV port injections.

Locking the Shield

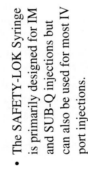

- After completing your injection, hold syringe with needle pointed away from you.

- Grasp the syringe flanges with one hand and position other hand over safety shield.

- Twist safety shield to loosen from syringe barrel by breaking seal.

- Push safety shield forward over needle until you hear an audible click. A slight twisting action may facilitate locking.

- The safety shield is now locked firmly in place.

Discarding the Used Syringe

- Proceed to nearest sharps collector and discard.

- All sharps should be safely discarded after use in an approved sharps collector.

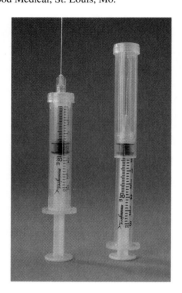

Figure 7-11 *Monoject safety syringes.*
Courtesy Sherwood Medical, St. Louis, Mo.

Skin antiseptic

Before an injection is administered, the skin must be cleaned with an antiseptic. The most commonly used is isopropyl alcohol placed on a clean cotton ball or a prepackaged sterile alcohol sponge.

Medications and diluents

Most medications for parenteral use are in an aqueous solution or in a suspension, although some are in an oil solution or in a suspension, and a few are in tablet or powdered form. When a sterile hypodermic tablet or powdered drug is to be dissolved before parenteral use, sterile water for injection or sterile normal saline is used as the diluent. The type and amount to be used are indicated on the container in which the drug is supplied.

Medication solutions are supplied in single- or multiple-dose form. Those for *single use* are supplied (1) in syringes or cartridges that are prefilled by the manufacturer, (2) in an ampule, a small glass container with a constricted neck that is to be broken off when the drug is to be used, or (3) in a single-dose vial.

Containers with *multiple doses* of a medication are called vials. These are small bottles containing from 10 to 50 ml of a drug solution. Vials are usually covered with a soft metal cover and have a rubber, self-sealing stopper. At the time of use, this rubber stopper is cleansed with an alcohol sponge and then punctured with the needle to inject air and withdraw an equal amount of drug (Figure 7-14). Procedures to withdraw solutions from an ampule and vial are discussed under the procedure "Administration of an Intramuscular Injection."

RECONSTITUTION OF A POWDERED DRUG

Some medications deteriorate or remain stable for only a short period of time when mixed in certain solutions. These medications are supplied as a powder in a sterile field. This powder has to be made into a solution before the medication can be administered. Sometimes a special diluent is provided with the medication; at other times sterile water or sterile normal saline is used to reconstitute the medication. *Reconstitution* is the process of adding a liquid to a powdered drug in preparation for administration. The manufacturer's directions for reconstituting the medication must be followed precisely to avoid overdosing or underdosing the patient. When the powder and diluent are mixed, the solution should appear clear (or cloudy if it is a suspension) without any clumps of powder left in it. Read the manufacturer's description of the medication to be certain if it should appear clear or cloudy. Examples of drugs supplied in a powdered form that need to be reconstituted before use include potassium; penicillin G; and the measles, mumps, and rubella vaccination.

Procedure for Reconstituting a Powdered Drug for Administration

1. Using a syringe and needle, insert the needle through the cleansed rubber stopper of the vial containing the diluent.
2. Withdraw the amount of liquid diluent that is to be added to the powdered drug. (See step 6 in the procedure for Administration of an Intramuscular Injection for the steps to take to withdraw a solution from a vial.)
3. Add this liquid to the vial containing the powdered drug.
4. With the needle above the fluid level in the vial, withdraw an amount of air equal to the amount of liquid diluent just added.
5. Remove the needle from the vial.
6. Discard the syringe and needle in the used sharps container.
7. Roll the vial between your hands. This mixes the liquid with the powdered drug.
8. Observe the solution obtained to make sure that all of the powdered drug has been mixed and dissolved. The solution should be clear (or cloudy if it is a suspension).
9. Label a multiple-dose vial with the date and time of preparation, the expiration date, the dilution/ strength of the medication prepared, and your initials. Labeling as stated is very important because reconstituted drugs are stable for only a short period of time.
10. Store any remaining drug according to the manufacturer's directions. Some drugs may have to be placed in a refrigerator.

SELECTION OF SYRINGE AND NEEDLE SIZE

The smaller the amount of medication to be given, the smaller the size of syringe to use. In special circumstances such as the administration of insulin, it is essential that an insulin syringe be used. For measuring a very small amount of drug, use a tuberculin syringe, which is a 1-cc syringe marked in tenths (0.1) and hundredths (0.01) of a cubic centimeter on one side of the scale and minims on the other side.

Figure 7-12 *A, Monoject system of safety with Monoject syringes and needles.*
Courtesy Sherwood Medical, St. Louis, Mo.

A

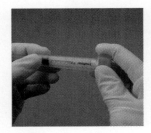

1. Select desired size from convenient Monoject dispenser. Color-coding makes it quick, easy. Check sterility (see that the heat stake has not been-broken).

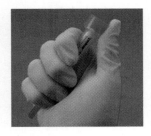

2. Open hard pack by breaking heat stake. Press area of cap directly above heat stake with thumb. Or lightly grasp and twist cap. Or tap cap against hard surface. Then remove cap.

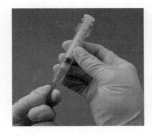

3. Hold sleeve firmly with one hand; then push needle sheath with other hand until syringe end protrudes from sleeve about 1 inch.

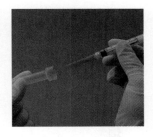

4. Remove syringe and needle from sleeve.

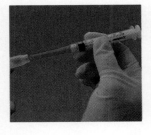

5. Reverse sleeve so small opening is facing the needle sheath end of syringe.

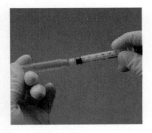

6. Firmly insert needle sheath into sleeve. Hold sleeve in stationary position. Then twist syringe clockwise to seat needle.

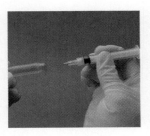

7. Pull syringe with attached needle straight out of needle sheath. Keep the sleeve containing sheath nearby. It's your Mini-safety platform or Mini-container.

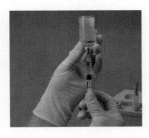

8. Insert needle into medication vial and draw prescribed amount of medication. You're ready to resheath with virtually no change of needlestick.

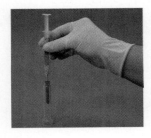

9. Resheath filled syringe in Mini-container. It's perfect for single-use situations.

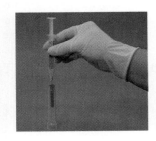

10. Or use handy Stat Tray. Holds two syringes and their Mini-containers. Fits conveniently on patient tray tables and unit dose carts.

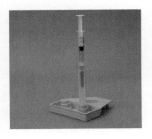

11. After administration, resheath contaminated needle into Mini-container, Stat, or Monotray Medication Tray using just one hand. Your hands don't get near the needle.

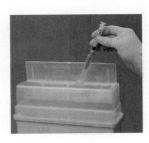

12. Discard entire unit into a puncture-resistant Monoject Sharps Container. That's the Monoject System of Safety.

Figure 7-12—cont'd B, *Monoject safety syringe.*

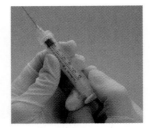 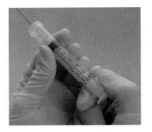 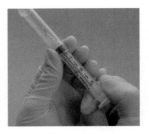

After giving the injection, hold syringe flanges and push safety shield forward over the needle. You will hear a click. The shield is now locked over the needle. Discard the whole unit into the sharps container.

Figure 7-13 A, *Various-sized needles;* **B,** *needle point and bevel.*

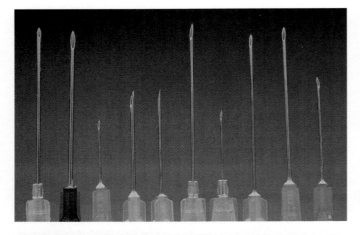

Needles with large lumens (for example, 18 to 20 gauge) are required when the medication to be injected is oily or very thick. Needles with small lumens (for example, 23 to 25 gauge) are used for aqueous, or thin, "watery" solutions.

The site and route of the injection help determine the length of the needle that you should use. The patient's muscle size and thickness of overlying fatty tissue must be taken into consideration when giving an intramuscular injection.

Shorter needles with a large-gauge number may be used on children and very thin patients; longer needles may be required for obese patients to ensure that the needle reaches muscular or subcutaneous tissue.

Figure 7-14 *Drugs supplied in liquid form.* **Left to right**: *Cartridge; vial; ampule.*

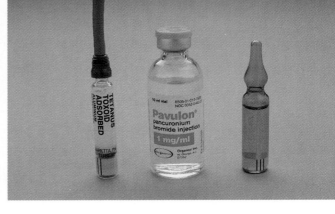

To restate, consider the following when selecting a needle for an injection:

- The patient's age and weight
- The condition and turgor (resiliency) of the tissue
- The route of administration
- The site to be used for the injection
- The thickness of the medication
- The thickness of both the muscle and fatty tissue

Common sizes of syringes and needles used for various injections are shown in Table 7-11.

ANATOMIC SELECTION OF THE INJECTION SITES
Intramuscular Injections

The main objective when administering an intramuscular medication is to inject it deep into the muscle for gradual and optimal absorption into the bloodstream. The usual amount of solution to be given by this method is 2 to 5 ml, *except* to the middeltoid, where the usual amount is 0.5 to 2 ml. It is recommended to divide a 4- or 5-ml dose in half, using two different sites for injecting the medication. Identification of suitable sites for an injection is based on the use of definite anatomic landmarks, located by palpation. Four anatomic sites commonly used follow.

TABLE 7-11

Common Sizes of Syringes and Needles and uses

Type of Injection	Size of Syringe	Size of Needle	Example for Use
Subcutaneous	2, 2½, or 3 cc	½ in. or ⅝ in., 23- or 26-gauge	Immunizations, heparin
Intramuscular	2 to 5 cc	1½ in. (1 in. for thin or small patients, 2-3 in. for obese patients), 21- or 22-gauge 1½ in., 20-gauge	Analgesics, vitamins, various antibiotics, and hormones Penicillin and thick solutions
Intradermal	1 cc	¼ in., ½ in., ⅜ in., 26- or 27-gauge	Schick, Dick, tuberculin, and allergy skin tests
Insulin	³⁄₁₀ cc, ½ cc, .5 cc, or 1 cc calibrated in units	½ in. or ⅝ in., 27- to 29-gauge	Insulin
Intravenous	10, 20, or 50 cc	1¼ in., 1½ in., 22-gauge 1 to 1½ in., 18-, 19-, 20-, or 21-gauge	Penicillin IV drip, transfusions Glucose, blood tests

Gluteus Medius or Dorsogluteal

The most common site for intramuscular injections, this is located in the upper outer quadrant (UOQ) of the buttock. Have the patient assume a prone position, toes pointed inward, with the buttock clearly exposed. This position allows for best relaxation of the muscles and best exposure of the area. Injecting a needle into a tense muscle causes pain. Undergarments must be completely removed. Under no circumstances must you deviate from using the correct technique. Palpate for and then draw a diagonal line from the greater trochanter of the femur to the posterior superior iliac spine. The injection is to be given *well above and outside* of this diagonal line. The upper limit of the site is an area several inches below the iliac crest. These landmarks must be palpated to ensure the correct location for the injection. Extreme care must be taken to locate the correct site to avoid hitting the sciatic nerve or the superior gluteal artery (Figure 7-15).

Middeltoid Area

This site is located on the upper, outer aspect of the arm, below the lower edge of the acromion and above the axilla. Although there is easy access to this site when the patient is standing, sitting, or in a prone or supine position, the actual area that can be used for the injection is limited, because there are major vessels, nerves, and bones to be avoided in the upper arm. Therefore it is recommended to limit the use this of site for injections because this small area can tolerate only small amounts of medication and infrequent injections. In addition, patients often experience more pain and tenderness in this area (Figure 7-16).

It is often a preferred site by some for giving vaccinations and some lipid-soluble analgesics, but it is generally not considered to be the first choice for other drugs.

Ventrogluteal area (von Hochstetter's site)

Growing in recognition for use, this site is removed from major blood vessels and nerves. To locate this site, have the patient in a supine or side position. Palpate for the greater trochanter of the femur, the iliac crest, and the anterior superior iliac spine. Then place the palm of your right hand on the patient's left greater trochanter and your index finger on the anterior superior iliac spine and move your middle finger posteriorly along the iliac crest as far as possible. (Do this with your left hand when injecting into the patient's right side.) A V space is now formed between your index and middle finger. The injection is to be given in the middle of this V space (Figures 7-17 and 7-18).

Vastus Lateralis*

This thick muscle on the upper side of the leg is also being used more frequently because it is free of major blood vessels and nerves. With the patient in a supine position, locate this site by palpating the greater trochanter of the femur and the lateral aspect of the patella. Divide the distance between these two landmarks into thirds. The needle is to be inserted into the middle third of this area (Figures 7-19 and 7-20).

Subcutaneous injections

The objective of a subcutaneous (sc) injection is to deposit a relatively small amount of an aqueous solution under the skin for fairly rapid absorption into the bloodstream. The amount of the solution given by this method should not exceed 2 ml. To avoid overdistention of the tissues, the medication should be administered slowly. The most common and preferred sites for a subcutaneous injection are these:

---

*When intramuscular injections are administered to children, both the ventrogluteal and the vastus lateralis sites are recommended.

Figure 7-15 A, *Gluteus medius IM injection site;* B, *dorso-gluteal-adult; posterior view of gluteal region and thigh;* C, *dorsogluteal-pediatric; posterior view of gluteal region and thigh.*

Figure 7-16 *Middeltoid IM injection site.* A, *Deltoid—adult; lateral view of shoulder and arm;* B, *deltoid—pediatric; anterior view of shoulder and arm.*

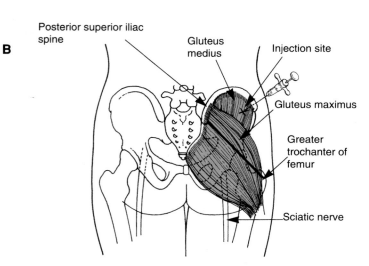

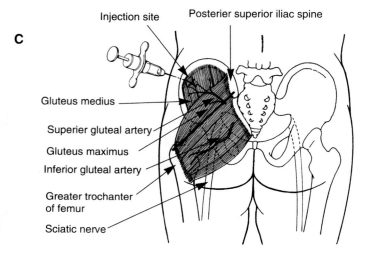

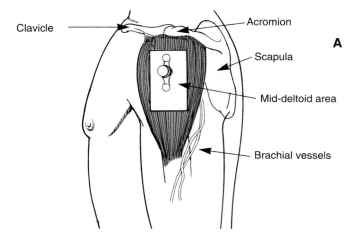

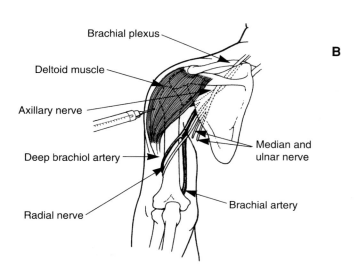

* Outer surface of the upper arm, usually halfway between the shoulder and elbow
* Lateral aspect of the thigh
* Upper two thirds of the back

Additional sites that may be used, especially when the medication it is self-administered, as a diabetic may do, include:

* Areas on the abdomen
* Front aspect of the thigh

When frequent subcutaneous injections are given, sites of administration should be rotated to prevent the damage of a tissue, excessive pain, and possible disfigurement (Figure 7-21).

Intradermal Injections

The objective of the intradermal injection is to inject a minute amount of solution between the layers of the skin. The

Figure 7-17 A, *Ventrogluteal IM injection site;* **B,** *ventro-gluteal—pediatric; lateral view of gluteal region and thigh.*

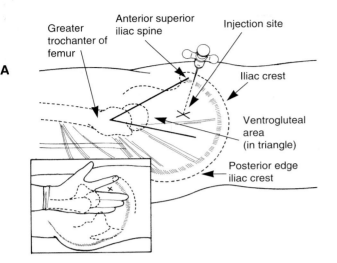

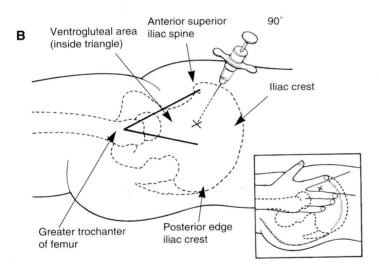

Figure 7-19 A, *Vastus lateralis IM injection site;* **B,** *vastus lateralis—pediatric; anterior view of the thigh.*

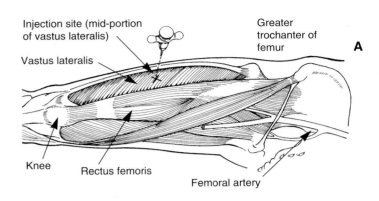

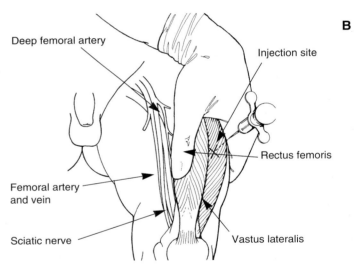

Figure 7-18 *Ventrogluteal area on a 130-pound boy.*

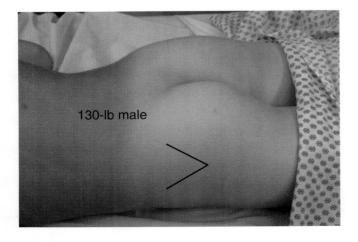

amount of drug given by this method is usually 0.1 ml to 0.3 ml. A tuberculin syringe (see Figure 7-9) is used because of the fine calibrations, which provide the best means for measuring minute amounts of a drug. Drugs must be administered slowly in this method; they produce a small, pale bump on the skin when given correctly.

The most common and preferred site for intradermal injections is the ventral surface of the forearm, approximately 4 inches below the elbow. The lateral and posterior sides of the arm can also be used if and when required because they can be easily observed for reactions to the drug injected and they also can be kept free of irritation from clothing. Intradermal injections are used for various skin tests to determine allergies (sensitivities) to drugs and various other foreign substances such as food substances, dust, and grass; to determine

Figure 7-20 A, *Vastus lateralis area on 135-pound female;* B, *Vastus lateralis area on 180-pound male.*

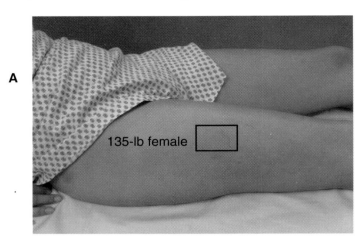

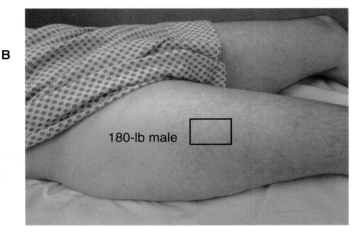

Figure 7-21 *Subcutaneous injection sites.*

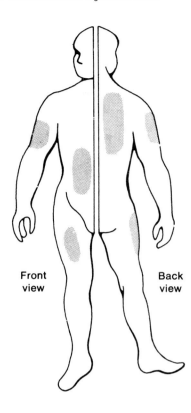

the patient's susceptibility to an infectious disease, such as tuberculosis (the Mantoux text) and diphtheria (the Schick test); or to aid in the diagnosis of infectious diseases. In addition to their frequent use for these tests, intradermal tests are used in the diagnosis of parasitic infections such as schistosomiasis and fungal diseases.

Because intradermal injections are used for skin tests, the procedure for administering the injection is discussed and outlined as follows. For more information on intradermal injections, see Unit Eight. Preparation of the syringe and needle and withdrawal of the drug into the syringe are the same as for the IM and sc injections, except that a ³/₈- or ¹/₂-inch, 26- or 27-gauge needle, and a tuberculin syringe are used. The needle is inserted, bevel facing up, only about ¹/₈-inch (or until just the bevel is under the surface of the skin).

Administration of an Intradermal Injection
Assemble the following equipment:
- Alcohol sponge or skin antiseptic and cotton ball
- Tuberculin syringe because fine calibrations are needed (0.5 or 1.0 ml) (see Figure 7-9)
- Needle ³/₈ or ¹/₂ inch, 26- or 27-gauge (see Figure 7-7)
- Solution to be injected
- Disposable single-use exam gloves

In addition to the rules listed on pages 265 to 268, the following apply to injections:
1. Select the injection site carefully. You must avoid major blood vessels, nerves, and bones.
2. Use only sterile, preferably disposable, syringes and needles (Figure 7-22).
3. Select the correct size of syringe according to the amount of medication to be given and the appropriate size and length of needle, depending on the type of solution to be given and the size and condition of the patient.
4. Insert the needle, using the correct angle (Figure 7-23).
5. After inserting the needle, but before injecting the medication, always pull the plunger back to determine if you have entered a blood vessel (except when injecting heparin or insulin subcutaneously or when giving a drug intradermally).
6. If you have entered a blood vessel, you may withdraw the needle a bit, redirect, and again insert the needle. Pull the plunger back to determine if you have entered a second blood vessel, or some recommend removing the needle and beginning the procedure over again as stated in No. 7.
7. If a large amount of blood returns in the syringe when you pull back on the plunger, remove the needle and begin the procedure again, using new medication, syringe, and needle.
8. Rotate injection sites on patients receiving frequent injections.
9. Aseptic technique must be used when administering all injections.

10. OSHA's Universal Precautions Standards state: "Gloves shall be worn when it can be reasonably anticipated that the employee may have hand contact with blood, other potentially infectious materials, mucous membranes, and nonintact skin; when performing vascular access procedures; and when handling or touching contaminated items or surfaces." Therefore wearing gloves for administering an injection is highly recommended by most professionals. You have to make this decision on the basis of each situation and patient and according to agency policy. The employer must have gloves readily accessible for your use if you decide to wear gloves for administering injections.

11. Dispose of used needles and sharps into the puncture-resistant containers immediately.

12. Allow refrigerated drugs to warm to room temperature before injecting (unless otherwise instructed by the manufacturer's literature).

13. Allow the skin disinfectant to dry before giving the injection. If the skin is not dry before the injection is given, some of the disinfectant can be forced into subcutaneous tissue and cause more discomfort to the patient.

14. To help in reducing pain to the patient, insert and remove the needle quickly.

Figure 7-22 *Prepackaged tray of sterile intradermal syringes for allergy testing.*

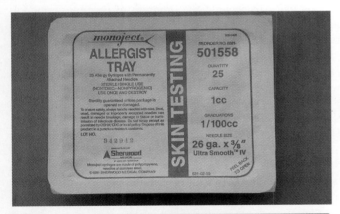

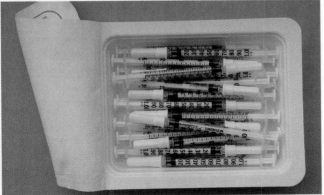

15. Inject the medication slowly. Rapid injection can cause sudden distention of the tissue and more discomfort.

MANTOUX TEST FOR TUBERCULOSIS

The standard test recommended by the American Lung Association to help detect infection with *Mycobacterium tuberculosis* is the Mantoux test. The Mantoux test is performed by injecting intradermally exactly 0.1 ml of tuberculin purified protein derivative (PPD). This dose contains 5 tuberculin units (TU) or tuberculin PPD. The reaction is read 48 to 72 hours later. Only induration is considered when interpreting the test results.

GUIDELINES FOR PREVENTING NEEDLESTICKS

1. Slow down and *think* when using or disposing of needles.
2. *DO NOT recap* needles unless absolutely necessary. If necessary, place cap on table top before inserting needle (insert needle into cap without holding cap) (Figure 7-24).
3. When using syringes that have a safety shield, learn how to use them proficiently before you use them. After giving an injection, slide the cover over the needle and lock it in place (see Figures 7-6, 7-10, and 7-11).
4. Never put a needle down—dispose of it promptly in approved container.
5. Never put needles or other sharp instruments in trash cans, your pocket, or linen containers.
6. Never leave needles or other sharp instruments on counter tops, examination tables, or disposable procedure trays.
7. Never push a needle into the sharps container with your hand. If the needle does not go into the opening easily, use a large syringe to push it in.
8. Never try to remove a needle or syringe from the sharps container.

Figure 7-23 *Angles of insertion for parenteral injections.*

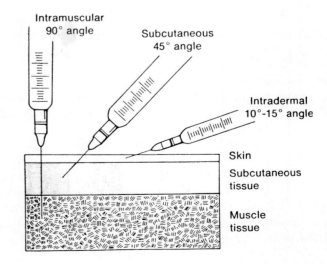

Figure 7-24 *When you have to cap a needle, place needle cap on its side on a flat surface. Insert needle into cap without holding the cap. Secure the cap on the needle by pushing it against a vertical surface such as a closet door or the wall. Keep your other hand behind your back during this procedure. This technique has been approved by OSHA.*

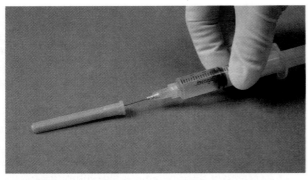

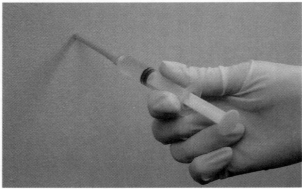

9. Pick up improperly discarded needles with extreme caution and dispose of them in the nearest sharps container. Do not attempt to cap the needle; use tongs or forceps to pick up sharps. Wash your hands after you dispose of the needle.

There are more than two dozen needlestick-prevention devices on the market. Hospitals and health care agencies are starting to test and adopt some of the new technologies. When you encounter any of these for use, make sure that you are proficient in the technique for using the device before you use it so that the purpose of the device and technique are ensured.

CAUTION: Some authorities believe that some of the devices may even increase needlesticks by giving the user a false sense of security and a feeling that he or she does not have to be vigilant about proper technique. *There is no substitution for proper technique. This must not be forgotten regardless of any device on the market.*

If a reusable injector and medication in a prefilled sterile cartridge-needle unit are used, the method for giving the medication is basically the same as when using a disposable or reusable syringe. After use, you should clean the reusable injector with an antiseptic solution. Sterilization is not required since the injector does not come in direct with the patient.

USING THE TUBEX INJECTOR

For the procedure for using this newer type of injector and sterile cartridge-needle unit, see Figure 7-25.

INSULIN INJECTIONS

Insulin is a hormone produced in the body by the beta cells of the islands of Langerhans in the pancreas. It is secreted in response to increased levels of glucose in the bloodstream. Insulin takes part in the regulation of the processes necessary for the metabolism of proteins, fats, and carbohydrates and regulates the metabolism of glucose. Insulin lowers blood glucose levels and aids in the transport of glucose from the blood to the muscle cells and other tissues. Insulin deficiency results in hyperglycemia and can also result in diabetes mellitus.

Insulin preparations are used to treat all Type I (insulin-dependent, formerly called juvenile-onset diabetes) diabetes patients and some Type II (noninsulin-dependent formerly called mature or adult-onset) diabetes patients whose blood glucose levels are acutely elevated (as may be seen during an infection or trauma), who become pregnant, or who need insulin only until they lose enough weight, *or* for Type III—gestational diabetes.

Insulin use is a type of replacement therapy; it restores the ability of the cells to use glucose as an energy source and to correct the metabolic derangements seen in the different types of diabetes. The goal is to mimic the body's normal production and use of insulin. Special regimens are designed for each patient according to his or her needs. In addition to taking insulin, the patient must be educated about diabetes; the special care, diet, and treatment needed; and the complications that can occur if the program of therapy is not followed diligently. It is highly recommended that the patient's family also receive diabetic education so that they can provide support to the patient and care if needed in time of emergency. (See also Insulin Reaction and Diabetic Coma in Unit Seventeen).

Insulin Preparations and Concentrations

Different types of insulin preparations and concentrations are available. The most common types are listed in Table 7-12. In the United States, the most common concentration of insulin is U-100 (100 units of insulin per milliliter). However, U-500 is also available (see Figure 7-8 for different types of insulin syringes).

Injection Sites and Factors That Influence Absorption of Insulin

Insulin is administered by a subcutaneous injection given into the abdomen, arms, thighs, and buttocks.

Insulin absorption rates and timing can vary for a patient. Insulin is absorbed at different rates, varying with the injection site. For example, the timing of insulin injected into the thigh can vary as much as 50% from the same amount of insulin given into the abdomen, resulting in variable insulin

Text continues on page 294.

Figure 7-25 *Technique for using the Tubex Injector (closed injection system). Method of administration is the same as with conventional syringe. Remove needle cover by grasping it securely; twist and pull. Introduce needle into patient, aspirate by pulling back slightly on the plunger, and inject.*

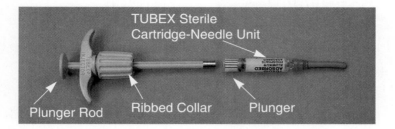

TUBEX Sterile
Cartridge-Needle Unit

Plunger Rod   Ribbed Collar   Plunger

HOW TO LOAD

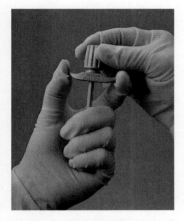

1. Turn the ribbed collar to the "OPEN" position until it stops.

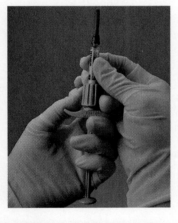

2. Hold injector with the open end up and fully insert the TUBEX sterile cartridge-needle unit.

Firmly tighten the ribbed collar in the direction of the "CLOSE" arrow.

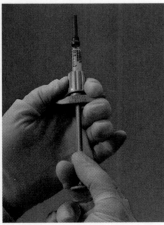

3. Thread the plunger rod into the plunger of the TUBEX sterile cartridge-needle until slight resistance is felt.

The injector is now ready for use in the usual manner.

HOW TO UNLOAD AND DISCARD USED UNIT

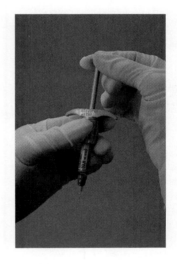

1. Do not recap the needle. Disengage the plunger rod.

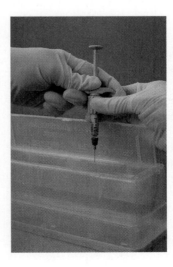

2. Hold the injector, needle down, over a needle disposal container and loosen the ribbed collar. Tubex cartridge-needle unit will drop into the container. The TUBEX Injector is reusable; do not discard.

ADMINISTRATION OF AN INTRAMUSCULAR INJECTION

Equipment

Appropriate-sized sterile needle and syringe, depending on amount and type of drug to be given (usually a 2- or 3-cc syringe, and a 21- or 22-gauge, 1½-inch needle) *or* hypodermic metal syringe when the medication is supplied in a prefilled sterile cartridge-needle unit such as a Tubex hypodermic metal syringe.

A 23-gauge, 2-inch needle may be used when administering the drug into the deltoid muscle.
Sterile alcohol sponges
Medication ordered
Small tray
Disposable single-use exam gloves

PROCEDURE	RATIONALE
1. Wash your hands. **Use appropriate personal protective equipment (PPE) as dictated by facility.**	
2. Assemble the equipment.	
3. Prepare the syringe and needle for use. When using a separate syringe and needle, remove them from the wrappers and leave the cover (sheath) on the needle intact. Grasping the hub of the needle and the barrel of the syringe, attach the hub of the needle to the tip of the syringe. Secure by turning the hub ¼ inch clockwise. Avoid touching the tip of the syringe and the open end of the hub of the needle with your fingers.	*The tip of the syringe and the open end of the needle are to remain sterile.*
4. Compare the physician's order with the label on the medication.	*These must be the same. At times you may have to calculate the dosage to be given.*
5. Check the label of the medication three times during the preparation of the medication to ensure that you have the correct medication and strength: • When removing the medication from storage area • When filling the syringe • When replacing the medication in the storage area	*The same medication is often supplied in different strengths.*
6. Take an alcohol sponge to cleanse the rubber stopper of the vial or the neck of the ampule; then discard this sponge. Withdraw medication into the syringe.	*Cleansing helps prevent the introduction of microorganisms into the vial and prevents contamination of the needle.*
If an ampule is used: a. Tap the tip of the ampule to dislodge any medication there. b. Cleanse the neck at the marked line. c. Hold the ampule; with your other hand, cover the top end with a sponge, and break the top off going away from you (Figure 7-26). The medication is now ready for use. d. Remove the needle cover (sheath). Do not touch the opening of the ampule with the needle. e. Insert the needle into the ampule (Figure 7-27). f. Pull back on the plunger of the syringe to withdraw the required amount of medication. g. Remove the needle from the ampule. h. Replace the needle cover (sheath) over the needle, using the one-handed method (see Figure 7-24) or a recapping device.	*The sponge is used to protect your fingers when the top is broken off.* *The needle is contaminated if it touches the outside or entrance of the ampule. In this instance, you must obtain another sterile needle for use.*

ADMINISTRATION OF AN INTRAMUSCULAR INJECTION—cont'd

PROCEDURE	RATIONALE
i. Place this unit on a small tray.	
j. Check the label, and then discard the ampule or keep the ampule with the syringe until after the medication has been administered, and then discard both in the used sharps container.	*Keeping the ampule with the syringe containing the drug is good for identification purposes.*
k. Proceed to the patient, carrying this medication and a sterile alcohol sponge on the small tray.	

If a vial is used,

PROCEDURE	RATIONALE
a. Take the syringe and pull the plunger back to obtain a measured amount of air equal to the amount of medication to be withdrawn from the vial.	
b. Remove the needle cover.	
c. Insert the needle through the cleansed rubber stopper, keeping it above the solutions (Figure 7-28, A).	
d. Push the plunger of the syringe down to the bottom of the barrel (see Figure 7-28, A).	*This gives air replacement, which prevents the creation of a vacuum in the vial when the medication is withdrawn. If a vacuum is created, it makes it difficult to withdraw the medication. Do not inject more air than is required because the pressure in the vial then forces the solution into the syringe, making it difficult to obtain an accurate dosage*
e. Invert the vial; have the vial and syringe at eye level (see Figure 7-28, B).	*Keep the vial and syringe at eye level to ensure correct measurement of the drug withdrawn.*
f. With the needle opening in the solution, pull the plunger of the syringe back gently until the required amount of medication has been obtained (see Figure 7-28, B).	
g. Remove any air bubbles in the syringe by tapping the barrel with your fingertips until all of the air bubbles have disappeared (Figure 7-28, C). Check again to make sure that you have the required amount of drug in the syringe before removing the needle from the vial.	
h. Remove the needle from the vial.	
i. Replace the needle cover over the needle, using a recapping device or a one-hand method.	*Prevent contamination of the needle.*

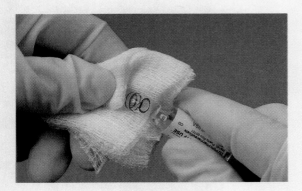

Figure 7-26 *Technique for breaking top off ampule.*

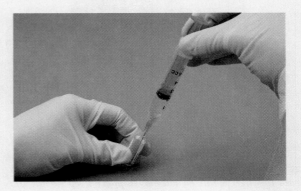

Figure 7-27 *Insert needle into ampule and pull back on syringe plunger to withdraw the medication.*

ADMINISTRATION OF AN INTRAMUSCULAR INJECTION—cont'd

PROCEDURE	RATIONALE
j. Place the filled syringe with the covered needle on a small tray.	*Ensure that the correct medication will be administered.*
k. Check the label on the vial, and replace it in the correct storage area.	
l. Proceed to the patient, carrying the medication and a sterile alcohol sponge on the small tray.	
7. Identify the patient, and explain the procedure.	*Correct patient identification is crucial. Explanations help gain the patient's cooperation and relaxation.*
8. Select the injection site and position the patient accordingly, exposing the site clearly. Refer to Anatomic Selection of Injection Sites, page 278. Your view of and accessibility to the injection site must not be obstructed by the patient's clothing or any drape sheet. Be sure that you have ample lighting when administering the injection.	
9. Don disposable single-use exam gloves.	
10. With the alcohol sponge, cleanse the injection site, starting at a central point and moving out to an area approximately 2 inches square; allow it to dry.	
11. Remove the needle cover.	
12. Hold the syringe with the needle facing upward; slowly push on the plunger until a tiny drop of medication comes to the needle tip.	*This helps get rid of air bubbles, which must be expelled from the syringe before injecting the medication. Also, the tiny drop of medication obtained at the top of the syringe ensures that the needle is clear and not plugged.*
13. Using the index finger and thumb of your nondominant hand, spread or tense the skin around the injection site. For the deltoid and vastus lateralis sites grasp the skin. This technique works best on these muscles.	*Spreading the skin will make the skin taut. This make needle insertion easier.*

A

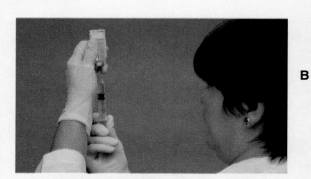

B

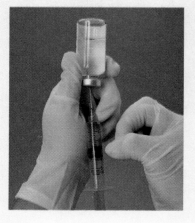

C

Figure 7-28 *Withdrawing medication from vial. A, Insert needle through cleansed rubber stopper; keep needle above level of solution; push plunger down; B, hold syringe at eye level to ensure correct measurement of medication; C, keep syringe in a vertical position tap barrel to remove any air bubbles.*

ADMINISTRATION OF AN INTRAMUSCULAR INJECTION—cont'd

PROCEDURE

For the deltoid and vastus lateralis sites grasp the skin. This technique works best on these muscles.

14. Using your dominant hand, hold the syringe and needle as if you were holding a pencil, with the bevel of the needle facing up (Figure 7-29, A). Your index finger and second finger may surround the top part of the needle hub with your thumb placed on the end of the syringe; or all three fingers may surround the bottom end of the syringe near the needle, but not touching the needle.

15. With a quick thrust, insert the needle at a 90-degree angle to about three fourths of the needle length. Do not hit the skin with the hub of the needle (Figure 7-29 B). Hold the needle perpendicular to the skin, and insert quickly in a dartlike thrust.

16. Steady the syringe with your dominant hand. Using your other hand, pull back on the plunger to see if any blood can be aspirated into the syringe (Figure 7-30). If you have entered a blood vessel, withdraw the needle slightly, redirect, and reinsert; then pull back on the plunger again to check for blood. Some recommend completely withdrawing the needle if a blood vessel is entered and beginning the procedure again with a new needle, syringe, and medication.

17. Continue to steady the syringe with your dominant hand. With your other hand, push on the plunger *slowly* to inject the medication.

18. Using your nondominant hand, apply pressure at the injection site with the alcohol sponge, and quickly remove the needle with your dominant hand (the hand that has constantly been on the syringe and needle unit).

RATIONALE

Aspiration must be done to check if you have entered a blood vessel.

Injection of the medication slowly allows the solution to disperse into the tissues. Discomfort caused by pressure will result if the medication is injected too quickly.

Applied pressure and the quick withdrawal of the needle reduces discomfort and the risk of medication leaking into the subcutaneous tissues and possibly forming abscesses.
NOTE: By keeping your dominant hand in constant contact with the syringe and needle unit, rather than switching hands after inserting the needle as some suggest (that is, inserting the needle with your dominant hand, then changing hands and steadying the syringe with your nondominant hand, then using your dominant hand to aspirate and push on the plunger), you help prevent further discomfort to the patient and tissue irritation that may occur if the syringe is jiggled or moved during a hand change.

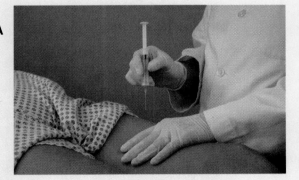
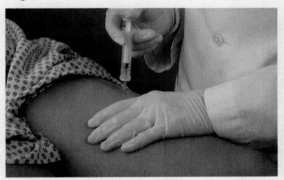

Figure 7-29 A, *Giving intramuscular injection. Hold syringe and needle in pencil or dartlike grip; insert at 90-degree angle.* **B,** *Insert at 90-degree angle with a quick thrust. Do not hit skin with hub of needle.*

ADMINISTRATION OF AN INTRAMUSCULAR INJECTION—cont'd

PROCEDURE	RATIONALE
19. Massage the injection site. Move the tissue as you massage, not merely the sponge (Figure 7-31). If rapid absorption is desired, continue to massage the area for about 2 minutes.	*Massaging the area helps spread the medication in the tissue.*
20. Help the patient assume a comfortable and safe position.	
21. Observe the patient for any unusual reactions such as a rash or shock.	
22. Inform the patient if he or she is free to leave or if the physician requires additional consultation time.	
23. Place a disposable needle and syringe in a puncture-resistant container without breaking or recapping the needle. The needle box should be in the room or as close as possible to the area of use (Figure 7-32). After using a reusable syringe and needle, flush tap water through both until clean. Separate the needle, barrel, and plunger, and place each in a designated cleansing solution until ready to prepare all for sterilization.	*To protect the physician, medical assistant, and janitorial staff. Needle recapping and disposal are frequent causes of needlesticks.*
24. Remove gloves.	
25. Wash your hands.	

26. Record the procedure on the patient's chart.	*Charting example:*
	June 3, 19____, 4 p.m.
	    Penbritin-S 500 mg IM in ROQ [right outer quadrant] of buttock, for respiratory tract infection.
	    Brook Thomas, CMA

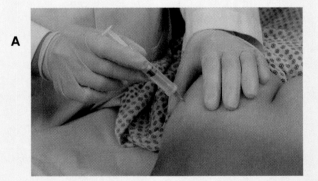

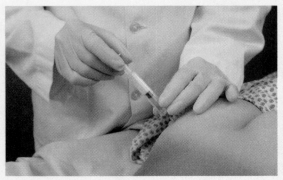

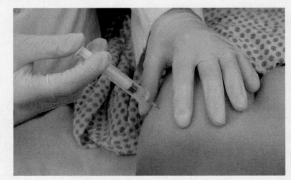

Figure 7-30 A, *Insert needle with a quick thrust. Do not hit skin with hub of needle.* **B,** *Pull back on plunger to determine if the needle entered a blood vessel.* **C,** *Intramuscular injection technique.*

ADMINISTRATION OF AN INTRAMUSCULAR INJECTION—cont'd

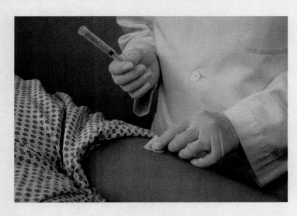

Figure 7-31 *After the injection has been administered, massage and cleanse injection site with sponge to remove any blood or medication that might be present.*

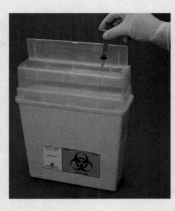

Figure 7-32 *Puncture-resistant containers marked "Bio–hazard" must be used to dispose of used syringes.*

TABLE 7-12

Insulin Preparations

Type (Classification)	Onset of Action*	Peak Action*	Duration of Action*
1.Regular (short-acting))	Within 1 hour (15-60 minutes)	2 to 4 hours	5 to 8 hours
2. Semilente (short-acting)	30 to 60 minutes	4 to 6 hours	8 to 12 hours
3. Lente (intermediate-acting)	1 to 4 hours	6 to 10 hours	12 to 24 hours
4. NPH (intermediate-acting)	1 to 4 hours	6 to 10 hours	12 to 24 hours
5. Human Ultralente (intermediate-acting)	1 to 4 hours	6 to 10 hours	12 to 24 hours
6. Animal Ultralente (long-acting)	3 to 6 hours	14 to 20 hours	24 to 36 hours
7. 70/30: mixture of NPH (70%)— and Regular (30%)	See timing for each above.		

* Approximate ranges only.
Insulin should be stored in a refrigerator. Some bottles that are currently used can be stored at room temperature out of direct sunlight for 1 month. Read the manufacturer's directions carefully.
Regular insulin should be clear. All other types should be uniformly cloudy after rolled in your hands before use. DO NOT use the insulin if it looks clumpy or stays in precipitation after you roll it in your hands.

INTRAMUSCULAR Z-TRACT TECHNIQUE

The alternate intramuscular injection technique is called the **Z**:-tract technique. It can be used for an iron injection, which may cause irritation of subcutaneous tissue and discoloration from leaking medications, or when complete absorption of the medication by the muscle tissue is crucial. The preferred site for this technique is the upper outer quadrant of the buttock.

In this technique the tissue is pulled down and toward the median before, during, and after the injection. When the tissue is released, the needle track that is created is a **Z** pattern rather than the straight needle track that is created in other intramuscular injections. The **Z** pattern tract keeps the medication deep in the muscle and prevents seepage up through the tissues.

Use a 2-inch needle if the patient weighs approximately 200 pounds. If you don't use a needle 2 inches long on a patient of this weight, you will need to insert the needle its full length and then indent the tissue with the hub of the needle to ensure deep muscle penetration.

Use a 1 1/4- to 1 1/2-inch needle if the patient weighs around 100 pounds. Use a 3/4 to 1-inch needle on children weighing around 50 pounds.

Follow steps 1 through 12 as outlined on pages 286 to 288, under Administration of an Intramuscular Injection, *except* that you should change needles after you have drawn the medication into the syringe. This eliminates the chance of medication left in the needle leaking into the tissue during the injection or of an extra "needle's worth" of medication being given. This minute extra amount of drug is of less concern with adult patients than it is with children, for whom even minute quantities of drug may be significant. Now use the following procedure.

PROCEDURE

13. Move the skin downward and toward the median.

14. Insert the needle at a 90-degree angle while maintaining traction on the tissue.

15. Extend the thumb and index finger of the hand that is displacing the tissue to support the base of the syringe and aspirate by pulling back on the plunger with your other hand.
Maintain traction on the tissue. If blood appears, select a new site and use a new needle.

16. Inject slowly and smoothly while maintaining traction on the tissue.

17. Wait 10 seconds; then withdraw the needle and immediately release the skin, creating a **Z** pattern, which blocks any infiltration of the medication into the subcutaneous tissue.

18. DO NOT MASSAGE THE INJECTION SITE. If bleeding occurs, gently wipe the area with a dry sterile cotton ball or gauze.

19. Advise the patient not to exercise or wear tight clothing immediately after the injection.

20. Continue with steps 20 through 26 on page 290, Administration of an Intramuscular Injection.

RATIONALE

The skin and subcutaneous tissue of an average adult moves about 1 to 1.6 inches. The underlying muscle within the selected injection site remains stationary.

You may damage subcutaneous tissue and cause pain if traction is released while the needle is in place.

Waiting provides time for the medication to disperse into the muscle and gives the muscle time to relax.

This minimizes the change of the medication spreading into other layers of tissue.

ADMINISTRATION OF A SUBCUTANEOUS INJECTION

Equipment

Sterile needle and syringe; usually a 2-cc syringe, 1/2 or 5/8-inch, 25-gauge needle (a 23- or 27-gauge needle could be also be used)
Sterile alcohol sponges
Medication ordered
Small tray to transport prepared medication to the patient
Disposable single-use exam gloves

Preparation of the needle, syringe, and medication follows the same procedure that was outlined under Administration of an Intramuscular Injection. Remember to wash your hands before beginning the procedure, check the medication label three times, measure dosage accurately, identify the patient and explain the procedure, position the patient, and select the injection site correctly before administering the medication.

Follow steps 1 through 12 as outlined under the intramuscular injection technique on pages 320 to 323 and then continue as follows.

PROCEDURE

13. Grasp the skin surrounding the injection area between your thumb and index finger, or spread the skin and hold it taut.

14. Hold the barrel of the syringe between your thumb and the other fingers of your dominant hand, letting the hub of the needle rest on your index finger. The bevel of the needle should be facing upward.

15. Insert the needle at a 45-degree angle into the skin, using a quick, forward thrust (Figure 7-33). The needle should be inserted almost to its full length. Do not touch the skin with the hub of the needle.

16. Release the skin.

17. Keep your dominant hand on the syringe for support. With your other hand, pull back on the plunger to see if you aspirate any blood. Refer to steps 16 through 23, Administering an Intramuscular Injection, for full explanations of the remaining steps.

18. Inject the medication slowly.

19. With an alcohol sponge, apply gentle pressure to the injection site, and quickly remove the needle.

20. Massage the injection site with the alcohol sponge, and observe the patient for any unusual reaction.
    NOTE: *Do not* massage the injection site after administering allergy injections or heparin. Only apply pressure for these injections.

21. Leave the patient safe and comfortable, providing any further instructions.

RATIONALE

The decision of which method to use depends on the size of the patient and the size of the needle. You may grasp the skin on small, very thin, or dehydrated patients; you may spread the skin on large, well-nourished patients. Whichever method you use, be sure that you enter subcutaneous tissue when inserting the needle.

Applying gentle pressure prevents the skin from being pulled along with the needle.

Massaging the tissue after giving heparin can cause dispersal of the heparin, resulting in a hematoma.

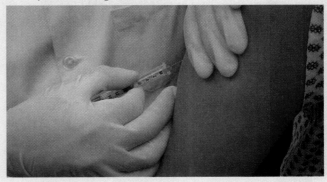

Figure 7-33 *Technique for administering a subcutaneous injection. Insert needle at a 45-degree angle.*

ADMINISTRATION OF A SUBCUTANEOUS INJECTION—cont'd

PROCEDURE

22. Remove and dispose of used equipment properly. Do *not* recap the needle. Place disposable syringe and needle in a puncture-resistant container for used sharps. See No. 23, page 290.

23. Remove gloves.

24. Wash hands.

25. Record the procedure on the patient's chart.

RATIONALE

Charting example:
June 2, 19____, 2 p.m.
Thiomerin [a diuretic] 1 ml, sc in left upper arm.
Kathy Kron, CMA

---

effects and blood glucose levels. Therefore *rotating injection sites is no longer recommended*. However, *it is recommended* that each injection site be about 1 inch from the last site used in the *same body area* (that is, if given in the abdomen, the next injection would be given in the abdomen 1 inch away from that site). This method not only prevents tissue damage, but it increases the predictability of the effects of the insulin. Each site should not be used more than once every 30 days.

Other factors that affect the absorption rate of insulin include the following:

• Angle and depth of the injection
• Vascularity of the injection site
• Physical activity (for example, jogging after an injection into the thigh)
• Temperature (for example, increased after jogging or taking a hot bath)

The abdominal sites are preferred because absorption from these sites is rapid and unaffected by exercise. The arms are the second sites that provide the fastest absorption rate of insulin, followed by the thighs and buttocks. These last three areas are acceptable, especially for pregnant patients and for those who are taking more than two injections per day. For patients who wish to use more than the abdominal sites and who are taking more than two injections per day, the recommendation is to be consistent in the use of one area for each injection time. For example, insulin taken before breakfast would always be given in the abdomen, and insulin taken before lunch would always be given in the arm.

Procedure For Insulin Injections

1. Insulin should always be given 30 minutes *before* a meal.
2. Each injection site should be 1 inch away from the last site used.
3. Cleanse skin with alcohol and allow it to dry before inserting the needle.
4. Inject at a 90-degree angle *unless* the patient is very thin; then inject the needle at a 45-degree angle.
5. Insert the needle *quickly*. This minimizes discomfort.
6. If you grasped the tissue to insert the needle, let go of the skin before you inject the insulin. Pressure from the grasp can lead to insulin leakage.
7. Inject the insulin slowly. This allows tissue expansion and minimizes pressure that could cause leakage of some of the insulin.
8. Withdraw the needle quickly. Quick withdrawal minimizes a track for insulin leakage.
9. *Do not* rub the injection site after withdrawing the needle. Rubbing the injection site can vary the absorption rate.
10. *Do not* use the same site more than once every 30 days.
11. *Do not* rotate injection sites.
12. When mixing Regular Insulin with a longer-acting insulin, you must follow the manufacturer's recommendation, which states that you must always first draw up the clear Regular Insulin into the syringe, and then draw up the second insulin (for example, NPH).

Procedure for Reconstituting a Powdered Drug for Administration

1. Using a syringe and needle, insert the needle through the cleansed rubber stopper of the vial containing the diluent.
2. Withdraw the amount of liquid diluent that is to be added to the powdered drug.
3. Insert the needle through the cleansed rubber stopper of the vial containing the diluent and withdraw the amount of liquid needed. (See step 6, Administration of an Intramuscular Injection, for the steps to take to withdraw a solution from a vial.)
4. Add this liquid to the vial containing the powdered drug.
5. Remove the needle from the vial.
6. Discard the syringe and needle in the used sharps container.
7. Roll the vial between your hands. This mixes the liquid with the powdered drug.
8. Observe the solution obtained to make sure that all of the powdered drug has been mixed and dissolved. The solution should be clear (or cloudy if it is a suspension).
9. Label a multiple-dose vial with the date and time of preparation, the expiration date, the dilution/strength of the medication prepared, and your initials. Labeling as stated is very important because reconstituted drugs are stable for only a short period of time.
10. Using a new syringe and needle, insert the needle into the reconstituted medication and withdraw the desired amount of medication to be given to patient.
11. Using gloves, place a new needle on the syringe and select an appropriate site for injection.
12. Insert the needle into the appropriate injection site and withdraw the plunger to observe for any blood return. If blood return is noted, remove the needle/syringe and apply pressure with gauze to the site to control any bleeding. Select an alternate injection site.
13. If no blood is noted on aspiration of plunger, repeat step 12; inject medication slowly, remove the needle/syringe, and apply pressure with gauze.
14. *Do not* recap the needle, but place the used needle/syringe directly in the sharps container.
15. Place any soiled gauze or gloves in biohazard trash.
16. Store any remaining drug according to the manufacturer's directions. Some drugs may have to be placed in a refrigerator.

CONCLUSION

Having completed this unit, you should be able to discuss the laws regulating the distribution and administration of medication, in addition to the responsibilities and rules governing the administration of all types of medication. Certain legal stipulations are set forth that a physician must meet before using narcotics. You should be familiar with the special laws of your state and know how you can best help your physician comply with the state and federal laws applying to the dispensing, administering, and prescribing of medications, including narcotics and controlled substances. Knowledge of and familiarity with resource reference books on drugs are necessary to ensure adequate knowledge of any medication you are required to administer. Numerous references provide information on improved medication techniques and current pharmacologic products.

Check with your instructor for additional assignments and reference sources in areas of your own particular interest and need.

A variety of ways in which medications may be administered has been discussed in this unit. You must be able to describe all nine routes of administration and demonstrate your ability to administer an intramuscular and a subcutaneous injection. When you think you are competent, arrange with your instructor to take the performance tests. You are expected to accurately demonstrate your ability to prepare for and administer subcutaneous and intramuscular injections to a patient, in addition to identifying the equipment used and the care of such equipment after use.

Read and define the italicized terms that have been presented in this unit.

Addiction and habituation of many drugs are major health problems in present-day society. To add to this problem, many use *crude drugs* rather than *pure drugs*, which may exert increasing *toxicity* in those who partake. Many individuals are unaware of the many *side effects* that drugs may produce such as drug *tolerance* or the more severe reaction of *anaphylactic shock*. *Chemotherapy* used correctly in medical situations can produce marvelous results. But at times there are *contraindications* to administering certain drugs to a patient. *Drug idiosyncrasies or side effects* may occur in patients receiving certain drugs. It is vital that you report this information to the physician so that this particular *prophylactic treatment may be altered*.

A *cumulative action of a drug* may be desired at times and at other times, contraindicated; thus any prolonged drug therapy must be monitored closely for various medical reasons.

The *HHS, FDA,* and *DEA* are all governmental agencies involved with the regulations controlling the commerce and administration of drugs.

Useful pharmacology book resources include the *PDR* and *USR-NF*. Familiarity with these sources is vital when knowledge of approved drugs, their dosages, actions, and contraindications is sought.

When you take an inventory of the *stock supply of drugs* in the office, you must discard *outdated drugs* and reorder a new supply. At times you may receive medications in a *unit dose*. An accurate inventory of all medications on hand is the responsibility of the medical assistant. Always know the drug before administering it to a patient. It is also important for a medical assistant to be familiar with drugs that have been *dispensed, administered,* or *prescribed* to the patient by the physician.

CASE STUDY

The Physician's Desk Reference (PDR) is a vital resource manual found in every health provider's office. Understanding its use is important to all health providers, including medical assistants. It is published annually, and product updates are released periodically. Using the following information for a fictitious drug, using the same format as the PDR, be prepared to discuss the italicized terminology.

Fictitious drug: DriplessNosey

Caution: *Federal law prohibits dispensing without prescription* (see BNDD statues).

Description: Each *tablet* contains 60 mg of haltitnow and 20 mg of thatisenuf in an outer *press-coat* for immediate release and 110 mg of isaidstop in an *extended-release core*. . . .

Clinical pharmacology: DriplessNosey is a *histamine H₁-receptor antagonist*, chemically and pharmacologically distinct from other *antihistamines*. . . .

Indications and usage; DriplessNosey is indicated for the relief of symptoms associated with seasonal *allergic rhinitis* such as sneezing, *rhinorrhea, pruritus,* lacrimation, and *nasal congestion*. . . .

Contraindications: DriplessNosey is contraindicated in nursing mothers, patients with severe *hypertension* or severe *coronary artery disease*. . . .

Warnings: DriplessNosey should be used *judiciously* (no addiction reported) and sparingly in patients with hypertension, *diabetes mellitus,* or severe CAD. . . .

Precautions: DriplessNosey should be used with caution in patients with *hyperreactivity* to *ephedrine* or previous anaphylactic reaction.

Adverse reaction: In *double-blind parallel,* controlled studies in over 300 patients...compared to extended-release *pseudoephedrine,* adverse reactions reported for greater than 1% of the patients...were not clinically different from those reported for patients receiving DriplessNosey. . . .

Overdosage: Acute overdosage with DriplessNosey tablets may produce clinical signs of *CNS stimulation* or depression. . . .

Dosage and administrations: Adults and children 12 years and older: one tablet swallowed whole, morning and night with water.

How applied: DriplessNosey containing 60 mg of haltitnow and 10 mg of thatisenuf in an outer press-coat for Case immediate release and 10 mg of isaidstop.

REVIEW QUESTIONS

1. Explain what a drug is; list three uses and four sources from which drugs are derived.
2. Describe the difference between the trade name and the generic name of a drug, and give two examples of each.
3. Describe the difference between the following three classifications of drugs: (a) controlled substances, (b) prescription drugs, (c) nonprescription drugs.
4. List one use for each of the following: (a) analgesics, (b) anticoagulants, (c) antidotes, (d) antiseptics, (e) bronchodilators, (f) diuretics, (g) emetics, (h) hemostatics, (i) miotics, (j) narcotics, (k) tranquilizers, (l) vasodilators, (m) insulin.
5. List seven parts of a prescription.
6. Drugs are supplied in either a solid or liquid form. List five types of solid preparations and five types of liquid preparations.
7. Describe how and where medications should be stored.
8. When the label of a medication is torn and soiled so that the name of the drug cannot be clearly identified, what should you do with it?
9. List the information that must be kept on the office record for Schedule II controlled substances after they have been administered to a patient in the office.
10. List and briefly describe 12 routes by which medications can be administered.
11. List the five rights of proper medication administration. List one additional right added by many medical authorities.
12. When preparing medication to be administered, the label should be checked three times. List the three times when you should read the label of the medication.
13. Discuss at least ten rules and responsibilities that you must be concerned with when administering medications.
14. Discuss five factors that influence dosage and drug action.
15. List six reasons for administering a medication by injection.
16. Discuss dangers involved and areas to avoid when giving medication by injection.
17. When asked to give a patient a subcutaneous injection, what size needle and syringe will you use? What sizes would be used for an intramuscular injection? Into which body sites would you administer each of these injections?

18. You have inserted the needle into the patient's right gluteus medius. As you withdraw the plunger of the syringe, a large amount of blood returns. What does this indicate, and what would be your next action?
19. The following orders have been written by the physician for patients. Using the abbreviation lists, transcribe these orders into English.
    a Compazine 15 mg × 12 caps
       Sig ī cap po, tid, ac & hs, prn
    b. Digoxin 0.25 mg × 30 tabs
       Sig ī cap po, od
    c. Digoxin 0.25 mg × 30 tabs
       Sig ī tab po, bid for 10 days, then ½ tab bid po for 10 days
    d. Benadryl 50 mg × 8 caps
       Sig i cap po, qid for 2d
    e. Naprosyn 500 mg × 60 tabs
       Sig - tab po bid pc
    f. Vitamin B$_{12}$ 200 mcg, IM, qd
    g. Ampicillin 500 mg × 28 caps
       Sig 500 mg po, q6h for 7 days
    h. Amoxi 500 mg po, qd for 7 days
    i. Tetracycline 250 mg × 28 caps
       Sig i po, 1 hr ac c̄ H$_2$O
    j. Keflin 0.5 gm IM stat and then q6h for 7 days
    k. Regular insulin 1 vial 100 IU/cc
       Sig 20 IU sc, ac and 40 IU, hs, sc
    l. Demerol 200 mg IM stat
    m. Seconal 50 mg po, hs, may repeat × 1, prn
20. Solve the following problems to determine the amount of drug that is to be administered.
    a. Give ASA gr 10 po; bottle reads 5 gr/tablet
    b. Give Compazine 10 mg IM; ampule reads 5 mg/ml
    c. Give ascorbic acid 0.5 g po; bottle reads 500 mg/tablet
    d. Give Kantrex 15 gr IM; bottle reads 1 g=3 ml
    e. Give Maalox 1 ounce. How many ml do you give?
    f. Give tetracycline 500 mg, po; bottle reads 250 mg/capsule
    g. Give Valium 5 mg po; bottle reads 10 mg/tablet

PERFORMANCE TEST

In a skills laboratory, a simulation of a joblike environment, the medical assistant student will demonstrate skill and knowledge in preparing for and administering medication safely and efficiently by accomplishing the following without reference to source materials. For these activities, the student needs a person to play the role of the patient to demonstrate the correct positioning of the patient and to locate the correct anatomic site to be used for the injection. An artificial limb may be used for performing the actual injection. Time limits for the performance of each procedure are to be assigned by the instructor (see also page 52).

1. Intramuscular injection in one of the four sites discussed in this unit; IM injection using the **Z-Tract** technique.
2. Subcutaneous injection in the upper, outer part of the arm.
3. Loading and using a Tubex injector with a prefilled sterile cartridge-needle unit for an IM injection.
4. Reconstituting a powdered drug for administration

The student is expected to perform the above skills and record the procedures on the patient's chart with 100% accuracy.

Diagnostic Allergy Tests and Intradermal Skin Tests

COGNITIVE OBJECTIVES

On completion of Unit Eight, the medical assistant student should be able to:

1. Define and pronounce the terms listed in the vocabulary.
2. Discuss the nature, causes, signs, and symptoms of allergies.
3. List methods used for the diagnosis and treatment of allergies.
4. Describe and differentiate between the following test:
   a. Patch test
   b. Scratch test
   c. Intradermal skin test
   d. Mantoux test for tuberculosis
   e. Tine tuberculin test
5. Describe how to determine the results for each of the tests given in No. 4.

TERMINAL PERFORMANCE OBJECTIVES

On completion of Unit Eight, the medical assistant student should be able to:

1. Select the correct equipment and supplies needed to perform diagnostic allergy and intradermal skin tests.
2. Correctly perform and read and record the results of the following tests:
   a. Patch test
   b. Scratch test
   c. Intradermal skin test
   d. Mantoux test for tuberculosis
   e. Tine tuberculin test
3. Prepare the patient and the equipment, and administer an intradermal injection in the correct body site.

   The student is to perform these activities with 100% accuracy.

The consistent use of universal precautions is required by all health care professionals in all health care settings as a method of infection control. It is assumed that these precautions are used in all of the following procedures. Review Unit One if you have any question on methods to use, as the methods/techniques will not be repeated in detail in each procedure presented in the unit.

Be sure to consult the latest guidelines issued by the Centers for Disease Control and Prevention and consult with infection control practitioners when needed to identify specific precautions that pertain to your particular work situation.

ALLERGIES

The study and diagnosis of allergies are closely related to the field of immunity (review pages 174 to 176). When a foreign agent (antigen) enters the body, antibodies are produced that attack and render the antigen harmless. This reaction is part of the body's natural defense mechanisms. However, in some instances, when the same antigen enters the body again, the antibodies, rather than protecting the body, set up an antigen-antibody reaction, producing harmful or uncomfortable results such as the signs and symptoms of an allergy.

An allergy is the abnormal individual hypersensitivity to substances (allergens) that are usually harmless. Allergens, substances capable of inducing hypersensitivity, can be almost any substance in the environment. Examples of allergens to which patients have become sensitive are dust, animal hairs, plant and tree pollens, mold spores, soaps, determents, cosmetics, dyes, food, feathers, plastics, and even some valuable medicines. When the allergen is in contact with or enters the body, it sets off a chain of events that brings about the allergic reaction. The allergen in itself is not directly responsible for the allergic reaction. An allergy does not develop on the first contact with the allergen, but can develop on the second contact or even years later after repeated contact with the allergen.

Signs and symptoms of allergies include sneezing, stuffed-up and running nose, watery eyes, itching, coughing, shortness of breath, wheezing, rashes, skin eruptions, slight local edema, and also mild-to-severe anaphylactic shock, which can be fatal unless treated.

DIAGNOSIS AND TREATMENT OF ALLERGIES

For the physician to correctly treat the patient's condition, the allergen responsible for the reaction

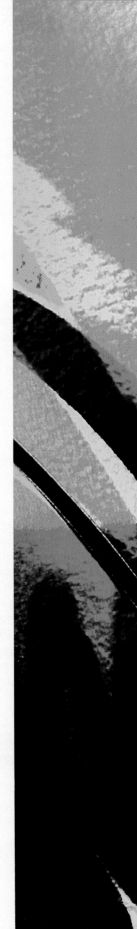

Allergen (al´-er-jen)—Any substance that induces hypersensitivity.

Allergy (al´ er-je)—An unusual and increased sensitivity (hypersensitivity) to specific substances that are ordinarily harmless.

Anaphylaxis (an″ah-fi-lak´ sis)—An usual or hypersensitive reaction of the body to foreign protein and other substances; frequently caused by drugs, foreign serum (for example, tetanus), and insect stings and bites.

Atopy (at´ o-pe)—A hypersensitive state that is subject to hereditary influences (for example, hay fever, asthma, and eczema).

Contact dermatitis—Dermatitis caused by an allergic reaction resulting from contact of the skin with various substances (for example, poison ivy, or chemical, physical, and mechanical agents).

Dermatitis (der″mah-ti´ tis)—Inflammation of the skin.

Induration (in″du-ra´ shun)—An abnormally hard spot; a process of hardening.

Vesicle (ves´ i′kl)—A circular, blisterlike elevation on the skin containing fluid.

Wheal (hwel)—A temporary, round elevation on the skin that is white in the center and often accompanied by itching.

must be identified. After obtaining a detailed case history from the patient, the physician may order one of three skin tests: (1) patch test, (2) scratch test, or (3) intradermal test. You may do these tests or prepare the equipment and assist the physician with the procedure. The principle involved is that when a minute amount of various suspected allergens is applied to the skin in these tests, a mild allergic reaction occurs at the site of the offending allergen without causing any serious symptoms.

As many as 20 to 30 tests may be necessary before the offending allergen or allergens are identified. Control tests using the diluent without the active allergen are essential in each type of testing. Positive reactions at the other test sites can be compared with the appearance at the control site to verify that they are a true allergic reaction and not merely an irritating reaction to the diluent or trauma to the skin area. Ready-made bottled preparations of allergen materials or diagnostic sets with vials containing up to 39 various allergens are available for testing.

Once the offending allergen has been identified, the first step in treatment is to avoid it. At times a special diet may have to be designed for the patient, or special antiallergic cosmetics may have to be used. When the allergen is animal hair, the patient has to avoid the animal and may have to give away a household pet. Patients with hay fever or asthma often have to move to a different locale or plan a trip to a place free from the offending pollen during certain seasons of the year. Often patients can be cured of allergies by receiving a series of desensitization treatments. For these treatments patients are given the allergen(s) in gradually increasing amounts to reduce their sensitivity to those substances or to build up their resistance to the point of immunity. Allergies that are resistant to cure may be controlled with certain medications such as antihistamines, epinephrine, aminophylline, and cortisone preparation.

PATCH TEST

Formerly used to detect tuberculosis, the patch test has been proven to be unreliable for that use. Today the patch test is most often used to diagnose skin allergies, especially contact dermatitis. This is the simplest type of skin test. To determine tissue hypersensitivity, gauze is impregnated with the substance to be tested and then applied and left in contact with an intact skin surface for 24 to 72 hours (usually 48 hours).

SCRATCH TEST

In the scratch test, one or more scratches are made in the skin, and a drop of the substance to be tested is placed in the scratch and left for 30 minutes. The scratch test is frequently used for detecting types of allergies. Kits to be used for this test come in various sizes with various numbers of allergens. Some physicians may keep multiple-dose bottles of allergens for common allergies rather than using the test kits. The history obtained from the patient usually indicates the type and number of tests to be performed. *A physician must be in the office or clinic when this test is done because the patient could experience respiratory distress or anaphylaxis.*

Text continues on page 305.

PATCH TEST

Equipment
Antiseptic sponge to cleanse the skin or an alcohol sponge
Containers with the allergen(s) to be tested

Small gauze dressings(s) and square of plastic wrap *or* commercially prepared protective covering patches
Adhesive or paper tape

PATCH TEST—cont'd

PROCEDURE	RATIONALE
1. Check physician's order.	
2. Wash your hands. **Use appropriate personal protective equipment (PPE) as dictated by facility.**	
3. Assemble supplies.	
4. Identify and prepare the patient. a. Explain the procedure. b. Provide a patient gown if needed. c. Position in a comfortable sitting position with the arm exposed and well supported, or the back exposed if the patch is to be applied there.	*Explanations help gain the patient's cooperation, help alleviate fear of the unknown, and help the patient relax.*
5. Cleanse the skin site to be used, and allow it to dry. The anterior forearm or the upper back are frequent test sites. The forearm is the preferred site for adults, and the back is the preferred site for children.	
6. Place a drop or two of the specific allergen on the gauze dressing; cover this with a square of plastic wrap.	
7. Place the gauze on the skin site and attach with tape. Commercially prepared covering patches come ready to be applied and do not need the plastic wrap covering.	
8. Write the name of the test substance on the tape, or write a number on the tape and in the patient's record with the name of the allergen used.	*When a positive reaction occurs, it is vital that the correct allergen be identified. Correct record-keeping is a must. As many as 20 to 30 patches may be applied at one time on the back.*
9. Instruct the patient. Explain to the patient that, if intense itching occurs, he or she should remove the patch and contact the physician immediately for further instructions. Also tell the patient to avoid wetting or scratching the test site until the patch is removed so that the allergen is not spread over a large area.	*The patch is to be kept in place for varying lengths of time, depending on the allergen used and the physician's order (minimum 24 hours) up to 72 hours. Frequently it is left in place for 48 hours.*

10. Record the test on the patient's record.	*Charting example:*
	 August 4, 19____, 1 p.m.
	    Patch tests done on forearm X2.
	       Ari Sabir, CMA

11. Remove the patch at the specified time and read the results (observe the reaction). Discard the patch in a designated covered container. The test result is negative when there is no reaction on the skin; the test result is positive when the skin is reddened (erythematous) or swollen, or when vesicles are present.	
12. Instruct the patient when and if to return for another appointment.	
13. Leave the treatment room clean.	
14. Wash your hands.	

15. Record the reaction on the patient's record	*Charting example:*
	 August 6, 19____, 1 p.m.
	    Skin patches removed.
	    Results of the test—negative.
	       Ari Sabir, CMA

SCRATCH TEST

Equipment

Commercially prepared kit with needles for each test and the allergen solutions, either in a capillary tube or bottle; when the prepared kit is not used, you will need the bottles containing the allergens to be tested and 26-gauge needles (a lancet or a dull sterile knife may also be used)

Two small towels

Washable ink pen

Toothpick or medicine dropper (to be used when the substance is provided in a bottle)

Patient gown

Disposable single-use exam gloves

PROCEDURE

1. Check physician's orders.

2. Wash your hands. **Use appropriate personal protective equipment (PPE) as dictated by facility.**

3. Assemble the equipment.

4. Identify and prepare the patient:
   a. Explain the procedure.
   b. Ask the patient to disrobe to the waist and put the gown on with opening in back.
   c. Position the patient in a prone position (face down) on the examining table with the back exposed, *or* sitting with the arm well supported and exposed.

5. Don gloves. Wash the back (or arm) with soap and water; dry thoroughly.

6. Write test numbers 2 inches apart on sections of the skin to correspond with the allergen container numbers. Use a pen with washable ink.

7. Make a $1/8$-inch, superficial scratch with the needle supplied in the kit *or* with a 26-gauge needle *or* with a dull, sterile knife. Do not penetrate the skin or cause bleeding.

8. Place a drop of the allergen on the scratch. For solutions supplied in a capillary tube, break the tube in two and allow the solution to drop onto the scratch. For solutions supplied in separate bottles, use a toothpick end or a medicine dropper to pick up a drop of the solution and drop it onto the scratch. If the first scratch as a control test site, place a drop of normal saline on it.

9. Make each additional scratch with a separate needle. Use a clean toothpick or medicine dropper for each solution to be tested.

10. Allow the allergen solution to set for 30 minutes with the back or arm exposed to the air. Provide for the patient's comfort.

11. Wipe the excess solution from each scratch separately.

12. Read the results (observe the skin reactions). NOTE: You may also read the test results 24 hours later to check for delayed reactions. You may have the physician check the results with you.

RATIONALE

Explanations help gain the patient's cooperation and help the patient relax.

The skin must be thoroughly cleansed and dried before the scratches are made. Gloves protect you against contamination.

Each allergen container is numbered to correspond with the numbered section on the skin to eliminate the possibility of incorrect readings.

Use only a minute quantity of the allergen solution to avoid severe allergic reactions. When placed on the scratch, some of the solution is absorbed into the deeper layers of tissue.

Make sure that the patient is not chilled; provide extra covering over areas of the body not used for testing.

Avoid spreading the solution in one scratch to another scratch.

Test results are interpreted as:
* NEGATIVE: No reaction has occurred after 30 minutes.*
* POSITIVE: The appearance of redness or swelling or a wheal at the test site. Positive results are designated as slight (1 +), moderate (2 +), or marked (3 +).*

SCRATCH TEST—cont'd

PROCEDURE	RATIONALE

13. Give the patient further instruction:
   a. To dress and feel free to leave
   b. To return in 24 hours for a delayed reaction reading
   c. To schedule a future appointment for consultation	

14. Remove used supplies from the treatment room; dispose of in designated covered containers for used supplies and laundry; needles must be put in a rigid, puncture-resistant container used for contaminated sharps. Leave the treatment room clean and neat.	
15. Remove gloves and wash your hands.	

16. Record the test and results on the patient's chart.	*Charting example:*
	   August 4, 19___, 1 p.m.
	     20 scratch test administered. Results—positive to dust, cat hair, and plant pollen. Negative to other substances.
	     Mary Donovan, CMA

ADMINISTRATION OF AN INTRADERMAL INJECTION

Equipment

Alcohol sponge or skin antiseptic and cotton ball
Tuberculin syringe because fine calibrations are needed (0.5 or 1 ml)

Needle $3/8$- or $1/2$-inch, 26- or 27-gauge (see Figure 7-7)
Solution to be injected
Disposable single-use exam gloves

PROCEDURE	RATIONALE
1. Wash your hands. **Use appropriate personal protective equipment (PPE) as dictated by facility.** Steps 1 through 11 listed here correspond to steps 1 to 11, Administration of an Intramuscular Injection, pages 286 to 288.	
2. Assemble the equipment.	
3. Prepare the syringe and needle for use.	
4. Compare the physician's order with the medication label.	
5. Check the medication label three times during preparation: when removing drug from the storage area, before measuring the desired amount, and when replacing container in the storage area.	
6. Cleanse the vial rubber stopper, insert the needle, and withdraw the needed amount of solution into the syringe.	
7. Identify the patient and explain the procedure.	*Explanations help to reassure and relax the patient.*
8. Select the injection site, and position the patient comfortably. For intradermal injections, use the dorsal surface of the forearm, about 4 inches below the elbow. In patients over 60 years of age, inject the solution into the area over the trapezius muscle (on the back), just below the acromial process (Figure 8-1).	*For patients over 60 years of age, loss of skin turgor in the area can contribute to bruising or to extravasation of the testing solution.*

ADMINISTRATION OF AN INTRADERMAL INJECTION—cont'd

PROCEDURE

RATIONALE

9. Don gloves. Cleanse the injection site with the alcohol sponge and allow to dry thoroughly.

Gloves provide protection against possible contamination.

10. Remove the needle cover.

11. Expel any excess air that may be entered the syringe.

12. Stand in front of the patient. With your nondominant hand, grasp the middle of the patient's forearm on the posterior side, and pull the anterior skin taut.

Pulling the skin taut allows for easier insertion of the needle.

13. Hold the barrel of the syringe between your thumb and other fingers of your dominant hand; have the bevel of the needle facing upward.

14. Insert the needle into the skin at a 10- to 15-degree angle (see Figure 8-1 and Unit Seven). The angle used to insert the needle is almost parallel to the skin. Insert the point of the needle into the most superficial layers of the skin.

15. Inject the solution slowly. NOTE: This type of injection does not require aspiration before the solution is injected. As the drug is injected, a small pale bump will rise over the point of the needle in the skin. If the injection is given subcutaneously (that is, no bump forms), or if a significant part of the solution leaks from the injection site, repeat the test immediately at another site at least 2 inches (5 cm) away.

16. Withdraw the needle, and wipe the injection site gently with the alcohol sponge. Do not apply pressure or massage the skin.

The medication must not be dispersed into the underlying tissues.

17. Observe the patient for any unusual reaction such as general febrile reaction, faint feeling, and shock.

18. Position the patient for safety and comfort, and provide further instructions. If the patient feels faint, have him or her lie down or sit for a few minutes.

Ensure that no unusual reaction occurs.

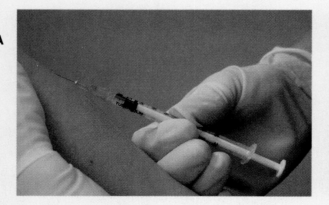
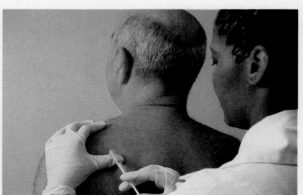

A   B

Figure 8-1   A, *Administering an intradermal injection at a 10- to 15-degree angle on dorsal surface of forearm, about 4 inches below elbow; B, administering intradermal skin test over the trapezius muscle just below the acromial process on elderly patients.*

ADMINISTRATION OF AN INTRADERMAL INJECTION—cont'd

PROCEDURE	RATIONALE

19. Tell the patient when the test results will be read. Schedule a future appointment when necessary. The patient may be dismissed if the results are not read until a day or two later. If the test result is to be determined within the next half hour or so, let the patient rest comfortable and safely. The skin reaction is read at various times, depending on the test done. Check with the physician or the literature that accompanies the drug used. Most allergy skin tests are read within 20 to 30 minutes, the Mantoux test for tuberculosis is read within 48 to 72 hours, and other tests are read at varying times within 48 hours.

20. Remove and dispose of the used syringe and needle correctly. Place a disposable syringe and needle in a puncture-resistant, disposable container without breaking or recapping the needle. Flush reusable syringes and needles with water, separate them, and place them in a designated cleaning solution until prepared for sterilization (see Unit Five).

21. Remove gloves.

22. Wash your hands.

23. Record the procedure on the patient's chart. When several skin tests are given, record the site of each injection and the name of the substance injected.

This avoids confusion when the results are read.

24. Read the skin reaction. Many tests are read as either positive or negative, depending on the amount of redness (erythema) or hardening (induration). For some tests the areas of redness or induration must be measured in millimeters. Follow the directions provided with the test solution.

25. Record the reaction on the patient's chart.

Charting example:
August 5, 19___, 4 p.m.
    Reaction of Mantoux test given August 3, 19___, 4 p.m. is negative.
        M.E. Burgdorf, CMA

INTRADERMAL SKIN TESTS

In intradermal (intracutaneous) tests, a small amount of the substance under study is injected into the substance of the skin. These tests are used to determine allergies, to determine the patient's susceptibility to an infectious disease, and to diagnose infectious diseases such as tuberculosis (the Mantoux test) and diphtheria (the Schick test). For all these tests the general rules for administering injections apply (refer to pages 280 to 283, Intradermal Injections and Instructions for Administering Injections). Commercial trays of prepackaged sterile syringes are available for intradermal allergy tests.

TUBERCULOSIS

Tuberculosis (TB) is an infectious disease caused by the tubercle bacillus *Mycobacterium tuberculosis* and generally transmitted by inhaling or ingesting infected droplets. It usually affects the lungs, although other organs such as the kidneys, bones, and joints can be affected. With early diagnosis and appropriate treatment, TB can usually be cured. In 1989 the Department of Health and Human Services predicted that by the year 2010 tuberculosis would be eliminated. Unfortunately the opposite is occurring; the cases of TB are increasing. Even more alarming, there is an increase in tuberculosis cases that are resistant to the common anti-TB drugs used to cure this disease. Officials associate much of the increase to the growing incidence of HIV (human immunodeficiency virus) disease, which leaves individuals much more susceptible to the disease. Other risk factors include poor nutrition, poor and crowded living conditions, homelessness, high stress, and substance abuse.

MANTOUX TEST

The standard test recommended by the American Lung Association to help detect people exposed to and infected with *M. tuberculosis* is the Mantoux test (also called the tuberculin or purified protein derivative (PPD) skin test or intermediate [5 TU]). The Mantoux test is performed by injecting intradermally exactly 0.1 ml of tuberculin PPD. This dose contains 5 tuberculin units (TUs) of tuberculin PPD. The reaction is read 48 to 72 hours later. Only induration is considered when interpreting the test results. The Mantoux test should only be given to patients who have never had a positive PPD test in the past. Additional exposure to the tuberculin may cause skin necrosis at the site of the intradermal injection.

Equipment
- Alcohol sponge
- Tuberculin syringe (0.5 or 1.0 ml) with a $^3/_8$- or $^1/_2$-inch, 26- or 27-gauge needle
- Tuberculin PPD, 5 TU (intermediate) strength
- Disposable single-use exam gloves

Procedure

Follow the intradermal injection technique described in previous paragraphs, measuring 0.1 ml of tuberculin PPD 5 TU into the syringe for administration. Record the date, time, manufacturer, lot number, amount of PPD administered, site and route of administration, and your signature.

Reading Mantoux Skin Reactions
- Read 48 to 72 hours after the injection.
- Consider *only* induration (area of hardened tissue) when interpreting the results.
- Measure the diameter of induration transversely (lying in crosswise direction) to the long axis of the forearm and record in millimeters.
- Disregard erythema (redness) of less than 10 mm.
- Disregard erythema greater than 10 mm if induration is absent because the injection may have been made too deeply. In this case, repeat testing.

Interpreting Tuberculin Reaction

Positive reaction. Induration measuring 10 mm or more indicates hypersensitivity to the tuberculin PPD and is interpreted as positive for present or past infection with *M. tuberculosis*. A positive reaction does not necessarily signify active disease. Further diagnostic procedures must be performed before a diagnosis of TB is made. A chest x-ray film should be performed because it will show evidence of disease in an otherwise asymptomatic patient. Patients who have productive coughs should have sputum smears and bacteriologic cultures for the presence of acid-fast bacilli (AFB) tested. TB is suspected if a smear is AFB positive but is not excluded if AFB are not present, since only 50% to 80% of patients with TB of the lung have AFB-positive smears. A diagnosis of TB is confirmed when the culture demonstrates the growth of *M. tuberculosis*. A confirmed diagnosis may take 6 to 8 weeks because it takes weeks for this bacteria to grow in a culture.

Doubtful reaction. Induration measuring 5 to 9 mm means that retesting may be indicated using a different test site.

Negative reaction. Induration of less than 5 mm indicates a lack of hypersensitivity to the tuberculin; thus tuberculosis infection is highly unlikely.

NOTE: The Centers for Disease Control and Prevention (CDC) has recommended that 5 mm or more induration should be the value used to interpret this skin test in HIV-positive individuals because, when it is interpreted in HIV-infected individuals using the standard 10-mm induration measurement, it has been found to be less reliable.

NOTE: To detect people who have been exposed to TB but test negative to the PPD skin test because they have very low antibody levels to the tuberculin, a second PPD test, called a booster dose, should be given 1 week after the first test.

TINE TUBERCULIN TEST

The intradermal tine tuberculin test provides a convenient *screening* method for skin tuberculin reactivity in individuals and in large population groups. It does not diagnose TB. The reactivity of this test is comparable to, or more potent than, the intermediate-strength Mantoux test (5 TU) administered intradermally. The disposable tine unit used for this test consists of a stainless steel disk, with four tines or prongs 2 mm long attached to a plastic handle. The tines have been dipped in a solution of old tuberculin containing stabilizers and then dried. The entire unit is sterile as long as the plastic cap is not removed (Figure 8-2, *A*).

Figure 8-2 A, *Tine unit for tuberculin testing;* **B,** *administering the tine tuberculin test.*

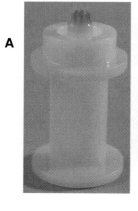
A

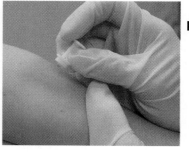
B

ADMINISTRATION OF THE TINE TUBERCULIN TEST

Equipment

Disposable single-use exam gloves
Alcohol sponge (acetone, ether, or soap and water can also be used

Tine unit
Millimeter ruler (supplied with tine unit)

PROCEDURE

1. Wash your hands. **Use appropriate personal protective equipment (PPE) as dictated by facility.**

2. Assemble the equipment.

3. Identify the patient and explain the procedure.

4. Don gloves, explain what is to occur and how it may feel.

5. Expose the patient's forearm, cleanse the skin with the alcohol sponge, and *allow the skin to dry thoroughly.* The preferred site for the administration of this test is the volar surface of the upper third of the forearm, over a muscle belly. Avoid hairy areas and areas without adequate subcutaneous tissue such as over a tendon or a bone.

6. Remove the protective cap on the tine unit while holding the plastic handle.

7. With your nondominant hand, grasp the upper third of the patient's forearm on the posterior side firmly and stretch the anterior skin tightly (Figure 8-2, B).

8. With your dominant hand, apply the disk by puncturing the skin. Hold approximately 1 second before withdrawing.

9. Discard the tine test unit in the appropriate rigid, puncture-resistant sharps disposal container. The tine test unit must *never* be reused.

10. Instruct the patient when to return for the reading of the test results. Tests should be read in 48 to 72 hours.

11. Remove gloves.

12. Wash your hands.

13. Record the test on the patient's medical record.

RATIONALE

Explanations help gain the patient's cooperation and alleviate any apprehension.

The protective cap is removed to expose the four impregnated tines.

A firm grasp of the patient's forearm is necessary because the sharp momentary sting from the tine unit may cause the patient to jerk the arm and cause scratching.

Sufficient pressure must be exerted so that the four puncture sites and a circular depression of the skin from the plastic base are visible on the patient's skin.

Charting example:
August 27, 19__, 11 a.m.
  Tine test administered in left forearm. Patient to return August 29, 19__, 11 a.m. for reading of the reaction.
  Sissy Block, CMA

ADMINISTRATION OF THE TINE TUBERCULIN TEST—cont'd

PROCEDURE

14. Read the reaction in a good light with the patient's forearm slightly flexed. Tests should be read in 48 to 72 hours. The extent of induration is the sole criterion; erythema without induration is insignificant. Determine the size of the induration in millimeters by inspecting the site and palpating with gentle finger stroking. Measure with a millimeter ruler the diameter of the largest single reaction around one of the puncture sites (Figure 8-3).

15. Record the time and results on the patient's record.

RATIONALE

Interpretation of tuberculin test reactions as recommended by the American Lung Association follow.

- *POSITIVE REACTION: Induration measuring 5 mm or more. The significance of this test and the management of the patient are the same as for one who reacts with 10 mm or more of induration to the standard Mantoux test. Further diagnostic procedures must be considered, such as a chest x-ray film, laboratory examinations of sputum and other specimens, and confirmation using the Mantoux method. Chemotherapy should not be started solely on the basis of a single positive tine test.*
- *DOUBTFUL REACTION: Induration of 2 to 4 mm. Patients in this group should have a Mantoux test done, and management should be based on the Mantoux reaction.*
- *NEGATIVE REACTION: Induration of less than 2 mm. Patients in this group do not need to be retested unless they are in contact with a tuberculosis case or if there is suggestive clinical evidence of the disease.*

Charting example:
  August 29, 19___, 11 a.m.
    Results of the tine test administered August 27, 19___, at 11 a.m. are negative.
    Sissy Block, CMA

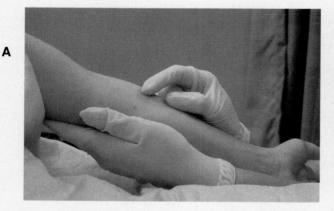
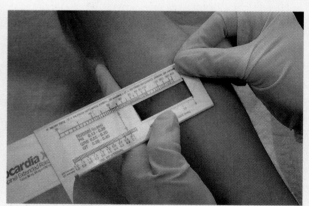

Figure 8-3 *Reading the reaction of a tine tuberculin test.* **A,** *Palpate the area for presence of induration.* **B,** *Using a millimeter ruler, measure the largest single reaction around one of the puncture sites.*

CONCLUSION

You have now completed the unit on Diagnostic Allergy Tests and Intradermal Skin Tests. When you are familiar with the contents of this unit, arrange with your instructor to take a performance test. You are expected to demonstrate accurately your skill in preparing for and performing all of the procedures outlined in this unit.

REVIEW OF VOCABULARY

Read the following report and define the italicized terms. Ms. Amy Fenster came to the office with an obvious case of *contact dermatitis*. Patient stated that she had been working in her garden when the signs and symptoms started and thinks that poison ivy may be the *allergen*. Patient has no other known *allergies*; and has never experienced *anaphylaxis* nor any previous dermatitis.

Family history includes the presence of various *atopies* in both her mother and father.
Further studies will include a *scratch test*, in addition to a *Mantoux test* that is required by her present employment.
A. *Wheal*, MD

CASE STUDY

Read and discuss the following italicized terminology.
1. A 7-year-old male presents today for evaluation of suspected *allergies*. *Intradermal* (*intracutaneous*) tests to inject a substance to determine the patient's *susceptibility* to particular *allergens* were performed on the patient. Past history reports *wheals* on abdomen.
2. In 2 weeks a *screening* test for *skin tuberculin reactivity* is scheduled for employees. Order *Tuberculin PPD* and *tuberculin syringes* (0.5 or 1 ml) with a 3/8- or 1/2-inch, 26- or 27-gauge needle.
3. A 24-year-old female presents with a *dermatitis* consisting of a series of *vesicles* the size of dimes filled with clear, yellowish fluid located on her anterior thighs. In addition, she has *signs* and *symptoms* of *allergies*, including *wheezing* and itching. She has a past history of *hypersensitivity* to many *environmental allergens*, including tree *pollens*, *spores*, and detergents. She was placed on *antihistamines* and *cortisone* preparation in the past.

REVIEW QUESTIONS

1. Define the term allergy, and list six signs and symptoms of an allergy.
2. A patch test is left in place for a minimum of __ hours, up to a maximum of __ hours.
3. List two body sites that are frequently used to apply a patch test. Which is the preferred site for adults? For children?
4. Describe how you would read and record the results of:
   a. Patch test
   b. Scratch test
   c. Mantoux test
   d. Tine tuberculin test
5. What body site would you use to administer an intradermal injection?
6. Why don't you massage the skin after administering an intradermal injection?
7. Where would you administer the tine tuberculin test? What is the purpose of this test?
8. Why are control tests essential in each type of allergy skin test?

PERFORMANCE TEST

In a skills laboratory, the medical assistant student will demonstrate skill in performing the following activities without reference to source materials. Time limits for the performance of each procedure are to be assigned by the instructor (see also page 60).
1. Select and prepare the supplies and equipment and then perform the following procedures:
   a. Patch test
   b. Scratch test
   c. Intradermal skin test (intradermal injection)
   d. Mantoux test
   e. Tine tuberculin test
2. Read and record the results of the above tests.

The student is expected to perform these skills with 100% accuracy.

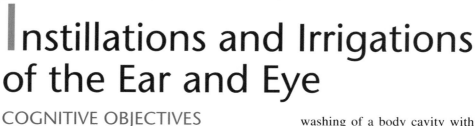

Instillations and Irrigations of the Ear and Eye

COGNITIVE OBJECTIVES

On completion of Unit Nine, the medical assistant student should be able to.

1. Define and pronounce the terms listed in the vocabulary.
2. Describe how to instill drops into the ear and eye, and explain the reason for the actions taken.
3. Describe how to irrigate the ear and eye, and explain the reasons for the steps taken.
4. Explain the difference between an instillation and an irrigation.
5. List:
   a. Two purposes for an ear instillation
   b. Four purposes for an eye instillation
   c. Four purposes for an ear irrigation
   d. Four purposes for an eye irrigation

TERMINAL PERFORMANCE OBJECTIVES

On completion of Unit Nine, the medical assistant student should be able to:

1. Demonstrate the proper procedure for performing an ear instillation and irrigation.
2. Demonstrate the proper procedure for performing an eye instillation and irrigation.

The above activities are to be performed with 100% accuracy 95% of the time.

The consistent use of universal precautions is required by all health care professionals in all health care settings as a method of infection control. It is assumed that these precautions are used in all of the following procedures. Review Unit One if you have any question on methods to use as the methods/techniques will not be repeated in detail in each procedure presented in the unit.

Be sure to consult the latest guidelines issued by the Centers for Disease Control and Prevention and consult with infection control practitioners when needed to identify specific precautions that pertain to your particular work situation.

You may be asked to perform ear and eye instillations and irrigations. These procedures differ slightly. An instillation is the dropping of a fluid into a body cavity; an irrigation is the flushing or washing of a body cavity with a stream of fluid. Observe practices of medical asepsis (as outlined in Unit Five) when performing these procedures. If there is an open wound in the area being treated, use sterile technique.

To understand ear and eye instillations and irrigations and to be of most help to the patient and physician, you should be familiar with the anatomy and physiology of these two special sense organs. It is suggested that you review these topics before studying and practicing the procedures in this unit. The ear is diagrammed in Figure 9-1; the eye is diagrammed in Figures 9-2 and 9-3.

EAR INSTILLATION

When solutions are instilled into the ear, keep in mind that the direction of the external ear canal in adults differs from that in children. To straighten the ear canal so that the medication will be effective, slightly different techniques are used for each age group.

Use medical aseptic technique when instilling solutions into the ear, since the outer ear is not sterile. However, if the tympanic membrane is not intact, you must use sterile technique. To lessen discomfort for the patient, warm the medications slightly before using. Solutions that are either too cold or too hot may cause a feeling of dizziness in addition to pain. You can warm a bottle of eardrops by placing the bottle in a plastic bag to protect the label, and then placing the bag and bottle in a basin of warm water for a few minutes. You can check the temperature of the medication by placing a drop or two on your inner wrist; it should feel warm, not hot.

Ear instillations are performed to:

1. Soften cerumen (ear wax) so that it can be removed easily later.
2. Instill an antibiotic solution to combat an infection in the ear canal or eardrum.

EAR IRRIGATION

An ear irrigation is the washing out of the external auditory canal with a stream of fluid. It is performed to:

1. Cleanse the external auditory canal (external acoustic meatus).
2. Relieve inflammation of the ear.

Figure 9-1 *Diagram of the ear.*
From Thibodeau GA: Anatomy and Physiology, ed 2, St. Louis, 1993, Mosby.

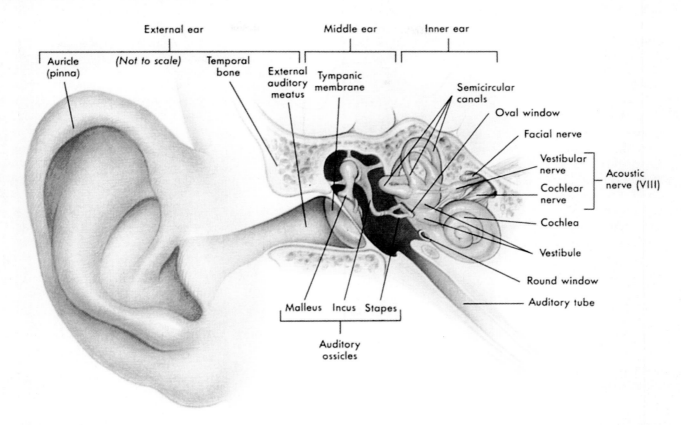

3. Dislodge impacted cerumen or foreign bodies from the external auditory canal.
4. Apply antiseptics to combat infection.
5. Apply heat to the tissues of the ear canal.

Before an irrigation is done, ask the patient if he or she has a history of drainage from the ear and if he or she has ever had a perforation or other complications from a previous irrigation. If the answer to either question is "yes," notify the physician before giving this treatment. Also, before the irrigation, visually examine the ear canal with an otoscope. When the purpose of the irrigation is to cleanse the ear canal or to remove cerumen or foreign bodies, also perform a visual examination after the irrigation to determine if the results are satisfactory.

When this procedure is done, take extreme care to prevent injury to the tympanic membrane and the spread of any infection to the mastoid cavity.

EYE INSTILLATION

Eye instillations are performed to:
1. Dilate the pupil of the eye.
2. Constrict the pupil of the eye.
3. Relieve pain in the eye.
4. Treat eye infections; relieve inflammation.
5. Anesthetize the eye.
6. Stimulate circulation in the eye.

Medications instilled into the eye are supplied either in a sterile liquid form as eyedrops or in a sterile ointment form.

EYE IRRIGATION

Eye irrigations are performed to:
1. Relieve inflammation of the conjunctiva.
2. Remove inflammatory secretions.
3. Prepare the eye for surgery.
4. Wash away foreign material or injurious chemicals.
5. Provide antibacterial and antifungal effects.

Figure 9-2 *External structure of the right eye.*

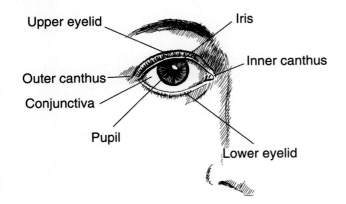

VOCABULARY

Auricle (aw'ri-kl)—The outer projection of the ear; also known as the pinna (pin'nah).

Canthus (kan'thus)—The inner canthus is the angle of the eyelids near the nose; the outer canthus is the angle of the eyelids at the outside corner of the eyes (see Figure 9-3).

Cerumen (se-roo' men)—Ear wax secreted by the glands of the external auditory meatus.

Conjunctiva (kon"junk-ti ' vah)—The delicate membrane lining the eyelids and reflected onto the front of the eyeball.

External ear—Includes the auricle, or pinna, and the external auditory meatus.

External auditory meatus (me-a 'tus)—The canal or passage leading from the outside opening of the ear to the eardrum. Also called the external acoustic meatus.

Miotic (mi-ot'ik)—A medication that causes the pupil of the eye to contract.

Mydriatic (mid"re-at' ik)—A medication that causes the pupil of the eye to dilate.

Ocular (ok'u-lar)—Pertaining to the eye.

Ophthalmic (of-thal'mik)—Pertaining to the eye.

Ophthalmology (of"thal-mol"o-je)—The study and science of the eye and its diseases.

Otic (o'tik)—Pertaining to the ear.

Otology (o-tol'o-je)—The study and science of the ear and its diseases.

Otoscope (o'to-skop)—An instrument used for visual inspection of the ear.

Tympanic (tim-pan' ik) membrane (TM)—The eardrum; it serves as the membrane that separates the external auditory meatus from the middle ear cavity.

Figure 9-3 *Diagram of the eye.*
From Thibodeau GA: *Anatomy and Physiology,* ed 2, St. Louis, 1993, Mosby.

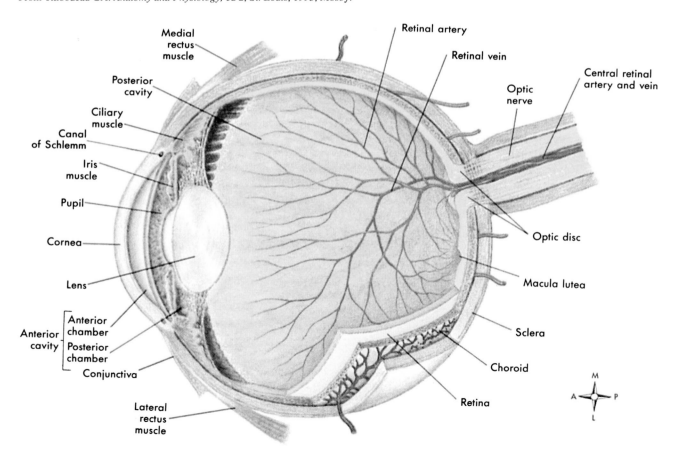

EAR INSTILLATION

Equipment

Prescribed medication and eardropper
Cotton balls

PROCEDURE	RATIONALE
1. Check the medication order carefully (that is, the name and amount of medication and which ear requires treatment).	*Avoid medication errors.*
2. Wash your hands. **Use appropriate personal protective equipment (PPE) as dictated by facility.**	
3. Assemble supplies.	
4. Read the medication label carefully three times, and check with the order. warm the solution.	*The label must be checked to avoid the possibility of any mistake*
5. Identify the patient, and explain the nature of the procedure and the purpose.	*Prevent giving a drug to the wrong patient. Explanations help gain the patient's full cooperation.*
6. Place the patient in a sitting or side-lying position.	
7. Don disposable single-use exam gloves.	
8. Instruct the patient to tilt the head toward the unaffected side.	
9. Stand at the patient's head.	
10. Withdraw the medication into the dropper, and examine the dropper for any defects.	*A safe vehicle must be used to administer the medication*
11. Straighten the external ear canal. For adults, gently pull the top of the earlobe upward and backward (Figure 9-4). For children, gently pull the bottom of the earlobe downward and backward.	*The direction of the external ear canal differs in adults and children.*
12. Place the tip of the dropper just slightly inside the external meatus (external ear canal), and instill the correct amount of medication. Do not touch the ear canal. Position the dropper so that the drops are instilled along the side of the ear canal.	
13. Instruct the patient to keep the head tilted or to remain on the unaffected side for a few minutes.	*This position prevents leakage of the medication from the ear and helps the medication flow through the inside of the ear to the infected eardrum.*
14. Place a cotton ball over the opening of the ear only if ordered.	
15. Discard unused medication in the dropper, and replace the dropper into the bottle, avoiding contamination. When the dropper is contaminated, it must be replaced with a clean dropper.	*A cotton ball is placed over the ear opening only when ordered, as it may absorb some of the medication and prevent the desired action on the ear tissue. Also, cotton balls may prevent drainage from escaping when present.*
16. Remove and discard gloves.	
17. Provide for the patient's safety and comfort. Give further instructions as required.	
18. Return supplies to designated area.	

EAR INSTILLATION—cont'd

PROCEDURE

19. Wash your hands.

20. Record the procedure on the patient's chart.

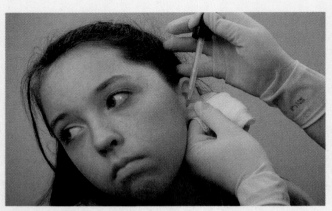

Figure 9-4 *Instillation of eardrops.*

RATIONALE

Charting example:
  October 10, 19____, 11 a.m.
    5 gtt Cerumenex instilled to left ear. Cotton ball placed in external ear canal and left for 15 minutes, then left ear irrigated with warm normal saline. Large amount of cerumen returned.
      Sarah Dolan, CMA

EAR IRRIGATION

Equipment

Drapes: towel, and a small rubber sheet, if available, or a waterproof pad
Kidney or ear basin for drainage
Syringe—either a metal ear syringe (such as a Pomeroy syringe), an Asepto bulb syringe (Figure 9-5), or a rubber bulb syringe
Warm sterile solution/medication as ordered by the physician, in a container; solutions commonly used include:
  Normal saline
  Sterile water
  Antiseptic solutions
    Amount: 500 to 1000 ml, as ordered
    Temperature: 100° F (approximately 38° C) (near body temperature)

Sterile cotton balls
Sterile applicators
Disposable single-use exam gloves

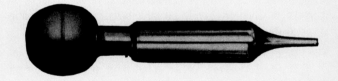

Figure 9-5 *Asepto bulb syringe.*
Courtesy Becton-Dickinson, Division of Becton, Dickinson and Co., Rutherford, N.J.

PROCEDURE

1. Follow the procedure as outlined for an ear instillation in steps 1 through 5:
   a. Check the medication order.
   b. Wash your hands. **Use appropriate personal protective equipment (PPE) as dictated by facility.**
   c. Assemble the supplies.
   d. Check the solution/medication label three times; warm solution.
   e. Identify the patient, and explain the procedure and purpose.

RATIONALE

EAR IRRIGATION—cont'd

PROCEDURE	RATIONALE
2. Position the patient sitting with the head slightly tilted toward the affected side.	This position allows gravity to help the irrigating solution to flow from the ear to the basin.
3. Place a small rubber sheet (when available) and a towel over the patient's shoulder.	Protect the patient's clothing from any drainage.
4. Instruct the patient to hold the kidney or ear basin under the ear and firmly against the neck (Figure 9-6).	The basin provides a receptacle to receive the irrigating solution and to prevent it from running down the patient's neck.
5. Cleanse the outer ear and external auditory meatus as necessary (to remove any discharge or debris present) with the irrigating solution or normal saline.	Cleansing the outer parts of the ear is necessary to prevent the introduction of foreign materials into the ear canal during the irrigation.
6. Test the temperature of the solution by putting a few drops on the inner aspect of your wrist and on the patient's wrist. The solution should feel warm.	Warm solutions are more comfortable for the patient. Cold or too hot solutions may cause more discomfort and a feeling of dizziness. Anxiety is reduced when the patient knows the temperature of the solution.
7. Fill the syringe with the irrigating solution; expel any air present.	Air forced into the ear canal produces excessive discomfort for the patient.
8. Straighten the ear canal by gently pulling the earlobe downward and backward for infants and children; upward and backward for adults.	Straightening the ear canal allows the irrigating solution to reach all areas of the canal.
9. Place the tip of the syringe at the opening of the ear. With the tip pointing upward and toward the posterior end of the canal, gently direct a steady slow stream of solution against the roof of the canal. Use only enough force to accomplish the purpose of irrigation (see Figure 9-6).	Direct the solution at the roof of the canal to prevent injury to the tympanic membrane, to prevent pushing material further into the canal, and to facilitate directing the inflow and outflow of the solution.
10. Do not obstruct the opening of the ear canal with the syringe tip.	
11. Observe the returning solution to see if anything is removed such as cerumen, a foreign object, or discharge.	The solution must be able to flow freely in and out of the ear canal.
12. Observe the patient for any signs of discomfort or dizziness. If these occur, discontinue irrigation and report to the physician. Irritation to the semicircular canals may cause dizziness and nausea. Have a glass of water for the patient.	Water may help to reduce any dizziness.
13. Continue the irrigation until the desired results appear or the prescribed amount of solution has been used.	

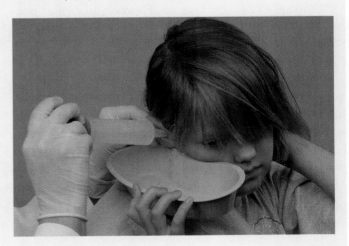

Figure 9-6 *Ear irrigation. Have patient hold kidney or ear basin under ear and against the neck. Head should be tilted toward the affected side. Pull earlobe up and backward. Place tip of syringe in ear pointing up and back, and gently direct a steady slow stream of solution against the roof of the ear canal.*

EAR IRRIGATION—cont'd

PROCEDURE	RATIONALE
14. On completion of the treatment, dry the external ear with a cotton ball; dry the neck when required.	*Drying promotes patient comfort.*
15. Have the patient keep the head tilted toward the affected side or lie on the affected side for a few minutes.	*This allows any remaining solution in the ear canal to escape from the ear.*
16. Remove the soiled towel and rubber sheet (if used). Give further instructions as indicated. Patient may resume normal level of activity.	*Provide for the patient's safety and comfort.*
17. Return supplies to designated area. Remove and dispose of gloves.	
18. Wash your hands.	

19. Record the procedure on the patient's chart.	*Charting example:*
	October 11, 19___, 12 p.m.
	   Left ear irrigated with normal saline. Large amount of cerumen returned. Patient stated that he felt much relief on completion of the irrigation.
	      Jane Evans, CMA

EYEDROP INSTILLATION

Equipment

Sterile eyedropper
Sterile medication, *or*
Sterile medication in bottle with sterile eyedropper

Cotton balls or tissue
Disposable single-use exam gloves

PROCEDURE	RATIONALE
1. Check the medication order carefully (that is, the name and amount of medication and which eye requires medication). Know the abbreviations: OD—right eye (ocular dexter) OS—left eye (ocular sinister) OU—both eyes	*Avoid medication errors.*
2. Wash your hands. **Use appropriate personal protective equipment (PPE) as dictated by facility.**	
3. Assemble supplies.	
4. Read the medication label carefully three times, and check with the order.	*The label must be checked to avoid the possibility of any mistake, because an error could have serious results.*
5. Identify the patient, and explain the procedure and the purpose. Warn the patient that the medication may feel cold and to avoid flinching or squeezing the eye when it is instilled.	*The patient must be identified to avoid giving the drug to the wrong patient. Explanations help gain the patient's full cooperation.*
6. Have the patient assume a supine or a sitting position with the head tilted slightly backward.	
7. Don disposable single-use exam gloves.	

EYEDROP INSTILLATION—cont'd

PROCEDURE	RATIONALE
8. Stand at the patient's head.	
9. Withdraw medication into the dropper. Examine the dropper carefully for any defects.	*A safe vehicle must be used for administering the medication.*
10. Using the index and middle finger over a tissue, draw the lower lid down gently, *or* draw the lower lid down with index finger, and the brow up with the middle finger; have the patient look up (Figure 9-7). Do not touch any part of the eye during the procedure except the lower lid—especially in patients who have had eye surgery.	*The tissue prevents your fingers from slipping when instilling the drops.*
11. Hold the dropper parallel to the eye about $1/2$ inch away from the inner canthus (the inner angle of the eyelids near the nose), and instill the drop(s) into the center of the conjunctival sac of the lower lid (see Figure 9-7).	*To avoid injuring the eye, never point the dropper toward it; never allow the dropper to touch the eyeball or the eyelids. Be extremely careful to support the head well if the patient is restless or jerking the head.*
12. Instruct the patient to close the eyelids and move the eye, but not to squeeze the eyelids.	*This movement helps distribute the medication over the eyeball; squeezing would cause some of the medication to be forced out.*
13. Wipe off the excess medication that overflows onto the cheek or eyelids with cotton balls or tissue.	
14. Discard the unused solution, and replace the dropper into the bottle without touching the sides or outside of the bottle with the dropper.	*Avoid contaminating the dropper. When the dropper is contaminated, a new bottle of eyedrops must be ordered.*
15. Provide for the patient's safety and comfort. At times an eye pad may be applied as a dressing over the eye for protection (Figure 9-8).	
16. Return supplies to designated area.	
17. Wash your hands.	

18. Record the procedure on the patient's chart.	*Charting example:*
	    Oct. 9, 19___, 10:30 a.m.
	    Neosporin Ophthalmic Solution 2 gtts given in OD.
	    Nancy Brown, CMA

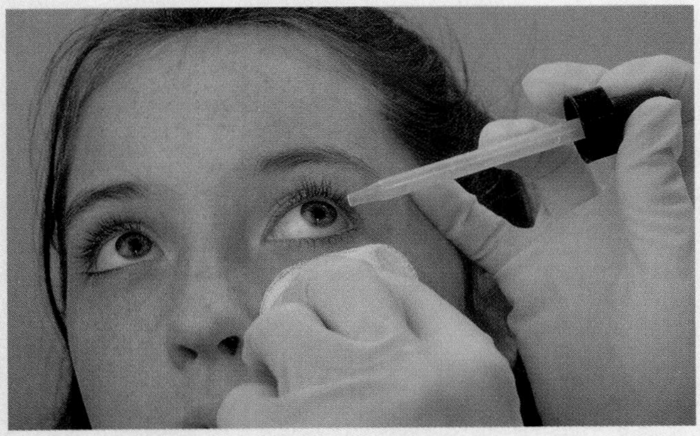

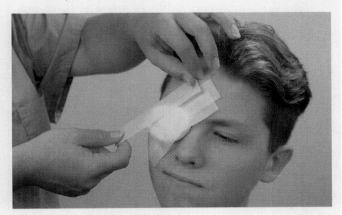

Figure 9-7 *Instilling eyedrops. Hold eyedropper parallel to eye to avoid injury to eye of patient.*

Figure 9-8 *Application of eye pad.*

EYE OINTMENT INSTILLATION

Equipment

Sterile eye ointment in tube
Cotton balls or tissue
Disposable single-use examination gloves

PROCEDURE

Same as for instilling eyedrops *except*:

1. Gently squeeze a thin strip of ointment from the tube along the lower lid without touching the lid.

   NOTE: When instilling eyedrops and ointment at the same time *instill the eyedrops first*, ointment last.

   If the patient's eyedropper or tube touches the eyelid and is contaminated, do not use it again until it is resterilized.

   Discard the contaminated tube unless it is being used by only one patient.

RATIONALE

EYE IRRIGATION

Equipment

Towel
Sterile eyedropper for small amounts of solution; rubber bulb or Asepto syringe for larger amounts of solution; sterile eye cup for home use
Small basin for solution

Sterile cotton balls
Kidney basin to catch the solution
Sterile solution as ordered by the physician, usually boric acid or normal saline, 30 to 240 ml (2 to 8 ounces) at 98.6° F (37° C) (that is, near body temperature)
Disposable single-use exam gloves

PROCEDURE

1. Check the medication order carefully (that is, the name and amount of solution to be used and which eye is to be treated). Know the abbreviations:
   OD—right eye
   OS—left eye
   OU—both eyes

2. Wash your hands. **Use appropriate personal protective equipment (PPE) as dictated by facility.**

3. Assemble supplies.

4. Check the label of the solution three times.

5. Identify the patient, and explain the procedure and the purpose of the irrigation. Instruct the patient not to squeeze the eyes during the treatment.

6. Have the patient assume a lying or sitting position with the head tilted backward and toward the side being treated.

7. Place or have the patient hold the kidney basin in position to receive the solution from the eye. Place a towel under the basin (Figure 9-9).

8. Don disposable single-use exam gloves if the patient's eye is infected.

RATIONALE

Prevent drug errors (see Unit Seven).

Gain the patient's cooperation by providing an explanation and adequate instructions.

The head is tilted to the side so that the solution does not run toward the inner canthus of the eye or over to the unaffected eye, which could then result in cross-infection (when the eye treated is infected).

Avoid getting the solution on the patient or on the examining table when the patient is lying down.

Gloves protect your hands from exposure to pathogens.

EYE IRRIGATION—cont'd

PROCEDURE	RATIONALE
9. Stand in front of or at the side of the patient.	
10. Cleanse the eyelid with a cotton ball moistened with the irrigating solution. Start at the inner canthus and wipe toward the outer canthus.	*All materials (crusts, discharge, and so on) on the lids or lashes must be washed away before exposing the conjunctiva.*
11. Fill the irrigating dropper or syringe with the solution. Warm solutions are most comfortable to the patient (that is, the solution temperature should be close to normal body temperature).	
12. Pull the lower lid down gently and the brow up. Instruct the patient to look up, but not to squeeze the eyelids (Figure 8-8). Do not apply pressure over the eye. If the patient has had intraocular surgery, do not ask the patient to look up, because this may cause injury.	*Supporting the eyelids minimizes blinking and exposes the upper and lower conjunctival membranes for irrigation. Pressure on the internal eye structures could cause injury.*
13. Holding the dropper or syringe parallel to the eye, squeeze the solution into the eye, allowing it to flow away from the nose. Hold the dropper or syringe ½ inch from the eye, and allow the solution to flow in a steady stream, but at low pressure (see Figure 9-9).	*The solution is directed away from the nose so that it does not enter the nasolacrimal duct or spill over into the unaffected eye, which could result in transmission of an infection, if it is present. Too much pressure may be injurious to the eye tissues.*
14. Do not allow the dropper or syringe to touch the eye or eyelids.	*Prevent injury to the eye. Dropper or syringe becomes contaminated if it touches the eye.*
15. Continue the procedure until the eye is free of secretions, or the desired results occur, or the prescribed amount of solution has been used.	
16. Gently dry the eye and cheek with sterile cotton balls; discard the cotton balls in designated container.	*Remove excess solution. Provide for the patient's comfort.*
17. Provide for the patient's safety and comfort; provide further instructions as indicated; allow the patient to rest for a few minutes.	
18. Observe the drainage in the basin, then discard. Discard soiled disposable items; return reusable items to designated area for used supplies.	
19. Remove gloves is you have worn them.	
20. Wash your hands.	

21. Record the procedure, the type and amount of solution used, and the results on the patient's chart.	*Charting example:*
	    October 11, 19___, 1 p.m.
	        OD irrigated with 100 ml 5% boric acid.
	        Redness in OD has markedly decreased.
	        Patient stated that the treatment felt soothing.
	        Patient instructed to continue treatments at home for 1 week, as ordered by Dr. McArthur, and then to return for examination.

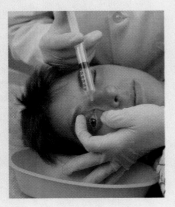

Figure 9-9 *Eye irrigation. Hold dropper or syringe parallel to eye, squeeze solution into eye at inner canthus, allowing it to flow away from the nose.*

CONCLUSION

When you have practiced the procedures outlined in this unit and feel competent with your knowledge and skills, arrange with your instructor to take the performance test. You will be expected to prepare for and perform ear and eye instillations and irrigations.

When treating the eye, keep in mind that it is a delicate sense organ that must be treated gently. Solutions and medications instilled into the eye should be applied to the lower conjunctiva and *not* on the corneal surface.

When irrigating the ear, you must gently direct a steady slow stream of solution against the roof of the canal to prevent injury to the tympanic membrane, to prevent pushing material further into the canal, and to permit the solution flow in and out of the ear freely.

REVIEW OF VOCABULARY

Using the information presented in this unit and other reference sources of your own choice, define the following terms.

TERMS PERTAINING TO THE EAR

1. *Auricle*
2. *Cerumen*
3. *External acoustic meatus*
4. *Semicircular canals*
5. *Pinna*
6. *Tinnitus*
7. *Otopyorrhea*
8. *Otitis media*
9. Audiometer
10. *Meniere's syndrome*
11. *Tympanic membrane (TM)*
12. *Otoscope*
13. *Otology*
14. *Myringoplasty*

TERMS PERTAINING TO THE EYE

1. *Canthus*
2. *Cataract*
3. *Pupil*
4. *Conjunctivitis*
5. *Mydriatic*
6. *Miotic*
7. *Presbyopia*
8. *Glaucoma*
9. *Hyperopia*
10. *Errors of refraction*
11. *Ophthalmoscope*
12. *Lacrimal duct*
13. *Intraocular*
14. *Cornea*

CASE STUDY

Children commonly insert small objects into their ears and up their noses. These foreign bodies may be removed in the physician's office, an ambulatory surgical center, or outpatient department of the hospital if general anesthesia is required. The following is an example of an operative note dictated at the conclusion of a procedure performed on a young child. Read it and be prepared to discuss the italicized terminology.

OPERATIVE REPORT

PATIENT: Busy Beaver

PREOPERATIVE DIAGNOSIS: *Foreign body bilaterally* of the ear canal and right *serous otitis media*.

POSTOPERATIVE DIAGNOSIS: Same.

OPERATION: Removal of foreign body both ears, *cerumen*, and right *myringotomy*.

FINDINGS: The *external ear* was examined for signs of inflammation or trauma. Examination of the *external auditory meatus* revealed a piece of dry popcorn in the right ear; was removed and myringotomy was done; gluelike fluid was aspirated. A piece of Styrofoam was removed from the left ear canal. The *tympanic membrane was normal*.

REVIEW QUESTIONS

1. Explain the difference between an instillation and an irrigation.
2. State the reason for pulling an adult's earlobe upward and backward when giving an ear instillation or irrigation.
3. List three reasons why an ear irrigation is done with a steady, slow stream of solution and not a fast, high-pressure flow.
4. Explain how cerumen can be softened for later removal.
5. Explain to Mrs. Sanson how she should instill eardrops into her 5-year-old son's left ear.
6. Describe the position you would have Mr. John Rogan assume for an ear irrigation. Explain the reason for your answer.
7. The physician has asked you to prepare Nancy Lilly for an eye irrigation. List the supplies you would need, and explain how you would prepare and position Nancy for this procedure.
8. List four purposes for which an eye irrigation may be performed.
9. Explain how you would put eye ointment into Connie Hepworth's eye.
10. When eyedrops and eye ointment are both ordered for the patient at the same time, which agent would you instill into the eye first?
11. Name the region of the eye into which eyedrops should be instilled.

PERFORMANCE TEST

In a skills laboratory, the medical assistant student, with a partner, will assemble supplies and demonstrate the correct procedure for the following without reference to source materials. Time limits for the performance of each procedure are to be assigned by the instructor (see also page 52).

1. Ear instillation
2. Ear irrigation
3. Eye instillation
4. Eye irrigation

The student is expected to perform these skills and record the procedures on the patient's chart with 100% accuracy.

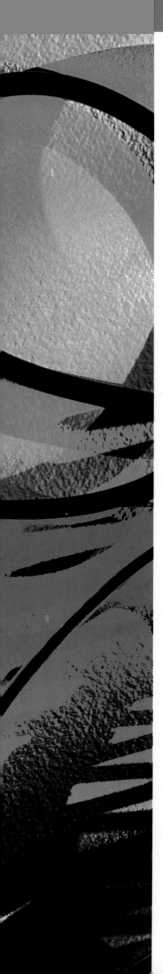

Laboratory Orientation

COGNITIVE OBJECTIVES

On completion of Unit Ten, the medical assistant student should be able to:

1. State the importance of the information gathered from clinical laboratory tests.
2. List and discuss three formats that may be used to organize the recordings of various diagnostic procedures.
3. State the reason why most laboratory tests are performed in a commercial clinical laboratory rather than in a physician's office or in a health care agency.
4. List six types of workers in a clinical laboratory, indicating the basic functions/responsibilities of each.
5. List six specialized departments common to all clinical laboratories and describe the function of each department.
6. List five additional special departments that may be part of some clinical laboratories and describe the function of each department.
7. Discuss the medical assistant's responsibilities when dealing with a clinical laboratory.
8. List seven items that are to be included on laboratory requisition that accompanies a specimen to the laboratory.
9. List three reasons for the performance of diagnostic studies.
10. Discuss the organization of diagnostic reports that are to be placed in the patient's chart.
11. Discuss the concept and the purpose of quality control in the laboratory.
12. List 20 safety rules that should be followed when using laboratory equipment and chemicals, and when around specimens.

TERMINAL PERFORMANCE OBJECTIVES

On completion of Unit Ten, the medical assistant student should be able to:

1. Demonstrate safe practices when working with laboratory equipment and specimens.
2. Demonstrate proficiency in using a microscope.
3. Identify by name the parts of a microscope.
4. Demonstrate proficiency in using a clinical centrifuge

The student is to perform these objectives with 100% accuracy 95% of the time.

The consistent use of universal precautions is required by all health care professionals in all health care settings as a method of infection control. It is assumed that these precautions are used in all of the following procedures. Review Unit One if you have any question on methods to use, as the methods/techniques will not be repeated in detail in each procedure presented in the unit.

Be sure to consult the latest guidelines issued by the Centers for Disease Control and Prevention and consult with infection control practitioners when needed to identify specific precautions that pertain to your particular work situation.

Medical practice is based on information obtained from various sources. Unit Two discussed information obtained from a patient history and from a general or specific physical examination. Another important source of information to help diagnose and treat disease processes is gathered from clinical laboratory tests. It is important to remember that the physician evaluates all data gathered before a diagnosis is made or treatment initiated. Frequently, information from a combination of sources is required because one source may not be sufficient (see Appendix B). Repeat tests may be needed to confirm initial findings and establish the progress of a disease process or its elimination.

Scientific and technologic discoveries have aided medicine tremendously by making accessible abundant data on numerous types of body specimens with a speed and accuracy that previously were not available. Laboratory medicine can determine changes in the chemical or physical characteristics of body fluids, excretions, and tissues and in turn reflect changes in the anatomy and physiology of various organs. Changes noted may indicate a disease process at the site from which the specimen was obtained (for example, a wound culture may identify the presence of bacteria and an infectious process). At other times, the changes in the characteristics of the specimen may indicate a disease process in another part of the body (for example, the presence of excessive sugar in the urine may indicate diabetes mellitus, a disorder in carbohydrate metabolism, and not a disorder of the urinary system; elevated levels of certain blood enzymes may indicate a heart attack or a liver disease).

VOCABULARY

Vocabulary terms are presented in the specific sections to which they apply throughout this unit.

Thus, with laboratory techniques, specific data concerning the status of certain body functions and conditions may be determined. Normal values for the physical and chemical characteristics of body substances have been predetermined; each technique used has its own normal value ratio. Deviations from these set norms aid in the diagnosis and treatment of abnormal disturbances in body function and structure.

THE TYPICAL LABORATORY

Initially, many clinical laboratory procedures were performed in the physician's office. Over the years, as numerous tests have been developed that are more time-consuming and require more specialized equipment, specially trained personnel have become necessary. Although many physicians still perform basic routine tests in their offices, they usually find it more economical, efficient, and accurate to have most tests performed by the trained personnel in a hospital or a private or public health department laboratory.

There are various types of workers in a clinical laboratory. These may include a physician who is certified as a pathologist acting as the director of the laboratory; medical technologists, who are trained at a college for 4 years (who may also have a 1 year internship) and are able to perform specialized tests; medical technicians, trained for 2 years at a junior or community college, who assist and perform tests under the supervision of the medical technologists. A cytotechnologist, trained for 2 years at a college (plus a 1 to 2 year program in cytotechnology), is a highly specialized worker who examines cells and tissues microscopically for the presence of cancer. A histologic technician, trained for 1 or 2 years in a technical training program, is also a specialized worker who is involved with the preparation of various types of tissues for microscopic examination performed by the pathologist. The clinical laboratory assistant, usually trained at a technical level or below that of a 2-year college program, performs basic and routine tests under the direct supervision of the medical technologist or the director of the laboratory. Frequently, medical technologists become specialized in one or two fields in the clinical laboratory and devote all their working time to the area of their expertise.

All clinical laboratories have certain specialized departments in common. They are divided into areas on the basis of function and types of tests performed. These areas usually include hematology, urinalysis, serology, blood banking, medical microbiology, and clinical chemistry. Parasitology and examination of feces may be special departments or they

VOCABULARY

Bacteriology (bak-te″-re-ol′o-je) The study of bacteria.
Virology (vi-rol′ -o-je)—The study of viruses.
Mycology (mi-kol′ o-je)—The study of fungi.
Rickettsiology (ri-ket″si-ol′o-je)—The study of rickettsiae.
Protozoology (pro″to-zo-o′o-je)—The study of protozoa, the simplest forms of animals.
Phycology (fi-kol′je)—The study of algae.
Parasitology (par′ah-si-tol′o-je)—The study of parasites. These may be protozoans or even larger organisms that have microscopic stages in their development.

may be included in one of the other departments. Some laboratories may also have special areas for histology, mycology, immunochemistry, and cytology.

Hematology deals with the study of blood. Examination for the total cell number, the types and number of different cells, cell morphology (shape and size), and the important aspects of the functions of blood, in addition to coagulation studies, are all part of hematology (see also Tables 13-1 and 13-2).

Urinalysis deals with the examination of the physical, chemical, and microscopic properties of urine (see also Tables 12-1, 12-2, 12-4, and 12-5 to 12-7).

Serology involves laboratory tests that examine blood serum. Reactions involving antibodies and antigens are observed and used to determine various types of infections such as tests for infectious mononucleosis (Monospot). The tests for pregnancy, hepatitis B surface antigen, and syphilis are also serology tests, since they involve immunologic reactions (see also Table 13-2).

Blood banking deals with the processing of blood and blood products that will be used for transfusions. It is also known as immunohematology because antigen-antibody reactions are involved in the typing of blood (see also Table 13-2).

Medical microbiology deals with isolation and culture, microscopic identification, and biochemical tests to detect microorganisms that cause disease. Depending on the classification of the microorganisms under investigation, the field of medical microbiology is generally divided into areas of specialization that include the following (see also Tables 12-7 and 13-2).

Parasitology may be an area apart from microbiology. Stool and blood specimens are examined for the presence of eggs or parts of a variety of roundworms, tapeworms, and flukes.

Clinical chemistry examines body fluids such as blood, urine, and cerebrospinal fluid for any change in their chemical content. Glucose and electrolyte levels are determined, as well as the presence of uric acid or urea in the urine or blood (see also Tables 12-1, 12-2, 12-4, and 13-2).

Histology involves the study of specimens of tissue from any source in the body. Form and structural changes are observed microscopically.

Immunochemistry is the study of the chemistry involved with immunity.

Cytology involves the microscopic study of cells to detect any abnormal or malignant changes. Examples include the Pap test and chromosome studies.

COST CONTAINMENT

Cost containment is a factor that must be considered when ordering or performing laboratory tests. Generally speaking, it is least expensive for the patient if simple routine laboratory tests are performed in the physician's office or health care agency. There are two reasons for this. First, the physician can collect and perform simple laboratory tests with relative ease on samples collected when the patient is in the office. Second, the physician or health care agency can avoid the costs of extensive laboratory equipment and the high salary of laboratory technicians or technologists. The next least expensive situation for patients is for the physician to obtain the sample in his or her facility and forward it to a commercial laboratory or to refer patients directly to a commercial laboratory to have the test performed. The larger the laboratory or organization, the less expensive the procedure is for the patient, because large laboratories perform tests on a large volume of samples using more sophisticated equipment. The specialized instruments available in large laboratories can perform multiple tests at the same time, thereby reducing the cost to each patient. The most expensive situation for patients is for the physician to refer them to a hospital laboratory to have the required test performed because the general high cost of operating a hospital must be shared by all departments. An example follows. When a laboratory test is performed in the physician's office or in a health care agency, it may cost the patient $10. When the same test is performed at a commercial clinical laboratory it may cost the patient $15, and when the test is performed at a hospital laboratory it may cost $20. Thus, when laboratory tests other than the very simple procedures that the physician can easily perform in his or her facility are ordered, it is suggested that patients be referred to a commercial laboratory that is qualified and with which the physician has established a business relationship. This is the most cost-efficient procedure to follow. It is also important that the patient be referred to a laboratory that accepts payment under the his or her insurance plan.

LIASION AND RESPONSIBILITIES OF THE MEDICAL ASSISTANT WITH LABORATORIES

You have certain responsibilities when dealing with a laboratory. These include a basic knowledge of the various tests available, proper collection and handling of specimens that are to be forwarded to a laboratory, instruction to the patient

when preparing for certain tests (see Units Six and Eleven), and the handling of completed reports as they return to the office. To help prevent errors, good communication among all parties involved is vital. When you are not sure of the procedure for collecting or handling a specimen or what instructions are to be given to the patient, never hesitate to contact the laboratory for this information. By doing this, you avoid errors and inconvenience to the patient, who would have to return to give another specimen if the initial procedure had been performed incorrectly.

Correct labeling of the specimen and completing the laboratory requisition are other important responsibilities. Always label the container in which the specimen has been collected with the date, the patient's name, and the source of the specimen. On the laboratory requisition that accompanies the specimen, include the following:

- The patient's full name, age, sex, and address
- The physician's full name (also address when sending specimens to outside laboratories)
- Date the specimen was collected, date the specimen was sent to the laboratory if this differs from the date of collection, and time the specimen was collected
- Source of the specimen
- Test(s) required*
- Possible diagnosis when feasible (this alerts the laboratory for specifics for which to watch)
- Medications or treatments the patient is receiving that may interfere with test results

At times the physician requires test results immediately. In these situations the STAT (immediately) should be checked off on the laboratory requisition or printed in large bold letters on the requisition. Some laboratories provide you with "STAT" stickers. Place them on the specimen container *and* on the lab requisition.

Most laboratories provide specific requisitions for the various types of tests that are to be performed in different areas of the laboratory (see sample requisitions in Units Eleven and Thirteen). Be certain that you use the correct requisition for the test(s) requested on the specimen. For example, a blood specimen is sent to the hematology department when the test ordered is a complete blood count; therefore you must complete the hematology requisition. A cytology requisition is sent with a cervical smear for a Pap test.

In addition, many labs provide you with manuals that include the names of the tests that they perform; the normal values or normal ranges for each test; patient preparation; supplies needed; the amount and type of specimen required;

---

*At times, more than one test is performed at the same time to study a specific organ, body system, or disease or to be used as a screening process. This grouping of specific tests is referred to as profiles or panels. They provide the physician with an overview of the patient's status that a single test could not provide (for example, a kidney function profile that may entail 12 different tests or a cardiac profile that may entail 10 different tests). Different laboratories may include different tests in their profiles/panels as discussed in Unit Thirteen under Automation in the Clinical Laboratory.

and instructions for the proper handling, storage, and transporting of the specimen for each test.

Medical assistants should know the normal ranges of test results so that, when abnormal results are reported, they can be brought to the physician's attention immediately. Depending on the policy of the office or health agency, you may circle or underline abnormal results in red. This helps to bring them to the physician's attention quickly. In many cases, computerized reports automatically identify abnormal results on the report. Frequently, physicians sign or put a check on a laboratory report after viewing it. This gives you an indication that it may be filed in the patient's chart. *Never* file a report before it has been reviewed by the physician. To hasten the physician's awareness of abnormal test results, many laboratories report these by telephone immediately and forward the written report later, signed by the laboratory worker who performed the test. Accuracy in reporting test results cannot be stressed enough because frequently the diagnosis and treatment for a patient are contingent on these reports.

DIAGNOSTIC AND THERAPEUTIC PROCEDURES

Earlier in this book it was stated that the physician arrives at a diagnosis by using and reviewing multiple factors and information obtained on the patient's condition (that is, the physician uses various studies to arrive at a diagnosis). Three reasons for diagnostic studies follow.

1. To determine (diagnose) the condition from which the patient is suffering so that treatment, if feasible, may be initiated.
2. To discover disease in its early stage before the patient experiences any signs or symptoms. This is called screening. Screening for disease often permits the cure of the disease because treatment can be started in the early stages of the disease process (for example, cancer), or early treatment can delay the progression of the disease (for example, hypotension).
3. To evaluate past or ongoing treatment received by the patient.

As the field of medical science continues to expand, newer and more accurate and sophisticated techniques are continually made available to help physicians diagnosis disease processes. Diagnostic procedures and studies include, but are not limited to, physical examinations, surgical intervention, and laboratory technology. Other procedures used when diagnosing and treating disease processes require some elaboration. These involve the areas of radiology (roentgenology), the specialized field of nuclear medicine, special skin tests, physical medicine and physiotherapy, and electrocardiography.

To completely understand all these diagnostic and therapeutic procedures, special courses of study are necessary. Nevertheless, the following units expose you to various additional tests that the physician may order for a patient. (Physical examinations, minor surgery, and special skin tests were discussed in preceding units of this book.) It is hoped that the descriptions of the following diagnostic and therapeutic studies and procedures help you understand the nature and purpose(s) of the numerous clinical entities available to health care practitioners for the treatment and care of patients.

Various studies, related vocabulary, and procedures are presented, along with special patient preparation when it is required. *It is important to remember that you are not expected to also be a laboratory, x-ray, nuclear medicine, or electrocardiography technician or a physical therapist, but that you are expected to be familiar with the vocabulary and the nature and purpose(s) of diagnostic or therapeutic procedures and studies performed by these specialists.* At times you may be called on to assist with procedures performed by these medical specialties or to perform the more routine and simplified procedures such as routine urinalysis, skin tests, the application of hot or cold, and electrocardiograms. Additional medical assistant responsibilities may be to explain the nature and purpose of the procedure to the patient, to give the patient special instructions when needed, to record the procedure on the patient's medical record, and to file or store the reports and films received after the test or treatment has been completed.

This unit and Units Fourteen and Fifteen present an opportunity for students to design their own step-by-step procedures and performance checklists. Appendix B gives a summary of studies used for diagnosing conditions affecting body organs and systems.

ORGANIZING THE RECORDINGS OF DIAGNOSTIC PROCEDURES

A patient's medical record should be maintained in an organized manner to facilitate easy accessibility to the information. Regular-sized paper or preprinted forms are customarily used when recording all information relevant to the patient's care. If you receive reports on small sheets, affix them to standard-sized sheets before filing them in the patient's medical record.

Various methods are used when filing laboratory reports in a patient's medical record. Some office or health agencies have a certain order for compiling medical records, so that the laboratory report papers follow or precede other entries. One common method uses a special standard-size sheet of paper designated specifically for staggering these reports (Figure 10-1).

One of three formats can be used for recording and organizing information and test results in the patient's record: the source-oriented format, the integrated format, or the problem-oriented format.

In the *source-oriented* medical record, all reports are filed chronologically according to their specialty (for example, all laboratory reports are filed together, x-ray film reports are filed together, and electrocardiogram records are kept together). The latest information is placed on top, since it is the most important for the patient's current care and treatment.

Figure 10-1 *Laboratory report records. Place the first report on the lower portion where indicated. Place each additional report on top of the preceding one, allowing the bottom $^1/_2$ inch of each report to be visible. This area is where the date is recorded. The most recent report is on top, allowing for quick review of each current information.*

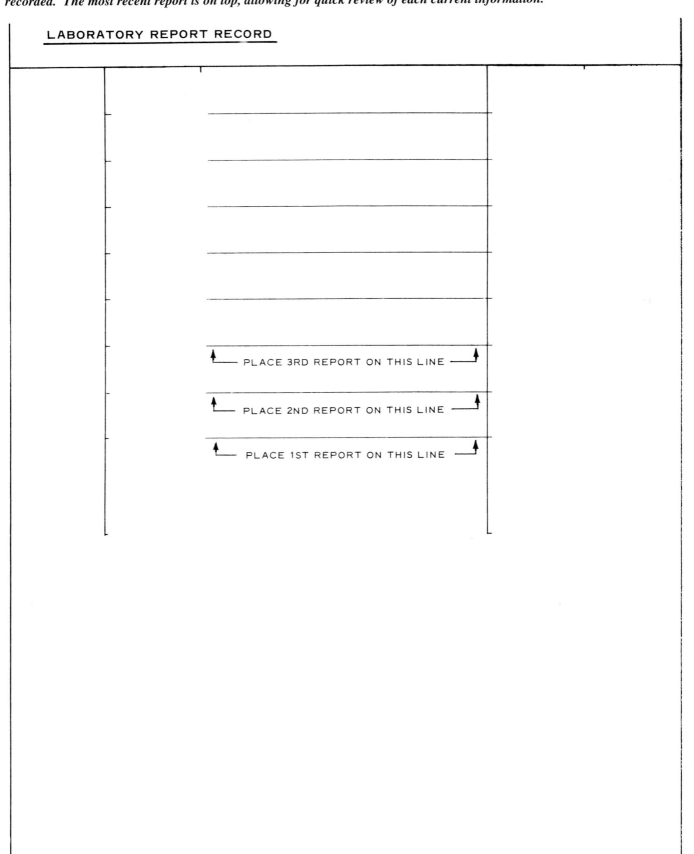

LABORATORY REPORT RECORD

PLACE 3RD REPORT ON THIS LINE

PLACE 2ND REPORT ON THIS LINE

PLACE 1ST REPORT ON THIS LINE

Figure 10-1—cont'd *Laboratory report records.*

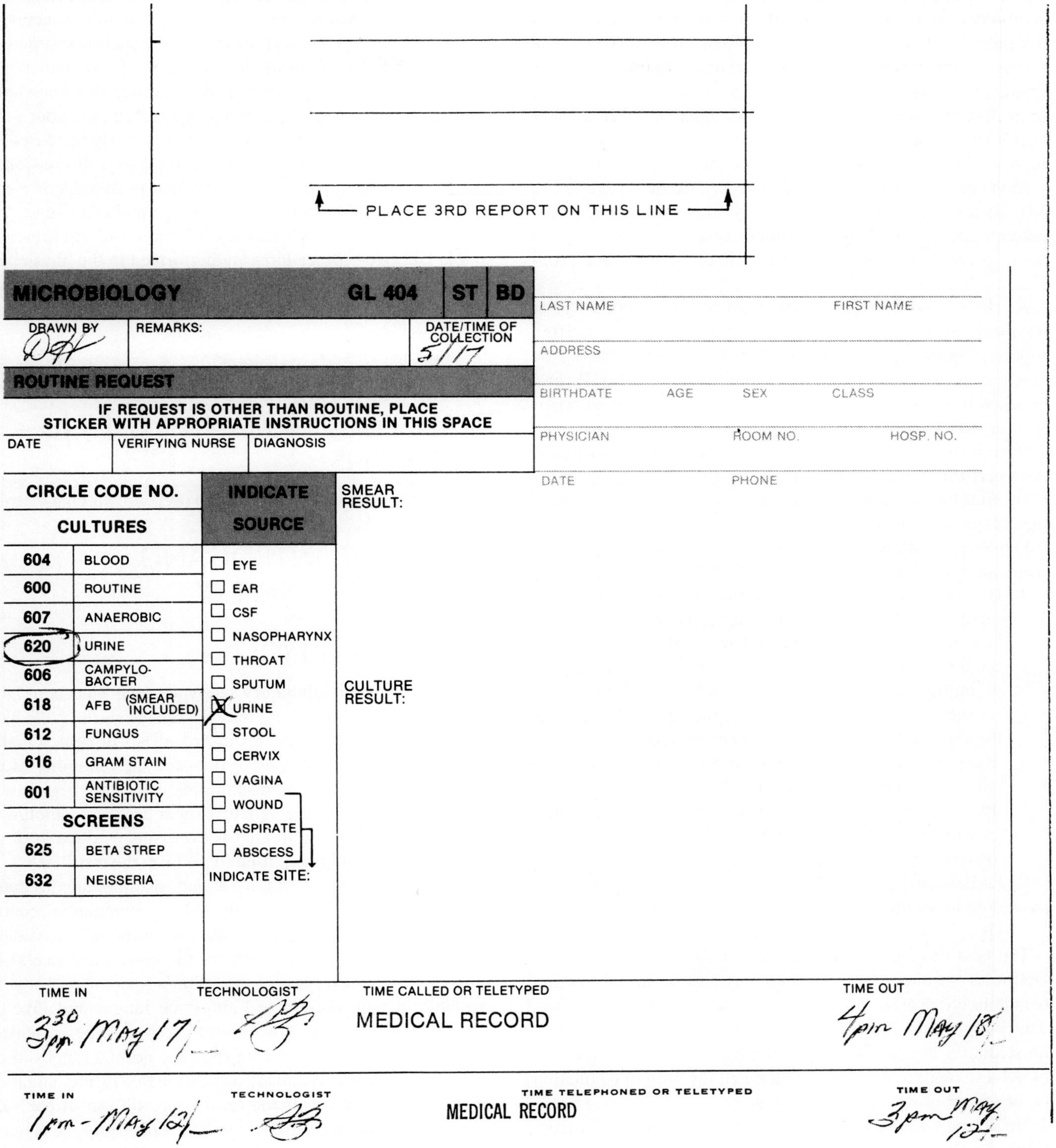

PLACE 3RD REPORT ON THIS LINE

MICROBIOLOGY		GL 404	ST	BD

DRAWN BY	REMARKS:		DATE/TIME OF COLLECTION
DH			*5/17*

ROUTINE REQUEST

IF REQUEST IS OTHER THAN ROUTINE, PLACE STICKER WITH APPROPRIATE INSTRUCTIONS IN THIS SPACE

DATE	VERIFYING NURSE	DIAGNOSIS

LAST NAME   FIRST NAME

ADDRESS

BIRTHDATE   AGE   SEX   CLASS

PHYSICIAN   ROOM NO.   HOSP. NO.

DATE   PHONE

CIRCLE CODE NO.		INDICATE	
CULTURES		**SOURCE**	

SMEAR RESULT:

Code	Culture	Source
604	BLOOD	☐ EYE
600	ROUTINE	☐ EAR
607	ANAEROBIC	☐ CSF
(**620**)	URINE	☐ NASOPHARYNX
606	CAMPYLO-BACTER	☐ THROAT
618	AFB (SMEAR INCLUDED)	☐ SPUTUM
612	FUNGUS	☒ URINE
616	GRAM STAIN	☐ STOOL
601	ANTIBIOTIC SENSITIVITY	☐ CERVIX

CULTURE RESULT:

	SCREENS	☐ VAGINA
		☐ WOUND
625	BETA STREP	☐ ASPIRATE
632	NEISSERIA	☐ ABSCESS
		INDICATE SITE:

TIME IN	TECHNOLOGIST	TIME CALLED OR TELETYPED	TIME OUT
3³⁰pm May 17		**MEDICAL RECORD**	*4pm May 18*

TIME IN	TECHNOLOGIST	TIME TELEPHONED OR TELETYPED	TIME OUT
1pm - May 18		**MEDICAL RECORD**	*3pm May 18*

In the *integrated record,* all information is recorded in strict chronologic order as the physician sees the patient, gives care, and orders various tests (that is, the physician dates and enters the patient's history, physical examination results, and the treatment given and ordered; the laboratory, electrocardiogram, and x-ray film reports are filed in the medical record immediately following the physician's notes for this particular situation; progress notes and future laboratory or x-ray reports continue to be entered in strict chronologic order).

In the *problem-oriented medical record* (review pages 62 to 64), all test results (laboratory, x-ray film, and physical) are entered and recorded in the Objective part of the progress notes, preceded by the number and title of the particular problem.

At times, a radiologist's office, an outside laboratory, or hospital telephones test results before mailing a written report. The information received in this manner should be labeled as a verbal report and recorded accurately and attached to the patient's medical record until the actual report is received.

You must ensure that all reports are received for diagnostic tests performed on the patient outside the physician's office. Only after the physician reviews them should you file them in the patient's medical record.

Develop a follow-through procedure for pending reports from outside sources. Usable methods include the following:

1. Use individual sheets for laboratory tests, x-ray film reports, electrocardiograms, and consultations from outside sources; they can be kept in separate files or in a binder. Each entry should be made on a separate line, giving the date, patient's name, and the test(s) ordered. As the reports are received, enter the date and check off the entry to indicate that it has been received.

2. Keep the patient's medical record in a special file until all outstanding reports have been received.

3. Place the patient's record back in the usual file with a colored flag attached to indicate that reports are yet to be received.

Regardless of the method, use a consistent follow-through procedure to ensure that all test results are received on a regular basis.

The next three units are devoted to information on the collection of various types of specimens and on urinalysis and hematology because urine and blood are the two most abundant body fluids and provide a wealth of information on an individual's health. Reference tables for various urine and blood tests with related information and the normal evaluation ranges for their results are also presented.

No attempt is made in this book to give detailed instructions for the procedures involved when performing all of these laboratory tests, since *most* **must** *only be performed by* certified laboratory personnel or physicians. The purposes of the following information and Units Eleven through Thirteen are to prepare you for performing basic routine procedures that may be done in the physician's office or health care agency and to make you aware of some of the many laboratory tests, the special equipment, and the supplies that are available, along with the normal ranges for test results. You are expected to know how to collect and handle specimens. When applicable, you must also know the special instructions to give to the patient before the collection of a specimen, and the normal test results expected. By attaining this knowledge and these skills, patient care can be enhanced, and your value to the physician, patient, and laboratory is vastly increased.

The remainder of this unit is devoted to a discussion of quality control and laboratory safety and of two major pieces of laboratory equipment, the microscope and centrifuge. You should be familiar with this information and equipment if simple laboratory procedures are performed in the physician's office or health care agency and also when specimens and blood samples are to be prepared for transport to a commercial laboratory.

COLLECTING, HANDLING, TRANSPORTING, AND STORING SPECIMENS

See Unit Eleven, page 340, and also review Unit One.

QUALITY CONTROL AND LABORATORY SAFETY

QUALITY CONTROL

Quality control and laboratory safety are vital aspects of laboratory technology. They are directly related to the collection, handling, processing, and testing of all specimens. Quality control involves methods used to ensure the reliability of the tests performed and tests results obtained. This begins with proper preparation of the patient, proper care and handling of specimens as discussed in Unit Eleven, and evaluation of the techniques and equipment used to perform the tests.

Even the smallest laboratory should use methods to determine the accuracy of test results. Many commercial control products are available to check the reliability of test products and results. These products test for the same substance(s) for which you would be testing a patient's specimen. They are available in both normal and abnormal ranges and give the range of valid results. You should use both types to ensure test accuracy. Results differing from the normal ranges of the control indicate that your test is inaccurate. In this situation, repeat the control test. If the results are still out of the valid control range, do not use these supplies for testing specimens from patients until the problem has been identified and corrected. Machines must be calibrated frequently to ensure that they are working properly. Many are calibrated automatically with the aid of a computer. Keep a record of the results and dates of all the control tests you run. State laws usually require the records (see Figures 12-3 through 12-6 and Controls for Routine Urinalysis on page 395 in Unit Twelve.)

Controls provide the laboratory worker with the capability to evaluate the changes and/or errors that are commonly associated with routine clinical chemistry. The controls should be used to establish confidence that the variables that cause errors are in check or within a range of acceptability as established by the laboratory. Guidelines have been established to aid the laboratory to initiate a quality control program using solutions of known values. By understanding the trends established by responsible interpretation of control values, better results are obtained with clinical procedures. Controls are tested often, usually in duplicate, to control laboratory error. By realizing that quality control assesses the sources of variables, from specimen transporting to recording of results, better values are obtained—with a high degree of confidence in the procedures used. An example of controls used for routine urinalysis is given in Unit Twelve, pages 396 to 398.

LABORATORY SAFETY

Laboratory testing involves certain safety hazards such as exposure to strong chemicals and infectious materials. Thus it is most important that laboratory workers use safe, proper techniques when around and using laboratory equipment, chemicals, and specimens. The following *safety rules* are to assist you to work in a safe manner. Also review Unit One, Universal Precautions—OSHA's Blood-Borne Pathogens Standards.

General

- Do not eat, drink, or smoke in the laboratory.
- Use protective equipment such as rubber gloves, eye goggles, and apron when required.
- Keep pens, pencils, and fingers away from your mouth.
- Wash your hands *frequently and thoroughly*. **Use appropriate personal protective equipment (PPE) as dictated by facility.**
- If you are pregnant, you should not be exposed to potential or known pathogenic agents.
- If you are inexperienced, you should be well supervised.
- When you have an open wound or an eczematous skin condition, you should not handle pathogenic material unless the risks involved can be avoided by protective equipment.
- Process specimens from known infectious material separately from other specimens. Disinfect nondisposable equipment used for these specimens after use. Place all used disposable equipment in biohazardous waste containers.
- Clean your work area with a disinfectant at the end of the day and at least one other time during the day.

Chemicals and Reagents

- Current inventory control is important. Discard chemical reagents in accordance with their expiration dates.
- Store labeled chemicals and reagents under nonreactive conditions with respect to light, moisture, and temperature. Follow the manufacturer's recommended storage procedures.
- You must not pipette by mouth. Mouth pipetting is prohib-

ited under OSHA's Universal Precautions. Use a commercial pipetting device.
- You must use disposable gloves when handling specimens and disinfectants and when cleaning automatic blood-analyzing equipment.

Equipment

- Clean automatic blood- and serum-analyzing systems after each use according to the manufacturer's directions.
- Unplug electric appliances before cleaning or washing them.
- Unplug major appliances when lights stay dim or unusually bright.
- Use properly grounded 3-pronged UL-approved, double-insulated electrical equipment.
- Discard materials used to wipe machine parts during operation and cleaning with other biohazardous waste.
- Do not wear loose-fitting clothing when working around a bunsen burner.
- Do not use bunsen burners near areas where oxygen is in use or where flammables are stored.
- Know emergency fire procedures if use of a bunsen burner is required.
- Do not leave bunsen burners unattended when they are lit.
- Position centrifuges in areas where their vibrations do not cause items to fall off nearby shelves.
- Always balance the load in a centrifuge to avoid damage to the equipment and injury to yourself.
- Cover centrifuges when in use.
- Take care when loading and unloading a centrifuge to avoid spilling the specimens.
- Turn the centrifuge off before opening the lid (if it is not equipped with an interlocking device).

Glassware

- Take a regular inventory of all glassware. Discard all chipped or cracked pieces.
- Handle and store all glassware carefully to avoid breakage.

Identification of Materials (Chemicals and Reagents)

- Label *all* materials clearly. Replace soiled labels immediately.
- Do not use, but discard any unlabeled item according to Material Safety Data Sheets (MSDSs) in your area.
- When affixing a label, moisten it with a damp sponge. Do not lick the label.
- Make sure that poisons, corrosives, and flammable materials are labeled as such. Have a proper storage area for these items away from other solutions that you may have in the office or clinic. Consult the Environmental Protection Agency and the Hazard Communications Act in your area regarding regulations concerning MSDSs, labeling requirements, and posting of notices. These materials must be placed in special, approved containers when being transferred from the storage area to the work space.

THE MICROSCOPE

The microscope (Figure 10-2) is a precise scientific instrument used in the laboratory when an enlarged image of a small (microscopic) object is required. When using the microscope, details of structure not otherwise distinguishable are revealed. Microscopes vary greatly in quality. For maximum efficiency, the operation of a microscope must be studied carefully. Complete instructions for assembling and using the microscope are provided by each manufacturer. Read these instructions completely before you use the microscope for laboratory procedures.

PARTS OF THE MICROSCOPE
Eyepieces

Eyepieces fit into the eyepiece tubes. The eyepieces in common use today are marked 5 ×, 6 ×, or 10 ×. The 10 × eyepiece has the greatest magnifying power. Because the exterior surface of the eyepiece is exposed, it is likely to become dusty; therefore it should be carefully cleaned before use. You can clean it with a special lens paper or with a soft cloth.

Nosepiece and Objectives

The microscope is provided with a revolving nosepiece into which the various objectives are screwed. Care must be used

Figure 10-2 A, *Nikon Labophot microscope;* **B,** *Nikon Optiphot microscope.*
Courtesy Nikon Inc., Instrument Division, Garden City, N.Y.

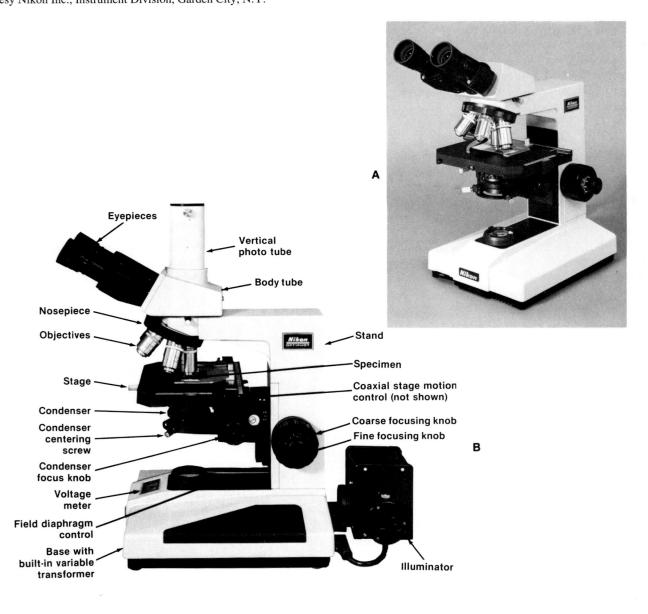

in properly attaching the objectives to the nosepiece. Follow the procedure provided by the manufacturer of the microscope. The objectives make up the lens system on the nosepiece. *Never* at any time force the objective or allow its lower end (the lens) to touch the metal stage. Lenses are very expensive and are easily damaged by contact with any other objects—slides, cover glasses, specimens.

Objectives have different magnifying powers. The following are commonly used (see Table 10-1):
- The lowest power objective, marked 16 mm or 10 ×
- The intermediate power (frequently called the high dry power) marked 4 mm, 43 ×, or 45 ×
- The highest power, the oil-immersion objective, marked 1.8 mm, 97 ×, or 100 ×

In becoming familiar with the different objectives, remember that the low power is the shortest of the three objectives, whereas the oil immersion is the longest of the three. Another point of differentiation is the size of the opening in the smaller end of the objectives. The objective with the widest lens is the lowest power, and conversely the one with the smallest lens is the highest power, the oil-immersion lens. Some examples of magnification power follow.

Arm or Stand
The arm or stand (see Figure 10-2) is used for carrying the microscope. When carrying the microscope, place one hand on the arm and support the base of the microscope with your other hand.

Body Tube
The body tube directs the path of light from the light source to the eyepieces.

Stage
The stage is the flat heavy part on which slides are placed for examination. On the stage are found two slide clips. In place of these clips, it is more convenient to apply an attachable mechanical stage, which is used to move the slides more precisely. This mechanical stage is almost indispensable in laboratory work, especially when the work requires high-power magnification.

Substage
Fitting into the opening on the stage and immediately below it is the substage. This part holds the *substage condenser*, a necessity in microscopic work. Its purpose is to direct, focus, and condense the light on the object under examination. For best results, focus the proper amount of light onto the object by lowering and raising the substage by means of the pinion adjustment (or condenser focus knob). On the lower part of the substage condenser is found the *shutter or diaphragm*. This shutter or diaphragm is to close off light or to admit more light. Since the amount of light required varies, adjustment of the substage in connection with specific uses of the microscope is described in a later paragraph.

Eyepiece	Objective	Magnification
5 ×	10 ×	50
10 ×	10 ×	100
5 ×	45 ×	225
10 ×	45 ×	450
5 ×	100 ×	500
10 ×	100 ×	1000

TABLE 10-1

Microscope Objectives and Uses

Objective	Focal Length	Power	Uses
Low power	16 mm	10 × 10	Initial focusing Initial light adjustment Initial scanning of urine sediment and blood smears Manual counting of white blood cells
High power	4 mm	43× *or* 45 ×	Study of cells and sediment in more detail Study of wet preparations such as urine sediment Manual counting of red blood cells
Oil immersion	1.8 mm	97 × *or* 100 ×	Viewing of very small structures Viewing blood films such as the differential white blood cell count or the reticulocyte count Viewing microorganisms Viewing a Gram stain to identify different types of bacteria

Other Parts of the Microscope

The larger of the two knobs, the *pinion head or coarse-focusing knob*, is used for coarse adjustment of the microscope. The smaller knob, the *fine-focusing knob*, is used in fine adjustment and focusing. These two knobs are important because they must be used every time the instrument is used. When you are looking for the field, you must always lower the head of the microscope by means of the coarse adjustment. You then use the fine adjustment. This is absolutely essential when using high-power magnification. Another part of the microscope is the *light source or illuminator*, which is part of the illumination or light system providing a source of light for viewing a slide. You can direct the light precisely to obtain the clearest possible image. The light source is a built-in lightbulb (illuminator) located at the base of the microscope directly under the center of the stage. The light is directed to the condenser above it, which directs/condenses the light on the object under examination. Two other parts of the illumination or light system are the condenser and the diaphragm. These parts were explained under the heading "Substage."

Care, Cautions, and Maintenance

1. When carrying the microscope, hold it by the arm with one hand, supporting the bottom of the microscope base with the other.
2. Handle the microscope gently, taking care to avoid sharp knocks.
3. Do not try to adjust the microscope yourself if you do not fully understand its mechanism. You may throw the instrument out of balance and adjustment or damage the lens by hitting it on the stage.
4. Never force the adjustment knobs if they do not turn easily. They may need oiling or simple adjustment.
5. Never force a high-powered objective on a microscope slide. Doing so may break the slide, scratch the objective, or damage the lens.
6. Be sure that the lens of the objective is clean before attempting to do microscopic work. Do not leave dust, dirt, or finger marks on the lens surfaces. To clean the lens surfaces, remove dust with a soft-haired brush or gauze. Use a soft cotton cloth, lens tissue, or gauze lightly moistened with absolute alcohol (methanol or ethanol) only for removing finger marks or grease. For cleaning the objectives and immersion oil, use only xylene. For cleaning the surface of the entrance lens of the eyepiece tube, use absolute alcohol. Observe sufficient caution in handling alcohol and xylene.
7. Avoid the use of any organic solvent (for example, thinner, ether, alcohol, or xylene) for cleaning the painted surfaces and plastic parts of the instrument. Mild soap and water may be used on these parts.
8. Avoid the use of the microscope in a dusty place or where it is subject to vibrations or exposed to high temperatures, moisture, or direct sunlight.
9. To avoid the possibility of impairing its operational efficiency and accuracy, never attempt to dismantle the instrument

10. Attention must be given to protecting the objective lenses. Never leave immersion oil on the objective when the instrument is not being used. Before you put the microscope away, rotate the nosepiece so that the low-power objective is in position.
11. Remove the eye lens at regular intervals to clean out the dust and dirt particles that may have collected there.
12. When the microscope is not in use, cover it with the accessory vinyl cover and store it in a place free from moisture and fungus. It is especially recommended that you keep the objectives and eyepieces in an airtight container containing desiccant (a substance that promotes dryness).
13. Contact the salesperson for any serious problems you may have with the instrument.

SPACE FOR USING THE MICROSCOPE

The microscope should be kept set up and ready for use. However limited the office laboratory area is, sufficient space must be allotted exclusively for the use of the microscope. It need be no more than a shelf wide enough to accommodate the equipment. Added to this should be a convenient seat of *proper height*. A kitchen stool will suffice. Trying to work with the microscope handicapped by improper relationship between the height of the worktable and stool is fatiguing and may lead to unreliable work.

USE OF THE MICROSCOPE (FIGURE 10-3)

Place the material to be examined under the microscope on a glass slide. Place the slide on the microscope stage and fasten it with the clips or hold it in place by the mechanical stage. Using the lowest power objective and a 10 × eyepiece, slowly lower the microscope head by using the coarse-focusing knob. When you find the field, adjust the light by raising or lowering the pinion attached to the substage. Next, open or close the diaphragm to admit just the proper amount of light to give a clear, distinct field. To make the field of vision clear, use the fine-adjustment knob. From this point on, you can obtain a higher power of magnification by changing the objective.

PROPER ADJUSTMENT OF ILLUMINATION

The problem of obtaining maximum efficiency of illumination remains. Two factors enter into this problem: the light itself and the manipulation of the diaphragm, which controls the amount of light admitted to the condenser.

To know when the illumination has been properly adjusted, place a slide on the microscope and focus the low-power lens on it. Remove the ocular and look down the tube of the microscope at the lenses of the objective. If shadows appear in this field, try to eliminate them by raising and lowering the condenser.

The most difficult part of illumination seems to be the proper manipulation of the iris diaphragm. Two cardinal principles should be remembered. First, the lower the power of

Figure 10-3 *Technologist using microscope.*

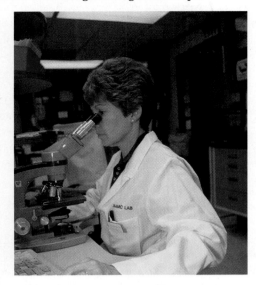

the objective used, the more the light should be cut. In using the 16-mm lens to examine urine sediment or to count leukocytes, close the diaphragm almost completely; when the 4-mm objective is brought into play, the opening should be slightly increased; and, when using the oil-immersion objective, the diaphragm may be opened wide. Second, the more brilliantly stained the object being viewed, the more light you can admit. As an example, if a differential blood count is being made with the 4-mm lens (the high dry power), the diaphragm may be at least half open; whereas during the examination of urinary sediment, especially if seeking hyaline casts, the light should be cut almost completely off. If this is not done, these hyaline structures will not be seen. *The diaphragm should be constantly adjusted while an examination is being made to get the most revealing picture. It is controlled by a little lever below the condenser. You should learn to seek this out and manipulate it subconsciously, since the fine adjustment is kept in constant use while focusing. If you are having trouble with an examination and things are not seen as clearly as they should be, examine the amount of light being admitted. The trouble is not infrequently caused by improper adjustment of the diaphragm.*

FOCUSING

In the microscopes illustrated in Figure 10-2, a coarse- and a fine-adjustment control are seen; the larger, coarse-adjustment knob is placed behind the smaller, which is for fine adjustment. The coarse adjustment is for finding the relative focus; the fine adjustment is for bringing out the details clearly. *Do not use these interchangeably.* Using the coarse adjustment for fine focusing results in broken cover glasses and slides; *trying to find a field with the fine adjustment places too much strain on it and quickly wear it out.*

Place a slide on the stage and bring the low or high dry power objective down until it almost touches. Then, while looking into the microscope, slowly raise it with the coarse adjustment until the image is seen. Using the fine adjustment,

bring out the details as described. It is a good plan never to turn the fine adjustment more than two thirds of one revolution. It is frequently desirable to keep the slide moving on the stage while attempting to focus. If this is not done, you may find that you are trying to focus on a spot where there is no material.

If it is impossible to obtain a clear image although the illumination has been found satisfactory, rotate the eyepiece. If the blur is seen to rotate, the eyepiece is the source of the trouble. Remove it and wipe it thoroughly. Clean the upper portion frequently because it becomes soiled from contact with the eyelashes. In the event that the difficulty is not in the ocular, it is possible that the back of the objective has become fogged. This is not an infrequent occurrence if the instrument has been brought into a warm room from a cold one. Again, it is possible that the objective has been dipped into some fluid—immersion oil or water—and this has dried and caused fogging. Water can be removed with moistened lens tissue, and the lens can then be polished dry. If oil has dried on the lens, remove it cautiously with the smallest possible amount of xylene, and wipe away the excess of this reagent lens tissue.

Never focus down while looking through the microscope. This is inviting disaster to slides and cover glasses, as well as possible damage to the lens. Observe from one side when you do focus down.

USE OF OBJECTIVES

Of the three objectives, which are designated 16 mm, 4 mm, and 1.8 mm respectively, the 16-mm is the shortest in length and has the widest lens. The objective is used for low-power work, principally examining urine sediment, counting leukocytes, and inspecting the counting chamber of red cells for irregularity of distribution (*but only an expert should use it for counting these cells*). The 4-mm lens, the high dry, is mostly used for close inspection of the urinary sediment, counting red blood cells, and making routine differential blood cell counts.

Always use a cover glass when using the high dry power objective for examining urinary sediment. Do not dip the lens into the fluid without this protection. When using the 4-mm objective for differential blood counts, spread a thin film of immersion oil on the slide, over the stained blood, before making the examination.

The oil-immersion lens (1.8 mm) is used for obtaining the highest magnification in a conventional light microscope. Used with the eyepiece that gives a magnification of 10 diameters (marked 10 ×), the object as seen is about 1000 times its actual size. To use this lens, place a drop of oil (such as Junol) on the slide and focus down with coarse adjustment until the tip of the lens just touches the oil. Now, look through the microscope and focus upward very slowly with the coarse adjustment. When the object is seen, bring it into proper detail by use of the fine adjustment. This lens is used for all types of bacteriologic work, for seeking parasites, and for all other purposes demanding high magnification (see also Table 10-1).

PRACTICAL POINTERS FOR MICROSCOPE USE

If a single-tube microscope is used, learn to work with both eyes open. Squinting or closing one eye causes unnecessary strain. If much work is done, frequently shift from one eye to the other.

If you wear glasses, learn to do microscopy without them if possible. The instrument will focus to compensate for your visual defects if you are nearsighted or farsighted. On the other hand, if astigmatism is your difficulty, you have to wear glasses, since this difficulty cannot be corrected by the microscopic lens.

CENTRIFUGES

Centrifuges are motorized devices that rotate at a high speed (Figure l0-4). The speed is stated as *revolutions per minute (rpm)*. Centrifuges are used to separate components of varying densities contained in liquids by spinning them at high speeds. Through centrifugal (moving away from a center) force, heavier or solid components move to the lower part of the container, and lighter substances move to the upper part of the container. By this process the two substances, solid material and fluid supernatant, are separated. The supernatant is the clear upper portion of the mixture after it has been centrifuged.

Centrifuges are used in every department of a clinical laboratory. In a physician's office or health care agency, centrifuges are used if a microscopic analysis of urine is performed and also when serum is required for hematology or blood chemistry laboratory tests.

Numerous types of centrifuges are available. Each must be selected according to the intended use. Centrifuges commonly used in a physician's office or clinic are table models. One type is used for routine blood and urine separations (see Figure 10-4), and another type is used for microhematocrit applications. The speed at which these centrifuges operate varies from 3200 rpm for the routine blood and urine separations to 11,500 to 15,000 rpm for the microhematocrit centrifuges. Use special centrifuge tubes in the centrifuges for serum or urine separations. These tubes are either conical or round-bottomed and made of a special quality glass. You can also put some Vacutainer tubes used for blood collection into the centrifuge. Use capillary tubes in the microhematocrit centrifuges. It is important that you always use tubes that are the correct size and strength for the required application.

In the centrifuge there are special centrifuge cups with rubber cushions that are used to hold the tubes containing the blood or urine samples. Be certain that the cushions are at the bottom of the holders before you place the tubes into them.

PLACEMENT OF TUBES IN THE CENTRIFUGE

When you place a tube containing a specimen into the centrifuge, you must counterbalance it with a tube of similar design and weight. The other tube must be placed directly

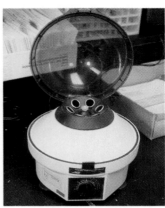

Figure 10-4 *Centrifuge used for blood and urine separations.*

opposite the tube containing the specimen and should contain a liquid of equal weight. Water can usually be used for this purpose (Figure 10-5). If you do not balance the load in a centrifuge, severe vibration of the centrifuge may occur, and you may lose the specimens. *Do not* use tubes that are cracked or badly scratched because they may break under the stress of the centrifugal force. If breakage does occur, immediately turn the centrifuge off. Don rubber gloves and clean the centrifuge cushion and cup. You must clean these areas before using the centrifuge again to avoid additional breakage of tubes.

OPERATING THE CENTRIFUGE

When you operate the centrifuge, you must close the cover. (Many newer models will not work if you do not close the cover.) If you are using an older model centrifuge, *do not* open the cover until the rotor has completely stopped. Do *not* brake sharply when using centrifuges that operate with hand brakes. Always use tubes that are the correct size and strength for the required application. Electrical appliances such as the centrifuge should have three-pronged grounding plugs, and sufficient grounded outlets should be available. Frequent lubrication, calibration, and cleaning are required for the proper operation of all centrifuges. Specific instructions for operating each centrifuge are provided by the manufacturer. Read these instructions completely and carefully before you operate any centrifuge.

Figure 10-5 *Placing specimen tubes in centrifuge.*

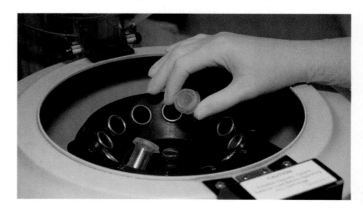

CONCLUSION

With the advances in the knowledge of physiology and improved technology, scientific, diagnostic and therapeutic procedures have increasingly become valuable aids to the physician and the patient. From all the diagnostic and therapeutic procedures presented in the preceding units and Units Eleven through Sixteen, it can be readily seen that modern medicine offers many methods to physicians for arriving at a diagnosis and treating disease processes. The functional and structural alterations of body tissues, organs, and systems in disease can be studied and treated. Great strides have been made, and even greater achievements are expected as the mysteries of scientific research continue to unfold. At the opposite end of the spectrum from the concept of disease is health. For the body to remain healthy, the functions of the body systems must be normal. A primary requirement for survival of the human organism is the maintenance and safeguarding of the anatomic and physiologic equilibrium of the individual cells that make up the sum of the body and its parts.

Numerous sources are available for expanding your knowledge on the topics discussed in the following units. Check with your instructor for additional enrichment assignments and references in areas of your own particular need and interest.

REVIEW OF VOCABULARY

Using the information presented in this unit and other reference sources of your own choice, read and define the italicized terms.

All clinical laboratories have certain specialized departments in common. They are divided into areas on the basis of function and types of tests performed. These areas usually include *hematology, urinalysis, serology, blood banking, medical microbiology,* and *clinical chemistry. Parasitology* and examination of feces may be special departments or they may be included in one of the above. Some laboratories may also have special areas for *histology, mycology, immunochemistry,* and *cytology.*

Correct labeling of a specimen and completing a laboratory requisition are important duties of the medical assistant when sending specimens to outside laboratories.

One of three formats can be used for recording and organizing information and test results in the patient's record: the *source-oriented format, the integrated format, or the problem-oriented format.*

Special care must be given to the microscope and centrifuge when using these pieces of equipment for laboratory work.

CASE STUDY

If the medical office uses the services of an outside laboratory for processing specimens received in the office, it is the medical assistant's responsibility to develop a good working relationship and to adhere to the policies and procedures of such a contract. Read the following information and discuss its implication on small practices. Discuss the italicized terminology used in the typical laboratory. The objectives of the *Clinical Laboratory Improvement Amendments of 1988* (CLIA) are to increase *documentation*, quality control process (QA), *proficiency testing* (PT), and quality of staff, for "essentially all laboratories that test *human specimens* for the purposes of *diagnosis* and/or treatment." These include *hematology, urinalysis, serology, blood banking,* and *medical microbiology.*

REVIEW QUESTIONS

1. State the importance of the information gathered from clinical laboratory tests.
2. List six specialized departments common to all clinical laboratories. Describe the function of each department.
3. Describe the medical assistant's responsibilities when dealing with a commercial clinical laboratory.
4. List seven items that are to be included on a laboratory requisition that accompanies a specimen to the laboratory.
5. Describe how reports would be filed in the source-oriented record.
6. List seven safety rules that should be adhered to when working with laboratory equipment and specimens.
7. State how you should carry a microscope.
8. State what type of tubes should be used in a centrifuge.

PERFORMANCE TEST

In a skills laboratory, a simulation of a joblike environment, the medical assistant student is to demonstrate the correct procedure for the following without reference to source materials.

1. Demonstrate proper use and care of a microscope.
2. Demonstrate proper use and care of a centrifuge.
3. Given sample laboratory requisitions and physician's orders, correctly complete each requisition to be sent to the laboratory along with a specimen.
4. Demonstrate the use of safety rules when working with laboratory equipment and specimens.
5. Demonstrate the use of commercial control products to check the reliability of test products and test results.

The student is expected to perform the above skills with 100% accuracy 90% of the time.

Collecting and Handling Specimens

COGNITIVE OBJECTIVES

On completion of Unit Eleven, the medical assistant student should be able to:

1. Define and pronounce the vocabulary terms listed.
2. Discuss the proper care, handling, transporting, and storage of all specimens.
3. List the information that must be included on a laboratory requisition when sending a specimen for examination.
4. Explain how a specimen should be prepared for transportation through the mail to an outside laboratory.
5. List the purposes, basic equipment, and supplies required and the medical assistant's usual assisting responsibilities for each procedure described in this unit.
6. Discuss the definition of "fasting" with reference to the collection of a specimen from a patient.
7. Discuss steps and precautionary measures that should be used to prevent infection from a specimen.
8. Discuss techniques and methods that must be used to prevent contamination of a patient specimen.
9. State and define seven types of urine specimens, and discuss at least 10 general facts relating to the collection of urine for examination.
10. Discuss the hemoccult slide test for stool specimens, stating why and how it is done; the special diagnostic diet that the patient may be on before and during the test; and medications that would interfere with the test.
11. Differentiate between upper and lower respiratory tract specimens.
12. Differentiate between a smear, a culture, and a culture medium.
13. Briefly discuss the Gram stain and the culture and sensitivity tests performed for bacteriologic studies.
14. List seven types of smears that may be done to detect vaginal disorders and diseases.
15. Discuss patient care before and after a lumbar puncture.
16. State the cause and list at least four common signs and symptoms of a strep throat infection. Discuss complications that could result if not treated in the early stages of infection.
17. Discuss an example of a screening laboratory test that may be used to diagnose strep throat while the patient is in the physician's office or clinic.
18. Briefly discuss the causes, signs and symptoms, diagnostic methods used, treatment, and complications that can result for the sexually transmitted diseases discussed in this unit.

TERMINAL PERFORMANCE OBJECTIVES

On completion of Unit Eleven, the medical assistant student should be able to:

1. Demonstrate correct technique and proper communication to the patient for collecting the following specimens, preparing them to be sent to the laboratory, and completing the appropriate requisition form for the tests that are ordered:
   a. Urine specimen
   b. Stool specimen
   c. Sputum specimen
   d. Throat culture
   e. Nasopharyngeal culture
   f. Wound culture
   g. Vaginal smears and cultures
2. Demonstrate the correct technique for making a smear for cytology studies and a smear for bacteriology studies.
3. Demonstrate the correct technique for performing a Ventrescreen Strep A diagnostic test that is used to diagnose strep throat.
4. Demonstrate the correct procedure for performing a Gram stain.
5. Demonstrate the correct procedure for performing a hemoccult slide test on a stool specimen.
6. Demonstrate the correct technique for inoculating a culture medium with a specimen obtained on a cotton-tipped applicator.

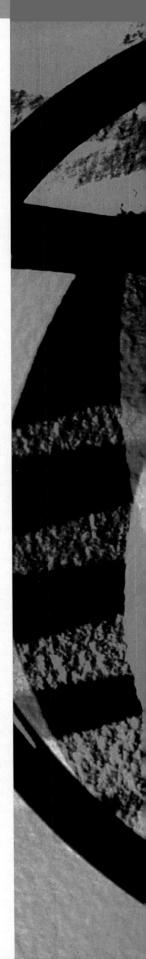

7. Demonstrate the proper procedure for assisting with a lumbar puncture.
8. Demonstrate the correct method for recording information on a patient's medical record after the specimen has been sent to the laboratory.
9. Demonstrate the correct method for completing various types of laboratory requisition forms that accompany a specimen that is sent to the laboratory.

The student is to perform these objectives with 100% accuracy 95% of the time.

The consistent use of universal precautions is required by all health care professionals in all health care settings as a method of infection control. It is assumed that these precautions are used in all of the following procedures. Review Unit One if you have any questions on methods to use as the methods/techniques will not be repeated in detail in each procedure presented in the unit.

Be sure to consult the latest guidelines issued by the Centers for Disease Control and Prevention and consult with infection control practitioners when needed to identify specific precautions that pertain to your particular work situation.

The science of laboratory technology is becoming increasingly sophisticated in methods used to process specimens obtained from a patient. Thus it is rare, if not obsolete, that you will be required to perform the actual tests on collected specimens in a physician's office or health agency, other than simple tests that may be performed several times a day such as a routine urinalysis. The Clinical Laboratory Improvement Amendments (CLIAs) of 1988 have established three categories of laboratory tests on the basis of the complexity of the test. To perform tests under each category, the laboratory must meet certain personnel standards. Each state may establish stricter standards. These regulations in each state determine which laboratory tests that you can perform. Most physicians use the services of professional laboratories that perform tests under controlled conditions and use expensive equipment that is impractical for the physician's office. Frequently the patient is referred to a clinical laboratory, where the specimen is obtained and processed and the results prepared for report to the physician. At other times, you must collect the specimen or assist the physician when obtaining the specimen. Once the specimen has been properly obtained, your responsibility is to ensure that it is preserved and labeled correctly for submission to the laboratory for examination. Therefore it is imperative that you know how to collect various types of specimens and prepare a smear or culture from the specimen, so that specimens arrive at the laboratory in good condition for processing. When collecting specimens, you must also be aware of any special preparation that is required by the patient, ensure that the patient is thoroughly informed and understands the instructions (for example, collect the first morning specimen, or fast 12 hours before collection of the specimen), ascertain that this preparation has been followed, and be certain that the correct equipment is used for the specimen obtained. Most professional laborato-

ries furnish manuals on request that outline the specific requirements for each study to be performed. In this unit you learn techniques for obtaining and for helping the physician obtain different types of specimens, smears, and cultures, in addition to the care and handling of specimens.

Before beginning this unit, review the infectious disease process, Universal Precautions, infection control, and medical and surgical aseptic techniques presented in Units One, Five, and Six.

VOCABULARY

Aerobe (a′ er-ob)—A microorganism that lives and grows in the presence of free oxygen.
Aerobic (aero′ bic)—Capable of living and functioning in the presence of free oxygen.
Bacteriology (bak-te″-re-ol′ o-je)—The study of bacteria.
Bacteriolysis (bak-te ″re-ol ′ i-sis)—The destruction of bacteria.
Biochemistry (bi-″-o-ken′ is-tre)—The study of chemical changes occurring in living organisms.
Culture (kul′ tur)—The reproduction or growth of microorganisms or of living tissue cells in special laboratory media (the material on which the organisms grow) conducive (to promote) to their growth. Various types of cultures include the following:
Blood culture—Used in the diagnosis of specific infectious diseases. Blood is withdrawn from a vein and placed in or on suitable culture media; then it is determined whether or not pathogens grow in the media. If organisms do grow, they are identified by bacteriologic methods.
Gelatin culture—A culture of bacteria on gelatin.
Handing drop culture—A culture in which the bacteria are inoculated into a drop of fluid on a coverglass, and then mounted into the depressor on a concave slide.
Negative culture—A culture made from suspected material that fails to reveal the suspected microorganism.
Positive culture—A culture that reveals the suspected microorganism.
Pure culture—A culture of a single microorganism.
Smear culture—A culture prepared by smearing the specimen across the surface of the culture medium.
Stab culture—A bacterial culture made by thrusting a needle inoculated with the microorganisms under examination deep into the culture medium.
Streak culture—A bacterial culture in which the infectious material is implanted in streaks across the culture medium.
Tissue culture—The growing of tissue cells in artificial nutrient medium.
Type culture—A culture that is generally agreed to represent microorganisms of a particular species.

Culturette—A commercially prepared bacterial culture collection/transport system, consisting of a sterile plastic tube with applicator. Modified Stuart's transport medium is held in a glass ampule at the bottom end to ensure stability of medium at the time of use. Transport medium is released only after the sample is taken, by crushing the ampule. A moist environment (not immersion) is maintained up to 72 hours to preserve the specimen (see Figure 6-7).

Culturette II culture collection system—Identical to the Culturette, with the exception that the plastic tube contains two applicators and the ampule contains twice the medium (1 ml) (see Figure 6-7).

Anaerobic Culturette culture collection system—This system offers the same basic properties of the Culturette, plus a standardized and dependable anaerobic environment for transport of anaerobic bacteria. Once released, the transport medium maintains an anaerobic environment for up to 48 hours. Many laboratories request that the anaerobic culture system be used when taking a wound culture.

Culture medium—A commercial preparation used for the growth of microorganisms or other cells. (Types of culture media are described in this unit.)

Cytology (si-tol′ o-je)—The study of the structure and function of cells.

Dysplasia (dis-pla′ ze-ah)—An abnormal development of tissue.

Fixation of a smear—Spraying with or immersing a slide into a special solution, or drying the slide over a flame, or air drying to harden and preserve the bacteria for future microscopic examination.

Histology (his-tol′ o-je)—The study of the microscopic form and structure of tissue.

Incubation (in-ku-ba′ shun)—When pertaining to bacteriology, this term refers to the period of culture development.

Inoculate (i-nok″i-lat)—In microbiology, this refers to the introduction of infectious matter into a culture medium in an effort to produce growth of the causative organism.

Macroscopic (mak-ro-skop′ ik) examination—An examination in which the specimen is large enough to be seen by the naked eye.

Medical microbiology—The study and identification of pathogens, and the development of effective methods for their control or elimination (see also Unit Five).

Microorganism (mi-kro-or′ gan-ism)—A minute, living body not visible to the naked eye, especially a bacterium or protozoan; these are viewed with a microscope.

Microscopic (mik-ro-skop′ ik) examination—An examination in which the specimen is visible only with the aid of a microscope.

Pathogen (path′ o-jen)—A disease-producing substance or microorganism.

Pathogenic (path′ o-jen′ ic)—Pertaining to a disease-producing microorganism or substance.

Serologic (se-ro-loj′ ik) test—A laboratory test involving the examination and study of blood serum.

Smear (smer)—Material spread thinly across a slide or culture medium with a swab, loop, or another slide in preparation for microscopic study.

Specimen (spec′ i-men)—A small part or sample taken to show kind and quality of the whole (for example, a specimen of urine, blood, or other body excretions) or a small piece of tissue for macroscopic and microscopic examinations.

Sputum (spu′ -tum)—A mucous secretion from the trachea, bronchi, and lungs ejected through the mouth, in contrast to saliva, which is the secretion of the salivary glands.

Stool (stool)—Body waste material discharged from the large intestine; synonym: feces, bowel movement

Swab (swob)—A small piece of cotton or gauze wrapped around the end of a slender stick used for applying medications, cleansing cavities, or obtaining a piece of tissue or body secretion for bacteriologic, examination; synonym, cotton-tipped applicator.

Urine (u′ rine)—The fluid containing certain waste products and water that is secreted by the kidneys, stored in the bladder, and excreted through the urethra.

Viable (vi′ ah-bl)—Able to maintain an independent existence.

SPECIMENS

Samples of body fluids, secretions, excretions, or tissues can be removed from a patient's body for laboratory study. These materials, once removed, are called *specimens*. Serologic, biochemical, and microscopic tests can be performed on all body specimens. These tests provide a means for evaluating the patient's health status and identifying pathogenic microorganisms and other abnormalities present. Once the suspected cause of a disease process is determined, appropriate methods of treatment can be provided.

INSTRUCTIONS TO THE PATIENT AND SPECIAL PREPARATION

It is important that a specimen be collected at the onset of a disease or condition and, when possible, before the administration of any antibiotics when an infectious process is suspected. Frequently the active participation of a patient is required to obtain a specimen; therefore you must give appropriate instructions. Explain the procedure that is to be used in collecting the specimen (such as urine, sputum, or stool) completely and accurately.

Some tests require special preparation by the patient, and again you must give the appropriate instructions, along with an explanation of the necessity for following these instructions. An informed patient usually is more cooperative in following specific directions, which in turn facilitates accurate tests results. Special preparation usually means a modification in diet or a period of fasting before the specimen collection, or medication restrictions. The time of day the specimen is to be collected may be specific; that is, the first morning urine is to be collected. Fasting means abstaining from *all* food, gum, cigarettes, and fluids except water for usually 12 to 14 hours before the specimen is collected. Fasting specimens are generally collected in the morning for the patient's convenience.

Some medications interfere with test results. When feasible, a patient may be advised by the physician to discontinue the medication for 48 to 72 hours before certain urine tests and for 4 to 24 hours before some blood tests. When it is not medically advisable for the patient to go without the medication for any length of time, a notation must be made on the laboratory requisition as to what drug and the amount of drug that the patient is taking. This alerts the laboratory to the presence of the drug. At times the laboratory may be able to use a different method of testing that would not be altered by the presence of the medication. For women, the use of vaginal medications, douches, or the time of the menstrual flow should be avoided when vaginal specimens are to be obtained.

It is frequently advisable to write out the specific directions for patients so they have an accurate reminder of the special requirements for each test to be performed in addition to the time and date of the test. For some tests you may have preprinted instruction forms to give to the patient.

CARING FOR, HANDLING, TRANSPORTING, AND STORING SPECIMENS

Essential considerations to remember with regard to each specimen follow. See Vocabulary for types of collection and transport systems used.

1. *Review and follow the Centers for Disease Control and Prevention Universal Precautions in Unit One. Universal Precautions* is an approach to infection control. According to the concept of Universal Precautions, all human blood and other body fluids such as semen, vaginal secretions, cerebrospinal fluid, pleural fluid, pericardial fluid, peritoneal fluid, amniotic fluid, saliva in dental procedures, any body fluid that is visibly contaminated with blood, and all body fluids in situations in which it is difficult or impossible to differentiate between body fluids are treated as if known to be infectious for HIV, HBV, and other bloodborne pathogens. Wear gloves for handling specimens at all times.

2. *The specimen must be properly labeled and placed in the correct container.* Place each specimen in the proper container or solution that is designed for the type of material collected with the lid fastened securely. Label the container with the specimen with the patient's name, the date, the source of the specimen, and the attending physician's name.

Place specimens of blood or other potentially infectious materials containers that prevent leakage during collection, handling, processing, storage, transport, or shipping. Label of color-code these containers before they leave your facility unless you place them in red bags or red containers which may substitute for labels. The label must bear the legend *BIOHAZARD* and must be fluorescent orange or orange-red or predominantly so, with lettering or symbols in a contrasting color. Affix the labels as close as possible to the container by adhesive, wire, string, or other method that prevents their loss or unintentional removal. You must also affix these warning labels to refrigerators and freezers that contain blood or other potentially infectious materials (Figure 11-1).

3. *The specimen must be protected when it is sent to outside laboratories or through the mail.* Most outside laboratories provide specific instructions for the transportation of specimens to them. You must place and secure specimens that are sent to outside laboratories through the mail in a proper transport container. This special container protects and preserves the specimen for examination. Close the container securely and wrap it in a protective covering such as corrugated cardboard or cotton, which absorbs shock or possible leakage. Place the wrapped specimen container in a watertight metal container (Figure 11-2), which is then placed with a laboratory requisition into a stiff cardboard mailing container that has shock-resistant insulating material (Figure 11-3). The outside of this container must have a label that identifies it as a medical specimen.

4. *The specimen must be uncontaminated.* To prevent addition of microorganisms to the specimen obtained from the patient, use sterile containers, sterile applicators, or other sterile devices, as well as clean or sterile techniques to collect the specimen.

Figure 11-1 *Biohazard label in fluorescent orange or orange-red with lettering or symbols in a contrasting color.*

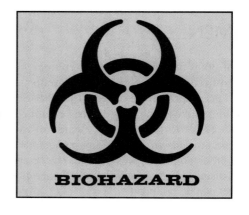

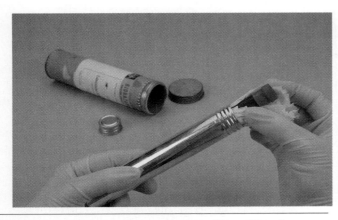

Figure 11-2 *Wrap specimen container for mailing in corrugated cardboard or cotton and place in watertight metal container.*

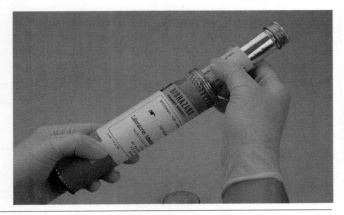

Figure 11-3 *Place watertight metal container containing specimen and laboratory requisition into a stiff cardboard mailing container.*

a. Do *not* use cracked or broken containers and applicators.
b. Use only regulation tops or plugs on stopper bottles and test tubes. Do *not* use cotton balls or gauze as a substitute. Many laboratories now use plastic-capped tubes, screw caps, and metal closure tubes; special vials or tube with rubber stoppers are used for transporting suspected anaerobic organisms.
c. Discard plugs or the inner surface of tops that come in contact with an unsterile surface.
d. Fill containers only half-way. Do not allow the top or plug to become wet, either from the specimen or other sources, in order to prevent contamination to the specimen and to personnel handling it.
e. Do not spill specimen material on the outside of the container or on any surface. If outside contamination of the primary container occurs, place the primary container into a second container that prevents leakage during handling, processing, storage, transport, or shipping, and label or color-code it as discussed in No. 2. This is for the protection of everyone handling the specimen or near the area. If a specimen is accidentally spilled, call the laboratory

to inquire how to destroy the pathogens that may be in the specimen and what to use. You must clean the work area immediately. A disinfectant such as a 1:10 dilution of sodium hypochlorite (household bleach) or Bytech solution is frequently used to clean the area.

5. *Spills of blood and other body secretions:* Clean spills up promptly. Wear gloves to clean up large spills; use paper towels, which should be placed in an infectious waste container. Then use 5%/25% sodium hypochlorite (household bleach) diluted 1:10 to disinfect the area. Do not place sodium hypochlorite directly on large amounts of protein matter (for example, urine, stool, blood, or sputum), to protect the employee from noxious fumes. You may order a 1:10 dilution of bleach for the office or clinic from a hospital pharmacy.
6. *Laboratory procedures* should be adopted to prevent the formation of aerosols. Biologic safety cabinets (Class I or II) and other primary containment devices (for example, centrifuge safety cups) are advised whenever you conduct procedures that have a high potential for creating aerosols or infectious droplets. Follow other standard laboratory safety practices.
7. *The specimen must contain living organisms collected from the proper source and reach the laboratory in a condition suitable for culturing, incubating, or examining.* Specimens collected for a smear or culture may be taken from any body opening, whether natural, surgical, or accidental; for example, material may be collected from the ear, eye, nose, throat, urethra, vagina, rectum, or a wound. Body fluids such as urine, blood, and cerebrospinal fluid, as well as samples of tissue (biopsy), may also be obtained. To make sure that the pathogens remain viable (living), send all specimens to the laboratory for processing without delay. If there is a delay, keep most specimens in a refrigerator for a few hours. Generally you may store swabs from the throat, rectum, and wounds, as well as fecal (except when feces are to be examined for the presence of parasites) and sputum samples, in a refrigerator for several hours. Spinal fluid may contain organisms that are sensitive to cold; therefore place this specimen in a bacteriologic incubator.

Swabs of infectious matter must be prevented from drying before they are processed in the laboratory. Sometimes the sterile swab is moistened with a broth, or placed into tubes containing broth or a selected holding medium to prevent drying of the specimen. The broth is used to keep the air around the swab moist and is *not* a culture medium.

Use special procedures for preservation and growth when an anaerobic organism (one able to live in the absence of oxygen) is believed to be the causative agent. Processing these specimens *immediately* is vital to maintaining the organism in a viable state. When there is a delay, you may place inoculated culture plates in a candle jar (see Figure 11-18) and then send them to the laboratory.

Urine specimens should be examined or sent to the laboratory immediately. If this is not possible, you must refrigerate them (see Nos. 8 and 9 under General Facts Relating to Urine Collection, which follows later in this chapter, and also Unit Twelve).

Most *blood specimens* must be examined within 8 hours or less from the time they were collected, and preferably, within 2 to 4 hours from the time they were collected. Blood for bacteriologic studies must be collected in special containers and must not be left unattended for any length of time. These specimens must be examined as soon as possible. Blood drawn for an electrolyte panel should be refrigerated if it is not tested immediately. Other blood samples may be left standing on the counter for 2 to 4 hours before testing, although some results may vary if the blood is left standing for 2 or more house (see Unit Thirteen)

When a specimen is to be examined in the physician's office or clinic, you should test, culture, or examine it microscopically immediately.

8. *The specimen should be handled and transported in an upright position and should not be shaken.* Remember that failure to successfully identify pathogens may result from improper collection, care, and handling techniques.

9. *Avoid and prevent contamination to yourself and other personnel who will be handling the specimen.* All specimens obtained for microbiologic study are presumed to contain potentially dangerous pathogens. Always keep in mind the possibility of spreading the infectious pathogen, know the necessary protective measures that must be adhered to (as listed), and use excellent aseptic technique when obtaining the specimen. Disposable single-use exam gloves must be worn for handling all specimens. In addition:
   a. *Do not* eat, drink, or smoke while handling specimens because you could transmit pathogens to yourself by hand-to-mouth contact.
   b. *Do not* lick the label that will be placed on the specimen container.
   c. Wear gloves to cover any cut or scratch that you have.
   d. If you accidentally touch some of the specimen collected, immediately wash the contact area thoroughly with an antiseptic soap. If the contact area was on a cut or scratch, apply tincture of iodine or another antiseptic solution to the area. Report the incident to your supervisor or employer.
   e. At the end of each work day, clean the work area with a disinfectant solution.

10. *A laboratory requisition to accompany the specimen must always be filled out completely and accurately.* The following information must be included:
   a. Date (time of day if relevant; for example, an early morning specimen)
   b. Name of the patient, address, age, and sex
   c. Name of the attending physician and address
   d. Source of the specimen
   e. Name of laboratory test(s) to be performed
   f. A notation if the patient is already taking antibiotics. (False-negative results could be obtained if the antibiotic has suppressed the growth of the microorganism(s).

Additional information depends on the type of specimen obtained and may include the following:.
   g. Clinical history
   h. Previous normal or abnormal results
   i. Previous surgery
   j. X-ray film treatment
   k. Clinical diagnosis

For vaginal and cervical specimens, the following, if applicable, are also added:
   l. Hormone treatment
   m. Date of last menstrual period (LMP)
   n. Postpartum
   o. Postmenopausal
   p. Pregnant
   q. DES child (that is, if the mother took DES [diethylstilbesterol] when pregnant with the patient)

11. All specimens from all patients, whether known to be infected or not, should be handled with caution (see also Unit One).

URINE SPECIMEN COLLECTION

A specimen of urine is collected to perform a urinalysis (u"ri-nal' i-sis), which is an analysis of the physical, chemical, and microscopic properties of urine. The result of these examinations help determine renal (kidney) functions of the body, which in turn helps the physician diagnose and provide the appropriate treatment required for a disease process.

Many types of tests are used in analyzing the urine to determine whether it contains abnormal substances indicative of disease (see Unit Twelve for urinalysis procedures). The most significant substances normally absent from urine and detected by a urinalysis are protein, glucose, acetone, blood, pus, casts, and bacteria.

TYPES OF URINE SPECIMENS
Random or Spot Specimen

To collect a random or spot specimen, the patient voids at any time of the day or night, collecting a portion of the urine in a clean container.

Fasting Specimen

To collect a fasting specimen, the patient voids 4 or more hours after ingestion of food and discards this urine. The next voided specimen is collected and regarded as the fasting specimen.

First Morning Specimen

To collect a first morning specimen, the patient voids and discards the specimen before going to bed. On arising the next morning. the patient collects the first morning specimen.

Urination (u-"ri-na' shun), voiding, micturition (mik"tu-rish' un)—The act of passing urine from the body.

Diuresis (di"ur-re' sis)—An abnormal, increased secretion of urine as seen in diabetes mellitus, diabetes insipidus, or when large amounts of fluid have been drunk; this can be artificially produced by drugs with diuretic properties.

Enuresis (en"u-re' sis)—The involuntary excretion of urine, especially at night during sleep; bedwetting; most frequently seen in children with either physical or emotional problems.

Frequency—The need to urinate frequently.

Incontinence (in-kon' ti-nens)—The inability to refrain from the urge to urinate. This may occur in times of stress, anxiety, anger, postoperatively, or from obstructions that prevent the normal emptying of the urinary bladder, spasms of the bladder, irritation caused by injury or inflammation of the urinary tract, damage to the spinal cord or brain, or from the development of a fistula (an abnormal tubelike passage) between the bladder and the vagina or urethra.

Urgency—The need to urinate immediately.

Postprandial Specimen

To collect a postprandial specimen, the patient voids after eating and collects this specimen.

Midstream Specimen

To collect a midstream specimen, the patient start to void into the toilet or bedpan; then, without stopping the process of voiding, a portion of the urine is collected in a clean container. The last part of the urine flow is passed into the toilet or bedpan.

Clean-catch Specimen

To collect a clean-catch specimen, the patient washes the external genitalia with soap and water or some mild antiseptic solution. Then a midstream urine specimen is collected in a clean, dry container or in a sterile container if the specimen is being collected for bacterial examination. This yields a specimen with limited contamination by skin bacteria.

Multiple-glass Specimens

The multiple-glass test is performed on men to evaluate a lower urinary tract infection. The man must have a full bladder because three samples of urine are collected. To collect a multiple-glass specimen, the patient washes the area around the urinary meatus with an antiseptic solution. He then voids about 100 ml (approximately 3½ ounces) into a clean, dry container. This specimen contains microorganisms and sediment "washed" from the urethra. Without interrupting the voiding process, he then voies another 100 ml of urine into a second clean, dry container. This specimen contains microorganisms and sediment representative of that in the bladder and kidney. Then the man stops voiding, and the physician gently massages

the prostate gland. After this, the third urine specimen is collected in a clean, dry container. This last specimen contains secretions from the prostate gland.

Timed Specimens (24-hour Specimen)

To collect a timed specimen, the patient discards the first morning specimen and then collects all urine for exactly 24 hours. (See No. 12, under General Facts Relating to Urine Collection.) Other timed specimens could be for 12 hours or as requested by the laboratory for specific examinations.

Drug Screen Specimen (Urine Toxicology Screening)

A random urine specimen may be collected. Only a small amount of urine is needed. For some tests the laboratory uses only 7 drops, but you should collect at least 1 ml. Always check with the laboratory for their requirements. Obtain as much information about the type and amount of drug taken and the time it was consumed. If the test is for medicolegal testing purposes, the patient must sign a *consent form.*

A specific type of urine collection can provide optimum information when performing certain tests; for example, postprandial urine can be used for testing sugar content, and first morning specimens can be used for testing protein content.

GENERAL FACTS RELATING TO URINE COLLECTION

1. To minimize bacterial and chemical contamination, use only clean, dry, or sterile collection containers. Disposable containers are ideal.

2. The early morning urine specimen is the most concentrated; therefore, if at all possible, this is the specimen that should be obtained for simple routine testing. The concentration of urine varies during a 24-hour period, partly as a result of the patient's food and water intake and level of activity.

3. A freshly voided specimen is adequate for *most* urinalysis when the first morning specimen cannot be obtained, although collection of a clean-catch midstream specimen is the method of choice.

4. To collect a freshly voided specimen in the office, give the patient a clean, wide-mouthed bottle, and instruct her or him to void directly into it. Inform the patient how much urine you want in the bottle (that is, up to what point in the bottle you want collected). Usually 2 to 4 ounces is sufficient.

5. When urine is required for bacterial cultures, collect a clean-catch midstream specimen in a sterile container and submit it to the bacteriology laboratory department as soon as possible for testing.

6. Ask patients if they are taking any medications and what type, and if they are on a special diet, because certain medications and diets affect the findings of a urinalysis. NOTE: A note of medications and/or special diet should be recorded on the laboratory requisition and the patient's chart (see Table 12-5). When feasible, the physician may advise the patient to stop taking the medication for 48 to 72 hours before the test.

7. Inquire if a female patient is menstruating when a urine specimen is collected because, if blood is found in the urine, it may be from the vaginal canal rather than from the urinary tract. A note of this must also be recorded, and another specimen may be required when the patient has finished menstruating.

8. Voided specimens should not be left standing at room temperature because they become alkaline as a result of contamination by urea-splitting bacteria from the environment. Explain to the patient that refrigeration of the specimen is necessary if collected at home, until time to submit it for analysis. If examination is delayed in your office or the laboratory, the specimen should also be refrigerated.

9. Microscopic examination of urine should be performed within 1 hour after collection. Waiting for longer than 1 hour causes dissolution of cellular elements and casts and bacterial overgrowth, unless the specimen was obtained under sterile conditions.

10. When more than one specimen is required, number each specimen according to its sequence.

11. If the patient is to collect the specimen at home, you should have explained the following procedure previously.

a. Use a thoroughly clean, 3- to 4-ounce container in which to collect the specimen.

b. Boil the container that will be used for the collection for 20 minutes before using it.

c. Do not use a container that has held drugs or other solutions that may make the specimen unsuitable for examination. Medical facilities that have specimen containers readily available may provide them to the patient.

12. When a 24-hour specimen is required, it is vital that the patient understand the procedure. *All* urine must be collected within a 24-hour period.

a. The first early-morning specimen is discarded.

b. All subsequent specimens are collected, including the first early-morning specimen the next day.

c. The last specimen is collected 24 hours after collection was started.

d. Urine is collected in a clean bottle into which a preservative has been added. (Preservative is prescribed by the laboratory.) This bottle must be refrigerated or kept cold by placing it in a bucket of ice. Instruct the patient not to shift the contents of the container, and if male, not to void directly into the container.

CLEAN-CATCH, MIDSTREAM, VOIDED SPECIMEN

Equipment

Antiseptic solution or antiseptic wipes (such as povidone-iodine wipes) *or* soap and water
Washcloth
Sterile gauze sponges 4 × 4 inch

Sterile specimen container (with cover) NOTE: Commercially prepared kits for collecting a midstream specimen are available. These kits contain a sterile specimen container and label, antiseptic wipes, and absorbent tissues.
Tissues
Laboratory requisition
Disposable single-use exam gloves (if you will be handling specimen)

PROCEDURE

1. Wash your hands. **Use appropriate personal protective equipment (PPE) as dictated by facility.**

2. Assemble supplies and equipment.

3. Identify the patient, and explain the procedure.

   For a female patient:

   a. Ask patient to wash her perineal area using soap, water, and washcloth; separate labia and cleanse the area around the urinary meatus.

   b. Repeat step (a) using water and 4 × 4-inch sponges. NOTE: Rather than using soap and water, the patient may wash herself with 4 × 4-inch sponges soaked with a mild antiseptic solution such as povidone-iodine.

RATIONALE

Explanations help gain full cooperation from the patient, which is required to obtain a specimen successfully.

Careful cleansing is necessary to obtain a satisfactory specimen. The urethral orifice is colonized by bacteria. Urine readily becomes contaminated during voiding.

It is important to remove all the soap because a soap residue changes the results of the specimen analysis.

CLEAN-CATCH, MIDSTREAM, VOIDED SPECIMEN—cont'd

PROCEDURE

c. Instruct patient to start voiding into the toilet and, after she has voided for a few seconds, to move the specimen container into the urinary stream to catch the midstream specimen in the sterile container. Instruct the patient to fill the container no more than three-fourths full.

d. Instruct the patient to finish voiding into the toilet bowl. Provide tissues for the patient to wipe herself and to wash the outside of the container if spillage should occur after collecting the specimen.

For a male patient:

a. Instruct the patient to take the penis, retract the foreskin (if uncircumcised) to expose the urinary meatus, and cleanse thoroughly with soap and water using the washcloth.

b. Repeat step (a) using 4 × 4 inch sponges and water. NOTE: Rather than using soap and water, the patient may wash himself with 4 × 4 inch sponges soaked with a mild antiseptic solution such as povidone-iodine.

c. Instruct the patient to start voiding into the toilet and, after he has voided for a few seconds, to move the specimen container into the urinary stream to catch the midstream specimen. Instruct the patient to fill the container no more than three-fourths full.

d. Instruct the patient to then finish voiding into the toilet. The patient is to avoid collecting the last few drops of urine.

4. Have the patient signal you when the specimen has been obtained, or instruct the patient where to place the specimen container.

5. Send properly labeled specimen, with the correct laboratory requisition, to appropriate laboratory; or refrigerate it until it can either be tested or sent to the laboratory (Figure 11-4). Do not allow a urine specimen to stand at room temperature for any length of time. It is best to put a cover on the container.

6. Don single-use disposable exam gloves.

7. Perform the urinalysis if this is required of you. See Unit Twelve for this procedure.

8. Remove gloves.

9. Wash your hands.

10. Record on the chart the appropriate information. Always record on the chart if the urine appeared abnormal (for example, if blood appeared to be present or if the urine was cloudy). Record the results if you have performed the analysis (as described in Unit Twelve).

RATIONALE

This helps wash away urethral contaminants.
You need approximately 2 to 4 ounces of urine for analysis.

Careful cleansing is necessary to obtain a satisfactory specimen. The urethral orifice is colonized by bacteria. Urine readily becomes contaminated during voiding.

It is important to remove all soap because a soap residue changes the results of the specimen analysis.

This helps cleanse the urethral canal.
You need only 2 to 4 ounces for the analysis.

Prostatic secretions may be introduced into the urine at the end of the urinary stream.

An unrefrigerated urine specimen becomes worthless.

Avoid contamination.

Charting example:
   February 25, 19___, 4 p.m.
      Clean-catch urine specimen obtained and sent to the laboratory for routine UA [urinalysis].
      Betty Bittinger, CMA

CLEAN-CATCH, MIDSTREAM, VOIDED SPECIMEN—cont'd

URINALYSIS		G/L 410		ST	SP	LAST NAME		FIRST NAME

URINALYSIS — PLEASE PRINT – PRESS HARD

REMARKS: — TIME OF COLLECTION:

ADDRESS

ROUTINE REQUEST — ROUTINE – SPECIMENS NOT ACCEPTED AFTER 4:00 P.M. — PRE-OP – SPECIMENS NOT ACCEPTED AFTER 8:00 P.M.

BIRTHDATE AGE SEX CLASS

IF REQUEST IS OTHER THAN ROUTINE, PLACE STICKER WITH APPROPRIATE INSTRUCTIONS IN THIS SPACE

PHYSICIAN

DATE VERIFYING NURSE DIAGNOSIS

DATE PHONE

CODE
800 — ROUTINE URINALYSIS (INCLUDES ALL TESTS LISTED)

CODE			CODE		
	COLOR		820	WBC/HPF	
	CHARACTER		M	RBC/HPF	
836	SPECIFIC GRAVITY	1.0	I	BACTERIA /HPF	
	pH		C R	MUCUS /LPF	
830	PROTEIN		O	EPITHELIAL CELLS/LPF	
814	GLUCOSE		S C	CRYSTALS /LPF	
818	KETONES		O	CASTS /LPF	
822	OCCULT BLOOD		P	OTHER:	
814	REDUCING SUBSTANCES		I		
815	GALACTOSE		C		

TIME IN TECHNOLOGIST TIME CALLED OR TELETYPED TIME OUT

Figure 11-4 *Sample urinalysis laboratory requisition that is sent with urine specimen to the laboratory.*

STOOL SPECIMEN COLLECTION

A stool specimen is collected for macroscopic, microscopic, and chemical examination to help diagnose the presence of parasites and ova, occult blood, fecal urobilinogen, pus or mucus, membranous shreds, worms, infectious diseases, foreign bodies, and to detect the amount of fat being eliminated and various disorders of metabolism.

The stool is examined macroscopically for its amount, consistency, color, and odor. Normal color varies from light to dark brown, depending on urobilin content, a product formed from bilirubin. Various foods, medications, and conditions affect the color of the stool. For example, when a person has ingested the following, the color of the stool may be affected:

- Meat protein—The stool may be dark brown.
- Spinach—The stool may be green.
- Beets—The stool may be red.
- Cocoa—The stool may be dark red or brown.
- Bismuth, iron, or charcoal—The stool may be black.
- Barium—The stool may be milky white.

In conditions in which a patient is having upper gastrointestinal bleeding, the stool is tarry black; in lower gastrointestinal bleeding, it is bright red bloody; and in biliary obstruction, it is clay colored. Other clinical conditions in which the stool has certain characteristics include the following:

- Steatorrhea (excess fat in the feces due to a malabsorption state caused by disease of the intestinal mucosa or pancreatic enzyme deficiency)—The stool appears bulky,

greasy, foamy, foul in odor, and gray or clay-colored with a silvery sheen.
- Chronic ulcerative colitis—Mucus or pus may be visible in the stool.
- Constipation, obstipation, and fecal obstruction—The stool appears as small, dry, rocky-hard masses.

As with most specimens, a fresh specimen is absolutely necessary and should be obtained before the administration of antibiotic therapy. Stool containing barium, mineral oils, or magnesia is usually unsuitable for diagnosis.

To best demonstrate parasitic infection, three fresh specimens collected on three different days are usually required. These must be sent to the laboratory immediately so that the parasites can be observed under the microscope while they are fresh, viable, and warm. Stool for occult blood testing should not be more than 1 hour old.

Some laboratories now prefer the new collection system that no longer requires that specimens be warm. The specimens are placed into two separate vials, each containing a special preservative, and then are to be sent to the laboratory as soon as possible.

When forwarding the specimen to a hospital or large laboratory, send specimens to be tested for occult blood to the hematology laboratory, specimens for culture and acid-fast bacilli to the bacteriology laboratory, and specimens for parasites and ova to the parasitology laboratory. Accompany all specimens with the appropriate clinical laboratory slips with accurate and completed information.

VOCABULARY

Bowel movement—The elimination/excretion of fecal material from the intestinal tract.

Constipation (kon-sti-pa′ shun)—A condition in which the waste material in the intestine is too hard to pass easily, or in which bowel movements are so infrequent that discomfort results.

Diarrhea (di-a-re′ a)—Rapid movement of fecal material through the intestine, resulting in poor absorption and producing frequent, watery stools.

Excrete—To eliminate useless matter such as feces and urine.

Excreta (ek-skre′ tah)—Waste material excreted or eliminated from the body. Feces, urine, perspiration, and also mucus and carbon dioxide (CO_2) can be considered excreta.

Excretion (ek-skre′ shun)—The elimination of waste materials from the body. Ordinarily, what is meant by excretion is the elimination of feces, but it can refer to the material eliminated from any part of the body.

Feces (fe′ sez)—Body waste excreted from the intestine; also called stool, excreta, or excrement.

Flatulence (flat′ u-lens)—Excessive formation of gases in the stomach or intestine.

Flatus (fla′ tus)—Air or gas in the stomach or intestine.

Guaiac (gwi′ ak) **test**—The preferred chemical test to determine the presence of occult blood in feces.

Melena (mel-e′ nah)—Darkening of stool by blood pigments.

Obstipation (ob′ sti-pa′ shun)—Extreme constipation caused by an obstruction.

Occult blood—Obscure or hidden from view.

Occult blood test—A microscopic or a chemical test performed on a specimen to determine the presence of blood not otherwise detectable. Stool is tested when intestinal bleeding is suspected but there is no visible evidence of blood in the stool.

Parasite (par′ ah-sit)—An organism that lives on or in another organism, known as the host, from which it gains its nourishment (for example, fungi, bacteria, and single-celled and multi-celled animals).

Stool—The fecal discharge from the bowels (see also feces).

Lienteric stool—Feces containing much undigested food.

Urobilinogen—A colorless compound formed in the intestines by the reduction of bilirubin.

STOOL SPECIMEN

Equipment

Stool specimen container of waxed paper with a lid of glass or of plastic
Wooden tongue depressor or spatula
Clean bedpan with cover
Label for container
Small plastic bag
Laboratory requisition
Disposable single-use exam gloves

PROCEDURE

1. Wash your hands. **Use appropriate personal protective equipment (PPE) as dictated by facility.** Obtain a clean bedpan with a clean cover to give to the patient for use.

2. Identify the patient. Explain to the patient that a stool specimen is needed and that a bedpan must be used. Have the patient empty the bladder first if required, as urine should not be collected in the bedpan with the stool specimen.

3. Prepare the label for the specimen container. Fill out the laboratory requisition accurately and completely. You can do this while the patient is collecting the specimen.

4. Don gloves.

5. After the patient has used the bedpan, cover it and remove it to your work area. Provide means for the patient to wash the hands.

RATIONALE

Explanations help gain the patient's full cooperation, which is essential for proper specimen collection.

STOOL SPECIMEN—cont'd

PROCEDURE	RATIONALE
6. Transfer a portion (1 to 2 teaspoons) of the stool into the specimen container by using the clean tongue depressor or spatula as a spoon. Place the lid on the container securely. Be sure that there is no toilet tissue in the stool specimen. Do not smear the specimen on the edge or outside of the container. You may scrape the tongue depressor or spatula only on the inside of the container to rid it of feces.	
7. Place the tongue depressor or spatula in the plastic bag, and wrap it securely for proper disposal. *Do not* throw it in the wastebasket. You should have a special container for used equipment such as this.	*The wastebasket may be contaminated with infectious disease organisms.*
8. Empty and clean the bedpan. Avoid contaminating yourself or your work area. *Before* emptying the bedpan, observe the feces for anything that appears abnormal to you; if so, report it at once.	
9. Remove gloves.	
10. Wash your hands thoroughly.	
11. Label the container, and attach the correct completed laboratory requisition to the container (Figure 11-5). The purpose of the examination must be stated on the requisition.	
12. Send or take the labeled specimen to the laboratory immediately. If there is a delay, try to place the specimen for parasite examination in a warm place until it can be delivered to or picked up by the laboratory. Refrigerate specimens for other examinations until delivered to the laboratory. NOTE: If more than one specimen is to be sent, indicate No. 1, No. 2, and so on. A stool specimen should be warm when it arrives in the laboratory for examination. This is especially important when looking for parasites so that they may be examined under the microscope while viable, fresh, and warm. Specimens for tests other than parasite detection can generally be refrigerated for a few hours when not sent immediately to the laboratory.	
13. Wash your hands again.	*Because of the chance of having disease organisms on your hands, wash them again to be safe.*
14. Record on the patient's chart. If relevant, describe the appearance of the stool when charting.	*Charting example:* *Feb. 27, 19__, 10 a.m.* *Stool specimen No. 1 sent to laboratory for ova and parasites, and fat content examinations.* *Connie Hanks, CMA*

STOOL SPECIMEN—cont'd

FECES - SEMEN

	FECES – SEMEN LABORATORY	DATE

Feb. 27, 19__.
Patient's name
Physician's name and
address

Routine Feces Consists Of • Gross Description • Ova & Parasites • Occult Blood
☐ CULTURE REQUIRED (ALSO SUBMIT BACTERIOLOGY REQUEST)

☐ ROUTINE FECES   ☐ UROBILINOGEN (QUAL.)   ☐ SEMEN ANALYSIS   ☐
☑ OVA & PARASITES   ☑ FAT (QUAL.)   ☐
☐ OCCULT BLOOD   ☐ STARCH   ☐
☐ BILE PIGMENT (QUAL.)   ☐ TRYPSIN   ☐

COMMENTS: *Stool spec #1*

FECES – SEMEN

FINDINGS	STOOL EXAMINATION		FINDINGS			FINDINGS	SEMEN ANALYSIS
	COLOR			OVA & HELMINTHS	PARASITES		APPEARANCE
	CONSISTENCY			DIRECT			VOLUME (cc)
	MUCUS			CONC.			COUNT 100-150 M/cc
	PUS CELLS			TROPHOZOITES	AMEBAE		RBC
	RED BLOOD CELLS			CYSTS			WBC
	BENZIDINE	OCCULT BLOOD		NEUTRAL FAT	Fats		CRYSTALS
	GUAIAC			STARCH			% MOTILITY (INIT.)
	UROBILIN	BILE PIGMENT		TRYPSIN			MORPHOLOGY
	BILIRUBIN						
	UROBILINOGEN (QUAL.)						

ADDITIONAL RESULTS:

DATE	TECHNOLOGIST'S SIGNATURE

Figure 11-5 *Sample laboratory requisition for fecal specimen*

HEMOCCULT SLIDE TEST ON A STOOL SPECIMEN

The Hemoccult slide test is a rapid, noninvasive, convenient, and virtually odorless method for detecting the presence of fecal occult (hidden) blood, as an aid to diagnosis of various gastrointestinal conditions, including polyps, peptic ulcers, hemorrhoids, hiatal hernia, and cancer of the colon or rectum. This test is performed:

- During routine physical examinations
- In newly admitted hospital patients
- In postoperative patients
- In newborn infants
- In screening programs for colorectal cancer

Because Hemoccult tests require only a small stool specimen, offensive odors are minimized, and storage or transport of large stool specimens is unnecessary. Figure 11-6 contains more information, special instructions for the patient, and the equipment and procedure for performing this test. The American Cancer Society recommends that a stool blood test be performed every year on patients ages 50 years and older. This test indicates hidden (occult) blood in feces, which may be an early indicator of colorectal cancer. The risk of developing colorectal cancer increases after age 50 for both men and women. Anyone with personal or family history of colorectal cancer, ulcerative colitis, polyps in the colon or rectum, or a personal history of inflammatory bowel disease has a higher chance of developing this cancer.

The American Cancer Society estimates that 155,000 people will develop colorectal cancer this year. When colorectal cancer is detected in its early stages, up to 85% of these people may be treated successfully. When cancer is detected after symptoms appear and it has spread to other parts of the body, only 46% to 58% may be treated successfully. Thus earlier detection could save thousands of lives each year (see also Figure 4-22).

Millions of people have the Hemoccult screening test performed each year *because* early detection and treatment of colorectal cancer has proven effective in saving lives.

Figure 11-6 A, *Hemoccult slides procedure;* **B,** *reading and interpreting the Hemoccult Test;* **C,** *on-slide performance Monitor feature;* **D,** *Hemoccult Tape Preparation and Development.* **E,** *Hemoccult II Slides.* **F,** *Hemoccult II Dispensapak with on-slide performance monitors.* **G,** *Instructions to the patient for collecting fecal specimens for Hemoccult II slide test and Hemoccult II procedure.*
Courtesy SmithKline Diagnostics, Inc., Sunnyvale, Calif.

Hemoccult Single Slides are convenient for use when single stool specimens are to be tested.

Hemoccult II Slides, in cards of three tests, are designed so your patient can collect serial specimens at home over the course of three bowel movements. After the patient collects the specimens, the Hemoccult II test may be returned to a laboratory, a hospital, or a medical office for developing and evaluation. Serial fecal specimen analysis is recommended when screening asymptomatic patients (**B** and **D**).

Hemoccult Tape is designed to complement Hemoccult slides and is best suited for "on-the-spot" testing for occult blood during rectal or sigmoidoscopic examinations. The Hemoccult test and other unmodified guaiac tests are *not recommended* for use with gastric specimens.

SUMMARY, EXPLANATION AND LIMITATIONS OF THE TEST

The Hemoccult test is a simplified, standardized variation of the guaiac test for occult blood. It contains specially prepared guaiac-impregnated paper and is ready for use without additional preparation.

When a small stool specimen containing occult blood is applied to Hemoccult test paper, the hemoglobin comes in contact with the guaiac. Application of Hemoccult Developer (a stablized hydrogen peroxide solution) creates a guaiac/peroxidase-like reaction which turns the test paper blue within 60 seconds if occult blood is present.

The test reacts with hemoglobin released from lysed cells. When blood is present, hemolysis is promoted by substances in the stool, primarily water and salts. Typical positive reactions for occult blood are shown under READING AND INTERPRETATION OF THE HEMOCCULT TEST. As with any occult blood test, results with the Hemoccult test cannot be considered conclusive evidence of the presence or absence of gastrointestinal bleeding or pathology. *Hemoccult tests are designed for preliminary screening as a diagnostic aid and are not intended to replace other diagnostic procedures such as proctosigmoidoscopic examination, barium enema, or other x-ray studies.*

BIOLOGICAL PRINCIPLE

The discovery that gum guaiac was a useful indicator for occult blood is generally credited to Van Deen. The test depends on the oxidation of a phenolic, compound, alpha guaiaconic acid, which yields a blue-covered, highly conjugated quinone structure. Hemoglobin exerts a peroxidase-like activity and facilitates the oxidation of this phenolic compound by hydrogen peroxide.

REAGENTS

Natural guaiac resin impregnated into standardized, high-quality filter paper.
A developing solution containing a stabilized dilute mixture of hydrogen peroxide (less than 6%) and 75% denatured ethyl alcohol in aqueous solution.

PERFORMANCE MONITORS

The function and stability of the slides and Developer can be tested using the on-slide Performance Monitor. Both a positive and negative Performance Monitor are located under the flap and below the specimen windows on the back of the Hemoccult II and Hemoccult single slides.

The positive Performance Monitor contains a hemoglobin-derived catalyst which, upon application of Developer, will turn blue within 10 seconds.

The negative Performance Monitor contains no such catalyst and should not turn blue upon application of Developer.

The Performance Monitors provide additional assurance that the guaiac-impregnated paper and Developer are functional. In the unlikely event that the Performance Monitors do not react as expected after application of Developer, the test results should be regarded as invalid. The manufacturer will provide further assistance should this occur.

Precautions

- For *In Vitro* Diagnostic Use.
- Because this test is visually read and requires color differentiation, it should not be interpreted by people who are color-blind or visually impaired.
- Patient specimens and all materials that come in contact with them, should be handled as potentially infectious and disposed of with proper precautions.

Hemoccult Slides (yellow and green card)

- Do not use after the expiration date which appears on each slide.

Hemoccult Developer (yellow label and bottle cap)

- Hemoccult Developer is an irritant and is flammable.

Avoid contact with eyes and skin. If developer comes in contact with eyes or skin, rinse promptly with water. Do not leave uncapped or expose to heat.

- Do not use after expiration date on the bottle.

IMPORTANT: Use Hemoccult Developer (yellow label and cap) only with Hemoccult slides and tape. *Do not interchange Hemoccult with Hemoccult SENSA test reagents, which are identified by blue and green packaging.*

Storage and Stability

Store Hemoccult test components at controlled room temperture, 15 - 30°C (59 - 86°F), in original packaging. Do not refrigerate or freeze.

Protect Hemoccult slides from heat and light. Do not store near volatile chemicals (e.g., iodine, chlorine, bromine, or ammonia).

Store Hemoccult Developer at 15° to 30°C (59° to 86°F); protect from heat. Keep bottle tightly capped when not in use to prevent evaporation.

Sample Collection

The Hemoccult test requires only a small fecal sample. The sample is applied as a **thin smear** to the guaiac paper of the Hemoccult slide or tape using the applicator stick provided. The sample may be collected from the toilet bowl with the aid of a container, toilet tissue, or collection tissue (provided with Hemoccult II Dispensapak™ Plus).

Hemoccult slides may be prepared and developed immediately, or prepared and stored for up to 14 days at controlled room temperature, 15-30° (59-86°F), before developing.

Patients using the Hemoccult II test should be instructed to return all slides to the physician or laboratory immediately after preparing the last test.

IMPORTANT NOTE: *Current U.S. Postal Regulations prohibit mailing completed test slides in standard paper envelopes. Physicians who wish their patients to return slides by mail, must instruct their patients to use only U.S. Postal Service approved mailing pouches.**

Fecal samples **should not be collected** if hematuria or obvious rectal bleeding, such as from hemorrhoids, is present. Pre-menopausal women must be instructed to avoid collecting fecal samples during or in the first three days after a menstrual period.

Since bleeding from gastrointestinal lesions may be intermittent, *fecal samples for testing should be collected from three consecutive bowel movements or three bowel movements closely spaced in time.* To further increase the probability of detecting occult blood, separate samples should be taken from two different sections of each fecal specimen.

INTERFERING SUBSTANCES

In general, patients should not ingest foods, drugs, vitamins or other substances which can cause false-positive or false-negative test results for at least 48 hours before and continuing through the test period. Aspirin and other non-steroidal anti-inflammatory drugs should be avoided for at least seven days prior to and continuing through the test period.

Foods that can cause false-positive test results include red meat (beef, lamb) as well as processed meats and liver. In addition, some raw fruits and vegetables which are high in peroxidase, can cause false-positive results when fecal samples are tested immediately after collection. However, plant peroxidases are relatively unstable and when slides are developed several days after sample preparation, as is the case in a typical take-home or screening situation, even large quantities of raw fruits and vegetables have been observed to have no significant effect on test results.

Substances which irritate the gastrointestinal tract and cause bleeding, such as aspirin, corticosteroids, indomethacin, zomepirac, naproxen, tolmetin, phenylbutazone, reserpine, anticoagulants, antimetabolites, cancer chemotherapeutic drugs, and alcohol in excess may produce positive test results. However, because acetaminophen has not been observed to cause susstantial gastrointestinal tract bleeding, the use of acetaminophen is not expected to significantly affect test results.

The application of antiseptic preparations containing iodine, such as povidone iodine mixtures, to the anal area can also cause false-positive results.

False-negative test results can be caused by ascorbic acid (vitamin C) intake of more than 250 mg/day or by the consumption of excessive amounts of vitamin C enriched foods, such as citrus fruits and juices.

PROCEDURE

Materials Supplied: (see Panel E)

- Hemoccult Slides (or tape in plastic dispenser)
- Hemoccult Developer (yellow label and cap)
- Applicator sticks
- Patient envelopes with instructions for diet and sample collection
- Mailing Pouch for returning completed slides†
- Collection tissues†
- Hemoccult Product Instructions

*Mailing Pouches are included in HemoccutIII Dispensapak Plus and may be ordered separately; refer to ORDERING INFORMATION.

†In Dispensapak# Plus configuration only.

Figure 11-6—cont

A. PROCEDURE: HEMOCCULT SLIDES

Identification	**Preparation**	**Development of Test**	**Development of Performance Monitors**
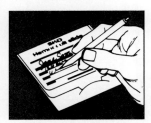	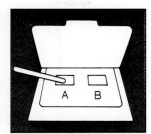	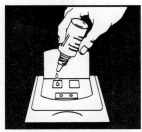	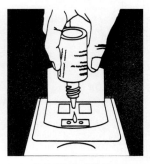

Identification

Write, or have patient write his or her name, age, address, phone number, and date specimen was collected in space provided on front of each slide.

Preparation

1. Collect small stool sample on one end of applicator.
2. Apply thin smear inside box A.
3. Reuse applicator to obtain second sample from different part of stool. Apply thin smear inside box B.
4. Close cover. Return slide to physician.
CAUTION: Protect from heat.
5. If testing immediately, wait 3-5 minutes before developing. Otherwise, store slides as directed for up to 14 days until ready to develop.

Development of Test

1. Open flap in back of slide and apply two drops of Hemoccult Developer to guaiac paper directly over each smear.
2. Read results within 60 seconds.
ANY TRACE OF BLUE ON OR AT THE EDGE OF THE SMEAR IS POSITIVE FOR OCCULT BLOOD.

Development of Performance Monitors

1. Apply ONE DROP ONLY of Hemoccult Developer between the positive and negative Performance Monitors.
2. Read results within 10 seconds.
A BLUE COLOR WILL APPEAR IN THE POSITIVE PERFORMANCE MONITOR, AND NO BLUE WILL APPEAR IN THE NEGATIVE PERFORMANCE MONITOR, IF THE SLIDES AND DEVEL-

IMPORTANT NOTE: Follow the procedure exactly as outlined above. Always develop the test, read the results, interpret them and make a decision as to whether the fecal specimen is positive or negative for occult blood BEFORE you develop the Performance Monitors. Do not apply Developer to Performance Monitors before interpreting test results. Any blue originating from the Performance Monitors should be ignored in the reading of the specimen test results.

B. READING AND INTERPRETATION OF THE HEMOCCULT TEST

Negative Smears*	**Negative and Positive Smears***	**Positive Smears***
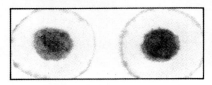	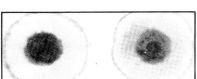	

Specimen report: negative
No detectable blue on or at the edge of the smears indicates test is negative for occult blood.

Specimen report: Positive
Any trace of blue on or at the edge of one or more of the smears indicates test is positive for occult blood.

c. On-Slide Performance Monitors Feature*

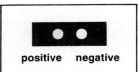

positive   negative

A blue color in the positive Performance Monitor will appear within 10 seconds if test system is functional.

No blue color will appear in the negative Performance Monitor if the test system if functional.

Neither the intensity nor the shade of the blue from the positive Performance Monitor should be regarded as an indication of what the blue from a positive fecal specimen should look like.

*The illustrations are an artist's rendition. Each specimen illustration is of two smears from a single stool specimen as displayed on a single Hemoccult test slide. A reaction on Hemoccult Tape may appear as any one of the illustrated smears.

D. Hemoccult Tape

Preparation	**Development**	
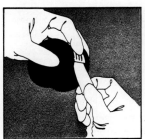	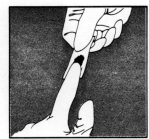	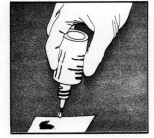

1. Apply two drops of Hemoccult Developer to side opposite smear.
2. Read results on side opposite smear within 60 seconds.
ANY TRACE OF BLUE ON OR AT THE EDGE OF THE SMEAR IS POSITIVE FOR OCCULT BLOOD.

1. Tear strip of tape from dispenser.

2. Apply thin smear of fecal sample. Wait 3 to 5 minutes.

Figure 11-6—cont

E. SATISFACTORY LIMITS OF PERFORMANCE; EXPECTED RESULTS

Results with the Hemocult test are visually determined. The Hemoccult guaiac test paper should be observed for color change within 60 seconds after Developer has been applied.

This reading time is important because the color reaction may fade after two to four minutes.

If any trace of blue on or at the edge of the smear is seen, the test is positive for occult blood. For typical positive reaction, see READING AND INTERPRETATION OF THE HEMOCCULT TEST.

NOTE: Because this test is visually read and requires color differentiation, it should not be read by the visually impaired.

The function and stability of the Hemoccult slides and Developer can be tested using the on-slide Performance Monitors. The Hemoccult Tape may be tested by applying a drop of diluted whole blood (1:5,000 in distilled water) to an unused portion of the tape. Add Developer to opposite side. If any blue appears, the guaiac-impregnated paper and Developer are functional.

F. INSTRUCTIONS TO THE PATIENT FOR COLLECTING FECAL SPECIMENS FOR THE HEMOCCULT II SLIDE TEST

Hemocult slides are used routinely to check the intestinal tract.
Please follow these instructions carefully.

Before beginning the Test Procedure, please read Sample Collection Instructions. For accurate test results, it is important to follow the diet below for at least 48 hours before collecting the first stool sample. Remain on this diet until you have completed all three slides.

1. Use a ball-point pen to write your name, age and address on the front of each slide.
2. After a bowel movement, open the front of Slide 1. Use one applicator to collect a small stool sample from the toilet bowl.
3. Apply sample inside Box A. Collect a second sample from a different part of the stool using the same applicator. Apply this sample inside Box B. Discard applicator in a waste container. Do not flush wooden applicator.
4. Close the cover flap. Fill in the date on the front of the slide; place slide in the paper envelope; allowing slide to air-dry overnight.
5. Repeat Steps 2-4 for your next 2 bowel movements. After last completed slide has air-dried overnight, immediately return all slides to your doctor or laboratory. NOTE: Current U.S. Postal Regulations prohibit mailing completed test slides in a standard paper envelope. If you wish to return your slides by mail, ask your doctor for a U.S. Postal Service approved mailing pouch.

G. SAMPLE COLLECTION INSTRUCTIONS

Do not collect samples during, or until three days after your menstrual period, or while you have bleeding hemorrhoids or blood in your urine.

Do collect samples from three consecutive bowel movements or three bowel movements closely spaced in time.

Do protect slides from heat, light, and volatile chemicals (e.g., iodine or bleach).

Do keep slides closed when not in use

Do follow the Special Diagnostic Diet Instructions (below) for 48 hours before proceeding.

Special Diagnostic Diet Instructions
Foods To Eat

- Well-cooked, pork, poultry, and fish
- Any cooked fruits and vegetables
- High-fiber foods (e.g., whole wheat bread, bran cereal, popcorn)
If following any part of the Special Diagnostic Diet is a problem, talk to your doctor.

Foods, Vitamins, And Drugs To Avoid

- Red meat (beef, lamb), including processed meats and liver
- Any raw fruits and vegetables (especially melons, radishes, turnips and horse-radish)
- Vitamin C in excess of 250 mg per day
- Aspirin or other nonsteroidal anti-inflammatory drugs (avoid for 7 days prior to and during the testing period)

(Text material adapted with permission of SmithKline Diagnostics, Inc., Sunnyvale, Calif.)

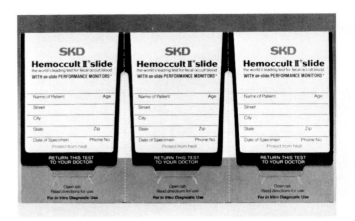

E

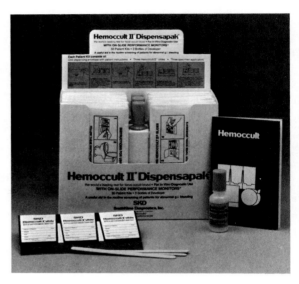

F

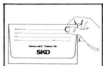
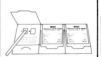

1. Fill in patient information on Hemoccult II* test. Give kit to patient.

2. **Patient,** at home, opens a cover flap and applies thin stool smear to Box A, a second smear from a different site to Box B. Patient performs procedure for three consecutive bowel movements.

3. **Patient** returns prepared slides to doctor's office or lab.

4. **Doctor or medical assistant** applies two drops of Developer on the back of the slide directly over each smear.

5. **Doctor or medical assistant** reads results within 60 seconds. Any trace of blue on or at the edge of the smear is positive for blood.

6. **Doctor or medical assistant** applies ONE DROP ONLY of Developer between the positive and negative Performance Monitors*. A blue color will appear within 10 seconds in the positive Performance Monitor, no blue in the negative Performance Monitor, if the slides and Developer are functional.

G

RESPIRATORY TRACT SPECIMENS

SPUTUM SPECIMEN COLLECTION

Sputum specimens are examined to help determine the presence of infectious organisms or to identify tumor cells in the respiratory tract. The laboratory findings provide relevant information to the physician when making a diagnosis and initiating treatment.

Other specimens that may be obtained if a patient is unable to produce sputum include tracheal aspirates collected by aspiration with a suction catheter, and bronchial washings and transtracheal aspirates collected by the physician or a pulmonary technician. These specimens are of more value diagnostically than sputum, since they are not likely to become as contaminated with oropharyngeal flora. Nevertheless, because sputum is easy to collect and causes little discomfort to the patient, it is usually the first type of lower respiratory tract specimen to be obtained for examination and culture.

Procedures ordered on sputum specimens when sent to the laboratory include direct smears, routine culture and sensitivities, cultures for acid-fast bacilli (tuberculosis), fungus cultures, and sputum cytology (exfoliative cytology), which is performed to identify tumor cells.

Periodic sputum examinations may also be done on patients receiving antibiotics, steroids, and immunosuppressive agents for prolonged periods, since these agents give rise to opportunistic pulmonary infections.

When you collect sputum specimens, it is essential that you understand the physician's order. For example, if the order states "sputum cultures × 3," this means that you should collect three different specimens at different times or on 3 successive days. This order *does not* means that you collect one specimen and divide it into three different containers. Even though these specimens would each be cultured, the findings will show that they were duplicates; thus the whole procedure would have to be repeated.

VOCABULARY

Exfoliative cytology—Microscopic examination of cells desquamated (shedding) from a body surface as a means of detecting malignant change.

Expectorate—The ejection of sputum and other materials from the air passages.

Hemoptysis (he-mop′ -ti-sis)—Coughing up blood as a result of bleeding from any part of the respiratory tract. The appearance of the secretion in true hemoptysis is bright red and frothy with air bubbles.

Immunosuppressive agents—Drugs that inhibit the formation of antibodies to antigens that may be present.

Saliva (sah-li′ vah)—The enzyme-containing secretion of the salivary glands in the mouth.

SPUTUM SPECIMEN

Equipment

Disposable single-use exam gloves, lab coat, and face shield or eye protection
Sterile specimen container
Glass jar for acid-fast bacilli culture

Cardboard sputum container may be used for other studies
Label
Laboratory requisition
Plastic bag and tape

PROCEDURE	RATIONALE
1. Wash your hands. **Use appropriate personal protective equipment (PPE) as dictated by facility.** Don gloves and lab coat, and assemble the supplies.	*This lab coat is to be worn only when collecting specimens. This protects your uniform.*
2. Identify the patient, and explain the procedure. Give the sterile specimen container to the patient. Instruct the patient not to touch the inside of the container with the hands. Put face shield on. If feasible, the specimen should be collected in the morning before eating or drinking. Usually a minimum of 5 ml of sputum is required by the laboratory for testing.	*Obtain freshly expectorated sputum.*
3. Instruct the patient to cough deeply and expectorate directly into the container, avoiding contamination to the outside of the container with the sputum.	*Sputum (lung and bronchial specimen) is produced by a deep cough. You do not want a specimen of saliva from the mouth.*

PROCEDURE

4. Label the container, and indicate test(s) required on the laboratory requisition (Figure 11-7). Accurate, complete information is always required: data, time, patient's name, type of specimen, test(s) to be performed, name of attending physician and, when available, the probable diagnosis.

5. Send the specimen to the laboratory.
   a. Secure the sputum container lid with tape.
   b. Place the container in a plastic bag, and attach the laboratory requisition.
   c. Place all into a secure transport container for delivery to an outside laboratory. Specimens for culture and cytology should be sent to the laboratory within 30 minutes of collection. Refrigerate the specimen when it is not sent to the laboratory immediately.
      NOTE: Specimens must be as fresh as possible, except when accumulation over a specific length of time is ordered. Clearly mark on the label if the specimen is a 24-hour collection.

6. Remove gloves, lab coat, and face shield.

7. Wash your hands.

8. Record on chart. Note any abnormal quality that you may have observed such as sputum that appears to be blood-tinged.

RATIONALE

Any delay can cause organisms to multiply, which would result in misleading findings.
Refrigerate to prevent bacteria overgrowth.

If a 24-hour specimen is to be obtained, instruct the patient to wrap a paper towel around the jar and secure it with a rubber band. Always keep the lid of the container closed except when in use.

Avoid contamination.

Charting example:
   February 25, 19____, 8 a.m.
      Sputum specimen obtained; sent to laboratory for C&S [culture and sensitivity].
      Marjory Alvory, CMA

THROAT AND NASOPHARYNGEAL CULTURES

Upper respiratory secretions most often obtained for examination are throat and nasopharyngeal cultures.

The throat is defined as the area of the body that includes the larynx and pharynx, passageways that link the nose and mouth with the respiratory and digestive systems. A sore throat is caused by inflammation, irritation, or infection of tissue in one or more of the areas in the pharynx or larynx. The common cause of throat infection is the invasion of the tissues by bacteria, such as streptococci, staphylococci, or pneumococci. Inflammation and discomfort in the throat are often caused by tonsillitis, as well as by just an overuse of the voice or excessive smoking.

Throat cultures are performed to determine the presence and the type of microscopic organism that is the cause of an infection. They are frequently ordered for patients suspected of having streptococcal pharyngitis and also for those with suspected cases of pertussis (whooping cough), diphtheria, and gonococcal pharyngitis. The nasopharynx (na′zo-far′ings) is the part of the pharynx above the soft palate that is connected with the nasal cavities, and provides a passage for air during breathing.

Usually nasopharyngeal cultures are ordered on infants and children (when a sputum specimen cannot be obtained) who are suspected of having whooping cough, pneumonia, or croup. They may also be ordered for patients suspected of being carriers of pathogenic organisms that cause meningitis, diphtheria, scarlet fever, pneumonia, rheumatic fever, and other diseases.

Cultures should be obtained before antibiotic therapy is started because antibiotics may interfere with the growth of the microorganism in the laboratory.

Text continues on page 358.

SPUTUM SPECIMEN—cont'd

MICROBIOLOGY		GL 404	ST	BD	LAST NAME		FIRST NAME

DRAWN BY	REMARKS:		DATE/TIME OF COLLECTION

ADDRESS

ROUTINE REQUEST

BIRTHDATE   AGE   SEX   CLASS

IF REQUEST IS OTHER THAN ROUTINE, PLACE STICKER WITH APPROPRIATE INSTRUCTIONS IN THIS SPACE

PHYSICIAN   ROOM NO.   HOSP. NO.

DATE	VERIFYING NURSE	DIAGNOSIS

DATE   PHONE

CIRCLE CODE NO.	INDICATE	SMEAR RESULT:
CULTURES	**SOURCE**	
604 BLOOD	☐ EYE	
(600) (ROUTINE)	☐ EAR	
607 ANAEROBIC	☐ CSF	
620 URINE	☐ NASOPHARYNX	
606 CAMPYLO-BACTER	☐ THROAT	
	☑ SPUTUM	CULTURE RESULT:
618 AFB (SMEAR INCLUDED)	☐ URINE	
612 FUNGUS	☐ STOOL	
616 GRAM STAIN	☐ CERVIX	
(601) ANTIBIOTIC SENSITIVITY	☐ VAGINA	
SCREENS	☐ WOUND	
	☐ ASPIRATE	
625 BETA STREP	☐ ABSCESS	
632 NEISSERIA	INDICATE SITE:	

MICROBIOLOGY PLEASE PRINT • PRESS HARD

TIME IN	TECHNOLOGIST	TIME CALLED OR TELETYPED	TIME OUT

MEDICAL RECORD

Figure 11-7 *Sample laboratory requisition for sputum specimen for culture and sensitivity tests.*

THROAT CULTURE

Equipment

Sterile cotton-tipped applicator(s) in a sterile culture tube(s) or Culturette(s) (Figure 11-8)
Clean tongue depressor
Laboratory requisition(s)
Disposable single-use exam gloves

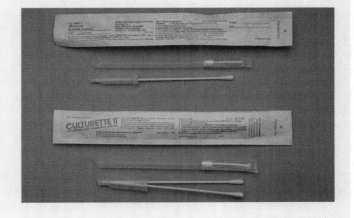

Figure 11-8 *Culturette II and Culturette bacterial collection/transport systems. See Vocabulary, page 359, for an explanation of these systems.*
Courtesy Marion Scientific Corp., Kansas City, Mo.

THROAT CULTURE—cont'd

PROCEDURE	RATIONALE

PROCEDURE

1. Wash your hands. **Use appropriate personal protective equipment (PPE) as dictated by facility.**

2. Assemble the required equipment.

3. Identify the patient, and explain the procedure. Tell the patient that you are going to swab the back of the throat with the cotton-tipped applicator to obtain a specimen that will then be examined in the laboratory.

4. Have the patient assume an upright sitting position facing you. The area where you are working should be well lighted. You may use an examination light that is positioned to give maximal illumination of the patient's throat.

5. Don gloves.

6. Ask the patient to open the mouth as wide as possible, to extend the tongue, and to say "ah."

7. Remove the sterile, cotton-tipped applicator(s) from the culture tube or from the Culturette tube. There are commercially prepared culture tubes in which the applicator stick is secured in the lid of the tube.

8. Depress the patient's extended tongue with the tongue blade until the back of the throat is clearly visible (Figures 11-9 and 11-10). Place the tongue blade over two thirds of the tongue.

9. Using the cotton-tipped applicator, swab the area at the very back of the throat on both sides. Pay particular attention to swabbing any red, raw, or raised bumps along the side and any areas coated with pus. Take care not to swab the tongue, but only the part of the throat from which the specimen should be obtained. Saliva must be avoided. Heavy mucus draining down the back of the throat from the nose is also undesirable culture material.

10. Remove the applicator quickly but gently, and place it into the culture tube, securing the lid. If a Culturette has been used, release the transport medium by crushing the ampule with your finger.

    NOTE: On occasion, two cultures are required—one each from the right and left tonsillar areas. Use two culture tubes with applicators when doing this, and label each specifically. Use a quick, downward stroke, first on one side and then, with another applicator, on the opposite side. Keep the tongue depressed while obtaining both specimens.

11. Remove the tongue blade, and discard into covered waste container.

12. Attend to the patient's comfort; you may reposition the patient if necessary.

13. Remove gloves.

14. Wash your hands.

RATIONALE

Avoid contamination.

This helps determine the cause of the patient's sore throat.

Saying "ah" helps relax the patient's throat muscle and minimizes the gag reflex.

This helps prevent the patient's tongue from touching the applicators as you are obtaining the throat specimen.

Saliva dilutes the specimen, leads to overgrowth of nonpathogens, or inhibits the growth of the pharyngeal flora.

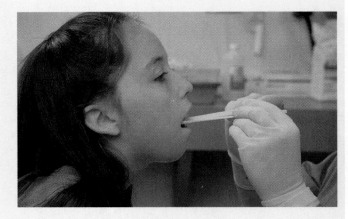

Figure 11-9 Obtaining a throat culture.

THROAT CULTURE—cont'd

PROCEDURE

15. Label the culture tube(s) completely and accurately: patient's name, doctor's name, date, and source of culture.

16. Complete and attach the appropriate laboratory requisition. The information in No. 15 is to be included, as well as the type of examination required.

17. Send the culture tube to the laboratory. Avoid delay. In the laboratory the culture is transferred by the technician to a culture medium.

18. Record on chart.

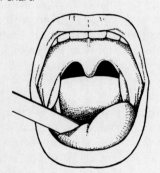

RATIONALE

Your specimen must not dry out before the laboratory can transfer it to a culture medium.
A culture medium enables growth of the infectious organism for future examination.

Charting example:
　February 27, 19___, 1 p.m.
　　Throat culture obtained and sent to laboratory for C&S [culture and sensitivity].
　　　Marcia Edwards, CMA

Figure 11-10 *Area of the mouth in which to swab for the throat culture.*

NASOPHARYNGEAL CULTURE

To obtain a better specimen with more organisms, you may induce the patient to cough by taking a throat culture first. Coughing can force organisms from the lower respiratory tract up to the nasopharyngeal area.

PROCEDURE

1. Obtain a throat culture first (if desired).

2. Insert a sterile cotton-tipped applicator through the nose into the nasopharyngeal area.

3. Gently rotate the applicator to obtain the specimen.

4. Remove the applicator, and place it into the sterile culture tube; secure the lid.

5. Label and send the specimen to the laboratory with the correct laboratory requisition.

6. Record the procedure on the patient's chart.

RATIONALE

To prevent the drying of the specimen on the applicator, avoid delay.

Charting example:
　February 27, 19___, 1 p.m.
　　Throat and nasopharyngeal specimens obtained and sent to the laboratory for C & S [culture and sensitivity].
　　　Abby Nelson, CMA

STREPTOCOCCUS SCREENING

A very common infection, especially in children and young adults, is streptococcal pharyngitis, commonly referred to as strep throat. This infection is caused by the Group A beta-hemolytic streptococcus. These pathogens are the most common bacterial agent associated with infections of the upper respiratory tract and of the skin. Common signs and symptoms of strep throat include a sore throat, fever, chills, swollen lymph nodes in the neck, and, on occasion, nausea and vomiting. The tonsils are often covered with a white or yellow exudate, and the throat is diffusely red. Treatment generally includes penicillin, or erythromycin for patients allergic to penicillin. Prompt diagnosis and treatment of strep throat is important because complications such as rheumatic fever, otitis media, acute glomerulonephritis, or sinusitis may develop.

Several commercial kits can be used to screen for the Group A streptococcus in 4 to 8 minutes. The tests used in the physician's office or clinic most frequently include the Ventrescreen(R) Strep A, the QTEST(TM) Strep A, the Icon(TM) Strep A, and the Testpack Strep A. A throat specimen is needed to perform all of these tests. The manufacturer's directions for each test must be followed precisely to ensure accurate and reliable results. (See also Gram stain on page 361).

Ventrescreen Strep A

The Ventrescreen Strep A enzyme immunoassay uses a solid-phase (antibody-coated tube) to detect group A streptococcal antigen directly from throat swabs or from culture plates. The quality of the test result depends on the quality of the throat swab specimen collected. Obtain specimens by following standard throat swab collection methods, *using the swabs provided with the Ventrescreen kit.* If you are not doing the test in your facility, all throat swab specimens should be transported to the laboratory and tested within 5 days after collection. The Ventrescreen Strep A test does not depend on the specimen containing viable organisms.

Handling swab specimens. Since group A streptococcus is an infectious agent, follow standard precautions for infectious agents such as wearing disposable rubber gloves while handling swab specimens. Swabs may be disposed of according to the usual procedure of your facility.

Procedure and interpreting test results. Immediately following the final reaction in the tube, hold the tube against a white background to interpret the results. Patient samples that exhibit a blue color are considered positive. Colorless samples are considered negative.

WOUND CULTURE

When it is suspected that a wound is infected, a wound culture is done to determine the presence and the type of microorganism that is causing the infection. Cultures can be obtained from wounds on any part of the body.

The procedure for obtaining a wound culture is described on pages 257 to 262 in Unit Six.

SMEARS FOR CYTOLOGY STUDIES

CYTOLOGY SMEARS

Equipment

Sterile cotton-tipped applicators or Ayer spatulas (number depending on the number of smears to be obtained)

Frosted-end glass slide(s)

Fixative spray such as Cyto-Fix (a water-soluble antiseptic), Spray-Cyte, or bottle of fixative solution (solution of 95% isopropyl alcohol preferred; however, formalin 10% may also be used)

Cardboard or plastic slide holder, rubber band, and envelope provided by the laboratory if the slide is to be mailed

Laboratory requisition

Disposable single-use exam gloves

PROCEDURE

1. Wash your hands. Use appropriate personal protective equipment (PPE) as dictated by facility.

2. Write the patient's name and the date on the frosted end of the slide.

3. Don gloves.

Provides protection for yourself from possible contamination.

CYTOLOGY SMEARS—cont'd

PROCEDURE

4. When a physician has obtained the specimen on the applicator or spatula, be prepared to hold the slide while the physician makes the smear.

    or

    Take the applicator from the physician with your dominant hand, grasping the distal end of the stick.

5. Hold the glass slide between your thumb and the index finger of your nondominant hand.

6. Starting near the unfrosted end of the slide, spread the specimen longitudinally along the slide by rotating the applicator in the opposite direction of spreading motion (that is, when spreading the specimen from right to left over the slide, rotate the cotton applicator clockwise (Figure 11-11)).

7. Spread the specimen onto the slide evenly and moderately thin so that individual cells can be identified under a microscope.

8. Discard the applicator in a biohazardous waste container.

9. Fix the smear by immediately spraying it with the fixative spray or by immersing it in the bottle of fixative solution obtained from the laboratory. This should be done within 4 seconds. Spray 5 to 6 inches away. With a continuous flow, make a stroke from left to right, then right to left. Allow to dry 4 to 6 minutes.

10. Remove gloves. Wash your hands.

11. Send the smear in the designated container to the laboratory for cytologic tests with the correct and completed requisition (Figure 11-12).

    NOTE: If you are to mail the slide to a particular laboratory, place the slide inside the cardboard slide holder provided, once the fixative is dry. Close it with a rubber band.

    Fill out the requisition, giving the patient's name, age, LMP (last menstrual period), hormonal or other medication or treatment, pertinent clinical data, and history of any previous atypical Pap smears if this is a vaginal or cervical smear. Insert the slide and requisition into the envelope provided, seal, and mail (see Figure 4-19).

    In the laboratory, the smear will be incubated for a prescribed time (24 to 72 hours) at 37° C (98.6° F) or room temperature, because excessive heating of the smear destroys the microorganisms. To identify specific organisms, the laboratory personnel will use various staining procedures and then examine the smear microscopically.

RATIONALE

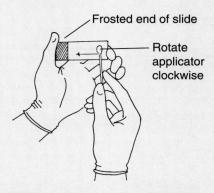

Frosted end of slide

Rotate applicator clockwise

Figure 11-11 *Making a smear for cytology studies.*

Use fixative spray to prevent drying and death of cells.

CYTOLOGY SMEARS—cont'd

CYTOLOGY—SURGICAL PATHOLOGY REQUISITION. SEE BACK PAGE FOR INSTRUCTIONS

FOR LAB USE ONLY

CYTOLOGY - SLIDE NUMBER _____

PREVIOUS SMEARS: ☐ NO ☐ YES GRADE _____

PERTINENT HISTORY: (MUST BE COMPLETED)

| LMP | HORMONES | LAST PREG. | PREGNANT NOW? ☐ YES ☐ NO | IRRAD-IATION | SURGERY? | POST-MENOPAUSAL |
| / / | | | | | | |

MISCELLANEOUS FINDINGS

TEST	MANY	MOD-ERATE	FEW	NONE
RBC				
WBC				
TRICHOMONAS				
CANDIDA				
BACTERIA				
ENDOCERVICAL CELLS				

ESTROGEN EFFECT
HIGH / MODERATE / LOW / ATROPHY / INVALID DUE TO INFLAMMATION

MATERIAL SOURCE
☐ CERVIX ☐ GASTRIC ☐ VAGINA ☐ BREAST ☐ SPUTUM ☐ CSF ☐ URINE ☐ FLUID OTHER ____

DATE & TIME OF COLLECT ____

HORMONAL PROFILE
PB / I / S / MI
☐ SPECIMEN UNSATISFACTORY
EXCESSIVE INFLAM.
SCANTY ☐ DRIED ☐ EXUDATE ☐

PLEASE PRINT
LAST NAME / FIRST NAME
ADDRESS
BIRTHDATE / AGE / SEX / CLASS
PHYSICIAN / ROOM NO. / HOSP. NO.
DATE / PHONE
NAME OF INSURANCE CO.
NAME OF INSURED & I.D. NO.
ATTACH MEDI-CAL STICKER TO GREEN COPY
CHARGE TO: ☐ PATIENT ☐ PHYSICIAN
☐ NEGATIVE ☐ ABNORMAL SEE REPORT BELOW

TECHNOLOGIST/ PATHOLOGIST ____

TIME IN — TIME OUT

GENERAL INSTRUCTIONS:
1. Fill out history
2. Label all specimen containers and slides with patient's FULL name.
3. Deliver sputum, fluid and urine specimens within 1 hour of collection; REFRIGERATE until delivery

CERVICAL/VAGINAL PAP SMEAR
1. Prepare 1 or 2 smears of material from scraping of cervical canal and/or cervical os.
2. Place slides in fixative* immediately for a minimum of 10 minutes.

SPUTUM
1. Obtain first morning, deep-cough specimen.
2. Instruct patient to rinse mouth with water before stimulating cough.
3. Collect specimen in container with tightly fitted lid.
4. 50% Alcohol may be added as a preservative if specimen cannot be delivered to laboratory within 2 hours of collection.

BREAST (Nipple Secretion, Cyst Fluid)
1. Prepare 1 or 2 direct smears on a Dakin all-frosted slide.
2. Place slides in fixative* immediately.

BRONCHIAL WASH / PERICARDIAL FLUID / PERITONEAL FLUID / PLEURAL FLUID
1. Collect fluid in vacuum bottle or Vacu-Bag.

GASTRIC WASH Contact Cytology 24 hours in advance for detailed instructions.

SPINAL FLUID
1. Collect 5 to 7 ml of fluid.

URINE
1. Collect 1st morning, clean catch specimen. A catherized specimen is suggested from female patients.

FLUIDS DELIVER TO LAB IMMEDIATELY

* Fixative in bottle can be obtained in Cytology Lab.

Figure 11-12 *Sample laboratory requisition for cytology studies.*

SMEARS FOR BACTERIOLOGY STUDIES

BACTERIOLOGY SMEARS

The procedure for making a smear for bacteriology studies is the same as that for cytology smears (Steps 1 to 8, pages 358 and 359), *except* to fix the smear.

PROCEDURE	RATIONALE
9. Place the smear on a flat surface and allow to air dry for approximately a half hour.	Air drying allows the specimens cells to dry slowly.
10. Grasp the slide with forceps, and pass it quickly through the flame of a Bunsen burner three or four times to *heat fix* the slide. *Do not* overheat the slide because this will distort the cells present.	Microorganisms are destroyed with the heat and attached to the slide so that they will not wash off when the slide is stained in preparation for examination.
11. Forward the slide to the laboratory in the container provided with the completed laboratory requisition.	

GRAM STAIN

Once a smear is sent to the laboratory, it will be treated in various ways so that visualization or microorganisms under a microscope is possible. A method commonly used to identify bacterial organisms is the Gram stain. This staining method permits the classification of bacteria into four groups: gram-positive or gram-negative rods and gram-positive or gram-negative cocci. The technique involves the treatment of the smear with Gram crystal violet, Gram iodine solution, 95% ethyl alcohol-acetone decolorizer, and safranin counterstain, after which the forms and structure of the microorganisms can be visualized. Bacteria are differentiated on the basis of their color reaction to the above stains. Gram-positive organisms stain purple (for example, staphylococci, streptococci, and pneumococci). Gram-negative organisms are decolorized with the alcohol-acetone solution and retain only the red color of the counterstain, safranin (for example, gonococci, meningococci, and *Escherichia coli [E. coli]*). Such a classification has important clinical implications because it immediately narrows down the differential diagnosis, thus guiding treatment until additional tests such as culture and sensitivity are completed. The type of groups in which bacteria are arranged, such as chains, pairs, and clusters, can also be seen on the Gram stain. This is another important guide for treatment.

The Gram stain is usually followed by a culture and sensitivity test to help determine definitive diagnosis and appropriate treatment of an infectious process.

Frequently the physician will want to start antibiotic therapy for an infectious process before the culture and sensitivity test results are available. In this case the results of the Gram stain are most useful. With the results of the Gram stain, the physician can start a reasonable antibiotic regimen on the basis of past experience as to what drug(s) work against the identified microorganism. For example, this protocol is used when it is suspected that the patient may have streptococcal pharyngitis (strep throat) caused by a group A beta-hemolytic streptococcus. This type of streptococcal pharyngitis most frequently affects young children between the ages of 3 and 15 years and young adults. Early diagnosis and treatment of this condition is important because it can be followed by serious conditions such as rheumatic fever or glomerulonephritis.

GRAM STAIN

Equipment

Smear on a glass slide that has been *heat fixed*
Slide forceps
Straining rack
Wash bottle containing distilled water
Gram crystal violet

Gram iodine solution
95% ethyl alcohol-acetone decolorizer
Safranin counterstain
Bibulous paper pad (absorbent paper pad)
Disposable single-exam gloves

GRAM STAIN—cont'd

PROCEDURE

1. After making the smear and heat fixing it as described above, place the slide on the straining rack, smear side facing up.

2. Cover the slide with Gram crystal violet. Allow it to react for 1 minute (Figure 11-13, *A*).

3. Grasp the slide with slide forceps and tilt it about 45 degrees to allow the Gram crystal violet to drain off (Figure 11-13, *B*).

4. Rinse the slide thoroughly with distilled water for about 5 seconds (Figure 11-13, *C*).

5. Replace the slide on the staining rack.

6. Cover the smear with Gram iodine solution, allowing it to react for 1 to 2 minutes.

7. Grasp the slide with the slide forceps and tilt it to a 45-degree angle to allow the Gram iodine solution to drain off.

8. Rinse the slide in this position with distilled water from the wash bottle for 5 seconds.

9. With the slide still tilted at a 45-degree angle, slowly pour the alcohol-acetone solution over it. This decolorizes the smear. Gram-positive bacteria are resistant to decolorization and retain the Gram crystal violet stain. These bacteria remain purple. Gram-negative bacteria are now clear or colorless because they are unable to retain the stain.

PROCEDURE

10. Rinse the slide with distilled water for 5 seconds.

11. Replace the slide on the staining rack, cover it with the safranin counterstain, and allow it to react for 30 to 60 seconds. The gram-negative bacteria must be counterstained to be seen under the microscope. The safranin counterstain stains them pink or red.

12. Grasp the slide with the slide forceps and tilt it to a 45-degree angle to allow the safranin counterstain to drain off.

13. Rinse the slide thoroughly with distilled water for 5 seconds.

14. Blot the smear dry between the pages of the bibulous paper pad with the smear side facing down. Do not rub the slide because you could rub the smear off the slide (Figure 11-13, *D*).

15. The slide is now ready to be examined microscopically. Position the slide on the microscope using the oil-immersion objective. Adjust the microscope for the examination of the smear, ensuring that the slide was prepared properly (Figure 11-13, *E*). (Refer to Unit Ten for instructions on using a microscope.)

16. Notify the physician that the smear is ready to be examined.

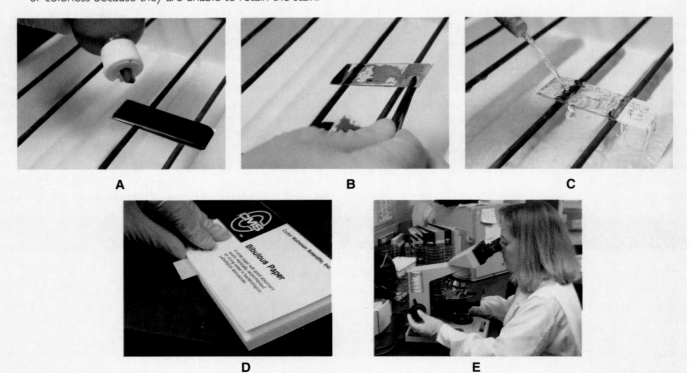

Figure 11-13 *Gram stain procedure.*

BACTERIAL CULTURE AND SENSITIVITY (C&S) TESTING

Bacteria may be identified by means of a culture. A specimen is put on a culture medium that is conducive to the growth of microorganisms (Figure 11-14). The culture is then incubated for 24 to 48 hours to allow for the growth of the microorganisms. After this period, the appropriate tests are performed to identify the microorganisms present. Most frequently, the identification of a specific microorganism is accompanied by a sensitivity study. A sensitivity study determines the sensitivity of bacteria to antibiotics. The disc-plate method is most commonly used clinically (Figure 11-15). This method measures the inhibition of growth of a microorganism, on the surface of an inoculated culture medium plate, by an antibiotic diffusing into the surrounding medium from an impregnated disc. The organism is reported as being sensitive, intermediate, or resistant to the antibiotic. The results obtained from a C&S provide the physician with information used to determine which antibiotic can be used to destroy pathogens causing a patient's infectious condition.

CULTURE MEDIA

A *culture medium* is a sterile, commercial preparation used for the growth of microorganisms or other cells. The most commonly used media are broths (liquids), gelatin (solid), and agar (solid). The liquid media are usually prepared in test tubes; solid media are prepared in test tubes on in Petri dishes or plates (round, flat, covered dishes) (see Figure 11-14).

Liquid media (broths) may be used for the growth of most organisms and for studying the production of gas, odor, and Ph changes. Solid media (agar and gelatin base) are used for the growth of organisms, which then allows for the observation of colony size, shape, and color.

The classification of media according to their function and content follows:

- *Enrichment media.* These contain substances that inhibit the growth of various bacteria. They are used especially to isolate organisms that grow in the intestines and to prepare cultures from stool specimens. Examples include chocolate agar and blood agar.
- *Selective media.* These contain substances that suppress the growth of some organisms while enhancing the growth of others. They are used for the examination of stool and sputum specimens (for example, mannitol salt agar and the modified Thayer Martin media, which are used mainly for suspected gonorrhea specimens and sometimes for detection of meningitis).
- *Differential media.* These contain substances that are used to distinguish between one microorganism and another. They are used to differentiate between forms of colony growth; for example, MacConkey agar is used for routine culturing of stool specimens, and eosin-methylene blue (EMB) agar is used for routine culturing of urine specimens.

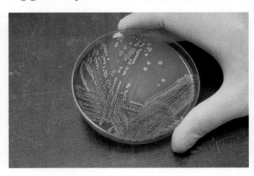

Figure 11-14 *Blood agar culture media contained in a Petri dish showing growth of bacterial colonies.*

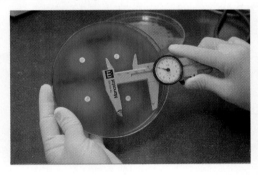

Figure 11-15 *Disc-plate method for sensitivity test. Microorganism being tested is inoculated on the agar medium. Paper discs containing antibiotics are placed on the medium. Clear zones represent inhibition of growth of the microorganism by the specific antibiotic. Zone size is significant. If zone size is smaller than prescribed for clinical effectiveness, the microorganism is reported to be resistant to the drug. Growth around the impregnated disc indicates that the organism cannot be destroyed or inhibited by that antibiotic. When the microorganism is sensitive to the antibiotic, there is a clear zone around the impregnated disc, indicating that the antibiotic was effective in destroying the organism.*

Culture media are stored in a refrigerator and warmed to room temperature before being used. If the culture media are cold when used, the microorganisms placed on them will be destroyed. Petri plates are placed in the refrigerator with the media side facing up. Commercial plates come packaged in plastic bags that prevent the media from drying out. These plates have an expiration date on them. If the expiration date has passed, these plates must not be used.

VAGINAL SMEARS AND CULTURE COLLECTION

To assist the physician in diagnosing various gynecologic conditions (for example, cancer of the uterus or cervix, dysplasia, infections, sexually transmitted diseases, and estrogen levels), smears and cultures for cytologic and bacteriologic tests are obtained from the vagina, cervix, and sometimes the rectum. Some of the more common gynecologic laboratory tests include the Pap smear, vaginal smears for trichomoniasis and candidiasis (moniliasis) (common vaginal infections),

Text continues on page 367.

INOCULATING A CULTURE MEDIUM

Equipment

Sterile cotton-tipped applicators in a sterile tube, or Culturettes

Culture medium—this varies with the type of specimen collected and the laboratory's preference; for example, Thayer Martin (TM) culture medium is used most frequently for vaginal, cervical, and rectal cultures

Bunsen burner and match
Sterile wire loop in container
Candle jar (See Figure 11-18)
Disposable single-use exam gloves

PROCEDURE	RATIONALE
1. Wash your hands. **Use appropriate personal protective equipment (PPE) as dictated by facility.** Don disposable, single-use exam gloves.	*Prevent contamination.*
2. When you or the physician has obtained the specimen, remove the top cover lid of the culture plate and place it upside down on a flat surface.	*Placing the lid in this manner avoids contamination to the inner surface of the lid, which covers the culture.*
3. Inoculate the culture plate by rolling the applicator in a large **Z** pattern on the culture medium (Figure 11-16).	*This pattern provides adequate exposure of the organisms on the medium.*
4. Discard the applicator in a covered container for waste materials.	
5. Replace the cover lid on the culture plate.	
6. Obtain the wire loop and the Bunsen burner.	
7. Light the burner, and place the wire loop over the flame until it is red hot.	*Heating the loop destroys unwanted organisms. If these organisms were not destroyed, a contaminated growth of organisms would be found in the culture medium.*
8. Allow the loop to cool.	*If the loop is too hot, it destroys the organisms that were inoculated on the medium.*
9. Remove the lid of the plate, placing it upside down on a flat surface.	
10. Cross-streak the inoculated medium with the wire loop. With moderate pressure, crisscross the Z with the wire loop (Figure 11-17). Cross-streaking may be done in the laboratory.	*Cross-streaking spreads the organisms and isolates the colonies from the few contaminants that occasionally grow on selective media.*
11. Replace the lid on the culture plate.	
12. Reflame the loop to destroy any organisms that were picked up during the streaking process.	
13. Return the loop to the storage place. Store the loop with the wire extending out of the container.	*Protect the delicate wire so that it is not be destroyed.*
14. Label the cover plate with the patient's name, date, and source of specimen.	

INOCULATING A CULTURE MEDIUM—cont'd

PROCEDURE

15. Place the culture plate in a candle jar, with the medium on the top side of the plate (Figure 11-18).

    NOTE: A candle jar is a large, gallon jar with a candle burning in it. The lid is tightly closed after the culture plate has been placed in it. When the oxygen in the jar is depleted, the candle goes out. An appropriate carbon dioxide environment is thus established. The gonococcus bacteria grows best in an environment enriched with carbon dioxide. Each time you place a culture plate in this jar or remove a plate, the candle must be relit.

16. Remove gloves.

17. Wash your hands.

18. Send the culture plate in the candle to the laboratory for incubation, along with the appropriate laboratory requisition completed correctly. The jar is kept at room temperature for 35° to 36° C (95 to 96.8° F). Incubation period is usually 20 to 24 hours. After this period, the laboratory worker will examine the culture growth.

19. Record the procedure completely and accurately.

20. NOTE: Following the determination of the type of organisms that has grown on a culture plate, sensitivity tests are usually performed to determine the appropriate antibiotic to use for treatment. The organism grown is subjected to a special plate containing various samples of antibiotics. After a period of incubation, this plate is examined. When no growth is observed around a particular antibiotic sample, this indicates that the particular drug is effective in destroying or controlling the infectious organism causing the disease process in the patient (see Figure 11-15).

RATIONALE

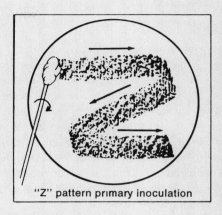

"Z" pattern primary inoculation

Figure 11-16   *Method for inoculating culture medium.*
From Criteria and techniques for diagnosis of gonorrhea, US Department of HEW/Public Health Service, Centers for Disease Control and Prevention, Atlanta, Ga.

Charting example:
   February 20, 19___, 5 p.m.
      Cervical and rectal specimens obtained by Dr. Edwards.
      Culture made and sent to the laboratory for C & S.
         Judy Dansie, CMA

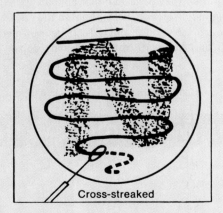

Cross-streaked

Figure 11-17   *Cross streaking inoculated medium with sterile wire loop.*
From Criteria and techniques for diagnosis of gonorrhea, US Department of HEW/Public Health Service, Centers for Disease Control and Prevention, Atlanta, Ga.

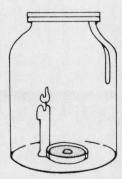

Figure 11-18 *Inoculated culture medium plate placed in a candle jar for incubation. The jar provides an environment in which bacterial colonies can grow.*

vaginal smears to determine estrogen levels, and smears and cultures for sexually transmitted diseases (STDs) (for example, gonorrhea, herpes simplex virus type II, and *chlamydia trachomatis*) (Table 11-1).

GENERAL INSTRUCTIONS

1. Instruct the patient not to douche or use vaginal medication or have sexual intercourse for 24 hours before having a specimen taken (some physicians request abstinence for 48 hours or up to 3 days before the specimen is obtained).
2. Do not collect vaginal or cervical smears when a woman is menstruating, because the blood cells that are produced during that period can invalidate the microscopic readings.
3. Avoid doing a Pap smear for at least 6 weeks if the cervix has been cauterized and for a longer period if the woman has undergone radiation therapy because these procedures cause distortion to the cervical cells.
4. Call the laboratory for specific instructions when in doubt on how to collect a particular specimen. Many laboratories provide all the necessary equipment and instructions.
5. Always wash your hands extremely well before and after assisting with any of these procedures. **Always wear gloves when obtaining and handling ALL specimens.**
6. General preparatory and assisting techniques required are the same as those outlined for assisting with a pelvic examination (see page 100).
7. Always adhere to proper and accurate procedures to help the physician make a correct diagnosis and initiate the best treatment possible. It is your responsibility to see that specimens are handled and labeled correctly after the physician has collected them.

PAPANICOLAOU SMEAR OR TEST (PAP SMEAR)

This is probably the most common vaginal and cervical smear done, since the specimen is easily obtained at the same time that a woman is having a pelvic examination. The Pap test is used to detect cervical or uterine cancer. The American Cancer Society recommends the following:

- All asymptomatic women age 18 to 40, and those under 18 who are sexually active, have a Pap test annually for three negative examinations. After three or more consecutive satisfactory normal annual examinations, the Pap test may be performed less frequently at the discretion of the physician.

- All asymptomatic women age 40 and over have a Pap test annually for three negative examinations. After three or more consecutive satisfactory normal annual examinations, the Pap test may be performed less frequently at the discretion of the physician.
- Women who are at high risk of developing cervical cancer because of early age of first intercourse, multiple sexual partners, or other risk factors may need to be tested more frequently.
- A pelvic examination should be done as part of a general physical examination every 3 years from age 20 to 40 and annually thereafter.*

Refer to Figure 11-19 on page 370 and Pelvic Examination with a Pap Smear, pages 100 to 105, for more specific information about the procedure, method, and assisting techniques used when obtaining this smear for examination.

Vaginal Secretions for Hormone Evaluation

Used to determine a woman's estrogen level, the specimen is obtained from the midlateral vaginal wall on a cotton-tipped applicator or spatula. A smear is then made and sent to the laboratory.

Smear for Trichomoniasis Vaginitis

Trichomonas is a genus of parasitic protozoa that occurs in vaginal secretions, causing a vaginal discharge, pruritus (itching), and sometimes a burning sensation when voiding. When trichomoniasis is diagnosed, specific medication such as Flagyl will be prescribed for treatment. This organism is generally passed from one person to another through sexual contact; therefore the patient's partner, who may be a carrier of the infection but is presenting no symptoms, should also be treated.

When obtaining a smear to diagnose this condition, follow the procedure for assembling equipment and preparing and assisting the patient as outlined for obtaining a Pelvic Examination with a Pap Smear in Unit Four, *except* that a vaginal aspirator may be used rather than an applicator to collect the vaginal discharge, depending on the physician's preference. Follow steps 1 through 13(b) as outlined on pages 100 to 105, and then perform the following steps.

*The American Cancer Society: Cancer-related checkup, 1992.

SMEAR FOR TRICHOMONIASIS VAGINITIS (WET MOUNT METHOD)

PROCEDURE

1. Wearing disposable, single-use exam gloves, place a small amount of normal saline on a slide. The physician obtains a vaginal specimen by saturating the cotton-tipped applicator with the vaginal discharge (or collects the fluid with the vaginal aspirator).

2. You or the physician then dip the saturated cotton-tipped applicator into the saline solution on the slide (or place the fluid in the aspirator into the saline).

RATIONALE

SMEAR FOR TRICHOMONIASIS VAGINITIS (WET MOUNT METHOD)—cont'd

PROCEDURE	RATIONALE
1. Wearing disposable, single-use exam gloves, place a small amount of normal saline on a slide. The physician obtains a vaginal specimen by saturating the cotton-tipped applicator with the vaginal discharge (or collects the fluid with the vaginal aspirator).	
2. You or the physician then dip the saturated cotton-tipped applicator into the saline solution on the slide (or place the fluid in the aspirator into the saline).	
3. Discard the applicator in a covered container for waste disposal.	
4. Place a coverglass over the depressed section in the middle of the slide. A *coverglass* is a small, thin piece of glass that covers the saline and the specimen obtained on the glass slide so that any movement of the live cells can be viewed when the slide is examined under a microscope.	
5. Send the smear to the laboratory at once. If the *Trichomonas* organism is present, the laboratory technician will observe a moving, flagellated organism when the slide is viewed under the microscope.	*If the organism is present, it has to be identified immediately.*
6. Assist the patient as required.	
7. Assemble used equipment and dispose of it according to office or agency policy. Refer to steps 14 to 25 as outlined in the pelvic examination procedure, pages 100 to 105.	
8. Remove gloves.	
9. Wash your hands. Resupply clean equipment as necessary.	
10. Record on the patient's chart accurate and complete information.	*Charting example:* *February 9, 19——, 1:15 p.m.* *Vaginal smear for Trichomonas obtained by Dr. Rouse. Specimen sent to the laboratory immediately.* *Patient sent home with a prescription to be filled, pending positive test results from the lab.* *Mike King, CMA*

Smear for Candidiasis (Monilial Vaginitis)

Monilia, now commonly referred to as *Candida*, is a yeast-like fungus. Referred to simply as a yeast infection by the general public, it is often in the female's vagina without causing any symptoms; and at other times it produces an uncomfortable white, cheesy or curdlike vaginal discharge, itching, and irritation of the vulva.

Yeast infections are not commonly transmitted by sexual contact; the organisms are found everywhere. Frequently, infections tend to recur. The treatment generally includes the use of vaginal suppositories or creams that the physician prescribes. The procedure for obtaining this smear is identical to the one just described for trichomoniasis, *except* that the following three steps should be done first.

1. Place a small amount of saline on a slide.

2. Add (mix) 10% potassium hydroxide (KOH) to the saline.

3. Proceed as was described in steps 2 through 9 in the preceding box.

NOTE: If the *Candida Monilia* organism is present on the smear, the laboratory technician will observe the branching arms of the fungus when it is viewed under a microscope.

Smears and Cultures to Detect Gonorrhea

Gonorrhea is a highly contagious, sexually transmitted disease caused by the bacterial organism, *Neisseria gonorrhoeae,* or the gonococcus. Symptoms in a man usually occur within 1 week after exposure; a woman experiences no early symptoms. A man has a burning sensation when

TABLE 11-1

Sexually Transmitted Diseases

	Acquired Immune Deficiency Syndrome (AIDS)	Cervicityis	Chlamydia	Genital Warts/ Condyloma
What is it?	An infection by a virus that damages the body's ability to fight infections Most at risk: • Gay and bisexual males • I.V. drug users • Recipients of certain blood products • Sexual partners of these groups • Infants born to mothers at risk	An infection of the cervix due to gonorrhea, chlamydia or herpes	An infection by a microorganism • In women, can cause cervicitis, urethritis and PID • In men, may cause non-gonococcal urethritis (NGU) or infection of the prostate and epididymis	Warts caused by a virus called the human papiloma-virus (HPV)
How do you get it?	• Sexual contact with semen, blood or vaginal secretions of someone with AIDS • Sharing unsterile I.V. needles	• Sexual contact with someone who carries the organisms	• Sexual contact with someone who carries the organism	• Skin-to-skin contact with genital warts
How long after contact will it infect your body? (even if you don't have symptoms)	2 weeks-6 months: symptoms may not develop for 2-6 years	Gonorrhea: 3-5 days Chlamydia: 1-3 weeks Herpes: 2-20 days	1-3 weeks	1-6 months
What are the symptoms?	• Constant fatigue • Unexplained fever, chills, or night sweats • Unexplained weight loss greater than 10 pounds • Unexplained swollen glands • Pink/purple flat or raised blotches on or under skin • Constant diarrhea • Persistent white spots in mouth • Dry cough, shortness of breath	• Green, yellow or white vaginal discharge in some women • Light bleeding or spotting after intercourse • Occasionally mild pelvic pain or painful intercourse • MOST WOMEN HAVE NO SYMPTOMS	WOMEN: • Pelvic pain, painful or frequent urination • Vaginal discharge • Bleeding after intercourse • MANY WOMEN HAVE NO SYMPTOMS MEN: • Discharge from the penis • Painful urination • MAY HAVE NO SYMPTOMS	• Small, painless, cauliflower-like bumps that grow around the sex organs or rectum • There might be slight itching, burning, or irritation, especially with many sores • Warts may be found on the cervix (inside the vagina) where the woman may not notice them
How to know for sure?	• Symptoms reviewed by a clinician • Exam performed • Tests performed	• Pelvic exam to look at cervix • Sample of cervical discharge examined under microscope and sent for lab tests	• Sample of discharge examined under a microscope and sent for lab tests	• Sores examined
How is it treated?	There is no known cure for AIDS. Treatments focus on the secondary diseases which take advantage of the body's inability to fight infection. AIDS patients should consult a counselor for long-range health planning.	• Gonorrhea treated with ampicillin or similar antibiotic • Chlamydia treated with tetracycline or similar antibiotic • Usually both drugs are given to treat both organisms	• Tetracycline or similar antibiotic	Can be removed by: • Burning them off with chemicals, electric current, or laser • Freezing them off • Minor surgery (only if nothing else works)
What can happen if you don't take care of it? What should you do if you think you might have it?	• Persons with AIDS can develop certain life-threatening diseases which healthy persons with functioning immune systems can ward off • If a woman has AIDS, she can pass the virus to her fetus who can then develop AIDS • Can spread infection to sexual partner(s)	• Gonorrhea and chlamydia can spread to cause pelvic inflammatory disease (PID) • Infertility (inability to have children) • All 3 organisms can be passed to newborn at birth • Can spread organisms to sexual partner(s)	• Severe infection of the reproductive organs • Infertity (inability to have children) • If a woman has cervical chlamydia when she gives birth, the infection can be passed to newborn • Can spread infection to sexual partner(s)	• They can grow larger in size, or spread to new areas and become harder to remove • Cervical warts are associated with abnormal pap smears, and can lead to more serious problems • If a woman has cervical or vaginal warts when she gives birth, they can be passed to newborn • Can spread warts to sexual partner(s)
What should you do if you think you might have it?	1. Go to your doctor, local health department, VD or family planning clinic for tests and treatment. GO AS SOON AS POSSIBLE. 2. If you have an infection, be sure to contact all of your recent sexual partners, so that they can be tested and treated. 3. Avoid sexual contact until you've taken all of your medication and all symptoms are gone. You might have to return to your doctor or clinic for a test to be sure that your infection is cured.			

Table 11-1—cont'd

Sexually Transmitted Diseases

Gonorrhea	Herpes	Inflammatory Disease (PID)	Syphilis	Uethritis	Vagionitis
An infection by a bacteria In women, can infect the cervix, urethra, uterus & tubes In men, can infect the urethra, prostate and epididymis	An infection by a virus	An infection of the uterus, tubes and pelvic organs due to gonorrhea, chlamydia, or other bacteria	An infection from a bacteria	An infection of the urethra due to gonorrhea, chlamydia, trichomonas, or other organisms • In men, urethritis without gonorrhea is called NGU (nongonococcal urethritis)	An infection of the vagina that has many causes Most common infections: • yeast • trichomonas • gardnerella
• Sexual contact with someone who has gonorrhea	• Sexual contact with someone who has herpes • Direct contact with a herpes sore, or discharge from a sore • Herpes can be spread a few days before a sore appears and for a week after the skin has healed	• Sexual contact with someone who carries the organisms	• Sexual contact with someone who carries the organisms • Any contact with a syphilis sore	• Sexual contact with someone who carries the organisms	• Sexual contact with someone who carries the organisms • Yeast infections can also occur in women who have not had sexual contact
1-10 days	Usually 2-20 days	Varies: organisms can be carried in cervix for months before PID develops	10-90 days	Gonorrhea: 3-5 days NGU: 1-3 weeks	Varies
WOMEN: • Pelvic pain, painful urination, vaginal discharge or fever • 8 OUT OF 10 WOMEN WITH GONORRHEA HAVE NO SYMPTOMS MEN: • Painful urination • Drip or discharge from the penis • May have no symptoms	• Painful blisters that break into open-sores • Sores usually appear on or near the mouth, sex organs, or rectum. They may be found on a woman's cervix (inside her vagina) where She may not notice them • Sores will dry up and disappear in 5-21 day	• Lower abdominal pain, painful intercourse, burning on urination, heavy periods or irregular bleeding, fever, chills • SOME WOMEN HAVE MILD OR NO SYMPTOMS	• EARLY STAGE: A painless sore on the mouth, sex organs, or elsewhere on the body. If you don't treat it, the sore will go away in a couple of weeks, but syphilis is still present in the body • Many people with syphilis do not notice the sores	WOMEN: • Painful or frequent urination MEN: • Painful or frequent urination • Drip or discharge from penis	• Change in vaginal discharge (more than usual, different color, bad odor) • Itching or burning in or near vagina • Painful urination
• Sample of discharge examined under a microscope and sent for lab tests	• Sores examined • Fluid may be taken from a sore and sent to a lab • Blood test may be taken	• Pelvic exam to feel uterus and tubes • Sample of cervical discharge examined under a microscope and sent for lab tests • Blood tests • Pregnancy test to exclude ectopic pregnancy	• A doctor may take a sample from a sore and look at it under a microscope • A blood test will be taken • If the first blood test is negative, another may be necessary in 6 weeks	• Sample of urethral discharge or urine is examined under a microscope and sent for lab tests	• Sample of discharge examined under a microscope
• Penicillin or similar antiobiotic	• Once infected, the virus stays in your body. There is no known care for herpes • Acyclovir is used to treat outbreaks or can be used continously for up to 6 months to prevent new outbreaks	• Ampicillin or similar antibiotic followed by tetracycline or doxycycline • Bedrest and "pelvic rest"	• Penicillin or other antibiotic medicine	• Gonorrhea treated with ampicillin or similar antibiotic • Chlamydia treated with tetracycline or similar antibiotic • Usually both drugs are given to treat both organisms	Depending on type of infection: • Vaginal creams, tablets, douches • Oral antibiotic medicine
• Severe infection of the reproductive organs • Infertility (inability to have children) • Heart trouble • Skin disease • Arthritis (joint problems) • If a women has gonorrhea when she gives birth, the infection can be passed to newborn • Can spread infection to sexual partner(s)	• The sores will go away on their own but they can return, often when you are ill or under stress • If a woman has herpes sores when she gives birth, the infection can be passed to newborn, causing it serious illness or death • Can spread infection to sexual partner(s)	• Pelvic abcess, which may require surgery • Infertility (inability to have children) • Repeat episodes of PID Chronic pelvic pain • Increased risk of tubal pregnancy • Can spread organisms to sexual partner(s)	SECOND STAGE • (6 weeks-4 months after contact): new sores, rash, fever, hair loss, body aches, sore throat, enlarged lymph nodes THIRD STAGE • (years later): damage to heart, blood vessels, brain, eyes • A pregnant woman with syphillis can pass it on to the unborn child, causing it severe damage or death	• In men, urethritis organisms can infect the reproductive organs • Infertility (inability to have children) • Can spread organisms to sexual partner(s)	• Extreme discomfort which will get worse • Can spread to sexual partner(s)

Reproduced with permission of Planned Parenthood, Alameda/San Francisco, revised 1989.

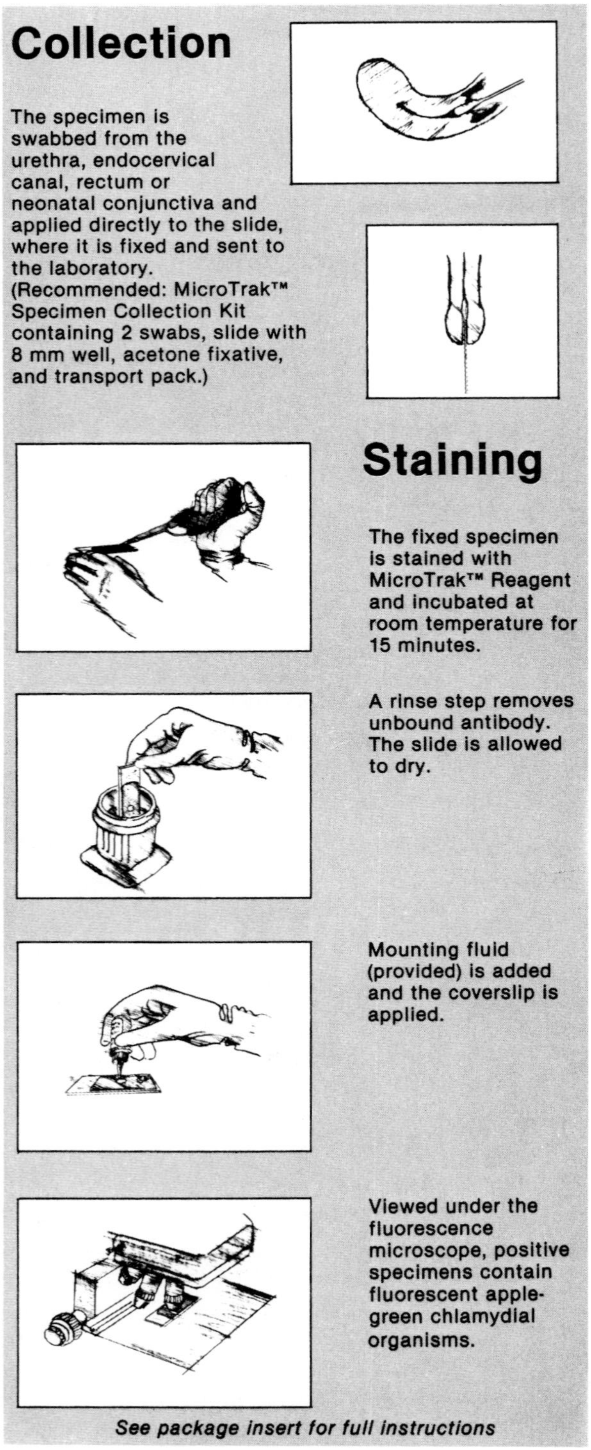

Collection

The specimen is swabbed from the urethra, endocervical canal, rectum or neonatal conjunctiva and applied directly to the slide, where it is fixed and sent to the laboratory. (Recommended: MicroTrak™ Specimen Collection Kit containing 2 swabs, slide with 8 mm well, acetone fixative, and transport pack.)

Staining

The fixed specimen is stained with MicroTrak™ Reagent and incubated at room temperature for 15 minutes.

A rinse step removes unbound antibody. The slide is allowed to dry.

Mounting fluid (provided) is added and the coverslip is applied.

Viewed under the fluorescence microscope, positive specimens contain fluorescent apple-green chlamydial organisms.

See package insert for full instructions

Figure 11-19 Procedure for Chlamydia Trachomatous Direct Specimen Test.
Courtesy MicroTrak/Syva Co., Palo Alto, Calif.

voiding and a whitish fluid discharge or pus from the penis. Women may experience pain in the lower abdomen, with or without a whitish vaginal discharge or a burning sensation when voiding. Penicillin and other antibiotics or the sulfonamide drugs are all effective treatment. Cure for gonorrhea occurs relatively rapidly, although the patient is not considered cured until cultures taken of the discharge are negative for 3 to 4 weeks. Although gonorrhea is contracted through sexual contact, the gonococcus bacteria can infect the eyes (gonorrheal conjunctivitis), a break in the skin, or an open wound. Thus the importance of preventing contamination to yourself and others with specimens obtained from patients suspected of having gonorrhea cannot be overemphasized. Avoid touching your eyes, always wear gloves and then wash your hands extremely well after assisting the physician when a specimen is obtained.

Procedure. For direct smears to be examined, urethral, endocervical, and vaginal specimens are collected and smeared evenly and moderately thinly on two glass slides and then fixed and dried for 4 to 6 minutes (as described previously). Some physicians may obtain a specimen from the anal canal and also from the oropharynx, a common local source for disseminated gonococcal infection. The anal specimen is obtained by inserting a sterile, cotton-tipped applicator approximately 1 inch into the anal canal. The applicator is moved from side to side; 10 to 30 seconds are allowed for absorption of the organisms on the applicator. A smear is then made and fixed. The oropharynx culture is obtained by swabbing the posterior pharynx and tonsillar crypts with a cotton-tipped applicator.

When a culture is desired, two sterile, cotton-tipped applicators or Culturettes are used to collect the specimen. One is placed in a sterile culture tube or Culturette. The second applicator with the specimen is streaked across a special culture medium such as the Thayer Martin medium. Both specimens are sent to the laboratory together.

CHLAMYDIA TRACHOMATIS: THE DIRECT SPECIMEN TEST*

The Chlamydiae are a large group of obligate (able to survive only in a particular environment), intracellular parasites closely related to gram-negative bacteria. There are two species: *Chlamydia trachomatis,* primarily a human pathogen; and *Chlamydia psittaci,* primarily an animal pathogen.

The chlamydial infections of trachoma, inclusion conjunctivitis, and lymphogranuloma venereum have been recognized and studied for many years. However, the chlamydiae have only recently been identified as important etiologic agents in sexually transmissible diseases. The prevalence of these chlamydia-related diseases and the population at risk are thought to exceed those of gonorrhea. *C. trachomatis,* the

*Courtesy MicroTrak/Syva Co., Palo Alto, Calif.

nation's **most common sexually transmitted disease,** is now known to cause urethritis, epididymitis, proctitis, cervicitis, pelvic inflammatory disease, infant pneumonia, and conjunctivitis. It has also been implicated in Reiter's syndrome and prematurue birth. In both sexes, the infection *may be asymptomatic.*

Females risk the most serious complication of chlamydial infection—acute salpingitis—and they can pass the infection to their newborn infants and sexual partners. Because of these risks, specific diagnosis of *C. trachomatis* in the large population of asymptomatic females is critical.

In addition to being undetected in large proportions of the female population, the organism is masked in another large population: men and women who have gonorrhea. Often chlamydia cannot be differentiated from gonorrhea on the basis of symptoms alone. The result—gonorrhea is treated, but the *C. trachomatis* goes undetected. Moreover, *Chlamydia* and gonorrhea may require different antibiotic treatment.

The common thread running through all of these aspects, and the most significant element in terms of control, has been the difficulty of diagnosis. Clinically visible signs (for example, macroscopic appearance of cervix, amount of vaginal discharge) are not specific for chlamydial infection, nor are cellular changes seen on Pap smears. Tissue culture, although extremely sensitive and specific, requires a considerable technical and financial commitment and, hence, is unavailable to most physicians. Also, results from tissue cultures are not available until 4 to 6 days later.

Current efforts to control chlamydial infections have been limited by this lack of adequate diagnosis. Asymptomatic and recurrent infections have gone undetected, and coinfections have been treated inappropriately.

PRACTICAL SCREENING: THE DIRECT SPECIMEN TEST*

Screening for chlamydial infections in asymptomatic women requires a diagnostic method that is less costly, less complex, and more available than tissue culture. *The MicroTrak(TM) Direct Specimen Test* meets these criteria, while retaining the sensitivity and specificity of tissue culture.

Using monoclonal antibodies labeled with fluorescein, the direct specimen test can detect and identify the smallest forms of the organisms, elementary and reticulate bodies, in direct urethral or cervical smears. Diagnosis can be made within 30 minutes after specimen receipt in the laboratory. No cell culture is required.

Procedure. As simple a procedure for a physician to perform as a Pap smear, the cervix (or, in the male, the urethra) is swabbed to remove a smear specimen. The specimen is rolled onto a glass slide fixed with methanol and sent to the laboratory at room temperature. In the laboratory, the slide is stained with the MicroTrak antibody solution, causing *Chlamydia,* if present, to appear as individual, bright apple-green pinpoints on a background of reddish cells when viewed through a fluo-

rescence microscope, a typical item available in most large laboratories. MicroTrak Mounting Fluid contains photobleaching retardant to inhibit fading of fluorescence during examination of the specimen (see Figure 11-19).

This simple test design allows specific diagnosis of *C. trachomatis* in exactly the screening situations that must be tapped: prenatal clinics, family planning clinics, gynecologic offices, and abortion clinics. Further, any routine pelvic examination during which a Pap smear is taken can now be seen as an opportunity to screen for *C. trachomatis*. In populations of women under 25 years of age, in which *C. trachomatis* is about 40 times more prevalent than abnormal cytology, the rationale for such Pap/MicroTrak(TM) testing is apparent. With the rapid results afforded by the new test, physicians can prevent further spread to sexual partners or neonates by beginning specific treatment immediately, even while patients are still in the clinic. Follow-up testing to document cure also becomes more convenient.

These advances will undoubtedly contribute to a more targeted therapy and an eventual reduction in the number of chlamydial infections. Similar applications of monoclonal antibody technology are being developed for herpes simplex virus, gonorrhea, and other infectious diseases. The promise for improved diagnosis in these areas is equally great.

HERPES SIMPLEX VIRUSES: DISEASES, DIAGNOSIS, AND TYPING*

Herpes simplex viruses (HSVs) are ubiquitous among humans. Once acquired, HSV can remain latent in the regional sensory ganglia and, when reactivated, move back along the sensory nerves to produce recurrent infections. HSV infections include genital lesions, cold sores, pharyngitis, ocular keratitis, and encephalitis.

The viruses are classified as type 1 or 2 according to their genetic and antigenic composition. Although each type has been associated with a characteristic pattern of infection (oral HSV 1 and genital HSV 2), the site of infection is not an accurate predictor of the virus type. For example, HSV 1 is now suspected to cause a significant proportion of primary genital herpes.

Specific diagnosis of HSV infection is required in many situations, including infections of neonates, immunocompromised patients, or individuals suspected of having herpes encephalitis. In addition, specific diagnosis is useful in the counseling of sexually active individuals. Typing may be useful in (1) prognosis, since it has been reported that the recurrence rate of genital HSV 1 infection is less than that of genital HSV 2; (2) treatment, since it has been reported that they antiviral activity of chemotherapeutic agents can differ between the two HSV types; and (3) epidemiologic research, in which an association of HSV infection with other disease processes such as cervical carcinoma is being studied.

*Courtesy MicroTrak/Syva Co., Palo Alto, Calif.

Virus isolation in tissue culture is routinely used for diagnosing HSV infections. Although tissue culture amplifies small numbers of infectious organisms for detection, it requires special facilities and 1 to 7 days before a result can be reported. Culture has stood as a generally recognized reference method, but recovery is recognized to be less than 100%.

Direct examination of viral antigen in cells obtained from lesions provides results more rapidly. A poorly prepared slide can be rapidly identified so that another specimen can be obtained promptly. However, it must be recognized that viral antigen is identified by stained specimens, and no direct association with infectivity can be made.

Several laboratory methods of typing HSV have been reported, including plaque size, pock size on chorionic membrane, neutralizational, ELISA, restriction endonuclease analysis, BVDU [E-5-(2-bromovinyl)-2′-deoxyuridine] sensitivity, and immunofluorescence.

THE SYVA MICROTRAK HSV 1/HSV 2 DIRECT SPECIMEN IDENTIFICATION/ TYPING TEST AND CULTURE CONFIRMATION/TYPING TEST*

The Syva MicroTrak HSV 1/HSV 2 Direct Specimen Identification/Typing Test can provide typing results within 30 minutes of specimen receipt. The test can easily be used for the identification and typing of HSV in clinical specimens taken directly from external lesions (Figure 11-20, *A* and *B*).

Cell culture must be initiated at the same time the direct specimen is taken. This allows recourse to the culture results if a direct specimen is negative or inadequate for analysis.

Procedure. Samples are taken by swabbing the base of the lesion with two Dacron-tipped swabs simultaneously. One swab is used to apply the specimen directly to a dual-well

*Courtesy MicroTrak/Syva Co., Palo Alto, Calif.

Figure 11-20 A, *Syva MicroTrak specimen collection kit;* **B,** *HSV 1/HSV 2 Direct Specimen Identification/Typing Test.*
Courtesy Micro Trak/Syva Co., Palo Alto, Calif.

A
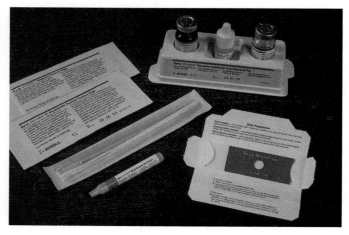

microscope slide, which is then air dried and fixed with acetone. The other swab is placed in a transport medium, and both specimens are sent to the laboratory. Monoclonal antibodies that react specifically with HSV 1 or HSV 2 have been

Procedure

B

Collection

The specimen is swabbed from the base of the lesion and applied directly to two slide wells, which are then fixed and sent to the laboratory. (Recommended: MicroTrak™ Specimen Collection Kit containing 2 swabs, slide with 8 mm wells, acetone fixative, and transport pack.)

Samples of poor quality may result in false negative determinations. A sample for isolation in cell culture must therefore be taken at the same time as the direct specimen. This allows recourse to the culture if a direct specimen is negative or inadequate for analysis.

Staining

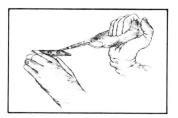
One fixed specimen is stained with HSV 1 Reagent and the other is stained with HSV 2 Reagent. The slide is incubated either at room temperature for 30 minutes or at 37°C for 15 minutes.

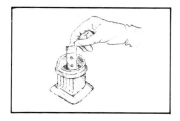
A rinse step removes unbound antibody. The slide is allowed to dry.

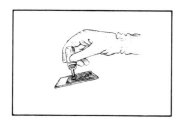
Mounting fluid (provided) is added and the coverslip is applied.

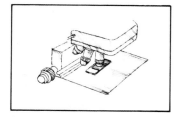
Viewed under the fluorescence microscope, positive cells display characteristic fluorescent apple-green staining. (Specimen quality is checked by evaluating the counterstained cells.)

prepared and labeled with fluorescein isothiocynate. At the laboratory, one well on the dual-well slide is stained with HSV 1 Reagent and the other well with HSV 2 Reagent.

The labeled antibodies bind specifically to their respective viral antigens, and rinse step removes unbound antibody. When slides are viewed under a fluorescence microscope, cells that are positive for the particular viral type show apple-green fluorescent staining that is characteristic of infection with HSV 1 and HSV 2, as demonstrated in the positive control wells; negative cells show only counterstaining, as demonstrated in the negative control wells. The absence of positive cells in the specimen wells should be interpreted cautiously.

In the culture procedure, the transport medium is inoculated into two tissue culture tubes. After the specimens have been cultured, cells are transferred to two slide wells, air dried, fixed with acetone, and tested with the Syva MicroTrak HSV 1/HSV 2 culture confirmation/typing reagents.

LUMBAR PUNCTURE

A lumbar puncture (LP) is the insertion of a thin, hollow needle into the subarachnoid space of the spinal canal, usually between the third and fourth (L-3 and L-4) or between the fourth and fifth (L-4 and L-5) lumbar vertebrae to withdraw cerebrospinal fluid (CSF) or to inject air or a radiopaque contrast medium into this space. This procedure, also referred to as a spinal puncture or a spinal tap, is done under aseptic conditions for both diagnostic and therapeutic purposes.

For diagnostic purposes, an LP is done to:
* Obtain a specimen of CSF for laboratory examination (for example, microscopic examination to determine the presence of white blood cells, red blood cells, neoplastic cells, and microorganisms; chemical determinations for sugar and protein; and serology tests to detect syphilis and certain viral infections).
* Determine the presence of an obstruction to the flow of the CSF.
* Measure the pressure within the cerebrospinal cavities.
* Inject air into the subarachnoid space for certain x-ray film examinations of the skull such as a pneumoencephalogram.

For therapeutic purposes, an LP may be performed to relieve cerebrospinal pressure or to remove pus or blood from the subarachnoid space. It is also necessary for the injection of a spinal anesthetic. The patient must sign a consent form before an LP is performed.

LUMBAR PUNCTURE

Equipment

A sterile prepackaged or disposable set containing the following:
  Lumbar puncture needles, 20- to 22-gauge, 3 to 5 inches long (size may be specified by the physician)
  Three-way stopcock
  Needles, 22-gauge, 1 1/2-inch and 25-gauge, 1/2-inch; and a 3-ml syringe for injecting a local anesthetic
  Spinal fluid manometer for measuring CSF pressure
  Local anesthetic—usually 1% lidocaine (Xylocaine) 10 mg/ml, or procaine
  Three sterile gauze sponges, 2 × 2 inch
  Sterile drape towel
  Sterile fenestrated drape (drape sheet with an open window or hole in it)
  Three swab sticks (stick with a small sponge on the end)
  Three sterile test tubes fitted with snap-top or screw-on caps, for the collection of the CSF
  Small sterile container for antiseptic solution, which is used on the patient's skin
  Adhesive bandage or gauze and tape for dressing at site of puncture when the needle is withdrawn.
Additional supplies needed:
  Sterile gloves
  Local anesthetic, if not on sterile tray
  Skin antiseptic such as Betadine
  Soap and water
  Blood pressure cuff (may be used if a Queckenstedt test is to be performed)
  Laboratory requisition
  This is a sterile procedure; excellent aseptic technique must be adhered to to avoid any possibility of introducing microorganisms into the spinal canal. It is more frequently done in a hospital or clinic where the patient may rest, lying flat for at least 6 hours after the procedure has been completed.

PROCEDURE

1. Wash your hands. **Use appropriate personal protective equipment (PPE) as dictated by facility.**

2. Assemble the required supplies and equipment.

RATIONALE

LUMBAR PUNCTURE—cont'd

<table>
<tr><td align="center">**PROCEDURE**</td><td align="center">**RATIONALE**</td></tr>
<tr><td valign="top">

3. Identify the patient and explain the procedure. Ensure that the consent form has been signed. Explain what is to occur and how it may feel. You may explain to the patient that there is no danger of injury to the spinal cord, since it does not extend past the second lumbar vertebra and the physician will be inserting the needle at a location that is lower than that level.

</td><td valign="top">

Explanations help alleviate some fear of the unknown, thus allowing the patient to relax somewhat and cooperate during the procedure.

</td></tr>
<tr><td valign="top">

4. Have the patient void; save a specimen if required. A full bladder only makes the patient more uncomfortable.

</td><td></td></tr>
<tr><td valign="top">

5. Provide a patient gown, and have the patient disrobe completely. The gown should be put on with the opening in the back.

</td><td></td></tr>
<tr><td valign="top">

6. Summon the physician into the room.

</td><td></td></tr>
<tr><td valign="top">

7. Using aseptic technique, open the sterile glove pack and the outer wraps of the LP tray for the physician. The physician dons the sterile gloves and prepares the supplies on the tray for use. The tray and all contents are sterile on all surfaces.

</td><td></td></tr>
<tr><td valign="top">

8. Position the patient on the side with a pillow under the head. The knees must be drawn up toward the chest, and the head bent forward as close as possible to the knees.

</td><td></td></tr>
<tr><td valign="top">

9. Cleanse the skin with soap and water at and around the site to be entered; then prepare (swab) this area with the antiseptic solution by taking a sterile swab stick soaked in the desired antiseptic solution. It is best to start at the area that will be punctured and cleanse and prepare in a circular outward fashion. The physician may choose to do the skin preparation after donning sterile gloves. In this case, you pour the antiseptic solution into the small sterile container on the tray.

   After the skin is prepared, the physician drapes the area with the fenestrated drape and the towel.

</td><td valign="top">

Because the patient's skin is the most likely source of contamination, it must be disinfected before the puncture is done.

</td></tr>
<tr><td valign="top">

10. Assist the physician as required. When using a stock supply of local anesthetic solution, hold the vial, check the label, and repeat the name and dosage of the drug aloud so that the physician hears what you are saying. Then hold the vial so that the physician can also read the label before withdrawing the solution into the needle and syringe. This step is omitted if the drug ampule is supplied on the tray, because the physician alone checks the label and withdraws the drug.

</td><td></td></tr>
<tr><td valign="top">

11. Help the patient maintain the correct position. Explain to the patient the importance of remaining very still. You may stand on the side facing the patient's front and hold onto the back of the knees and shoulder. Tell the patient to breathe slowly and deeply through the mouth. Using the 3-ml syringe with the 25-gauge needle, the physician administers the local anesthetic. For deep infiltration, the 22-gauge, 1 1/2-inch needle is used. The usual dose of lidocaine is 1 to 2 ml.

</td><td valign="top">

Supporting the patient helps prevent sudden moves that (1) make it more difficult for the physician to insert the spinal needle, or (2) cause the needle to break, or (3) cause trauma to the surrounding tissues.

</td></tr>
</table>

LUMBAR PUNCTURE—cont'd

PROCEDURE

12. Once the spinal needle is in place, instruct and help the patient to slowly straighten the legs (this prevents a false increase in intraspinal pressure), and to breathe normally (that is, not to hold the breath or strain). The spinal puncture needle is introduced into the L3-4 or L4-5 interspace, which is below the level of the spinal cord. To take a pressure reading, the physician attaches the stopcock to the spinal needle and the manometer into the stopcock. At this time you may be asked to record the pressure reading.

13. Don gloves and be ready to receive the specimens of CSF once the physician has obtained them. Check that the caps are secured tightly; stand tubes upright, after securing the caps on tightly. Approximately 2 ml of fluid is collected in each of the three test tubes for observation, comparison, and analysis. Normal CSF is clear, colorless, and sterile.

14. Date and label the tubes, CSF No. 1, No. 2, and No. 3, respectively.
If asked to assist with a Queckenstedt test, which is done when a spinal tumor is suspected, follow this procedure.

15. Place a blood pressure cuff around the patient's neck and inflate it to a pressure of 22 mm Hg (the physician attaches the manometer).

or

You may be asked or compress the jugular veins for 10 seconds and then release either the cuff or your own pressure on the jugular veins.

Normally, there is a rapid rise in pressure of the CSF when the veins are compressed and a rapid return to normal when compression is released. When the pressure rises and falls slowly, this indicates a blockage caused by a lesion or tumor that is compressing the spinal subarachnoid pathways.

These pressure readings are done at 10-second intervals and measured each time the veins are compressed.

16. Note any unusual reaction in the patient (for example, a change in patient's color, respiratory rate, or pulse rate). If you do note any of these changes, inform the physician in a manner that does not alarm the patient.

17. After the needle is withdrawn, you may place an adhesive bandage or gauze dressing over the puncture site.

RATIONALE

Numbering of the tubes is important to the laboratory because it considers the contents of tube No. 3 to be the cleanest specimen. This specimen is used by the laboratory for bacteriology and microbiology examinations. The first specimen obtained (tube No. 1) contains the first amount of fluid obtained. Because this is the first amount of fluid obtained after the needle punctured the skin, it is considered by the laboratory to be the most likely specimen to be contaminated.

LUMBAR PUNCTURE—cont'd

PROCEDURE	RATIONALE
18. Assist the patient as required. It is highly advisable to keep the patient lying flat for 6 to 12 hours (up to 24 hours is recommended) to help avoid headaches. If this procedure was done in the office or clinic, keep the patient lying flat for as long as possible before sending him or her home. Encourage the patient to take a liberal amount of fluids. Inform the patient of any special instructions. Frequently glucose or saline is administered intravenously to a patient with a severe headache. An ice cap and aspirin may also be given to alleviate a headache.	
19. Label and send specimens obtained to the laboratory with the completed requisition. Spinal fluid is to be stored in an incubator, *not* a refrigerator.	*Spinal fluid may contain organisms that are sensitive to cold.*
20. Return to the examining room to assemble all used supplies and equipment, dispose of them properly, and replace with clean equipment as necessary.	
21. Remove gloves.	
22. Wash your hands.	
23. Do any recording required of you accurately and completely. NOTE: Physicians may wish to vary the procedural details according to their technique and judgment.	*Charting example:* *February 11, 19___, 2 p.m.* *Lumbar puncture done by Dr. Cox. Three CSF specimens sent to lab for examination. Opening pressure reading was 250 mm H_2O. Spinal fluid appeared slightly blood tinged.* *Patient had no complaints at this time and is resting quietly in the office bed.* *Susan Oliver, CMA*

CONCLUSION

When you have practiced the procedures in this unit sufficiently, arrange with your instructor to take the Performance Test. You are expected to demonstrate accurately your ability to prepare for and to assist with all the procedures outlined in this unit and to perform some of them. In addition you are expected to identify accurately the supplies and equipment by the proper name when questioned by your instructor.

REVIEW OF VOCABULARY

The following are samples of information seen on various patient charts. Read them and define the italicized terms.

1. Chief complaint: *Diuresis* and *frequency* for the past 2 months. Laboratory data: urine specimen obtained for C&S, and a routine urinalysis. Results: C&S showed no growth and no cells; *routine urinalysis*— sugar 4 plus ; acetone, moderate.

2. History: This 35-year-old white female accountant has approximately nine *bowel movements* a day times 4 months, increased by activity and eating either fatty or sugary foods. The *stools* are loose and have no form. There is some mucus in the stools and some *melena.* She had problems with *constipation* up until 4 months ago. Stools are extremely foul smelling. *Tarry stools* were followed with *guaiac tests; occult blood stools* were noted. Question of *GI bleeding.*

3. History: This 54-year-old gentleman stated that he first coughed up some bright red blood in his *sputum* about 3 weeks ago. The *hemoptysis* occurred again 1 week ago. He has a chronic cough and has smoked two packs of cigarettes daily for the past 15 years.

   Sputum exfoliative cytology: There was a single group of highly atypical cells present, with nuclear features strongly suggestive of malignancy, although the nuclei are partially obscured by the blood and show some degenerative changes.

4. This patient was first seen 1 week ago, at which time she complained of lower abdominal pain and *dysuria.* The patient also indicated that she had noted progressive *vaginal discharge* during the past week. The patient had previously been followed in the *GYN* clinic at City Hospital because of repeated *Pap smears* that showed *dysplasia* consistent with malignancy. A cervical biopsy was done, but the pathology specimen showed no malignancy. *Vaginal and endocervical smears* were obtained and sent to the lab for *Trichomonas* and *Monilia examinations.* Treatment pending positive laboratory results.

5. This patient complained of severe, persistent pain in the lower back radiating down the right leg. After a complete examination was done, this patient was referred to the x-ray film department for a *myelogram.*

6. *Rectal, cervical, and throat cultures* showed no *gonorrhea.*

7. *Vaginitis,* secondary to the steroid treatment. The patient has had well-documented *Candida* growth in her vaginal mucosa and has been treated with Mycostatin suppositories.

PATHOLOGY REPORT

The following is a pathology report received in the physician's office after the patient had surgery because of an abnormal Pap smear and postmenopausal bleeding. After reading this, you should be able to discuss the contents with your instructor. A dictionary or other reference book may be used to define terms that are not familiar to you.

PATIENT: Pat Lewis
DATE OF BIRTH: 7-09-27
DATE RECEIVED: 12-12-94
PREOPERATIVE DIAGNOSIS: Abnormal Pap smear, postmenopausal bleeding.
POSTOPERATIVE DIAGNOSIS: Same.
SOURCE OF TISSUE: A, D&C; B, Cold cone biopsy.
OPERATION: Biopsy.
GROSS DESCRIPTION: **A**, Specimen consists of bits of glistening mucoid pink-to-reddish material, totaling about 1 cm in aggregate. Totally embedded in one cassette. **B**, Specimen consists of a somewhat cone-shaped piece of pink, rubbery tissue, 1.8 cm in maximum diameter and varying from 1 to 1.7 cm in height. A widely patulous, round external os, 1 cm in diameter, occupies the cervical aspect.
MICROSCOPIC DESCRIPTION: **A**, Sections show one intact fragment of endometrial tissue with a single nonsecretory gland and compact stroma, along with fragments of glandular tissues lined usually by low-columnar, inactive cells. A rare gland shows slightly taller lining and some perinuclear vacuoles within the cytoplasm. **B**, Sections show a moderately severe chronic and subacute cervicitis and endocervicitis with many of the endocervical glands located in the exocervical tissues and opening almost up to the surface. Some of these glands are lined by atypical reactive cells. The overlying squamous epithelium shows thickening and areas of parakeratosis and rather marked hyperkeratosis. Occasional granular cell layer is present, and the epithelium is infiltrated with occasional inflammatory cells. The endocervical mucosa is denuded, covered with fibrin and fresh blood. Stroma shows infiltrated chronic inflammatory cells along with an occasional lymphoid follicle. No evidence of malignancy.
DIAGNOSIS: **A**, Fragments of nonsecretory endometrial glands. **B**, Severe chronic and subacute cervicitis and endocervicitis, conization.
M.L. McArthur, MD

CASE STUDY

Read the following policy and procedure for the care of specimens (*urine, blood, stool*), and be prepared to discuss the procedure and italicized terms.

PURPOSE: To describe the manner in which *specimens* should be handled.

POLICY: Extreme care should be taken when handling all specimens, including *histology* specimens, to ensure they reach the laboratory in proper condition and are clearly identified. Proper *incubation* and *inoculation* medium for accurate processing of specimens is essential. Physical equipment such as a *microscope* for viewing *microorganisms* must be in working order.

PROCEDURE: The following procedures should be followed in the handling of specimens.

1. Specimens should be placed in a separate pan to avoid loss at the operative field.

a. Use the proper container for transport of specimens: *formalin or formaldehyde, saline, dry specimen cup with top, or a dry, disposable impervious towel.*

b. Gloves will be used when handling specimens.

c. Avoid handling specimen after it is placed in specimen pan.

2. Procedure for cultures:

a. *Culture tubes (gelatin, hanging drop, negative/positive, pure, smear, sputum, stab, streak, tissue and type cultures)* should be available.

b. A *microbiology* test form is completed and sent to the laboratory.

3. An error could cause an inaccurate *diagnosis*, improper *therapy*, or reoperation.

a. Use *markers* identified as right and left for *bilateral specimens*.

REVIEW QUESTIONS

1. List four types of materials that can be obtained from a patient's body for laboratory examination.

2. What is meant by "special preparation" of the patient before collecting a specimen?

3. List three types of specimens for which active participation of the patient is required.

4. After obtaining a throat culture, you accidentally drop the lid of the culture tube on the floor. What action would you take before sending the specimen to the laboratory?

5. What specimens should be kept refrigerated if you cannot send them to the laboratory immediately, and why do you refrigerate them?

6. Itemize all the information that should be written on a laboratory requisition when submitting a specimen to the laboratory for examination.

7. You have obtained a wound culture and have sent it to the laboratory for a C&S. Explain what types of testing will be performed on the culture and the purpose of these tests.

8. Why is it important for you to wash your hands before and after obtaining any type of specimen from a patient?

9. List information that you should provide to patients when they are collecting a urine specimen at home.

10. Explain the procedure for fixing a smear; state the value and use of smears.

11. Explain the procedure for inoculating culture media.

12. In what position would you place a patient who is to have a vaginal smear taken? Why?

13. When a physician is doing a lumbar puncture on the patient, where would the spinal needle be inserted, and why at this location?

14. List and compare the three classifications of culture media as described in this unit.

15. What is the purpose of performing an occult blood test on a stool specimen?

16. List three substances that may affect the color of a stool specimen.

17. What is the purpose(s) of obtaining a sputum specimen from a patient? Describe the explanation that you would give to a patient who is to collect a sputum specimen.

18. Name two common vaginal infections that are diagnosed by means of vaginal smears.

PERFORMANCE TEST

In a skills laboratory, a simulation of a joblike environment, the medical assistant student is to demonstrate skill and knowledge in performing the following procedures without reference to source materials. For these activities the student needs a person to play the role of the patient. Time limits for the performance of each procedure are to be assigned by the instructor (see also page 52).

1. Given an ambulatory patient and the appropriate supplies, prepare for, give explanations to the patient for, and obtain the following: (a) urine specimen, (b) stool specimen, (c) sputum specimen, (d) throat culture, (3) nasopharyngeal culture, (f) wound culture.

2. Given an ambulatory patient and the required equipment, prepare for, give explanations to the patient for, and assist with the following procedure:
   a. Vaginal smears and cultures
   b. Preparing a smear from the specimen obtained by the physician
   c. Lumbar puncture

3. Having obtained the above specimens, smears, and cultures, complete the appropriate laboratory requisition form, forward all to the laboratory for examination, and record the procedure on the patient's chart.

4. Given the required supplies, demonstrate the correct procedure for staining a smear using the Gram stain.

5. Given the required supplies, demonstrate the proper procedure for performing a hemoccult slide test on a stool specimen.

6. Given the required supplies, demonstrate how to inoculate a culture medium.

The student is expected to perform the above with 100% accuracy 95% of the time.

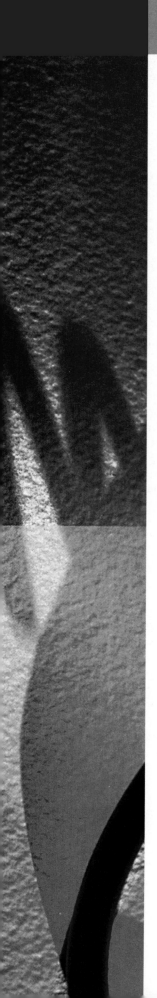

Urinalysis

COGNITIVE OBJECTIVES

On completion of Unit Twelve, the medical assistant student should be able to:

1. Define and pronounce the vocabulary terms listed.
2. Briefly describe the formation of urine, list the main normal components of urine, and give a description of normal urine.
3. Define "routine urinalysis," listing the three basic categories into which it is divided, along with the major observations and examinations made in each category.
4. Describe the fourth category of tests that may now be included in a routine urinalysis.
5. Describe the standard procedure to follow when performing a routine urinalysis.
6. Identify normal and abnormal findings obtained on a complete urinalysis. Relate the abnormal findings to the most probable or possible causes.
7. Describe a reagent strip that is used for doing chemical tests on a urine specimen.
8. Explain how reagent tablets are to be stored.
9. Discuss the advantage and use of the Dipper and Dropper quality control systems for the chemical analysis of urine.
10. List the organized and unorganized sediment that may be present in a urine specimen, indicating if they are normal or abnormal findings.
11. Identify urine tests other than those performed on a routine urinalysis.

TERMINAL PERFORMANCE OBJECTIVES

On completion of Unit Twelve, the medical assistant student should be able to:

1. Demonstrate the correct procedure for performing a physical and chemical analysis of a urine specimen.
2. Demonstrate the correct procedure for preparing a urine specimen for a microscopic examination.
3. Demonstrate the correct procedure for testing a urine specimen for the presence of glucose, acetone, and bilirubin using the Clinitest, Acetest, and Icotest reagent tablets.
4. Demonstrate the correct procedure for testing a clean-catch midstream urine specimen for bacteriuria using the Microstix-3 reagent strip.
5. Demonstrate the correct procedure for testing a urine specimen for the presence of glucose using the Tes-Tape.
6. Demonstrate the correct methods for using the Dipper and the Dropper quality control systems.
7. Demonstrate the correct procedure for testing a urine specimen to determine a pregnancy.
8. Demonstrate the correct procedure for testing urine for phenylketonuria (PKU).

The student is expected to perform these objectives with 100% accuracy.

The consistent use of universal precautions is required by all health care professionals in all health care settings as a method of infection control. It is assumed that these precautions are used in all of the following procedures. Review Unit One if you have any questions on methods to use as the methods/techniques will not be repeated in detail in each procedure presented in the unit.

Be sure to consult the latest guidelines issued by the Centers for Disease Control and Prevention and consult with infection control practitioners when needed to identify specific precautions that pertain to your particular work situation.

URINARY SYSTEM: FORMATION AND COMPONENTS OF NORMAL URINE

The organs of the urinary system include the two kidneys, two ureters, one bladder, and one urethra (see also Unit Eighteen). Urine is formed in the kidneys and passes through the ureters into the bladder, where it remains until the individual voids; then it is excreted through the urethra. The kidneys, located in the retroperitoneal cavity (which means they lie behind the peritoneum), lie anterior and lateral to the twelfth thoracic and first three lumbar vertebrae; they are relatively small, approximately $4^1/2$ inches long, 2 inches wide, and $1^1/4$ inches thick. Being highly complex and discriminatory organs, they help maintain the state of homeostasis in the internal environment by selectively excreting or reabsorbing various substances according to the needs of the body. From your studies in anatomy and physiology, you should

VOCABULARY

Acetonuria (as″t-to-nu′re-ah) or ketonuria (ke″to-nu′re-ah)—The presence of acetone or ketone in the urine.

Albuminuria (al-bu″mi-nu′re-ah)—The presence of serum albumin in urine.

Anuria (ah-nu′re-ah)—The absence of urine.

Bacteriuria (bak-te″re-u′re-ah)—The presence of bacteria in urine.

Dysuria (dis-u′re-ah)—Painful or difficult urination.

Glucosuria (gloo″ko-su′re-ah) or glycosuria (gli″ko-su′re-ah)—Abnormally high sugar content in urine.

Hematuria (hem″ah-tu″re-ah)—The presence of blood in urine.

Oliguria (ol″i-gu′re-ah)—Scanty amounts of urine.

Polyuria (pol″e-u′re′ah)—Excessive excretion of urine.

Proteinuria (pro″te-in-u′re-ah)—An abnormal increase of protein in urine.

Pyuria (pi-u′re-ah)—The presence of pus in urine.

Qualitative tests—Used for screening purposes. These tests provide an indication as to whether or not a substance is present in a specimen in abnormal quantities. A qualitative test does not determine the exact amount of a substance present in a specimen. Color charts are usually used to interpret qualitative tests. *Sometimes they are called semiquantitative tests.* Results are reported in terms such as trace; small amount; moderate; large amount; or 1 +, 2 +, 3 +, and so on; or simply as positive or negative.

Quantitative tests—More precise tests. They determine accurately the amount of a specific substance that is present in a specimen. A high level of skill is required to perform these tests on sophisticated equipment. Results are reported in units such as grams (g) per 100 milliliters (ml), or milligrams (mg) percent, or milligrams per deciliter (dl).

recall the nephron unit, which is the functional unit of the kidney. Each kidney has approximately 1,000,000 nephron units working together to selectively retain or excrete the substances passing through them. Blood, entering the kidneys by way of the renal arteries, eventually reaches the nephron unit for this process to occur. Approximately 1200 ml (30 ml = 1 fluid ounce) of blood flows through the kidneys each minute. This represents about one fourth of the total blood volume in an adult. As blood enters the glomerulus of the nephron, water and the low-molecular-weight components of the plasma filter through to Bowman's capsule, then to Bowman's space, and on through the various parts of the tubules. It is in the tubules that reabsorption of some substances, secretion of others, and the concentration of the urine occur as mechanisms for conserving body water. Many components of the plasma filtrate such as water, glucose, and amino acids are partially or completely reabsorbed; and potassium, hydrogen ions, and other substances are secreted. On the average, nearly all the water that passes through this network is reabsorbed; approximately 1 liter (1000 ml) or so is secreted as the largest component of urine (Figure 12-1). The main normal components of urine follow:

1. Water—About 95% of urine is water.
2. Nitrogenous waste substances or the organic compounds (that is, urea, uric acid, and creatinine).
3. Mineral salts or the inorganic compounds such as sodium chloride, sulfates, and phosphates of different kinds.
4. Pigment—Derived from certain bile compounds, it gives color to the urine.

Many physiologic changes in the body can lead to an upset in the normal functions carried out by the kidneys. Urine, which is continuously formed in and excreted from the body, provides important information with regard to many diseases and disorders. Accordingly, it is widely studied as an aid in diagnosis, in monitoring the course of treatment of disease, and also in providing a profile of the patient's health status. Urine has been referred to as a mirror that reflects activities within the body and, as such, provides much varied information as a result of many chemical, physical, and microscopic measurements. The analysis of urine can provide information about the whole body, as well as its many parts. Kidney disorders modify the composition of urine and may also affect many other body functions. The study of urine may also reflect the situation in which kidney function is normal but other parts of the body are functioning incorrectly.

ROUTINE URINALYSIS

A routine urinalysis, or basic urinalysis as it is often called, can be easily and quickly performed. It is a basic test, but it provides the physician with a tremendous amount of information when a disease process is present. This test can help confirm or rule out a suspected diagnosis. All patients having a physical examination or entering the hospital for treatment have a urinalysis performed. Frequently it is a routine test for many patients seen in the physician's office or clinic and is repeated annually or as frequently as necessary to evaluate the patient's health status.

A routine urinalysis is divided into three basic categories. (A fourth category—detection and semiquantitation of bacteriuria—can now also be done easily in the microbiology and urinalysis laboratories). These categories, the major observations, and the examinations for each follow.

1. General physical characteristics and measurements
   a. Appearance
   b. Color
   c. Odor
   d. Quantity
   e. Specific gravity

Figure 12-1 A, *Coronal section through right kidney.*
A and B from Anthony CP: *Textbook of Anatomy and Physiology*, ed 13, St. Louis, 1990, Mosby.

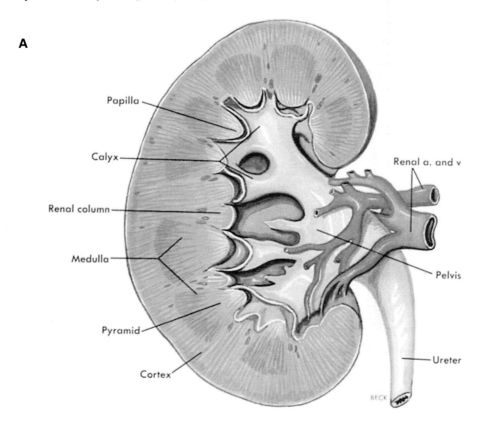

A

- Papilla
- Calyx
- Renal column
- Medulla
- Pyramid
- Cortex
- Renal a. and v
- Pelvis
- Ureter

BECK

2. Chemical examinations
   a. Reaction (pH)
   b. Protein
   c. Glucose
   d. Ketone
   e. Bilirubin
   f. Blood
   g. Nitrate
   h. Uribilinogen
   i. Special tests when indicated, such as for pregnancy, phenylketonuria, and porphyrinuria
3. Microscopic examination of centrifuged sediment
   a. Cells (epithelial, red, and white blood cells)
   b. Casts
   c. Bacteria
   d. Parasites and yeasts
   e. Spermatozoa
   f. Crystals
   g. Artifacts and contaminants
4. Detection and semiquantitation of bacteriuria
   a. Culture plate methods—this requires the special facilities and personnel of a microbiology laboratory. Tests should be done immediately, or the specimen should be refrigerated.
   b. Nitrite test and culture strip methods—this can now be done in the urinalysis laboratory.

STANDARD PROCEDURES

A freshly voided random urine specimen is collected in a dry, clean container. (Review types of urine specimens outlined in Unit Eleven; also review Unit Ten.) This specimen should be examined within 1 hour to avoid changes or deterioration to the contents. If the examination cannot be performed within this time, the specimen should be refrigerated at 5° C (41° F) to preserve the specimen.

When you are doing the examination, the *first* procedure is to note the physical characteristics of the urine; the *second* is to measure the specific gravity; the *third* is to perform a series of chemical tests; and the *fourth* is to prepare the specimen for the microscopic examination. This fourth step is accomplished by centrifuging 10 to 12 ml of a thoroughly mixed urine specimen; the residual sediment is resuspended in 0.25 to 1 ml of urine on a slide for the microscopic examination. The remainder of the urine specimen should be kept until all the procedures are completed, in case any of the tests have to be repeated, or if other special tests have to be performed.

Tests performed on a random specimen of urine are *qualitative*. Only the concentration of a substance in this particular specimen can be measured. The total amount of a substance excreted can be measured only when urine is collected over an accurately measured period of time, such as when collecting a 24-hour specimen.

Figure 12-1—cont'd *Coronal section through right kidney.*
B, *Nephron unit with its blood vessels. Blood flows through nephron vessels as follows: intralobular artery - afferent arteriole - glomerulus efferent arteriole - efferent arteriole - peritubular capillaries (around tubules) - venules - intralobular vein.*

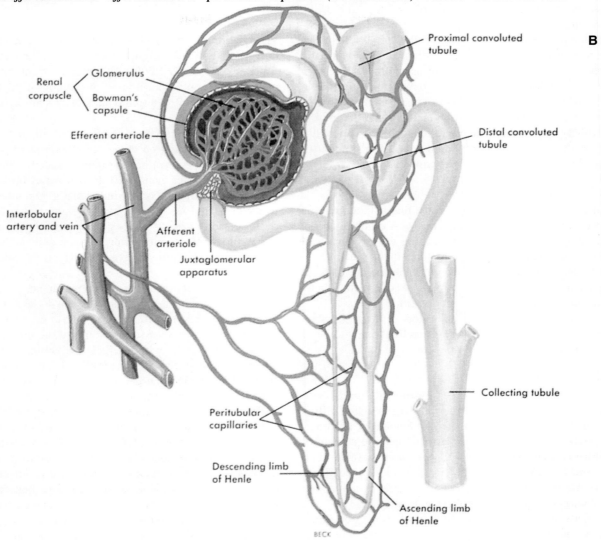

GENERAL PHYSICAL CHARACTERISTICS AND MEASUREMENTS
Appearance

The appearance is generally the first observation made about a urine specimen by virtue of just handling the specimen.

Normal, fresh urine is usually transparent or clear. If the specimen is alkaline, it may appear white and cloudy because of the presence of carbonates and phosphates, but it will clear when a small amount of acid is added to the urine. Urate crystals may be present in an acid urine, giving the specimen a pinkish, cloudy appearance, which usually clears on heating to 60° C (140° F). Both of these appearances are normal.

Abnormal cloudiness in urine may be seen in patients who have a urinary tract infection. This may be caused by the presence of pus cells, leukocytes, and bacteria or by the alkalinity of the urine. Also important to note when observing the appearance of urine is the presence of any sediment (solid particles) in the urine. The presence of red blood cells, white blood cells, or casts in large amount could indicate renal disease or bladder or urinary tract infection.

Color

Normal fresh urine color ranges are described as straw-colored, yellow, or amber, the result of the presence of the yellow pigment, urochrome. The concentration of normal urine determines the degree of the color: highly concentrated urine is dark; dilute urine is pale. Various other factors affect the color of urine (for example, medications, dyes, blood, and food pigments). In many disease states color changes are caused by the presence of pigments that normally do not appear.

Medications such as multivitamins may make the urine a very pronounced dark yellow; nitrofurantoin (Furadantin) (used in the treatment of urinary tract infections) may make the urine brown; and phenazopyridine (Pyridium) (an analgesic used for relief of pain, frequency, urgency, and other discomforts arising from irritation of the lower urinary tract mucosa) produces a red-orange discoloration of the urine. The presence of hemoglobin in the urine may make it red-brown; bile pigments may turn urine yellow to yellow-brown or greenish. Melanins (dark pigments that occur abnormally in certain tumors), when excreted in urine, cause it to turn brown-black if left standing. If the patient is eating large amounts of carrots, the urine may turn a bright yellow. In hepatitis the urine may be a pronounced orange (when the urine is shaken, even the bubbles are orange if the patient has hepatitis). Also, when an individual eats a fair amount of rhubarb, the urine may be red to red-brown.

Odor

Normal urine has a characteristic aroma that is thought to be caused by the presence of certain acids. An ammonia-like odor develops when urine is left standing for any length of time, because of the decomposition of urea in the specimen.

Urine containing acetone, as seen in patients with diabetes mellitus, may have a fruity odor. Urinary tract infections may cause the urine to be foul smelling or putrid.

Although you usually record the odor of the urine when performing a routine analysis, it is generally thought to be of little significance in diagnosing a patient's condition.

Quantity

The normal quantity of urine voided by an adult in a 24-hour period varies somewhat, depending on the individual's fluid intake, the temperature and climate, the amount of fluid output through the intestines (as in diarrhea), and the amount of perspiration. The average quantity is about 1500 ml and ranges from 750 to 2000 ml. The quantity voided by children is somewhat smaller than the amount excreted by adults, but the total volume is greater in proportion to body size.

To measure the quantity of urine, pour the specimen into a large graduate cylinder and record the quantity in cubic centimeters or milliliters. The amount recorded is reported as urine quantity per unit of time (usually 24 hours). Measuring the quantity of urine output is an important aid in diagnosing conditions or diseases related to polyuria, oliguria, or anuria.

Anuria is the absence of urine. At times it may be described as the diminution of urine secretion to 100 ml or less in 24 hours. This may be seen in shock, severe dehydration, and urinary system disease.

Oliguria is the diminution of urinary secretions to between 100 and 400 ml in 24 hours, more commonly defined as scanty amounts of urine. This is seen in drug poisoning, deep coma, and cardiac insufficiency and after profuse bleeding, vomiting, diarrhea, and perspiration. Oliguria is also present with decreased fluid intake and with an increased ingestion of salt.

Polyuria is an excessive excretion of urine. This occurs in diabetes mellitus, diabetes insipidus, chronic nephritis, and following the use of diuretic medications or an excessive intake of fluids. It also may be present during periods of anxiety or nervousness.

Dysuria is painful or difficult urination, symptomatic of many conditions such as cystitis, prolapse or the uterus, enlargement of the prostate, and urethritis.

Specific Gravity

The specific gravity or urine is its weight compared with the universal standard weight of an equal amount of distilled water (expressed as 1.000). This measurement indicates the relative degree of concentration of dilution of the specimen, which in turn helps determine the kidney's ability to concentrate and dilute urine.

Normal specific gravity of urine is generally between 1.010 and 1.030, depending on the concentration of the urine. The first morning specimen has the highest specific gravity, generally being greater than 1.020. It then varies throughout the day, depending largely on the individual's fluid intake.

Abnormally low specific gravity values may be seen in patients who have diabetes insipidus, pyelonephritis, glomerulonephritis, and various kidney anomalies. In these conditions, the kidneys have lost effective concentrating abilities.

Abnormally high values are seen in patients with diabetes mellitus, congestive heart failure, hepatic disease, and adrenal insufficiency. The specific gravity is also elevated when the patient has lost an excessive amount of water through the gastrointestinal tract, as with diarrhea and vomiting, or through the skin during excessive perspiration. High amounts of glucose and protein in the urine, as seen in patients with diabetes mellitus, also increase this value.

There are several methods by which the specific gravity of urine can be measured. The newest and easiest method is by using one of three of the Ames Company's Multistix reagent strips. The strip is dipped into the urine specimen and then is compared with the color chart. The test trip reflects specific gravity as it changes color from blue (low specific gravity) through shades of green to yellow (high specific gravity). (See also *Chemical Examinations of Urine Using Reagent Strips.*)

Specific gravity can also be measured by using a refractometer—Total Solids (TS) Meter—a delicate, hand-held instrument that requires calibration daily. Only 1 to 2 drops of urine are required when using this meter.

Procedure for Determining the Specific Gravity of Urine (Refractometer)

1. Clean and dry the surface of the prism and cover, and close the cover.
2. Using an eye dropper, place a drop of urine at the notched end of the cover (Figure 12-2, *A,*). The urine should be drawn over the prism by capillary action.
3. Pointing the meter toward a light source, rotate the eyepiece to focus on the calibrated scale (Figure 12-2, *B*). You will observe a light and a dark area (Figure 12-2).
4. Read the results on the specific gravity scale at the line that divides the light and dark areas (Figure 12-2, *C*). The specific gravity of this specimen is 1.020.
5. Record the results.
6. Clean the prism with a damp cloth and dry it.

Figure 12-2 A *to* C, *Using a refractometer to determine the specific gravity of urine.*

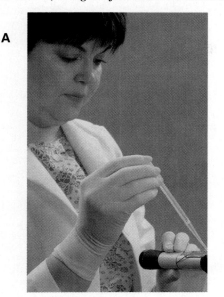

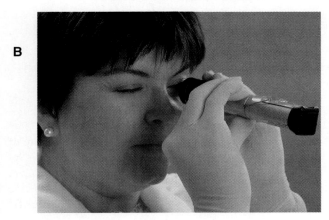

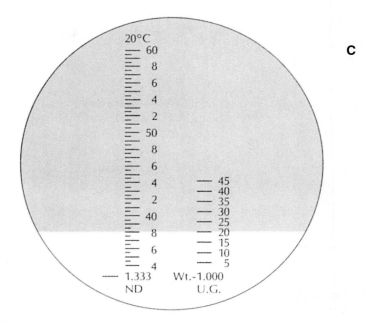

The specific gravity of urine can also be determined by using a urinometer, a weighted, bulb-shaped instrument that has a stem with a scale calibrated from 1.000 to 1.040. The procedure for using the urinometer follows.

The urinometer should be placed in distilled water and checked daily to test its reliability. If it does not read 1.000 when in the distilled water, the urinometer must be replaced. Also, if an unusually high reading is found when testing a urine specimen, remove the urinometer and rinse it under cool water to remove all urine residual; test in distilled water, and then retest the urine specimen. These extra steps are important in case someone had previously left an unclean urinometer, which would lead to abnormal test results when used again.

CHEMICAL EXAMINATION OF URINE USING REAGENT STRIPS

Chemically impregnated reagent strips have virtually replaced older, more cumbersome methods for performing a urinalysis. They provide an easy and rapid method for obtaining the results of tests done in a routine or basic urinalysis; thus they are especially practical and convenient for use in a physi-

cian's office or clinic. In addition to these strips, other special paper tapes, chemical tablets, selectively treated slides, and simplified culture tests are available for special examinations.

The pH of urine and several other components can be easily and rapidly determined with the use of a variety of specially prepared reagent strips and a color chart. The reagent strip is a clear plastic strip with up to 10 pieces of colored filter paper attached, each used to identify different components in the urine. Every piece of filter paper is impregnated with various chemicals and changes color when dipped in the urine. Color changes on the filter papers depend on the presence and amount of the substance that is being measured.

The most complete reagent strip is the Multistix 10 SG,* which is used for determining the pH and specific gravity, as well as the presence and amount of urobilinogen, nitrite, blood, bilirubin, ketone, glucose, protein, and intact and lysed leukocytes (white blood cells) in urine. There are various other Multistix reagent strips available. The Multistix product name includes a number suffix that indicates the number of

*Ames Co., Inc., Elkhart, Ind.

DETERMINING THE SPECIFIC GRAVITY OF URINE (URINOMETER)

Equipment (Figure 12-3)
One 5-inch high glass cylinder
One urinometer

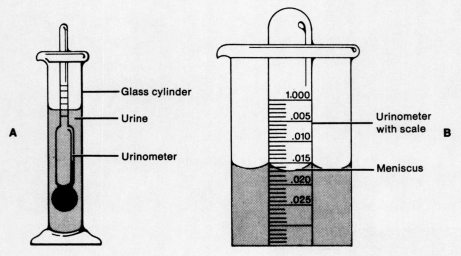

Figure 12-3 **A,** *Items for determining specific gravity of urine;* **B,** *urinometer scale for determining specific gravity of urine. Specific gravity as shown would be 1.017.*

PROCEDURE

1. Wash your hands. **Use appropriate personal protective equipment (PPE) as dictated by facility.** Assemble the equipment and don disposable single-use exam gloves.

2. Pour well-mixed urine into the cylinder to the three-quarter mark (to within 1 inch from the top of the cylinder). Have the cylinder on a flat surface.

3. Place the urinometer in the urine, and spin it gently (Figure 12-4, A). The urinometer floats in the urine.

4. Place the cylinder so that the lower line of the meniscus is at eye level (Figure 12-4, B). The meniscus is a crescent-shaped structure appearing at the surface of a liquid column.

5. Read the specific gravity by noting the point where the lower middle part of the meniscus crossed the urinometer scale. Do not allow the urinometer to touch the sides of the cylinder.

6. Discard the urine. Rinse the urinometer and cylinder with water. Wipe the urinometer dry before using it again.

7. Remove gloves and wash your hands.

8. Record the reading.

RATIONALE

When there is insufficient urine to float the urinometer, the specific gravity cannot be read. You would then simply record "Quantity insufficient."

An inaccurate reading results if the urinometer touches the sides of the cylinder.

Charting example:
   Oct. 10, 19___, 9 a.m.
      Urine specific gravity 1.017
      D. Day, CMA

DETERMINING THE SPECIFIC GRAVITY OF URINE (URINOMETER)—cont'd

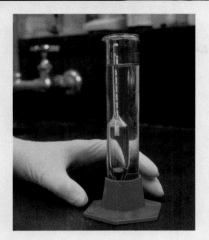

A

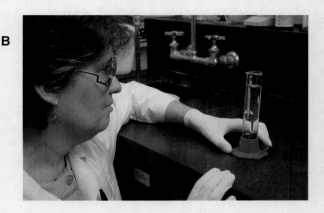

B

Figure 12-4 A, *Place urinometer in the urine and spin it gently.* **B,** *To read specific gravity, place the cylinder so that the lower line of the meniscus is at eye level.*

urine tests on the strip. In addition, strips that test specific gravity have an SG suffix.

Reagent strips are supplied in dark plastic bottles containing 100 strips with directions for use (Figure 12-5, *A*). The color chart and specified times used to read the results of the tests are presented on the sides of the bottle. Both open and unopened product expiration dates are established for these strips to ensure maximum product quality. Always check the expiration date before using.

Because the pH of urine is usually determined as part of a complete urinalysis, it is desirable to use a multiple reagent strip such as one of the Multistix or one of the other reagent strips. Table 12-1 shows the wide range of Ames reagent strips and tablets that are readily available for use.

Procedure for Using a Reagent Strip

1. Don disposable single-use exam gloves.
2. Dip the test areas of the strip into a freshly voided urine specimen (Figure 12-6, *A*); remove immediately and tap to remove excess urine (Figure 12-6, *B*).
3. Compare the test areas to the appropriate color chart on the bottle at the specified times (Figure 12-6, *C*).
4. Remove gloves and wash your hands.
5. Record the results.

For best results, reading urine tests at the proper time is critical. Multistix reagent areas are designed to be read from the bottom up. After removing the Multistix 10 SG reagent strip from the urine, read the results at the following specified times (see Figure 12-5, *B*):

Glucose—read at 30 seconds
Bilirubin—read at 30 seconds
Ketone—read at 40 seconds
Specific gravity—read at 45 seconds
Blood—read at 50 seconds
pH—read at 60 seconds
Protein—read at 60 seconds

Figure 12-5 A, *Multistix 10 SG reagent strips;* **B,** *Multistix 10 SG chart used for determining amounts of 10 factors when performing urinalysis.*
B Courtesy Ames Co., Inc, Elkhart, Ind.

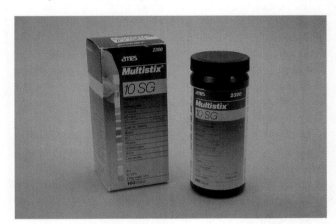

A

B

TABLE 12-1

Rapid Reagent Tests for Routine and Special Urinalyses

Reagent Test	Substances Determined	Technique*
N-Multistix	pH, protein, glucose, ketones, bilirubin, blood, nitrite and urobilinogen	Use fresh, uncentrifuged urine. Preservatives may be added. Dip reagent strip in specimen, remove, and compare each reagent area with corresponding color chart on bottle label at the number of seconds specified.
Multistix	pH, protein, glucose, ketones, bilirubin, blood, and urobilinogen	As above
Multistix 10 SG	Glucose, bilirubin, ketone, specific gravity, blood, pH, protein, urobilinogen, nitrite, leukocytes	As above
Multistix 9	Glucose, bilirubin, ketone, blood, pH, protein, urobilinogen, nitrite, leukocytes	As above
Multistix 9 SG	Glucose, bilirubin, ketone, specific gravity, blood, pH, protein, nitrite leukocytes	As above
Multistix 8	Glucose, bilirubin, ketone, blood, pH, protein, nitrite, leukocytes	As above
Multistix 8 SG	Glucose, ketone, specific gravity, blood, pH, protein, nitrite, leukocytes	As above
Multistix 7	Glucose, ketone, blood, pH, protein, nitrite, leukocytes	As above
Uristix 4	Glucose, protein, nitrite, leukocytes	As above
Multistix 2	Nitrite, leukocytes	As above
N-Multistix SG	Glucose, bilirubin, ketone, specific gravity, blood, pH, protein, urobilinogen, nitrite	As above
Bili-Labstix	pH, protein, glucose, ketones, bilirubin, and blood	As above
Labstix	pH, protein, glucose, ketones, and blood	As above
Hema-Combistix	pH, protein, glucose, and blood	As above
Combistix	pH, protein, and glucose	As above

Courtesy Ames Co. Inc., Division Miles Laboratories, Inc., Elkhart, Ind. 1986.
See package inserts for proper procedures.

Urobilinogen—read at 60 seconds
Nitrite—read at 60 seconds
Leukocytes—read at 2 minutes
For screening positive from negative specimens only, all reagent areas except leukocytes may be read between 1 and 2 minutes.

The addition of a leukocyte test to dry reagent strips may reduce the need for microscopic analysis. Chemical testing for leukocyte esterase detects lysed white blood cells that cannot be detected microscopically. Since leukocyte esterase will be present hours after sample collection, false negatives are reduced.

Microscopic analysis of urine is not indicated when negative findings are obtained for leukocytes, nitrite, protein, and occult blood. Time-consuming microscopics can be reduced to those specimens for which positive chemical results suggest that more specific information is needed.

URINE CHEMISTRY ANALYZERS FOR USE WITH REAGENT STRIPS

The Ames Multistix reagent strips are also designed for use with instrumentation, such as with the Ames Clinitex 200 semi-automated urine chemistry analyzer for moderate to

Table 12-1—cont'd

Rapid Reagent Tests for Routine and Special Urinalyses

Reagent Test	Substances Determined	Technique*
N-Uristix	Protein, glucose, and nitrite	As above
Uristix	Protein and glucose	As above
Clinistix	Glucose	As above
IAlbustix	Protein	As above
Hemastix	Blood	As above
Microstix-nitrite	Nitrite	As above
Urobilistix	Urobilinogen	As above, but preferably using a 2 hour urine specimen collected in early afternoon (between 2 and 4 PM).
Microstix-3	Bacteriuria	Dip culture-reagent strip in specimen for 5 seconds, remove, read nitrite test area after 30 seconds. Insert and seal strip in sterilized plastic pouch provided, incubate for 18 to 24 hours. Compare color densities on total and Gram-negative culture pads with chart provided, without removing strip from pouch. Incinerate pouch with strip still sealed inside. (Some facilities may autoclave the pouch and then dispose of according to their policies).
Ictotest	Bilirubin	Place 5 drops of urine on the special mat. Cover with the reagent tablet. Flow 2 drops of water onto tablet Compare the color reaction with the color chart.
Diastix	Glucose	Use fresh, uncentrifuged urine. Do not use preservative containing formaldehyde. Dip reagent strip in specimen, remove, and compare with color chart on bottle label.
Ketostix	Ketones (principally acetoacetic acid)	As above, but urine must be at least at room temperature at the time of testing.
Keto-Diastix	Glucose and ketones (principally acetoacetic acid)	As above for Diastix and Ketostix.
Clinitest	Reducing substances, including sugars	Add Clinitest tablet to test tube containing mixture of 5 drops of urine and 10 drops of water. Spontaneous boiling occurs; after it stops, compare color in tube with color chart.
Phenistix	Phenylpyruvic acid (phenylketonuria, or PKU)	Use fresh, uncentrifuged urine. Dip reagent strip in specimen, remove, and compare with color chart on bottle label.

Courtesy Ames Co. Inc., Division Miles Laboratories, Inc., Elkhart, Ind. 1986.
See package inserts for proper procedures.

large–volume urine testing (Figure 12-7) or the Clinitek 20 urine chemistry analyzer for small to medium–volume urine testing (Figure 12-8). These instruments are semi-automated and are designed to *read* the reagent strips. Readings are standardized for improved precision through the elimination of visual color discrepancies and operator and environmental variables. Both of these analyzers are easy to use. Directions for use are supplied with the instruments, and they must be followed explicitly. To ensure quality control, daily calibration is recommended for these analyzers. (See also Unit Ten for additional information on quality control.)

Clinitek 10

When the Clinitek 10 analyzer is turned on, the feed table automatically moves out to the *load* position; then the instrument goes through a self-test cycle. After this cycle is completed, the name of the Ames strip programmed to be read is displayed (see Figure 12-8).

After properly immersing the reagent strip in urine and removing the excess urine by blotting, slide the strip onto the feed table, pad-side up, within 10 seconds after pressing the *Start* button. Be sure that the tip of the strip lies flat on the table and is touching the end stop of the feed table insert.

Figure 12-6 A *to* C, *Using a reagent strip.*

A

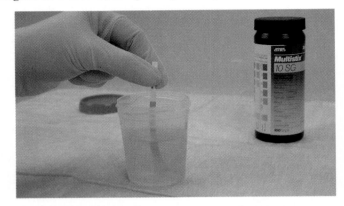

B

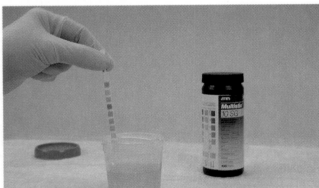

C

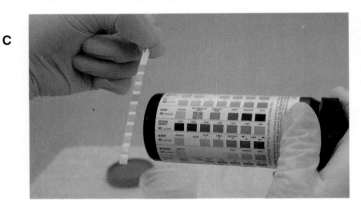

Figure 12-7 *Clinitek 200 semi-automated urine chemistry analyzer for moderate to large–volume urine testing. It is designed to read Strips. Results are printed on a paper printout.*
Courtesy Ames Co., Inc., Elkhart, Ind.

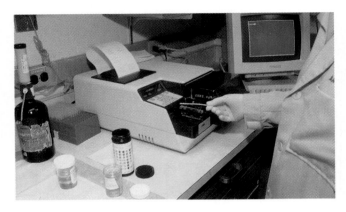

Figure 12-8 *Clinitek 10 urine chemistry analyzer. A semi-automated instrument designed to read the reagent strip. Results show up on the display panel.*

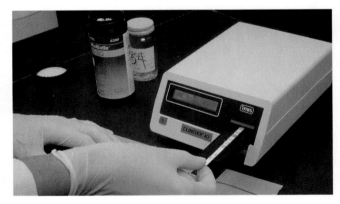

Record the test results shown on the display panel; then remove and discard the used reagent strip.

SIGNIFICANCE OF TEST RESULTS

Multistix 10 SG reagent strips (see Figure 12-5) may provide diagnostically useful information about the status of carbohydrate metabolism, kidney and liver function, acid-base balance, bacteriuria-pyuria, and many other conditions.

Reaction (pH)

pH is the symbol for the hydrogen-ion concentration that expresses the degree of acidity or alkalinity of a solution. The pH is measured on a scale ranging from 0 to 14:7 is neutral, 0 to 7 is acidic, and 7 to 14 is alkaline. Usually freshly voided normal urine from patients on normal diets is acidic, having a pH of 6.0, although normal kidneys are capable of secreting urine that may vary in pH from 4.5 to slightly higher than 8.0.

Excessively acid urine may be obtained from patients on a high-protein diet or who are taking certain medications such as vitamin C or ammonium chloride, and from patients who are retaining a large amount of sodium. In the conditions of uncontrolled diabetes mellitus and acidosis, the patient's urine is also very acidic.

Alkaline urine is seen in patients who have ingested a large meal and in those who consume a diet high in milk and other dairy products, citrus fruits, and vegetables. Certain medications such as sodium bicarbonate help produce alkaline urine. Urinary tract infections, specimens contaminated by bacteria, and specimens left standing for any length of time also produce highly alkaline urine (Table 12-2).

VOCABULARY

Acetonuria (as"e-to-nu're-ah) or ketonuria (ke"to-nur're-ah) is the presence of acetone or ketone bodies in the urine. This is an important symptom in diabetes mellitus. Ketonuria is also seen in patients whose carbohydrate intake is decreased such as with fasting or anorexia, in gastrointestinal disturbances, and following general anesthesia.

Albuminuria (al-bu-mi-nu-re-ah) is the presence of serum albumin or serum globulin in the urine. It is usually a sign of renal impairment; however, it can also occur in healthy individuals following vigorous exercise.

Bacteriuria (bak-te"re-u're-ah) is the presence of bacteria in the urine. A positive nitrite test is indicative of a urinary tract infection.

Bilirubinuria (bil"i-roo"bi-nu're-ah) is the presence of bilirubin in the urine. This occurs in liver disease, bile duct obstruction, and cancer of the head of the pancreas.

Glucosuria (gloo'ko-su're-ah) or glycosuria (gli"ko-su're-ah) is abnormally high sugar content in the urine. The major cause of this is diabetes mellitus. Other common causes of glucosuria include an excessive carbohydrate intake, pain, excitement, liver damage, shock, and sometimes general anesthesia. Ingestion of large amounts of vitamin C may interfere with glucose testing and produce a false positive result.

Hematuria (hem"ah'tu-re-ah) is the presence of blood in the urine. The urine may be slightly blood tinged, grossly bloody, or a smoky brown color. This is symptomatic of injury, disease, or calculi in the urinary system. Certain drugs such as anticoagulants or sulfonamides may also cause hematuria.

Proteinuria (pro'te-in-ure-ah) is an abnormal increase of protein in the urine. This is an important indicator of renal disease. Also it is seen in congestive heart disease, constrictive pericarditis, multiple myeloma, and toxemia of pregnancy. Functional proteinuria is seen in fever, excessive exercise, emotional stress, exposure to heat or cold, and fad diets.

Protein

Normal urine may contain protein, mostly albumin, after exposure to cold, excessive muscular activity, or ingestion of large amounts of protein (see Table 12-2).

Glucose

Normal urine does not contain any detectable glucose unless the concentration of blood glucose exceeds 160 to 180 mg/100 ml; at that point, glucose begins to spill into the urine (see Table 12-2).

Ketone

Normally ketone bodies do not appear in urine unless the patient is on a carbohydrate-deficient diet or a diet that is extremely rich in fat content (see Table 12-2).

Bilirubin

Normally, no bilirubin appears in the urine (see Table 12-2).

Blood

A few red blood cells noted in urine when examined under the microscope are normal. The Multistix 10 SG does not determine the number of red blood cells present, but provides an indication of the presence of occult blood conditions (see Table 12-2).

Nitrite

Normal urine should yield negative results; a positive result is a reliable indication of significant bacteriuria (see Table 12-2).

Urobilinogen

Normal urine contains a small amount of urobilinogen. Biliary obstruction leads to the absence of urobilinogen in the urine; reduced amounts are seen during antibiotic therapy; and increased amounts of urobilinogen in the urine are present in liver tissue damage and in congestive heart failure (see Table 12-2).

Leukocytes

Positive results are clinically significant. Positive and repeat trace results indicate that further testing of the patient and/or sample is needed, according to the medically accepted procedures for pyuria.

Specific Gravity

See page 384 and Table 12-2.

TESTS FOR GLUCOSE, ACETONE, AND BILIRUBIN USING CHEMICAL REAGENT TABLETS
Clinitest*

When the presence of glucose is determined by use of reagent strip, a more quantitative determination may be required. This can be accomplished by using the Clinitest reagent tablet 5-drop method (Figure 12-9).

1. Don disposable single-use exam gloves.
2. Place 5 drops of urine into a test tube.
3. Rinse dropper; add 10 drops of water to the test tube.
4. Add one Clinitest tablet to the test tube.
5. Wait 15 seconds while the spontaneous boiling occurs; this is the normal action seen when the tablet is added to the urine and water mixture. Do not touch the bottom of the test tube because intense heat is generated during this reaction.

*Ames Co., Elkhart, Ind.

TABLE 12-2

Urine Profile of Differential Disease Findings*

Multistix Urine Reagent Strip Tests	Renal	Hepatic	Pancreatic	Gastrointestinal	Cardiovascular	Other
pH	Renal tubular acidosis—D; Bacterial infections—I; Chronic renal failure—I		Diabetic acidosis—D	Diarrhea—D; Pyloric obstruction—I; Vomiting—I; Malabsorption—N or D	Congestive heart failure—N	Dehydration—D; Starvation—D; Low-carbohydrate diets—I; Acetazolamide therapy—I; Metabolic acidosis—D; Metabolic alkalosis—I; Emphysema—D
Protein	Nephrotic syndrome—I; Pyelonephritis—I; Glomerulonephritis—I; Kimmelstiel-Wilson syndrome—I; Malignant hypertension-I				Benign hypertension—I; Congestive heart failure—I; Subacute bacterial endocarditis—I	Toxemia of pregnancy—I; Gout—I; Brown-spider bite—I; Acute febrile state—I; Carbon tetrachloride poisoning—I; Electric-current injury—I; Potassium depletion—I; Orthostatic proteinuria—I
Glucose	Lowered renal threshold—I; Renal tubular disease—I		Pancreatitis-I; Diabetes mellitus—I	Alimentary glycosuria—I	Coronary thrombosis—I	Pheochromocytoma—I; Hyperthyroidism—I; Acromegaly—I; Shock—I; Pain—I; Excitement—I
Ketones		von Gierke's disease (glycogen storage disease)—I	Diabetic acidosis	Vomiting—I; Diarrhea—I		Starvation—I; Low-carbohydrate diets—I; Eclampsia—I; Trauma—I; Chloroform or ether anesthesia—I
Specific gravity	Glomerulonephritis—D; Pyelonephritis—D	Hepatic disease—I	Vomiting—I; Diarrhea—I		Congestive heart failure	Hyperthyroidism—I; Diabetes insipidus—D; Fever—I

Nitrite	Urinary tract infection		
Bilirubin	Complete and partial obstructive Jaundice—I Viral and drug—induced hepatitis-I	Carcinoma of the head of the pancreas—I	Congestive heart failure in the presence of jaundice—I	Recurrent idiopathic jaundice of pregnancy—I Noxious fumes—I Chlorpromazine hepatitis—I
Blood	Hematuria in: Acute nephritis Passive congestion of the kidneys Calculi Malignant papilloma Renal carcinoma Nephrotic syndrome Polycystic kidneys	Hemoglobinuria in: Kimmelstiel-Wilson syndrome	Hematuria in: Diverticulosis of the colon	Hematuria in: Chronic infections Chronic phenacetin ingestion Sulfonamide therapy Sickle-cell disease Hemoglobinuria in: Severe burns Hemolytic anemias Transfusion reaction Sudden cold Eclampsia Allergic reactions Multiple myeloma Alkaloids— poisonous mushrooms
	Cirrhosis—I Hematuria in: Cirrhosis (impaired prothrombin function)		Hematuria in: Bacterial endocarditis Hemoglobinuria in: Intravascular hemolysis Hypertension with renal involvement	
Urobilinogen	Obstruction of the bile duct—D Liver cell damage—I Cirrhosis—I	Carcinoma of the head of the pancreas—D	Suppression of the gut flora—D (antibiotic therapy)	Congestive heart failure—I Extravascular hemolysis—I
				Noxious fumes—I Hepatitis associated with infectious mononucleosis—I Thalassemia—I Pernicious anemia—I Hemolytic anemias—I Chlorpromazine hepatitis—D

Courtesy Ames Co., Inc., Division Miles Laboratories, Inc., Elkhart, Ind
These findings are characteristic of the conditions listed, but are not necessarily found consistently in all cases. Definitive diagnosis must rely upon clinical acumen and the results of other indicated procedures.
N, normal; I, increased; D, decreased.

Figure 12-9 *Clinitest procedure. A, Place 10 drops of water into test tube containing 5 drops of urine. B, Add 1 Clinitest tablet to test tube. C, Compare contents in test tube with color chart.*

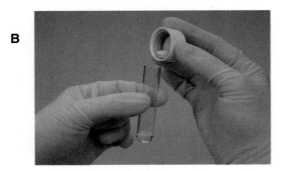

A

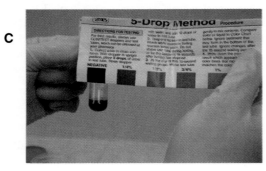

B

C

Test Result	Color Change	Interpretation
Negative (0%)	Dark blue	No glucose present*
Trace (¹/4%)	Green	250 mg/dl*
1 + (¹/2%)	Olive green	500 mg/dl
2 + (³/4%)	Green-brown	750 mg/dl
3 + (1%)	Tan	1000 mg/dl
4 + (2%)	Orange	2000 mg/dl

1 deciliter (dl) = 100 milliliters (ml).

NOTE: The use of this method is not advisable for patients receiving the drugs nalidixic acid (NagGram), cephalothin (Keflin), cephalexin monohydrate (Keflex), cephaloridine (Loridine), probenecid (Benemid), or large amounts of ascorbic acid because they may cause a false positive. The preferred method in these situations is testing the urine by the Tes-Tape method discussed later in this unit.

A modification of the above standard (5-drop) procedure is the Clinitest reagent tablet 2-drop method, also used for quantitative determination of reducing sugars, generally glucose, in urine. Directions for use are identical to the standard procedure, *except* use 2 drops of urine and 10 drops of water. For this specific tablet, the results are identified by comparing the contents in the test tube with a color chart having seven color blocks ranging from dark blue through green and tan up to orange. The results are interpreted and recorded as 0, trace, ¹/2%, 1%, 2%, 3%, or 5% or more.

Acetest*

To detect the presence of acetone and acetoacetic acid in urine, you may use the Acetest reagent tablet.

1. Don disposable single-use exam gloves.
2. Place one tablet on a clean piece of paper, preferably white (Fig. 12-10, *A*).
3. Place 1 drop of urine on the tablet (Figure 12-10, *B*).
4. At 30 seconds, compare the test results with the color chart. Colors will range from buff to lavender to purple. The four color blocks indicate negative, small, moderate, or large concentrations being present (Figure 12-10, *C*).
5. Remove gloves and wash your hands.
6. Record the results.

NOTE: This tablet may also be used to test serum, plasma, or whole blood. Serum or plasma ketone readings are made 2 minutes after application of the specimen to the tablet. When testing whole blood for ketones, apply the specimen to the tablet, wait 10 minutes, and then remove clotted blood and read the results immediately.

Ictotest*

To detect liver function, a simple test on urine to determine the presence of bilirubin may be done with the use of the Ictotest reagent tablet.

1. Don disposable single-use exam gloves.

*Ames Co., Elkhart, Ind.

6. Once the boiling stops, shake the tube gently and compare the color of the contents with the color chart that accompanies the bottle of tablets. Do not wait longer than 15 seconds to compare the colors because results seen after this period are invalid. There are six color blocks ranging from dark blue (indicating a negative reading) through green and tan up to orange, which is read as 2% or 4+ , indicating the presence of large amounts of sugar. The results are interpreted and record as negative, trace, 1+ , 2+ , 3+ , or 4+ , or 0%, 1/4%, 1/2%, 3/4%, 1%, or 2%.

Observe the solution in the test tube carefully during the reaction and the 15-second waiting period to detect rapid, pass-through color changes caused by large amounts of sugar (over 2%). Should the color *rapidly* pass through green, tan, and orange to a dark green-brown, record as over 2% (4+) sugar without comparing the final color development with the color chart.

7. Remove gloves and wash your hands.
8. Record the results.

Figure 12-10 *Using the Acetest reagent tablet to detect the presence of acetone and acetoacetic acid in urine.* **A,** *Place tablet on clean paper.* **B,** *Place 1 drop of urine of the tablet.* **C,** *Compare contents in test tube with color chart.*

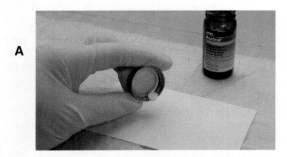

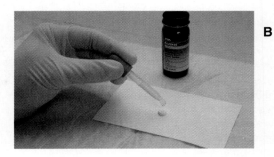

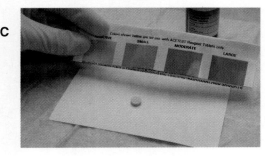

2. Place 5 drops of urine on the piece of special mat that is provided with the tablets.
3. Place a tablet in the center of the wet area.
4. Put 2 drops of water on the tablet.
5. Determine any color change on the mat around the table within 30 seconds, and compare with the color chart. The presence of a blue or purple color indicates a positive reaction.
6. Remove gloves and wash your hands.
7. Record the results.

Summary

These three reagent tablets and the reagent strips must be kept in the bottles in which they are supplied, with the cap secured tightly. Exposure to the air or moisture for any length of time causes them to deteriorate, and they would then be unfit to use for testing urine. Do not remove the desiccants from the bottles. A desiccant is an agent usually provided in a small pack in the bottle. Its function is to help keep the tablets or reagent strips dry. Store at temperatures under 30° C (86° F). Do not store in a refrigerator. Do not use after the expiration date indicated on the bottle.

CONTROLS FOR ROUTINE URINALYSIS

The various qualitative (or semiquantitative) tests for urinary pH, protein, blood, glucose, ketones, bilirubin, nitrite, urobilinogen, and specific gravity should be checked from time to time, using solutions containing known quantities of these substances. Two convenient quality control systems to help determine if tests are properly performed and interpreted are available: the Dipper and the Dropper, Quantimetrix urine dipstick controls. They are particularly valuable in instituting a quality control system or making an existing system more convenient by the use of ready-made controls.

Implementation of a quality control program is essential to ensure accuracy of urinalysis results. Performance of dipsticks and reagent tablets should be validated by testing with known positive and negative controls. Daily monitoring of control values establishes intralaboratory parameters for accuracy and precision of the test method. The Dipper and the Dropper Quantimetrix Urine Dipstick controls (Tables 12-3 and 12-4) are intended to be used to validate the performance of the Multistix, Chemstrip, and Rapignost dipsticks for both visual and instrument readings and as a control for confirmatory tests such as Acetest, Clinitest, and Ictotest reagent tablets, and for hCG methods. Each laboratory should establish its own standards of performance. Quality Control data logs (Table 12-5) such as the one provided with the Dipper should be maintained for all urine dipstick and reagent tablet tests. Each kit contains a summary of the controls, instructions for use, and the expected values that should be obtained when using the controls with the different products.

TEST FOR GLUCOSE USING THE TES-TAPE*

The Tes-Tape is a roll of paper that is treated specifically for the analysis of glucose in urine. It comes packaged in a small plastic dispenser, with directions for use and a color chart for comparing the test results printed on the sides.

Instructions for Use

1. Don disposable single-use exam gloves.
2. Tear off $1^1/_2$ inches of Test-Tape paper (Figure 12-11, *A*).
3. Dip one end of tape into the urine specimen, and remove (Figure 12-11, *B*).
4. Wait 1 minute; then compare any color change on the tape with the color chart on the dispenser (Figure 12-11, *C*). If the tape indicates 3+ or higher, make a final comparison 1 minute later.
5. Remove gloves and wash your hands.
6. Record the results.

MICROSCOPIC EXAMINATION OF CENTRIFUGED URINE SEDIMENT

The third part of the routine urinalysis is the microscopic examination of the sediment present in the urine. The purpose

*Eli Lilly and Co.; Indianapolis, Ind.

Text continues on page 400.

Urine Dipstick Control Kit

THE DIPPER

Product Description

The Quantimetrix Urine Dipstick Controls are supplied liquid, ready-to-use, requiring no reconstitution or dilution. They are prepared from human urine fortified to target levels with selected compounds that produce the desired reaction when tested by the methods indicated below in the **Intended Use** section. Preservatives including sodium azide have been added to inhibit microbial growth.

Intended Use

Control materials having known component concentrations are an integral part of diagnostic procedures. Daily monitoring of control values established intralaboratory parameters for accuracy and precision of the test method. The Quantimetrix Urine Dipstick Control is intended to validate the performance of the **Multistix, Chemstrip** ane **Rapignost** dipsticks, and as a control for confirmatory tests such as **Acetest, Clinitest,** and **Ictotest** reagent tablets, and for hCG methods.

FOR IN VITRO DIAGNOSTIC USE ONLY

Procedure for Dipstick Testing

NOTE: Each tube of the Level 1 Control can be used as a normal control for dipsticks.

Each tube of the level 2 Control can be used as an abnormal control for dipsticks.

1. Remove the controls from the refrigerator and allow them come to room temperature.
2. Immerse the dipstick in the control vial as if it were a patient specimen. **(Chemstrip users see limitations section).**
3. Read the urine dipsticks, visually or with an instrumental reader, in accordance with the manufacturer's instructions.
4. Immediately recap the controls and return them to 2-8 C when not in use.

Procedure for hCG Testing

NOTE: The tubes of Level 1 Control marked hCG negative are to be used as a negative control for hCG methods. The tube of Level 1 Control marked hCG positive is to be used as a positive control for hCG methods.

1. Remove the controls from the refrigerator and allow them to come to room temperature.
2. Use the Level 1 hCG positive and negative controls as if they were patient specimens in accordance with the hCG test kit manufacturer's instructions.
3. Immediately recap the controls and return them to 2°-8°C when not in use.

Storage and Stability

1. The Urine Dipstick Control Kit should be stored at 2°-8° C when not in use. **Do not freeze.**
   Discard the control if turbid or any evidence of microbial contamination is present.
2. When stored at 2°-8° C the controls are stable until the expiration date stated on the label or 20 immersions, whichever occurs first.
3. The level 1 Controls are suitable for use as positive and negative controls for hCG methods until the expiration date, **even after 20 uses as a dipstick control.**

Expected Values

For **Visual readings,** the expected ranges have been established from interlaboratory data by comparing the dipstick reaction that occurs with the controls to the color comparison chart with multiple lots of each manufacturer's dipsticks or reagent tablets.

For **instrument readings,** the expected ranges have been established from interlaboratory data from multiple lots of each manufacturer's dipsticks. Each laboratory should establish its own precision parameters.

For **specific gravity,** the expected ranges by refractometer have been established from the interlaboratory data.

For **total protein confirmation,** the Urine Dipstick Control may be used with the sulfosalicylic acid method at the user's discretion. This method has not been validated in our laboratory.

For **hCG,** the positive and negative results were obtained by testing each lot number of the Level 1 control with multiple lot numbers of at least ten different hCG test kits of various sensitivities.

Limitations

Any future changes made by the manufacturer of a test method may give different values from the indicated range. Detailed information on the limitations of each test method is included in the limitations section of the manufacturers' package insert.

Rapignost Users: Colors produced by the **urobilinogen** and **bilirubin** reactions on the Rapignost Dipstick with the Urine Dipstick Control are not characteristic of those shown on the manufacturer's label. The Urine Dipstick Control is *not* recommended for visual use for **urobilinogen** and **bilirubin.**

Chemstrip Users: Loss of sensitivity of the bilirubin reactions, resulting in a **negative** response for **bilirubin,** may occur **prior** to 20 immersions of the Chemstrip Dipstick in each tube of Level 2 control. Therefore, it is recommended that the Urine Dipstick Control be transferred directly onto the Chemstrip Dipstick rather than immersing the dipstick into the Level 2 control.

Clinitest tablet test: Use of the Level 2 Urine Dipstick Control with the Ames Clinitest tablets for reducing sugars may give an atypical color response. Due to purple and orange color formation in the foam, a murky green to a Clinitest assay for the Urine Dipstick Control are best interpreted as a positive or negative response. A clearer color representation is achieved if the tube is not swirled during or after the boiling reaction.

WARNING AND PRECAUTIONS
POTENTIAL BIOHAZARDOUS MATERIAL
Contains human urine. The FDA recommends that such samples be handled at the Center for Disease Control's Bio-Safety Level 2.
DISPOSE OF PROPERLY
Sodium azide may form metal azides in plumbing and pose a threat of explosion.

From Poon R, Hinberg I: Reflectometric evaluation of Quantimetrix urine dipstick controls, Clin Chem 35:6, 1989.

Table 12-3—cont'd

Urine Dipstick Control Kit

	Ames MULTISTIX			
	VISUAL		**CLINITEK**	
ANALYZE	Level 1 Lot No. 44091 N or P	Level 2 Lot No. 44092	Level 1 Lot No. 44091 N or P	Level 2 Lot No. 44092
Glucose	Negative	100 (tr) - 250 mg/dl	Negative	100 (tr) - 250 mg/dl
Bilirubin	Negative	small (+) - lg (+++)	Negative	small (+) - lg (+++)
Ketones	Negative	5(tr) - 80(lg) mg/dl	Negative	5(tr) - 40(mod) mg/dl†
Specific Gravity	1.025 - >1.030	1.010 - 1.015	1.025 - >1.030	1.010 - 1.015
Blood	Negative	mod (++) - lg (+++)	Negative	small (+) - lg (+++)
pH	5.0 - 6.0	6.0 - 7.0	5.0 - 6.0	6.0 - 7.0
Protein	Negative	trace -100(++) mg/dl	Negative	trace -100(++) mg/dl
Urobilinogen	Normal	1 - 4 mg/dl*	Normal	1 - 4 mg/dl
Nitrite	Negative	positive	Negative	positive
Leukocytes	Negative	mod (++) - lg (+++)	Negative	mod (++) - lg (+++)

*For non-numbered Multistix SG and N-Multistix SG dipsticks visual or Clinitek readings are 8 -#12 Eu/dl for urobilinogen in Level 2.
†Clinitek 200 and 200# instruments may give an occasional reading of # 80. Clinitek 2000 instrument gives readings of 40 - #160.

	Behring RAPIGNOST			
	VISUAL		**RAPIMAT**	
ANALYZE	Level 1 Lot No. 44091 N or P	Level 2 Lot No. 44092	Level 1 Lot No. 44091 N or P	Level 2 Lot No. 44092
Leukocytes	Normal	25 - 75 Leuk/ml	0.00 - 20 Leuk/ml	25 - 75 Leuk/ml
Nitrite	Negative	Positive	0.00 mg/dl	0.05 mg/dl (+)
pH	5 - 6	6 - 7	5 - 6	6 - 7
Blood	Negative	(+) - (++)	0.00 Ery/ul	10(+) - 60(++)Ery/ul
Protein	Negative	30 - 100 mg/dl	0.00 mg/dl	30 - 100 mg/dl
Glucose	Normal	50 - 500 mg/dl	0.00 mg/dl	50 - 500 mg/dl
Ascorbic Acid	Negative	Negative	Negative	Negative
Ketones	Negative	(+) - (+++)	0.00 mg/dl	100(++)-300(+++) mg/dl
Urobilinogen	Normal	*	0.00 mg/dl	4 - 12 mg/dl
Bilirubin	Negative	*	0.00 mg/dl	0.00 mg/dl
		*See Limitations		

	Boehringer Mannheim CHEMSTRIP VISUAL	
ANALYZE	Level 1 Lot No. 44091 N or P	Level 2 Lot No. 44092
Leukocytes	Negative	Trace - (++)
Nitrite	Negative	Positive
pH	5 - 6	6 - 7
Protein	Negative	30(+) - 100(++) mg/dl
Glucose	Normal	1/10 - 1/2
Ketones	Negative	mod (++) - lg (+++)
Urobilinogen	Normal	1 - 8 mg/dl
Bilirubin	Negative	(++) - (+++)*
Blood	Negative	10 - 250 Ery/ul
Specific Gravity	1.015 - 1.020	1.005 - 1.015
		*See Limitations

Additional Available Tests		
Test	Level 1 Lot No. 44091 N or P	Level 2 Lot No. 44092
Acetest	Negative	Small - mod
Clinitest	Negative	1/4 - 1/2%*
Ictotest	Negative	Positive
Specific Gravity (Refractometer)	1.019 - 1.025	1.007 - 1.012
Total Protein (Sulfosalicylic acid)	Negative	Positive† *See limitations †See expected values

HcG	Lot No. 44091 N	Lot No. 44091 P*
(method sensitivity # 50 mIU/ml)	negative	positive

Multistix, Clinitek, Acetest, Clinitest, and Ictotest are trademarks of Miles Laboratories Inc. Diagnostics Division, Elkhart, Ind 46515.
Rapignost and Rapimat are trademarks of Behring Diagnostics Inc., Somerville, N.J. 08876.
Chemstrip is a trademark of Boehringer Mannheim Diagnostics, Indianapolis, Ind. 46250.

TABLE 12-4

Urine Dipstick Control Kit

THE DROPPER

Product Description

The Quantimetirx Urine Dipstick Controls are supplied liquid, ready-to-use, requiring no reconstitution or dilution. They are prepared from human urine fortified to target levels with selected compounds that produce the desired reaction when tested by the methods indicated below in the Intended Use section. Preservations including sodium azide have been added to inhibit microbial growth.

Intended Use

Control materials having known component concentrations are an integral part of diagnostic procedures. Daily monitoring of control values establishes intralaboratory parameters for accuracy and precision of the test method. The Quantimetrix Urine Dipstick Control is intended to validate the performance of the Multistix, Chemstrip, and Rapignost dipsticks, and as a control for confirmatory tests such as Acetest, Clinitest, and Ictotest reagent tablets, and for hCG methods.

FOR IN VITRO DIAGNOSTIC USE ONLY

Procedure

1. Remove the control from the refrigerator and allow to come to room temperature.
2. Remove cap and invert bottle. While holding dipstick, gently squeeze the sides of the dropper bottle, and touch the tip of the bottle to the dipstick. Draw across all of the reagent pads. Turn dipstick on its side and drain excess control onto absorbent material.
3. Read the urine dipsticks, visually or with an instrumental reader, in accordance with the manufacturers' instructions.
4. Wipe off dropper tips and recap controls. Return them to 2°-8° C when not in use. Discard the controls if turbid or any evidence of microbial contamination is present.

Storage and Stability

1. The Urine Dipstick Control Kit should be stored at 2°-8° C when not in use. Do not freeze.
2. When stored at 2°-8° C the controls are stable until the expiration date stated on the label.

Expected Values

For **visal readings,** the expected ranges have been established from interlaboratory data by comparing the dipstick reaction that occurs with the controls to the color comparison chart with multiple lots of each manufacturers' dipsticks or reagent tablets.

For **instrument readings,** the expected ranges have been established from interlaboratory data from multiple lots of each manufacturers' dipsticks. Each laboratory should establish its own precision parameters.

For **specific gravity,** the expected ranges by refractometer have been established from interlaboratory data.

For **total protein** confirmation, the Urine Dipstick Control may be used with the sulfosalicylic acid method at the user's discretion. This method has not been validated in our laboratory.

For **hCG,** the positive and negative results were obtained by testing each lot number of the Level 1 control with multiple lot numbers of at least ten different hCG test kits of various sensitivities.

Limitations

Any future changes made by the manufacturer of a test method may give different values from the indicated range. Detailed information on the limitations of each test method is included in the limitations section of the manufacturers' package insert.

Rapignost users: Colors produced by the urobilinogen and bilirubin reactions on the Rapignost Dipstick with the Urine Dipstick Control are not characteristic of those shown on the manufacturer's label. The Urine Dipstick Control is not recommended for visual use for urobilinogen and bilirubin.

Clinitest tablet test: Use of the Level 2 Urine Dipstick Control with the Ames Clinitest tablets for reducing sugars may give an atypical color response. Due to purple and orange color formation in the foam, a murky green to a purple color response may occur. Therefore, results of the Clinitest assay for the Urine Dipstick Control are best interpreted as a positive or negative response. A clearer color representation is achieved if the tube is not swirled during or after the boiling reaction.

*See also page 397.

WARNING AND PRECAUTIONS
POTENTIAL BIOHAZARDOUS MATERIAL
Contains human urine. The FDA recommends that such samples be handled at the Center for Disease Control's Bio-Safety Level 2.
DISPOSE OF PROPERLY
Sodium azide may form metal azides in plumbing and pose a threat of explosion.

Quantimetrix Corporation, 4955 West 145th Street, Hawthorne, Calif. 90250.

TABLE 12-5

THE **dipper™** URINE DIPSTICK CONTROL QC Quantimetrix QUALITY CONTROL LOG **dropper**

DATE _____ URINE DIPSTICK CONTROL LEVEL _____ LOT # _____ EXPIRATION DATE _____

DATE	Reagent Strip — Lot#	DIPSTICK TESTS										CONFIRMATORY TESTS								ADD. TESTS			INITIAL
		Leukocytes	Nitrites	Urobilinogen	Protein	pH	Blood	Specific Gravity	Ketones	Bilirubin	Glucose	Protein	Method / Lot #	Ketones	Method / Lot #	Glucose	Method / Lot #	Bilirubin	Method / Lot #	HCG	Method / Lot #	Specific Gravity / Refractometer	
Assayed Value																							

of this examination is to identify the type and the approximate number of formed elements present, which in turn helps the physician determine the presence of a disease process. The sediment in urine is usually classified as organized or unorganized sediment. *Organized sediment* includes red blood cells, white blood cells, epithelial cells, casts, bacteria, parasites, yeast, fungi, and spermatozoa. *Unorganized sediment* is usually chemical and includes crystals of various components and other amorphous (having no definite shape) material. The urine specimen to be used in the microscopic examination must be freshly voided, preferably a clean-catch voided specimen, and examined without excessive delay so that cellular deterioration is prevented. Microscopic examination of urine is performed after the urine is centrifuged. Centrifugation produces a solid portion called sediment.

Figure 12-11 A *to* C; *Test for glucose in urine using Tes-Tape.*

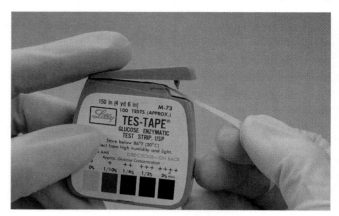

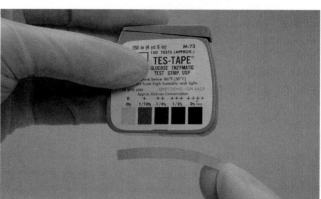

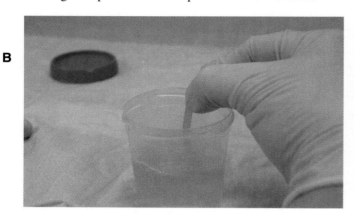

PREPARATION AND MICROSCOPIC EXAMINATION OF SPECIMEN

Equipment

Disposable single-use exam gloves
Laboratory coat (used only when working with specimens)
Eye protection (optional)
Fresh urine specimen
Conical centrifuge tubes

Clinical centrifuge
Droppers
Glass slides
Coverglass
Microscope
See Unit Eleven for information on microscopes and centrifuges.

PROCEDURE

1. Don disposable single-use exam gloves.

2. To obtain the sediment, place 10 to 15 ml of thoroughly mixed urine in a centrifuge tube and centrifuge for 5 minutes at the standard speed of 1500 revolutions per minute (rpm).

3. Pour off the supernate fluid (Figure 12-12, A). The supernate is the clear upper liquid in the tube after it has been centrifuged.

PROCEDURE

4. Allow the several drops of urine that remain along the side of the tube to flow back down into the sediment, then tap the tube with your finger to mix the contents.

5. Place a drop of this sediment on a slide and cover with a coverglass. The slide is now ready to be examined (Figure 12-12, B).

6. Position the slide on the microscope stage (Figure 12-12, C).

PREPARATION AND MICROSCOPIC EXAMINATION OF SPECIMEN—cont'd

PROCEDURE

7. Remove gloves and wash your hands.

8. Adjust the low-power objective of the microscope and examine the slide for casts in at least ten different fields; then examine for other elements that are present in just a few fields. Reduce the light to a minimum by almost completely closing the diaphragm beneath the stage on the microscope, and scan the entire slide to obtain an overall picture of the sediment. You must vary the intensity of the light source on the microscope so that correct identification of the various components may be obtained.

9. Next adjust the microscope to the high-power objective to identify the specific types of cells such as red blood cells, white blood cells, crystals, and other elements present in the sediment. Further identification of the various types of casts should also be done at this time.

PROCEDURE

10. Estimate the approximate number of the various structures identified. Casts are counted per low-power field; epithelial cells, white blood cells (WBCs), and red blood cells are reported in terms of cells per high-power field (hpf) (for example, 10 to 15 WBCs/hpf). To determine the number of elements present, count the number of each type seen in at least ten fields. The average of this number is then used for the reported value. The other elements (crystals, bacteria, parasites, and spermatozoa) are reported as none, rare, occasional, frequent, many, or numerous.

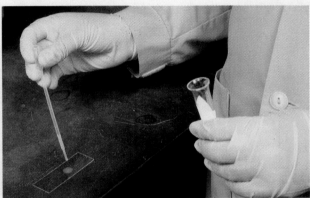

B

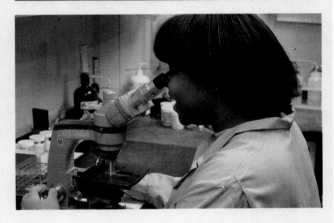

C

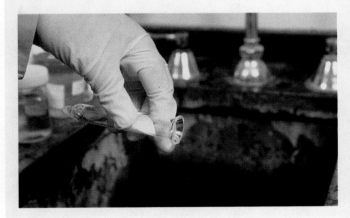

A

Figure 12-12 A *to* **C,** *Microscopic examination of urine.*

There is no easy way to learn how to identify these structures (Figure 12-13). A great deal of practice and training is required to master this skill. Reference charts and books should always be used without hesitation. *Usually this examination is performed by laboratory personnel; on occasion the physician may do it in the office or clinic laboratory. It is not commonly your responsibility to do the actual examination, although there may be instances when you may be required to prepare the slide for the examination* (Figure 12-14, *A* and *B*).

Significance of Microscopic Test Results

Normal urine sediment contains a limited number of formed elements. The presence of one or two white and red blood cells and a few epithelial cells per high-power field is usually not considered abnormal. At times an occasional hyaline case may also be considered to be a normal finding. Mucous threads in moderate amounts are normal.

Organized sediment (Tables 12-6 and 12-7)

1. Cells
   a. Red blood cells: The presence of more than one or two red blood cells per high-power field is an abnormal finding. This may be caused by a variety of kidney and systemic diseases, as well as by trauma to the urinary system, violent exercise, or possible contamination from menstrual blood. Hemorrhagic dis-

Figure 12-13 *Atlas of urine sediment.*
Courtesy Ames Co., Elkhart, Ind.

Crystals found in acid urine (×400)

 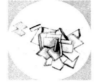

Uric acid | Amorphous urates and uric acid crystals | Hippuric acid | Calcium oxalate | Tyrosine needles Leucine spheroids Cholesterin plates | Cystine

Crystals found in alkaline urine (×400)

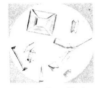 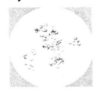 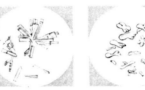

Triple phosphate Ammonium and magnesium | Triple phosphate going in solution | Amorphous phosphate | Calcium phosphate | Calcium carbonate | Ammonium urate

Sulfa crystals

Sulfanilamide | Sulfathiazole | Sulfadiazine | Sulfapyridine

Cells found in urine

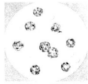   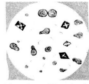

RBC and WBC | Renal epithelium | Caudate cells of renal pelvis | Urethral and bladder epithelium | Vaginal epithelium | Yeast and bacteria

Casts and artifacts found in urine (×400)

     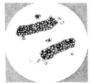

Granular casts fine and coarse | Hyaline cast | Leukocyte cast | Epithelial cast | Waxy cast | Blood cast

    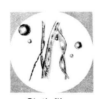

Cylindroids | Mucous thread | Spermatozoa | *Trichomonas vaginalis* | Cloth fibers and bubbles

Figure 12-14 *Laboratory requisitions for urinalysis.*

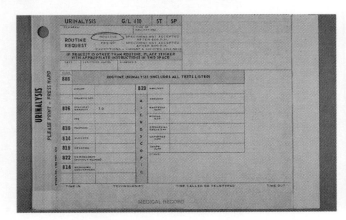
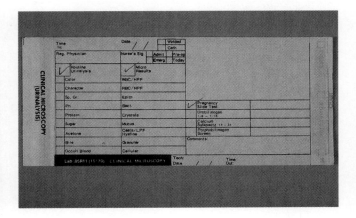

eases such as hemophilia may also produce hematuria. The presence of red blood cells in the urine must always be reported because this is a significant finding.

b. White blood cells (leukocytes): The presence of large numbers of white blood cells in the urine usually indicates the presence of a bacterial infection in the urinary tract and/or pyuria. Pyuria (pi-u're-ah) is the excretion of urine containing pus. This indicates renal disease that may be either infection or lesions in the bladder, urethra, ureters, and kidneys.

c. Epithelial cells: The presence of large numbers of renal and bladder-type epithelial cells is abnormal and should always be reported. The presence of a large number of renal-epithelial cells may indicate degeneration of the renal tubules. Proteinuria and casts are frequently seen in this condition.

2. Casts

a. It is essential that casts be correctly identified because the presence of these structures is a most significant laboratory finding. Inflammatory disorders or damage to the glomerulus, tubules, or general renal tissue are usually associated with the presence of casts and are usually accompanied by albuminuria.

b. The various types of casts include red blood cell, white blood cell, epithelial cell, hyaline, granular, and waxy and fatty casts.

3. Bacteria (see Table 12-9): Normal urine does not contain bacteria unless the specimen was contaminated by improper collection techniques and handling, or by vaginal secretions in the female. The presence of numerous bacteria in the urine may indicate a urinary tract infection. A true infection can be differentiated from contamination if the specimen also contains white blood cells.

4. Yeasts and parasites:

a. Yeast may be seen as a contaminant in the urine of females who have vaginal moniliasis, or it may indicate a urinary moniliasis, especially in patients who have diabetes mellitus.

b. Parasites seen in the urine are usually contaminants from vaginal or fecal excretions.

5. Spermatozoa: Spermatozoa may appear as contaminants in the urine. They frequently are present in urine after sexual intercourse or nocturnal emissions.

Unorganized sediment (Tables 12-8 and 12-9)

1. Crystals

a. The type and quantity of crystals in the urine vary with the pH of the specimen. Normally, most crystals are of little importance and will form in urine as it cools.

b. Crystals seen in normal acid urine are uric acid, amorphous urates, hippuric acid, and calcium oxalate. Crystals seen in normal alkaline urine include triple phosphate, ammonium, magnesium, calcium phosphate, calcium carbonate, and ammonium urate. Abnormal crystals found in acid urine include cholesterin, cystine, leucine, and tyrosine.

2. Artifacts and contaminants: These include hair, cloth fibers, mucous threads, and other contaminants. It is important to differentiate these structures from other elements in the sediment that may indicate the presence of a disease process.

DETECTION AND SEMIQUANTITATION OF BACTERIURIA

When obtaining a urine specimen for bacteriologic examination, you should collect a clean-catch midstream specimen in a sterile container (refer to Unit Eleven for this procedure). The first voided specimen of the day should be used whenever possible because bacteria will be more numerous. The examination should be done within 1 hour from the time of collection. When this is not possible, refrigerate the specimen to prevent the growth of microorganisms, and test the specimen within 8 hours. *Never* add a preservative to a urine specimen that is to be used for bacteriologic culture tests because the preservative destroys the viability of most of the bacteria that may be present.

Text continues on page 407.

TABLE 12-6

Cells in Urine Sediment

Type	Presence in Normal Urine	Possible Causes of Abnormal Amounts Of Cells in Urine
Red blood cells	0 to 5 cells /hpf (depending on preparation of urinary sediment)	Inflammatory diseases Acute glomerulonephritis Pyelonephritis Hypertension Renal infarction Trauma Stones Tumor Bleeding diseases Use of anticoagulants
White blood cells	0 to 8 cells/hpf (depending on preparation of urinary sediment)	Pyelonephritis Cystis Urethritis Prostatis Transplant rejection (manifested by lymphocytes in urine) Tissue injury accompanied by severe inflammation (manifested by monocytes in urine) Inflammation, immune mechanisms, and other host defense mechanisms (manifested by histiocytes in urine)
Squamous epithelial cells	Often present, depending on collection technique	Vaginal contamination
Transitional epithelial cells	Moderate number of cells present	Disease of bladder or renal pelvis Catheterization
Renal tubular epithelial cells	Present in small numbers; higher numbers in infants	Acute tubular necrosis Glomerulonephritis Acute infection Renal toxicity Viral infection
Cytomegalic inclusion bodies	Not normally present in urine	Cytomegalic inclusion disease
Tumor cells	Not normally present in urine	Tumors of • Renal pelvis • Renal parenchyma • Ureters • Bladder

Courtesy Boehringer Mannheim Diagnostics, Indianapolis, Ind.

TABLE 12-7

Casts in Urine Sediment

Type	Description	Possible Causes
Hyaline casts	Colorless, transparent Low refractive index	Normal urine Strenuous exercise Acute glomerulonephritis Acute pyelonephritis Malignant hypertension Chronic renal disease
Red blood cell casts	Red cells in hyaline matrix Yellow-orange color High refractive index	Acute glomerulonephritis Lupus nephritis Severe nephritis Collagen diseases Renal infarction Malignant hypertension
White blood cell casts	Neutrophils in hyaline matrix High refractive index	Acute pyelonephritis Acute glomerulonephritis Chronic renal disease
Epithelial cell casts	Renal tubular epithelial cells in hyaline matrix High refractive index	Glomerulonephritis Vascular disease Toxin Virus
Granular casts	Opaque granules in matrix	Heavy proteinuria (nephrotic syndrome) Orthostatic proteinuria Congestive heart failure with proteinuria Acute or chronic renal disease
Waxy casts	Sharp, refractile outlines Irregular "broken off" ends Absence of differentiated structures	Severe chronic renal disease Malignant hypertension Kidney disease resulting from diabetes mellitus Acute renal disease
Fatty casts	Fat globules in transparent matrix	Nephrotic syndrome Diabetes mellitus Mercury poisoning Ethylene glycol poisoning
Broad casts	Larger diameter than other casts	Acute tubular necrosis Severe chronic renal disease Urinary tract obstruction
Mixed casts	Combination of any of the above	Any of the above, depending on cellular constituents

Courtesy of Boehringer Mannheim Diagnostics, Indianapolis, Ind.

TABLE 12-8

Urinary Crystals

Type of Urine	Type of Crystals	Description of Crystals	Significance When Found in Urine
Normal acid urine	Amorphous urate	Colorless or yellow-brown granules (pink macroscopically)	Nonpathologic
	Uric acid	Occur in many shapes; may be colorless, yellow-brown, or red-brown; and square, diamond shaped, wedge shaped, or grouped in rosettes	Usually nonpathologic; in large numbers, may indicate gout
	Calcium oxalate	Octahedral or dumbbell shaped; possess double refractive index	Usually nonpathologic; may be associated with urine stasis or chronic urinary tract infection
Normal alkaline urine	Amorphous phosphates	Small, colorless granules	Nonpathologic
	Triple phosphates	Colorless prisms with three to six sides ("coffin lids") or feathery, shaped like fern leaves	Usually nonpathologic; may be associated with urine stasis or chronic urinary tract infection
	Ammonium biurate	Yellow-brown "thorny apple" appearance or yellow-brown spheres	Nonpathologic
	Calcium phosphate	Colorless prisms or rosettes	Usually nonpathologic; may be associated with urine stasis or chronic urinary tract infection
	Calcium carbonate	Usually appear colorless and amorphous; may be shaped like dumbbells, rhombi, or needles	Usually nonpathologic; may be associated with inorganic calculi formation
Abnormal urine	Tyrosine Leucine Cystine	Thin, dark needles, arranged in sheaves or clumps; usually colorless, but may be pale yellow-brown	Liver disease or inherited metabolic disorder
	Hippuric acid Bilirubin	Yellow-brown spheres with radial striations	Liver disease or inherited metabolic disorder
	Cholesterol	Clear, hexagonal plates	Cystinuria
	Creatine	Star-shaped clusters of needles, rhombic plates, or elongated prisms; may be colorless or yellow-brown	Usually nonpathologic
	Aspirin	Delicate needles or rhombic plates; red-brown in color; birefringent	Bilirubinuria
	Sulfonamide	Colorless, transparent plates with regular or irregular cornet notches	Chyluria, urinary tract infections, nephrotic syndrome
	Ampicillin	Pseudohexagonal plates with positive birefringence	Destruction of muscle tissue due to muscular dystrophies, atrophies, and myositis
	X-ray media	Distinctive prismatic or starlike forms; usually colorless; show positive birefringence	Ingestion of aspirin or other salicylates
		Yellow-brown dumbbells, asymmetric sheaves, rosettes, or hexagonal plates	Ingestion of sulfonamide drugs
		Long, thin, clear crystals	Parenteral administration of ampicillin
		Long, thin rectangles or flat, four-sided, notched plates	X-ray procedure with contrast media

Courtesy Boehringer Mannheim Diagnostics, Indianapolis, Ind.

TABLE 12-9

Microorganisms and Artifacts in Urine

Microorganisms/Artifacts	Significance When Found in Urine
Bacteria	More than 100,000 bacteria/ml indicates urinary tract infection
	10,000 to 100,000 bacteria/ml indicates that tests should be repeated
	Less than 10,000 bacteria/ml may signify urine in which any bacteria are due to urethral organisms or contamination
	Bacteria accompanied by white blood cells and/or white cell or mixed casts may indicate acute pyelonephritis
Fungi	May indicate contamination by yeasts from skin and hair
	May indicate diabetes mellitus or urinary tract infection
	Candida albicans may occur in patients with diabetes mellitus or in the contaminated urine of female patients with candidal vaginitis
Parasites and parasitic ova	Usually indicate fecal or vaginal contamination and should be reported
	Trichomonas may be found in patients with urethritis and in the contaminated urine of women with trichomonas vaginitis
	Pinworm is a common contaminant and should be reported
Spermatozoa	Nonpathologic
Urinary artifacts	Nonpathologic
Hair	May result from improper urine collection, improper slide preparation, or outside contamination
Starch from surgical gloves	
Pollen grains	
Bubbles	
Oil droplets	
Fibers	
Talc	
Dust	
Threads	
Glass particles	

Courtesy Boehringer Mannheim Diagnostics, Indianapolis, Ind.

CULTURE PLATE METHODS

This technique requires the special facilities and trained personnel of a microbiology laboratory. There the identification and precise quantitation of bacterial species will be ascertained. If the specimen is not cultured immediately, refrigeration is mandatory.

NITRITE TEST AND CULTURE STRIP METHODS

A chemical test using a reagent strip, as discussed under the chemical examination of urine, is used for the nitrite test. The culture strip method, a simplified semiquantitative culture test, provides greater precision than is possible with the nitrite test. Frequently used are the Microstix-3 reagent strips. This is a three-way bacteriuria test. The strip contains three pads: (1) a nitrite reagent pad, (2) a dehydrated culture media pad that favors the growth of all types of bacteria commonly seen in urinary tract infections, and (3) a dehy-drated culture media pad that supports growth of only gram-negative bacteria. A thermostatically controlled incubator specifically designed for use with the Microstix-3 is available. It is small, about the size of an average textbook, and relatively inexpensive; therefore it is very practical for use in a urinalysis laboratory in a physician's office or clinic.

Procedure for Using the Microstix-3 Reagent Strip

1. Don disposable single-use exam gloves.
2. Remove the strip from the wrapper; avoid contact of the test areas with anything.
3. Dip the strip in the urine specimen for 5 seconds and remove.
4. Read the nitrite test area 30 seconds later. Any degree of a pink color indicates the presence of 10^5 or more organisms per milliliter of urine.

5. Insert the strip in the sterile plastic pouch provided, and seal.
6. Incubate the pouch for 12 to 18 hours.
7. Read the results without removing the strip from the transparent pouch. Compare the color densities on both culture pads with the chart provided. Magenta spots on the pads indicate bacterial locations.
8. Remove gloves and wash your hands.
9. Record the results and dispose of the still-sealed pouches by incineration (*or* autoclave pouches and then dispose of according to agency policy).

OTHER URINE TESTS

PROTEIN DETERMINATIONS

Bence Jones protein is the name of an abnormal protein in the urine that is frequently seen in patients who have multiple myeloma and a few other abnormalities. This protein is characterized by the fact that, during special testing methods (the Bence Jones Protein Test), it precipitates (separates from the liquid) when urine is heated, but disappears once the urine is cooled. Many believe that this is not a very sensitive test because it can miss detecting small amounts of the Bence Jones protein or other similar types of abnormal protein. Thus many laboratories have discontinued using this test and are now doing the urine-protein electrophoresis. This test determines the relative concentration and also the type of abnormal protein present in the urine. It can be performed on a random urine specimen, although it is preferable to collect a 24-hour specimen in most cases.

HORMONE DETERMINATIONS

These urine tests help detect metabolic and endocrine conditions or disorders. One common test performed is the pregnancy test in which urine is tested for the presence of the human chorionic gonadotropin (hCG) hormone. A wide range of tests are used for this purpose. Many are slide tests that provide results within a few minutes. Complete instructions for use are provided with the test equipment when purchased. Although these tests are highly reliable, incorrect results may be obtained at times because of the presence of protein or blood in the urine or when the urine is too dilute. For most reliable results, the urine should have a specific gravity of at least 1.015. The first morning specimen is preferred for testing.

PREGNANCY TEST

To determine if a woman is pregnant, blood or urine can be tested for the presence of the hCG hormone (Figure 12-15). Blood tests called radioisotope or radioimmunoassay (RIA) tests are more sensitive than urine tests. They use a radioactive substance to determine the presence of hCG in the blood. These tests can identify a pregnancy 7 days after conception. RIA tests take 1 to 2 hours to process in the laboratory. In the physician's office or clinic, urine tests are more commonly used to detect pregnancy. The urine pregnancy tests use an antigen-antibody response to determine the presence of hCG. Antibodies to the hCG bind with the HCG to produce either a clumping of cells or a color change that indicates pregnancy. Urine tests for pregnancy are usually recommended at least 2 weeks after the first missed menstrual period. A first voided morning specimen is preferred for testing because it usually contains the greatest concentration of hCG. The patient must be given a clean urine container and an explanation of how to collect the specimen. If the specimen is collected at home, direct the patient to keep the specimen in the refrigerator until she can bring it to the office or lab for testing.

Before the test is done, the specific gravity of the specimen must be measured. If the specific gravity is less than 1.010, the results of the hCG test may be false-negative because the urine is too dilute for testing. For the most reliable results, the urine should have a specific gravity of at least 1.015. The protein content should also be checked and noted if positive because protein can affect test results. It must be remembered that these tests are used to diagnose a pregnancy but they do not necessarily indicate a normal pregnancy.

QUALITY CONTROLS

Positive and negative controls should be performed routinely to check the reliability of the reagents and your technique. Commercial controls can be obtained, or you may use the urine from women who are known to be pregnant and those who are not pregnant. Check the expiration dates on the supplies so that outdated materials may be discarded and replaced with new supplies.

PHENYLKETONURIA

Phenylketonuria (PKU) is an inherited disease that must be diagnosed early to avoid serious brain damage and mental retardation. A blood test may be performed 2 to 3 days after birth to aid in a diagnosis of PKU. Two urine tests can also be performed to diagnose or recheck the results of the first test. Urine tests for PKU are generally performed on the infant's first checkup 6 weeks after birth. These tests cannot be used before the sixth week of life because if performed earlier they will produce invalid results. The two urine tests are the Phenistix test (see Table 12-1) using a reagent strip and the Diaper test, using 10% ferric chloride, both to determine color changes from the urine. PKU and the blood and urine tests performed are discussed further under Pediatric Examination in Unit Four.

PHENISTIX TEST

1. Press a Phenistix test reagent strip against a diaper containing urine *or* dip a Phenistix reagent strip into a urine specimen.
2. Compare color changes on the reagent strip with the color chart on the reagent strip bottle. A green color reaction indicates probable PKU.

Figure 12-15 *Procedures for using a one-step pregnancy test.*
Courtesy Pacific-Biotech, Inc., San Diego, Calif.

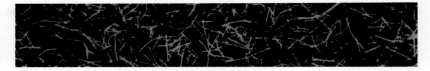

HCG-URINE
One-Step Pregnancy Test

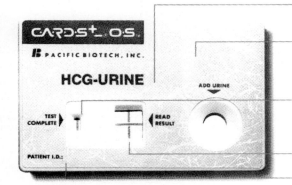

Label clearly identifies type of test—no potential mix-ups if other CARDS®OS® assays are also being performed.

Unique Reaction Unit functions as a stable workstation that is easy to handle and will not tip over.

"TEST COMPLETE" signal appears in approximately 5 minutes. This procedural control confirms the test is finished and the system has worked properly.

Easy-to-read result stays visible for record keeping or patient keepsake.

Markable space for writing patient information.

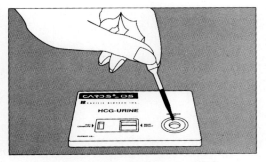

Use the dropper provided to add urine into the sample well. **Walk away.**

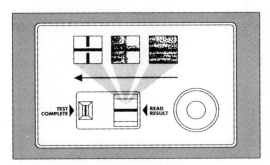

During the next few minutes, a blue color will be seen moving from right to left through the "READ RESULT" window.

Read the result anytime after the signal appears in the "TEST COMPLETE" window.

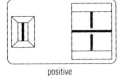

positive

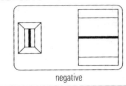

negative

DIAPER TEST

1. Drop 10% ferric chloride on a diaper that contains fresh urine.
2. Read the results. A green spot on the diaper is considered to be a positive result. This indicates the possibility of PKU.

MULTIPLE-GLASS TEST

The multiple-glass test is performed on men to evaluate a lower urinary tract infection. See Unit Eleven for the procedure used to collect three specimens for this test.

OTHER TESTS

Numerous other tests can be performed on urine to aid the physician when diagnosing and treating a patient's condition. It is not in the scope of this book to discuss all of them in detail. *Most must be performed in a laboratory by qualified personnel.* See Table 12-10 for additional urine tests, the average normal values, and the type of specimen that is required for testing.

URINE PREGNANCY TEST—WAMPOLE 2-MINUTE SLIDE TEST

Equipment

Timer
Pregnancy kit, which includes:
  Antiserum reagent
  Antigen reagent
  Clean glass slide with one or more raised circles on it
  Disposable stirrer
  Disposable pipet with rubber bulb

A good light source that the slide can be observed under the urine specimen
Disposable single-use exam gloves
Laboratory requisition

PROCEDURE	RATIONALE
1. Wash your hands. **Use appropriate personal protective equipment (PPE) as dictated by facility.** Assemble equipment.	
2. Remove reagents from the refrigerator and allow them to warm to room temperature.	*To ensure accurate results, all the fluids must be at room temperature.*
3. Don disposable single-use exam gloves	
4. Make sure that the urine specimen has been allowed to warm to room temperature if it had been stored in the refrigerator. If the urine is cloudy, centrifuge it and use the supernate for the test. The supernate is the clear upper portion of a mixture after it has been centrifuged.	
5. Using the disposable pipet, place 1 drop of clear urine within one of the circles on the clean glass slide. The slide must be clean. Do not let the pipet touch the slide.	*Dirty slides can cause errors.*
6. Add 1 drop of the antiserum reagent to the drop of urine. Hold the dropper at a 90-degree angle to the slide. Do not touch the urine with the dropper. Adding the reagents to the urine in the correct order is vital.	*If the order is changed, the results can be inaccurate. Holding the dropper at a 90-degree angle allows you to squeeze out a standard size drop.*
7. To mix the antigen reagent well, shake the bottle. Add 1 drop to the slide in the same circle with the urine and antiserum. Hold the reagent dropper at a 90-degree angle when adding the drop to the slide. Do not touch the specimen with the dropper.	*Avoid contamination.*
8. Mix the reagents and urine with the stirrer. Spread the mixture over the entire circle.	
9. Gently rock the slide for exactly 2 minutes. Set your timer. This rocking motion must be slow. Have the slide under a good light so that you can observe any agglutination (clumping together of cells).	
10. Read the slide at 2 minutes. *If agglutination occurs,* the test is considered *negative* for pregnancy. Agglutination is recognized as a granular appearance to the solution. The test must be read at exactly 2 minutes.	*After 2 minutes, evaporation may occur and give the appearance of agglutination. Before 2 minutes, agglutination may occur and can be read as a negative result.*
11. If agglutination *does not* occur, the test is considered *positive* for pregnancy. Absence of agglutination is observed as a smooth, opaque suspension.	

URINE PREGNANCY TEST—WAMPOLE 2-MINUTE SLIDE TEST—cont'd

PROCEDURE

12. Thoroughly wash the glass slide, wipe dry, and replace in storage area. Return reagents to the refrigerator.

13. Remove your gloves and wash your hands before returning supplies to the storage area.

14. Record the results on the patient's chart. Include the date of the patient's last menstrual period (LMP) (see Figure 12-14, B).

RATIONALE

Charting example:
   Oct. 10, 19__ - 8 p.m.
     Pregnancy slide test - positive
     LMP - August 26, 19__
      M.L. Johnson, CMA

TABLE 12-10

Average Normal Values for Urine Determinations*

Test	Average Normal Value	Type of Specimen
Addis Count	WBC 1,800,000	12-hour
	RBC 500,000	
	Casts 0-5000	
Albumin		
Qualitative	Negative	Random
Quantitative	10-100 mg/24 hr	24-hour
Aldosterone	2-23 mg/24 hr	24-hour, refrigerated
Amino acid nitrogen	100-290 mg/24 hr	24-hour, refrigerated, collected in thymol
Ammonia	20-70 mEq/24 hr	24-hour
Ammonia nitrogen	0.14-1.47 g/24 hr	24-hour
Bence Jones Protein	Negative	First morning specimen
Bilirubin	Negative	Random
Blood, occult	Negative	Random
Calcium		
Sulkowitch	Positive 1+	Random
Quantitative	100-250 mg/24 hr on an average diet	24-hour
Catecholamines	100-230 mg/24 hr	24-hour, preserve with 1 ml concentrated H_2SO_4
Chloride	110-250 mEq/24 hr	24-hour
Concentration test	Specific gravity of 1.025 or higher	Withholding fluids for the day before the test
Coproporphyrin	20 m/100 ml	Random
Random	Adults: 50-200 mg/24 hr	24-hour, preserve with 5 g Na_2CO_3
24-hour	Children: 0-80 mg/24 hr	
Creatine	Men: 0-40 mg/24 hr	24-hour
	Women: 0-100 mg/24 hr	
	Higher in children	
Creatinine	Men: 1-1.9 mg/24 hr	24-hour
	Women 0.8-1.7 g/24 hr	
Dilution test	Specific gravity of 1.001 to 1.003	After 1200 ml water load
Estrogens	Men: 4-25 mg/24 hr	24-hour, refrigerate
	Women: 4-60 mg/24 hr	

Courtesy Ames Co., Division of Miles Laboratories, Inc., Elkhart, Ind., 1986. After Davidson I, Henry JB: Todd-Sanford clinical diagnosis by laboratory methods, Philadelphia, 1969, Saunders, and Goodale RH, Widmann FK: Clinical interpretation of laboratory tests, Philadelphia, 1969, Davis.

Table 12-10—cont'd

Average Normal Values for Urine Determinations*

Test	Average Normal Value	Type of Specimen
Glucose		
Qualitative	Negative	Random
Quantitative	130 mg/24 hr	24-hour
Hemoglobin	Negative	Random
17-hydroxycorti-costeriods	Men: 5.5-14.5 mg/24 hr Women: 5-13 mg/24 hr	24-hour, tranquilizers interfere
17-ketosteroids	Men: 8-15 mg/24 hr Women 6-11.5 mg/24 hr Children: 5 mg/24 hr	24-hour, tranquilizers interfere
Ketones	Negative	Random
Lead	100 μg/24 hr	24-hour, collect in lead-free bottle
Osmolality		
Normal fluid intake	500-800 mOsm/kg water	Random
Full range	38-1400 mOsm/kg water	Random
pH	4.6-8	Random
Phenylpyruvic acid	Negative	Random
Phosphorus	0.9-1.3 g/24 hr	24-hour
Porphobilinogen	Negative	Random
Potassium	25-100 mEq/24 hr	24-hour
Pregnanediol	Men: 0-1 mg/24 hr Women: 1-8 mg/24 hr Children: Negative	24-hour, refrigerate
Pregnanetriol	Men: 1-2 mg/24 hr Women: 0.5-2 mg/24 hr Children: <0.5 mg/24 hr	24-hour, refrigerate
Protein		
Qualitative	Negative	Random
Quantitative	10-150 mg/24 hr	24-hour
Bence Jones	Negative	First morning specimen
Sodium	110-260 mEq/24 hr	24-hour
Specific gravity		
Random	1.002-1.030	Random
24-hour	1.015-1.025	24-hour
Sugars	Negative	Random
Tritratable acidity	200-500 ml of 0.1 NaOH/24 hr	24-hour, preserve with toluene
Urea nitrogen	6-17 g/24	24-hour
Uric acid	250-750 mg/24 hr	24-hour
Urobilinogen		
Semiquanti-tative	0.3-1 Ehrlich units/2 hr	2-hour afternoon spcimen
Quantitative	1-4 mg/24 hr	24-hour, collect in dark bottle with 5 g Na_2CO_3, refrigerate
Uroporphyrin	10-30 μg/24 hr	24-hour, collect in dark bottle with 5 g Na_2CO_3
VMA (Vanilman-delic acid)	1-8 mg/24 hr	24-hour, preserve in 3 ml 25% H_2SO_4; no coffee or fruit for 2 days before test
Volume Adults	600-1500 ml/24 hr	24-hour

Courtesy Ames Co., Division of Miles Laboratories, Inc., Elkhart, Ind., 1986. After Davidson I, Henry JB: Todd-Sanford clinical diagnosis by laboratory methods, Philadelphia, 1969, Saunders, and Goodale RH, Widmann FK: Clinical interpretation of laboratory tests, Philadelphia, 1969, Davis.

CONCLUSION

Having completed the unit on Urinalysis, practice the procedures. When you think that you know the equipment and steps of the procedures, arrange with your instructor to take the performance tests. You are expected to demonstrate accurately your ability to prepare for and perform all of the procedures that have been presented.

REVIEW OF VOCABULARY

The following is a sample of recorded patient information using words that have been presented in this unit. Read it and define the italicized terms.

This patient, a 45-year-old man, was first seen in my office today with the chief complaint of *dysuria* for the past month. The patient stated that this was associated with *polyuria*, gross *hematuria*, weakness, back pain, and a high fever. He has never experienced *oliguria* and stated that he drinks copious amounts of water daily. One week ago he had an attack of dyspnea and coughing. The urinalysis today revealed marked *proteinuria, glycosuria,* and *ketonuria; specific gravity* of 1.030. *Microscopic* examination revealed *white cells* of 15 to 20/high-power field (hpf) and *red cells* of 10 to 15/hpf. *Pyuria* was also detected in large amounts. Further study and examination were recommended for this patient. He will be admitted to the hospital at the end of this week.

M. Crossett, MD

CASE STUDY

Read and discuss the following underlined terminology.

1. Patients often report symptoms of *dysuria, pyuria,* and *hematuria* associated with bladder infections. *Glycosuria* is often detected on routine *urinalysis* during pregnancy. Urinalysis poses few concerns for the preoperative assessment of most healthy patients; however, the patient with *diabetes mellitus* is at increased risk for *morbidity* and *mortality*. The stress of an operation can send a *labile* diabetic patient into *insulin shock or ketoacidosis, albuminuria,* and *anuria*.

   Normal *regimen* of dietary intake of calories and *insulin* or *oral hypoglycemic* agents are interrupted when a diabetic patient requires surgery. What is the significance of preoperative and postoperative urinalysis for this special needs patient?

2. Using the following urinalysis report, discuss the values.

URINALYSIS

SOURCE	RANDOM
COLOR	Straw
CLARITY	Slightly cloudy
SPECIFIC GRAVITY	1.010
pH	7.5
ALBUMIN	Negative
GLUCOSE	Negative
KETONES	Negative
UROBILINOGEN	0.2
OCCULT BLOOD	Negative
LEUKOCYTE ESTER	Negative
RED CELLS	4
SQUAMOUS EPITHELIUM	42
BACTERIA	Small amount

REVIEW QUESTIONS

1. List the four major components of normal urine.
2. Why and when is a routine urinalysis performed?
3. List five physical characteristics of urine and eight chemical examinations that are part of a routine urinalysis.
4. List and classify urine microscopic sediment as either organized or unorganized sediment.
5. Indicate if the following urinalysis results are normal or abnormal findings:
   - a Specific gravity of 1.035
   - b. Red
   - c. Glucose 4+
   - d. Acetone, negative
   - e. Numerous bacteria
   - f. Foul odor
   - g. Cloudy
   - h. Quantity, 3500 ml in 24 hours
   - i. pH 6.5
   - j. Protein, trace amounts
   - k. Ketones, large amount
   - l. Blood, negative
   - m. Urobilinogen 0.1 to 1, small amount
   - n. Nitrite, positive
6. List two conditions or diseases in which each of the following may be detected:
   - a. Albuminuria
   - b. Glucosuria
   - c. Acetonuria
   - d. Bilirubinuria
   - e. Hematuria
   - f. Bacteriuria
   - g. Polyuria
   - h. Oliguria
   - i. Anuria
   - j. Dysuria
   - k. Excessively acid urine
   - l. Excessively alkaline urine
   - m. Very low specific gravity
7. Name three items used for measuring the specific gravity of urine.
8. Differentiate between normal and abnormal sediment and contaminants that may be observed during a microscopic examination of urine.
9. You are asked to perform the chemical analysis on a urine specimen and find the bottle of reagent strips on the refrigerator with the cap removed. Is this the proper storage method for these reagent strips? Would you use one of these strips to perform the tests? Explain the reason for your answer.
10. A urine specimen that was collected at 10 a.m. for a microscopic examination was placed in your laboratory on the shelf. It is now 3 p.m.. What would you do with this specimen? Explain the reason for your answer.
11. Describe two tests for determining bacteriuria and three tests for determining glucosuria.
12. To determine if a woman is pregnant, urine may be tested to detect the presence of which hormone?

PERFORMANCE TEST

In a skills laboratory, a simulation of a joblike environment, the medical assistant student is to demonstrate skill in performing the following procedures without reference to source materials. For these activities the student requires a fresh urine specimen or a synthetic preparation of the same. Time limits for the performance of each procedure are to be assigned by the instructor (see also page 52.)

1. Given a fresh urine specimen and the required supplies, perform a routine physical and chemical analysis on the specimen and record the results; then prepare the specimen for a microscopic examination.
2. Given a fresh urine specimen and the required supplies, perform a Clinitest, Acetest, Ictotest, and pregnancy test and record the results.
3. Given a fresh urine specimen and Tes-Tape, test the urine for the presence of glucose and record the results.
4. Given a fresh clean-catch midstream urine specimen and a Multistix-3 reagent strip, perform a semiquantitative culture test and record the results.
5. Given a Dipper or Dropper urinalysis control kit, determine if the test reagent strips are reacting properly.
6. Given a Phenestix test reagent strip test a urine specimen for PKU,

The student is expected to perform the above activities with 100% accuracy.

Hematology

COGNITIVE OBJECTIVES

On completion of Unit Thirteen, the medical assistant student should be able to:*

1. Define and pronounce the listed vocabulary terms and define the listed laboratory abbreviations.
2. List the components of blood; state where each is formed in the body and the functions of each.
3. Differentiate between granulocytes and agranulocytes.
4. List body sites used for obtaining capillary and venous blood for testing. List body sites to avoid when obtaining blood samples.
5. State three types of specimens that can be obtained from a venous blood sample.
6. Identify the use of different vacuum blood collection tubes by tube top color.
7. Explain the difference between a collection tube with an additive and one without an additive, indicating the preferred use for each.
8. List twelve factors that should be considered before performing a venipuncture.
9. List the general order of draw when more than one tube of blood is to be obtained during a venipuncture for various different tests.
10. Discuss how a blood specimen should be handled after collection.
11. Discuss patient preparation for blood tests.
12. List at leave five blood tests that require the patient to be in a fasting state before having a blood sample drawn.
13. Give the laboratory results on blood tests that are presented in this unit, determine if they represent normal values, and relate the abnormal findings to the most probable or possible causes.
14. Describe the steps for performing a blood glucose test using a blood glucose meter.
15. State three elements of quality assurance for blood glucose testing.
16. State seven possible causes of inaccurate blood glucose readings when using blood glucose meters.
17. Discuss the advantages of the Accu-Chek III and One Touch blood glucose meters used in monitoring blood glucose levels.
18. Describe the steps for performing a blood cholesterol test using the AccuMeter.
19. State the three levels of cholesterol results and explain how each is classified.
20. State the two most routinely used systems for blood grouping and typing. List the blood types in each group and explain what the typing indicates.
21. State why it is important for a person who is to receive a blood transfusion to receive the same blood group that he or she has.
22. Discuss why it is important in pregnancy to identify cases in which the mother has Rh 2 blood and the father has Rh plus blood type.
23. List six blood tests that are performed for a complete blood count (CBC) and the normal values for each.
24. List blood tests that would be listed under the following classifications: hematology, chemistry, serology, thyroid function tests.
25. Explain the terms multiphasic tests, test panels, and profiles.
26. Discuss automation in the clinical laboratory and the advantages this provides.

TERMINAL PERFORMANCE OBJECTIVES

On completion of Unit Thirteen, the medical assistant student should be able to:

1. Demonstrate the correct procedure for obtaining a blood sample from a patient by performing a skin puncture using (a) a lancet and (b) a Penlet II.
2. Demonstrate the correct procedure for obtaining a blood sample from a patient by performing a venipuncture using (a) a syringe and needle and (b) a vacutainer needle and holder, and vacuum tube.
3. Demonstrate the correct procedure for obtaining multiple blood samples using the vacutainer holder and needle, and evacuated blood collection tubes.
4. Demonstrate the correct procedure for using (a) the Unopette system and (b) the Microtainer capillary whole blood collector.
5. Demonstrate the correct procedure for performing (a) a copper sulfate relative density test used for screening anemia and (b) hematocrit on capillary blood.

*It is suggested that you review Unit Ten before proceeding with this unit.

6. Demonstrate the correct procedure for determining the presence of glucose in blood by using (a) Dextrostix, (b) the Accu-chek III and Bg Chemstrip, and (c) One Touch II Blood Glucose meter and test strip.

7. Demonstrate the correct procedure for performing a blood cholesterol test using the AccuMeter.

8. Demonstrate the correct method for recording information relevant to the above procedures and findings.

The student is expected to perform these objectives with 100% accuracy.

The consistent use of universal precautions is required by all health care professionals in all health care settings as a method of infection control. It is assumed that these precautions are used in all of the following procedures. Review Unit One if you have any questions on methods to use as the methods/techniques will not be repeated in detail in each procedure presented in the unit.

Be sure to consult the latest guidelines issued by the Centers for Disease Control and Prevention and consult with infection control practitioners when needed to identify specific precautions that pertain to your particular work situation.

Hematology, the study of blood, covers vast areas and numerous tests. Today, in the physician's office or health care facility, most of the tests are performed by a trained laboratory worker, or blood samples are obtained and then sent to a larger clinical laboratory for testing. At other times, the patient is sent directly to the laboratory to have the blood sample drawn. Most laboratories use automated equipment when performing many of the tests. These modern advances in laboratory technology have made it possible to obtain quick and accurate results on a relatively small sample of blood.

For the most part, it is not your duty to perform blood tests, other than a few simple ones. Depending on the laws of the state in which you practice, you may be called on to perform a skin puncture or a venipuncture to obtain blood samples for testing at a clinical laboratory. Even though you may not do these procedures, it is important that you be familiar with the equipment and supplies that are needed, so that you are capable of assisting the physician as required or explaining the procedure to a patient. These procedures, supplies, and some of the routine and basic blood tests are discussed in this unit.

BLOOD COMPONENTS, FUNCTIONS, AND FORMATION

Blood, a type of connective tissue, is composed of a clear, yellow, liquid portion, the plasma, in which the cellular or formed elements are suspended and which makes up about 55% of the blood by volume. The remaining 45% consists of the formed elements, which are RBCs, WBCs, and platelets. The average adult has approximately 5 to 6 quarts of blood.

Blood has at times been referred to as the "river of life," because it is by way of this special tissue that numerous substances are transported to all the cells in our body for nourish-

VOCABULARY

Ailutination (ah-gloo"tin-na' shun)—A clumping together of cells, as of blood cells or bacteria. An example is when red blood cells (RBCs) clump together as a result of an incompatible blood transfusion.

Agranulocyte (a-gran'u-lo-sit")—A white blood cell (WBC) with a clear or nongranular cytoplasm. There are two types, monocytes and lymphocytes.

Anemia (ah-ne'me-ah)—There are various forms of anemia, but broadly speaking it is a lack of RBCs in the circulating blood or a reduction of hemoglobin or both. Anemia is thought of as a symptom of a disease or disorder; it is not a disease.

Anisocytosis (an-i"-so-si-to'sis)—A state of abnormal variations in the size of RBCs in the blood.

Blood dyscrasia (dis-kra'ze-ah)—An abnormal or diseased condition of the blood.

Electrolyte (e-lek'tro-lit)—Substances that separate into electrically charged particles, positive or negative, when dissolved in water; thus they are capable of conducting an electric current. They play an important part in maintaining fluid balance, in normal metabolism function, and in the functions of cells in the body. EXAMPLES: sodium, potassium, calcium, magnesium, chloride, and bicarbonate.

Electrophoresis (e-lek"tro-fo-re'sis)—A laboratory method used to diagnose certain diseases by analyzing the plasma protein content.

Erythrocytosis (e-rith"ro-si-to'sis)—Increased numbers of RBCs (erythrocytes).

Granulocyte (gran'u-lo-sit")—A WBC having granules in its cytoplasm. These types of WBCs are neutrophils, basophils and eosinophils.

AggBand-form granulocyte—A granular WBC in a stage of development.

Hemoglobin (he"mo-glo'bin)—A protein in an RBC that carries oxygen and carbon dioxide. The pigment in hemoglobin is what gives the blood its red color. The protein in hemoglobin is globin; the red pigment is heme. For the body to make hemoglobin, it must have iron, which is derived from the food we eat.

Hemolysis (he-mol'i-sis)—The destruction of RBCs with the release of hemoglobin into the plasma.

Hyperbilirubinemia (hy"per-bil"i-roo"bi-ne'me-ah)—Increased or excessive levels of bilirubin in the blood.

Hypercalcemia (hi"per-kal-se'me-ah)—Increased or excessive levels of calcium in the blood.

Hypercholesterolemia (hi'per-ko-les"ter-ol-e'me-ah)—Excessive levels of cholesterol in the blood.

Hyperchromia (hi'per-kro'me-ah)—An abnormal increase of the hemoglobin levels in RBCs.

Hypercythemia (hy'per-si-the'me-ah)—An excessive number of RBCs in the circulating blood.

Hyperemia (hi′per-e′me-ah)—An excessive amount of blood in a part.

Hyperglycemia (hi″per-gli-se′me-ah)—Excessive amounts of glucose in the blood.

Hyperkalemia (hi″per-kah-le′me-ah)—An excessive level of potassium in the blood.

Hypernatremia (hi′per-na-tre′me-ah)—An excessive amount of sodium in the blood.

Hyperoxemia (hi″per-ok-se′me-ah)—A condition in which the blood is excessively acidic.

Hyperproteinemia (hi″per-pro″te-i-ne′me-ah)—An excessive amount of protein in the blood.

Hypo (hi′po)—A word part meaning an abnormal decrease or deficient amounts. If you replace this word element and definition for the word element "hyper" in all of the preceding terms (except in hyperemia and hyperoxemia), the correct meaning will be defined.

Hypoxemia (h′pok-se′me-ah)—A deficient amount of oxygen (O_2) in the blood.

Ischemia (is-ke′me-ah)—A deficient amount of blood in a body part as a result of an obstruction of a functional constriction of a blood vessel.

Isocytosis (i″so-si-to′sis)—A state in which cells are equal in size; refers especially to equality of size of RBCs.

Leukemia (lu-ke′me-ah)—A malignant disease of various types that is classified clinically as acute or chronic, depending on the character and duration of the disease; and myeloid, lymphoid, or monocytic, depending on the cells involved. This disease affects the tissues of the lymph nodes, spleen, and/or bone marrow. Symptoms include an uncontrolled increase of WBCs, accompanied by a decrease in RBCs and platelets. This results in anemia and an increased tendency to infection and hemorrhage. Other classic symptoms include pain in bones and joints, fever, and swelling of the liver, spleen, and lymph nodes. The precise cause is unknown.

Leukocytosis (lu″ko-si-to′sis)—An increased number of circulating WBCs.

Leukopenia (lu″ko-pe′ne-ah)—A deficient number of circulating WBCs.

Macrocyte (mak′ro-sit)—The largest type of red blood cell; seen in cases of pernicious anemia (vitamin B_{12} deficiency) and folic acid deficiency.

Microcyte (mi′kro-sit)—An abnormally small RBC, found in cases of iron-deficient anemia and thalassemia.

Mononucleosis (mon″-o-nu″kle-o ′sis)—An abnormal increase of the mononuclear WBCs in the blood.

Infections mononucleosis—Also called glandular fever, is an acute infectious disease, caused by the Epstein-Barr virus.

Phagocytosis (fag″o-si-to′sis)—The process by which WBCs destroy and engulf or ingest harmful microorganisms.

Poikilocytosis (poi″ki-lo-si-to′sis)—The presence of RBCs in the blood that show abnormal variations in shape.

Polycythemia (pol″e-si-the′me-ah)—An abnormally increased amount of RBCs or hemoglobin.

Reticulocyte (re-tik′u-lo-sit)—A nonnucleated immature RBC. Generally, of all the RBCs in the circulating blood, less than 2% are reticulocytes.

Septicemia (sep″ti-se′me-ah)—A condition in which there are toxins or bacteria in the blood.

Serum (se′rum)—The clear, straw-colored liquid portion obtained after blood clots; it consists of plasma minus fibrinogen, which is removed in the process of clotting.

Thrombocyte (throm′bo-sit)—A blood platelet.

Thrombocythemia (throm″bo-si-the′me-ah)—An increased number of platelets in the circulating blood.

Thrombocytopenia (throm″bo-si″to-pe′ne-ah)—A decreased number of platelets in the circulating blood.

Uremia (u-re′ me-ah)—A toxic condition in which there are substances in the blood that should normally be eliminated in the urine.

Venipuncture (ven″i-pungk′ tur)—Puncturing a vein to collect a blood specimen or to administer medication.

Vitamin K—A vitamin that is essential for the formation of prothrombin and the normal clotting of blood. A deficiency may result in hemorrhage because of a prolonged prothrombin time.

ment and function, and waste products are in turn carried to certain body systems for disposal. It is a transportation system in our body, helping also in the maintenance of acid-base, electrolyte, and fluid balance of the internal environment.

Plasma, which is 90% water, acts as the carrier for the formed elements and other substances, which include blood proteins, carbohydrates, fats, amino acids (proteins), mineral salts (the electrolytes), hormones, enzymes, gases, antibodies, and waste products such as urea and uric acid.

The prime function of *RBCs or erythrocytes* is to transport oxygen from the lungs to the body cells and carbon dioxide from the cells back to the lungs to be exhaled. Each RBC contains a protein substance, hemoglobin (Hgb, or Hb), which gives red color to blood and also transports the oxygen and

carbon dioxide to and from the body cells. Anemia is the result of too few RBCs in the circulating blood, or RBCs with reduced amounts of hemoglobin, or both.

The five types of *WBCs or leukocytes* are classified into general groups, the granular and agranular. *Granular* WBCs, sometimes called polymorphonuclear leukocytes, include the eosinophils, basophils, and neutrophils. They are characterized by their heavily granulated cytoplasm and segmented nuclei. The *agranular* leukocytes are the monocytes and lymphocytes, both having a solid nucleus and a clear cytoplasm. The prime function of WBCs is to protect the body against infection and disease; some fight invading bacteria by their phagocytic activity (destroying and ingesting harmful microorganisms), and others play an important role in producing immunity to disease. Infection in the body is indicated when there is a marked rise in the WBC count. In leukemia, the WBC count is also greatly increased.

Platelets (thrombocytes), the smallest of the formed elements in the blood, play a vital role in initiating the clotting process of blood. Thrombocytopenia may be accompanied by bleeding.

All blood cells are produced in hemopoietic (blood-forming) tissue. The agranular WBCs are produced mainly in lymph nodes and other lymphoid tissues. Granular WBCs, RBCs, and platelets are produced in the red bone marrow or myeloid tissue of bones such as the femur, humerus, sternum vertebrae, and cranial bones.

OBTAINING BLOOD SAMPLES

TYPES AND SOURCES

For most routine hematologic studies, there are two sources of blood for testing. *Capillary or peripheral blood* is obtained by performing a skin puncture on the palmar surface of the fingertip or on the ear lobe. For infants, the skin puncture is done on the plantar surface of the great toe or heel. You *must* avoid areas that are cyanotic, scarred, traumatized, edematous, and heavily calloused. A minimal amount of blood, just a few drops, is obtained by this method, but it is sufficient to perform some of the routine tests, such as the complete blood count (CBC), some coagulation studies, and some of the chemistry tests.

The second source for obtaining blood is a vein. This is called *venous blood*, and the procedure by which it is obtained is called a *venipuncture*. The most common sites for obtaining blood by this method are the basilic and cephalic veins located in the antecubital area of the arm, which is at the inner aspect of the arm opposite the elbow. This is the more common method for obtaining a blood sample and is the method that must be used when larger amounts of blood are needed to perform several different tests. When blood cannot be obtained from a vein in the antecubital space because of stenosed or collapsed veins or if the patient has plaster casts on both arms, alternative sites to use are the veins on the top of the hand, in the wrist, or even in the foot. In extreme situations, blood may be obtained from the femoral vein. This site must be used *only* by physicians.

Three types of specimens can be obtained from a venous blood sample.

1. *Serum.* Serum is obtained from a sample collected in a tube *without* an additive. Serum is most frequently used for most blood chemistry tests, pregnancy tests, viral studies, and the HIV antibody test.

2. *Whole blood.* Whole blood is obtained by collecting the blood sample with a tube *with* an anticoagulant additive. This specimen is most frequently used for hematology tests such as the CBC, coagulation studies, blood glucose, and some other blood chemistry tests that vary with the laboratory's preferences.

3. *Plasma.* Plasma is obtained from whole blood collected in a tube *with* an anticoagulant additive and then centrifuged. Centrifugation causes the specimen to separate into three layers. The top layer is plasma, the middle layer contains WBCs and platelets, and the bottom layer contains RBCs. Hematology tests and some chemistry tests are performed on this type of specimen.

At times, special blood studies such as blood gases are ordered. In these circumstances, *arterial blood* (blood from an artery, usually the brachial or femoral) rather than venous blood is required. A physician or qualified laboratory personnel *must* obtain this blood sample. A situation in which this may be necessary in the physician's office is when an emphysemic patient has an acute episode of shortness of breath. The physician may draw arterial blood for blood gases while the patient is still breathing room air; then if oxygen is administered to the patient, the physician draws another arterial blood sample for examination. In the latter case, it is important to indicate on the laboratory requisition how many liters of oxygen were administered to the patient so that this can be considered when the tests results are interpreted.

Commercial kits with required supplies are available. The blood sample must be collected in a heparinized vacuum tube or heparinized syringe. Heparin is used because unclotted blood is needed for analysis. Most labs require the needle to be removed from the syringe and the syringe to be capped with a rubber stopper. The specimen must be free from air contact because exposure to air affects the blood gases. Recapping or needle removal *must* be accomplished through the use of a mechanical device or a one-handed technique (see Unit Seven). The specimen must be placed in ice for delivery to the laboratory. This maintains the viability of the blood as close to body conditions as possible. The specimen must be delivered to the laboratory as soon as possible, preferably within 5 to 10 minutes, for accurate testing to occur.

COLLECTION TUBES AND PROPER HANDLING OF A VENOUS BLOOD SAMPLE

Because of the multitude of tests that can be performed on a blood sample, certain requirements must be met when collecting and handling the sample. Using excellent technique, you will collect the samples in either a plain tube without additives or in a tube that contains anticoagulant additives. *The type of test to be performed, as well as the laboratory's preference, will govern this choice.*

Tubes Without Additives

Generally speaking, a tube without an additive is used when you want a clot to form to obtain *serum* for testing. Once collected, the blood is left standing in an upright position at room temperature, usually for 10 to 30 minutes, to allow a clot to form. To separate the serum from the clot, the sample is then centrifuged for 10 minutes. After this, serum is removed from the tube and is ready for testing.

When serum is required for testing, it is more convenient to use a *serum separator tube* to collect the blood sample (Figure 13-1, *A* and *B*). Once collected, the sample is left standing at room temperature for 10 to 30 minutes and then centrifuged for 10 minutes. After centrifugation, a jellylike substance forms between the clot and the serum in the tube. The sample can then be sent to the laboratory in this tube. This sample is used most frequently for most blood chemistries (varying with the laboratory's preference), serology tests, and for Rh factor testing (see Unit Ten for instructions for using a centrifuge).

Tubes with Additives

Tubes containing EDTA anticoagulant additive are recommended for use when doing hematology studies. The WBCs and platelets are best preserved in this type of tube, and better red cell morphology results will be obtained. The additive has no adverse effects on the blood sample when a sufficient quantity of blood is obtained. Problems arise if too little blood is drawn into tubes containing anticoagulant additives. Misleading results and therefore incorrect diagnoses occur (for example, the hematocrit is lowered and poor RBC morphology results because the RBC shrinks and produces a false appearance). All tubes with anticoagulant additives must be filled with blood.

A tube containing an anticoagulant additive such as heparin prevents the blood from clotting. Depending on methods used by the laboratory when performing certain tests, this is generally the preferred tube to use when collecting a sample for blood chemistries, and especially for potassium levels. Do not use this type for hematology studies because the heparin additive distorts the cells and leads to false results.

There are several other additives used in tubes for collecting venous blood. It is important that the correct tube, plain or with an additive, be used. Most laboratories supply these tubes with directions indicating which to use for various tests. *They are not interchangeable and must not be confused.*

Vacutainer System

Rather than using the conventional syringe, needle, and test tube when obtaining blood samples, newer, more convenient systems consisting of a disposable needle, a holder, and vacuum tubes are available. One such unit is the Vacutainer system, which consists of a holder-needle combination or separate needle and holder, and evacuated glass tubes containing a premeasured vacuum to provide a controlled amount of blood draw. The tubes have color-coded stoppers that indicate the type of test that they are best suited for, and are supplied plain or with additives, sterile or nonsterile (Figure 13-2). (The trend today is to use sterile tubes for all collections.) All are

---

Figure 13-1 A, *Vacutainer evacuated blood collection system.* **B,** *Serum separation tube (SST) used for various tests performed on serum.* **C,** *Sterile Vacutainer serum tubes of various sizes without additives used for chemistry tests, serology tests, blood typing, and other tests.*

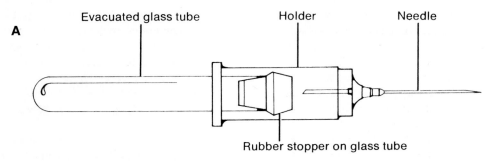

A

Evacuated glass tube   Holder   Needle

Rubber stopper on glass tube

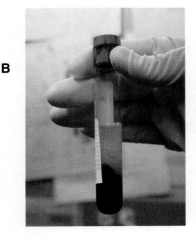

B

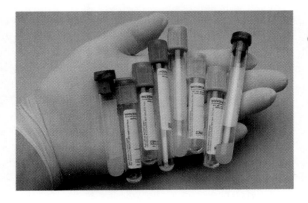

C

Figure 13-2 *Vacutainer tube guide.*

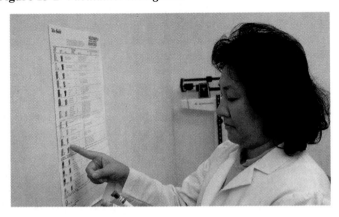

available in a variety of sizes, the most common being 3-, 5-, 7-, 10-, and 15-ml capacities. Vacutainers are supplied in packages with labels that indicate the additives present in the tubes, the expiration date, and the approximate draw amount (see Figure 13-1, *C*).

The most frequently used vacuum tubes, classified according to the tube top color, additive content, average amount of blood drawn, and recommended use, are found in Table 13-1.

When you are to draw more than one tube of blood, the general order of draw is as follows:

- First draw—blood culture tubes (for example, sterile tubes with no additive; blood should be transferred to a culture medium with 5 minutes)
- Second draw—tubes with no additives (for example, red tops)
- Third draw—coagulation tests (for example, blue tops)
- Last draw—tubes with additives (for example, lavender, green, and gray tops)

After blood has been drawn, the tubes without an additive are *not* to be inverted or shaken, but are to be centrifuged as discussed previously. Tubes that contain an additive should be gently inverted 8 to 10 times to mix the blood with the additive. *Do not shake these types* because vigorous mixing may cause hemolysis. The amount of blood drawn varies according to the size of the tube used.

TABLE 13-1

Frequently Used Vacuum Tubes

Tube top Color	Additive	Average Amount of Blood Drawn	Common Blood Determinations
Red (most common)	No additive	10 ml	Used for tests done on serum-Blood bank tests, e.g., blood typing (ABO and Rh factor) and cross-matching; serology tests; serum pregnancy test; most blood chemistries; immunology tests; viral studies; AIDS antibody (HIV antibody)
Lavender	EDTA (Ethylenediamine tetraacetic acid, an anticoagulant)	5 ml	Used for tests done on whole blood or plasma-hematologic tests including a CBC, WBC, RBC, hematocrit, hemoglobin, platelet count, reticulocyte count, and sedimentation rate
Blue	Sodium citrate (an anticoagulant)	5 ml	Used for tests done on whole blood-coagulation studies including prothrombin time (PT), partial thromboplastin time (PTT), and thrombin time (TT)
Green	Sodium heparin	5 ml	Used for tests done on whole blood or plasma-blood chemistry tests, especially potassium levels, electrolytes, blood gases
Gray	Potassium oxalate and sodium fluoride	5 ml	Used for tests done on whole blood or plasma-blood glucose; blood alcohol; the coagulation study activated clotting time (ACT)
Gray and red (mottled top; serum separation tube)	Silicone serum separation material	5 ml	Used for tests done on serum—can be used for every test where you want the blood to clot **DO NOT USE FOR BLOOD BANK TESTS.**
Yellow	Sterile Sodium polyanetholesulfonate	5 ml	Used to collect whole blood for microbiology tests (blood culture tests)

Amount and Handling of the Specimen

The amount of venous blood to be drawn is 3 to 30 ml, varying with the test(s) to be performed. The blood must be collected in the correct tube. The tube must be at room temperature. Consult your laboratory for the exact amounts that are needed for each specific test that is to be performed. Frequently 1 to 2 ml more blood than required is drawn to avoid having a patient return for a second collection if the first battery of tests does not turn out.

A blood specimen must be tested on the same day of collection. When serum is needed for the test, it *must* be separated from the blood within 30 to 45 minutes after the sample has been collected. Blood collected in a tube containing an anticoagulant *must* be mixed gently with the anticoagulant immediately after collection.

Depending on the test(s) to be performed, blood should be examined within 8 hours or less from the time it was collected, and preferably within 2 to 4 hours from the time that it was drawn. Blood for bacteriologic studies must be collected in special containers and must not be left standing for any length of time. These specimens must be examined as soon as possible. Blood drawn for an electrolyte panel should be refrigerated if it is not tested immediately. Other blood samples may be left standing on the counter for 2 to 4 hours before testing, although some results may vary if the blood is left standing for 2 or more hours. On request, your laboratory will provide schedules that list specific sample requirements for each test they perform. The quality of a test is diminished if a blood sample stands for a long time before being tested; for example, glucose levels will decrease within a couple of hours, and potassium levels will rise if serum is allowed to stand on the cells; the sedimentation rate will be lowered if left standing for over 2 hours, and the bacteria count will increase.

When the specimen is to be sent to an outside laboratory, wrap it in protective materials and place it into the appropriate transport or mailing container. Always include the correctly completed laboratory requisition with the specimen.

Labeling

As with all specimens, you must accurately identify blood samples; label them with the patient's name, the date, your initials, and any other information required by the laboratory; and forward adequate amounts the laboratory as soon as possible. You should also indicate on the laboratory requisition the time the sample was drawn. To prevent errors, patient identification on the collection tube must be identical to that on the requisition.

Patient Preparation for Blood Tests

There are very few blood tests that require any special patient preparation. Generally, special preparation means that the patient should fast (that is, abstain from all solid foods and liquids) for up to 14 hours before the blood sample is drawn. This is required because food substances may alter the reliability of the test results. Water may be taken before some tests. The laboratory will provide you with specific directions.

Usually you are to instruct the patient to take nothing by mouth (NPO) after midnight the night before the test is to be done. The tests for which the patient has to fast should be scheduled for the early morning to minimize the inconvenience that abstaining from food or fluids may cause the patient.

The principal tests that require the patient to fast beforehand include fasting blood sugar; glucose tolerance test; any type of lipid analysis such as cholesterol and triglycerides because fats from a meal flood the bloodstream and dramatically raise the triglycerides and thus the results would be meaningless; and the sequential multiple analysis (SMA-12, SMA-18, SMAC-20 and SMAC-24), a series of 12, 18, 20, and 24 blood chemistries. Some laboratories also request that the patient be fasting before all enzyme and electrolyte tests. At other times fasting will be done according to the individual orders of the physician. Care must be taken to provide the patient with correct and adequate instructions in these situations.

Some medications such as steroids, salicylates or diuretics interfere with test results. When feasible (that is, when health permits), the physician may advise a patient to discontinue medications for 4 to 24 hours or up to 3 days before some blood tests. When it is not medically advisable for the patient to go without the medication for any length of time, you must note on the laboratory requisition what drug and the amount that the patient is taking. This alerts the laboratory to the presence of the drug. At times the laboratory may be able to use a different method of testing that would not be altered by the presence of the medication. Other tests require timed samples; this is, samples may be collected every hour for 3 consecutive hours, as in a glucose tolerance test. Patients must be made aware of these requirements.

It is frequently advisable to write out the specific directions for patients so that they have an accurate reminder of the special requirements for each test to be performed, in addition to the time and date of the test. For some tests you may have preprinted instruction forms to give the patient. Make sure that the patient understands the reasons for any special instructions. An informed patient usually is more cooperative in following specific directions, which in turn facilitates accurate test results.

Recording

Proper recording on the patient's chart is essential. This includes the date, time, sample(s) obtained, test(s) to be performed, and when and how the sample was sent to the laboratory (see also Care, Handling, Transporting, and Storing Specimens in Unit Eleven).

VENIPUNCTURE TECHNIQUE

Venipuncture is the preferred method for obtaining blood samples and must be used when a larger amount of blood is required for testing. From 3 to more than 30 ml may be drawn by this method. To spare the patient the pain of unsuccessful punctures, consider the following before doing a venipuncture.

Venipuncture (Troubleshooting) Tips

1. Ask the patient if he or she has any preference as to which vein you should puncture. Patients often know where their better veins are and which sites should be avoided.
2. Palpate the vein before inserting the needle to determine if the vein is patent (open, unobstructed).
3. Use a sturdy-walled vein for the puncture. The walls of sturdy veins feel firm when you touch them, and will exhibit elasticity and resilience when pressure is carefully applied.
4. If unable to get into a vein in the antecubital space, check for different sites such as veins in the wrist or hand.
5. Fragile veins are usually narrow veins. If you must puncture these veins, use a 23- rather than a 21- gauge needle.
6. For small or fragile veins you may use the butterfly technique using a butterfly needle and tubing. Insert the needle into the vein. When you see blood starting to flow into the tubing, insert the needle at the other end of the tubing into the vacuum tube. Leave the needle in position until the desired amount of blood is obtained.
7. Do not use a weak-walled vein. These veins are soft to the touch and lack the elasticity of a sturdy vein.
8. Do not use sclerosed veins. These veins resistant to pressure, even if they do look like good veins.

9. Do not use vacuum apparatus to draw blood from a small or constricted vein because this causes the vein to collapse.
10. For obese patients, put the tourniquet on fairly tight and feel for a vein deep in the antecubital space. There may be a deep vein in the center of this area. Be careful not to puncture an artery if going into deep tissue. If you find and feel an artery, you will feel it pulsate. A vein will feel like a tube and you will not feel it pulsate. You may also check the veins in the wrist to use for the venipuncture site on an obese patient.
11. For children, have the parent leave the room before you do the venipuncture. Have someone assist you with the child. Another person can hold the child, hold his or her arm secure, and also talk to him or her. Do the procedure quickly. When someone is supporting the child and distracting his or her mind off of the needle, you are better able to perform the venipuncture quickly.
12. For the elderly. It is sometimes advisable to have someone hold the arm for support because the patient could move his or her arm and this could interfere with the tests. This is especially important if the patient is comatosed.
13. ALWAYS explain who you are and what you will be doing, even if the patient has passed out or is comatosed, because he or she may still be able to hear you or feel the needle prick.

VENIPUNCTURE USING A SYRINGE AND NEEDLE

Equipment

70% alcohol and sterile cotton sponges; or disposable alcohol sponges
Sterile cotton sponges
Tourniquet
Sterile disposable needle, usually 1-inch, 1¼-inch, or 1½-inch, 21-gauge
Sterile disposable syringe, either 5, 10, 20, or 30 ml, depending on the amount of blood to be obtained

Test tube(s) with proper patient identification, with or without additive, depending on the test that is to be performed; or a vacuum tube (*rather than the syringe and test tube, or vacuum tube, you may use the Vacutainer system with appropriate tube[s], needle, and holder; see Figure 13-1.*)
Adhesive bandage
Disposable single-use exam gloves

PROCEDURE

1. Wash your hands. **Use appropriate personal protective equipment (PPE) as dictated by facility.**

2. Assemble required equipment.

3. Identify the patient, and explain the procedure.

4. Have the patient sit with the arm well supported in a downward position (Figure 13-3).

5. Prepare equipment for use: attach the needle to the syringe (or to the Vacutainer holder [see Figure 13-1, A]), leaving the needle shield in place. Label the collection tube with the patient's name, the date, and the time (Figure 13-4).

RATIONALE

Explanations help gain the patient's cooperation.

This avoids movement by the patient.

If you are drawing blood from more than one patient, it is best to label the tubes after you have drawn the blood. Often when tubes are prelabeled, people have a tendency to use the wrong tube if they are in a rush or under pressure.

VENIPUNCTURE USING A SYRINGE AND NEEDLE—cont'd

PROCEDURE	RATIONALE

PROCEDURE

6. Select the site for venipuncture by palpitating the antecubital space. This site is located on the inner aspect of the arm, opposite the elbow. You must avoid the artery. At the antecubital site, the basilic and cephalic veins are used for drawing blood samples.

7. Don gloves.

8. Apply the tourniquet around the patient's arm 3 to 4 inches above the elbow (Figure 13-5). The tourniquet must have enough tension to stop venous flow. Palpate the vein again (Figure 13-6). You may ask the patient to open and close the hand several times to help produce engorgement of the vein in the arm. The radial pulse should still be palpable.

9. Swab the venipuncture site with an alcohol sponge. Do not palpate the venipuncture area after cleansing with alcohol.

10. Remove the needle shield.

11. Using your nondominant hand, draw the skin over the puncture site until tense. Gently and slowly insert the needle at a 15-degree angle through the skin into the vein (Figure 13-7).

12. Having entered the vein using your dominant hand, now use your nondominant hand to slowly pull on the plunger of the syringe to withdraw blood. As soon as blood starts to flow into the syringe, release the tourniquet (Figure 13-8; see Figure 13-10). Make sure that you do not move the needle and syringe after entering the vein.

RATIONALE

Do not tie the tourniquet too tight because that obstructs arterial blood flow.

Countertension immobilizes the vein and exerts tension in the opposite direction to that of the needle. Thus the needle goes in more easily and less painfully. You retain better control over the needle when the vein is immobilized by the countertension.
The bevel of the needle should be facing upward so the sharpest point of the needle is inserted first.

If you withdraw the blood too rapidly, you may cause the vein to collapse, and thus will be unable to obtain the required sample. Keep in mind that a nontraumatic venipuncture produces the most reliable results, because any tissue injury can falsely elevate some results such an enzyme levels.

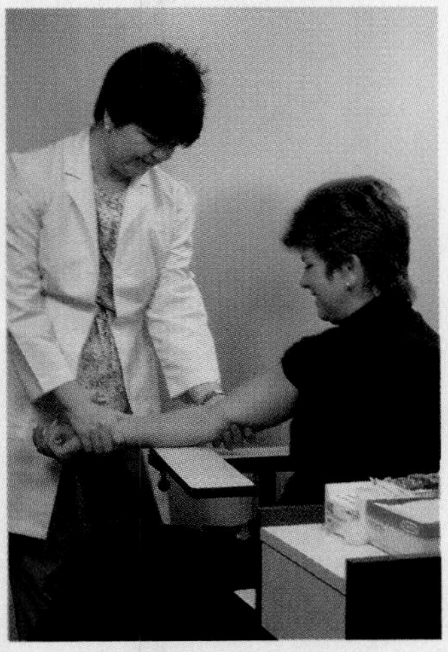

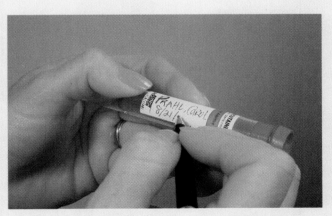

Figure 13-3 *For a venipuncture, have the patient sit with the arm well supported in a downward position.*

Figure 13-4 *Label the collection tube with the patient's name, the date and the time.*

VENIPUNCTURE USING A SYRINGE AND NEEDLE—cont'd

PROCEDURE

13. When you have obtained the required amount of blood, place a dry sterile sponge over the puncture site and withdraw the needle, using a straight, downward motion. The tourniquet must be off before the needle is withdrawn.

14. Apply pressure with a sterile sponge over the puncture site for a few minutes; you may have the patient elevate the arm at this time. Do not apply pressure to the puncture site until the needle is completely removed. You may ask the patient to hold the sponge over the puncture site and apply the pressure.

15. Inject blood into the test tube(s) (Figure 13-9). NOTE: When injecting blood into a vacuum tube from a syringe and needle system, leave the needle on the syringe, and gently insert the needle through the rubber stopper on the tube. The vacuum inside draws the required amount of blood into the tube. When using different tubes for multiple samples, first inject blood into the tubes that do not contain any additives, then into the coagulation tubes, and then into the tubes containing an additive.

16. Cap the tubes. Those that contain an additive should be gently inverted 8 to 10 times to mix the blood with the additive. Do not shake these tubes. Do not mix blood in the plain tubes (that is, tubes without an additive). Vigorous mixing may cause hemolysis.

17. Apply an adhesive bandage to the puncture site if desired.

18. Discard disposable syringe and needle in puncture-resistant containers designated for disposal. (If you have used a nondisposable glass syringe rather than a disposable one, rinse it with cold water, separate the barrel and plunger, and soak in detergent and water) (see Figures 7-31 and 13-12).

19. Remove gloves.

20. Wash your hands.

21. Complete the laboratory requisition, and send it to the laboratory with the blood sample(s) obtained.

22. Record on patient's chart.

RATIONALE

Elevation prevents oozing of blood at the puncture site. Elevating rather than bending the arm helps to prevent possible bruising of the area.

Proper disposal aids in preventing needlesticks and infection and is required by the OSHA bloodborne pathogen standard.

Charting example:
May 18, 19_____, 1 p.m.
Venipuncture done on left arm.
Two samples sent to lab for a CBC and blood chemistries.
Charles Rubin, CMA

VENIPUNCTURE USING A SYRINGE AND NEEDLE—cont'd

A

B

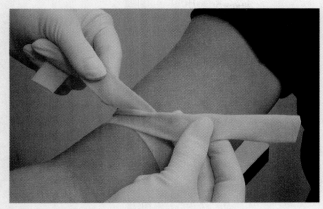
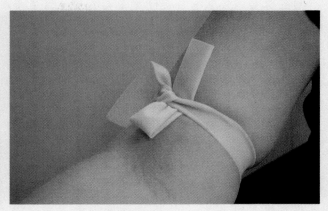

Figure 13-5 *A, Apply the tourniquet around the patient's arm 3 to 4 inches above the elbow. Cross the ends of the tourniquet and pull the ends away from each other to create tension. B, Secure the tourniquet by tucking the upper end into the band to form a half-elbow. The tourniquet must be tight enough to obstruct venous blood flow.*

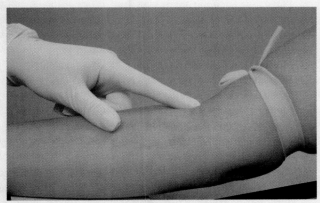
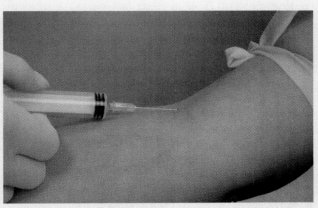

Figure 13-6 *Palpate the vein once again after the tourniquet has been positioned.*

Figure 13-7 *Gently and slowly, insert the needle at a 15-degree angle through the skin into the vein.*

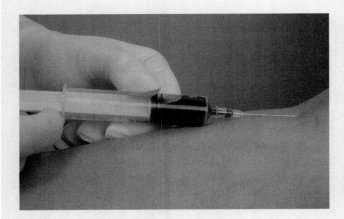
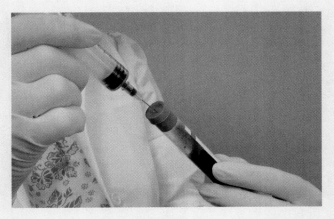

Figure 13-8 *After entering the vein, use your nondominant hand to slowly pull on the plunger of the syringe to withdraw blood. Release the tourniquet as soon as blood starts to flow into the syringe.*

Figure 13-9 *After obtaining the required amount of blood and removing the needle from the vein, inject blood into the test tube. When using a vacuum tube, leave the needle on the syringe and gently insert the needle through the rubber stopper on the tube.*

Venipuncture Using the Vacutainer Evacuated Blood Collection Tube(s) For Drawing Single and Multiple Blood Samples (see Figure 13-1, *A*).

1. Complete steps 1 through 5 as described in Venipuncture Using A Syringe and Needle, page 422.
2. Select the correct tube for the type of sample required and label it. Gently tap tubes that contain additives to dislodge any additive that may be trapped around the stopper.
3. Insert the tube into the holder up to the guideline; push the tube stopper onto the needle inside the holder.
4. Perform the venipuncture in the usual manner (steps 6 through 11 in Venipuncture Using a Syringe and Needle).
5. Place two fingers at the end of the holder; with your thumb, push the tube onto the needle to the end of the holder (Figure 13-10).
6. Release the tourniquet as soon as blood begins to fill the tube (Figure 13-10). Do not allow contents of tube to contact the stopper or the end of the needle during the procedure. NOTE: If blood doesn't flow into the tube or if the blood flow ceases before an adequate amount is collected, take the following steps:
   a. Check to see that the needle cannula is in the correct position in the vein.
   b. If a multiple sample needle is being used, remove the tube and place a new tube into the holder.
   c. Remove the needle and tube and discard. Start the procedure over again.

Continue with the steps 7 through 16 for single-sample collections and steps 7 through 18 for multiple-sample collections.

Single-sample collection

7. Remove the needle from the vein when the vacuum is exhausted and blood stops flowing into the tube (Figure 13-11).
8. Apply pressure with a sterile sponge to the puncture site, and have the patient elevate his or her arm for a few minutes to prevent oozing of blood (see Figure 13-11).

9. Remove the tube of blood from the holder.
10. For tubes that contain additives, *gently* invert eight to ten times to mix blood thoroughly with the additive. *Do not shake.*
11. Apply an adhesive bandage to the puncture site if required.
12. Discard the needle in a designated container (Figure 13-12).
13. Remove gloves.
14. Wash your hands.
15. Complete the laboratory requisition and forward with the blood sample to the laboratory.
16. Record on the patient's chart the date, time, procedure, and your signature.

Multiple-sample collection

Complete steps 1 through 6 (column 1).

7. Remove the tube from the holder when the vacuum is exhausted and the blood stops flowing. Keep the needle holder steady.
8. Place the second and succeeding tubes into the holder, puncturing the diaphragm of the stopper to initiate blood flow. Keep the needle holder steady. Tubes without additives are drawn first, then coagulation tubes, and then tubes with additives.
9. While blood is flowing into succeeding tubes, gently invert previously filled tubes that contain additives 8 to 10 times to mix the additive with the blood. *Do not shake.* Vigorous mixing may cause hemolysis.
10. Remove the needle from the vein when blood stops flowing into the last tube (see Figure 13-11).
11. Apply pressure with a sterile sponge to the puncture site (see Figure 13-11), and have the patient elevate the arm for a few minutes to prevent oozing of blood.
12. Remove the tube of blood from the holder. *Gently* invert the tube 8 to 10 times if it contains an additive. *Do not shake.*
13. Apply an adhesive bandage to the puncture site if required.

Figure 13-10 *Correct position of patient's arm and tube assembly to prevent possibility of backflow. Tourniquet is released as soon as blood begins to flow or before the needle is removed if taking multiple tubes.*

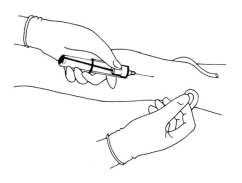

Figure 13-11 *Remove needle from vein when vacuum is exhausted and blood stops flowing into tube. Apply pressure with a sterile sponge to the puncture site.*

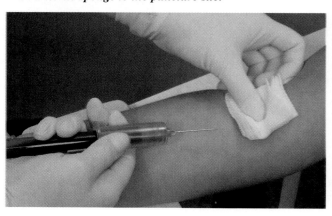

14. Discard the needle in a designated puncture-resistant container (see Figure 13-12). If using the Vacutainer needle container, insert the needle into the slot on the top of the container and twist the holder counterclockwise until the needle is detached and falls into the container. *The Vacutainer holder is reusable.*
15. Remove gloves.
16. Wash your hands.
17. Complete the laboratory requisition and forward it with the blood sample to the laboratory.
18. Record on the patient's chart the date, the time, procedure, and your signature.

FINGERTIP SKIN PUNCTURE

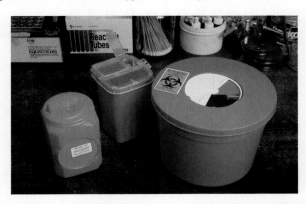

Figure 13-12 *Vacutainer-type needle disposal container.*

FINGERTIP SKIN PUNCTURE USING A LANCET

Equipment

A sterile disposable lancet

70% alcohol and cotton sponges; or disposable alcohol sponges

Clean blood pipette *or* capillary tube *or* Unopette *or* Microtainer (this piece of equipment varies with your agency's preference, with the test(s) to be performed on the blood sample, and with the methods used by the laboratory)

or

Disposable single-use exam gloves

A reagent strip if you are doing a simple test for blood glucose (see page 437)

PROCEDURE

1. Wash your hands. **Use appropriate personal protective equipment (PPE) as dictated by facility.**

2. Assemble equipment and supplies.

3. Identify the patient and explain the procedure.

4. Have the patient seated with the arm well supported.

5. . Select the lateral part of the tip of a *finger* or the *earlobe* for the puncture site; use the *heel* or *great toe* for an infant. Avoid the thumb and index finger.

6. "Milk" or gently rub the finger along the sides. If the patient's fingers are cold, you may rub them or apply a warm pack. You may also instruct the patient to dangle his or her hand toward the floor.

7. Clean the puncture site with an alcohol sponge; allow the area to dry. Do not blot or blow on the puncture site. Allow it to air-dry.

8. Don gloves.

9. Grasp the patient's finger on the sides near the puncture site with your nondominant thumb and forefinger.

RATIONALE

Explanations help gain the patient's cooperation.

This avoids movement by the patient.

The thumb and index finger are usually more calloused than the other fingers. Using the lateral part of a fingertip rather than the palm side lessens discomfort to the patient.

Rubbing the finger promotes circulation. Dangling the hand helps force blood into the finger.

FINGERTIP SKIN PUNCTURE USING A LANCET—cont'd

PROCEDURE

RATIONALE

10. Hold the lancet with your dominant fingers and make a quick in-and-out puncture on the side of the patient's fingertip. Hold the lancet at a right angle to the lines on the patient's finger (Figure 13-13). Lancets are usually designed so that you can make a puncture to a depth of 3 to 4 mm, which is sufficient to obtain drops of blood.

11. Wipe away the first drop of blood with a clean cotton sponge.

12. Apply gentle pressure above the puncture site to cause the blood to flow freely. Do not squeeze the finger.

13. Obtain the blood sample as required by the test to be performed. You may:

    a. Use the pipette to take up the blood sample. Take up the blood sample to the desired level in the pipette.

    b. Lightly touch the blood drop to the test pad on the reagent strip, and continue the test according to the individual test directions.

14. When more than one sample is needed, wipe the finger with a clean cotton sponge and obtain fresh drops of blood in each pipette. You may have to apply gentle pressure to the finger to obtain more blood.

15. When using bulb pipettes and Unopettes, make dilutions according to instructions for the specific test to be performed. Do not dilute blood collected in Microtainers and capillary tubes; send it directly to the laboratory for testing.

16. Apply pressure to the puncture site with a dry cotton sponge. You may have the patient apply pressure with a cotton sponge over the puncture site.

17. Discard lancet in sharps container. Any sponge with blood on it must be disposed of in a container for biohazardous waste.

18. Label the blood samples and laboratory requisition correctly, and forward to the laboratory for testing.

19. Remove gloves.

20. Wash your hands.

21. Record the patient's chart the date, time, procedure, and your signature.

The first drop of blood is not a desirable sample because it contains tissue fluid.

Squeezing the finger liberates tissue fluid, which in turn dilutes the blood and causes inaccurate results.

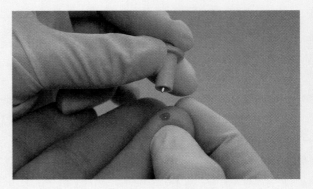

Figure 13-13 *Fingertip skin puncture technique using a lancet.*

Charting example:
   April 21, _____, 11 a.m.
      Finger puncture done on second finger, left hand. Blood sample sent to laboratory for a CBC (complete blood count).
         Ann Patterson, CMA

Fingertip Skin Puncture Using the Penlet II* (Figure 13-14)

Equipment

Penlet II disposable caps (see Figure 13-14)
Sterile lancet
70% alcohol and cotton sponges *or* disposable alcohol sponges
Disposable single-use exam gloves

Procedure

1. Wash your hands. **Use appropriate personal protective equipment (PPE) as dictated by facility.**
2. Assemble equipment and supplies.
3. Identify the patient and explain the procedure.
4. Have the patient seated with the arm well supported.
5. Load the Penlet II with a sterile lancet. Remove the Penlet II cap by pulling it straight off. Insert a new, sterile lancet into the lancet holder. The lancet will slide into the lancet holder easier if you *do not* line up the ridges on the lancet with the slots in the lancet holder. Inserting the lancet may automatically cock the Penlet II (Figure 13-14, *B* and *C*).
6. Select the lateral part of the tip of a finger for the puncture site.
7. "Milk" or gently rub the finger along the sides.
8. Clean the puncture site with alcohol sponge; allow the area to dry.
9. Don gloves.
10. Hold the end of the Penlet firmly with one hand, and with the other hand twist off the lancet protective disk (Figure 13-14, *D*).
11. Replace the Penlet II cap (Figure 13-14, *E*). The Penlet II Sampler includes two caps. The cap that comes attached to the Penlet II Sampler has a *single line* on the flat side and works well for children and most adults. The other cap has *two lines* on the flat side and works well for very thick or calloused skin or when a deeper puncture is needed (Figure 13-14, *F*).

12. Cock the Penlet II. Holding the lower portion of the Penlet II, pull out the dark gray sliding barrel until it clicks. If it does not click, the Penlet II may have been cocked when the lancet was inserted (Figure 13-14, *G*).
13. Grasp the patient's finger on the sides near the puncture site with your nondominant thumb and forefinger.
14. Place the Penlet II firmly against the side of the finger, with the cap resting on the finger (Figure 13-14, *H*).
15. Press the dark gray release button. The depth of penetration of the lancet depends on the amount of pressure with which the Penlet II is held against the skin. The greater the pressure, the deeper the puncture (Figure 13-14, *I*).
16. Complete this procedure by following steps 11 through 20 in the fingertip skin puncture technique using a lancet.
17. To remove the lancet from the Penlet II, take the cap off, insert the inside rim of the cap into the notched side of the lancet, and pull the lancet out. Grasp the dark gray T-shaped prongs. Point the lancet down and away from you. Pull back on the dark gray sliding barrel until the lancet drops out (Figure 13-14, *J*).
18. Remove gloves.
19. Wash your hands.
20. Put a clean cap on the Penlet and replace in the proper storage area. Clean with soap and water as needed.

UNOPETTE SYSTEM

The Unopette system consists of a disposable, self-filling diluting pipette and a plastic reservoir prefilled with a precise amount of diluent. These systems serve as a collection and dilution unit for microblood samples. Various types of Unopette systems are available that contain the appropriate diluting substances required for hematology and chemistry tests (Figure 13-15).

Figure 13-16 shows the Microtainer Capillary Whole Blood Collector.

*Lifescan, Inc., Mountain View, Calif.

Figure 13-14 A, *Penlet II automatic blood sampling pen for obtaining a skin puncture blood sample.*

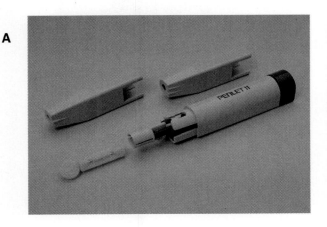

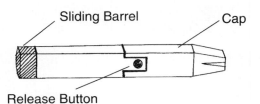

Figure 13-14—cont'd   B to J, *Technique for using the Penlet II puncture device.*

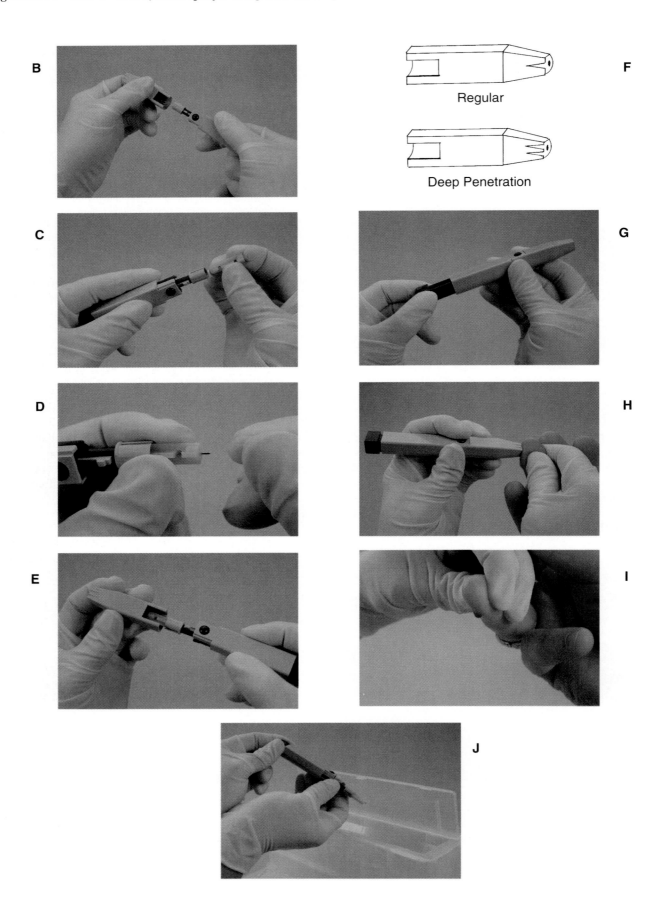

Figure 13-15 *Techniques for using the Unopette system for laboratory procedures.*
Courtesy Becton-Dickinson, Division of Becton, Dickinson & Co., Rutherford, NJ.

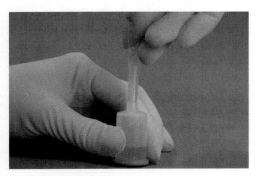

1. Puncture diaphragm
Using the protective shield on the capillary pipette, puncture the diaphragm of the reservoir as follows:

  a. Place reservoir on a flat surface. Grasping reservoir in one hand, take pipette assembly in other hand. Push tip of pipette shield firmly through diaphragm in neck of reservoir, then remove.

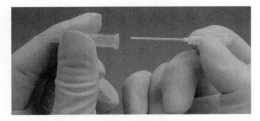

  b. Remove shield from pipette assembly with a twist.

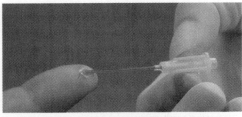

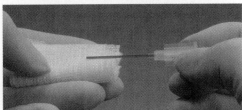

2. Add sample
Fill capillary with sample and transfer to reservoir as follows:

  a. Holding pipette almost horizontally, touch tip of pipette to sample . (See alternate methods in illustrations above.) Pipette will fill by capillary action. Filling is complete and will stop automatically when sample reaches end of capillary bore in neck of pipette.
  b. Wipe excess sample from outside of capillary pipette, making certain that no sample is removed from capillary bore.

  c. Squeeze reservoir slightly to force out some air. Do not expel any liquid. Maintain pressure on reservoir.

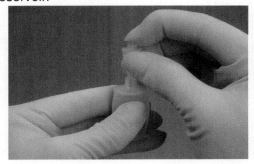

  d. Cover opening of overflow chamber with index finger and seat pipette securely in reservoir neck.
  e. Release pressure on reservoir. Then remove finger from pipette opening. Negative pressure will draw blood into diluent.

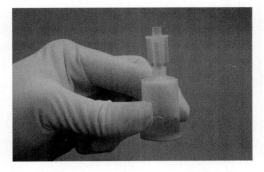

  f. Squeeze reservoir gently two or three times to rinse capillary bore, forcing diluent into, but not out of, overflow chamber, releasing pressure each time to return mixture to reservoir.

CAUTION: If reservoir is squeezed too hard, some of the specimen may be expelled through the top of the overflow chamber.

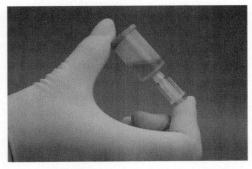

  g. Place index finger over upper opening and gently invert several times to thoroughly mix sample with diluent.

Figure 13-15—cont'd *Techniques for using the Unopette system for laboratory procedures.*

3. Count cells (option 1)

Mix diluted blood thoroughly be inverting reservoir (see 2g) to resuspend cells immediately prior to actual count.

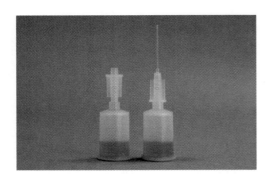

a. Convert to dropper assembly by withdrawing pipette from reservoir and reseating securely in reverse position.
b. Invert reservoir, gently squeeze sides and discard first three or four drops.

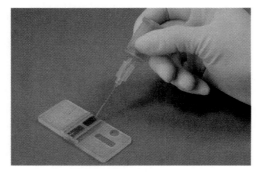

c. Carefully charge hemacytometer with diluted blood by gently squeezing sides of reservoir to expel contents until chamber is properly filled.

OR

3. Transfer contents (option 2)

Transfer thoroughly mixed contents of each reservoir to appropriately labeled test tubes or corresponding curvettes as follows:

a. Convert reservoir to dropper assembly by withdrawing pipette and reseating securely in reverse position as shown above.

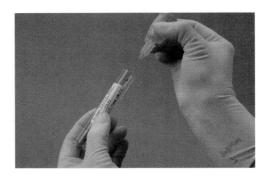

b. Place capillary tip into appropriately labeled test tube or cuvette which will accommodate 5.0 ml of reagent and squeeze reservoir to expel entire contents.

OR

3. Store diluted specimen (option 3)

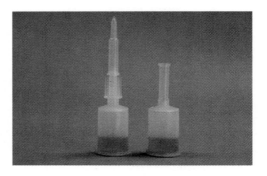

Cover overflow chamber with capillary shield or remove capillary and insert tip of shield firmly into reservoir opening. (Note time for which diluted specimen remains stable for each test.)

Figure 13-16 *Microtainer capillary whole blood collector.*
Courtesy Becton-Dickinson, Division of Becton, Dickinson & Co., Rutherford, NJ.

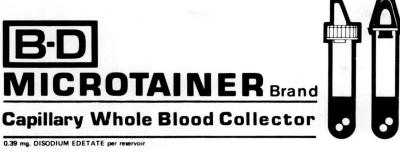

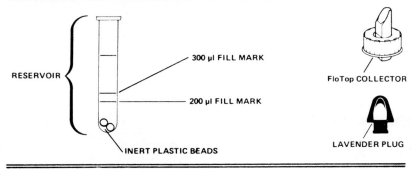

The MICROTAINER System for capillary whole blood samples provides a method for collecting, anticoagulating, storing and identifying the capillary blood sample... all in one unbreakable plastic tube.

ANTICOAGULANT

Each MICROTAINER Tube contains sufficient EDTA Na_2 (disodium edetate) to anticoagulate 300 microliters of capillary blood.

MIXING BEADS

Each MICROTAINER Tube contains two (2) inert plastic beads which aid in the dispersion of blood and anticoagulant for proper mixing of sample.

NON-INTERFERENCE WITH HEMATOLOGICAL DETERMINATIONS

Parallel comparisons of samples collected with the MICROTAINER Brand Capillary Whole Blood Collector and routine microcollection techniques have shown no significant differences for the following determination.[1]

WBC	MCH
RBC	MCHC
HGB	MCV
HCT	Platelets
Reticulocytes	
White Cell Differentials	

MICROTAINER Tubes for whole blood collections are to be used to collect and store capillary blood samples for outline hematological use. This system is composed of a one piece FloTop collector; a plastic tube containing an anticoagulant, EDTA Na_2 (disodium edetate), two (2) inert plastic mixing beads, and a lavender plug.

USERS SHOULD BE THOROUGHLY FAMILIAR WITH THE CONTENTS OF THIS PACKAGE INSERT PRIOR TO USE.

The FloTop collector directs the free flowing blood directly into the unbreakable plastic MICROTAINER tube. The tubes are marked at the 200 and 300 microliter (µl) levels which indicate the desired filling range.

When the appropriate sample has been collected, the FloTop collector is removed from the tube and is replaced with the lavender plug and gently inverted, 8 to 10 times, to insure adequate anticoagulation of the specimen. The stoppered tube is now provided with protection against contamination, evaporation and spillage.

The anticoagulated whole blood samples can be directly pipetted from the MICROTAINER Tube and assayed for routine hematological parameters.

BLOOD TESTS

The results obtained from laboratory examinations performed on blood samples, combined with other clinical information, help the physician in various aspects of patient care, such as screening for or diagnosing a condition, evaluating body functions, making therapeutic decisions, and monitoring therapy provided.

Numerous blood tests can be performed to aid the physician when diagnosing, treating, or evaluating a patient's condition. Some of these tests are performed on whole blood, whereas others are performed on blood serum. A few simple procedures that may be performed in the physician's office or health agency and a table of many common tests done frequently in laboratories by certified personnel with the aid of automated equipment follow on pages 452 to 467. The actual performance of these tests is usually not your responsibility, because in general *most state laws require that individuals performing laboratory procedures must be certified laboratory technicians or technologists, or physicians certified or licensed in the state of their practice.* Nonetheless, it is important for you to be familiar with the type of tests available and the normal values for each and to have an understanding of the significance of normal and abnormal results. When aware of this information, you can better understand and appreciate the diagnosis, treatment, and evaluation of patients under the physician's care; and you are of greater value to the patient, physician, and laboratory.

At times, basic screening tests are performed in the physician's office; more detailed tests and precise results are obtained from larger laboratories using automated equipment.

All tests have predetermined normal values or ranges that establish the limits within which the results indicate the absence of any pathologic condition. Normal ranges are established on the basis of the procedures and equipment used by the laboratory. It is important to keep this in mind when reviewing laboratory reports received on specimens obtained from the patients under your physician's care. Often you may obtain a list of normal blood values from the laboratory that performs the procedures.

Generally, hematology tests are done on whole blood, and serologic tests and blood chemistries are done on serum or sometimes on plasma. Blood banking and transfusion services use cells and serum for testing.

A conscientious medical assistant should be alert for new techniques that may be valuable to the physician in the office. Manufacturers provide brochures and catalogues with information on the latest developments. Medically oriented magazines are another good source for obtaining this information.

COPPER SULFATE RELATIVE DENSITY TEST FOR SCREENING ANEMIA AND A HEMATOCRIT

Gross screening tests to determine if a patient has a sufficient volume of RBCs can be done by performing a relative density test with a few drops of blood in a copper sulfate solution. This test can indicate if a patient may have a reduced capacity to produce RBCs, a problem with any blood loss, or an insufficient diet for the adequate production and functioning of RBCs. This test is based on the fact that RBCs are the heaviest portion of blood. The copper sulfate solution is prepared so that the density of this solution is equal to that of blood with 37% RBCs for women and 47% RBCs for men. These two figures are the normal lower limits for the percentage of RBCs in women and men, thus allowing you to divide all patients screened by this method into two groups—those above and those below the lower limit. When the results of this test indicate a volume of RBCs in the blood below the normal range, it should be followed by a more precise test (that is, a hematocrit). The hematocrit (Hct) represents the volume percentage of RBCs present in whole blood. The normal ranges for a hematocrit are women, 33% to 46%; men, 40% to 54%. Both of these tests are important aids to the physician when diagnosing and treating patients with anemia. They are relatively simple and can easily be performed in the physician's office or health agency.

RELATIVE DENSITY TEST

Equipment

Sterile alcohol swabs
Clean gauze pads
Sterile disposable lancets
Capillary tubes (heparinized and nonheparinized)
Copper sulfate (C_uSO_4) solution for anemia testing for women and men
Clean containers to hold the copper sulfate solution

Crito-seal clay trays or other sealing compound or sealing micro-hematocrit
Microhematocrit centrifuge
Microhematocrit reading card
Capillary bulbs (small rubber bulbs that fit over the capillary tube)
Disposable single-use exam gloves

PROCEDURE

1. Wash your hands. **Use appropriate personal protective equipment (PPE) as dictated by facility.**

2. Assemble and prepare equipment and supplies for use. Fill a container approximately two-thirds full with the copper sulfate solution. Cover the C_uS solution when not in use; do not expose it to direct sunlight or freezing temperatures or allow it evaporate. When doing multiple tests, change the solution after testing 15 patients.

3. Identify the patient and explain the procedure.

4. Don gloves.

5. . Perform a skin puncture on the fingertip (see steps 1 to 12 in Fingertip Skin Puncture Using a Lancet, pages 427 and 428).

6. Once blood flows freely, use a nonheparinized capillary tube to receive blood. Fill the tube to approximately three-quarters. You may hold the tube in a horizontal position or slightly lower when filling the tube (Figure 13-17).

RATIONALE

RELATIVE DENSITY TEST—cont'd

PROCEDURE

7. Apply pressure over the puncture site with a clean, dry gauze pad. Dispose of pad with blood on it in a container labeled for biohazardous waste. You may have the patient do this while you attend to the test.

8. Hold the capillary tube vertically over the container of copper sulfate to allow the blood to drop into the solution. If the blood does not drop into the solution, apply the capillary bulb to the tube, then squeeze the bulb to force blood into the solution (Figure 13-18, *A* and *B*).

9. Determine the test result. One of three reactions will occur:
   a. Blood drops through the solution without hesitating or rising.
   b. Blood hesitates and then drops through the solution.

   c. Blood hesitates, rises to the top of the solution, and eventually drops through the solution.

10. When a hematocrit is indicated:
    a. Swab the finger with a sponge, then "milk" the finger, and, using the same puncture site, obtain another blood sample in a heparinized tube. Fill calibrated tubes to the calibration line. Fill uncalibrated tubes to approximately three quarters (within 10 to 20 mm of the end of the tube).
    b. Seal the dry end of the tube with clay by sticking it into the Crito-seal clay tray (Figure 13-19).

    c. Place the tube into a slot in the microhematocrit centrifuge, with the sealed end down facing the outside of the centrifuge (sealed end toward the outer rim) (Figure 13-20). For balance, place another tube in a slot on the opposite side.
    d. Close and secure the lid of the centrifuge.
    e. Adjust the timer, and spin down for 5 minutes at the speed of 10,000 rpm.
    f. Using the scale provided on the centrifuge or the microhematocrit card, read the results as a percentage (Figure 13-21). Allow the centrifuge to come to a complete stop before you open the lid.
    g. Dispose of contaminated materials properly. Dispose of capillary tubes in puncture-resistant disposable sharps container labeled Biohazard. Any sponges with blood on them must be disposed of in a container for biohazardous waste.

RATIONALE

Result indication:
There are enough RBCs present in the blood. Record the results as "normal."
There may not be enough RBCs; a hematocrit should be performed.
There are probably not enough RBCs present; a hematocrit should be performed.

The tube must be sealed to prevent blood leaking from the tube in the centrifuge. Sealing is not necessary when using a self-sealing microhematocrit tube.
This tube position prevents leakage of blood when the centrifuge is turned on.

Centrifuging the blood samples causes the RBCs to settle at the bottom of the capillary tube.

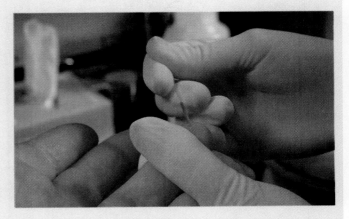

Figure 13-17 *Use a nonheparinized capillary tube to receive blood. Hold the tube horizontally to or slightly lower than the blood on the finger.*

RELATIVE DENSITY TEST—cont'd

PROCEDURE

11. Remove gloves.

12. Wash your hands.

13. Record the results.

A

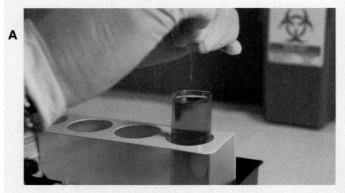

B

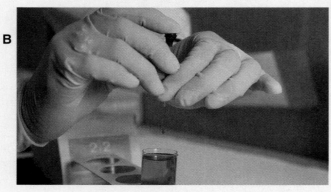

Figure 13-18 A, *Hold the capillary tube vertically over the container of copper sulfate to allow the blood to drop into the solution.* **B,** *Apply a capillary bulb to the tube if the blood does not drop into the solution, then squeeze the bulb to force blood into the solution.*

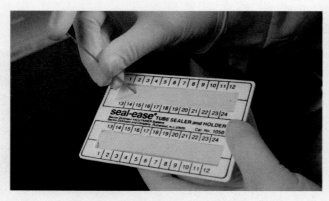

Figure 13-19 *For a hematocrit test, take the capillary tube filled with blood and seal the dry end with clay by sticking it into the clay tray.*

RATIONALE

Charting example:
    April 26, 19_____, 12 p.m.
        Skin puncture done on second finger, left hand. C_uSO_4
        test done, and hematocrit was indicated. Hct: 34%
            Anne Kaelberer, CMA
                                or
    CuS test indicated need for Hct.

    Hct: 34%

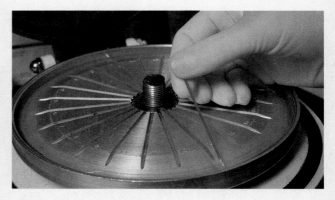

Figure 13-20 *Place tube into a slot in the microhematocrit centrifuge. The sealed end of the tube should face the outside of the centrifuge.*

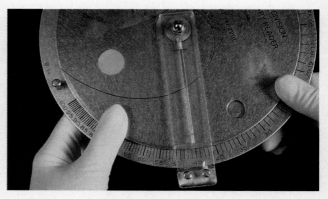

Figure 13-21 *Read the results, using the scale on the centrifuge or on a microhematocrit card or reader.*

BLOOD CHEMISTRIES

Some basic blood chemistries can be performed easily in the physician's office with the use of chemically impregnated reagent strips to determine the presence of blood glucose and blood urea nitrogen (BUN) (also see Table 13-2). (Blood glucose testing is more accurate than urine tests for glucose and is especially valuable in the management of diabetes.) In addition, there are compact and economical instruments on the market such as the *Ames Seralyzer Blood Chemistry Analyzer*. This instrument is a reflectance photometer that gives accurate quantitative results from blood serum or plasma for 15 routine diagnostic tests. Reflectance photometers measure light intensity to determine the exact amount of a substance present in a specimen. Blood chemistries, certain therapeutic drug assays (TDA), and electrolytes are determined using special reagent test strips. The blood chemistry analyzer is particularly useful in the physician's office when on-site testing is desirable so that test results can be viewed as an aid to prompt decision making, frequently while the patient is still in the office. Most tests require less that 15 minutes' elapsed time, averaging 2 minutes of operator time. Once the test strip is placed on the specimen table, you can read the test results on the digital display in less than 2 minutes. Complete instructions for specimen collection, preparation, and use are supplied with the instrument. *Always* check the expiration date on the container of reagent strips because outdated reagent strips may produce false or inaccurate test results.

Another easy-to-operate, in-office chemistry analyzer performing 16 tests using reagent strips is the *Reflotron* Plus System (Figure 13-22). The Reflotron Plus System has a keyboard for you to enter patient date and test information, and edit information to show patients how risks for certain conditions can be lowered by compliance with treatment recommendations. You place a drop of blood on the test pad on the reagent strip, insert the strip into the analyzer, and you have printed results in less than 3 minutes. The hard copy printer eliminates the change of transcription errors and simplifies record keeping. In addition, test profiles can be obtained (Figure 13-22, *C*). Profiles provide information on particular body system disorders or suspected conditions and also can be used for screening purposes or to monitor chronic conditions. Complete instructions come with the instrument, and you can call the manufacturer with questions you may have in reference to the testing procedures. (NOTE: In addition to performing blood chemistry tests, the Reflotron and other similar reflectance photometers give results for a hemoglobin test. The eliminates the tedious and less accurate manual procedures that have been used in the past (see also page 449, Hemoglobin).

BLOOD GLUCOSE
Test For Blood Glucose Using Dextrostix*

The Dextrostix is a reagent strip that measures blood glucose levels over a range of 45 to 250 mg/100 ml of blood (or 45 to

*Ames Co., Inc., Elkhart, Ind.

250 mg/dl). It is supplied in glass bottles that have a color chart on the side that is used for determining test results. Only fresh flood is to be used on these strips because plasma and serum give false results.

Procedure

1. Don single-use exam gloves.
2. Do a skin puncture on a fingertip. Allow a *large* drop of blood to form.
3. Place a large drop of blood on the test area of the strip. (This may be done by putting the strip on the blood over the puncture site.)
4. Wait 60 seconds exactly, holding the strip horizontally to avoid blood runoff from the test area.
5. Holding the strip vertically, wash the flood off, using a sharp stream of water from a wash bottle.
6. Compare the color on the test area with the color chart on the bottle. There are five color blocks representing 45, 90, 130, 175, and 250 mg/100 ml of blood.
7. Dispose lancet in puncture-resistant container used for sharps. Dispose test strip in container labeled "Biohazardous Waste."
8. Remove gloves.
9. Wash your hands.
10. Record the results.

NOTE: If you don't use enough blood, you will obtain lower values. If you overwash the strip, you can wash color off and obtain lower values.

To obtain more precise blood glucose results, the same manufacturer has marketed an instrument, the Eyetone Reflectance Colorimeter, to be used with the Dextrostix. From a precisely calibrated meter that covers the range of 10 to 400 mg/100 ml of blood glucose, rapid and accurate determination can be read. Complete instructions for use are provided with the instrument.

Blood glucose meters. There are many small, portable, easy-to-operate blood glucose meters on the market. Most use a specific reagent strip with a test pad area. When blood is applied to the test pad area, glucose in the blood reacts with the reagent in the test pad, and a color change occurs. This color change is read by the blood glucose meter as the concentration of glucose in the blood.

Timing of the test must be exact because both the amount of time the blood is on the test pad and the amount of glucose in the blood determine the test results. Newer meters begin timing automatically when blood is applied to the test pad, and/or they do not require wiping or blotting.

To obtain a blood sample, you need a lancet. There are many lancing devices on the market. The spring-loaded devices offer an advantage (that is, they provide a measured depth of lancet penetration for the finger puncture). Some manufacturers provide interchangeable endpieces that allow for different puncture depths (see Figure 13-14). You must not use endpieces or puncturing surfaces of the devices on more than one patient, or, if they are reusable, you must clean

Figure 13-22 A, *Reflotron Plus system;* **B,** *test results record;* **C,** *test profiles used to monitor chronic conditions.*
Courtesy Boehringer Mannheim Corp., Indianapolis, Ind.

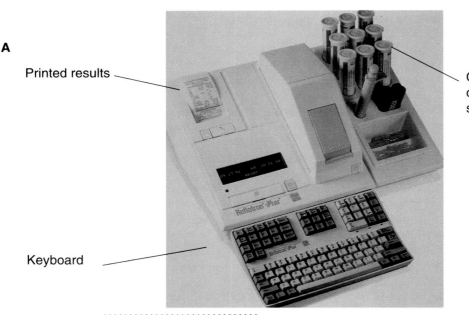

Test pad   Test strip

A

Printed results

Containers
of test
strips

Keyboard

16-test menu
Hemoglobin
Glucose
Cholesterol
Triglycerides
HDL
LDL (calculated)
Uric Acid
Bilirubin
SGPT (ALT)
SGOT (AST)
GGT
Amylase
BUN
Creatinine
Potassium
CK

B

```
******************************
09.17.93    AM    11:41:43
HEART HEALTH ASSESSMENT
        LOUIS KELLEY
******************************
CHOL        mg/dl   190.00
TG          mg/dl   150.00
HDL         mg/dl    38.00
SEX         M
AGE         45 years
SMOKING     No
DIABETES    No
CVD         Yes
ECG-LVH     No
SYSTOLIC    mmHg    145.00
DIASTOLIC   mmHg     98.00
LDL         mg/dl   122.00
CHOL/HDL RADIO       5.0
******************************
     FRAMINGHAM RISK
6 YR. CHD RISK       4.3%
RANGE        1.9% - 11.0%
CHD RISK MULT.       2.3
******************************
Hard  copy  test  results
```

An example of test results providing Heart Health Assessment which can be used to improve the effectiveness of your counseling efforts.

Run Total Cholesterol, Triglycerides and HDL Cholesterol tests.

Use the keyboard to input patient data at system prompt.

LDL and Total Cholesterol/HDL ratio calculated.

System calculates 6-year coronary heart disease (CHD) risk based on Framingham Study tables. CHD Risk Multiplier expresses patient risk in relation to the minimum risk (1.0) of the sex-related age group.

16-test menu makes it easier to monitor chronic conditions

C

Lipid/Coronary Risk	Total cholesterol	Gastrointestinal Disorders
Total cholesterol	HDL cholesterol	Amylase
HDL cholesterol	LDL (calculated)	Total cholesterol
Triglycerides	Uric acid	GGT
LDL (calculated)	Glucose	SGPT (ALT)
Diabetes	BUN	SGOT (AST)
Glucose	Creatinine	Bilirubin
Triglycerides	Anemia	Potassium
BUN	Hemoglobin	Renal Disease
Creatinine	Arthritis/Musculoskeletal Disease	BUN
Monitoring Hypertension Therapy	CK	Potassium
Potassium	Hemoglobin	Creatinine
Triglycerides	Uric acid	

them with a bleach solution before reuse. This practice is followed to avoid the spread of infection.

Use each lancet only once and then discard it in the container for disposable sharps. *As with all procedures involving blood or bodily fluids, it is essential to follow the Universal Precautions presented in Unit One of this textbook.*

There are specific operating instructions for *each* blood glucose meter. You must follow them precisely. Errors in technique or in use of the meter can cause inaccurate test results. Inaccurate readings are most often the result of operator error. Common errors include inaccurate timing, too much or too little blood, inaccurate calibration of the meter, and incorrect timing or method of wiping the blood from the reagent strip. These meters are designed for use with capillary (whole) blood; using venous blood or serum causes inaccurate readings. Other possible causes of inaccurate readings include a dirty meter, a outdated reagent strip, high altitudes, a high or low ascorbic acid blood level, and a high or low hematocrit. Remember that every instrument has limitations. If the blood glucose levels do not confirm other patient data, or when the results will have a critical impact on the physician's decision for treatment, a laboratory glucose level should be obtained.

Quality assurance is very important when using blood glucose meters. This includes regular cleaning and maintaining the instrument, and using control solutions periodically to test the accuracy of the meter.

Test For Blood Glucose Using The Accu-CheckIII and Chemstrip bG*

The Accu-Check III is a battery-operated meter used to measure blood glucose (sugar). Chemstrip bG test strips are "read" by the Accu-Chek III to determine blood glucose levels. The Accu-Chek III provides blood glucose readings between 20 and 500 mg/dl. The Chemstrip bG may also be read visually without using the Accu-Chek III. The results obtained will be very close to those you get when using the Accu-Chek III. This equipment can be used in the physician's office or by the patient at home (Figure 13-23, *A* to *C*). The purpose of testing with Chemstrip bG at home is to measure the amount of blood glucose in the blood. The results of this test help the patient determine how much insulin, food, and exercise are needed to control diabetes.

Equipment

Accu-Chek III Blood Glucose Monitor with a battery
Vial of Chemstrip bG 50's (Cat. No. 00502)
Alcohol swab
Lancet or automatic finger skin puncture device
Dry cotton or rayon ball
Disposable single-use exam gloves

*Courtesy Boehringer Mannheim Corporation, 1992. Accu-Chek and Chemstrip are registered trademarks of Boehringer Mannheim GmbH, Indianapolis, Ind.

Procedure for programming the Accu-Chek III

1. Open the box containing the vial of Chemstrip bGs. The box contains the package insert, a vial of 50 reagent strips, and a calibration strip that is wrapped in paper. Carefully remove the paper cover from the strip. This is the calibration strip that is used to program your Accu-Chek III meter for the new vial of strips. (Be sure that you are using Chemstrip bG 50, Cat. No. 00502.)
2. Compare the lot number on the calibration strip to the lot number on the side of the Chemstrip^R bG vial. These numbers must match exactly before proceeding to the next stop.
3. Now you must program the meter. The step *must* be performed whenever you open a new vial of Chemstrip bG 50 test strips. *Programming of the meter is required only once per vial of test strips.* The capacity for memory enables the meter to retain the calibration curve until it is reprogrammed for use with a different vial of strips.
4. To start, place the meter with a batter in place on a flat surface with the calibration slot toward you.
5. Press the ON/OFF button once to turn the Accu-Check III on.
6. Open door. Door is to the left of the display; press on outside left edge.
7. Insert code strip smoothly. Do not hesitate or pull back. Monitor beeps when code strip is in place. The code in the monitor display must match code on the vial of strips you are using. If not, repeat steps 6 to 8 with code strip that came with the test strips you are using.
8. Close the door.
   LEAVE THE CODE STRIP IN THE MONITOR. You can now turn the monitor off, or go on to do a test (see Figure 13-23).

Procedure for testing blood glucose with the Accu-Chek III

1. Turn the meter on by depressing the ON/OFF button once. The numeral "888" will appear on the display, followed by a three-digit code.
2. Lay an unused Chemstrip bG test strip on a flat work surface with the rest of the pads facing up.
3. Don gloves.
4. Do a skin puncture on the patient's fingertip using a lanced or an automatic finger-puncture device.
5. Lightly squeeze the fingertip, let go; repeat several times until a large droplet of blood has formed.
6. Lightly though the blood to the test pads on the Chemstrip bG strip. Make sure to cover both yellow and white squares completely. *Do not smear the blood.* Apply pressure over the puncture site with clean, dry gauze pad or cotton ball.
7. Immediately press the TIME button. The meter will count to 60.
8. During the displays of 57, 58, 59 the Accu-Chek III will emit three high beeps and, at 60, one low beep.
9. When the display reads 60 seconds, wipe the blood from the test pads with a clean, dry cotton ball using gentle pressure. Do not leave any blood on the test pads.

Figure 13-23 **A** *and* **B,** *Accu-Chek and Chemstrip bG companion system for blood glucose testing;* **C,** *Accu-Chek III test guide.*
Courtesy Boehringer Mannheim Corp., Indianapolis, Ind. Accu-Chek and Chemstrip are registered trademarks of Boehringer Mannheim GmbH).

A

Display Screen

Test Strip Guide

ON/OFF button

Time button

Door covering RCL, Beep and SET buttons

Battery Compartment on back

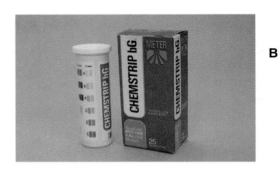

B

C

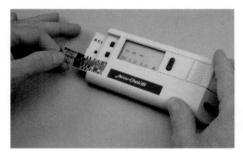

Insert code strip, pointed end first, as far as it will go.

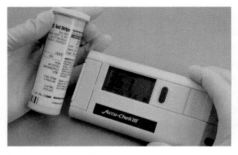

Turn monitor ON.
Check that code number in display matches code on test strip vial label.

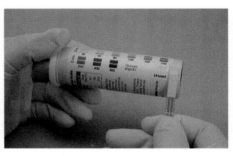

Remove unused test strip from vial and compare to "Unused" block on label. If strip pads are darker than label, follow directions in monitor *User's Manual.*

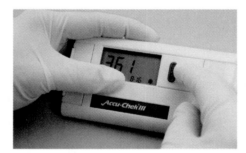

Press TIME button as soon as blood is on test strip.

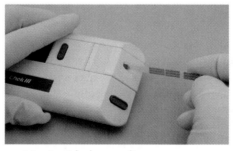

Insert test strip in monitor as soon as you wipe it. Result appears at 120 seconds.

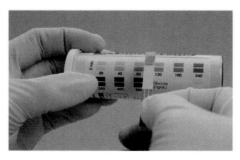

Compare colors on test pads to those on test strip vial label. If they do not agree, see "Problem Solving", page 18, in *Accu-Chek III User's Manual.*

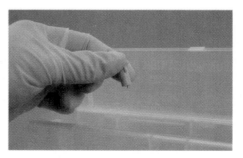

Carefully cover lancet and discard in a puncture-proof container.

10. The Accu-Chek III will continue to count to 120 seconds. While the meter is counting, turn the test strip on its side with the test pads *facing* the ON/OFF button, and insert the reacted test strip into the test strip adaptor. *The strip must be inserted before the display reads 120* (see Figure 13-23).

11. When the display reads 120, a high beep will be emitted, followed by the blood sugar value display in the milligrams per decaliter. Read the blood sugar value on the display screen.

    NOTE: If "HHH" appears on the display screen, the blood sugar level is over 500 mg/dl, or the strip was not prepared correctly. Wait an additional minute, then take the reacted test strip out of the meter and compare it to the color chart on the side of the Chemstrip bG vial to estimate results up to 800 mg/dl.

    If "LLL" appears on the display screen, the blood glucose value is lower than the reading range of the instrument (less than 10 mg/dl). Values below 20 mg/dl have not been confirmed clinically. Consult Troubleshooting Guide of the Accu-Chek III manual.

12. Record the test results.

13. Press the ON/OFF button to turn the Accu-Chek III off. Remove the test strip from the meter. Dispose of the lancet in biohazard container for used disposable sharps. Dispose of any sponge with blood on it and the test strip in container for Biohazardous waste.

14. Remove gloves and wash your hands.

How to change the battery in the Accu-Chek III monitor

1. Hold the Accu-Chek III face down in your hand.
2. Remove the battery compartment cover by placing your thumb on the grooved cover and sliding it toward you until it detaches from the instrument case.
3. Lightly press in and up on the edge of the battery to release it from the compartment. Tilt the instrument down until the battery slides out of the compartment.
4. Insert new battery, making sure the plus signs on the battery and monitor case match.
5. Place the battery compartment cover on the meter and snap it into place.

    NOTE: The compartment cover will not fit on the meter correctly if the battery is not inserted properly.

6. The meter will have to be reprogrammed before it is used.

How to clean the Accu-Chek III monitor

1. The outer casing may be wiped with a slightly dampened cloth and a *mild* household cleaning agent. Dry thoroughly. You should also clean the test strip guide each time you calibrate the meter.
2. Remove the guide from the meter by placing your thumb on the grooved surface above the test strip chamber and sliding the cover toward you. Slide the cover away from the meter.
3. Pinch together the two small black tabs located behind the beige chamber cover.

4. Slide the test strip guide out of the cover.
5. Clean the inner surfaces of the channel of the test strip guide with soap and water. You may scrub it with a toothbrush. Rinse and dry.
6. To disinfect it, soak for 2 minutes in 70% alcohol or a 1:10 solution of sodium hypochlorite (household bleach). Rinse guide in water and dry.
7. Also clean the window surfaces on the side of the guide. Air dry.
8. After the strip guide has dried completely, fold grey into black piece and replace in monitor. Slide test strip guide back into monitor until it snaps into place. (Be sure serial numbers on the strip guide and monitor match if you are cleaning more than one monitor).

Using the Glucose Control Solution

Glucose Control Solution should be used for the following reasons:

- To practice correct technique
- To check for test strip deterioration (vial left uncapped, exposed to excessive heat or cold)
- To verify the performance of the Accu-Chek III (results are lower or higher than expected and don't agree with how the patient feels)

Instructions (see Figure 13-23)

1. Place a drop of the Glucose Control Solution on the Chemstrip bG instead of blood. *Use only Glucose Control Solution designed for use with Accu-Chek III.*
2. Follow steps 7 through 13 of the blood-testing procedure.
3. Record your value and make sure it is within the control range listed in the package insert.

Reading the Chemstrip visually

1. Follow steps 2 through 6 of the Procedure for testing blood glucose with Accu-Chek III."
2. Immediately start timing for 60 seconds.
3. At the end of the first 60 seconds, using gentle pressure, wipe blood from the test pads with a clean, dry cotton ball. Put cotton ball in container for "Biohazardous Waste."
4. Now wait another 60 seconds.
5. Compare the two reacted colors on the test pads to the color chart on the Chemstrip bG vial.
6. If the test pad matches 240, wait an additional 60 seconds before making a final reading.
7. Sometimes the colors on the treated area of the test strip will match a color block on the chart exactly. Colors range from beige through various shades of blue and green. At other times, you will find that the reacted colors fall between color blocks.

For example:

The bottom (blue) square matches 180.
The top (green) square matches 240.
The results would be approximately 210.

$$180$$
$$\underline{+ \ 40}$$
$$420 \div 2 = 210 \text{ mg/dl}$$

8. NOTE: If the patient has eyesight problems, this test cannot be used by the patient without the use of the Accu-Chek III meter.
9. Continue with steps 12 through 14 under the section, Procedure for programming the Accu-Chek III.

How to avoid inaccurate readings

1. Always carefully place a large drop of blood onto the test pads of the Chemstrip bG. Do not smear or rub the blood into the test pads.
2. Always use a drop of blood that is large enough to adequately cover both test pads simultaneously.
3. Always use a cotton ball to remove blood from the test pads. Wipe the pads with two or three even strokes, using a clean area of the cotton ball.
4. Always use a watch with a second hand to monitor the reaction times.
5. Always discard Chemstrip bG test strips on the expiration date shown on the vial. Use of expired strips may result in inaccurate readings.
6. Always use the color chart from the vial that corresponds to the strips. Use of a different vial color chart may result in inaccurate readings.
7. Do not cut or alter the strips in any way.

Storage of the Chemstrip bG

Chemstrip bG may be damaged if the strips are exposed to heat, light, or moisture. You should follow these suggestions:

- Keep the Chemstrip bG strips in the original vial. Do not transfer the strips into any other container.
- Store at room temperature under 86° F (30° C). Do not freeze.
- Always keep the vial capped tightly.

How to tell if the Chemstrip bG has spoiled

1. Check the expiration date, which is stamped on the side of every vial.
2. Throw away any strips you still have after the expiration date.
3. If in doubt, replace the strips with a new vial of Chemstrip bG.

Test for Blood Glucose Using the One Touch Blood Glucose Meters Monitoring Systems

One Touch blood glucose meters are portable, battery-operated meters that are used with One Touch test strips to measure glucose concentrations in whole blood in a simple 45-second procedure (Figures 13-24 and 13-25). The *One Touch* meter provides blood glucose readings between 0 and 600 mg/dl (0 and 33.3 mmol/L). Higher values are displayed as HIGH. This equipment can be used in the physician's office or by the patient at home. The purpose of testing with the One Touch at home is to measure the amount of blood glucose in the blood. The results of this test help the patient determine how much insulin, food, and exercise are needed to control diabetes.

The new One Touch system makes reliable blood glucose monitoring easier than ever. With One Touch, results can be achieved by touching the reagent pad just once—to apply blood—because no wiping or blotting is required. One Touch eliminates three major stumbling blocks to reliable monitoring: starting the test, timing the test, and removing the blood. The opportunity for procedural error is virtually eliminated. To perform the test, insert the test strip into the meter, press the Power button, then apply a blood sample to the test spot on the reagent pad at any time. At this point the meter takes over, starting the test automatically when it detects blood on the reagent pad. No blood removal, timing, wiping, blotting, or washing is required. Test results appear in just 45 seconds. The One Touch meter provides a stable platform for the test strip while you are applying the blood sample. The test spot is smaller, so less blood is required and the wider test strip is easier to handle.

An added feature for convenience is that the One Touch system is the first to provide "conversational" messages in plain English to guide you through the test. Messages and results are shown on a large, easy-to-read display. With each test, numerous system self-checks are automatically performed to ensure that the meter is working properly. In addition, 250 previous results can be easily recalled from its memory.

See Figure 13-24 for the procedure for using the *One Touch Basic* blood glucose meter. Easy-to-follow prompts guide you through three simple steps. You see accurate results in just 45 seconds. See Figure 13-25 for the new *One Touch II* Meter. Accurate results are obtained in 45 seconds. Easy-to-read prompts in English, Spanish, or seven other languages guide you through the simple three-step procedure. The new One Touch II Meter detects most errors in blood sample size and application. It even notifies you when the meter must be cleaned. All of these meters are very easy to use in the physician's office or by the patient at home or work. When using these meters, you must read the Owner's Booklet for complete operating instructions and other important information.

All One Touch meters are supplied with an owner's booklet that provides detailed information and instructions for use.

Inaccurate test results may be obtained from the meters for any of the following reasons:

1. An inadequate amount of blood was placed on the test strip; the entire reagent pad must be completely covered.
2. The wrong test strips were used; *only* One Touch test strips can be used with the One Touch meters. Test strips must not be cut or altered in any way.
3. The One Touch test strips used were:
   a. Beyond their expiration date printed on each foil wrapper on the outer package label.
   b. Discolored before use (normal reaction pad is ivory-colored or light beige).
   c. Showing an abnormal color development during the test time (normal color development is blue/purple).
4. The One Touch test strip holder and window area are dirty.

Figure 13-24 *Abbreviated procedure, check strip procedure and steps for cleaning the One Touch Basic blood glucose monitoring systems.*
Courtesy Lifescan Inc., Mountain View, Calif.

ONE TOUCH®
BASIC™
BLOOD GLUCOSE MONITORING SYSTEM

Check Strip Procedure*

To check that the Meter is operating properly, the Check Strip must be used:
- At least once per day.
- After cleaning the Meter.
- If the Meter has been dropped.
- When results do not reflect how the user feels.
- When ✓ NOT OK REDO ✓ appears on the display.

STEP 1
Press On/Off Button.
- Last blood or Control Solution test result is displayed for 3 seconds.

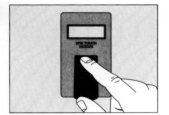

STEP 2
Insert Check Strip.
- While INSERT STRIP is displayed, insert Check Strip with Side 1 (purple) facing up.

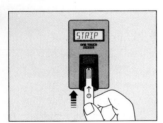

STEP 3
When APPLY SAMPLE appears, pull out the Check Strip.

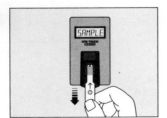

STEP 4
When INSERT SIDE 2 appears, turn the Check Strip over, with Side 2 (white) facing up, and insert Check Strip again.
- If ✓ 80 (example)
  ✓ OK

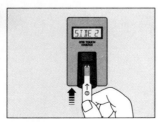
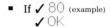

Cleaning the Meter*

STEP 1
Remove Test Strip Holder.

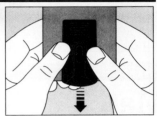

STEP 2
Wash and dry Test Strip Holder.

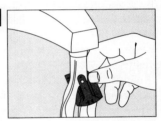

STEP 3
Clean Test Area. Use a cotton swab or soft cloth dampened with water to remove all blood, dirt, and lint from Test Area. **DO NOT USE:** Alcohol, cleansers with ammonia, glass cleaners, or abrasive cleansers.

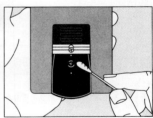

STEP 4
Dry Test Area with soft tissue or cloth. Remove any lint.

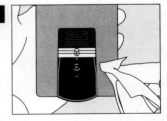

STEP 5
Replace Test Strip Holder.

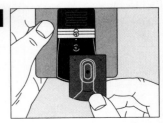

Figure 13-24—cont'd *Abbreviated procedure, check strip procedure and steps for cleaning the One Touch Basic blood glucose monitoring systems.*
Courtesy Lifescan Inc., Mountain View, Calif.

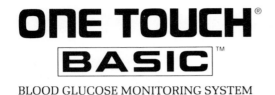

ONE TOUCH®
BASIC™
BLOOD GLUCOSE MONITORING SYSTEM

ABBREVIATED PROCEDURAL CHART*

STEP 1

Press On/Off Button.

- Last result, from either a blood glucose or Control Solution test, is displayed for 3 seconds.

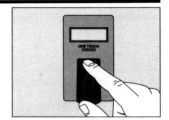

STEP 2

Match code numbers.

- Press C Button until code number on Meter <u>matches</u> code number on your current Test Strip package.

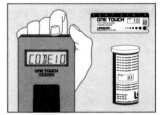

STEP 3

Insert Test Strip.

- While INSERT STRIP is displayed.

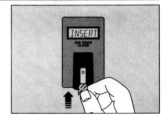

STEP 4

Obtain blood sample.

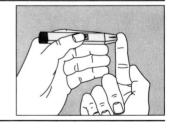

STEP 5

Apply blood sample to Test Spot.

- Check to make sure Meter is still on.
- Test Strip must be in Meter when you apply the blood.
- Blood should form a round, shiny drop and completely cover the Test Spot.

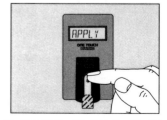

Figure 13-25 *One Touch II blood glucose meter.*
Courtesy Lifescan Inc., Mountain View, Calif.

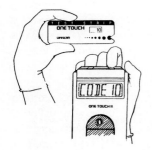

CODE and a number will appear on display. Press C Button until code number on Meter matches code number on your current Test Strip package.

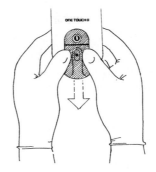

Hook bottom of Test Strip Holder to square notch at base of Meter. Push down on top of Holder until it snaps into place.

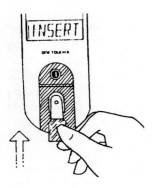

While INSERT STRIP is on the display, insert Test Strip with Test Spot facing up.

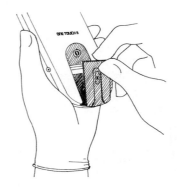

Remove Test Strip Holder. Place thumbs on raised dots. Slide Holder toward you to remove.

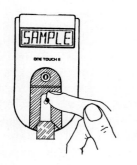

While APPLY SAMPLE is on the display and the Test Strip is in the Meter, apply blood sample to Test Spot. (NOTE: *Blood should form a round, shiny drop and completely cover the Test Spot.*)

5. The One Touch meter is out of calibration (for example, the calibration checkstrip result does not fall within the specified checkstrip range).
6. Inappropriate diagnostic use; One Touch test strips are for in vitro diagnostic use only.
7. Using the meter in intense direct sunlight may give low readings; shade the meter.

The Accu-Check III and the One Touch series of blood glucose meters are particularly valuable to diabetic patients who have to monitor their blood glucose levels closely. These meters can be used virtually anywhere. In many situations it is much easier for a person to obtain a small blood sample by a fingerprick than it is to obtain a urine sample. In addition a blood glucose level provides more accurate information than does a urine glucose level. Even the most accurate urine-testing method does not reflect the exact status of blood glucose at a given time. Factors that can affect urine tests include the ability of the kidneys to reabsorb glucose back into the bloodstream. Also, the urine may have passed from the kidney to the bladder hours before the urine is tested. Both of these situations would not reflect the correct blood glucose level. Urine tests also require you or the patient to compare colors on the test strip to colors on a color chart to determine the percentage of glucose. People with visual disturbances or color blindness cannot accurately use these methods and must rely on others to verify the results. The portable blood glucose meters eliminate these problems, and accurate results can be obtained.

Quality Assurance

Quality control is a key element of all laboratory tests. Quality assurance areas for blood glucose monitoring with *all* of the blood glucose meters include the following.

- Training and periodic retraining of both health care workers and patients who perform their own tests in techniques for obtaining a blood specimen and using the monitors.

*   Periodic verification with the laboratory of the accuracy of the meter.
*   Regular cleaning and maintenance of the monitor.

Quality control for the AccuMeter. Each cassette has two built-in controls to make sure it is working properly. The Test Working Indicator turns light purple as the reagents begin functioning. The Complete Indicator turns green when the test is complete. Both controls must work properly to ensure the validity of the test results.

Good laboratory practice recommends the testing of a control reagent each day that patients are tested. Each site should establish standards of performance.

AccuMeter Cholesterol Controls can be ordered from ChemTrak.

Troubleshooting. If you have any problems performing the ChemTrak AccuMeter Cholesterol Test, the suggestions below may be helpful.

IF	THEN
The cassette is cracked or otherwise damaged.	Do not use the cassette.
The Measurement Scale of the cassette is blue or yellow.	The cassette has been exposed to excessive moisture or heat and should not be used.
You are not sure if you have put enough blood into the Blood Well.	Add one or two more drops of blood. The blood must fill the well to the black circle. If it takes longer than 5 minutes to prick the finger and add blood, the results of the test may be erroneous.
You pulled the tab on the cassette without waiting 2 minutes after the addition of blood to the Blood Well.	Discard the cassette and start over. Put blood into the Blood Well, wait 2 minutes, and initiate the test by pulling the tab to the right until it clicks into place and the red line is visible.
The tab does not click into place after being pulled to the right.	The test will not start working until the tab shows the red line. Pull the tab again to the right.
After 20 minutes, the Test Working and/or the Complete Indicator(s) do not turn color.	The test result is not valid unless both internal controls function properly. Disregard the result. Discard the cassette and start over.
The matching *Cholesterol Result Chart* for the kit on hand is not available.	Use of an unmatched chart produces erroneous results. To obtain the matching *Cholesterol Result Chart*, call ChemTrak and specify the lot number of the AccuMeter Cholesterol Test on hand.

AccuMeter Cholesterol Test

The AccuMeter Cholesterol Test is a rapid, instrument-free enzyme assay for the in vitro quantitative determination of total cholesterol in whole blood. Cholesterol measurements are used in the diagnosis and monitoring of disorders involving excess cholesterol in the blood and of lipid and lipoprotein metabolism disorders. These conditions are often associated with coronary heart disease.

It is believed that lowering the mean value of cholesterol levels within the U.S. population will result in a reduction of the morbidity and mortality associated with coronary heart disease. This easy-to-use test system will assist medical professionals in the early identification and active monitoring of high-risk individuals.

Summary and Explanation of the Test

The AccuMeter Cholesterol Test is a fast, easy-to-use test system that combines the simplicity of visual result interpretation and proven enzymatic methods with the convenience of a cassette. The AccuMeter cassette is a self-contained chemical assay providing quantitative test results that are equivalent in accuracy, sensitivity, specificity, and reliability to complex, state-of-the-art, instrumented methods. The cassette combines a unique blood filtration device that separates plasma from RBCs and a mechanism that precisely meters sample volume. The assay is a solid-phase enzymatic method using a chromogenic complex for visual readout.

(A drop of fingerstick blood is put directly into the Blood Well near the bottom of the cassette [see figure]). After a few minutes, plasma is separated from whole blood by filtration. The tab is then pulled to initiate the reaction. Shortly thereafter the reagents start working, and a purple color appears in the Test Working Indicator. Over the next 15 minutes, a purple front advances up the Measurement Scale. The reaction is complete when a green color appears in the Complete Indicator. The test result is obtained by reading the height of the purple peak, as one would a thermometer, and determining the cholesterol concentration for a conversion chart.

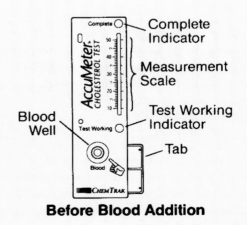

Before Blood Addition

AccuMeter Cholesterol Test

Equipment

Foil pouch containing an AccuMeter cassette and a desiccant packet
2 Lancet(s)
Alcohol pad

Gauze pad or clean tissues
Bandage
Procedure summary/Cholesterol result chart
Disposable single-unit exam gloves

PROCEDURE

1. Wash your hands. Use appropriate personal protective equipment (PPE) as dictated by facility.

2. Assemble and prepare equipment and supplies for use.

3. Identify the patient and explain the procedure.
   NOTE: IT IS *NOT* REQUIRED THAT THE PATIENT FAST FOR THIS TEST.

4. Have the patient seated for at least 5 minutes before taking the blood sample.

5. Don gloves. Perform a skin puncture on the fingertip. (See steps 1 through 11 in Fingertip Skin Puncture Using a Lancet, pages 427 and 428.) Use fresh whole blood obtained from a fingerprick. You need two or three large hanging drops for the test. You should complete fingerprick and blood addition within 5 minutes. Increase the blood flow to the fingers. Keep the hands below the heart, and warm them by gently rubbing or by using a warm compress.
   Choose the finger to be pricked. The ring or middle finger is recommended. *Avoid* pricking the center of the fingertip.
   Clean the chosen finger with alcohol and dry thoroughly with a sterile pad.

6. Wipe away the first blood with a sterile pad. Hold the puncture point downward. Gently massage the finger from the base to the puncture point. Apply pressure just below puncture point to form hanging drops of blood. Do not excessively squeeze the finger. If you have trouble making large drops, prick another finger.

7. Touch two to three hanging drops of blood to the bottom of the Blood Well. The Blood Well must be filled to the black circle. Do not worry about overfilling the Blood Well. For best results, add blood as quickly as possible. Do not take longer than 5 minutes to add the necessary amount of blood.
   It is essential that at least 2 to 3 large hanging drops of fingerstick blood ($\approx 40\mu l$) be added to the Blood Well. If sufficient blood cannot be obtained from the first fingerprick, a second finger should be pricked to complete the test.

RATIONALE

Sitting stabilizes the blood cholesterol.

Residual alcohol may interfere with the test.

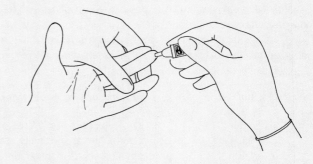

The first drop contains additional fluids from inside the finger. The blood that follows gives a more accurate result. Excessive squeezing and milking produce erroneous results. Hemolyzed samples should not be used. Residual alcohol may interfere with the test.

A low cholesterol value may be obtained if not enough blood is added to the cassette or if it has taken more than 5 minutes to add blood to the cassette.

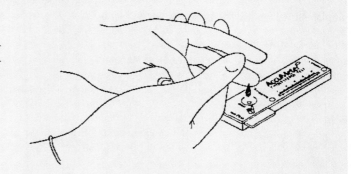

ACCUMETER CHOLESTEROL TEST—cont'd

PROCEDURE

8. WAIT 2 BUT NOT MORE THAN 4 MINUTES AFTER ADDING BLOOD BEFORE PULLING TAB.

9. Pick up the cassette in your left hand. Pull the tab firmly to the right with your other hand. Pull hard until the tab clicks into place. When the tab has been pulled out properly, a red line will be visible. The tab *can* be pulled very hard without breaking the tab or spilling blood.

10. Leave the cassette on a flat surface undisturbed for about 15 minutes. During the first few minutes, the Test Working Indicator will turn light purple. The test is complete and ready to read when the Complete Indicator turns green.

11. Read Results

Results are not valid unless the Complete Indicator is green and the Test Working Indicator is purple.

Read the result under good lighting. Find the peak of the purple color in the Measurement Scale. Read the peak at the farthest end of the color. The peak may resemble the tip of a feather. Read the mark to the left of the peak just as you would a thermometer. This is the test result number of the sample.

If an unusually low or high reading is obtained, repeat the test with a new cassette and a fresh fingerprick sample.

12. Evaluation of Results

The *Cholesterol Result Chart* is used to convert the color peak height to total cholesterol in milligrams per decaliter. Each *Cholesterol Result Chart* is specifically calibrated for the kit it accompanies. The lot number on the *Cholesterol Result Chart* must match the lot number of the cassette being used.

Find the test result number in the "Cassette Reading" column. Just to the right of the test result number on the chart is the cholesterol value of the sample.

RATIONALE

At least 2 minutes is needed for the blood to filter into the cassette.

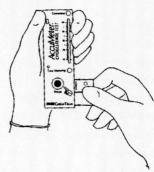

Samples must be obtained from free-flowing fingerstick blood.

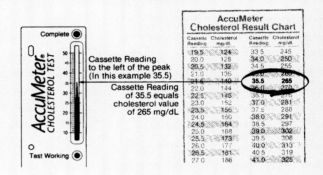

The test has been calibrated to measure cholesterol levels between 125 and 400 mg/dl. Patients with values below or above this level should be tested by another method. Elevated cholesterol levels should be confirmed by clinical laboratory method. Use of an unmatched chart produces erroneous cholesterol values.

Expected Values

The Expert Panel of the National Cholesterol Education Program (NCEP) has established guidelines for the Detection and Treatment of High Blood Cholesterol in Adults over 20 years of age to identify risk groups associated with various cholesterol levels. These levels are as follows:

NCEP Guidelines

Total Cholesterol	Classification
Less than 200 mg/dl	Desirable
200 to 239 mg/dl	Borderline high
240 mg/dl or greater	High

The Panel has made recommendations regarding the treatment of hypercholesterolemia. Recommendations include physician monitoring and changes in lifestyle to lower cholesterol values for individuals with values of 200 mg/dl or greater.

AccuMeter CHOLESTEROL TEST—cont'd

PROCEDURE

13. Dispose of contaminated materials properly. The used lancet should be placed in the disposable puncture-resistant sharps container. Place materials with blood on them in a container for "Biohazardous Waste."

14. Remove gloves.

15. Wash your hands.

16. Record the results.

RATIONALE

Charting example:
Dec. 22, 19_____, 2 p.m.
  Skin puncture done on second finger, left hand. AccuMeter Cholesterol test done. Results 186 mg.
    J.A. Lee, CMA

COMPLETE BLOOD COUNT: HEMATOLOGY TEST

Since the complete blood count (CBC) is the most common laboratory procedure ordered on blood, it is discussed more fully than other tests. A CBC gives a fairly complete look at the components in blood, providing a wealth of information on a patient's condition. The tests performed in a CBC include RBC count, hemoglobin (Hgb), hematocrit (Hct), WBC count, differential (Diff) white cell count, and a stained red cell examination (red cell morphology). The first four tests are quantitative measurements, and the last two are qualitative. All of these tests are performed on whole blood (Table 13-2).

RED CELL COUNT

The red cell count is the number of RBCs found in each cubic millimeter of blood. *Manual counting* may be used in some medical settings, but real care must be taken to minimize errors. *Determination with the automated counting equipment is considered more accurate.* Elevated red cell counts indicate polycythemia, or that the patient has moved to a location with a higher altitude where the air contains less oxygen. In the latter case, the body requires more red cells to carry sufficient oxygen to meet its needs. Decreased numbers of red cells are seen in patients with some form of anemia, after a hemorrhage, and also after the initial hemoconcentration of shock.

HEMOGLOBIN

A hemoglobin determines the oxygen-carrying ability of the blood. It is a simple and most efficient method to detect any

TABLE 13-2

Normal Values for a Complete Blood Count Performed on Whole Blood

Test	Values
Red cell count	
Females	4,000,000-5,500,000/ mm³ blood
Males	4,500,000-6,000,000/ mm³ blood
Hemoglobin	
Females	12-16 g/100 ml blood
Males	14-18 g/100 ml blood
Hematocrit	
Females	33% to 46%
Males	40%-54%
White cell count (females and males)	5000-10,000/mm³ blood
Differential	
Polymorphonuclear neutrophils	60%-70%
Monocytes	2%-6%
Lymphocytes	20%-40%
Eosinophils	1%-4%
Basophils	0.5%-1%
Morphology (stained red cell examination)	Normal

anemia (pernicious, iron deficiency, sickle cell) and the severity of the condition. It also helps the physician determine the effectiveness of treatments administered to the patient. A patient is considered anemic if the hemoglobin value is below 12 mg/100 ml. Low hemoglobin values are also caused by hemorrhage. Elevated concentrations of hemoglobin may be seen in severely burned or dehydrated patients. This is because the body has lost considerable amounts of fluid; thus the red cells are suspended in less fluid, and more hemoglobin is present in each 100 ml of blood.

HEMATOCRIT

The hematocrit, or packed-cell volume, represents the percentage of RBCs in the total blood volume. Elevated hematocrits are seen in patients with polycythemia; a low hematocrit is seen in anemia and leukemia. Generally the hematocrit and hemoglobin concentrations are related. Each 1% hematocrit contains 0.34 g of hemoglobin; the hematocrit should equal three times the hemoglobin within 3%. Thus, if a patient's hemoglobin is 14 g/100 ml, the hematocrit should fall between 39% and 45% ($14 \times 3 = 42$, and plus or minus 3 = 39% to 45%). Deviation from this relationship usually indicates the presence of red cells or abnormal size or hemoglobin content.

WHITE BLOOD CELL COUNT

The WBC count is the number of WBCs found in each cubic millimeter of blood. As with the red cell count, automated equipment now provides a more reliable count. A person's white count varies somewhat during a day because of exercise, emotional states, or digestion. Increases as great as 2000 WBC/mm^3 may be seen in these situations. Pathologically, the WBC count increases in infections and leukemia. Decreased WBC count may be caused by radiation therapy, immunosuppressive therapy (chemotherapy) for cancer and transplant patients, toxic reactions, measles, typhoid fever, and infection hepatitis. This is the result of a depression of the bone marrow's blood-forming centers.

DIFFERENTIAL WHITE CELL COUNT

The differential is a test that determines the percentage of each of the five different types of WBCs in the blood. Each type of white cell has a specific function. Together with the degree of increase or decrease in the total number of white cells and with the percentage of each type of white cell, the physician is able to make a more definite diagnosis. Characteristic abnormal numbers and types of white cells are seen in various diseases (Figure 13-26).

Neutrophils

The body's primary lines of defense against infection are the neutrophils. They seek and destroy any invading bacteria by the process of phagocytosis. Increased numbers of neutrophils are seen in conditions such as appendicitis, tonsillitis, pneumonia, abscesses, granulocytic leukemia, and meningitis. A decreased neutrophil count (neutropenia) is seen in mumps, hepatitis, measles, aplastic anemia, agranulocytosis, and also in patients who are taking certain drugs such as certain antibiotics, antihistamines, anticonvulsants, and sulfonamides. In these cases the decease in the neutrophils causes an increase in one of the other WBCs, especially in the lymphocytes. Thus one must know the actual value for each of the five types of WBCs to determine if this is the case.

Monocytes

The body's second line of defense against invasion by foreign substances is the monocytes. These are also phagocytes because they ingest any foreign particles or bacteria that the neutrophils are unable to. The monocytes also clean up any cellular debris that remains after an infection or abscess subsides. Increased numbers of monocytes are seen in patients who have tuberculosis, amebic dysentery, typhoid fever, Rocky Mountain spotted fever, subacute bacterial endocarditis, or monocytic leukemia or in those patients who are recovering from a bacterial infection. Conditions with decreased numbers of monocytes are difficult to indicate, since the normal count of the cells is so low.

Lymphocytes

The lymphocytes circulate through the body to destroy the toxic products of protein metabolism and to identify and produce antibodies against foreign cells. Recent studies are identifying new roles for these cells, especially in the field of immunology. Increased numbers of lymphocytes (lymphocytosis) are seen in viral diseases such as influenza, German measles, mumps, whooping cough, and infectious mononucleosis, as well as in lymphocytic leukemia. Decreased numbers are seen in patients who are taking cortisone, ACTH, and epinephrine. Other types of leukemia and radiation also cause lymphopenia.

Eosinophils and Basophils

Little is known about the eosinophils and basophils. It is thought that the eosinophils aid in detoxification by breaking down protein material and that they are associated with allergic reactions and production of antihistamine. Increased eosinophil counts are seen in patients who have hay fever, allergies, skin diseases, parasite infections, and asthma. Deceased counts are seen in patients who have increased levels of insulin, epinephrine, and ACTH. Stress following surgery may also cause eosinopenia.

Basophils are thought to produce heparin and histamine; thus some believe that they help prevent blood from clotting in inflamed tissues and play a role in clot breakdown. Increased basophil counts are seen in patients who have hemolytic anemias or chronic granulocytic leukemia and who have had their spleen removed (splenectomy) and exposure to radiation. Decreased conditions have not been identified.

ABNORMAL WHITE CELLS

The five types of white cells just discussed are all normal cells found in peripheral blood. In some disorders and diseases, immature neutrophils or atypical lymphocytes are seen. The immature neutrophils are myeloblasts, promyelocytes,

Figure 13-26 *Main types of leukocytes.* **A,** *Granulocytes-neutrophils: segmented neutrophils are round or oval cells. The cytoplasm is a lavender or pink color, with pinkish or lavender granules. The nucleus is segmented, having from two to 12 segments, but usually three or four, and it stains a purplish or lavendar color.* **B,** *Stab neutrophils are round or oval, with a cytoplasm similar in color to that of the segmented neutrophils. It contains fine granules that are pinkish or reddish violet. The nucleus is one continuous piece that looks like a flexible rod. It commonly forms letter shapes such as* **C, N,** *and* **U.** *The nucleus is colored a dark purple or lavender and occupies about one fourth of the cell.* **C,** *Juvenile neutrophils are round or oval, and cytoplasm is ususally a bluish pink, containing granules that may be definite or fine and of a purplish or reddish color. The nucleus is bean shaped, usually purplish in color, and usually occupies about half the cell (juvenile neutrophil also appears at bottom of panel B). Not shown, myelocyte neutrophil cytoplasm often takes an almost neutral stain, tinged with blue; and it, as well as the nucleus, is dotted with definite pinkish or purple granules. The nucleus is round or oval, ordinarily stains bluish purple, and takes up about two thirds of the cell.* **D,** *Granulocytes-eosinophils. Eosinophil cytoplasm has light blue tinges and is covered with coarse, round, or oval bright pink or red granules. The nucleus is usually segmented and stains a deep lavender to light blue.* **E,** *Lymphocyte cytoplasm is usually a bright blue and at times may be almost negligible, as the purple or lavender nucleus may take up almost the entire cell. Immature lymphocytes are larger than mature cells, having much more cytoplasm, which generally stains a very pale, glasslike blue. Occasionally a few pink granules may appear in the cytoplasm. The nucleus is usually round or oval but may be indented as well. It stains a purple or lavender color.* **F,** *Monocytes are the largest of all the white cells. Often they are quite irregular in shape and usually take a pale stain. The cytoplasm is usually a smoky blue-gray, sometimes sprinkled with a fine pink dust. The nucleus generally is kidney shaped or round, often lobulated, staining a lavender color.*

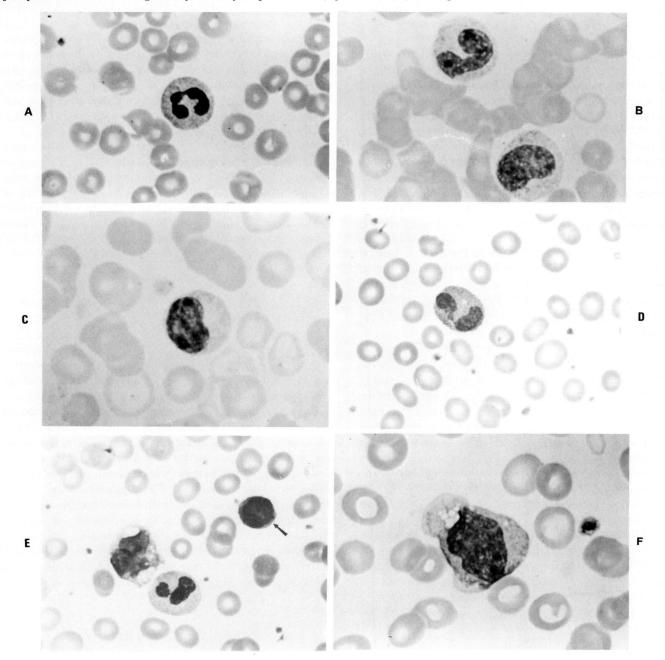

myelocytes, metamyelocytes, and band cells. You will see these terms on some laboratory reports included with a differential report.

STAINED RED CELL EXAMINATION

Using the same stained slide that was used for determining the differential, the laboratory technologist then examines the RBCs for any variation in size, shape, structure, color, or content. Anisocytosis, macrocytosis, microcytosis, and poikilocytosis are reported as slight, moderate, or marked.

SUMMARY

As you can see, the significant findings obtained from a CBC are numerous. Evaluation of these findings, along with the total clinical picture of a patient's condition, provides the physician with valuable information for screening, diagnosing, treating, or evaluating and monitoring the progress of treatment for patient care.

BLOOD GROUPS AND TYPES

Blood group and blood typing is the classification of blood on the basis of the presence or absence of antigens on the surface of the RBCs. The presence or absence of these antigens is determined by the individual's inherited genetic code. Several different blood groups have been identified. The importance of the blood groups depend on their clinical significance in maternal-fetal compatibility, blood transfusion therapy, organ transplantation, disputed paternity cases, and genetic studies. The two most routinely used systems for blood grouping and typing are the ABO system and the Rh factor or type. The ABO blood group is identified by the presence or absence of the A antigen and/or the B antigen on the surface of the RBC. The four blood types in this blood grouping are determined by and named for these antigens. They are type A, B, AB, and O. Corresponding antibodies, anti-A and anti-B agglutinins, can also be found in the plasma of some blood types (see Tables 13-3 and 13-4).

The Rh factor is an antigenic substance that is present in the RBCs of most people. Someone who has the Rh factor is referred to as Rh positive (Rh1); those that lack the factor in their RBCs are referred to as Rh negative (Rh2). 85% of the population is Rh1 . Rh stands for *Rhesus*. Because the Rh factor was discovered during studies on Rhesus monkeys in 1940, the factor was named using the first two letters of the word *Rhesus*.

Blood transfusions depend on the blood being classified as either Rh positive or Rh negative, and the ABO blood type classification. When receiving blood, it is vital that the recipient receive compatible blood (that is, blood that is the same type that the recipient has). If this does not occur, an antigen-antibody reaction can occur that could be harmful to the recipient. The reaction could result in mild to serious illness, anaphylaxis with severe intravascular hemolysis, or even

death. To safeguard against a reaction, donor blood is crossmatched (when time permits) with the recipient's blood to ensure that the two are compatible.

All pregnant women should have ABO and Rh typing performed during pregnancy. If the mother's blood is Rh2 further tests should be performed, and the father's blood type should be determined. If the father's blood is Rh1 , the mother's blood should be examined for the presence of Rh antibodies by the indirect Coombs test (see Table 13-2). If the first test is negative, it should be repeated at weeks 30 and 36 of pregnancy. If these results are negative, no risk is involved to the fetus. If the test results are positive, the Rh antibodies may find their way over to the fetus's circulation and cause hemolysis of the fetal RBCs. This causes what is commonly referred to as hemolytic disease of the newborn (HDN). To determine the severity of the hemolytic anemia in the fetus, an amniocentesis can be performed. The amniotic fluid is evaluated for the quantity of bilirubin present.

It is also important in pregnancy to identify cases in which the mother is Rh2 and the father is Rh1 . In these situations the mother should receive an injection of RhoGam (Rh immunoglobulin) within 72 hours of each delivery to prevent any fetal hemolytic problems in subsequent pregnancies. RhoGam prevents the mother's system from making Rh antibodies after the delivery.

In the medical laboratory, trained laboratory technologists can determine a person's blood type by doing either a slide test or a test tube test using commercially prepared antiserum. At times you may be required to obtain the blood specimen to be tested. In this case you should collect approximately 7 to 14 ml of venous blood in a red-top tube. Some laboratories may also want 5 ml collected in a lavender-top tube. (This may vary among laboratories.) Eating and drinking do not affect this test.

AUTOMATION IN THE CLINICAL LABORATORY

Within the past 20 to 25 years, clinical laboratories have been confronted with an ever-increasing workload. An answer to this problem has been sought in automated instrumentation. These specialized modular systems *automate* or *semiautomate* the time-consuming, step-by-step procedures formerly performed by manual analysis. With refinement of instrumentation, fast and accurate methods have been developed for reporting a wide variety of laboratory information on body fluids, which include whole blood, plasma, serum, urine, and cerebrospinal fluid. The human element of error is virtually eliminated, ensuring the absolute objectivity of measurement so important to accurate diagnosis and monitoring. *Multiphasic tests or test panels or profiles* consist of a battery of automated tests performed on the same specimen at the same time. It has been found that it is more useful and economical to subject every specimen to a battery or panel of automated tests than to limit the examination to one or two tests. Through this system of routine total blood counts and biochemical profiling, additional disease screening tests may be routinely performed. Most hematology panels in laboratories that have any volume at all are done on the Coulter systems or other systems such as the Technicon H-2. There are several different machines; most of them automate or at least semiautomate the whole process, using only 1 ml of blood. Tests results are obtained visually on a digital display or video screen or on a hematology printout card (Figures 13-27 to 13-

30). The latest state-of-the-art systems use laser technology. Laser counters in hematology such as the ELT-8 perform an automated CBC. The laser looks at the cells to determine the results. Traditionally the chemistry sections of laboratories are the most heavily automated. Most laboratories have at least some form of automation in chemistry if not in other departments. Frequently used biochemical panels are the SMA 12/60, SMA 18, SMA 20, SMAC 20 or 24. SMA stands for sequential multiple analysis, the C indicates that it is computer-assisted, and the numbers indicate the number of

Text continues on page 462.

Figure 13-27 *COULTER STKS, a fully automated hematology system for CBCs and white cell differentials. In addition to WBC data, the STKS reports comprehensive RBC and platelet profiles with histograms. In all, 20 parameters are provided.*

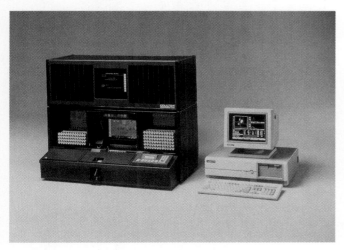

Figure 13-28 *The JT3 System provides a fully automated CBC, including the Coulter Histogram Differential with interpretive report, plus complete platelet and RBC profiles. Manual differentials are reduced by as much as 80%. Ideal for low-to-medium volume laboratory.*
Courtesy Coulter Corp., Miami, Fla.

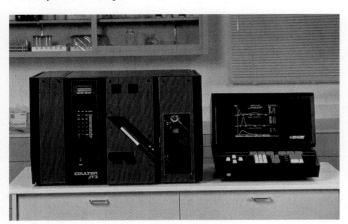

Figure 13-29 **A,** *Automated flow cytometry system capable of processing samples at rates greater than 100 samples per hour. The system has an automated sample preparation, a multi-sample autoloader and a high-speed flow cytometer.* **B,** *Histogram and report from the automated flow cytometer.*
Courtesy Coulter Corp., Miami, Fla.

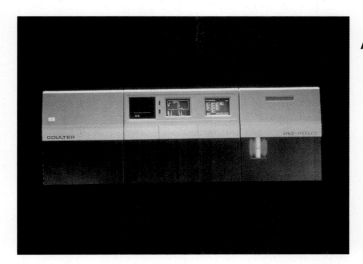

A

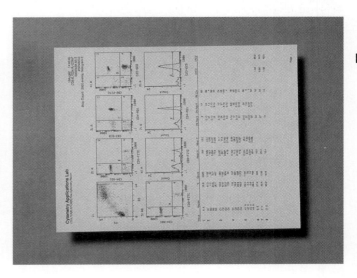

B

TABLE 13-3

Examinations Made on Blood

Test	Performed on	Normal Values*	Significance
Hematology blood tests			
1. Sedimentation rate (sedrate or ESR)	Whole blood	Wintrobe tubes: Female: 0-20 mm/hr Male: 0-9 mm/hr Wester: Female and male: 0-20 mm/hr	Increased in almost all infections, myocardial infarction, active rheumatoid arthritis, pulmonary infarction, shock, surgical operations, and pregnancy. Decreased in sickle cell anemia, polycythemia, cardiac decompensation, and newborn infants.
2. Microhematocrit (MCHC)	Whole blood	32%-36%	Same as for regular hematocrit.
3. Reticulocytes (immature RBC's)	Whole blood	0.5%-1.55% of all RBCs in peripheral whole blood	Increased when bone marrow is manufacturing RBC's at an increased rate. May be seen in patients with acute or chronic hemorrhage, or in sickle cell anemia. Normally elevated in infants and pregnant women. Decreased in aplastic and pernicious anemia.
4. Coagulation tests and platelets a. Bleeding time	Capillary whole blood	1-3 min	Increased time indicates platelet deficiency, which may be due to pernicious anemia, aplastic anemia, acute leukemias, hemorrhagic disease of the newborn, multiple myeloma, chronic lymphocytic leukemia, and Hodgkin's disease.
b. Clot retraction time	Venous blood	30-60 min	Prolonged time seen in primary or secondary thrombocytopenia due to aplastic or pernicious anemia, Hodgkin's disease, multiple myeloma, acute leukemia, and hemorrhagic disease of the newborn.
c. Coagulation or clotting time	Blood	Lee-White: 6-10 min Capillary tube: 3-7 min	Used as a measurement of the bility of blood to clot properly. May indicate that vitamin K or calcium levels are inadequate for clotting of blood.
d. Fibrinogen (quantitative)	Blood plasma	200-600 mg/100 ml	Increase seen in inflammatory processes, infections, pregnancy, menstruation, and after x-ray treatment. Decreases noted in liver diseases, anemia, and severe malnutrition.
e. Platelet count	Whole blood	200,000-400,000/mm³ blood	Decreased numbers may indicate disease of the spleen; also will cause bleeding.
f. Thromboplastin test	Whole blood	Abnormal thromboplastin formation	This test is used to differentiate blood coagulation abnormalities.

5. Prothrombin time (PT or Pro-Time)	Blood serum	70%-110% of control value	Prolonged time may indicate vitamin K deficiency, liver disease, or an excessive use of dicumarol in treatment. When anticoagulation therapy used, PT kept at from 2 to 2 1/2 times normal.
Blood chemistries			
1. Calcium (Ca++)	Blood serum	9-11.5 mg/100 ml or 9-11.5 mg/dl	Increased in chronic nephritis with uremia, bone tumors including metastatic cancer of bone, hyperparathyroidism, Addison's disease, adenoma of parathyroids, emphysema, cardiac decompensation.
2. Inorganic phosphorus (Inor phos)	Blood serum	3-4.5 mg/100 ml or 3-4.5 mg/dl	Increased in uremia, Bright's disease, excessive vitamin D intake, and hypoparathyroidism.
3. Glucose	Blood serum	80-120 mg/100 ml	Increased in diabetes mellitus. Decreased in hypoglycemia and after excessive insulin.
4. Blood urea nitrogen (BUN)	Blood serum	10-20 mg/100 ml or 10-20 mg/dl	Increased in some kidney diseases, for example, glomerulonephritis, pyelonephritis, acute tubular necrosis, and urinary obstruction from a tumor or stones. Also increased in dehydration, gastrointestinal bleeding, shock, and gout. Decreased levels seen in liver damage, malnutrition, protein deficiency, and overhydration.
5. Uric acid	Blood serum	2.5-8 mg/100 ml or 2.5-8 mg/dl	Increased in leukemia, gout, acidosis, toxemia, alcoholism, stress, lead poisoning, renal failure, diabetes mellitus.
6. Cholesterol	Blood serum	Up to 20 yr.: 120-230 mg/100 ml or mg/dl 30 yr.: 120-240 mg/100 ml or mg/dl 40 yr.: 140-240 mg/100 ml or mg/dl 50 yr.: 150-240 mg/100 ml or mg/dl 60 yr.: 160-240 mg/100 ml or mg/dl 100 yr.: 160-240 mg/100 ml or mg/dl	Increased in cardiovascular disease, atherosclerosis, liver disease with obstructive jaundice, nephrosis, diabetes mellitus, hypothyroidism, and in diets too high in saturated fat or cholesterol. Decreased in anemia, malabsorption, hyperthyroidism, and hepatic failure.

For many years, laboratories have reported a number of their test results in milligrams (mg) percent, or milligrams (mg) per 100 milliliters (ml) or 100 cubic centimeters (cm³). A newer method, used by many, is the use of a deciliter (dl); 1 dl = 0.1 L or 100 ml or 100 cm³. Thus in a report, mg/dl is the same as mg% or mg/100 ml. Keep in mind that test values may differ, depending on the methods and procedures used by the laboratory.

Table 13-3—cont'd

Examinations Made on Blood

NATIONAL GUIDELINES

Desirable: less than 200 mg/dl
Borderline High: 200 to 239 mg/dl
High: 240 mg/dl or higher.
Most physicians recommend that patients with levels higher than 200 take steps to reduce cholesterol to reduce the risk of coronary artery disease.

BLOOD LIPIDS, LIPID PROFILE

- Total lipids.
  400 to 1000 mg/dl
- Cholesterol:
  150 to 250 mg/dl
- Triglycerides:
  40 to 150 mg/dl
- Phospholipids:
  150 to 380 mg/dl
- Cholesterol lipoproteins:
  HDL: 45 mg/dl (men)
       55 mg/dl (women)
  VLDL: 25% to 50%
  LDL: 60 to 180 mg/dl

Increased LDL levels have been associated with coronary artery disease.
Increased HDL levels suggests a decreased risk of coronary artery disease.
These tests are also used to help determine dietary treatment for heart patients.

7. Total protein (TP)	Blood serum	6.0-8.0 g/100 ml or 6-8 g/dl	Increased in dehydration, malignancy, hepatic disease, infection. Decreased levels in overhydration, hepatic insufficiency, burns, malnutrition, nephrosis.
8. Albumin (Alb)	Blood serum	3.5-5.5 g/100 ml or 3.5-5.5 g/dl	Increase seen in dehydration. Decreased in overhydration, hepatic insufficiency, malnutrition, burns, nephrosis.
9. Total bilirubin (indirect)	Blood serum	0.2-1.2 mg/100 ml or 0.2-1.2 mg/dl	Increase seen in hemolysis, hepatic disease, obstructive jaundice, pulmonary infarct.

10. Alkaline phosphatase (Alk phos)	Blood serum	2-4.5 Bodansky units 4-13 King Armstrong units 20-90 IU/L	Increased in children and in women in the third trimester of pregnancy; in hepatic disease, obstructive jaundice, bone growth, osteoblastic bone tumors, peptic ulcer, and colitis. Decreased in hypothyroidism, anemia, malnutrition, pernicious anemia.
11. LDH (Lactic dehydrogenase)	Blood serum	90-200 IU/L	Increased in myocardial infarction, muscle necrosis, hemolysis, kidney infarct, liver disease, and cerebral damage.
12. AST (serum aspartate aminotransferase) formerly SGOT (serum glutamic oxaloacetic transaminase)	Blood serum	10-49 IU/L or 12 to 36 U/ml	Very high levels seen 24 hr after a myocardial infarction, in liver disease, complete biliary obstruction and jaundice with hepatic cirrhosis. Increased in skeletal trauma, hemolysis, cerebral damage. Lower levels seen in pregnancy, chronic dialysis, beri beri.

SMA 12/60 includes the preceding 12 chemistry tests

13. Serum alanine aminotransferase (ALT) formerly serum glutamic pyruvic transaminase (SGPT)	Blood serum	5 to 35 IU/L	Increased in liver dysfunction. AST and Alt levels are frequently compared. The AST/ALT ratio is usually greater than 1 in alcoholic cirrhosis, metabolic tumor to the liver, and liver congestion. Ratios below 1 may occur in patients with viral hepatitis, acute hepatitis, and infectious mononucleosis.
14. Serum phosphate (phosphorus)	Blood serum	Adults: 2.5 to 4.5 mg/dl Children: 3.5 to 5.8 mg/dl	Increased in renal failure, hypoparathyroidism, or increased dietary intake. Decreased in inadequate dietary intake, chronic antacid ingestion, hyperparathyroidism, and hypercalcemia.

Table 13-3—cont'd

Examinations Made on Blood

Test	Performed on	Normal Values*	Significance
15. Potassium	Blood serum	23.5 to 5.5 mEq/L	**Increased** in internal bleeding, renal failure, cell damage, acidosis, and Addison's disease. **Decreased** in chronic stress, diuretic administration, severe burns, diarrhea, starvation, pyloric obstruction, severe vomiting, liver disease, and malabsorption.
16. Chloride	Blood serum	96 to 110 mEq/L	**Increased** in anemia, eclampsia, dehydration, hyperventilation, and Cushing's syndrome. **Decreased** with severe vomiting, severe diarrhea, severe burns, ulcerative colitis, and pyloric obstruction.
17. Triglycerides	Blood serum	40-140 mg/100 ml or 40-140 mg/dl	Increased in diets too high in saturated fat or cholesterol. High level is a risk factor for heart attack. Decreased in anemia.
18. CPK (creatine phosphokinase)	Blood serum	1-10 U 0.2 to 1.42 U (two methods)	Increased in myocardial infarction, pulmonary edema, pulmonary infarction, DTs, and muscular dystrophy.
19. Creatinine	Blood serum	0.7-1.7 mg/dl	Increased in nephritis and impaired kidney function.
20. Icterus index	Blood serum	3-8 U	Used to discover early jaundice and for a liver function test.
Serology (Certain special blood tests are covered in this item)			
1. STS (serologic test for syphilis) includes;			
a. Fluorescent treponemal antibody (FTA)	Blood serum	Negative	
b. Rapid plasma reagin (RPR)	Blood serum	Negative	Used to confirm diagnosis of syphilis if VDRL or RPR is positive.
c. VDRL (Venereal Disease Research Laboratory)	Blood serum or plasma	Negative	Both are screening tests for syphilis. Sometimes false positive results are obtained. Positive results confirmed with the FTA.
2. Special human antibodies a. Coombs direct	Blood serum	Negative	Used to test newborn's blood for erythroblastosis fetalis. Also used in blood cross matching.

b. Coombs indirect	Blood serum	Negative	Used to detect blood incompatibilities when cross matching; also to detect Rh incompatibility in maternal blood before delivery by demonstrating anti-Rh antibodies.
c. Heterophil antibody (MonoSpot test)	Blood serum	Concentrated to 1/28	Elevated in infectious mononucleosis and serum sickness.
d. LE test (lupus erythematosus)	Whole blood	Negative	A slide test for antinucleoproteins found in systemic LE.
3. Bacterial and viral antibodies			
a. ASO (antistreptolysin) titer	Blood serum	To 400 U/ml	Increased values seen in rheumatic fever, and acute glomerulonephritis caused by hemolytic streptococcus.
b. Bacterial agglutinations Dysentery Brucellosis Paratyphoid A & B Typhoid O & H Typhus fever Leptospirosis	Blood serum	No agglutination	Certain infections caused by viruses, bacilli, rickettsiae, and spirochetes, produce antibodies in the serum, which in turn cause agglutination (clumping) of these organisms.
c. Widal test	Blood serum	Negative	A test to diagnose typhoid and paratyphoid fevers.
4. Rheumatoid factors			
a. Latex slide agglutination	Blood serum	1:40 is uppermost serum dilution	Positive in rheumatoid arthritis and in some connective tissue diseases.
b. RA (rheumatoid arthritis) test	Blood serum	Negative	Results positive in 85%-90% of patients with rheumatoid arthritis.
Thyroid function			
1. T_3 uptake (resin uptake/radioassay)	Blood serum	25%-35%	Increased in hyperthyroidism; decreased in hypothyroidism.
2. T_4 total thyroxin radioimmunoassay (T_4/RIA)	Blood serum	5.2-12.2 mg/dl	Decreased level of T_3 and increased level of T_4 if a woman is taking birth control pills. The free thyroxin index is done in this case to confirm normal thyroid function.

Table 13-3—cont'd

Examinations Made on Blood

Test	Performed on	Normal Values*	Significance
3. T₃; T₄ ratio	Blood serum		
4. Free thyroxin index (includes total T₄)	Blood serum	0.5-1.7	
Other tests			
1. Glucose tolerance test (standard test)	Blood serum	(Results per 100 ml blood) Fasting blood glucose: 80 mg – 120 mg After ingesting test doses of glucose: 30 min – 150 mg 60 min – 135 mg 2 hr – 100 mg 2 1/2 hr – 80 mg	Used to detect abnormalities in carbohydrate metabolism such as occur in diabetes mellitus, hypoglycemia, and adrenocortical and liver dysfunction. In diabetes, fasting blood sugar (FBS) is around 120 mg/100 ml or higher. After 1 hr, level rises over 180 mg/100 ml, and does not return to normal in 2 and 3 hr specimens. Normally blood sugar will return to normal after 2 hr.
2. Glucose tolerance sum (GTS)			In older patients, diabetes is sometimes hard to diagnose. Some physicicans will use the GTS. They will add the FBS, 1/2 hr, 1 hr, and 2 hr values obtained from the glucose tolerance test. If the sum of these values is less than 500 mg, the patient is not considered diabetic. When the sum is over 800 mg, the patient is considered diabetic.. Various other tests will be done to confirm this diagnosis and rule out liver disease, chronic diseases, or potassium depletion.
3. Blood culture	Sample of blood grown on culture media	No growth after incubation period	Growth on culture media indicative of blood stream infection or septicemia.
4. Bone marrow	Marrow aspirated from iliac crest or sternum, then placed on a slide and stained for examination	Various primitive cells are found	Abnormal cell findings may indicate a blood disorder such as leukemia.

Test	Specimen	Normal Values	Significance
5. Blood typing	Whole blood or blood serum	One of the following: Type O-45% of the population (Universal donor) Type A-40% of the population Type B-10% of the population Type AB-5% of the population (Universal recipient) And either: Rh positive-85% of population Rh negative-15% of population	Must be done before a patient receives a blood transfusion, to ensure a compatible transfusion; also important in pregnancy to help prevent erythroblastosis fetalis.
6. Radioimmunoassay for serum pregnancy or HCG Beta subunit for pregnancy	Serum Serum or plasma Serum	Quantitative results: 1st wk: 20-60 mIU/ml 2nd wk: 60-200 mIU/ml 3rd wk: 200-2000 mIU/ml 2nd or 3rd mo: 20,000-200m000 mIU/ml 2nd trimester: 12,000-60,000 mIU/ml 3rd trimeser: 10,000-30,000 mIU/ml	Results reported as either positive or negative for pregnancy. A result of 5-15 mIU/ml may indicate an ectopic pregnancy. A result of less than 5mIU/ml would be considered negative for an ectopic pregnancy.
7. HIV antibody for AIDS NOTE: In many states it is a state regulation that the patient must sign a consent form before this test is performed.		Negative	A negative result indicates that the antibody is not in the blood. A positive result indicates that the antibody is in the blood.
8. Hepatitis B surface antigen and hepatitis B core antibodies		Negative	The surface antigen test (HBsAg) is used to determine if a person is a carrier of the hepatitis B virus. The test for antibodies shows when there is active virus replication and may sometimes be detectable when the surface antigen is not.

TABLE 13-4

ABO Blood Groups

Blood Type	Antigen Present on the Red Blood Cell	Antibody Present in the Plasma
Group A	A	B
Group B	B	A
Group AB Universal rcipient	A,B	None
Group O Universal donor	None	A,B

tests that are performed. Another panel is simply called a Chemistry Screening Panel 12, 20, or 24. The numbers indicate how many tests are to be performed. These are general terms that are used; the type of tests run in these panels vary with the laboratory and how they have programmed the automated equipment for use. All of these panels are screening

devices that allow the physician to focus on abnormal results for further study and investigation. Test results from the SMA systems are reported on an $8^1/_2$ 3 11–inch sheet of pre-calibrated vertical graph paper called a serum chemistry graph (SCG), on an SMA 12, or on a similar horizontal graph for the other systems (Figures 13-31 to 13-33). Rather than sending the physician the graph paper, many laboratories now have special computer printout forms that also record the results of the tests performed. The laboratory keeps the graph as its permanent record and sends the computer printout to the physician. One example of the computer forms used is a sheet divided into columns. In different columns the names of the tests, the normal values, and the results of the tests performed are recorded (see Figure 13-33).

Many *multiphasic tests, panels, or profiles* are devised to provide information on particular body system disorders or suspected conditions and also for screening purposes, some of which include a hepatobiliary profile, diabetes profile, cardiac screening, renal function, thyroid function, and arthritis. The grouping of specific tests provides the physician with an overall view of the patient's status that a single test could not provide. An example of a *cardiac profile*

Figure 13-30 *The compact Technicon H.3 hematology system provides accurate, comprehensive information on all cell types of clinical interest. It offers the choice of: CBC with platelets, CBC and full Diff plus RBC morphology and Lymphocyte subset analyses from a single aspiration of blood. Multiple report formats let the operator review a variety of results on the video screen, and any CRT data can be printed out on a graphics printer. The Technicon H-2 provides a standard computer interface. Results may be automatically transmitted "live" to a remote laboratory computer, reducing data handling, transcription effort, and potential errors.*
Courtesy Miles Inc., Diagnostics Division, Tarrytown, N.Y.

Figure 13-31 *Technicon RA-2X system is a chemistry analyzer that can be programmed with 100 different tests. For chemistry profiles, one can select up to 27 tests at a time from this extensive menu, including immunoassays and electrolytes. Results are displayed on the computer screen and printed out on the computer.*
Courtesy Miles, Inc., Diagnostic Division, Tarrytown, NY.

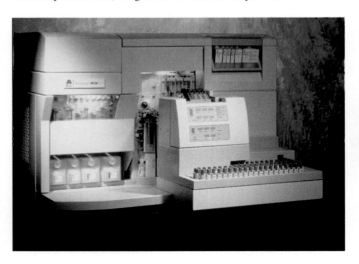

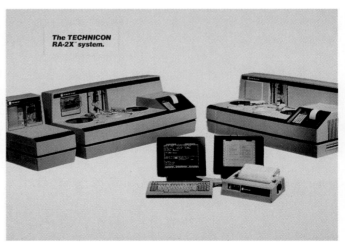

Figure 13-32 *The Serum Chemistry Graph displaying results from the SMA 12/60 on 12 biochemical tests. Results are presented in concentration terms on a precalibrated strip chart record. Normal test ranges for each parameter are printed as shaded areas; horizontal line crossing graph represents test results. Time from aspiration of given sample to finished chart is only 8 minutes—less time than it takes to complete any one of these test by any other methods.*
Courtesy Miles, Inc., Diagnostic Division, Tarrytown, N.Y.

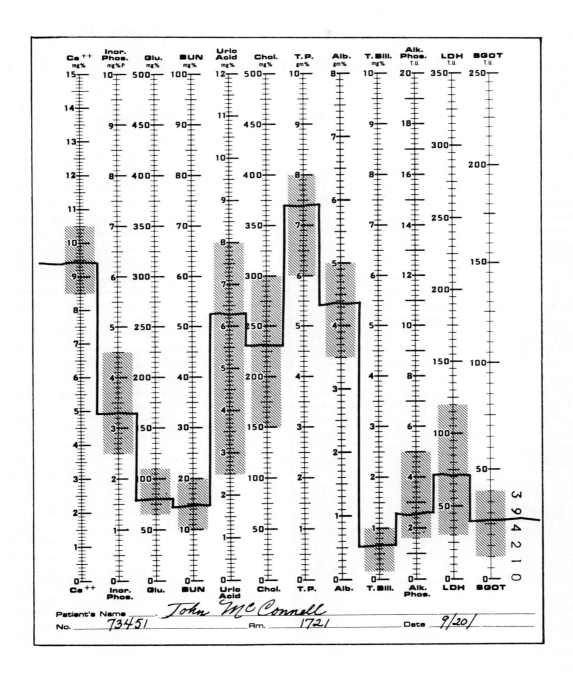

Figure 13-33 *Clinical laboratory computer-generated laboratory report.*

DATE & TIME RECEIVED	ACCESSION NUMBER
10/ 20/ 92 20: 45	
LOCATION	DATE REPORTED
	10/ 21/ 93

PHYSICIAN	PATIENT INFORMATION

TEST		RESULTS	REFERENCE RANGE	UNITS
TYPE AND XMATCH - PACKED CELLS				
Specimen Id is "1"				
BLOOD BANK UNIT NUMBER		Y34612		
UNIT STATUS		RELEASED		
COMPONENT		PACKED RBC		
PATIENT ABO AND Rh		O NEG		
ANTIBODY SCREEN		NEGATIVE		
DONOR ABO AND Rh		O NEG		
CROSSMATCH EXPIRES IN 72 HOURS, UNLESS BLOOD BANK IS NOTIFIED.				
CHEMISTRY 23 - PANEL A				
SODIUM		141	133-145	ME@/L
POTASSIUM		4. 0	3. 5-5. 5	ME@/L
CHLORIDE	HI	111	98-105	ME@/L
CO2 CONTENT		29	24-32	ME@/L
ANION GAP	LO	1	7-14	
BLOOD UREA NITROGEN	HI	31	10-20	MG/DL
CREATININE, SERUM/PLASMA	LO	0. 7	0. 9-1. 5	MG/DL
BUN/CREATININE RATIO	HI	44	12-20	MG/DL
GLUCOSE		110	80-125	MG/DL
FINAL Report		(Summary)	Page 1 of 2	

Figure 13-33—cont'd *Clinical laboratory computer-generated laboratory report.*

DATE & TIME RECEIVED	ACCESSION NUMBER
10/ 20/ 92 20: 45	
LOCATION	DATE REPORTED
	10/ 21/ 93

PHYSICIAN	PATIENTS INFORMATION

TEST		RESULTS	REFERENCE RANGE	UNITS
CHEMISTRY 23 - PANEL B				
CALCIUM, TOTAL, SERUM	LO	7. 4	8. 5-10. 5	MG/DL
PHOSPHORUS	LO	2. 8	3. 0-4. 6	MG/DL
URIC ACID	LO	3. 2	3. 5-7. 2	MG/DL
CHOLESTEROL	LO	123	151-240	MG/DL
TRIGLYCERIDE		121	58-258	MG/DL
LDH		217	118-242	IU/L
SGOT (AST)	HI	41	10-37	IU/L
SGPT (ALT)	HI	45	10-40	IU/L
GGTP	LO	8	11-51	IU/L
ALKALINE PHOSPHATASE		63	39-117	IU/L
BILIRUBIN, TOTAL		0. 3	0. 1-1. 5	MG/DL
ALBUMIN	LO	2. 4	3. 7-5. 2	G/DL
TOTAL PROTEIN	LO	3. 6	6. 0-8. 5	G/DL
ALBUMIN/GLOBULIN RATIO		2. 0	1. 0-2. 2	RATIO

FINAL Report   (Summary)   Page 2 of 2

Figure 13-33—cont'd *Clinical laboratory computer-generated laboratory report.*

DATE & TIME RECEIVED	ACCESSION NUMBER
10/ 20/ 92 20: 45	
LOCATION	DATE REPORTED
	10/ 21/ 93

PHYSICIAN	PATIENT INFORMATION

TEST		RESULTS	REFERENCE RANGE	UNITS
HEMOGRAM	LO	2. 9	4. 5-10. 5	CU. MM.
WHITE BLOOD COUNT	LO	2. 39	4. 40-5. 90	CU. MM.
RED BLOOD COUNT	LO	7. 4	14. 0-18. 0	GM/ 100 ML
HEMOGLOBIN	LO	22. 3	40. 0-52. 0	%
MEAN CORPUSCULAR VOLUME		93	80-100	fL
MEAN CORPUSCULAR HGB		31. 0	27. 0-32. 0	PG
MEAN CORPUSCULAR HGB CONC		33. 2	31. 0-36. 0	%
DIFFERENTIAL, WBC				
SEGMENTED NEUTROPHILS		57	38-80	%
LYMPHOCYTE		29	15-45	%
MONOCYTES		7	1-10	%
EOSINOPHILS		1	0-4	%
BAND NEUTROPHILS	HI	6	0-5	%
ANISOCYTOSIS	ABN	SLIGHT		
HYPOCHROMIA	ABN	SLIGHT		
PLATELET ESTIMATE	ABN	DECREASED		
PARTIAL THROMBOPLASTIN TIME				
PARTIAL THROMBOPLASTIN TIME		31.7	20. 0-40. 0	SECONDS
CONTROL PTT		30. 4	20. 0-40. 0	SECONDS
PROTHROMBIN TIME				
PROTHROMBIN TIME		12. 2	10. 0-13. 5	SECONDS
CONTROL PT		12. 0	11. 0-13. 0	SECONDS
FINAL Report		(Summary)		

(panel) may include an SGOT, SGPT, LDH, CPK, CBC, sedimentation rate, prothrombin time (PT), cholesterol, triglycerides, and potassium.

A *kidney function profile* may include total protein, albumin, globulin, A/G ratio, creatinine, BUN, BUN/creatinine ratio, sodium, potassium, chloride, uric acid, and cholesterol. A *liver function profile* may include alkaline phosphatase, LDH, SGOT, SGPT, total bilirubin, total protein, albumin, globulin, A/G ratio. See Table 13-2 for additional information on some of these tests and others. See also Figure 13-23, *C*; Figure 13-34.

QUALITY CONTROL AND LABORATORY SAFETY

See Unit 10, pages 328 and 329.

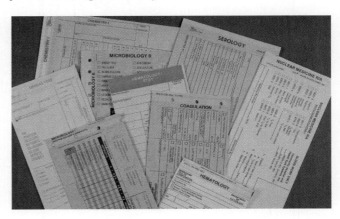

Figure 13-34 *Requisitions for laboratory work to be performed at a large laboratory.*

CONCLUSION

You have now completed the unit on hematology. Practice the procedures, and when you think that you know the equipment and steps of the procedures, arrange with your instructor to take the performance tests. You will be expected to demonstrate accurately your ability to prepare for and perform all of the procedures that have been presented.

REVIEW OF VOCABULARY

The following are samples of patient information from medical charts. In each, terms that have been presented in this unit are used. Read these and define the italicized terms. When laboratory values are given, determine if these are normal or abnormal results.

PATIENT NO. 1:

This patient has a history of various *blood dyscrasias*:

1990—*Anemia* and *anisocytosis*

1992—Both *hypernatremia* and *hypoglycemia* in different months

1993—*Septicemia* from undetermined causes

Present symptoms indicate *uremia* and *infectious mononucleosis*. Blood samples were obtained by *venipuncture* and sent to the laboratory for *multiphasic* tests.

PATIENT NO. 2:

Liver function studies showed minimal elevations of *SGOT* at 49.6 and 62 and then 41 units. *LDH* was not elevated, ranging at 100, 130, and 115. *Hypercholesterolemia* was revealed. *Serum electrolytes* showed slight *hypokalemia* of 3.4. With the use of potassium supplementation, the potassium rose to 4.1. The patient manifested some peripheral edema, which ultimately required the use of small doses of diuretics (Lasix 20 mg/day). This was thought to be the probable result of *hypoproteinemia*. *Serum albumin* was 3.0; total protein 6.4. *Bilirubin* remained minimally elevated at 1.4 and 1.2. *Alkaline phosphatase* was elevated at 278 and 288 IU/L (normal to 90). *CBC* showed a *hemoglobin* of 12.9 g, *hematocrit* of 37.6%, with *leukocytosis* of 14,000 and 13,500, and slight *poikilocytosis*. A *reticulocyte count* was 2.5%. *Prothrombin* time was 72%. *VDRL* was negative.

CASE STUDY

Blood component values are often essential to a *differentiated* medical diagnosis. Various blood *dyscrasias* are identified by their abnormal blood component values. Examples include *leukemia, infectious mononucleosis, septicemia,* and *thrombocytopenia.* You often perform a *venipuncture* to collect a specimen for analysis of blood. Using the sample hematology report below, discuss the underlined terminology. Define the abbreviations.

WBC	8.7
RBC	4.76
HGB	14.5
HCT	42.6
MCV	90
MCH	30.5
MCHC	34.0

PLATELET COUNT	257
ABS NEUT COUNT	5.0
ABS LYMPH COUNT	2.5
ABS MONOCYTE COUNT	1.0
MATURE NEUTROPHILS	58
LYMPH, NORMAL	29
MONO12	
RBC MORPHONUCLEARS	NORMAL

REVIEW QUESTIONS

1. Define blood.
2. List the WBCs that are classified as granulocytes and those that are classified as agranulocytes.
3. When asked to obtain a blood sample for a battery of 12 blood chemistry tests, what method and body site would you use to obtain this sample?
4. You have obtained a skin puncture blood sample. What tests might you perform in the office on this sample?
5. The following blood report has been sent to your office. Indicate which test results are normal and which are abnormal.
   WBCs—15,000/mm^3
   Red blood cells—5.6 million/mm^3
   Diff
      Lymphocytes—55%
      Eosinophils—8%
      Neutrophils—65%
   SGOT—65 U/ml
   Alkaline phosphatase—85 IU/L
   Prothrombin time—90% of control
   Hematocrit—45%
   Uric acid—13 mg/100 ml
   BUN—18 mg/100 ml
   Cholesterol—160 mg/100 ml
   VDRL—negative
   Coomb's indirect—negative
   Latex slide agglutination—positive

6. The physician has ordered a VDRL, a CBC, SMA-12, and a triglyceride test for J.D. Would you give this patient any special instructions before having a blood sample drawn? Could you collect one sample of blood in one tube? Would you use plain tube(s) or tube(s) with an anticoagulant additive? Explain the reasons for your answers.
7. The physician suspects that a patient may have hypothyroidism. What blood tests might be ordered to help diagnose this patient's condition?
8. What simplified tests might you do in the office to determine the presence of sugar in the blood?
9. Sexually transmitted diseases are on a constant rise at the present time. Frequently a physician orders a blood test to detect the presence of syphilis or use one of these tests as a screening purpose for unsuspected cases. List three blood tests that may be performed to detect the presence of syphilis in a patient.
10. List the blood test(s) that a physician may order to help diagnose the following conditions and diseases:
      Liver disease
      Infection mononucleosis
      Myocardial infarction
      A diet too high in fat content
      Kidney disease
      Leukemia
      Chronic or acute infections
      Anemia
      Diabetes
      Rheumatoid arthritis
      Septicemia

REVIEW QUESTIONS—cont'd

11. List the tests performed when a CBC is ordered.
12. Define: multiphasic tests, test panel, and profile.
13. List three blood tests that require a patient to fast before the blood sample is drawn.
14. List the two most common veins used to obtain a blood specimen by venipuncture.
    State/describe the anatomic location of these veins. State how much blood may be drawn from the patient by this method.
15. List three blood tests that would usually require you to use a collection tube without an additive.
    State the color of the rubber stopper of the vacuum tube that you would use for this. Explain what you would do with this specimen after collection is completed (two steps).
16. State when you would use a collection tube with the additive EDTA. What color is the rubber stopper on this vacuum tube?

17. State when you would use a collection tube with the additive heparin. State the reason why you would not use this tube for hematology studies.
18. State four reasons why it is vital that the ordered blood test be performed within 8 hours or less once the blood sample has been drawn.
19. State when you would release the tourniquet on the patient when performing a venipuncture.
20. Describe what may happen if you withdraw blood too quickly when using a standard syringe and needle when performing a venipuncture.
21. State why you do not shake tubes containing an additive and blood specimen, and why you should just gently invert them 8 to 10 times.

PERFORMANCE TEST

In a skills laboratory, a simulation of a joblike environment, the medical assistant student is to demonstrate the correct procedure for the following without reference to source materials. For these activities, the student needs a person to play the role of a patient *or* an artificial appliance representing a human arm and hand, and a blood sample. Time limits for the performance of each procedure are to be assigned by the instructor (also see page 52).

1. Given the required supplies and equipment, obtain blood samples from the patient by performing a fingertip skin puncture and a venipuncture. Then record these procedures on the patient's chart.
2. Having obtained a capillary blood sample in a nonheparinized capillary tube, perform a copper sulfate relative density test and record the results on the patient's chart.

3. Having obtained a capillary blood sample in a heparinized capillary tube, perform a hematocrit test using the microhematocrit centrifuge and record the results on the patient's chart.
4. Given a blood sample and a Dextrostix, test the sample for the presence of glucose and record the results on the patient's chart.
5. Having obtained a blood sample by performing a fingertip skin puncture, test the blood for the presence and amount of glucose using an Accu-Chek II and a Chemstrip bG, using a One Touch II blood glucose meter and a test strip.

The student is expected to perform the above skills with 100% accuracy.

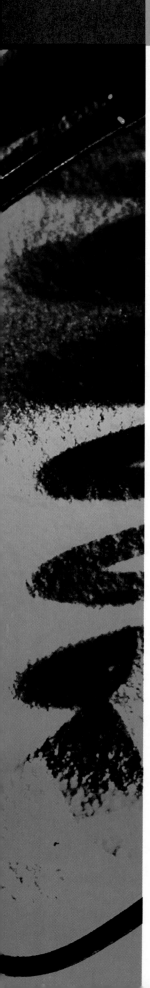

Diagnostic Radiology, Radiation Therapy, and Nuclear Medicine

COGNITIVE OBJECTIVES

On completion of Unit Fourteen, the medical assistant student should be able to:

1. Define and pronounce the terms listed in the vocabulary and text of this unit.
2. Explain the medical specialties of diagnostic radiology, radiation therapy, and nuclear medicine, listing examples of procedures performed by each.
3. Explain the nature and purpose of the diagnostic and therapeutic procedures outlined in this unit.
4. Define the term contrast medium as used in radiology; state the function of contrast media and list at least three examples of these.
5. List and explain the nature of at least 10 radiologic procedures that use contrast media.
6. Discuss and distinguish between the special techniques of mammography, xeroradiography, thermography, positron emission tomography (PET), tomography, computed tomography (CT), ultrasound, magnetic resonance imaging (MRI), digital radiography, and radiation therapy.
7. List and explain four basic positions used for proper exposure of the body part during radiography.
8. State and discuss the dangers, hazards, and safety precautions relevant to x-ray equipment and procedures.
9. List seven side effects that may be experienced by patients receiving high levels of radiation therapy.
10. List three body changes that may occur with overexposure to radiation.
11. Discuss the medical assistant's responsibilities relevant to radiologic procedures.
12. List at least eight x-ray examinations that do and eight that do not require special patient preparation.
13. Describe and discuss the possession, care, and storage of reports and x-ray films received in the physician's office.
14. Describe and discuss the steps involved in the processing of x-ray films.

TERMINAL PERFORMANCE OBJECTIVES

On completion of this unit, the medical assistant student should be able to:

1. Demonstrate proficiency in communicating proper preparation for x-rays to the patient.
2. Identify and demonstrate safety hazards and precautionary measures relevant to x-ray equipment.
3. Demonstrate the care and storage of the finished product when received in the physician's office.
4. Prepare and assist the patient for radiologic procedures.
5. Position the patient correctly for different x-ray film exposures (if licensed to do so).

The student is to perform these objectives with 100% accuracy 95% of the time.

The consistent use of universal precautions is required by all health care professionals in all health care settings as a method of infection control. It is assumed that these precautions are used in all of the following procedures. Review Unit One if you have any questions on methods to use as the methods/techniques will not be repeated in detail in each procedure presented in the unit.

Be sure to consult the latest guidelines issued by the Centers for Disease Control and Prevention and consult with infection control practitioners when needed to identify specific precautions that pertain to your particular work situation.

RADIOLOGIC PROCEDURES

Radiology (ra"de-ol'o-je) is the specialty of medical science that deals with the study, diagnosis, and treatment of disease by using x-rays, radioactive substances, and other forms of radiant energy such as gamma rays, ultraviolet rays, alpha and beta particles, and sound and magnetic waves.

The procedures involved in radiology can be divided into three specialties: diagnostic radiology, radiation therapy (radiation oncology), and nuclear medicine.

VOCABULARY

Cassette (kah-set')—A light-proof aluminum or bakelite container with front and back intensifying screens, between which x-ray film is placed when used for x-ray examinations.

Density—The quality of being dense or impenetrable. In radiology density refers to how light or dark a film appears.

Detail—The sharpness of the radiograph image.

Enema (en'e-mah)—The introduction of a solution into the rectum; for an x-ray examination of the colon, a radiopaque solution is administered by enema.

Fluoroscope (floo'or-o-skop")—Equipment used during x-ray examinations for visual observation of the internal body structures by means of x-ray films. The body part to be viewed is placed between the x-ray tube and a fluorescent screen. As x-rays pass through the body, shadowy images of the internal organs are projected on the screen. Most fluoroscopic examinations require the use of a contrast medium to provide contrast (see page 472).

Fluoroscopy (floo"or-os-ko-pe)—Visual examination by means of an image intensifier.

Ionizing (i"on-i-zing) radiation—Radiant energy given off by radioactive atoms and x-rays.

Irradiate (i-ra"de-at)—To treat with radiant energy.

Irradiation (i-ra"de'shun)—Exposure to radiation; the passage of penetrating rays through a substance or object.

Oscilloscope (o-sil'o-skop)—An instrument for visualizing the shape or wave form of sound waves, as in ultrasonography, or of electric currents, as when monitoring heart action and other body functions.

Radiation (ra"de-a'shun)—Electromagnetic waves or streams of atomic particles capable of penetrating and being absorbed into matter. Examples of electromagnetic waves are x-rays, gamma rays, ultraviolet rays, infrared rays, and rays of visible light. Atomic particles are alpha and beta particles.

Radiograph (ra'de-o-gra") or roentgenograph (rent'gen-o-graf) or roentgenogram (rent'gen-o-gram")—The film or photographic record produced by radiography.

Radiography (ra"de-og'rah-fe)—The taking of radiograms.

Radioisotope (ra"de-o-i-so-top)—A radioactive form of an element consisting of unstable atoms that emit rays of energy or streams of atomic particles. Radioisotopes occur naturally, as in the case of radium, or can be created artificially, as in the case of cobalt.

Radiologist (ra"de-o'o-jist)—A physician specialist in the study of radiology.

Radiolucent (ra"de-o-lu'sent)—That which permits the partial or complete passage of radiant energy such as x-rays. Dense objects appear white on the x-ray film because they absorb the radiation. An example of this is bone.

Radionuclide (ra"de-o-nu'klid)—A radioactive substance.

Radiopaque (ra"de-o-pak')—That which is impenetrable by x-rays and other forms of radiant energy; matter that obstructs the passage of radiant energy such as lead, which is frequently used as a protective device.

Voltage (vol-tij)—The electromotive force measured in volts (the units of force for electricity to flow).

The equipment used for radiologic procedures is very expensive and sophisticated; thus most physicians requisition these examinations or therapy from outside sources such as a major treatment center, local hospital, or radiology office. However, some diagnostic radiology procedures, such as radiographs of the chest or skeletal fractures, may be performed in some larger offices or clinics or in physicians' offices in rural areas. It takes special training and great skill to do radiologic procedures and for physicians to accurately interpret the fluoroscopic, scanning, and x-ray images formed. Skilled radiologic technologists, called radiographers, prepare and position the patient and take the x-ray images. These individuals must be registered nationally to practice. In addition, those who practice in California, New York, and 28 other states must also be licensed or certified by the state. The radiologist, a licensed physician specially trained in radiology, reads and interprets the films, scanning images, and fluoroscopic images.

For medical assistants to be well qualified and able to contribute to total patient care, it is imperative that they know the varied techniques, the purposes, and the nature of the specialized and highly technical radiology procedures. Descriptions of various x-ray, fluoroscopic, and nuclear medicine studies follow.

X-RAYS

X-rays are also called roentgen rays, after the discoverer, Wilhelm Konrad Roentgen (1845-1923), a physicist at the University of Wârzberg, Germany, in 1895. They are a form of radiation that consists of energy waves of very short wavelength. It is this extremely short wavelength that gives x-rays the special power of penetration. Although not visible to the human eye, x-rays can be captured on film as a visible image and can also be seen fluroscopically by an image intensifier. The density of the matter at which x-rays are aimed and the voltage used determine the degree of penetration of x-rays.

X-rays, capable of penetrating the body completely or in varying degrees and also of changing the basic structure of cells of the body, are used beneficially in the diagnosis of conditions and in the treatment of tumors and other medical conditions such as blood malignancies.

Various types of equipment are used for radiologic procedures. The equipment used for diagnostic procedures is of lower voltage than that used for radiation therapy.

DIAGNOSTIC RADIOLOGY

By exposing body parts to x-rays, diagnostic radiologic procedures create images on films or views on the fluoroscope and/or on videotape or videodisc that enable the physician to view the internal structures and functions of the body to pinpoint disease or anomalies. The observations made are then interpreted by the physician-radiologist, who then dictates the findings and radiologic diagnosis. The findings interpreted from these procedures help the physician make a diagnosis or evaluate ongoing treatment; they are also used to determine the effectiveness of a treatment program after therapy has been completed. In addition to the routine chest or skeletal films, there are many special diagnostic procedures and techniques that reveal more specific information about the function and structure of an organ.

Fluoroscopy: Image Intensification

Fluoroscopy, an image intensifier-television system, is an x-ray examination using an instrument that permits visual observation of deep structures of the body. X-rays from the x-ray tube pass through the patient's body and project shadowy images of organs and bones through an image intensifier. This information is fed to television monitors so that images can be readily observed during the procedure. Videotape and/or videodisc systems can record these images. This allows for playback during the procedure or after it has been completed. A permanent recording of the fluoroscopic image can be made on 35-mm film. This is called *cinefluorography* and occurs simultaneously with television monitoring and/or image recording on a videotape and/or videodisc unit.

The major advantage of the fluoroscope over the usual type of x-ray film is that the action of organs, joints, or entire body systems can be observed in motion. The use of a contrast medium during fluoroscopy may be necessary in most procedures using this system.

Contrast Medium Techniques

A contrast medium is a radiopaque substance that is used in diagnostic radiology to permit a more accurate visualization of internal body parts and tissues in contrast to their adjacent structures.

Contrast media include liquids, powders, gas, air, or pills; these are administered orally, parenterally (by injection), or through an enema, each being specific for the examination of a particular organ or structure. The contrast medium opacifies the body part(s) under examination. Thus the structure and functions of the organ(s) can be observed and studied through x-ray films or fluoroscopy. Positive contrast media include barium sulfate and iodine compounds. Because these media have more density, they absorb more of the radiation. They will appear white on x-ray images. Negative contrast media include air, gas, and carbon dioxide. They appear black on x-ray images.

Barium sulfate. This is a chalky compound, now available commercially in a premixed, flavored (such as cherry) liquid or paste. X-ray departments may also buy the powder form and mix it with water to the desired consistency.

Barium sulfate is an opaque medium used for two main types of x-ray and fluoroscopic examinations of the gastrointestinal (GI) tract. A barium meal or upper GI series is the oral ingestion of the barium mixture to outline the esophagus, stomach, and, if ordered, the small intestine, depending on the physician's request. A barium enema (BE), or lower GI series, outlines the colon for study after the instillation of the barium mixture through an enema. On occasion, a third examination, a barium swallow, is done to outline the esophagus (after the oral ingestion of the barium mixture) (Figures 14-1 and 14-2).

Iodine compounds. Containing up to 50% and more iodine, these radiopaque contrast media are used for the following tests on various body systems. If the patient is allergic to iodine, these examinations should not be performed. Other diagnostic techniques may then be used. The iodinated contrast media used for these procedures interferes with thyroid

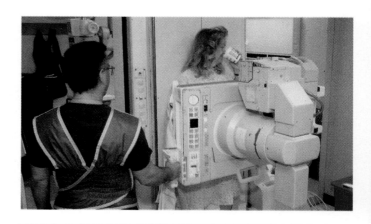

Figure 14-1 *Upper GI barium study done under fluoroscopic control by technologist.*

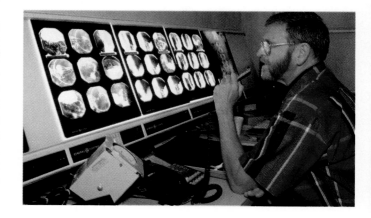

Figure 14-2 *Physicians viewing GI x-ray films.*

studies performed by the nuclear medicine department; therefore these procedures should not be performed when the patient is having thyroid function tests.

Air, oxygen (O_2), and carbon dioxide (CO_2). Since the introduction of computed tomography and magnetic resonance imaging (see pages 476 and 477), the frequency with which these negative contrast media have been used for cerebral pneumography (pneumoencephalography and pneu-moventriculography) in radiology departments has essentially disappeared. Still, at times these negative media can be used for examination of the spinal cord, joints, and in combination with barium sulfate during a barium enema. Oxygen is rarely used. Carbon dioxide is used most frequently because it is absorbed by the body faster than air or oxygen, thus limiting the duration of headaches that may follow a myelogram.

VOCABULARY

Angiogram—X-ray record of blood vessels after injecting a contrast medium through a catheter inserted in the appropriate vessel (arteriogram, lymphangiogram, phlebogram) (Figure 14-3).

Angiocardiogram—X-ray record of the heart and great vessels after injecting a contrast medium into a large peripheral vein or a chamber of the heart by direct heart catheterization.

Arteriogram—X-ray record of an artery or arterial system after injecting a contrast medium through a catheter inserted in an artery.

Arthrogram*—X-ray record of a joint after injecting a contrast medium into the joint, or after injecting air or other gas into the articular capsule. Air can be combined with an iodine compound for double contrast studies.

Bronchogram—X-ray record of the bronchial tree and lungs after instillation of a contrast medium into the bronchi via the trachea with a special instrument. This procedure is almost extinct since the introduction of the new, more sophisticated modalities.

Cerebral angiogram—X-ray record of the cerebral vessels after injecting a contrast medium into the common carotid artery; for x-ray records of the vessels in the posterior fossa or the occipital lobes, the medium is injected into the vertebral artery in the neck.

Cholecystogram†—X-ray record of the gallbladder after oral ingestion of radiopaque granules or tablets taken the evening before the examination.

Diskogram—X-ray record of the vertebral column after injecting a contrast medium into an intervertebral disk. This procedure is done infrequently.

Hysterosalpingogram—X-ray record of the uterus and fallopian tubes after injecting a contrast medium through the vagina into the uterus.

Intravenous cholangiogram*—X-ray record of the bile ducts after injecting a contrast medium intravenously. The contrast medium is excreted by the liver into the bile ducts; x-ray films are taken at intervals as the contrast medium is excreted through the hepatic, cystic, and common bile duct into the duodenum.

Intravenous pyelogram (IVP)—X-ray records taken at intervals after intravenous injection of a contrast medium at intervals to observe the excretion rate and the concentration of the dye in the renal pelves and the outline of the ureters and urinary bladder.

Lymphangiogram—X-ray record of the lymphatic vessels after the injection of a contrast medium into the lymphatic system.

Myelogram—X-ray record of the spinal cord after injection of a water-soluble or an oily contrast medium, air, or gas into the subarachnoid space through a lumbar puncture needle.

Retrograde pyelogram—X-ray record of the urinary tract after introduction of a contrast medium through a urinary catheter into the ureters and pelves of the kidneys.

Urogram—X-ray record of any part of the urinary tract after intravenous injection of a contrast medium. See also intravenous pyelogram.

Figure 14-3 *Vascular procedures suite. Patient is shown positioned for cerebral angiogram via femoral approach. Automatic injector and bilateral automatic film changers are used.*

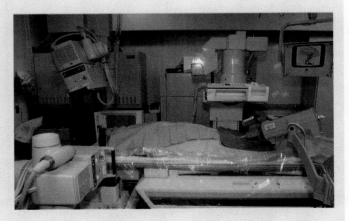

*These examinations are rapidly being replaced by magnetic resonance imaging (see page 477).

†In most facilities these procedures have been replaced by ultrasound examinations (sonography) of the gallbladder and bile ducts.

Mammography

Mammography, an x-ray examination of the breast to identify breast lesions or tumors, involves detection of radiodense tissue or calcifications. Mammography is the most effective method for detecting early and curable breast cancer.

Breast cancer is the leading cause of death in women under age 50, and second only to lung cancer as the leading cause of death for older women. According to the American Cancer Society, one out of every nine women in the United States will develop breast cancer at some point during her lifetime. According to specialists, "It has been shown very clearly that a tumor can be seen with a mammogram as long as 2 years before either the patient or the physician is able to feel that tumor. The woman therefore has a 2-year headstart on the treatment of her disease."

The new dedicated mammographic units (Figure 14-4) perform diagnostic x-ray examinations of the breast at radiation doses 5 to 10 times lower than the older units. Machines of this type provide enormous potential benefit for early cancer detection, and the minimal levels of radiation exposure have essentially removed any meaningful risk. Radiation physicists have estimated that the radiation risk of a low-dose mammogram may be equivalent to the lung cancer risk of smoking one cigarette. In addition, this "state-of-the-art" machine obtains magnified and grid images than can more optimally evaluate the young, dense, and small breast. Two films are taken from different angles: (1) the sitting or standing axillary, and (2) the sitting or standing craniocaudal views (Figure 14-5).

To achieve diagnostic x-ray images of the breasts at extremely low radiation doses, the breast must be compressed firmly by a clear plastic plate. Many women find this uncomfortable but tolerable. Some women find breast compression intolerable. For women with painful, tender breasts, it is suggested that they (1) schedule the examination during the time in the menstrual cycle when the breasts are least tender. This corresponds to the first 10 days of the cycle for many women;

(2) avoid caffeine-containing products such as coffee, tea, chocolate, cocoa, and soft drinks for 1 week before the examination; (3) verbally cooperate with the radiographer to mutually arrive at a degree of compression that is tolerable to them and consistent with the technical requirements of the examination. The patient should be asked not to wear any powder or deodorant on the day of the examination, as these products sometimes show up as artifacts on the x-ray images.

The American Cancer Society's *new* recommendations state that "women without symptoms of breast cancer ages 40 to 49 should have a mammogram every 1 to 2 years, and women age 50 and over, once a year. All women are advised that monthly breast self-examination is an important health habit." (see Unit Four). Women ages 20 to 39 should have a breast physical examination by a physician done every 3 years, and women age 40 and over should have it done yearly.

In cases in which a breast lump has been determined by a mammogram but is not clearly identifiable through palpation, a radiologist uses a *stereotactic Mammotest machine* to take "stereo" x-rays of the breast. With this machine, the radiologist can determine the exact location of a lesion within 1 mm of accuracy. A fine-needle aspiration (FNA) is then performed and evaluated by a cytopathologist. In a FNA a thin needle is inserted into the lump, and a cell specimen is withdrawn. The patient's physician is informed of the results within a matter of hours.

Xeroradiography

Xeroradiography uses a dry electrophotographic technique to produce images on specially treated Xerox paper. This system, used mostly for mammography, can also be used to obtain x-ray images in small areas in soft tissue and some bone. In general, xeroradiography compares favorably with the radiation dose the patient receives from other film-screen recording systems. The major advantages over a conventional film-screen system is its ability to outline or enhance the edges of a density (for example, bone, tumors, or foreign bodies such as glass).

Figure 14-4 *Mammographic unit.*

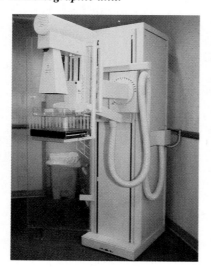

Figure 14-5 A, *Technologist positioning patient for right craniocaudal view of breast for mammography.*

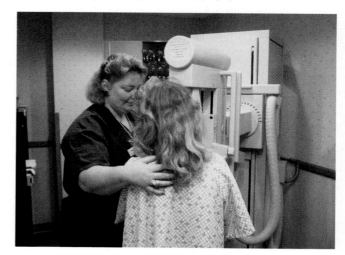

A

Figure 14-5—cont'd B, *x-ray film of female breast (mammography showing entire breast back to rib cage).*
Courtesy Picker Corporation, Cleveland, Ohio.

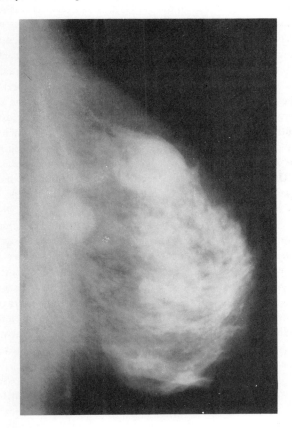

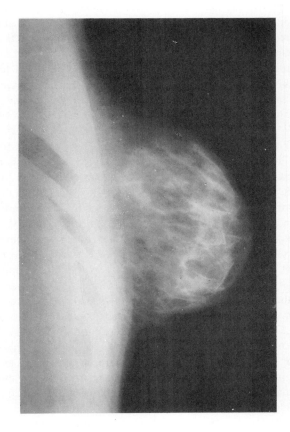

Thermography

Thermography is a heat-sensing technique used in the detection of breast tumors. Essentially, an apparatus makes a photographic image of the varying skin temperatures. Body areas that are warm appear light; cool areas appear dark; and medium-temperature areas appear gray on the thermogram. Localized skin temperature elevations such as occur over inflammatory or malignant lesions are then sharply delineated against the temperatures of the surrounding tissues.

Although research continues, the majority opinion is that thermography is not a sufficiently reliable procedure to use for screening or detecting breast cancer. Thus **it is not recommended and is seldom used now**, except in institutions continuing investigative work. X-ray mammography is the superior diagnostic tool for detecting breast cancer.

Tomography

Tomography, or section roentgenography, has a special ability to penetrate dense shadows. X-ray pictures are taken in sections at different depths in the patient's body, focusing on the plane of the structure to be studied. Structures in front of and behind the plane under examination are blurred out.

Because of this, tomography can be a valuable diagnostic procedure when a definitive diagnosis cannot be made from conventional radiographs. Used to demonstrate and evaluate a number of different disease processes, traumatic injuries, and congenital abnormalities, tomography can be used in any part of the body, but is most effective in areas of high contrast such as the lungs and bones. One of the most frequent uses is to demonstrate and evaluate benign and malignant processes in the lungs.

Although computed tomography (CT) and magnetic resonance imaging (MRI) (see the following paragraphs through page 477) have replaced the use of tomography to a great extent, there are still times when tomography is the examination of choice. Many hospitals do not have the CT and MRI units because of the high cost. In addition, the cost to the patient is much higher for a CT or MRI examination. Tomography can often provide a satisfying diagnosis or at least screen the patient for further evaluation by the more sophisticated modalities.

Positron Emission Tomography

Positron emission tomography (PET) is a computerized radiographic technique that uses radiopharmaceuticals (radioactive substances) to examine the metabolic activity of various body structures. The patient either inhales or is injected with a radiopharmaceutical. The computers and electronic circuitry of the PET device detect and convert gamma rays into color-coded images that indicate the intensity of the metabolic activity of the organ involved. Patients are exposed to very small amounts of radiation because the radioactive substances used are very short-lived. Presently PET is used predominately as a research tool to study blood flow and the metabolism of the heart and the blood vessels, and to determine local cerebral blood flow and the local cerebral metabolic rate of glucose. PET measures regional brain function that cannot be determined by any other diagnostic method, including CT and MRI. Current PET studies are used for patients with epilepsy, brain tumors, Alzheimer's disease, a stroke, spasmoid torticollis, and other movement disorders.

Computed Tomography (CT Scan)

The CT scanner, the developers of which were awarded the Nobel Prize for medicine in October 1979, has been a most significant breakthrough in medical technology.

CT is an advanced radiologic modality that provides valuable clinical information in the early detection, differentiation, and demarcation of diseases of the head and body. It often provides diagnostic information that cannot be obtained by any other method, especially in neurologic work.

Quick and noninvasive, the CT scan is particularly helpful in solving problems in which there is conflicting information from other radiologic or laboratory studies, and may be necessary for planning radiation therapy for certain tumor masses. Its use has frequently replaced some examinations such as echoencephalography (see Diagnostic Ultrasound) and others, many of which (for example, the pneumoencephalogram and arteriogram) carry greater risk and discomfort to the patient. In addition, CT does, in certain cases, replace procedures that would require the patient to be hospitalized. This technique is used for neurologic procedures; to detect cerebral abnormalities (for example, tumors, lesions, hematomas, and bleeding in the brains of newborn infants; to search for childhood cancer; to detect masses in the chest, abdominal, and pelvic cavities; to examine the liver, spleen, pancreas, kidneys, adrenal glands, pituitary gland, and optic nerve; and for a generalized survey for lymphoma or metastases [Figure 14-6]).

Machines called scanners (such as ACTA, CT/T, Synerview, Delta, Syntex) beam x-rays to scan the body site in a series of x-rays. The scanner combines the capabilities of traditional x-ray with that of a computer, providing an image of soft tissue in three dimensions. The x-ray tube and detector source rotate 360 degrees around the patient's head or body part being studied, taking multiple "slices"—cross-sectional readings. Thus every tissue and organ is x-rayed from all sides. As they pass through the body, the absorption rates of the x-ray are detected, and the density of the tissue is relayed to the computer. From the calculations performed by the computer, densities are translated into a picture of the body as if it were neatly cut into slices, each a fraction of an inch thick. This picture is projected on a screen for the radiologist to study (Figure 14-7).

The conventional x-ray film reveals only certain organs and tissues and requires multiple exposures to estimate the size and location of diseased areas. The CT scanner can distinguish nearly every type of tissue and more minute differences in the various tissues. CT can determine the size and location of any pathologic condition with great accuracy. When first developed around the mid seventies, CT scans were slow; but now many machines in use can complete a scan in 4 to 5 seconds, and a more sophisticated machine can complete a scan in 1 second. It takes 15 to 30 minutes or longer to complete all the slices required for a complete examination. Thus most CT scanners can only be used for 15 to 20 examinations during an 8-hour work day.

Minimal patient preparation is required for CT scans. Some facilities require the patient to have nothing by mouth for 4 hours before the examination if a contrast medium is used. For abdominal and pelvic scans, patient preparation is usually the same as that for a barium enema (see Table 14-3). When a contrast medium is not used, no patient preparation is required. A contrast medium, which is almost always used for a CT scan, can be administered orally or intravenously.

Research is continuing for a scanner than can make clear x-ray images of the fast-beating human heart. Some researchers are presently testing it as a noninvasive method to determine whether vein grafts installed in a coronary bypass surgery are

---

Figure 14-6 A, *Technologist positioning patient for head scan with CT total body scanner.* **B,** *Control room for the CT Scanner. The x-ray generation controls, scanning control console, and viewing monitors are found here. Main computer hardware is usually located in adjacent room.*

A
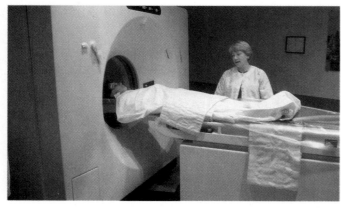

B
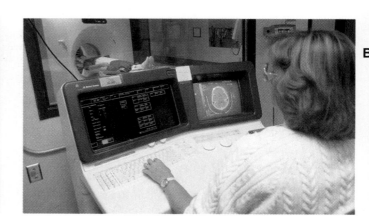

Figure 14-7 *Images from a CT head scan.*
Courtesy General Electric, Medical Systems, Milwaukee, Wisc.

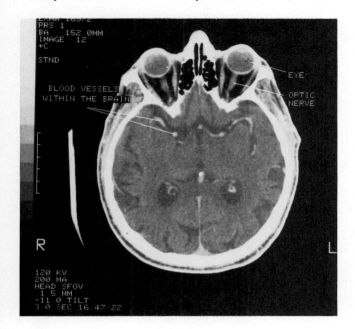

allowing blood to flow freely or have become closed and useless. The National Aeronautics and Space Administration (NASA) is also interested in this device because it may be valuable in detecting the loss of calcium in bones, a serious consequence of weightlessness in space travel.

Although the use of the CT scan is superior in numerous situations, at times the findings obtained do indicate the need for additional and invasive procedures so that a conclusive diagnosis can be established.

Magnetic Resonance Imaging

A newer and equally exciting form of imaging technique for examining the body is magnetic resonance (MR). MR is a computer-based, cross-sectional imaging modality that examines the interactions of magnetism and radio waves with tissue to obtain its images. Magnets, as the name suggests, are at the heart of this system. Many machines use super conducting magnets; the more powerful the magnets, the clearer the images produced.

There are major advantages to an MRI. It can examine properties of body tissue that have never before been visualized. Both anatomic and physiologic information can be obtained. No x-rays (that is, no ionizing radiation of any kind) are used to obtain the MR image. It is a painless and usually noninvasive technique. On a few occasions a contrast medium may be used. There are no known harmful effects to the patient when exposed to the current levels of magnetic field strength and radiowave energy transmission.

Magnetic resonance is used to detect tumors in soft tissues because even in early stages malignant tissue responds to the magnetic pull differently from normal tissue. No other imaging technique can detect such subtle differences in soft tissues. It is also used to examine the brain (it can distinguish

brain tumors from tiny blood clots and determine the chemical changes that cause dementia in the elderly); spinal cord tumors, cystic changes of the spine, and disk disease; the GI tract; the heart muscle, septal defects, and cardiac valve leaflets; the lungs; the extremities (but bone lesions and calcium within tumors are seen better with CT); and tumors of the liver and spleen; pelvic structures (for example, bladder tumors, neoplasms in the female genital tract). It may detect prostate tumors; and it can outline the kidneys, adrenal glands, and retroperitoneal structures such as lymph nodes (although there is limited evidence that MRI is superior to CT in this area).

However, MRI has its limitations. It can't see the hard part of the bones; thus we still need x-rays, CT, or other techniques to diagnose fractures and malformations in bones. Also, the strong magnetic field is potentially dangerous to patients with cardiac pacemakers and to those who have any type of metallic implants such as aneurysm clips on blood vessels within the skull or clips tying off other blood vessels. The pull of the magnets could slip the clips out of place, and vessels could be torn. *It is therefore important to check that the patient does not have a pacemaker or metallic implants before a MRI is scheduled.*

The image produced by the computer can be viewed on a television monitor. If desired, the images can be photographed for further study. These images can also be stored on a computer disc temporarily and then transferred to magnetic tape for permanent storage and retrieval (Figures 14-8, *A* to *C* and 14-9, *A* and *B*).

Digital Radiography

Digital radiography is the use of the conventional image intensifier-television system (fluoroscopy) in which the television signal is first digitized (information is stored in computer units called bits) and processed by the computer before the x-ray image is displayed on a standard television monitor.

The use of digital radiography has been successful in angiography. This procedure can replace the more complex and time-consuming procedure of arterial catheterization. Four advantages of this procedure are that it is safer for the patient, it is less painful, and it uses a lower x-ray dose and a much smaller amount of contrast medium

A contrast medium is injected through a catheter that is placed into a vein, preferably the basilic vein, or alternately in the cephalic vein or the superior vena cava. As the x-ray images are taken, they are formed electronically and displayed on the television monitor. At the same time, the image is stored on a videotape, videodisc, or digital disc.

Digital angiography is used for head and neck angiograms and images of the pulmonary arteries and cardiac structures. Hospitalization of the patient is not required.

As digital radiographic devices and procedures expand, traditional studies in which film processing has been used may gradually be replaced by digital image processing.

Quantitative digital radiography (QDR), using the most advanced technology available, is used to screen patients for osteoporosis by measuring bone density. QDR provides the

Figure 14-8 *MRI.* **A,** *Young child being assisted onto the table for an MRI procedure. People of all ages can have MR examinations.* **B,** *Patient being positioned for an MR scan of the head and neck.* **C,** *Control room for the MRI scanner. Technologists operating the MR equipment. Note the image of the brain produced by the computer displayed on the television monitor.*

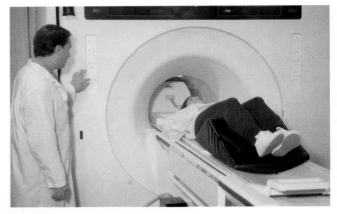

B

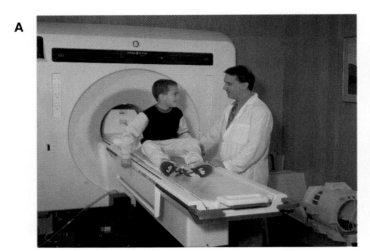

A

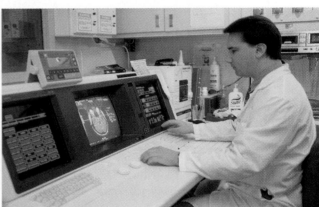

C

Figure 14-9 **A,** *Image from MRI head and neck scan.*

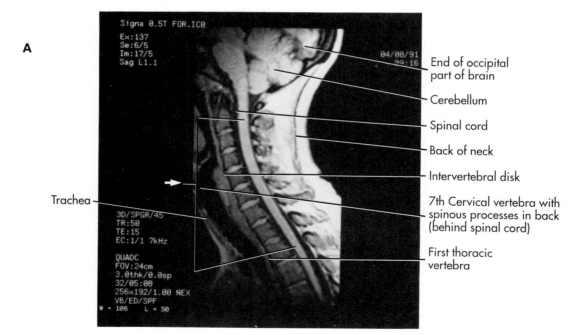

A

Trachea

End of occipital part of brain

Cerebellum

Spinal cord

Back of neck

Intervertebral disk

7th Cervical vertebra with spinous processes in back (behind spinal cord)

First thoracic vertebra

Figure 14-9 —cont'd B *Image from MRI knee scan.*
Courtesy General Electric, Medical Systems, Milwaukee, Wisc.

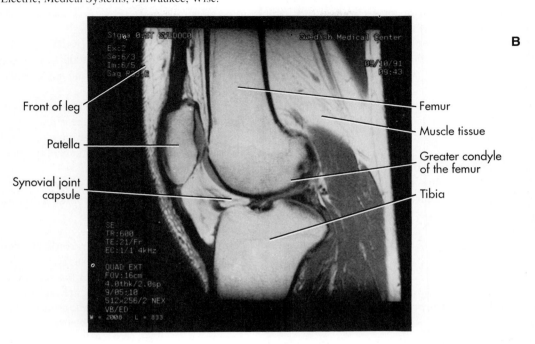

safest , quickest, most precise, and most reliable measurement of bone mineral content. It can be used to determine if osteoporosis is present and also is useful in following the effects of treatment for the disease. Cross-lateral and whole-body imaging can be obtained with the use of this examination.

Diagnostic Ultrasound

Diagnostic ultrasound, sometimes called diagnostic medical sonography or ultrasonography, does not utilize ionizing radiation to diagnose or treat disease, but uses very high frequency inaudible sound waves that bounce off the body to record information on the structure of internal organs.

In this examination, the patient's skin is covered with water, oil, or a special jelly that helps conduct the sound waves into the body. A special instrument emitting sound waves is placed and moved on or near the patient's skin. Sound waves pass through the skin, strike the body tissues, and pass an echo reflection back to the instrument. These ultrasonic echoes are then recorded on the oscilloscope as a picture of a series of dots. This record produced is called an echogram or sonogram. The method of image recording in which the data is stored on film, paper, video, or other recording material is sometimes called hard copy.

Ultrasound can be used to detect abnormalities in the heart (echocardiography), major blood vessels, kidneys, abdominopelivc cavity, breast (it is the best method for distinguishing between solid and fluid-filled lumps in the breast), scrotum, muscles, spine, and brain (echoencephalogram (EECG), although this has now been replaced by the CT scan, when available, because of the superiority of the CT images of the entire cranial vault versus very limited knowledge available from the EECG). It is also used to determine the presence of a pregnancy if other tests are unsuccessful; to differentiate between single and multiple pregnancies; to view placental position, various stages, and fetal positions during pregnancy; and for neonate examinations (Figure 14-10). In some procedures body structures, such as the diaphragm, cardiac or fetal heart motion, or other organ structures that move with respiration are visible as they change position in time.

Ultrasound has the advantages of being a painless, noninvasive procedure that does not expose the patient to ionizing radiation. After 30 years of use, physicians have found no evidence

Figure 14-10 *Obstetric ultrasound.*

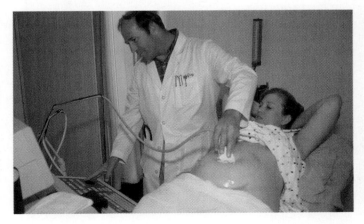

that diagnostic ultrasound causes any untoward biologic effect. Therefore it has generally been accepted as a safe technique.

Ultrasound is also used for treatment in physical medicine (by physical therapists) for deep muscle or tension pain. In this case a different machine with a different soundwave intensity is used. This is discussed in the physical therapy unit.

Other Diagnostic Radiologic Examinations

Abdomen. A survey film (flat plate) of the abdomen is ordered without the use of a contrast medium when abnormal conditions of the abdomen are suspected such as tumors, abscesses, enlarged or perforated organs, or hematomas.

In the plain survey, three films are often taken. The patient may be placed in the erect, supine, prone, or lateral decubitus position, depending on the suspected pathologic condition to be studied (Figure 14-11).

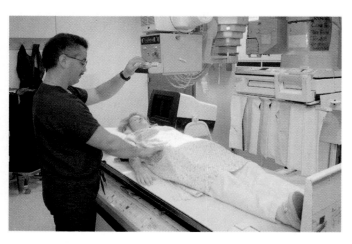

Figure 14-11 *Radiologic technologist performing routine radiographic work (for example, pelvis or abdomen) with overhead tube mount.*

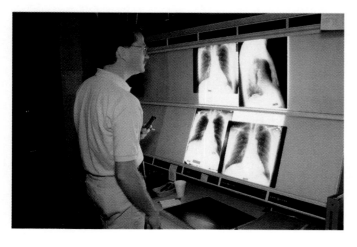

Figure 14-12 *Physician interpreting and dictating the results of a chest x-ray film.*

Routine chest x-ray film. An x-ray record of the chest is obtained with the patient in the posteroanterior erect position. Generally, a lateral view is also taken (Figure 14-12).

Kidney, ureter, bladder (KUB). A film of the abdomen is used to study the kidneys, flank area, gas patterns, abdominal wall, bones of the pelvis, and any unusual masses.

Skull series. A series of radiographs of the skull is used to determine cranial injuries or the effects of trauma to the head and neck. Computed tomography has replaced the use of these films, except in cases of severe trauma.

Paranasal sinus films. X-ray records are made of the paired sinuses within the frontal, ethmoid, sphenoid, and maxillary bones of the face.

Bone x-ray films. X-ray records are made of bones suspected of disease or trauma such as tumors and fractures or displacement. X-ray studies of the vertebral column are common. Radiographs of the neck are referred to as cervical x-ray films; those of the middle back are referred to as thoracic x-ray films; and those of the lower back are referred to as lumbosacral x-ray films.

RADIATION THERAPY

You should have some knowledge of radiation therapy, because patients who are to receive or have experienced it may ask you questions. When radiation is applied for treatment of cancer and various other conditions by x-rays, beta, and gamma rays and other radioactive substances, it is called radiation therapy, radiotherapy, or radiation oncology, the purpose being to administer a definite amount of radiation to a specific location to irradiate diseased cells. Radiation therapy alters the diseased cell so that it cannot reproduce and will eventually age and die, leaving no new cells behind. Only the most extreme dose of radiation kills the cells directly.

The amount of energy that is deposited within the tissue and the condition of the biologic system determine the effectiveness of ionizing radiation in living tissue. The radiosensitivity of most tissues depends on:

- The number of undifferentiated (lack or absence of normal cell differentiation) cells in the tissue.
- The degree of mitotic activity (cell division that produces new cells) of the tissue. It is during mitosis that human cells are most sensitive to radiation.
- The length of time that cells of the tissue continue to reproduce.
- The primary target of ionizing radiation is the DNA molecule in the human cell.

Certain tumors are more radiosensitive than others. Some that are highly radiosensitive include tumors of the ovaries and testes, lymphomas, Wilms' tumor of the kidney, retinoblastomas, and Hodgkin's disease. Those that are moderately radiosensitive include basal and squamous cell carcinomas of the skin and adenocarcinoma of the prostate.

Tumors that are *relatively* radioresistant include sarcomas of the bone, connective tissue, and muscle, and nerve tumors.

Certain sources of radioactivity are used for specific types or locations of cancer. Radium, for example, gives off rays (alpha, beta, and gamma) that affect the growth of tissue. In the form of seeds or needles (radium implants), radium can be implanted directly into a malignant tumor in the uterus or mouth for a prescribed period of time (possibly 3 to 4 days) to act on and destroy abnormal cells. This is called interstitial treatment. Permanent implant therapy may also be done using radon 222 seeds and iodine 125 seeds. These implants are left in the patient forever. Radioisotopes of cobalt can also be used for implantation, in addition to teletherapy or possible surgery. Teletherapy is radiation treatment administered by a radioactive isotope such as cobalt-60 or cerium-137, emitting high-energy gamma rays. These are housed in shielded units, similar to large x-ray units, which are placed at a distance from the patient. A beam of gamma radiation is aimed at the specific part of the body requiring treatment. Radiotherapy of this type is especially useful in the treatment of deep-seated malignancies not readily accessible for implantation. Radioisotopes are also available in a liquid form that can be used for local irradiation in the pleural or peritoneal cavities and also for the thyroid gland. The use of radiation therapy in cancer is based on the fact that cancer cells are more sensitive to x-rays and other radioactive substances than other cells in surrounding normal tissue.

Ionizing radiation affects both normal and diseased cells. The dose of radiation administered should be sufficient to treat the diseased area, but not so great that it would permanently damage the surrounding normal tissues. Treatment techniques are designed to deliver a precise dose to the tumor, while limiting the amount of radiation deliveredd to the uninvolved portions of the tissue. Greater damage occurs to the abnormal cells because more of these cells are undergoing mitosis and are more poorly differentiated. Normal cells have a greater capability of repairing the resulting damage than do malignant cells. Low-voltage x-rays are used to treat conditions that require only surface penetration such as skin lesions, whereas high-voltage radiation is used to treat deep-seated malignancies.

Effective treatment of cancer with radiation therapy depends on the following:

- The extent to which the disease has progressed
- The type of cells in the tumor
- The general health of the patient
- The location of the tumor
- The radiocurability of the tumor

For definitive treatment, the cancer must be in a tissue that is more radioresistant than the tumor.

Approximately 70% of all newly diagnosed cancer patients are treated with radiation therapy. Radiation therapy may be the only treatment used for some cancer such as cancer of the larynx, skin, oral cavity, nasopharynx, cervix (although surgery may be the preferred treatment for cancer of the cervix), Hodgkin's disease, and malignant lymphoma (chemotherapy may also be used here). Frequently surgical interventions or chemotherapy or a combination of the two are used in conjunction with radiation therapy for the treatment of cancer of the breast, uterus, lungs, and others. Other modalities such as CT and ultrasonography are used to locate the tumor(s) and to localize the boundaries of organs not involved. After therapy, these modalities can be used to record tumor regression and the effectiveness of the treatment program.

The advantageous role of radiation therapy for the treatment of cancer is well documented. It appears that it will continue to play an important and expanded role in the treatment of cancer.

NUCLEAR MEDICINE

Nuclear medicine is the medical specialty that deals with the diagnosis and treatment of disease processes with the use of radioactive substances, although it is used predominantly for diagnostic purposes. Radioactive pharmaceuticals are thought to be radionuclide, in which the nuclei of the atoms of that particular isotope are undergoing spontaneous disintegrations. These radionuclides are administered intravenously or orally to the patient, or a radioactive gas may be inhaled. Sophisticated measuring equipment and imaging devices that are interfaced with computers are used. A radiosensitive instrument known as a gamma camera or scintillation probe maps the area to be studied. To obtain the information desired, the gamma camera remains stationary over the organ of interest. This instrument records an image relating to the patterns of radioactivity concentrated within the organ being studied by this method. This image is called a scintigram or scintiscan and is used by the physician to diagnose tumors or other disease processes. The scintillation probe is used primarily in the evaluation of hyperthyroidism. The probe is placed in close proximity to the skin over the organ being studied and records the concentration of radioactivity within the organ by giving a numeric printout.

When a radionuclide is used to make a medical diagnosis, the physician refers to the concentration of radionuclides as being "hot spots" or "cold spots." If the radionuclide concentrates in an abnormality, it is known as a hot spot within the scan; or, if the tumor does not concentrate the radionuclide, it is known as a cold spot within the surrounding tissue that has concentrated the radioactive pharmaceutical. Hot spots or cold spots can both denote abnormality, depending on the organ being studied. All radionuclides used for diagnostic procedures are short-lived, which means that they remain radioactive only for a short time. Consequently, the radiation dose to the patient is small and usually does not cause any ill effects.

When radioisotopes are used in therapy doses, the effects are much like those seen when high-level radiation therapy is given to the patient. *The following are symptoms that may be seen when either radiation or radioisotope therapy is given:* loss of hair, shedding of skin, hemopoietic dysfunction, diarrhea, nausea, irritation of mucous membranes (such as in the mouth, throat, bladder, or vaginal), and chromosomal changes.

VOCABULARY

Scanning Studies Used for Diagnosis

Bone scan—Used to detect osteogenic sarcoma and its metastases, bone neoplasms, localized lesions for biopsy, osteomyelitis, and stress fractures; and to evaluate arthritis and Paget's disease.

Bone marrow scan—Used to detect hemolytic and iron deficiency, to detect decreased marrow function secondary to radiation therapy, and to measure the functional marrow reserve in patients on chemotherapy.

Brain scan—Used to detect, localize, or follow the course of suspected or proved vascular malformations, inflammatory diseases, abscesses, cerebrovascular accidents, metastatic brain tumor, and subdural hematomas.

Cardiac scan—Used to detect myocardial infarctions and blood flow related to cardiac stress testing and cardiac artery stenosis. Sometimes used to evaluate pericardial effusion and localized ischemic scar damage.

Cisternogram—Used to localize cerebrospinal fluid leaks, "normal pressure" hydrocephalus, and evaluation of the functional status of ventricular shunts. This procedure is done rarely.

Hepatobiliary scan—Used to detect gallbladder patency and functioning.

Kidney scan—Used to detect kidney disease, trauma, and tumors and to evaluate hypertension. Used to study patients with demonstrated or suspected sensitivity to iodinated radiographic contrast media.

Liver scan—Used to detect primary and metastatic malignancy, biliary obstruction, abscesses, and cysts; sometimes used for the evaluation of hepatitis or cirrhosis, hepatomegaly, jaundice, and rupture.

Lung perfusion—Used to detect a pulmonary embolus.

Lung ventilation—Used to detect a pulmonary embolus. This procedure is usually done with a lung perfusion. Ventilation is done first and may be followed with the lung perfusion.

Spleen scan—Used to detect splenomegaly and splenic rupture.

Thyroid scan—Used to detect hyperthyroidism and the localization of nodules. Preoperative and postoperative scans are done for patients with thyroid carcinoma.

White blood cell scan—Used to determine the source of an infection in questionable cases. The image shows the destination of many of the labeled white blood cells (that is, they show the site of the infection).

All scans can usually be done on an outpatient basis. You should be aware of any special preparation required of the patient before having the scan and the approximate length of time of each scan so that the patient can be briefed on what to expect. Tables 14-1 and 14-2 outline the most common scans and the time required for each. Similar reference sheets should be available in the physician's office for your reference when necessary. Your responsibilities relating to the diagnostic studies presented in this unit, as well as similar tables for x-ray examinations, are given on pages 486, 487, 489 and 490.

POSITION OF PATIENT FOR X-RAY STUDIES

Radiograms are made by directing beams of x-rays through the x-ray tube toward a specific body part. The body part to be radiographed must be positioned correctly between the film-containing cassette and the x-ray source. The body part to be filmed is positioned closest to the cassette.

When the physician orders x-ray film to be taken, and when radiologists interpret the film, they use special terms to designate the position or direction of the x-ray beam and the patient's position. Before the x-ray film is taken, markers are placed on the film-containing cassette to indicate the position used, the patient's identification, and the date (Figures 14-13 and 14-14).

Figure 14-13 *Samples of various lead numbers and letters in different heights and thicknesses for radiographing direct on x-ray film.*

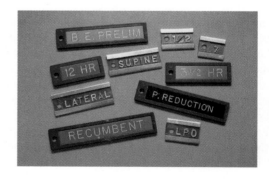

Figure 14-14 *Technologist placing cassette with patient in position to obtain an AP (anteroposterior) view*

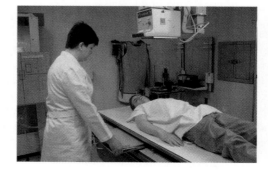

TABLE 14-1

Common Scans That Do Not Require Special Patient Preparation

Scan	Procedure	Approximate Time Required
Brain scan	IV (intravenous) injection and scan immediately. Wait 2 hr and take delayed scan.	Initial injection and flow study-15 min Delayed scan-45 min
Bone scan	IV injection done and wait 3 hr, then scan.	1 hr plus 3-hr interval
Bone marrow scan	IV injection and being scan in 15 min.	1 hr
Cisternogram	Injection into lumbar subarachnoid space via lumbar puncture.	Following injection, scans are done at 6, 24, 48, and 72 hr intervals
Kidney and/or spleen scan	IV injection and scan immediately. For some kidney scans, hydration of patient will be necessary.	45-60 min
Liver scan	IV injection and wait 15 min for scan.	45 min
Lung perfusion scan	Inject and scan immediately.	45 min
Lung ventilation scan	Patient inhales radioactive xenon gas. Serial films are taken for 30 min while patient breathes inert xenon gas.	40 min
Thyroid scan*	IV injection of Technitium 99m and scan; or patient is given Iodine-123 orally and scanned either immediately or 4 to 24 hr later, respectively.	45 min
White blood cell scan	Draw 50ml blood; label WBC with Indium III, then inject cells back into patient. Scan 24 hr later.	60 min

X-ray intravenous iodionated dyes will interfere with the thyroid studies and must not have been done within 3 months of study. Vitamins with iodine interfere with thyroid studies and must be discontinued for at least 2 weeks before study. Synthyroid or other thyroid medications must be stopped for at least 2 weeks before thyroid studies.

TABLE 14-2

Scans That Require Special Patient Preparation

Cardiac scans	If patient is going to have Thallium-201 heart scan, there should be NPO (nothing by mouth) for at least 3 hr before examination. Other cardiac scans need no special preparation.	
Thallium-201 heart scan	Injection IV and scan immediately. Scan is done with patient on a treadmill and at 85% stress. Delayed 6 and 24 hr films.	
Pyrophosphate heart scan	IV injection and scan immediately; then 1 1/2 and 3 hr delayed films.	30-45 min
Cardiac wall motion scan	IV injection and scan immediately.	30-45 min
Gallium scan	For tumor localization amd abscess. Patient is NPO for 6 hr before 24 hr examination. Does not have to be NPO for initial injection. Injection is given IV, and scans are taken at following times: 6 hr, 24 hr, 48 hr, 72 hr.	
Gallium scan of chest (only)	No preparation necessary; scan in 6 hr and 24 hr only.	
Gallius scan of abdomen (all orders should be obtained from physician)	NPO from midnight on evening of injection. Barium enema preparation evening of examination. Tap water enemas until clear on morning of 24-hr examination. Each day after 24 hr film, patient to have 30 ml milk of magnesia (light laxative) at hour of sleep to continue until examination is completed.	
Hepatobiliary scan	NPO 2 hr before. IV injection, then scan immediately.	60 min

VOCABULARY

Basic positions for proper exposure of body part

Anteroposterior (AP)—The x-ray beam is directed from front to back. The patient may be in a supine or standing position, having the back near the film and the front facing the x-ray tube (Figure 14-15).

Posteroanterior (PA)—The x-ray beam is directed from back to front. The patient is usually in an upright position, having the back facing the x-ray tube and the front near the film (Figure 14-16).

Lateral—The x-ray beam is directed from one side in the RL (right lateral) view, the right side of the body is near the film, and the x-ray tube is pointed toward the left side (Figure 14-17). For the LL (left lateral) view, the left side of the body is nearest the film.

Oblique—These views are often used to outline areas that would be hidden and superimposed in the AP/PA and lateral positions. The patient is turned at an oblique angle (Figure 14-18).

Terms to Describe the Patient's Position

Supine—The patient is lying on the back, with face up.

Prone—The patient is lying on the abdomen, face downward.

Recumbent—The patient is lying down.

Erect—The patient is standing either facing the tube or facing away from the tube.

Other Terms to Describe Direction of X-Ray Beam

Axial—The beam is angled.

*Mediolateral—The x-ray beam is directed from the midline toward the side of the part being filmed.

*Craniocaudal—The x-ray beam is directed from the superior to inferior (from head to toe).

Decubitus—The x-ray beam is directed horizontally with the patient lying down.

*This position is often used in mammography.

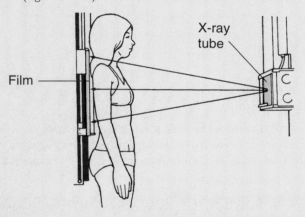

Figure 14-15 *Anteroposterior (AP): The x-ray beam is directed from front to back.*

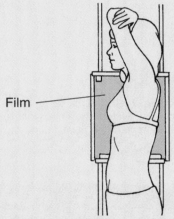

Figure 14-17 *Lateral: The x-ray beam is directed from one side.*

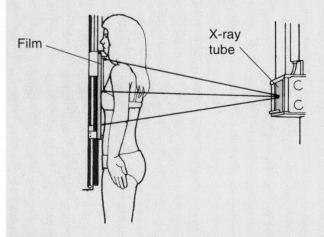

Figure 14-16 *Posteroanterior (PA): The x-ray beam is directed from back to front.*

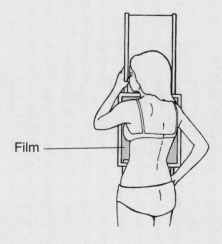

Figure 14-18 *Oblique: The x-ray beam is directed at an angle*

Factors That Affect Images

Kilovoltage

There are two reasons kilovoltage has a profound affect on density:

1. The amount ox x-rays produced is affected by tube kilovoltage.
2. The energy of the x-rays is affected by the kilovoltage. Kilovoltage determines the wavelength of radiation and thus its penetrating power. The greater the penetrating ability of the x-rays, the greater the amount of remnant radiation.

As mentioned earlier, the higher the kilovoltage, the greater the energy of the radiation, and more of the rays traverse the patient and exit on the other side to darken the film.

Milliamperage

The x-ray exposure rate is directly proportional to milliamperage. This is because milliamperage determines the amount of x-ray produced per unit time. With all factors remaining the same, the greater the milliamperage, the greater the amount of radiation produced. If the milliamperage is halved, the amount of x-rays is reduced by half. Thus the amount of remnant radiation is directly proportional to the milliamperage.

Distance

Distance as discussed here relates to the distance from the radiation source (that is, from the x-ray tube to the radiographic file). X-rays emerge from the tube and diverge, proceeding in straight paths. Because of the divergence, they cover an increasingly larger area as they travel farther away from the tube. The radiation emitted from the tube remains the same, but because a larger area is covered as the distance increases, the amount of radiation per square inch is reduced.

The intensity of x-rays reaching the film varies inversely with the square of the distance. Therefore, at twice the distance, the density is one fourth its original value; at half the distance, the density is four times greater.

The decrease in density at greater distances is solely a geometric factor relating to the divergent x-ray beam. The absorption of x-rays by intervening air is insignificant and can be totally disregarded.

From Gurley LT, Callaway WJ: Introduction to radiologic technology, ed 3, St. Louis, 1992, Mosby.

RADIOLOGIC DANGERS, HAZARDS, AND SAFETY PRECAUTIONS

DANGERS

X-rays do constitute a potential danger both to patients and health personnel; therefore proper precautions must be taken at all times.

Massive or excessive exposure to radiation can cause tissue damage and various side effects (see pages 480 and 481). The purpose of radiotherapy is to destroy tissue in diseased areas, but in diagnostic radiology exposure to radiation should be kept within safe limits because radiation has a cumulative effect over a period of time. That is, the radiation a person receives today adds to the last dose received, and these in turn will add to any future doses to accumulate a total radiation dosage. (Doses of radiation were measured in rads or rems or roentgens. According to the newer international standards set in the late 1980s, radiation units are now measured in gray (Gy), seivert (Sv), or coulomb/Kg. Rads = gray, rem = seivert, and roentgens = coulomb/Kg.)

Thus everyone should avoid all unnecessary radiation exposure. On the other hand, patients must be helped to realize the importance of any radiologic examination as an aid for the diagnosis and treatment of a disease process compared with the effects, if any, of the radiation dose that will be received. Newer machines and techniques have significantly reduced the amounts of radiation exposure compared with the same examination of 10 or more years ago.

When radiation goes beyond a safe limit, body tissues may begin to break down. Blood cells, skin, eyes, and reproductive cells are some of the tissues most sensitive to radiation. Overexposure to radiation can result in a lowered red blood cell and white blood cell count because of disturbances of bone marrow and other blood-forming organs; burns on the skin, and cancer; damage to the germinal cells in the ovaries and testes; and also damage to a fetus, especially in the first 3 months of pregnancy. Radiation also apparently predisposes individuals to the development of cataracts.

Studies have shown that massive and prolonged exposure to radiation can result in a higher incidence of cancer, especially of the lymph glands, and the various types of leukemia.

HAZARDS

Hazards of x-rays include the direct x-ray beam itself from the x-ray machine, which travels through an opening in the x-ray tube. Lead (which is able to stop x-rays from traveling) is in the x-ray tube housing to prevent the rays from escaping except through the opening.

A second hazard is scattered radiation of two types: *Leakage radiation* is radiation that may escape (leak) from the head of x-ray machines; this is dangerous to the operator. Therefore frequent inspection of all x-ray equipment is to be performed by a licensed radiation physicist. Once the primary beam of radiation strikes and reacts on the patient or anything else in its path, it is then called *secondary radiation*, which can be emitted in all directions. Secondary radiation is radiation that has deviated from its original path, being strongest close to the patient. Therefore distance is an important factor in radiation protection; that is, the farther one is away from the x-ray source, the better the protection one has from any form of radiation.

Lead screens or shields are used to separate x-ray personnel operating the controls of the machines from the patient receiving the radiation. These protect the personnel from secondary radiation. The walls of the x-ray room are also lined with lead, which absorbs secondary radiation when struck by it and thus prevents radiation from passing through the walls into adjacent areas, exposing others to the radiation. In most facilities, when x-ray machines are in use, a red light flashes on outside the room, indicating to others that radiation is being given and therefore not to enter the room. In some facilities there are interlocking devices by which the door won't open when radiation is being used. Sometimes these devices interact with the x-ray equipment so that the machines won't work unless the door is locked.

SAFETY PRECAUTIONS

X-ray personnel and medical assistants exposed to possible radiation can control the potential dangers by adhering to the following prescribed safety precautionary measures:

1. Have the equipment inspected frequently by a qualified person to ensure that there is no leakage of radiation.
2. Stay behind the lead shield in a lead-lined room when the x-ray machine is being used.
3. Wear a lead apron and protective rubber-lead gloves if it is absolutely necessary to hold the patient or to remain in the room during any radiologic procedure. On these occasions, always face the patient so that the lead apron is closest to the patient, or stay away from the patient. Never assume that you must hold or support the patient, and do not do this routinely. Certain techniques can be used to maintain the patient in the correct position.
4. Wear a film badge (Figure 14-19) on outer clothing at the neck at all times when your job involves exposure to any type of radiation, including exposure to radionuclides. A film badge is a small device that contains x-ray film that is sensitive to radiation and thus records the level and intensity of radiation exposure, which is measured in gray, seivert, or coulomb/Kg. These badges are to be submitted periodically (weekly in some facilities) to a film badge service for evaluation, thus providing a means for warning personnel when dangerous levels of radiation exposure are near.
5. Have a periodic blood count performed to determine if a blood dyscrasia is present. Blood counts do not measure the amount of radiation, but can indicate if there is any apparent radiation damage to blood cells.

To protect the patient from unnecessary radiation exposure, adhere to the following:

1. Before making arrangements for a patient to have an x-ray examination, routinely ask
   a. If and when the patient has had other x-ray studies or therapy and the nature of these.

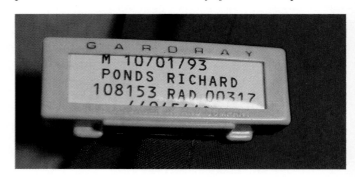

   b. If the patient has been exposed to any radiation for other reasons, such as in employment or an experimental situation.
   c. If it is possible that a female patient is pregnant. These inquiries are important because the patient may have received excessive doses of radiation, and further exposure at that time may be detrimental to the patient's health status. When it appears that the patient has been exposed to a large amount of radiation recently and when a woman suspects that she is pregnant, inform the physician, without alarming the patient, and before making arrangements for the x-ray studies. The physician may want to change the order for x-ray studies at that time. The physician weighs the facts: that is, how urgent is the need for the x-ray examination versus the risk to the patient or fetus who will receive the additional radiation exposure.
2. Position the patient correctly for the x-ray film if licensed to do so (unlicensed personnel should *not* position patients for x-ray procedures) and when this is one of your assisting duties. Accuracy of the film requires that the patient assume and maintain the correct position without moving during the exposure time. If this is not attained, film distortion results, thus requiring the patient to be exposed to additional radiation while a repeat film is taken.
3. Shield the patient's abdomen and reproductive organs with a lead apron when appropriate, especially patients who are pregnant, patients of childbearing age, and children.

MEDICAL ASSISTANT RESPONSIBILITIES

Your responsibilities relating to radiologic procedures used in the physician's office are to prepare the patient, provide reassurance when needed, and use the safety measures relevant to x-ray equipment. When the physician employs a radiographer, you may not do any of these functions.

When outside sources are used, you are responsible for calling the radiologist's office or hospital x-ray department to schedule the examination and for furnishing the patient's name, type of insurance, the referring physician's name, and the type of examination.

One of the most important communications between the medical assistant and radiology department involves the scheduling of multiple x-ray procedures that are ordered at one time for the patient. Consultation is needed to sequence the procedures so that they do not interfere with each other and to decide how many procedures can be done on the same day. You should give all the information to the radiology department so that they can schedule the examinations in proper sequence. The general rule is that examinations **not** using a contrast medium are done **before** examinations that do use a contrast medium; for example, a chest x-ray would be done before a barium enema. The patient is to take the physician's written requisition(s) to the x-ray department on the day of the examinations.

In either situation, before the scheduled date, patients should be informed of the appropriate amount of time that the examination will take so they can schedule other activities accordingly and not get unduly upset or surprised if the examination takes an hour or so. Also, certain x-ray examinations require special patient preparation the day before, the morning of the study, or both. To prepare the patient, you must know and go over the instructions orally with the patient to ensure that they are understood, and provide written instructions to be taken home. Many physicians' offices have preprinted individual instructions to be followed before x-ray studies, or they may use product literature provided by pharmaceutical companies for patient use. Written instructions are essential because oral instructions can easily be forgotten. Repeat examinations required because of poorly given or misunderstood instructions cause unnecessary radiation exposure and expense for the patient.

For the x-ray studies discussed in this unit, Tables 14-3 and 14-4 group those that do not require special patient preparation and those studies that do require individual patient preparation (listed as individual, because the specific preparation may vary among different radiology departments). The approximate amount of time required for each examination is also listed. Samples of individual patient preparations are given for common examinations. Similar reference sheets should be made available for you in the physician's office or clinic.

After the x-ray examination has been completed, you must check to ensure that a written report is received and then filed in the patient's chart after being reviewed by the physician and that the x-ray films, when sent to or when taken in the physician's office, are stored and handled correctly.

TABLE 14-3

X-ray Examinations That Do Not Require Special Patient Preparation

Examination	Time Required
Barium swallow	$^1/_2$ to $^3/_4$ hr
Arthrogram	1 1/2 hr
Diskogram, lumbar or cervical	1 hr
Hysterosalpingogram	1 hr
Lymphangiogram	6 hr
Mammogram	1/2 to 3/4 hr
Xeroradiography	Depends on area being studied
Thermography	Depends on area being studied(seldom used now)
Tomography	1 hr
Computed tomography	1 to 2 hr (no preparation if contrast medium not used)
Abdomen (flat plate)	20 min
Chest	20 min
KUB	10 min; 45 min when it includes intravenous urography
Skill series	20 to 30 min
Paranasal sinuses	20 to 30 min
Bone	15 min to 1 hr, depending on type and area being studied
Magnetic resonance imaging	1 hr (will vary with body part being examined)
Digital radiography	1 hr
Ultrasound of the gallbladder	1 hr

TABLE 14-4

X-ray Examinations That Require Special Patient Preparation

Examination	Time Required	Sample Preparation
Barium enema	30 to 60 min	Take 2 oz (4tbl) castor oil at 4:00 p.m. the day preceding x-ray examination (may be taken in grape juice or root beer). No solid foods on day preceding examination; just liquids such as fruit juice, clear soup, Jello, water, plain tea, or black coffee, but no milk products. NPO after midnight. No breakfast on day of examination. or Enemas till bowels are clear the evening before. NPO after midnight. Rectal suppository in the morning.
Barium meal (upper GI series)	30 to 60 min for stomach, but up to 90 min with small bowel examination; more films may be taken 6 hr or 24 hr later	Nothing to eat or drink after 10:00 p.m. the evening before examination. No breakfast, no fluids, and no cigarettes in the morning. Stomach must be empty. or Nothing to eat or drink after 8:00 p.m. Do not eat breakfast. No water. Report to x-ray office.
Angiogram Arteriogram Angiocardiogram Cerebral angiogram	1 to 3 hr 1 to 3 hr 2 hr 2 to 3 hr	No breakfast when any of these examinations are done in the early morning; or no lunch if they are done in the afternoon.
Bronchogram	1 hr	NPO
Myelogram	1 hr	NPO
Computed tomography	1 to 2 hr	NPO for 4 hr before if a contrast medium is used.
Cholecystogram (gallbladder series)	1 to 2 hr	Evening before x-ray examination, eat a light supper, consisting of nonfatty foods such as lean meat (small portion) and fresh vegetables cooked without butter and no eggs, mayonnaise, French dressing, fried or fatty foods. After supper swallow gallbladder tablets with water, taking one at a time. Eat nothing after evening meal. Water, however, may be taken in moderate amounts until bedtime. Do not take a laxative. Do not eat breakfast. Report to x-ray department. or Low-fat evening meal. Telepaque tablets the evening before. NPO after midnight.
Intravenous cholangiogram	3 hr	NPO
Intravenous pyelogram (IVP)	1 1/2 hr	Take 2 oz (4 tbl) of castor oil or 3 tablets Dulcolax at 4 p.m. the day before x-ray examination. Eat a light supper. Do not drink anything, even water, after midnight. Eat no breakfast, no fluids. or
Retrograde pyelogram	1 to 1 1/2 hr; usually done in operating room	Laxatives or enemas night before examination. NPO for 8 hr before examination
Pneumoencephalogram	2 to 4 hr	NPO
Pneumoencephalomyelogram	2 to 4 hr	NPO

Table 12-4—cont'd

X-ray Examinations That Require Special Patient Preparation

Examination	Time required	Sample Preparation
Ultrasonography Pelvic ultrasound	25 to 45 min up to 2 hr	Afternoon before the examination, take 3 Dulcolax tablets and 3 glasses of water to clear the bowel. On the day of examination, use a Dulcolax rectal suppository 3 hr before examination. Then take 3 to 4 glasses of water 45 min before the examination and do not urinate. A full urinary bladder is essential for this examination. *or* A full urinary bladder is essential. Please do not empty your bladder for 1 to 2 hr before examination. Drink 4 to 6 glasses of any liquid 45 min before examination. Use one Dulcolax suppository 3 hr before examination.
Abdominal ultrasound		Take 1 Mylicon tablet 4 times daily for 2 days before examination. Do not eat solid food after 8:00 a.m. on day of examination. You may take fluids as desired. *or* Take 10 oz. of citrate of magnesia and 3 glasses of water at noon the day before examination. Take 3 Dulcolax tablets at 6:00 p.m. with an additional 3 glasses of water. The evening meal should consist of clear fluids but no milk products. Have nothing other than liquids after midnight. Do not eat breakfast the day of examination.
Renal ultrasound Thyroid ultrasound		Drink 2 glasses of water 1 hr before examination. No preparation needed. Nothing in mouth 3 hr before examination. A full urinary bladder is essential. Do not empty your bladder for at least 1 hr before examination. Drink 4 to 6 glasses of any liquid 45 min before examination.

PREPARATION OF PATIENT AND ASSISTING WITH RADIOGRAPHS

PROCEDURE

1. Identify the patient, check if the special preparation was followed (when applicable), and explain the following:
   a. The value of the examination
   b. How the machine operates
   c. Whether it will hurt
   d. What clothing and other articles must be removed
   e. How to put on the patient gown (that is, with the opening in the front or back)
   f. What position will be required
   g. The importance of remaining still during the examination

RATIONALE

X-ray procedures performed in the office are used for diagnostic or screening purposes. If a required special preparation was not followed, the examination must be canceled and rescheduled. The patient can be told that x-ray examinations are painless, with the exception of those requiring the instillation of a contrast medium. On these occasions, an uncomfortable feeling can be expected, rather than pain. The patient is to remove clothes, watches, all metal, dentures, jewelry, and hairpins that may interfere with the accuracy of the x-ray film. These objects produce shadows on the film and may obscure details that should be observed.

The patient gown is usually put on with the opening in the back. For films of the breast, all clothing from the waist up is removed. The physician determines the position to be maintained by the patient; you tell the patient which position it will be (refer to page 484). Movement of the body during the examination causes distortion on the film. It is then necessary to repeat the examination, which provides additional radiation exposure for the patient.

PREPARATION OF PATIENT AND ASSISTING WITH RADIOGRAPHS—cont'd

PROCEDURE	RATIONALE
2. Drape the patient as necessary. Shield the abdominal regions with a lead apron, especially for patients who are pregnant, patients of childbearing age, or children.	*Drapes may be used to provide warmth and to protect the patient's modesty, but they are not to interfere with the body part being filmed.*
3. Reassure the patient as required. Radiographs are taken on either very sick patients or those who come in for diagnostic purposes, but they all must be given support and attention. Offer assistance to the patient when getting on and off the x-ray table. Remain calm and quietly cheerful.	*Careful and complete explanations to the patient help provide reassurance and reduce fear and confusion. Any reassurance of a nervous patient is helpful.*
4. Be empathetic and courteous; remain calm. The patient will be lying on or standing against a cold, hard plate. In an empathetic and courteous manner, emphasize the importance of remaining still in the proper position.	*Distortion on the film occurs unless the required position is maintained.*
5. When the examination has been completed by the physician or x-ray technician or radiographer, ask the patient to wait in the dressing room while the films are developed.	*The patient remains while films are developed to ensure that clear films have been obtained for study. This is much more convenient for everyone than to have the patient return later for retakes if the preliminary films are not clear.*
6. If it is necessary to obtain another film, explain to the patient that the physician requires another film for study.	*Careful communication is important because you must avoid creating fears in the patient that unnecessary exposure to radiation will result or that the individual taking the x-ray was incompetent, thus necessitating another film.*
7. Dismiss the patient after it has been determined that the films are satisfactory. If the x-ray film showed the presence of a fracture, make arrangements for immediate treatment. The physician will read the films later and notify the patient; *or* schedule a future appointment for a time when the physician can review the results with the patient.	

8. Record the procedure on the patient's chart.	*Charting example:*
	    August 1, 19—.
	        PA and lateral chest x-rays taken by Dr. Mouer.
	        Results—negative. Detailed report to follow.
	        Film No. 8179
	            Cassandra Quinn, CMA

PROCESSING X-RAY FILM

Previously processing x-ray film in a darkroom could be done by either manual methods or by mechanical methods using an automated film processor. Currently, because of the need for quality control procedures with emphasis on the developing equipment, state and federal guidelines require testing and consistency in developing, and only automated processing and developing meet these standards. The automated processing cycle produces a ready-to-read radiograph in as little as 90 seconds up to 10 minutes, depending on the processor used.

Three elements are required for proper automated processing. These include a processor, the correct film(s), and special chemicals. These components are designed to work together to produce a quality radiograph. Follow the manufacturer's recommendation for feeding the film into an automated processor. Usually you feed the film squarely into the processor and feed multiple films simultaneously. The processor transports, processes, and dries the film and replenishes and recirculates the processing solutions (Figure 14-20).

Figure 14-20 A, *Roller transport system of an automated x-ray film processor. Diagram showing how the roller transports films through the various sections of automated processor. The arrangement and number of components in the various assemblies may differ from model to model, but the basic plan is the same.* **B,** *Developing a radiograph using an automatic processor in the darkroom.*
A Reprinted courtesy of Eastman Kodak Co., Rochester, N.Y.

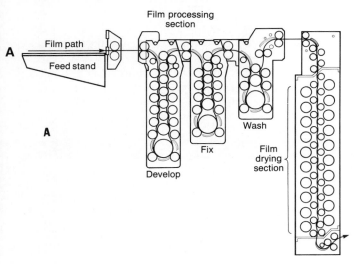

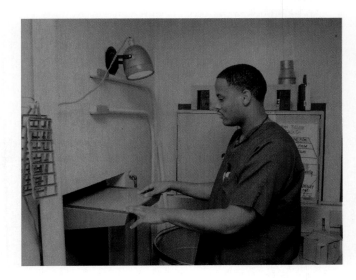

After the automated processing procedure has been completed, the radiograph is ready for viewing on an illuminated viewbox (see Figure 14-12) or is to be placed in a special file envelope labeled with the patient's name, the date, and the x-ray number when used.

STORAGE AND MANAGEMENT IN THE OFFICE

STORAGE OF X-RAY MATERIALS

When x-ray materials are used in the office, they require special storage attention. These supplies must be protected from damage caused by exposure to moisture, heat, and light. Film must be kept in a dry, cool place, preferably in a lead-lined box. The lead-lined box protects the film from any x-rays that may escape during filming.

When unexposed film is to be placed into a cassette for use, the film packets are to be opened only in the darkroom with only the darkroom light on. Before development, the exposed film obtained after the radiologic procedure is completed must also be stored in a lead-lined box to protect it from secondary radiation, which would spoil the radiograph recorded on the film.

X-ray developer solutions must also be stored in a moisture-free, cool location, because they are of extreme importance in the processing of quality radiographs.

OWNERSHIP OF X-RAY FILMS, REPORTS, AND RECORDS

Frequently there is much controversy over the ownership of medical records, reports, and x-ray films. The important thing to remember is that this type of property legally belongs to the medical facility where it is made or recorded. It does not belong to the patient. All x-ray films obtained on a patient are the sole property of the physician's office or hospital that performed the radiologic examination. Written x-ray reports from the radiologist are to be sent to the referring physician, but the actual films usually remain in the files of the office or hospital that did the filming. At times these films can be loaned out to the referring physician for further study, reference, or review as needed to confirm a diagnosis or to compare old films with current ones. At other times the radiologist's office routinely sends the films to the referring physician so that they may be kept as part of the patient's permanent medical record in the office, but they still remain as the legal property of the radiologist. Presently in a few states patients can request, pay for, and obtain copies of the original x-ray film.

Radiologic films are permanent records for current or future reference (as opposed to fluoroscopy, which can be viewed only at the time of the examination unless the procedure was recorded on a videotape or 35-mm film). Special file envelopes are available in which to keep exposed film. These envelopes must be labeled with the patient's name, the date, and the number, if and when used. (Some places file films by number rather than by the patient's name. In this case, the number *must* be recorded on the patient's medical record for a cross-reference.)

X-ray films placed in filing envelopes should be filed in a dry, cool storage area, preferably in a metal cabinet; ones no longer needed for current reference should be filed in a permanent storage file so that they are available for future reference.

CONCLUSION

This unit has given you an introduction to various diagnostic procedures used in the field of radiology. Your responsibilities in these fields, although limited, have been discussed. Numerous additional studies may be performed in these specialty areas of medicine for the diagnosis and treatment of disease processes. It is not within the scope of this book to discuss all of them in detail. There are various sources to which you may refer to expand your knowledge on these procedures. Check with your instructor for additional enrichment assignments and references in areas of your own particular need and interest. A tour through the radiology and nuclear medicine departments of a modern hospital, especially a large teaching hospital, would make you aware of the dramatic progress that has been made in these fields of medicine.

When you think that you know the information presented in this unit, arrange with your instructor to take a performance test.

REVIEW OF VOCABULARY

The following reports received in a physician's office pertain to some of the diagnostic examinations discussed in the preceding pages. Read these and be prepared to discuss the contents with your instructor. A dictionary or other reference books may be used to define the terms with which you are unfamiliar. In addition, it is suggested that you read more on these examinations elsewhere so that you may gain a more complete understanding of the procedures.

PATIENT NO. 1: Upper GI series
Preliminary film reveals no significant soft tissue or osseous abnormality.

There is a small, lesser-curvature antral ulcer measuring 7 mm at its neck and 4 mm deep. No mass is identified, and peristalsis passes through the area with ease. No abnormalities are seen of the distal esophagus, remaining stomach, duodenal bulb, duodenal loop, or proximal small bowel.

CONCLUSION: Small lesser curvature antral ulcer.

Follow up x-ray studies done by another physician
Comparison with previous study of 7-02-93 reveals near-complete clearing of the lesser-curvature antral ulcer. A tiny barium collection measuring about 2 to 3 mm remains in the same location with some adjacent thickened folds.

Duodenal bulb, duodenal loop, and proximal small bowel show no abnormalities.

Distal esophagus appeared normal without evidence of hiatus hernia or reflux.

Incomplete fusion of the L-5 spinous process demonstrated.

CONCLUSION: Near-complete clearing of the lesser curvature antral ulcer. L-5 spina bifida occulta.

PATIENT NO. 2: Barium enema
Following a water-cleansing preliminary enema, the colon was filled quite readily from rectum to cecum, including terminal ileum.

The descending colon is displaced quite strikingly forward and toward the midline in the region of the previously described soft tissue mass closely related to the lower pole of the left kidney. There is no mucosal distortion, and the deformity is mainly that of extrinsic pressure rather than an intrinsic or invasive lesion.

The only other abnormality is a small area of kinking with slight narrowing of the lumen in the proximal transverse colon just distally to the hepatic flexure. That portion of the colon is quite redundant, and this is most likely a kink at the site of redundancy and not a true lesion; however, if surgery is contemplated, direct palpation of this area is suggested. The colon is otherwise normally outlined, and so is the terminal ileum. It empties quite well.

CONCLUSION: Extrinsic pressure and displacement of the left colon by the previously described mass without evidence of any direct invasion. Small area of kinking and narrowing of the lumen at the proximal portion of the transverse colon, most likely normal and simply the result of local redundancy.

Otherwise normal study of the colon.

PATIENT NO. 3: Barium enema
This is compared with similar study of 8/26/93. On the preliminary film there is some barium in the pelvis from previous study. Gas pattern is unremarkable. The large bowel is filled in retrograde manner with barium. Free reflux into the terminal ileum was seen, and the appendix fills. There are a few diverticula deep in the sigmoid, which account for the retention of the barium seen on the scout film. The left colon now distends completely with no evidence of ischemic colitis and no residual stricture noted. The remainder of the colon is unchanged.

IMPRESSION: Normal barium enema without residual from the previously described ischemic colitis.

Diverticulosis of the sigmoid colon.

REVIEW OF VOCABULARY—cont'd

PATIENT NO. 4: Excretory urography with tomography
Preliminary examination demonstrates normal psoas and renal shadows.

There is an ovoid, homogeneous, increased density approximately 13 cm in maximum dimension in the left midabdomen.

Three calcified lymph nodes are in the right lower quadrant.

Opaque medium appears promptly and in good concentration demonstrating normal calyces, pelves, and ureters. The vesicle outline is normal, with minimal retention after voiding.

The left midabdominal mass moves independently from the lower pole of the left kidney, particularly noted in the erect position, and is separate from it. The mass has well-delineated margins and appears to be of homogeneous density. Ultrasound would readily distinguish a cystic from a solid lesion, separating such as a mesenteric cyst from a solid mesenchymal or epithelial tumor, or lymphoma. An ovarian tumor would be unusual in this location but possible.

CONCLUSION: Normal excretory urinary tract. Left midabdominal mass lesion, discussed above.

PATIENT NO. 5: Ultrasound consultation
CHIEF COMPLAINT: Right upper quadrant pain.

ULTRASOUND OF THE GALLBLADDER: The gallbladder is well seen. There is some slightly echogenic material in the dependent part of the gallbladder, but this is not definitely particulate, and there is no acoustic shadowing. Ducts are unremarkable.

IMPRESSION: The material in the gallbladder described above most likely represents sludge. This is not considered definitely abnormal.

PATIENT NO. 6: Chest x-ray report
In PA projection there is a mild dextroconvex curvature of the lower thoracic spine. The bony thorax is otherwise unremarkable.

The heart, vessels, and mediastinal structures are normal.

Clear lungs are well expanded with sharp costophrenic angles. There is no evidence of active disease.

PATIENT NO. 7: Facial bones x-ray report
The facial bones, including the orbits, are intact.

A smooth, 1×1.5–cm soft tissue opacity lies about the posterior aspect of the roof of the left maxillary sinus.

CONCLUSION: Facial bones negative for fracture.

Soft-tissue mass about the roof of the left maxillary sinus. The possibility of a blow-out fracture of the orbit might be considered and should be clinically correlated.

CASE STUDY

Medical personnel must have a proper respect for *radiation* and equipment such as the *fluoroscope*, *oscilloscope*, and the specialty of *radiography*. Read and discuss the following underlined terminology.

1. A 3-year old battered child was brought into the *MRI* facility for evaluation of her head *trauma* and suspected permanent *neurologic* damage, including blindness. *X-ray* had already confirmed a fractured skull, but thorough examination of the soft tissues of the brain were necessary to determine treatment and level of *disability*. Although MRI is a painless and *noninvasive* technique, it is essential the patient lie perfectly still; it poses immense problems for this *pediatric* patient. Because the child is frightened and in pain, it is necessary to administer an injection of *xanax* or *valium* to produce sleep for motionless study and positioning.

2. A 45-year-old male with an acute *exacerbation* of his chronic low back *syndrome* presents today for MRI study. On preparation of the patient for the study, he admits to being "scared to death" and finds it extremely uncomfortable to be positioned flat on his back with his arms at his sides and legs straight. He explains he does not feel he is able to lie still while the table moves him into the MRI unit, a tunnel-like apparatus.

3. A 30-year-old female is schedule for MRI evaluation of a suspected *pelvic mass*. As she is being positioned on the table and moved into the MRI unit, she experiences a major *anxiety attack* as a result of *claustrophobia*. Claustrophobic talk-throughs require a lot of *T.L.C.* In addition, she is very fearful of the loudness of the machine.

REVIEW QUESTIONS

1. Mrs. G.B. Emerson, a 46-year-old, 164-pound woman, has been scheduled for a barium enema and a cholecystogram. Mrs. Emerson does not understand why she must have these tests.

   Explain the nature and purpose of these tests to her and the special directions that she must follow before having these tests performed.

2. The physician has ordered a PA and lateral chest x-ray film to be taken on Mr. T. Rankin. Explain how the patient will be positioned when these films are taken.

3. Mrs. C.A. Lunatto has had extensive radiotherapy and now is experiencing diarrhea and some loss of scalp hair. List four other side effects that she may experience with continued radiation therapy.

4. Mr. K. Cole is suspected of having kidney disease. List five diagnostic studies that the physician may order to help diagnose the problem.

5. Ms. B. Milius has discovered several lumps in her breast while doing a breast self-examination and has now come to the physician for a checkup. List two studies that the physician may order for this patient to help diagnose the condition.

6. Mrs. Gwen Boyd is scheduled for ultrasound to determine if is she is pregnant, because other tests have proven unsuccessful. She feels apprehensive about having this test done and is fearful of the pain she expects to have during this test. Explain the nature and purpose of this test, indicating if pain is to be expected.

7. Explain the nature and purpose of CT. State the advantages of this technique and equipment over other types of radiologic examinations.

8. Explain the nature and purpose of magnetic resonance imaging. State the advantages of this technique over other types of radiologic equipment.

9. List four advantages of digital radiography.

10. What is a film badge, and why is it used?

11. List three ways to protect the patient from unnecessary radiation exposure when having x-ray examinations.

12. Discuss the medical assistant's responsibilities relevant to x-ray procedures performed in the physician's office; at an outside facility.

13. Describe how an x-ray film should be stored in the office.

14. Mr. B. Wingate had a myelogram performed last month and now is in your office, stating that he wants the x-ray films to take home. Define myelogram. Explain to Mr. Wingate why he cannot take the films home.

PERFORMANCE TEST

In a skills laboratory, a simulation of a joblike environment, the medical assistant student will demonstrate skill in performing the following activities without reference to source materials. Time limits for each of the following activities are to be assigned by the instructor (see also page 60).

1. Communicate proper preparation for x-ray procedures to the patient.

2. Prepare the patient for and assist the patient during an x-ray examination.

3. Position the patient for the AP, PA, LL, and RL x-ray exposure, *only* if licensed to do so.

4. Care for and store an x-ray film in the office.

5. Demonstrate safety hazards and precautionary measures relevant to x-ray equipment.

The student is expected to perform the above skills with 100% accuracy.

Physical Therapy

COGNITIVE OBJECTIVES

On completion of Unit Fifteen, the medical assistant student should be able to:

1. Define and pronounce the terms listed in the vocabulary.
2. Differentiate between physical medicine and physical therapy; a physiatrist and a physical therapist.
3. List 11 modalities and/or techniques used for treatments in physical therapy, indicating the nature and purpose or use of each.
4. Describe the differences between ultraviolet radiation, diathermy, ultrasound, and local applications of heat and cold.
5. State the physiologic reactions that occur with applications of heat and with applications of cold.
6. Discuss the principles of preparation and patient care for applications of heat and cold.
7. List examples of dry and moist applications of heat and cold, and describe how to apply these to a patient.
8. Outline the types and uses of traction, massage, and exercises.
9. Differentiate between electrotherapy and electrodiagnostic techniques, explaining the nature and purpose of each.
10. Identify the medical assistant's responsibilities relevant to physical therapy procedures.
11. Outline the steps for performance checklists for the application of heat and cold treatments and other physical therapy modalities listed in this unit.
12. Define and discuss the principles of body mechanics.
13. Discuss the safety precautions and techniques to use when helping patients get in and out of wheelchairs.

TERMINAL PERFORMANCE OBJECTIVES

On completion of Unit Fifteen, the medical assistant student should be able to:

1. Assemble supplies and equipment necessary to correctly apply applications of heat and cold.
2. Apply the various hot and cold applications, using safety precautions to avoid injury to the patient or yourself.
3. Demonstrate proficiency in communicating proper preparation of the patient for physical therapy treatments.
4. Discuss with the instructor the desired and undesired effects of applications of heat and cold.
5. Design a teaching-instruction program for the patient who will be using the following modalities at home:
   a. Heating pad
   b. Moist cold compress
   c. Hot water bottle
   d. Ice pack
   e. Hot moist compress
   f. Alcohol sponge bath
   g. Chemical hot pack
   h. Chemical cold pack
   i. Ice bag
6. Design a performance checklist to be used for the application of the following:
   a. Dry heat applications
   b. Dry cold applications
   c. Moist heat applications
   d. Moist cold applications
7. Demonstrate correct standing, lifting, and bending techniques.
8. Demonstrate safe techniques when helping a patient get in and out of a wheelchair.
9. Assist patients in learning how to walk with crutches, a cane, and a walker.
10. Determine the correct size of crutches, a cane, and a walker for a patient.

The student is to perform these activities with 100% accuracy.*

The consistent use of universal precautions is required by all health care professionals in all health care settings as a method of infection control. It is assumed that these precautions are used in all of the following procedures. Review Unit One if you have any questions on methods to use

*You should review Diagnostic and Therapeutic Procedures, as well as Organizing the Recordings of Diagnostic Procedures, in Unit Ten, pages 325 to 328, before proceeding with this unit.

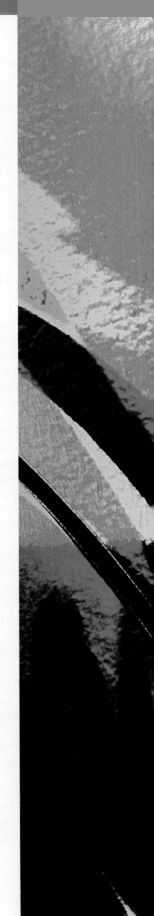

as the methods/techniques will not be repeated in detail in each procedure presented in the unit.

Be sure to consult the latest guidelines issued by the Centers for Disease Control and Prevention and consult with infection control practitioners when needed to identify specific precautions that pertain to your particular work situation.

Physical medicine or physiatrics (fiz′e-ah′triks) is the medical discipline that uses physical and mechanical agents in the diagnosis, treatment, and prevention of disease processes and bodily ailments. The therapeutic use of these agents in conjunction with patient education and rehabilitation programs (rather than by medicinal or surgical means) is called physical therapy (PT). Physicians who specialize in this field are physiatrists (fiz″e-ah′trist). *Physical therapists* (physiotherapists) are specially trained, licensed individuals skilled in the techniques of physical therapy (physiotherapy) and qualified to evaluate a patient's condition and complaints, to administer treatments and tests prescribed by a physician, and to evaluate the patient's progress and test results. Licensed physical therapists can treat patients without a physician's referral, and some do set up a private practice for this type of direct access for care.

The purpose and aim of physical therapy is to relieve pain, increase circulation, restore and improve muscular function, build strength, and increase the range of motion or mobility of a joint. Aside from treating patients with neuromuscular conditions, physical therapy is involved with a significant number of physical conditioning programs, particularly for patients with cardiac and pulmonary conditions. The primary objective of physical therapy is to promote optimum health and function. Chest therapy is also given to patients with pulmonary conditions to help clear secretions and keep the air passageways open and clear. Patient education is a major area in physical therapy (that is, physical therapists teach and train patients how to perform essential activities that they can do themselves for their condition and how to avoid recurrences of certain problems).

A great variety of modalities and techniques using the properties of heat, cold, electricity, water, light, mechanical maneuvers, and exercise are used in physical therapy. Generally speaking, physical therapy treatments are given by physical therapists or the physician; therefore your duties may be limited. However, if you work in a physician's office, you are often required to administer some types of physical therapy treatments under the direction and supervision of the physician. In addition, at the physician's request, you should be able to explain the nature and purpose of the treatment or test to the patient or provide adequate instructions to be followed by the patient at home. It is too often assumed that patients who are to use heat or cold applications at home know how to do so without assistance. You should ensure that these patients understand the dangers of using heat or cold to excess and the importance of using the correct solution at the proper temperature.

Some knowledge of the various modalities used in physical therapy is therefore a requirement for the well-trained medical assistant. The following pages are devoted to briefing you

VOCABULARY

Arthritis (ar-thri-tis)—Inflammation of a joint.

Bursitis (bur-si-tis)—Inflammation of a bursa. The most commonly affected is the bursa of the shoulder.

Conduction (kon-duk′shun)—The passage or conveyance of energy, as of electricity, heat, or sound.

Debridement (da-bred-ment)—The process of removing foreign material and dead tissue.

Hypothermia (hi-po-ther′me-ah)—Low body temperature.

Light therapy or phototherapy (fo′to-ther′ah-pe)—The use of light rays in the treatment of disease processes. By custom, this includes the use of ultraviolet and infrared or heat rays (radiation).

Modality (mo-dal′i-te)—Therapeutic agents used in physical medicine and physical therapy.

Psoriasis (so-ri-′ah-sis)—A chronic inflammatory recurrent skin disease characterized by scaly red patches on the body surfaces. The lesions are seen most often on knees, elbows, scalp, and fingernails. Other areas frequently affected are the chest, abdomen, palms of the hands, soles of the feet, and backs of the arms and legs. The cause is unknown, although a hereditary factor is suggested.

Sprain (spran)—A joint injury in which some fibers of a supporting ligament are torn or wrenched and partially ruptured, but continuity of the ligament remains intact. There may also be damage to the associated muscles, tendons, nerves, and blood vessels. A sprain is more serious than a strain.

Strain (stran)—An overexertion or overstretching of some part of a muscle.

Tendinitis (ten″di-ni′tis)—Inflammation of a tendon; one of the most common causes of acute pain in the shoulder.

on various physical therapy modalities and techniques used and their uses and purposes. Additional materials that may be studied or demonstrations for using the equipment are provided by the manufacturers of the modalities.

For any of the subsequent treatments that may fall within the scope of your job duties, you must implement the basic steps outlined in previous units for all procedures. You should now be able to organize the information that will be presented on various treatments into the following briefly stated procedural steps. These steps can also be used as a guideline for a performance test checklist.

1. Check the physician's order.
2. Wash your hands. **Use appropriate personal protective equipment (PPE) as dictated by facility.**
3. Assemble the equipment and supplies needed.
4. Identify the patient, and explain the nature and purpose of the treatment.
5. Prepare the patient: position correctly and comfortable, and drape as necessary.

6. Prepare supplies for use.
7. Proceed with the treatment, and time it accurately.
8. Observe the area to which the treatment has been applied frequently for desired or adverse reactions.
9. Remove the application used for the treatment.
10. Attend to the patient's safety and comfort; provide further instructions as indicated.
11. Properly care for the used equipment and supplies.
12. Wash your hands.
13. Record the treatment and the results obtained.
    Charting example:
        September 9, 19__, 9 a.m.
           Hot moist compress applied to a wound on the inner aspect of the right forearm at 105° F (40.8° C) for 20 minutes. On completion of the treatment, the skin appeared pink, and the wound appeared clean; no evidence of suppuration present. Dry dressing was applied. Patient stated that most of the pain was relieved and that the compress provided much comfort.
                                       Kim Worth, CMA

ULTRAVIOLET LIGHT

Ultraviolet rays are rays beyond the violet end of the visible spectrum. They are produced by the sun and by sun lamps. Although ultraviolet rays produce very little heat, they can cause tanning on the skin or a sunburn (redness, erythema) and are capable of killing bacteria and other microorganisms and activating the formation of vitamin D.

Ultraviolet rays (light) are used therapeutically in the treatment of acne, psoriasis, pressure sores, and wound infections. The purposes of this treatment are to stimulate growing epithelial cells and cause capillary hyperemia and to increase cellular metabolism and vascular engorgement (an excess amount of blood in the vessels), which increases the skin's defenses against bacterial infections.

Various forms of apparatus provide ultraviolet rays. Before receiving ultraviolet treatment, the patient's sensitivity must first be determined. This is done by exposing different areas of the patient's skin to different dosages of the rays for different time periods. The following day the patient returns so that the response can be determined. A little redness on the skin area is desired, but not a real burn. For example, if 20 seconds of exposure gives the maximum coloration to the skin that is wanted without giving any more, the treatment is started with a 20-second exposure period to the ultraviolet light; then, depending on the light used, the exposure time is usually increased by 10-second intervals. The number of treatments to be given depends on how well the patient is responding.

When this treatment is given, the light must be placed at least 30 inches away from the patient and directed *only* on the area(s) to be treated.

Timing of the exposure period *must be exact* because excessive exposure can cause severe sunburn up to second and third degree burns. Dark goggles should be worn by both the patient and the operator of the light to protect their eyes.

The patient *must never* be left unattended while being exposed to this light. If you are timing the exposure period and for some reason have to leave the room, you must disconnect the light and resume the treatment when you return. Some will turn off automatically, but it is still important for the operator to be present in the room when the patient is receiving this treatment to ensure that undesired burns do not result.

DIATHERMY

Diathermy is a heat-inducing wavelength that is part of the electromagnetic spectrum. It is the therapeutic use of a high-frequency current, the purpose being to generate heat within a part of the body. Diathermy works by inducing an electrical field, a conduction field in the tissues, and thereby heats the tissues and increases the circulation.

Diathermy is used in the treatment of muscular problems and sometimes for the treatment of arthritis, bursitis, and tendinitis.

The term diathermy is also applied to the many different machines available for this purpose.

Depending on the machine used, the applicator is generally placed at least 1 inch away from the patient's skin. The heating element of some machines has a spacer built into it (that is, there is a space between the outside cover on the unit and the actual heating element). With these machines, the element is placed directly against the skin, because it is the outside cover of the unit and not the actual heating element that is in contact with the skin. The built-in spacer of these machines provides the required distance between the skin and the heating element.

Other machines have pads on the applicators. When these machines are used, towels (1-inch thickness) are placed between the pad and the patient's skin.

When giving diathermy treatments, you must watch for desensitized skin areas because patients have to be able to feel the heat; otherwise they can get burned without realizing that they are getting burned. Areas of skin breakdown and other reactive areas such as inflamed areas must be avoided.

The electrical field of diathermy is attracted by metal. Therefore patients who have metal implants such as joint implants cannot receive diathermy treatments. In addition, patients cannot be wearing any jewelry or other metal objects such as buckles and hairpins and cannot be positioned on a metal table or chair, but must be on wooden furniture. If these practices are not followed, the patient may receive severe burns, because metal will become hot once the diathermy unit is turned on. Duration of the treatment is usually 15 to 20 minutes and should be timed carefully. It must be explained to the patient that a warm, comfortable feeling should be experienced and, if he or she becomes uncomfortable, to inform the operator of the unit. If the patient complains that the treatment is becoming too hot, it must be stopped to avoid burning the patient. To operate any of the diathermy units available, you must carefully follow the instructions for use supplied by the manufacturers of each unit. Currently diathermy is seldom used in many facilities. It has been replaced by ultrasound.

ULTRASOUND

Ultrasound is also part of the electromagnetic spectrum. Therapeutic ultrasound is a very specific part of the sound spectrum that provides acoustic vibration with frequencies beyond human ear perception. This form of treatment uses high-frequency sound waves to penetrate deep tissue layers. Sound waves transform into heat whey they reach deep tissues. (Ultrasound is also used for diagnostic purposes. Review page 479 in Unit Fourteen).

Ultrasound vibrates on a molecular level. The two effects obtained from ultrasound are a mechanical effect and a heating effect. The mechanical effect, the vibration that causes the heating, is most noticeable on connective tissues, such as tendons and ligaments. A heating effect is produced on almost all tissues with the exception of bone because bone reflects ultrasound (that is, ultrasound is reflected from bone).

Ultrasound is of value for the treatment of pain syndromes, to relax muscle spasm, to increase elasticity of tissues with collagen such as tendons and ligaments so that they will respond better to stretching, and to provide deep penetration of heat and stimulate circulation in small areas, as when used to increase blood supply to tissues in patients with vascular disorders. It is also used in breaking up calcium deposits and in loosening scars.

Ultrasound is applied by means of an applicator with a sound heat, approximately 2 inches in diameter, that extends off from the special machine. Since ultrasound is not conducted through the air, a conducting medium must be spread on the patient's skin over the area to be treated. Special gels are available for this; mineral oil can also be used, but it is not as effective. After the gel is applied to the skin, the operator of the machine holds the sound head and moves it in a steady, up-and-down and rotary motion over the skin. The applicator must be in motion when used to prevent internal burns or tissue damage. Special care must also be taken when this treatment is used on patients with implants such as joint implants because ultrasound tends to vibrate and loosen the implant. In addition, heat builds up in the metal (Figure 15-1). Ultrasound

---

Figure 15-1 *Ultrasound therapy applied to patient's shoulder in physical therapy.*

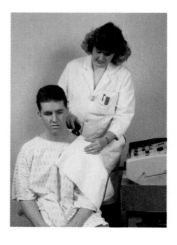

can also be applied under water for treatment of the hands and feet. The water then acts as the conducting medium for the ultrasound. The length of any treatment depends on the size of the area being treated, but is usually under 10 minutes. For example, ultrasound treatment to the lower back is applied for 6 to 7 minutes on one side. The minimal number of ultrasound treatments to be given to be effective varies from 5 to 12.

After use, the sound head should be cleansed with alcohol. Instructions for use of the ultrasound machines are supplied by the manufacturers and must be followed carefully.

LOCAL APPLICATIONS OF HEAT (THERMOTHERAPY) AND COLD (CRYOTHERAPY)

Dry and moist applications of heat and cold have been used universally as an effective means of treatment by individuals in the home and by physicians, nurses, medical assistants, and physical therapists, either in an office or hospital setting. Tolerance for the temperature changes that occur when heat or cold is applied to the body varies with the individual and also varies in different parts of the body. Generally, the areas of the skin more sensitive to these changes are those that are not usually exposed; the less sensitive areas are those that are exposed, usually having thicker and tougher layers of skin such as areas on the soles of the feet or the palms of the hands.

Once heat or cold is applied to the skin, certain physiologic reactions occur in the body; heat has the opposite effect to that of cold except for respiratory rate changes (Table 15-1).

Heat or cold modalities are to be placed on a bare body surface for only *short durations* usually 15 to 20 minutes. An important fact to remember is that the prolonged use of heat (more than 1 hour) produces reverse secondary effects (that is, blood vessels then constrict, thus decreasing blood supply to the area). The prolonged use of cold (more than 1 hour) also has a reverse secondary effect (that is, blood vessels dilate, thus increasing circulation and tissue metabolism). In other words, the immediate effect of heat applications is vasodilation, whereas the prolonged effect is vasoconstriction; and the immediate effect of cold applications is vasoconstriction, whereas the prolonged effect is vasodilation. Therefore heat applications should not be left in place for long periods of time. Cold applications can be used for longer periods than heat, depending on the desired effects. The physician usually indicates the temperature (that is, warm or hot, tepid, cool, cold, or very cold) and the time period to be used for the following applications of dry and moist hot and cold applications.

PRINCIPLES FOR PREPARATION AND PATIENT CARE

Because applications of heat and cold are common treatments, you should keep in mind the following principles regarding preparation and patient care:

TABLE 15-1

Physiologic Reactions Produced by Heat and Cold Applications

Body Function	Heat	Cold
Blood vessels in area	Dilated (increasing circulation)	Constricted (decreasing circulation)
Heat production	Decreased	Increased (by shivering)
Blood pressure	Lowered	Elevated
Respiratory rate	Increased	Increased
Tissue metabolism	Increased	Decreased
Muscle spasm	Relaxed	Reduced
Temperature	Increased	Reduced

1. Learn exactly where and for how long the application is to be placed on the patient's body.
2. Position the patient comfortably so that the treatment can be maintained for the designated time period.
3. Avoid accidents—be sure that the patient is positioned safely and will not fall. Place solutions in a convenient location and so that they will not spill.
4. Test the solution (with a bath thermometer) or the device you are using to be sure that it is at the exact temperature that the physician ordered or the recommended temperature for the method used.
5. Remove any dressings covering the area to be treated. (Review the procedure for a dressing change, pages 228 to 232. Apply a clean dressing, if ordered, when the treatment is completed.
6. Keep the application at the ordered temperature. Generally, compresses and packs cool off within 15 to 20 minutes and then have to be reheated and reapplied. If the temperature of the device or the solution changes, it will not accomplish its purpose and may even harm the patient.
7. Keep the patient warm during the application of heat; drape sheets or blankets can be used to cover the patient. When blood vessels dilate (as with the application of heat), more blood comes to the surface of the body, and the body is cooled by the surrounding air. Thus the patient can easily become chilled unless protected with covering.
8. Check the patient's skin frequently during the application to observe for any skin changes, as well as for any signs of burns or frostbite. Report any signs of burns or frostbite *immediately.*
9. Provide further instruction to the patient, as indicated, on completion of the treatment.

THERMOTHERAPY

Superficial heat treatments can be administered with dry or moist heat applications. These local heat applications are used to relieve pain, to promote muscle relaxation and reduce spasm, to increase circulation to an area to relieve congestion and swelling by dilating the blood vessels, and to speed up the inflammatory process to promote suppuration (pus formation) and drainage from an infected area. In addition, dry heat applications are used to dry and heal surgical incisions and sutures, perineal lacerations, and skin ulcers.

Dry Heat

Dry heat applications frequently used include the following:
- Infrared radiation (heat lamps)
- Electric light bulbs
- Electric heating pads
- Hot water bottles
- Chemical hot pack
- Aquamatic (K- or K-matic) pad with cover and heating unit

Infrared radiation is dry heat application by means of a heat lamp. The term infrared usually refers to the heat lamp. Infrared rays from these lamps provide surface heat and penetrate the skin to a depth of about 5 to 10 mm. At times, a plain gooseneck lamp is used, because the *incandescent light bulb* is a source of infrared rays. Heat lamps must be kept at least 2 to 4 feet away from the skin, varying with the type and intensity of the lamp used. The skin must be clean and free of any ointment or medicinal substances. The duration of the treatment is *usually 15 to 20 minutes*, because prolonged or intense application can lead to burning and blistering of the skin.

Place *electric heating pads* in a protective covering such as a towel or pillow case, and then apply them to a dry area. Never use them over moist or wet areas or dressings by means of which moisture could come in contact with the electricity. Instruct patients not to lie on the pad because burns could result. The heat selector switch is usually set on the low or medium setting and left for an accurately timed period. (The amount of heat and period of time to be applied are designated by the physician.)

When using a *hot water bottle*, it is essential to test the temperature of the water accurately with a thermometer before it is poured into the water bottle. Place hot tap water into a pitcher so that the temperature can be tested with a bath thermometer. Water not exceeding 125° F (32°C) is to be used. The accepted temperature ranges are from 115° to 125° F (46° to 52° C) for patients 2 years and older, and from 105° to 115° F (41° to 46° C) for children under 2 years and elderly patients. (The very young and the very old tend to be more sensitive to applications of heat and to cold.)

Fill the hot water bottle only about half full and expel the air before you seal it. This allows the bottle to be lighter and more pliable so that it can be molded to the area on which it is to be applied. The outside of the hot water bottle must be dry and then placed into a protective covering such as a pillowcase or towel before it is applied to the patient. This protective covering should remain dry unless the hot water bottle is placed over moist dressings to keep them warm (Figure 15-2).

Figure 15-2 A, *Test temperature of hot water before placing it into hot water bottle.* **B,** *Expel air from half-filled hot water bottle before using.* **C,** *Cover the hot water bottle before applying to patient.*

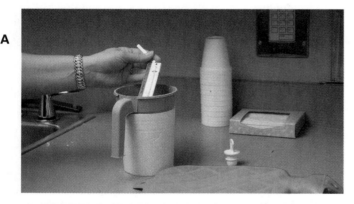

A

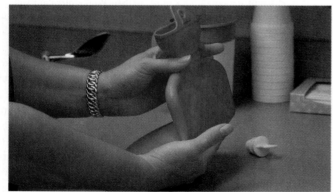

B

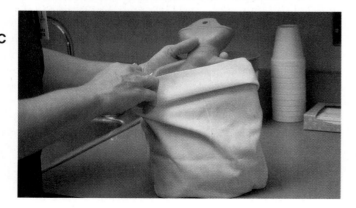

C

The patient should experience a feeling of warmth but not be uncomfortable; burns must be avoided. When the hot water bottle is left on for any length of time, it needs to be refilled with hot water so the desired temperature is maintained. After use, wash the hot water bottle thoroughly with warm water and detergent, rinse it, and allow it to dry before being stored. Store the bottle with the stopper in place and air inside to prevent the sides from sticking.

Disposable chemical hot packs are prepared commercially in various sizes and shapes. When they are activated, they provide a specific amount of heat for a specific amount of time. They are pliable so can fit the contour of any body part. Follow the manufacturer's directions to activate the chemical reaction that produces the heat. The directions are usually to deliver a sharp blow to the pack or to knead it. Cover the pack with a cloth before applying it to the patient's skin.

The *Aquamatic (K- or K-matic) pad* is a rubber pad of tubular construction that is filled to about two-thirds full with distilled water. The water is heated and kept at an even temperature by an electrical control unit. Cover the pad and place it around or over the body part or surface to be treated. It is usually left on the patient for 15 to 30 minutes. This pad is both more effective and safer than an electric heating pad or a hot water bottle because you can maintain a constant temperature by regulating the control unit (Figure 15-3).

Moist Heat Applications

Moist heat applications frequently used include the following:
- Hot soaks
- Hot compresses
- Hot packs

Hot Soaks

For a *hot soak*, the body part to be treated is immersed gradually (to allow the patient to become accustomed to the heat change) in tap water or a medicated solution of 105° to 110° F (41° to 44° C). Unless otherwise ordered, the body part is kept immersed for 15 to 20 minutes. This form of treatment can be used for heat application to the hands, arms, feet, or legs. The process of having the body from the neck down immersed in

Figure 15-3 *Aquamatic (K or K-matic) pad and heating unit used for dry heat application.*

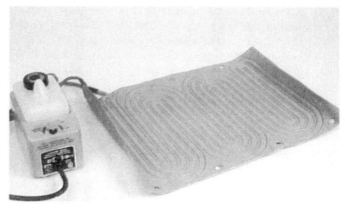

water in a special tank called the Hubbard tank, or the body or a limb immersed in a whirlpool tank, is more frequently referred to a hydrotherapy (see page 503). Soaks applied to open wounds require the use of sterile technique, a sterile container, and a sterile solution. The water or solution temperature should be maintained as much as possible throughout the treatment. You can do this by removing some of the solution every 5 minutes or so and adding more hot solution. Take care to avoid burning the patient when the hot solution is added. Add the hot solution to the container at the point farthest away from the patient's skin and stir it quickly into the cooler solution (Figure 15-4).

Position the patient comfortably to prevent strain or pressure on the area treated and also to prevent fatigue. Observe the patient's skin during the treatment for excessive redness, at which time remove the limb from the solution until it has cooled. Remember to record the observations made during the treatment on the patient's record. On completion of the treatment, dry the limb with a towel by patting, *not* rubbing. For an open wound, pat dry only the surrounding area. Do not allow the towel to touch the open wound. It is necessary to observe the area after the treatment because you must record this information on the patient's record. Soaks differ from compresses and packs in that soaks are used for shorter periods of time and usually at lower temperatures.

Hot moist compresses and packs. There are two basic differences between compresses and packs: (1) different materials are used for each, and (2) a pack is usually applied to a more extensive body area than a compress is.

A *compress* used for the application of moist heat is prepared by taking a soft square of gauze or similar absorbent material (a clean washcloth can also be used), soaking it in hot water, then wringing it out manually or with the use of forceps, to avoid excessive wetness. This material is then applied to a limited body area, such as the finger or a small area on the arm, for a designated period of time (Figure 15-5). *Dry compresses* are used to apply pressure or medications to specific restricted areas.)

Figure 15-4 *During a hot soak, add more hot solution to container at point farthest away from patient's skin and stir quickly into cooler solution.*

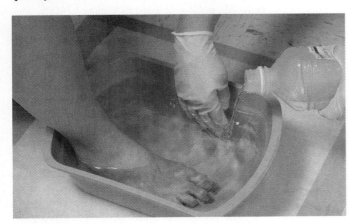

Figure 15-5 A, *Wring out hot compress to avoid excessive wetness before you apply it.* **B,** *Apply hot compress to body area.*

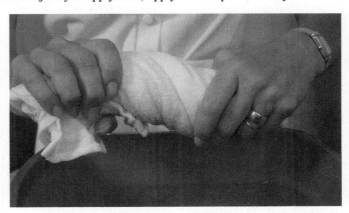

A

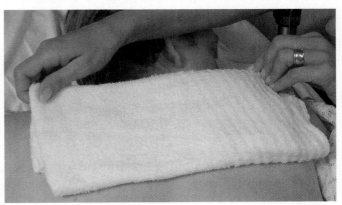

B

CRYOTHERAPY

Cryotherapy, the therapeutic use of cold, is applied with dry or moist cold applications. Cold applications are used to:

1. Prevent edema or swelling
2. Relieve pain or tenderness (cold produces a topical anesthetic effect)
3. Reduce the inflammation and pus formation (cold inhibits microbial activity in the early stages of the infectious process)
4. Control bleeding (the peripheral vessels constrict with the application of cold, resulting in a decreased blood flow)
5. Reduce body temperature

Cold is commonly used following strain, sprains, and bruises and also for muscle spasm and tenderness. Any type of acute injury responds fairly well to cold. During the acute phase of an injury when there may be bleeding in the area, you do not want to use heat. The old rule of thumb for treating such injuries was to apply cold for the first 24 hours, then apply heat. Currently, many health care practitioners frequently wait longer than 24 hours before using heat applications on patients, and often use cold continually when positive results are being obtained.

The physician should indicate the temperature to be used for cold applications. The temperatures of the water are described as follows:

- Tepid: 80° to 93° F (26.7° to 33.9° C)
- Cool: 65° to 80° F (18.3° to 26.7° C)

- Cold: 55° to 65° F (12.3° to 18.3° C)
- Very cold: Below 55° F (below 12.5° C)

The selection of the temperature to use depends on the following:

- Condition of the patient
- Sensitivity of the patient's skin
- Area to be covered
- Method to be used

The duration of the application depends on the temperature (for example, an ice massage is given for a shorter time period [5 minutes] than a cold compress or pack [20 or 32 minutes]). Colder temperatures can be tolerated best on small areas for short periods of time. It is usually considered dangerous to keep skin temperatures below 40° F (4.4° C) for long periods except when ice is used for anesthesia.

Dry Cold

Dry cold applications frequently used include the following:

- Ice bags
- Ice collars
- Chemical cold packs

Fill an *ice bag* one-half to two-thirds full with small pieces of ice; expel air from the bag by twisting the top and then capping (Figure 15-6). At this time check the bag for leaks. Small ice pieces reduce the amount of air spaces in the bag, which results in better conduction of cold and also allows the bag to mold better to the contour of the body part. Once the ice bag is sealed, dry it and place it in a protective covering, which provides comfort for the patient and absorbs moisture that condenses on the outside. For the ice bag to be effective, place it on the skin for 30 to 60 minutes, as designated by the physician. If the treatment is to be continuous, apply the ice bag for 30 to 60 minutes and then remove it for 1 hour. By doing the procedure in the manner, you allow the tissues to react to the immediate effects of the cold.

Check the patient's skin periodically for signs of decreased swelling or redness. When they are present, note signs of excessive coldness, which include mottled and pale skin, and excessive numbness in the body part. When or if this occurs, remove the ice bag and notify the physician.

Figure 15-6 *Expel air from ice bag by twisting the top and then the cap.*

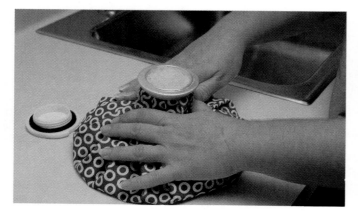

Ice collars are rubber or plastic modalities that are smaller than ice bags and look like a medium-sized rectangle. They are used on the neck, on small areas, or wrapped around a body part.

Chemical cold packs are rubberized, plasticized flat bags containing a chemical substance and a liquid. They are commercially prepared in various sizes and shapes and come with specific instructions that must be followed. Some are for one-time use. Others can be stored in a freezer for reuse. To activate the chemical reaction that produces the coldness, you must usually squeeze or knead the pack and then shake it to mix the contained granules and liquid. The pack remains cold for between 30 and 60 minutes, varying with the brand. Some packs are covered with a soft outer covering and/or wrap and therefore do not need an additional cover. Others have to be covered with a cloth before they are applied to the person's skin. They are pliable and can be molded to fit the contour of any body part (Figure 15-7, *A* and *B*).

Moist Cold

Moist cold applications frequently used include the following:

- Cold compresses
- Cold packs
- Ice massage
- Alcohol sponge baths

Moist cold compresses are generally applied to small areas, and cold packs are used on larger body areas, as are hot appli-

Figure 15-7 A, *Reusable chemical cold pack and cover;* **B,** *disposable chemical cold packs.*

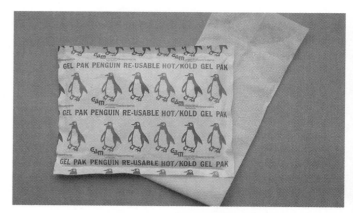

A

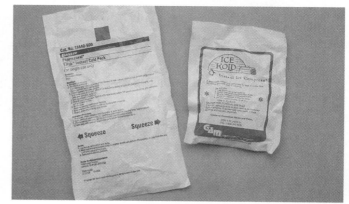

B

cations. Compresses may be used for treating a headache, a tooth extraction, or an eye injury. The area to which the compress is to be applied determines the type of material used. For example, a clean washcloth can be used on the head or face; surgical gauze dressings with a small amount of cotton filling can be used for eye compresses. Immerse the material used for the compress in a clean basin containing ice chips or small pieces of ice and a small amount of cold water. To avoid dripping, wring the material out manually or with the use of forceps and then place it on the skin for the time period designated by the physician (usually 20 to 30 minutes and then repeated every 2 hours). Change compresses frequently to maintain a cold application. Most patients will tell you when the compress no longer feels cold. Placing an ice bag over the compress helps keep the compress cold and reduces the number of times that it must be changed. Check the patient periodically during this treatment for any changes such as a decrease or increase in swelling or redness on the area or a decrease or increase of pain. On completion of the treatment, pat the skin dry if necessary. Record the treatment and observations on the patient's record.

Cold packs (ice packs) may be applied to a small area but are generally used on larger areas, such as an arm or leg. At times they can be applied to the whole body to lower the temperature. In this case, hypothermia pads or blankets may be used, rather than ice packs. These are used in hospitals with the patient under close observation for temperature and skin changes. Manufacturers of hypothermia units provide complete instructions for use, which must be followed precisely.

To apply a cold or ice pack, first wrap the extremity in wet toweling and then pack ice chips around it; place an additional towel over the ice to reduce the melting rate. Generally, these are applied for 20 to 30 minutes. Commercial cold packs are also available. These are kept in a freezer until used. They do not freeze stiff; thus they are pliable and can be molded to fit the contour of the body part.

Ice massage is simply massaging the area with ice. This can be as simple as freezing water in a paper cup and then rubbing it over the affected area for approximately 5 minutes (Figure 15-8).

Figure 15-8 *Ice massage is one form of cryotherapy that can be used to decrease pain. Use a chemical ice pack, or freeze water in paper cup, cover cup and rub it over affected area.*

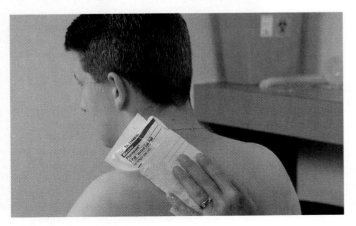

In the past, **alcohol sponge baths** were recommended and used frequently, both in hospital and at home, for reducing a patient's elevated temperature. Presently they are more commonly done in a home situation, because they have been replaced in many hospitals or health care facilities by hypothermia pads or blankets. A mixture of half alcohol and half tepid water is used for an alcohol sponge bath. Because alcohol vaporizes more quickly than water, heat is removed from the skin surface rapidly when this mixture is applied to the body in contrast to using just a cold bath.

An alcohol sponge bath should *not* exceed 30 minutes. Drape the patient with covers, and apply a hot water bottle to the feet to avoid excessive chilling and shivering. Apply an ice bag to the head to promote comfort and relieve a headache, if present. Expose only the area being sponged. You need two clean washcloths—while one is being used, the other is to be cooling in the alcohol-water solution. Sponge each extremity for approximately 5 minutes, the back and buttocks for 5 to 10 minutes, and the trunk and abdomen for 5 minutes. Moist, cool cloths can be placed over large superficial blood vessels in the neck, axilla, and groin during the procedure as additional aids to lower the body temperature. Record the temperature 30 minutes after the sponge bath to determine if the treatment has been effective.

You should caution patients *not* to use alcohol sponge baths indiscriminately because alcohol has a tendency to dry out the skin. In addition, if a fever does not break after the application of two or three alcohol sponge baths given in the home, the physician should be notified.

HYDROTHERAPY

Hydrotherapy is the use of water in the treatment of disease processes. Since these treatments are usually not performed in the physician's office, the patient is referred to a physiotherapy department in a hospital or to a physical therapist's office. On other occasions the patient may be instructed to apply hot or cold soaks, compresses, or packs at home.

Modalities used for hydrotherapy include the Hubbard tank, the whirlpool, and a larger pool, all with varying temperatures of hot or cold water, as designated by the physician for each patient's care.

These three modalities are used primarily to promote relaxation, circulation, and early motion (by exercising) of the injured body part. Other uses include those discussed previously under Local Applications of Heat, page 498. It is also used to cleanse and debride the skin (for example, in patients who have extensive burns). The Hubbard tank is a large tank in which the whole body can be immersed either in a sitting or lying position. It is basically a large whirlpool in which body exercises may also be done. The whirlpool is a tank of agitating water in which an arm, leg, or body can be immersed. The mechanical action of the water movement provides hydromassage, is very relaxing, and stimulates circulation. Body exercises cannot be done in the whirlpool tank because it is too small. The pool used in physical therapy is like a medium-sized swimming pool. Many types of exercises can be performed in the pool, because once in the pool, the effects of gravity can be reduced. For example, patients who are not strong enough to stand up alone can stand up in the pool because they are supported by the water. The water also produces a heating or cooling effect, depending on the temperature used.

PARAFFIN WAX HAND BATH

Another form of heat application used for patients with rheumatoid arthritis is the hot paraffin wax hand bath. The purposes of this treatment are to relieve pain, increase circulation, and decrease the duration of morning stiffness of the fingers, hands, and wrists. An advantage of this treatment over moist heat applications is the longer-lasting (2 to 3 hours) circulatory changes that it can produce. This procedure can be performed at home, in the physician's office, or in a physical therapy department. Special containers are available for storing and heating the wax; or in a home situation, a double boiler may be used. Melt seven parts of canning grade paraffin wax and heat to 126° F (52° C); mix with one part mineral oil. Rapidly dip the *dry* hand and wrist in the warm paraffin and remove. Do this repeatedly until a fairly thick coat of wax is allowed to harden. Cover the wax-covered area with a towel or aluminum foil or a newspaper, which acts as an insulator to help retain the head. Leave the wax (paraffin) in place for 15 to 20 minutes, then peel it off and replace it in the container for the next application. Put the fingers and wrist through range-of-motion exercises, because the heat relieves pain and thus enables the patient to exercise the fingers and wrist with greater mobility. NOTE: Be very careful that the hand and wrist are dry when placed in the warm paraffin wax. Moisture or water on the hand conducts heat much more quickly and will burn the area. Burns are prevented when the area immersed is dry and dipped and removed rapidly.

TRACTION

Traction is the process of pulling or drawing, as applied to the musculoskeletal system for dislocated joints, fractured bones, or diseased peripheral joints (for example, arthritic joints). This therapy may be used in the physician's office, but more frequently is applied by physical therapists. Traction devices can also be set up for home use. Traction is used to:
- Obtain and maintain proper position
- Correct or prevent a deformity
- Decrease or overcome muscle spasms
- Lessen or prevent contractures (an abnormal shortening of muscle tissue)
- Promote better movement of the area
- Lessen and prevent severe stiffening of peripheral joints
- Achieve relief of compression at vertebral joints

METHODS AND DEVICES
Weight or Static Traction

This method of traction is applied with weights of varied poundages that are connected to the end of a pulley mecha-

nism. For example, the patient's head is placed in a head harness, which is attached to a rope with weights on the end. The rope is attached to a pole or door top so that it stretches up over the head and then is displaced downward where the weights are attached. Units can be obtained for use at home (Figure 15-9).

Elastic Traction

Elastic traction is applied with elastic appliances that exert a pull on the affected limb.

Mechanical Traction

Mechanical traction is applied by means of units that give an intermittent type of traction. They are set to pull and hold a set amount of tension for a set period of time and then to relax for a set period of time. They continue to pull and relax as long as they are set (Figure 15-10).

Figure 15-9 *Weight or static traction as applied to head for cervical traction. The manufacturer's directions for use must be followed. The physician orderd the number of pounds of traction to use.*

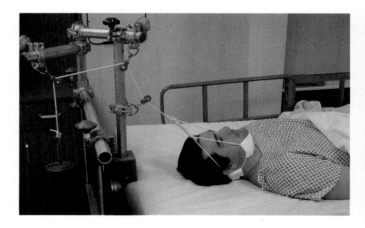

Figure 15-10 *Mechanical traction used for the cervical spine.*

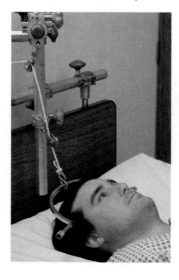

Manual Traction

Manual traction is applied by therapists using their hands to exert a pull on the affected part. In addition to other musculoskeletal problems, manual traction is frequently used to treat peripheral joint disease such as arthritic joints to distract (slightly separate) the joint surface in order to obtain more movement and prevent severe stiffening (Figure 15-11).

Skin Traction

Skin traction is applied by placing foam rubber pads or some other material, with a weight attached to the end along the sides of the affected limb. For support, this application is wrapped with elastic bandages.

Skeletal Traction

Skeletal traction is applied only in the hospital. Surgically installed pins and wires or tongs (for example, head tongs) are used to apply a pulling force directly on a bone.

MASSAGE

Massage was probably the first form of physical therapy. Individuals instinctively rub or massage an area after incurring an injury or bruise. After administering an injection, the injection site is rubbed, which is also a type of massage. Massage can be that simple, but it is also a highly skilled technique. Massage is a systematic and methodic pressure applied to bare skin by stroking, rubbing, kneading or rolling, tapping or pounding with the fingers or cupped hand, or by quick tappings with alternating fingertips. The type of massage used most frequently in the physician's office and clinics is stroking. Also tapotement, the pounding or cupping with a cupped hand on the back, is used on patients with chest congestion, because this helps loosen the secretions and clear the congestion (Figure 15-12). Other purposes of massage are to:

- Aid circulation by removing blood and waste products from injured tissues and by bringing fresh blood to the injured part, which helps the healing process

- Relax muscles and relieve spasms
- Reduce pain
- Help restore motion and function to the affected part
- Decrease swelling
- Reduce edema

To apply massage effectively, the therapist or assistant must be in a comfortable position to avoid straining, and the hands should be warm, to avoid discomfort to the patient. The patient must also be in a comfortable position so that beneficial results are more easily obtained.

EXERCISES

Therapeutic exercise is the performance of prescribed physical exertion to:

- Improve one's general health status
- Improve one's general health status after being afflicted with disabilities affecting the neuromuscular, skeletal, cardiovascular, integumentary, respiratory, and urinary systems, in addition to treatment for congenital defects, prenatal and postnatal care, and psychiatric problems
- Correct a physical deformity
- Improve muscle tone and strengthen muscles
- Restore the strength of muscles that have atrophied or weakened because of disease processes
- Restore motion after a fracture, injury, or any form of immobilization
- Aid circulation
- Improve coordination

Exercises may be performed in the physician's office or in physical therapy departments, or the patient may be given instructions and taught the exercises to be performed at home. Patients who are to do exercises at home must be *taught* how to do them and not just *told* what to do. Reasons for the exercise program must also be explained to the patient. The medical assistant responsible for these duties should have the patient perform the exercises while in the office until the motions involved are fully understood to ensure that the patient is capable of performing the prescribed exercise program.

Figure 15-11 *Manual traction applied by the therapist using the hands to exert a pull on the affected part.*

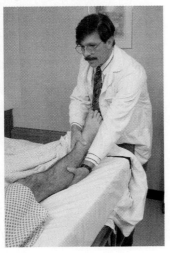

Figure 15-12 *Tapotement form of massage used on people with chest congestion. Cup your hands and pound or cup firmly and rapidly on the person's back over the lung area.*

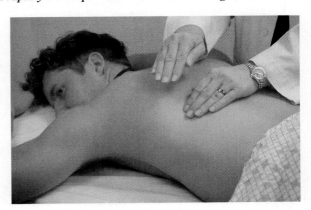

CLASSIFICATION
Active Exercises

All the motions involved in the exercise are performed totally by the patient and may involve the use of weights, pulleys, rubber balls, or similar appliances that the patient is to squeeze or manipulate.

Passive Exercises

In these exercises, movement to the part is done by another person or outside force without any voluntary participation from the patient (see Figures 15-14 to 15-16).

Aided Exercises

In these exercises, the patient is helped to move muscles that are too weak to move on their own strength. Exercises that are performed in a pool are also considered aided exercises.

Active Resistance Exercises

In these exercises the patient voluntarily applies pressure or movement of the part, and another individual applies resistance to the motion.

Range-of-Motion Exercises

These exercises are designed to assist joint mobility and normal functioning (for example, bending the fingers, twisting the wrist around in a normal motion, or rotation of the leg in a circumscribed fashion). They can be either active or passive exercises (Figures 15-13 to 15-16).

Figure 15-13 A, *Range-of-motion exercises for the upper extremities.*

A

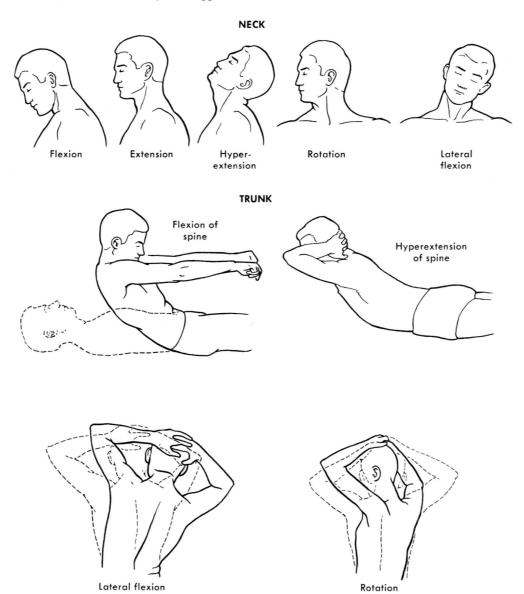

Figure 15-13—cont'd
A—cont'd *Range-of-motion exercises for the upper extremities.*

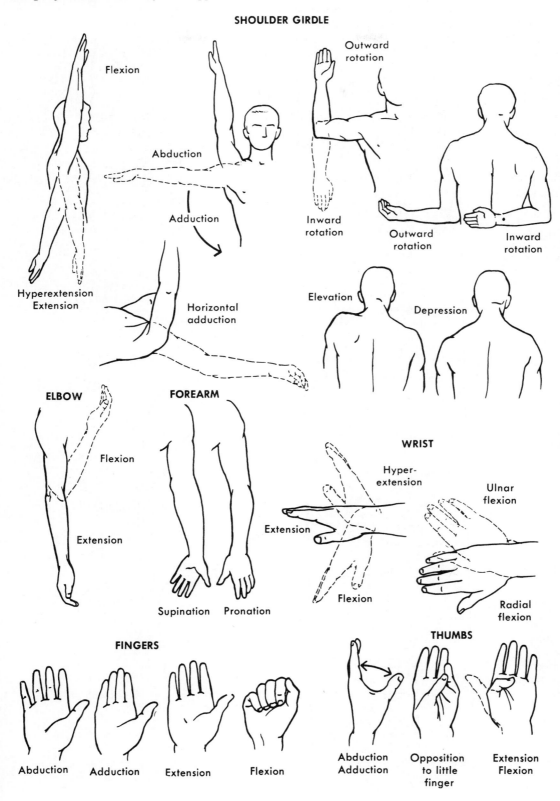

Figure 15-13—cont'd B, *Range-of-motion exercises for the lower extremities.*

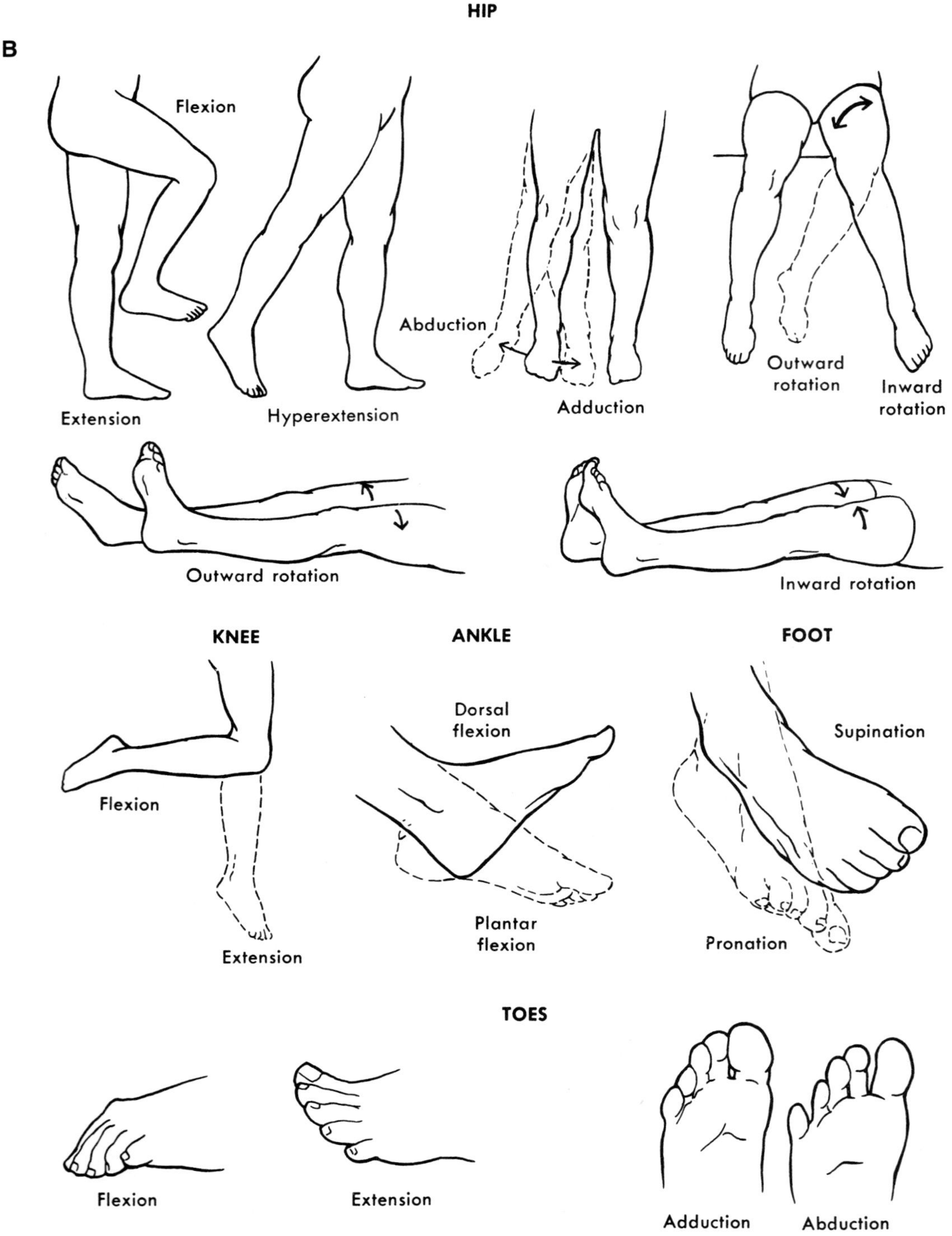

HIP

Flexion

Extension   Hyperextension   Abduction   Adduction   Outward rotation   Inward rotation

Outward rotation   Inward rotation

KNEE   **ANKLE**   **FOOT**

Flexion   Dorsal flexion   Supination

Extension   Plantar flexion   Pronation

TOES

Flexion   Extension   Adduction   Abduction

Figure 15-14 *Abduction of thumb and finger extension. **A,** Hold the patient's fingers straight with one hand. Bend the patient's thumb toward the palm with your other hand. **B,** Move the patient's thumb back, pointing away from the hand. Repeat this movement. **C,** Rotate the thumb (in a circle). Perform these exercises on both the good and weak hands.*

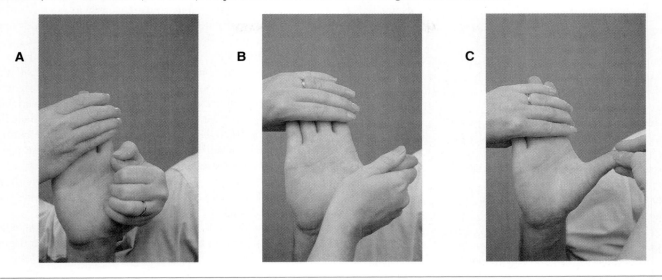

Figure 15-15 *Toe extension and flexion. **A,** Support patient's foot and pull up on the toes. **B,** Support patient's foot and push toes down.*

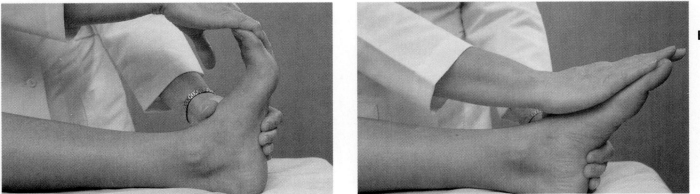

Figure 15-16 *Inversion of foot. **A,** Support patient's foot and turn whole foot outward. **B,** Support patient's foot and turn whole foot inward.*

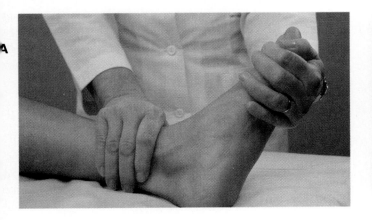
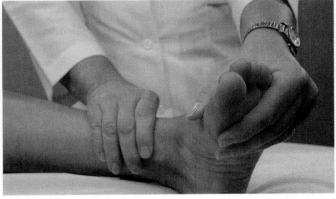

VOCABULARY

Joint mobility terminology

Abduction—Movement of a body part away from the midline of the body, as when moving the arm out to the side (see Figure. 15-14).

Abduction—Movement of a body part toward the midline of the body, as when bringing a raised arm down to the side of the body. The opposite of abduction.

Circumduction—Circular movement of a limb.

Extension—Movement of a joint that opens it or that increases the angle between the bones (see Figures 15-13 to 15-15).

Hyperextension—Extension of a limb or part beyond normal limits.

Flexion—Bending of a joint so that the angle between bones is reduced, as in bending the arm at the elbow or the leg at the knee or the toes. Opposite of extension (see Figures 15-13 and 15-15).

Dorsiflexion—Movement that bends a body part backward, as of the hand or foot.

Eversion—Movement that turns a body part outward; movement of the ankle that turns the foot outward.

Inversion—Movement that turns a body part inward; movement of the ankle that turns the foot inward (see Figure 15-16).

Pronation—Movement of the arm to have the palm facing downward.

Supination—Movement of the arm to have the palm facing upward. Opposite of pronation.

Rotation—Process of turning around an axis, such as seen in rotation of the head allowing the head to turn, extend, and flex.

External rotation—Outward rotation.

Internal rotation—Inward rotation.

BODY MECHANICS

Body mechanics is the way you handle yourself safely and effectively. Essentially it is how you hold yourself together to maintain good posture during function: when you are moving around, lifting, pulling, pushing, stooping, or carrying or when performing any type of manual labor. It is also how you use your body when sitting, standing, or lying down. Safe body mechanics include the principles of proper body alignment, balance, and movement. When you apply these principles, you minimize the amount of energy you expend, and you also improve your strength and flexibility when sitting, standing, and walking. An important aspect of using correct body mechanics is that you can prevent muscle and back fatigue, pain, strain, and injury.

Many individuals involved in the health care field often have to move and/or lift patients and equipment. Every time you lift, stand, sit, or even lie down, you are using your back.

Therefore it is crucial that you know how to use safe and effective methods for moving and lifting for your own protection and also so you can teach patients how to use these methods for their own safety and protection. These methods apply to all activities involving body movement and posture in everyday life. Safe and effective body mechanics keep the spine balanced in a healthy position when you stand, sit, or lie down. This means using the spine as a total unit whenever possible, and not as a series of loosely connected vertebrae. Try to keep your ears, shoulders, and hips in a straight line, and the neck erect, the pelvis tipped forward, and the buttocks and stomach tucked in during most activities. These proper movements are extremely important both on the job and at home. Good posture is necessary, since without it the overall spinal structure can be weakened and the back becomes more susceptible to injury.

You must develop, practice, and maintain correct standing, lifting, and bending habits. The following is a general guide for proper use of the body.

STANDING

Good posture and muscles help to keep your spine balanced when standing. Stand with your feet apart and one foot slightly in front of the other to provide a stable and wide base of support. When you have to stand for a long period of time with little movement, place one foot on a low stool to help keep your spine in balance and alternate now and again. Strain on the lower back is relieved by lifting the foot to return the spine to its natural curve. Don't twist or lean forward when standing and lifting; move your feet instead, and keep your upper body in line with your hips.

SITTING

For the least strain and injury to your back, keep the three normal curves of your spine (cervical, thoracic, and lumbar) in balanced alignment. The lumbar curve must accommodate the most weight and movement and is commonly the area of most complaints. Sit straight in a chair that supports your lower back or add a support to your lumbar curve by placing a pillow or a towel rolled up to 4 to 6 inches behind that area. When sitting on a stool, lean forward and rest your upper body lightly on your elbows and arms. *Don't* cross your legs. Crossed legs tilt the pelvis too far forward and aggravate bad backs. Always sit with your knees level with or slightly higher than your hips. Placing something under the feet such as a telephone book or a block of wood reduces back tension.

LIFTING TECHNIQUES

1. Assess the load before beginning to lift. Get help when in doubt about lifting alone.
2. Clear the area where the lift will take place (for example, move chairs out of the way).
3. Explain the procedure to the patient (when the load you will be lifting is a patient) and continue to communicate during the procedure so that the patient can work with and not against you.

4. Keep the weight as close to your body as possible when lifting rather than reaching forward.

5. Attain and maintain firm grip on the object or patient throughout the lift.

6. Keep your back straight and body weight over your feet (if possible). Don't bend the lower back at the lumbosacral area (Figure 15-17).

7. Use your leg muscles during the lift. Bend your knees sufficiently (not your waist) so that your large leg muscles are used.

8. Establish a firm, stable foot position. Place your feet 10 to 12 inches apart and point them in the direction of the lift. One foot may be placed in front of the other for balance (see Figure 15-17).

9. Move feet with the direction of the lift. You must avoid twisting your back. Think of your spine as a fused unit and make turning movements with your feet and entire body in the direction you are moving. Twisting or pivoting on fixed feet can injury your back.

10. Avoid jerking and jolting. Use even, smooth movements.

11. When two people are required to perform the lift, one person is to act as the leader. The leader should set and call the signals for beginning the lift and subsequent moves.

12. Bend your knees as much as possible when lowering the object or patient at the completion of the lift.

13. Use the appropriate type of lifting technique for the situation.

14 Use the "hip-bend" lift for loads that you must lift at a distance such as when helping or lifting a patient from the examining table or when getting something from a place that is hard to reach. Once again, get as close to the load as possible. Then put your buttocks out behind you, keeping your head and back in a straight line (this helps to balance and protect your spine). Then bend your knees (not your waist) and lift, using your leg, buttock, and abdominal muscles (Figure 15-18).

Remember that proper techniques are just as important when bending without lifting. Squat, don't bend (Figure 15-19).

Use both sides of your body when lifting, pushing, pulling, or carrying so that the weight does not pull your body into a strained position.

Pushing is easier on your back than pulling. When you push something, remember to bend your elbows, use your legs with one foot in front of the other, and keep the load close to your stomach when possible. Use a stool or ladder, if necessary when you must reach an item.

Wear comfortable, low-heeled shoes. Wearing high heels or clogs can throw your dynamic (functional or changing) posture off and make you compensate when trying to maintain balance.

By using proper body mechanics and maintaining a healthy posture, you can encourage a stabilized and pain-free back. A variety of exercises such as the partial sit-up and pelvic tilt can strengthen the lower back and abdominal muscles. Strengthening these muscles greatly facilitates correct posture and proper body mechanics. Physical therapists can provide

Figure 15-18 *The hip-bend lift for loads that are hard to reach.*

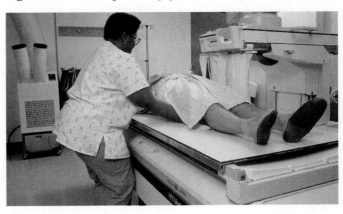

Figure 15-17 *Proper body mechanics. Keep your back straight and body weight over your feet when lifting.*

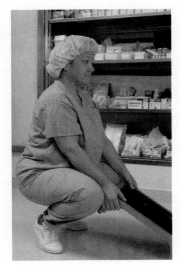

A

Figure 15-19 A *and* B, *Squat, don't bend.*

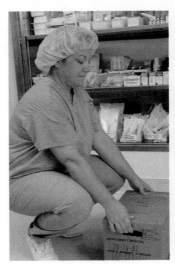

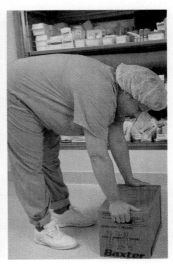

B

you with instructions for various back-strengthening exercises, *but* remember than an exercise program for back pain should not be initiated without a physician's recommendation.

WHEELCHAIRS

Wheelchairs are mobile chairs of various shapes and sizes that are equipped with large wheels and brakes. Some are moved around manually, and others are motorized. When a patient will be using a wheelchair for a long period of time or permanently, the physical therapist works with a medical product store to obtain a wheelchair that meets the patient's needs. The therapist provides the store with all of the patient's information such as size, disability, activities planned for the days ahead (for example, does the patient plan to go hiking in the wheelchair or use it just around the house), description of the patient's house and area where the chair will be used, what type of brakes are needed, and if the chair should have right- or left-handed propulsion.

Many patients who will be using the wheelchair forever are taught how to maintain it. For example, young patients who have spinal cord injuries are taught how to maintain the wheelchair just as they would be taught to maintain a bicycle (for example, how to fix a broken wheel or broken brakes). All patients are taught safety techniques for using a wheelchair such as how to lock and unlock the brakes, how to kick the footrest out of the way, how to operate the different pieces of the wheelchair, and how to maneuver it in and out of different spaces. The patient practices using the wheelchair in the hospital before going home to ensure safe functioning at home.

WHEELCHAIR TRANSFERS
Transferring a Patient from a Wheelchair

* Obtain help from another person if you think that you will be unable to accomplish the transfer safely for yourself and the patient.
* Use the strong muscles in your legs and not the weaker muscles in your back when transferring a patient.
* Always move the patient toward the strong side if one side is stronger than the other.
* Support the patient's strong side when assisting with the move.
* Position the wheelchair parallel to the examining table to where the patient will be moving.
* Explain the procedure to the patient.
* Lock the wheels (Figure 15-20, *A* and *B*).
  * Move the footrests out of the way (Figure 15-20, *B*).
  * Position a step stool near the examining table.
  * Stand facing the patient.
  * Have the patient move forward in the chair. Stay directly in front of the patient. This is important so that you don't twist because twisting hurts your back.
  * Bend down with your knees. *Do not* bend your back. Then put your arms under the patient's arms and your hands firmly over the patient's scapulae. Have the patient's hands rest on your shoulders (Figure 15-21, *A*).

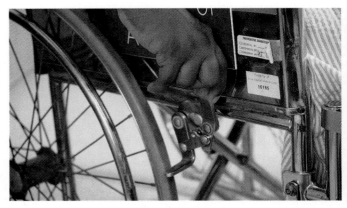
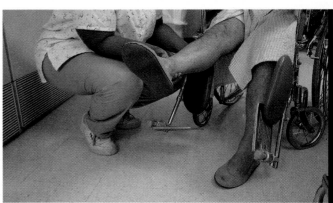

Figure 15-20 A, *Lock the wheels of the wheelchair before helping a patient getting in or out of it.* **B,** *Move footrests of wheelchair out of the way before a patient gets in or out of it.*

* Give a signal and lift upward so that the patient will rise to a standing position.
* Have the patient step up onto the stool and pivot with the back to the table (Figure 15-21, *B*).
* Ease the patient to a sitting position.
* Place one arm on the patient's shoulder and the other arm under the patient's knees (Figure 15-21, *C*).
* Using a *single* smooth move, raise the patient's legs onto the table and lower the head and trunk into the supine position.
* Attend to the patient's comfort and safety.

Transferring a Patient from the Examining Table to a Wheelchair

* Explain the procedure to the patient.
* Position the wheelchair parallel to the examining table.
* Lock the wheels and move the footrests out of the way (see Figure 15-20).
* Place one arm under the patient's shoulders and your other arm under the knees.
* Using a *single* smooth move, assist the patient to rise to a sitting position. At the same time, pivot a quarter of a turn so that the patient is sitting on the edge of the examining table with the feet dangling over the side.

Figure 15-21 A, *Assist patient out of wheelchair.* B, *Assist patient on to examining table. Have patient step up on stool and pivot with back to table.* C, *Assist patient to lie down on examining table. Place one arm on patient's shoulder and the other arm under patient's knees.*

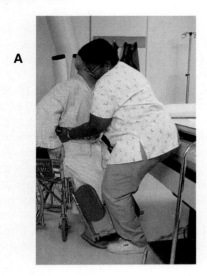
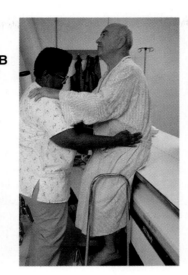
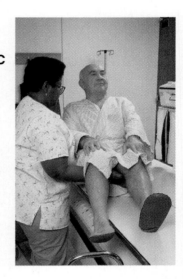

- Stand facing the patient.
- Put your arms under the patient's arms and your hands firmly over the patient's scapulae. Have the patient's hands rest on your shoulders.
- Give a signal, lift upward, and raise the patient to a standing position.
- Pivot a quarter of a turn so that the back of the patient's knees tough the edge of the wheelchair.
- Ease the patient into the wheelchair.
- Position the footrests and the patient's feet on them.
- Attend to the patient's safety and comfort.

CRUTCHES

Crutches are wooden or metal supports used to aid a person in walking. The most common types are the tall crutch, which reaches from the ground up to the axillae (axillary crutches), and the Lofstrand or Canadian crutch (forearm crutch), which is a shorter crutch. The Lofstrand or Canadian crutch is an aluminum tube with a hand bar on which the patient supports his or her weight and a metal cuff that fits around the forearm. The metal forearm cuff supports the patient when he or she has to let go of the handbar (for example, when grasping onto a handrail to climb stairs or when standing still). At the base of all crutches is a rubber tip that prevents slipping (Figure 15-22). The type of crutch used depends on the patient's disability. For example, if the patient has broken or sprained one ankle, axillary crutches are used. When the patient will be on crutches for a long time and/or has only limited mobility in the legs and/or is wearing leg braces, or when he or she is a paraplegic, forearm crutches may be used. Patients with severe arthritis who have poor use of their hands may use platform crutches. When using these crutches, patients use their forearms to lean on the crutches (Figure 15-23).

Figure 15-22 *Two types of crutches: axillary (left), and Lofstrand or Canadian (right).*

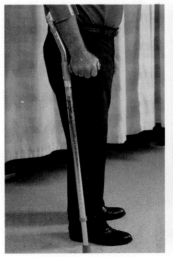
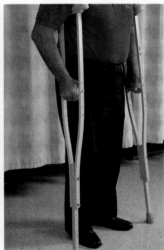

MEASURING FOR AXILLARY CRUTCHES

Axillary crutches should be measured for each patient so that they will not cause pressure on the axillae. To determine the correct crutch height, have the patient wear walking shoes and stand erect. Position the crutch tips 2 inches (5 cm) in front of and 6 inches (15 cm) to the side of each foot. Adjust the crutch length so that the position of the axilla bars are at least 3 finger-widths below the axilla. Adjust the handgrips on the crutches so that the patient's elbows are flexed at a 30-degree angle when the crutches are in place (Figure 15-24). The angle of elbow flexion can be verified by using a measuring device called a goniometer (Figure 15-25).

Figure 15-23 *Patient with platform crutches. Patient uses forearms to lean on crutches.*

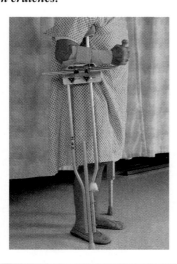

Figure 15-24 *Measuring crutches. Axilla bars should be three finger-widths below the axilla. Elbows should be flexed at a 30-degree angle when the patient's hands are on the handgrips.*

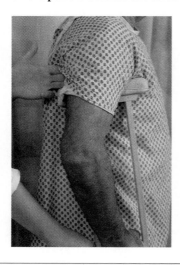

Figure 15-25 *Verifying elbow flexion of a 30-degree angle using a goniometer.*

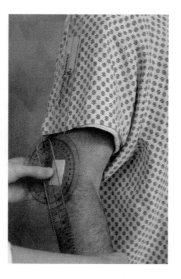

PATIENT TEACHING FOR USE OF CRUTCHES

Teaching the patient crutch-walking gaits may be your responsibility if a physical therapist is not available. *First,* you must instruct the patient in practicing correct standing posture, which is head and chest up, abdomen in, pelvis tiled inward, feet straight, and a 5-degree angle bend in the knee joint. Tell the patient *not* to look down at the feet.

The *basic crutch stance* is the tripod position (Figure 15-26). Have the patient stand erect with the feet slightly apart. Place the tips of the crutches 6 inches in front of and 6 inches to the side of the toes to provide a broad base of support and balance. This position forms a triangle in which a line drawn between the two crutch tips forms the base of the triangle and the patient's feet are the apex. Standing correctly is essential for maintaining balance. Have the patient practice standing with the support of the crutches to get familiar with them and to bear weight on the palms of the hand and not on the axillae. Check the distance between the axilla and the axilla bar on the crutch. It should be at least three finger-widths or about 2 inches.

You must teach the patient *not* to rest the body's weight on the axillary bars of the crutch for more than a few minutes at a time because pressure on the axillae will cause pressure on the brachial plexus. Excessive pressure on the brachial plexus can cause numbness and tingling and can lead to severe and sometimes permanent paralysis in the arms. Teach the patient to bear weight on the palms of hands (see Figure 15-28). Check the angle of the patient's arms. When the hands are on the handgrips and the crutches are in the walking position, the arms should be flexed at a 30-degree angle. Remind the

Figure 15-26 *The basic crutch stance is the tripod position.*

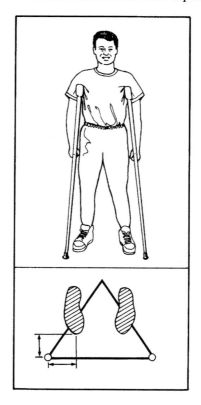

patient that the arms are to support the body weight, not the axilla. Teach the patient to take small steps at first (that is, to move the crutches only about 12 inches forward with each step). If larger steps are taken, the crutches could slide forward, and the patient could fall. Demonstrate the proper hand and arm position and gait before the patient tries to use the crutches. By doing this you help the patient understand how the crutches are to be used. Concentration on a normal rhythmic gait must be accomplished.

Teach the patient to check the crutches for cracks and the rubber tips for wear and loose fit. The tips should be kept dry. They should be replaced when they wear out. Wet or worn tips lessen surface tension and increase the likelihood of the patient falling.

SPECIAL CONCERNS
- For some patients, especially the elderly, additional arm strengthening exercises may be needed before they can use crutches adequately.
- Pediatric crutches must be used for children.
- Provide the patient with a list of medical supply stores where repairs or parts for the crutches can be purchased.
- Discuss ways that the patient's home could be modified for easier mobility (for example, the elimination of throw rugs or waxed floors).

GAITS
In crutch-walking gaits, each foot and crutch is called a point. For example, in a two-point gait, two points of the total of four (two crutches and two legs) are in contact with the ground when taking one step. The type of gait to be used depends on the patient's condition.

Standing
Before crutch walking begins the patient should assume the tripod position as discussed previously (see also Figure 15-26). From a sitting position, have the patient place the crutches in the hand on the strong side, move forward in the chair, grasp the arm of the chair with the other hand, and push himself or herself up to a standing position (Figure 15-27).

Two-point Gait
1. The first type of two-point gait is when you put both crutches ahead of you and hop forward with one foot (Figure 15-28). This is a nonweight-bearing gait.
2. The second type of two-point gait is contralateral walking and a reciprocal walk. Put your left crutch and right foot forward; then put your right crutch and left foot forward, and repeat (Figure 15-28).

This is partial weight bearing on each foot and used for patients who can bear weight on each leg.

Three-point Gait
This may be used when one leg is stronger than the other. Put your crutches forward and then bring the weaker leg through the crutches. Next bring the stronger leg forward, and then repeat, crutches out, then one leg, then the other leg. This is a partial weight-bearing gait (Figure 15-29).

Figure 15-27 *Using crutches to go from a sitting to a standing position.*

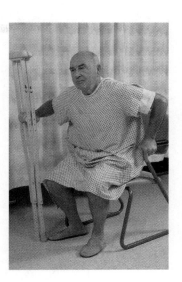

Figure 15-28 *Two-point gait.*

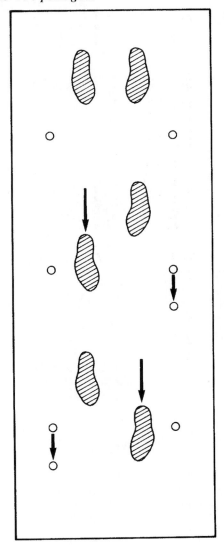

Figure 15-29 *Three-point gait.*

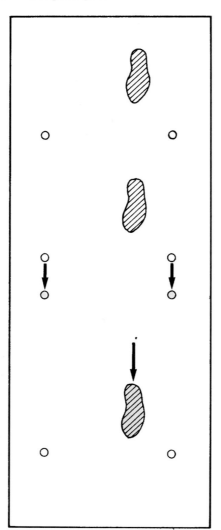

Figure 15-30 *Four-point gait.*

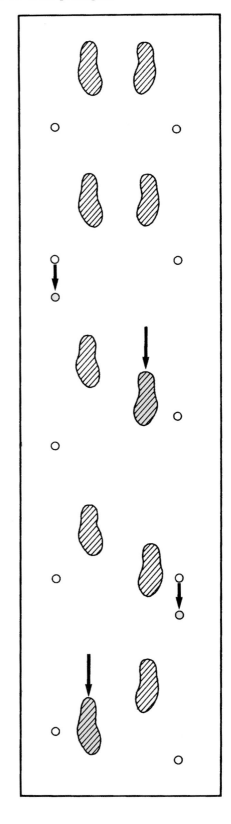

Four-point Gait

Put your right crutch forward, then the left foot, then the left crutch, and then the right foot, and repeat (Figure 15-30).

This is used for patients who can bear weight on the legs and also move each leg separately.

Swing-to Gait

Put the crutches forward and then swing the legs up to the same point (Figure 15-31).

Swing-through Gait

Put the crutches forward and then swing the legs past them (Figure 15-32).

The last two gaits are commonly used by paraplegics who are using forearm crutches, and by paraplegics who wear weight-supporting braces on their legs. They can also be used for people with generalized weakness in the legs.

Figure 15-31 *Swing-to gait.*

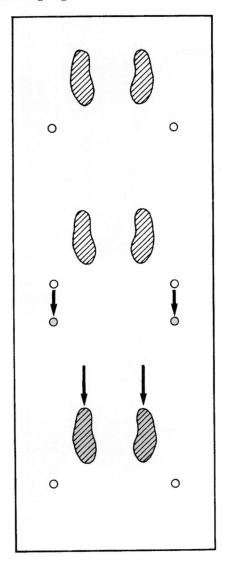

Figure 15-32 *Swing-through gait.*

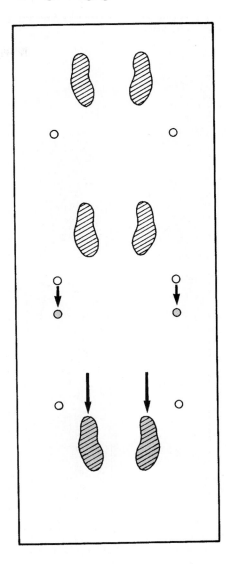

Sitting

To go from a standing position to a sitting position, teach the patient to:

1. Turn around and back into a well-supported chair until the legs touch the center of the chair seat.
2. Place the crutches in the hand on the opposite side of the affected leg or on the stronger side of the body.
3. Grasp the chair arm with the other hand and lower the body into the chair.

CANES

Canes of various sizes are made of aluminum or wood with a rubber tipped end that helps to prevent sliding and provides support. Patients who need help with balance or who have one-sided weakness may use a cane to provide additional support. The patient's needs determine whether a single-tipped or a four-point (quad) cane is needed (Figure 15-33).

To ensure maximum support, the cane length must be adjusted for each patient.

Instructions for Using a Single Crutch or Cane

1. Always hold a single crutch or cane on the *opposite* side of the injury. People normally walk contralaterally (that is, when the left arm swings out, the right leg goes out). Think of a crutch or cane as an extension of your arm. As your arm swings out, your opposite leg will go out. With the crutch or cane on the opposite side, it supports and takes the weight off of the injured leg (Figure 15-33, *B* and *C*).
2. Place the cane 6 inches in front of and slightly to the side of the foot on the *unaffected* side.
3. The hand grip should be at the level of the hip joint (at the level of the greater trochanter of the femur).

Figure 15-33 **A,** *Single-tipped and four-point (quad) canes;* **B,** *patient walking with a cane;* **C,** *patient walking with a single crutch.*

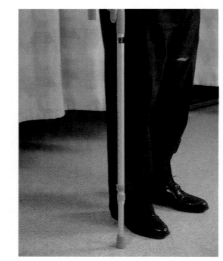

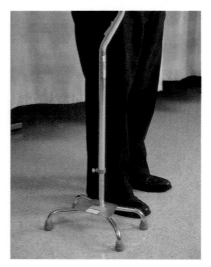

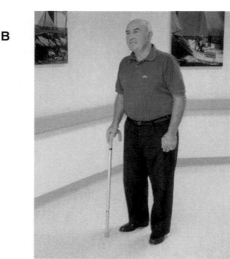

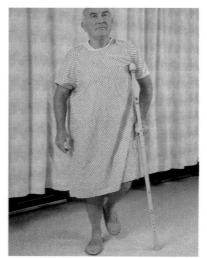

4. Flex the elbow slightly during weight bearing.
5. Simultaneously move the cane and *affected* leg forward 6 to 10 inches (this varies with the patient's condition) and bear weight on the *unaffected* foot.
6. Transfer weight to the *affected foot and cane* while moving the *unaffected* foot forward. The cane provides support for weight bearing on the affected leg.
7. Repeat the procedure, taking small steps.

WALKERS

Walkers are four-legged assistive devices made of aluminum. There are two types of walkers—the stationary walker, which has rubber tips on the legs; and the rolling walker, which has wheels on the four legs. Walkers are used by patients who need help when standing or walking, or who need help in maintaining balance. Patients who use walkers must have arms strong enough to bear partial weight.

Walkers are measured so that the height of the walker is just below the patient's waistline when the arms are flexed at a 30-degree angle while holding onto the handgrips.

To use the rolling walker, a patient just rolls it ahead as she or he walks with the walker. This type of walker can be dangerous for patients with balance or coordination problems. To use the stationary walker, the patient must lift it up and move it ahead a few inches, or slide it forward and then step into the open side of the walker. This sequence is then repeated for the desired distance (Figure 15-34).

ELECTROTHERAPY USING GALVANIC AND FARADIC CURRENTS

Galvanic current is a steady direct current (DC); faradic current is alternating current (AC) produced by induction. Both are currents of low voltage that are used for many therapeutic purposes. The basic use for galvanic and faradic currents is for muscle stimulation, used to retrain patients when they have had nerve injuries. For example, as the injured nerve regenerates, the body may have forgotten how to contract a muscle; thus frequently these treatments are given to remind them and help them function once again.

Figure 15-34 *Patient using a stationary walker. Note the height of the walker and the position of the patient's arms.*

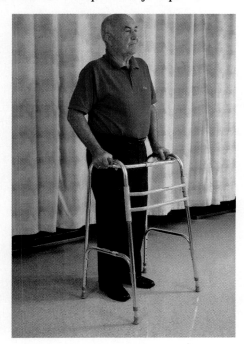

Galvanic stimulation (or faradic if it works) can be used just to maintain the contractility of the muscle while waiting for the nerve to regenerate. Once the nerve is cut or degenerates, or if the nerve itself does not conduct stimuli, galvanic current (direct current) is the only thing that can be used. Direct current works directly on muscle tissue even when there is no intact nerve. Faradic current (alternating current) cannot be used because it will not work on muscle tissue in this case. Galvanic current is also used for *iontophoresis* (i-on ′to-fo-re′sis). Iontophoresis or ionotherapy is the introduction of ions into the body through the skin by means of an electric current for therapeutic purposes. It is also used for the localized application of antiinflammatory drugs (for example, hydrocortisone applied to specific swollen or inflamed areas, rather than giving the drug by injection). (*Phonophoresis* is a similar modality using ultrasound instead of direct current.)

Faradic current is used mainly to stimulate weak muscles that have a normal nerve supply. This current causes contractions, which in turn increase blood supply to the muscle and thus help the muscle gain strength. Increased circulation also helps to decrease edema. Faradic current is also used to decrease pain as it helps to block pain sensations.

These treatments can be applied in various ways. To stimulate muscles, the current must be interrupted. This is accomplished by a hand interrupter or an interrupter that is built into the equipment. Basically, to apply these currents, two electrodes padded with cotton that has been soaked in salt water are placed over the area to be treated. The soaked pads prevent the occurrence of severe wounds. When small muscles are treated, a very small applicator can be used. This has a push button on it so that specific jolts of current can be given. This

apparatus can also be used when using what is called a surged current or a ramped current. These are currents that start out with nothing, then begin and increase up to a designated point, and then decrease. With these a smooth contraction and then a smooth relaxation is obtained. In addition to muscle stimulation, these currents can also be used on muscle spasms and on areas such as those around hematomas and bruises. Electrostimulation therapy is also used with biofeedback for muscle reeducation. The biofeedback machine allows the patient to hear the muscle contract and relax. This is especially helpful following surgery and for controlling chronic pain.

ELECTRODIAGNOSTIC EXAMINATIONS

Electrodiagnostic examinations used by physical therapy are performed by means of electrical stimulation applied to muscles and nerves. Various types of examinations are available, all having clinical value in the diagnosis and prognosis of some neuromuscular disorders. Two additional major electrodiagnostic examinations used for different clinical purposes are the electroencephalogram (EEG), which records the electrical impulses of the brain, and the electrocardiogram (EKG or ECG), which records the electrical action of the heart. The EKG is discussed in Unit Sixteen.

Electromyographic examinations specifically measure the electrical activity in a muscle as a result of nerve conduction. A needle electrode is introduced into a muscle belly to study muscle action potentials. It also measures just the general electrical excitability of the muscle cells. The recording obtained (the electromyogram) can be most specific diagnostically, since it not only tells you that something is wrong, but will point out exactly what is wrong. It helps distinguish any weakness from neuropathy from that of other causes.

Other examinations available test the reaction time of a muscle to a shot of electricity; the threshold is tested (that is, how much electricity it takes to get a reaction from the muscle). The results obtained are compared with normal levels. Any deviation or fluctuation from the established norm helps diagnose certain problems such as damaged nerve and muscle tissues.

Nerve conduction studies are performed to test the speed with which the nerve is conducting; again, this helps the physician diagnose.

Special electrodiagnostic equipment is used for each of these tests, which are generally performed by a physical therapist or a physician. You do not operate this equipment, but may be expected to keep it clean and ready for use. You may also be expected to explain the nature and purpose of the examination to the patient.

DISABILITIES AND THERAPY

To provide you with a broader insight into the various types of patient conditions that benefit from physical therapy, Table 15-2 lists common disabilities with the common physical therapy modalities used for each.

TABLE 15-2

Patient Education for Care of the Residual Limb

Patient conditions that benefit from physical therapy and occupational therapy. Occupational therapy uses activities to maximize a person's independence, prevent disabilities, and maintain health.

Disability	Therapy	Disability	Therapy
Amputations	Patient education for care of the residual limb. Bed positioning Exercise Crutch training Prosthetic care and training	Congenital defects	Exercise Functional training
Arthritis and other rheumatic diseases	Heat Hot paraffin wax bath Exercise Pool Transfer techniques *Occupational therapy:* Splinting (Figure 15-35), functional exercise, self-care instructions, such as dressing	Debility	Exercise Gait training
		Diabetes	Exercise
		Fractures of upper and lower extremity	Biofeedback and electrical stimulation therapy Exercise Gait training Modalities to control pain and edema, e.g., heat and/or cold applications
Burns	Hubbard tank Heat Exercise Whirlpool Massage Splinting	General Surgery	Graduated exercise program
		Heart surgery and pulmonary congestion	Bronchial hygiene that includes postural drainage and chest tapotement Breathing exercises Endurance exercises

Cardiovascular disease (Cardiac and Pulmonary Rehabilitation)	Bronchial hygiene
	   e.g., postural drainage, chest tapotement
	Graduated exercise program
	Occupational therapy:
	   Pacing activities:
	      work simplification
	      energy conservation
		Infectious diseases	Graduated exercise program

		Low back pain	Constant pelvic traction (in bed and in clinic)
			Intermittent pelvic traction
			Heat
			Massage
			Pool
			Exercise
			Body mechanics instruction
			Physical and occupational therapy:
			   Mobilization of soft tissues and joints-manual therapy
			   Ergonomics- assessment and modification
			   Industrial program for employee evaluation, work capacity, and modification training

Cerebral palsy	Exercise; neurologic facilitation exercises Functional training Occupational therapy: Self-care instruction, such as feeding and dressing		

Cerebrovascular accident (CVA)	Bed positioning
	Balance activities
	Bed mobility
	   Exercise-basic calisthenics→progress up to walking → running → riding bicycles
	Neurologic facilitation exercises
	Transfer techniques
	Gait training
	Occupational therapy:
	   Splinting, self-care instructions, such as dressing, training in one-handed activities
		Lymphedema (after CVA, mastectomy, or sprain)	Jobst Intermittent Pressure Pump
			Exercise

		Muscle spasm	Heat Cold Massage Exercise
		Muscle disease	Pool Exercise
		Multiple sclerosis	Adaptive equipment Ice baths for relief of spacticity Exercise Gait training Transfer activities Dressing training

Table 15-2—cont'd

Patient Education for Care of the Residual Limb

Disability	Therapy	Disability	Therapy
Neck pain	Occupational therapy Intermittent cervical traction or collars Constant vertical traction Heat Massage Exercise Ice Ultrasound Joint mobilization Also see "Low back pain"	Psychiatric problems (continued)	Pool Relaxation techniques Occupational therapy: Therapeutic crafts and remedial games
Osteoporosis	Bracing as indicated Exercise Graduated weight bearing Modalities for pain conrol	Pulmonary problems (emphysema, bronchitis, asthma)	Bronchial hygiene Breathing exercises Endurance exercises Outpatient pulmonary rehabilitation clinic Graduated rehabilitation with low flow oxygen Occupational therapy: Pacing activities: work simplification energy conservation
Parkinson's disease	Exercise Gait training Electrical stimulation	Renal failure and transplants	Graduated exercises Maintenance exercises
Peripheral nerve injuries	Exercise Splinting Occupational therapy Buerger's exercises	Scoliosis and other postural defects	Bracing Exercise Body mechanics Instruction Posture instruction
Peripheral vascular diseases	Gait training General exercises Bronchial hygiene	Spinal cord injuries	Bracing Exercise Gait training Transfer activities Wheelchair mobility *Occupational therapy:* Self-care instruction, such as dressing and splinting
Poliomyelitis	Exercise Gait training with braces Heat Pool		
Pressure sores and wound infections	Ultraviolet light (bacteriocidal) Bed positioning	Sprains	Heat Cold and compression Exercise Gait training Friction massage
Prenatal and postnatal situations	Exercise Breathing instruction		
Psoriasis	Ultraviolet light (bacteriocidal)		
Psychiatric problems	Exercise Heat		

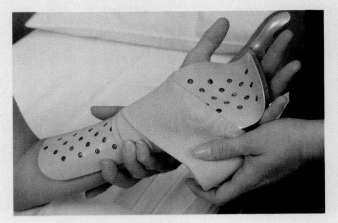

Figure 15-35 *Examples of splints as applied to patient's finger, wrist and forearm.*

CONCLUSION

You have now completed the unit on physical therapy. After you have practiced the procedures and are ready to demonstrate your skills and knowledge attained, arrange with your instructor to take a performance test.

There are various types of patient conditions and disabilities that benefit from physical therapy. Numerous other procedures, tests, and modalities are used in a physical therapy department. It is not within the scope of this book to discuss all of them in detail. A clinical experience or a field trip to a physical therapy facility would be most valuable to you; here you could see firsthand the use of the various modalities and techniques.

REVIEW OF VOCABULARY

The following are statements taken from patient charts. Read these and be able to explain the nature of the types of treatment each patient has received.

PATIENT NO. 1:

On January 14, the patient was working for the Webster Construction Co. in custodial activity. He was using a mop, and after pulling the mop through the wringer, he experienced right paralumbar pain. The next morning the patient couldn't move because of severe pain. He had an appointment at the Crossroads Clinic, and medications were prescribed. Later the patient saw Dr. Treadmill who recognized the problem as one involving compensation. Furthermore, Dr. Treadmill obtained x-ray films and prescribed physical therapy. Physical therapy involved massages, infrared therapy, ultrasound therapy, and pelvic traction. Temporary relief came from these measures. About 8 or 9 days ago, however, because the trouble persisted, the patient was referred to me.

The patient stated that the pain in the right lower extremity prevents work. It is "static," by which the patient means it is not worsening or improving.

The patient in formative years had an occasional "kink" in the back, but was never off work and never had professional attention.

PATIENT NO. 2:

Patient brought in a prescription to continue treatment for 3 more weeks. The physician thinks that physiotherapy is helping and will see the patient at the end of 3 weeks. Patient states pain is gradually decreasing. Treatment: hot packs; ultrasound at 1.5 w/cm^2 for 7 minutes to left low back; exercise as before. Patient does exercises well and reports that she continues them at home.

Will Kerrigan, RPT

CASE STUDY

Read the following *SOAP* note from a physical therapy evaluation and discuss the italicized terminology.

SUBJECTIVE: Patient states discouragement about having a second *stroke* and being unable to do things again after having made so much progress following his previous stroke. In addition, *arthritis* of hip and knee joints is significant. Nerve *conduction* studies of left shoulder reveal *bursitis*.

OBJECTIVE: Left lower extremity: Strength in the left lower extremity was as follows:

 Hip flexion: Poor + to fair −
 Knee extension: Good −
 Foot dorsiflexions: Trade

There was minimum extension *synergy* in the left lower extremity and hip extension and *adduction* primarily.

Right lower extremity: Strength was good to normal with normal tone present.

ASSESSMENT: Left lower extremity—Strength in the lower extremities bilaterally is normal. *ROM* is within normal limits. *Gait*—Patient *ambulates* with close supervision for long distances. Patient's gait is slightly unsteady, occasionally *listing* to the left and shuffling the left foot.

PLAN:

1. *Gait training* with supervision.
2. Mat activities for balance and coordination of lower extremity.

1. Define and state the purposes and time duration of application for each of the following:
   a. Ultraviolet light treatments
   b. Diathermy treatments
   c. Ultrasound treatments
   d. Application of moist and dry heat
   e. Application of moist and dry cold
2. How full should a hot water bottle be filled when applied to a patient? Why?
3. State the temperature of the water you would use when applying a hot water bottle to a 70-year-old male; to a 2-year-old child.
4. Define and discuss the principles of body mechanics.
5. Why should the patient's skin be checked frequently during any form of hot or cold application?
6. List five physiologic reactions produced by heat applications, and five produced by cold applications.

7. List five situations in which cold applications may be used for treatment.
8. List five situations in which hot applications may be used for treatment.
9. List two modalities used in hydrotherapy. Explain each briefly. List two uses for each.
10. List five uses or purposes of exercises.
11. Differentiate between active and passive exercises.
12. State three purposes of traction and three purposes of massage.
13. State two types of electrodiagnostic examinations, and explain each briefly.
14. Discuss the principles of electrotherapy using galvanic and faradic currents.

In a skills laboratory, the medical assistant student will demonstrate skill and knowledge in performing the following activities without reference to source materials. The student needs a partner to play the role of the patient. Time limits for the each of the following activities are to be assigned by the instructor (see also page 60).

1. To the outer aspect of the patient's right forearm, and to the inner aspect of the patient's left lower leg, prepare, apply, and remove the following:
   a. Hot water bottle
   b. Hot compress
   c. Ice bag
   d. Cold compress
2. Discuss the purpose and physiologic effects of hot and cold treatments with your instructor.
3. Demonstrate with a partner:
   a. Active exercises of the right arm
   b. Passive exercises to the right arm
   c. Active-resistant exercises to the patient's right hand
4. Using the information provided in this unit, correctly write out the procedural steps and a performance checklist for the following applications of heat or cold:
   a. Heating pad
   b. Hot water bottle
   c. Hot moist compress
   d. Hot soak
   e. Ice bag
   f. Ice pack
   g. Moist cold compress
   h. Alcohol sponge bath
   i. Chemical cold pack

5. Using the information you outlined in No. 4, design a teaching-instruction sheet for the patient to use at home for each of the hot and cold applications listed.
6. Demonstrate safe and effective body mechanics when lifting a patient or heavy object.
7. Assist patients to learn how to walk with crutches, and with a cane.
8. Assist patients to get in and out of a wheelchair.
9. Measure and determine the correct size of crutches, a cane, and a walker for a patient.

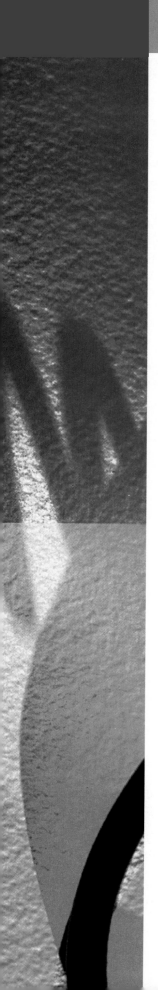

Electrocardiography

COGNITIVE OBJECTIVES

On completion of Unit Sixteen, the medical assistant student should be able to:

1. Define and pronounce the terms in the vocabulary and text of this unit.
2. Explain the cardiac cycle and conduction system of the heart.
3. Explain how the heartbeat is controlled.
4. List eight components recorded on the electrocardiogram (EKG) cycle, and relate these to the electrical activity of the heart.
5. State the normal time required for the cardiac cycle.
6. Describe electrocardiograph paper, and indicate the significance of each small block and each large block.
7. List four factors that are interpreted from an EKG.
8. Describe how to monitor an EKG for abnormal and erratic tracings.
9. Briefly define and discuss three types of each of the following: sinus rhythms, atrial arrhythmias, and ventricular arrhythmias. State possible causes of each.
10. List three types of common artifacts that may be seen on an EKG and the causes for each.
11. Describe electrodes and electrolytes, gel or paste, and state the purpose of each.
12. List the 12 leads recorded on a standard EKG; state the electrical activity that each is recording; and recognize each recorded lead by interpreting the identification code used.
13. Discuss the phrase, *standardizing the electrocardiograph*, indicating the importance of this. Illustrate and explain the universal standard of EKG measurement.
14. Discuss the concepts of the Phone-A-Gram, the computerized electrocardiograph.
15. Discuss the automatic electrocardiograph. State the advantages of this electrocardiograph.
16. Explain what ambulatory cardiac monitoring (Holter monitoring) is and state why it is performed.
17. List eight instructions that should be given to a patient who will be wearing a Holter monitor.
18. Explain what is involved in a treadmill stress test.
19. State four reasons for a stress EKG test.

TERMINAL PERFORMANCE OBJECTIVES

On completion of Unit Sixteen, the medical assistant student should be able to:

1. Demonstrate proficiency in communicating proper preparation of the patient for electrocardiography and in preparing the room and equipment.
2. Demonstrate the proper procedure for the application of the electrodes and lead wires to the patient for a standard 12-lead EKG and for a Holter monitor.
3. Locate and mark the six positions used to record the chest leads.
4. Demonstrate the proper procedure for recording the EKG with a standard electrocardiograph and the Phone-A-Gram system, mounting the finished product, and caring for the equipment after use.
5. Demonstrate the proper procedure for using a Holter Monitor.

The student is to perform these objectives with 100% accuracy 90% of the time (9 out of 10 times).

The consistent use of universal precautions is required by all health care professionals in all health care settings as a method of infection control. It is assumed that these precautions are used in all of the following procedures. Review Unit One if you have any questions on methods to use as the methods/techniques will not be repeated in detail in each procedure presented in the unit.

Be sure to consult the latest guidelines issued by the Centers for Disease Control and Prevention and consult with infection control practitioners when needed to identify specific precautions that pertain to your particular work situation.

The science and art of electrocardiography combine advanced electromedical technology with the science and art of medical practice. Present-day electrocardiographs present physicians with precise information by amplifying the minute electrical currents produced by the heart on a graphic record or tracing. This record or tracing is called an electrocardiogram, abbreviated EKG or ECG, defined simply as a graphic representation of the electrical activity (currents) produced by the heart during the

VOCABULARY

amplify (am'pli-fi)—To enlarge, to extend.

Arrhythmia (ah-rith'-me-ah)—A variation from the normal or an irregular rhythm of the heartbeat.

Atrium (a'tre-um)—One of the upper chambers of the heart. The right atrium receives deoxygenated blood from the body, whereas the left atrium receives oxygenated blood from the lungs. (The plural is *atria.*)

Cardiac (kar'de-ak) **arrest**—The sudden and often unexpected cessation of the heartbeat. Permanent damage of vital organs and death are probable if treatment is not given immediately.

Defibrillation (de-fi"bri-la'shun)—The application of electrical impulses to the heart to stop heart fibrillation or irregular contractions.

Electrocardiograph (e-lek"tro-kar-de-o-graf")—The instrument used in electrocardiology.

Fibrillation (fi"bri-la-shun)—A cardiac arrhythmia characterized by rapid, irregular, and ineffective electrical activity in the heart. Ventricular fibrillation is a common cause of cardiac arrest.

Myocardial infarction (MI) (mi"o-kar'de-al in-fark 'shun)—The death of cells in an area of the heart muscle due to oxygen deprivation, which in turn is caused by an interference of blood supply to the area. Commonly referred to as a "heart attack."

Myocardium (mi"o-kar-de-um)—The heart muscle.

Oscilloscope (o-sil'o-skop)—An instrument used to display the shape or wave form of the electrical activity of the heart and other body organs (comparable to a television screen).

Pacemaker (pas'mak-er)—The pacemaker of the heart is the sinoatrial (SA) node located in the right atrium.

Pericarditis (per "i-kar-di'tis)—Inflammation of the pericardium, the fibroserous sac enveloping the heart.

Rhythm strip—An EKG recording of a single lead that is used to determine the *rhythm* of the heartbeat, such as a fast, slow, regular, or irregular rhythm, and ventricular fibrillation. It is also used to determine if the patient is experiencing any type of heart block (for example, third-degree heart block). The rhythm strip gives a one-dimensional picture of the beating of the heart to demonstrate the rhythm of the heartbeat *only*, in contrast to the 12-lead EKG, which can show damage to the heart and other conditions. Data from the rhythm strip can be a useful screening tool because frequent runs of arrhythmias can be more easily observed. The rhythm strip can also be used to confirm the basic assessment made on the 12-lead EKG. Current use of the rhythm strip is to record Lead V_1, and possible Leads V_2 and V_5, although one could record any lead that is desired. Rhythm strips are frequently recorded from a continuous cardiac monitor in intensive care units in the hospital and by paramedics in the field in emergency situations.

Ventricle (ven'tri-kl)—One of the lower chambers of the heart. The right ventricle receives deoxygenated blood from the right atrium and pumps this blood through the pulmonary arteries to the lungs; the left ventricle receives oxygenated blood from the left atrium and pumps this blood out through the aorta to all body tissues.

Additional terms are defined within the text.

processes of contraction and relaxation. More precisely, the EKG records the amount of electrical activity, the time required for this activity to travel through the heart during each complete heartbeat, and the rate and rhythm of the heartbeat. Many physicians now include an electrocardiogram as part of a complete physical examination, especially for patients 40 years of age or older. It is also advisable to have an EKG or a treadmill stress EKG before any serious jogging or other exercise program is started (see "Treadmill Stress Test" at the end of this unit).

Frequently physicians have medical assistants take the EKG. To be valuable members of the health team, those who take EKGs must acquire related knowledge and develop skills (that is, they must know what they are doing, why and how to do it, and then do it well).

The following pages are designed to help you acquire this knowledge and skill by discussing the nature and purpose of the EKG, the equipment and materials needed, preparation of the patient and equipment, ways to monitor the record for abnormal and erratic tracings, procedure for taking the EKG, and mounting the record obtained.

Before going farther, it is suggested that you review the anatomy of the heart to maximize your understanding of electrocardiography (Figure 16-1).

Figure 16-1 A, *Your heart and how it works.*
Courtesy and by permission of the American Heart Association, Inc.

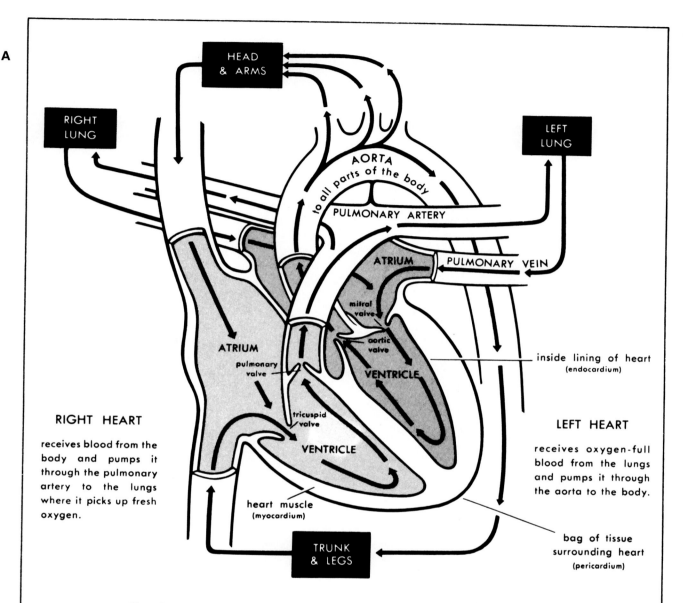

Your heart weighs well under a pound and is only a little larger than your fist, but it is a powerful, long working, hard working organ. Its job is to pump blood to the lungs and to all the body tissues.

The heart is a hollow organ. Its tough, muscular wall (myocardium) is surrounded by a fiberlike bag (pericardium) and is lined by a thin, strong membrane (endocardium). A wall (septum) divides the heart cavity down the middle into a "right heart" and a "left heart". Each side of the heart is divided again into an upper chamber (called an atrium or auricle) and a lower chamber (ventricle). Valves regulate the flow of blood through the heart and to the pulmonary artery and the aorta.

The heart is really a double pump. One pump (the right heart) receives blood which has just come from the body after delivering nutrients and oxygen to the body tissues. It pumps this dark, bluish red blood to the lungs where the blood gets rid of a waste gas (carbon dioxide) and picks up a fresh supply of oxygen which turns it a bright red again. The second pump (the left heart) receives this "reconditioned" blood from the lungs and pumps it out through the great trunk-artery (aorta) to be distributed by smaller arteries to all parts of the body.

Figure 16-1—cont'd B, *conduction system of the heart.*
From Goldberger AL, Goldberger E: *Clinical electrocardiography: a simplified approach*, ed 3, St. Louis, 1986, Mosby.

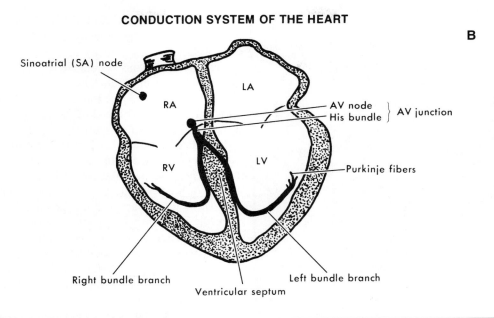

CONDUCTION SYSTEM OF THE HEART

THE CARDIAC CYCLE AND EKG CYCLE

The term *cardiac cycle* refers to one complete heartbeat, which consists of contraction (systole) and relaxation (diastole) of both atria and both ventricles. The many cells of the heart are arranged so they act together as one network or system. Throughout this network, two types of electrical processes, called *depolarization* and *repolarization*, are transmitted. When depolarization occurs, the cells are stimulated, and the myocardium (the heart muscle) contracts; as repolarization occurs, the myocardium relaxes. To understand the electrical activity of the heart, think of the heart as consisting of two separate cell networks, one being the atria and the other the ventricles. The two atria contrast simultaneously; then as they relax, the two ventricles contract and relax, rather than the entire heart contracting as a unit. Any disturbance in the processes of the cardiac cycle will cause a change in the electrical forces needed to maintain normal, rhythmic heartbeats and may produce an arrhythmia. Depending on the degree of disturbance, it could be a minor disruption of rhythm or a major life-threatening arrhythmia.

The atria and the ventricles are considered separately on the EKG. The waves or deflections recorded on the electrocardiograph paper represent the sequence of events that occur during the cardiac cycle. The normal EKG cycle consists of waves that have been arbitrarily labeled P, QRS, and T waves. Each wave corresponds to a particular part of the cardiac cycle (Figure 16-2). The *P wave* reflects contraction (depolarization) of the atria. The *QRS wave* (QRS complex) reflects ventricular recovery (repolarization of the ventricles). A *T wave* reflecting the repolarization of the atria is not visible, because it is obscured by the QRS wave. A T wave fol-

Figure 16-2 *Normal EKG deflections.*
From Conover MB: *Understanding electrocardiography*, ed 4, St. Louis, 1992, Mosby.

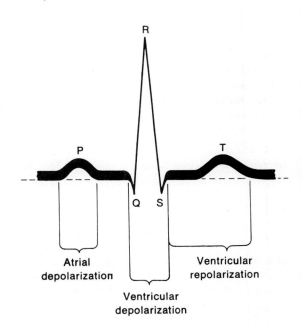

lows every QRS wave. Because the ventricles are much larger than the atria, the QRS and T waves are normally much larger than the P wave.

The *P-R interval* reflects the time it takes from the beginning of the atrial contraction to the beginning of the ventricular contraction. The P-R interval is measured from the beginning of the P wave to the beginning of the QRS complex (Figure 16-3).

Figure 16-3 *EKG intervals.*
From Conover MB: *Understanding electrocardiography*, ed 4, St. Louis, 1992, Mosby.

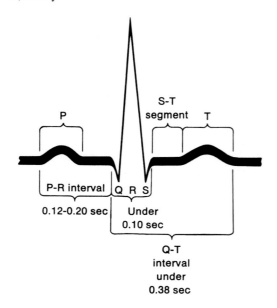

The *ST segment* reflects the time interval from the end of the ventricular contraction to the beginning of the ventricular recovery.

The *Q-T interval* reflects the time it takes from the beginning of the ventricular depolarization to the end of the ventricular repolarization. This interval gives a better picture of the total ventricular activity. It is measured from the beginning of the QRS complex to the end of the T wave.

The *baseline*, a flat horizontal line that separates the waves, may be seen to run the length of the EKG tracing. This is known as the isoelectric line. The waves of the EKG cycle will deflect either upward (positive deflection) or downward (negative deflection) from the baseline. This line is present when there is no current flowing in the heart. The baseline present after the T wave reflects the period when the entire heart is resting or in its polarized state.

Observing and measuring the configuration and location of each wave in relation to the other waves and baseline, the intervals and segments in each cycle, and the intervals and segments between each of the EKG cycles allows the physician to interpret and analyze the rate, rhythm, and conduction of the heart. Abnormalities detected in the EKG cycles help diagnose cardiac problems (for example, myocardial infarction [MI]), pericarditis, myocarditis, left ventricular hypertrophy, atrial and ventricular arrhythmias, nodal block, atrial and ventricular fibrillation, and a variety of other conditions such as acid-base imbalance, effects of various drugs, metabolic diseases, autonomic hyperactivity, and hyperventilation).

CONTROL OF THE HEARTBEAT: CONDUCTION SYSTEMS OF THE HEART

To understand the interpretation of an EKG, one must know the mechanism by which the heartbeat originates. Stimulation of the heartbeat originates in the sympathetic (acting to increase the heart rate) and parasympathetic (the vagus nerve, acting to slow the heart rate) branches of the autonomic nervous system. Although the heart is under the control of the nervous system, the myocardium (heart muscle) itself is capable of contracting rhythmically independently of this outside control. Despite this property of automaticity, impulses from the autonomic nervous system are required to produce a rapid enough beat to maintain circulation and life effectively. Without the nerve connection, the heart rate may be less than 40 beats per minute instead of the usual 70 to 90 per minute (average 80 beats per minute).

Specialized masses of tissue in the heart form the conduction system, regulating the sequence of events of the cardiac cycle. These include the sinoatrial (SA) node, the "pacemaker" of the heart, located in the upper right-hand corner of the right atrium adjacent to the opening of the superior vena cava; the atrioventricular (AV) node, located near the intraventricular septum in the inferior wall of the right atrium and near the tricuspid valve; the bundle of His (or atrioventricular bundle), located in the interventricular septum, which then divides into the left and right bundles; and the Purkinje fibers, which terminate in the ventricles.

The electrical impulse of the cardiac cycle travels first to the sinoatrial node, from which wavelike impulses are sent through the atria, stimulating first the right and then the left atrium; they eventually sweep over the heart.

When the atria have been stimulated, the impulse slows as it passes through the AV node. Slowing of the impulse at the AV node allows the resting ventricles (in diastole) to fill with blood from the atria. This wave of excitation (stimulation) then spreads down to the bundle of His, then to the right and left bundle branches, which then relay the impulse to the Purkinje fibers, an interlacing network terminating in the musculature of the ventricle. The Purkinje fibers distribute the impulse in the right and left ventricles, causing them to contract. Stimulation of the muscle of the ventricle begins in the intraventricular septum and moves downward, causing ventricular depolarization and contraction. Mechanically, the ventricles empty blood into the pulmonary (or lesser) circulation by way of the pulmonary artery and the right and left pulmonary branches, and into the systemic (or greater) circulation by way of the aorta. This stimulation or impulse must spread through the muscle of both atria and both ventricles before mechanical contraction can occur. To complete the cardiac cycle, the entire heart now relaxes momentarily, and then a new impulse is initiated by the SA node to repeat the whole cycle.

The electrical wave form that originates in the SA node and spreads throughout the heart then spreads through the body. From the body surface it is possible to pick up these electrical impulses and record them on specialized paper (the EKG) or display them on an oscilloscope (comparable to a television screen).

TIME REQUIRED FOR CARDIAC CYCLE

Each cardiac cycle takes approximately 0.8 second. With this time limit, there are 75 heartbeats per minute. When the heartbeats more than 75 times per minute, the cycle requires less time. Conversely, when the heartbeats less than 75 beats per minute, the cardiac cycle requires more than 0.8 second.

HEART SOUNDS DURING CARDIAC CYCLE

Typical sounds are elicited from the heart during each cardiac cycle. These sounds are described a *lubb dupp* as heard through a stethoscope. The first sound, *lubb* or systolic sound, is a longer and lower-pitched sound and is believed to be from the contraction of the ventricles and vibrations from the closing of the cuspid valves. The second sound, *dupp* (the diastolic sound), is shorter and sharper and occurs during the beginning of ventricular relaxation. It is thought to be due to the vibrations of the closure of the semilunar valves (pulmonic and aortic valves). Since these sounds provide information about the valves of the heart, they have clinical significance. Variations from normal in these sounds indicate imperfect functioning of the valves. Heart murmurs are one type of abnormal sound heard and may indicate stenosis or incomplete closing of the valves (valvular insufficiency). It is important to remember that the EKG does not record these sounds. They can be heard with a stethoscope that is put on the chest wall over the apex region of the heart.

ELECTROCARDIOGRAM

ELECTROCARDIOGRAM PAPER

To understand the significance of each wave and interval of various heights and widths recorded by an electrocardiograph, the medical assistant needs to know the significance of the small and large blocks on the EKG paper (Figure 16-4, *A*). On the horizontal line, one small block represents 0.04 second (Figure 16-4, *B*). On the vertical axis, one small block represents 1 mm. Since a large block is five small blocks wide and five deep, each small block represents 0.2 second (horizontal) and 5 mm (vertical).

Notice all the lines. Every fifth line (horizontal and vertical) is usually printed darker than other lines, producing blocks (squares) that are 5 mm × 5 mm. Thus two of the larger blocks equal 10 mm or 1 cm.

These measurements, accepted internationally, allow physicians to interpret cardiac time (rate) on the horizontal line and cardiac voltage on the vertical axis and thus determine if the electrical activity of the heart is within normal limits.

EKG paper is heat-sensitive and pressure-sensitive. When the machine is on and running, a heated stylus moves over the paper to record the cardiac cycles. Because it is pressure-sensitive, EKG paper must be handled carefully to avoid markings that would blemish the actual tracing.

INTERPRETATION

When the physician interprets an EKG, the following factors are usually determined:

- *Rate*—How many beats per minute; determined are the atrial rate and the ventricular rate.

- *Rhythm*—Whether the heart rhythm is regular or irregular; determined are the atrial rhythm and the ventricular rhythm.
- *Conduction time*—How long it takes for the impulse originating at the SA node to stimulate ventricular contraction (review the conduction system, page 528); determined are the P-R interval and the QRS duration.
- *Configuration and location*—Of each wave, the ST segment, the P-R interval, and sometimes the Q-T interval.

These findings are then recorded and reviewed by the physician to help establish a diagnosis or evaluate current treatment.

Because many physicians expect the medical assistant who takes a patient's EKG to monitor the graph for abnormal or erratic tracings, you should be aware of *heart rates and rhythms.*

In a normal EKG, all heartbeats consist of three major units, the P wave, the QRS complex, and the T wave; and they appear as a similar pattern, equally spaced.

Briefly, the rate of a particular rhythm may be determined from the EKG simply by noting the distance between two R waves. As seen in Figure 16-4, *A*, two large squares between R waves means that the rate is 150 beats per minute; three large squares between R waves means that the rate is 100 beats per minute. Similarly, four large squares between R waves indicates a heart rate of 75 beats per minute. To get this rate per minute, divide the number of large squares between the R waves into 300. NOTE: If the rhythm is irregular, counting the squares in a single R-R interval will give an approximate rather than the precise rate that would be obtained with a perfectly regular rhythm. To calculate heart rate when the rhythm is *irregular*, count the number of cycles in a 6-second strip and multiply by 10. The EKG paper is marked along the top in 3-second intervals. 15 large squares equals 3 seconds. 30 large squares equals 6 seconds (see Figure 16-2).

To determine if heart rhythm is regular or irregular, the distance between each P wave and then that between each R wave is measured. If the distance between all P waves is the same, atrial rhythm is regular; if the distance varies, rhythm is irregular. Similarly, if the distance between all R waves is the same, ventricular rhythm is regular; if not, it is irregular.

The term *normal sinus rhythm* refers to an EKG that is within normal limits. In normal sinus rhythm, the heart rate is 60 to 100 beats per minute, the rhythm is regular, P waves are present, QRS waves are of normal duration, and the P/QRS relationship and PR intervals are all within normal limits.

Common Rhythms

Sinus rhythms. Three arrhythmias that originate in the sinus or sinoatrial node are:

- *Sinus tachycardia*—A regular sinus rhythm of 100 to 180 beats per minute. It may be one of the first signs of congestive heart failure. It may also be seen when the patient has a fever; is anxious; has hypotension, hyperthyroidism, or chronic obstructive pulmonary disease; or is taking the drugs atropine or epinephrine.

Figure 16-4 *EKG paper with section enlarged.* **A,** *Number of large squares between recorded R waves indicate rate of heartbeat per minute;* **B,** *one large square enlarged.*

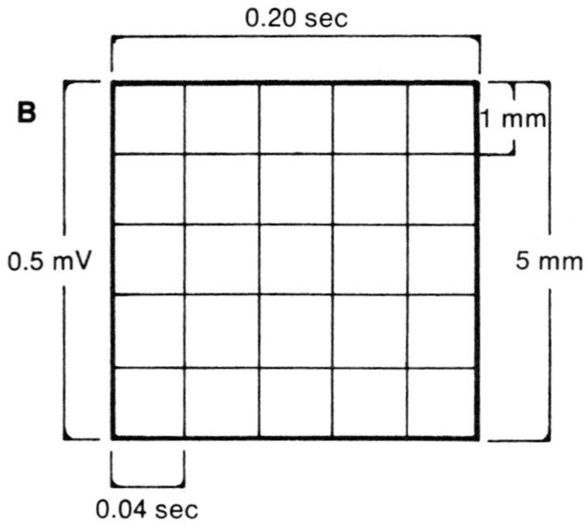

- *Sinus bradycardia*—A regular sinus rhythm of less than 60 beats per minute. This may be seen in a patient with hypothyroidism, in an athlete, or in a patient who is taking digitalis or propranolol.
- *Sinus arrhythmia*—An irregular sinus rhythm in which the cycle lengths vary. It is a normal response of the heart to respiration in which the rate increases with inspiration and decreases with expiration.

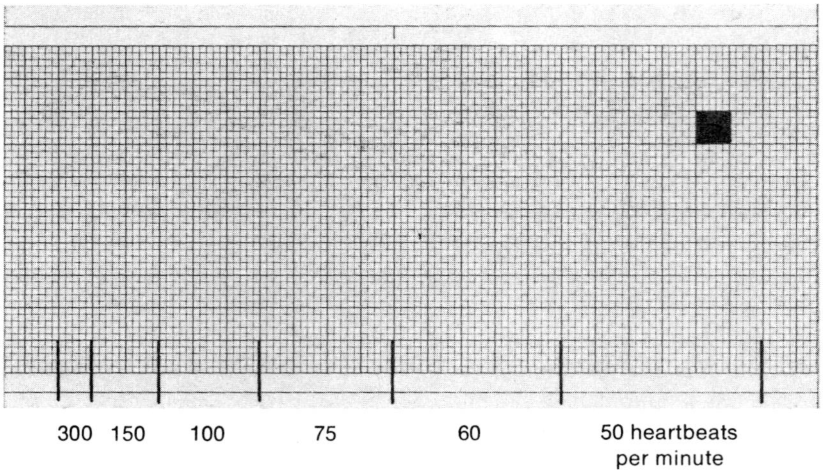

Atrial arrhythmias. Three arrhythmias that originate outside of the sinus node and above the branching portion of the bundle of His are:
- *Premature atrial contractions (PACs)*—An irregular rhythm resulting from a premature atrial contraction originating within the atria but outside of the sinus node. It may be caused by a variety of stimuli such as stress, caffeine, tobacco, hypoxia, electrolyte imbalance, congestive heart failure (in MI), or with digitalis toxicity.
- *Paroxysmal atrial tachycardia (PAT)*—A regular rhythm of 140 to 250 beats per minute. This often has a sudden onset and terminates suddenly. It can occur in a normal person or in one with heart disease. It also can be a sign of digitalis toxicity and can deteriorate into atrial flutter or fibrillation.

- *Atrial fibrillation*—An irregular rhythm of 150 to 200 beats per minute. This diagnosis is made because of an irregular ventricular rhythm and the absence of the P waves on the EKG. It is seen in patients with heart disease, pericarditis, mitral valve disease, hypertension, and pulmonary embolism.

Ventricular arrhythmias
- *Premature ventricular contractions (PVCs)*—An irregular rhythm with a distorted QRS complex and no P wave. PVCs are common after an MI or in heart disease and are often associated with an increased incidence of ventricular fibrillation or tachycardia, or sudden death. In people with normal hearts, PVCs are not associated with sudden death and are not treated. Anxiety, caffeine, and even anemia can cause PVCs.
- *Ventricular tachycardia*—A regular rhythm 75% of the time consisting of three or more PVCs at the rate of 120 to 250 beats per minute. Life-threatening ventricular tachycardia may lead to ventricular fibrillation. This is seen in patients with coronary artery disease or acute MI, digitalis toxicity, hypoxia, and anemia and with caffeine intake and also anxiety.
- *Ventricular fibrillation*—A disorganized activity in the

ventricles. Ventricular fibrillation is very serious because the heart quivers and twitches but does not pump blood into the body. There is electrical chaos in the ventricles. It is caused by MI or ischemia and can be preceded by a PVC or ventricular tachycardia. It can result in cardiac arrest and death.

Artifacts

Artifacts are defects (unwanted activity) on the electrocardiograph *not* caused by the electrical activity produced during the cardiac cycle. Since the EKG picks up and records every kind of electrical activity it can find, artifacts may appear, making the recording difficult to interpret. To remedy this situation, you should understand what causes artifacts and how they can be eliminated or greatly minimized, and use the correct recording technique.

There are several types of artifacts, the most common being somatic tremor (muscle movement), wandering baseline (baseline shift), and alternating current (AC) interference.

Somatic tremor.

These artifacts can be identified by the unnatural baseline deflections, ranging from irregular vibrations in amplitude and frequency (jagged peaks of irregular height and spacing) to large shifting of the baseline (Figure 16-5, A to C). Muscle movement, which is either voluntary or involuntary, produces artifacts caused mainly when the patient:

- Is tense and/or apprehensive.
- Moves or talks.
- Is in an uncomfortable position.
- Suffers from a nervous disorder that causes constant tremors such as Parkinson's disease.

The best way to avoid these patient-produced artifacts is to prepare the patient well, both emotionally and physically, preferably in a pleasant and relaxing atmosphere. The following will aid in patient preparation:

- Gain the full cooperation of the patient.
- Explain the procedure and what you will be doing.
- Position the patient comfortably, with limbs well supported.
- Offer assistance and reassurance as needed.
- Have patients suffering from a nervous disorder put their hands, palms down, under the buttocks or take a deep breath. This will help reduce artifacts (see also Preparation of Patient, page 534).

Wandering Baseline (Baseline Shift) (Figure 16-5, *B*).

Causes of this artifact include the following:

1. Electrodes that are applied too tightly or too loosely
2. Tension on an electrode as a result of an unsupported lead wire that is pulling the electrode away from the patient's skin
3. Too little or poor quality electrolyte gel or paste on an electrode
4. Corroded or dirty electrodes
5. Skin creams or lotions present on the area where the electrode is applied

To prevent artifacts, correct and attentive technique when applying the electrodes with the electrolyte gel or paste is a must. Wash the electrodes after each use and occasionally with kitchen cleanser, but *never* use steel wool. Electrolyte gels or pastes that are left on the electrode can cause corrosion, which makes the electrode a poor conductor of cardiac electrical currents. The tips of the lead wires must also be kept clean.

Figure 16-5 *EKG artifacts.* **A,** *Somatic tremor artifact;* **B,** *Wandering baseline.* **C,** *Alternating current artifact.*
Conover MB: *Understanding electrocardiography,* ed 4, St. Louis, 1992, Mosby.

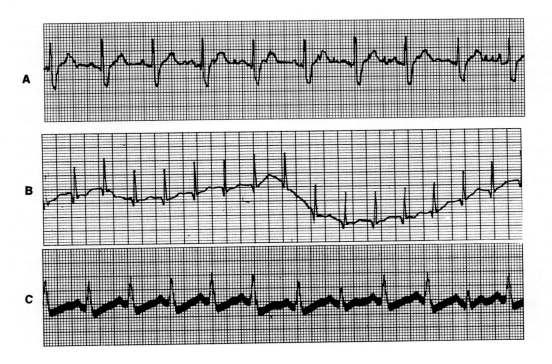

Ensure that the patient's skin where the electrodes will be applied is clean; if necessary, wash the area briskly with alcohol or the presaturated electrolyte pads before applying the electrode.

Alternating current interference. AC artifacts appear as a series of small regular peaks (or spiked lines) the EKG (Figure 16-5, *C*).

Alternating current (AC) is our standard source for electrical power. AC present in electrical equipment or wires can radiate or leak a small amount of energy into the immediate area. When a patient is present in this area, some of the AC may be picked up by the body, which in turn is detected by the electrocardiograph. Thus an EKG with AC artifacts results. Common causes of AC interference artifacts include the following:

1. Improper grounding of the electrocardiograph
2. Presence of other electrical equipment in the room
3. Electrical wiring in walls or ceilings
4. X-ray or other large electrical equipment being used in adjacent rooms
5. Lead wires crossed and not following the contour of the patient's body
6. Corroded or dirty electrodes
7. Faulty technique of the operator

To minimize or eliminate AC interference, correct technique is required. The EKG unit must be properly grounded. Check the instructions in the operator's manual supplied with each unit by the manufacturer. Newer units have three-pronged plugs that are inserted into a properly grounded, three-receptacle outlet. Older units may have a two-pronged plug. In this case a ground wire from the unit is connected to a suitable ground such as a cold water pipe.

Unplug other electrical equipment in the room. When x-ray equipment is being used in adjacent rooms, it may be necessary for you to wait until that procedure is completed or move to another room to record the EKG. Moving the patient table away from the wall may help minimize interference caused from electrical wiring. Lead wires must be straight and positioned to follow body contour; the line cord is to be away from the patient, and the unit should be near the patient's feet, not head. Electrodes must be cleaned after each use and occasionally should be scrubbed with a kitchen cleanser.

Additional Problems

When recording an EKG, one may encounter a few additional erratic tracings which may appear as follows:

- An indistinct tracing usually caused by (a) the stylus heat being too low, (2) a bent stylus, (3) incorrect stylus pressure, or (4) a broken stylus heating element, which results in no tracing
- A straight line but no tracing, caused by the patient cable not being plugged in correctly
- A break between complexes, caused by a loose or broken lead wire

When you cannot correct the cause of an artifact, inform the physician and call the manufacturer's or other repair service, according to office policy.

ELECTROCARDIOGRAM ELECTRODES AND ELECTROLYTES

Electrodes (also called sensors) are small metal plates placed on the patient to pick up the electrical activity of the heart and conduct it to the electrocardiograph. The standard 12-lead electrocardiograph has five electrodes: two to be attached to the fleshy part of the arms, two to be attached to the fleshy part of the legs, and one floating electrode that will be placed in six different positions on the chest when recording the chest leads.

In the machine, this electrical current is changed into mechanical action, which is recorded on the EKG paper by a heated stylus. To help conduct this electric current, an *electrolyte* is applied to each electrode. They are used because skin is a poor conductor of electricity. Electrolytes are available in the form of gels, pastes, or flannel materials presaturated with an electrolyte solution.

Once the electrodes are correctly secured to the patient with rubber straps, lead wires are fastened to them. These lead wires extend off the patient cable, which is attached to the electrocardiograph machine.

ELECTROCARDIOGRAM LEADS

The standard 12-lead electrocardiograph system records electrical activity from the frontal and horizontal planes of the body by using 12 leads as follows:

Standard Limb or Bipolar Leads

The first three leads to be recorded on a standard EKG are known as Lead I, Lead II, and Lead III. These are called bipolar leads, because each of them uses two limb electrodes that record simultaneously the electrical forces of the heart from the frontal plane; that is, Lead I records electrical activity between the right arm (RA) and left arm (LA); Lead II records activity between the right arm and left leg; Lead III records activity between the left arm (LA) and left leg (LL) (Figure 16-6, *A* and *B*).

The right arm is considered to be a negative pole, and the left leg a positive pole. The left arm will either be negative or positive, depending on the lead; in Lead I it is positive, in Lead II it is negative.

Upright (positive) deflections on the EKG indicate current flowing toward a positive pole; inverted (negative) wave deflections indicate current flowing toward a negative pole. For example, in Lead I, the flow of current will be from a negative to a positive pole; thus the wave deflections on the recording will be upright.

Augmented Leads

The next three leads are the augmented leads, designated as aV_R, aV_L, and aV_F. The aV stands for augmented voltage; the R, L, and F stand for right, left, and foot (leg), respectively. Augmented leads are unipolar and also record frontal plane activity.

Lead aV_R records electrical activity from the midpoint between the left arm and left leg to the right arm.

Lead aV_L records electrical activity from the midpoint between the right arm and left leg to the left arm.

Figure 16-6 A, *Lead triangle showing position of standard limb leads;* **B,** *lead triangle showing position of augmented leads.*

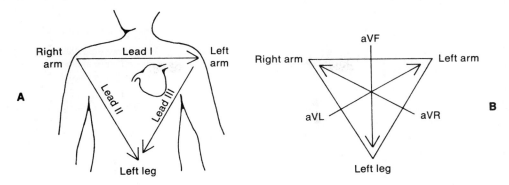

Lead aVF records electrical activity from the midpoint between the right arm and left arm to the left leg.

Chest or Precordial Leads

The last six leads of the standard 12-lead EKG are the chest or precordial leads. These leads are also unipolar and are designated as V_1, V_2, V_3, V_4, V_5, and V_6.

This third set of leads records electrical activity between six points on the chest wall and a point within the heart. To obtain these recordings, the chest electrode is to be moved to six predesignated positions on the chest. Figure 16-7 shows the location of these positions. It is imperative that the correct position be used for each lead recording.

All 12 leads discussed can be interpreted separately or in combination. Each lead presents a picture of a different anatomic part of the heart, thus allowing the physician to determine areas of damage or problem areas.

When doing an EKG, the machine automatically connects the proper electrode potentials for Leads I, III, III, aV_R, aV_L, and aV_F. To record the chest leads, the chest electrode must be moved manually to each of the assigned chest positions.

Suggested Codes for Marking Leads

Certain codes are used to identify each lead recorded. Without these codes it would be difficult to determine which lead was being interpreted, and it would be impossible to mount the recording with proper lead identification. An example of codes used is seen in Figure 16-7. On older machines the leads are coded (marked) by depressing the lead marker button. New machines automatically code for each lead as it is being recorded.

STANDARDIZING THE ELECTROCARDIOGRAPH

The diagnostic value of an EKG depends on an accurate recording. Standard techniques have been adapted to provide a recording that can be interpreted anywhere in the world, assuming the EKG machine used has been calibrated according to universal measurements.

The universal standard of EKG measurement is the following: 1 millivolt of cardiac electrical activity will deflect the stylus precisely 10 mm high (Figure 16-8). This is equal to 10 small blocks on the EKG paper.

Before any EKG is recorded, the machine must be standardized, (that is, it must be checked to determine it if is set to record according to the universal measurement).

To standardize the machine, turn the main power switch on. The stylus should be positioned to run along on one of the dark horizontal lines. Set the lead selector switch to STD and the record switch to RUN. Quickly depress and release the standardization button. The standardization mark should reach 10-mm high and 2-mm wide. It appears as an open-ended rectangle (the open end being along the baseline). A slight slant may be seen in the top right corner, which is normal; but any other deviation is not normal and must be corrected. To correct any deviation, turn the standardization adjustment knob and repeat the procedure until the correct standardization mark is obtained.

It is important to consult the instruction manual provided by the manufacturer of each EKG machine because the above procedure may vary slightly among the various machines on the market.

The universal standard for recording an EKG is at a speed of 22 mm per second. This can be increased on the machine to run the paper at 50 mm per second when segments of the EKG are close together or when heart rate is rapid. A notation of this *must* be made to alert the physician of this change to allow an accurate interpretation of the record.

PREPARATION AND PROCEDURE FOR OBTAINING ELECTROCARDIOGRAMS
Equipment

Bed or examining table (preferably without any metal attachments)
Linen sheet or blanket
Electrocardiograph with patient cable lead wires
Electrolyte gel *or* paste *or* presaturated electrolyte pads
Electrodes and rubber straps
Gauze squares
Patient gown

Preparation of Electrocardiograph Room

1. The room should be as far away as possible from all x-ray and other electrical equipment that may cause artifacts on the EKG.

Figure 16-7 *Leads of routine EKG.*
Courtesy The Burdick Corporation, Milton, Wisc.

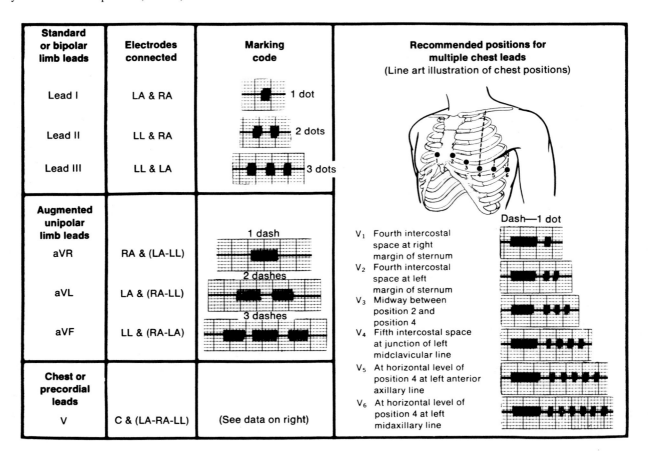

Standard or bipolar limb leads	Electrodes connected	Marking code	Recommended positions for multiple chest leads (Line art illustration of chest positions)
Lead I	LA & RA	1 dot	
Lead II	LL & RA	2 dots	
Lead III	LL & LA	3 dots	
Augmented unipolar limb leads			Dash—1 dot
aVR	RA & (LA-LL)	1 dash	V_1 Fourth intercostal space at right margin of sternum
aVL	LA & (RA-LL)	2 dashes	V_2 Fourth intercostal space at left margin of sternum
aVF	LL & (RA-LA)	3 dashes	V_3 Midway between position 2 and position 4
Chest or precordial leads			V_4 Fifth intercostal space at junction of left midclavicular line
V	C & (LA-RA-LL)	(See data on right)	V_5 At horizontal level of position 4 at left anterior axillary line
			V_6 At horizontal level of position 4 at left midaxillary line

Figure 16-8 *Universal standard of EKG measurement 10 mm (1 cm) high. This is equal to 10 small blocks on the EKG paper.*
From Goldberger AL, Goldberger E: *Clinical electrocardiography: a simplified approach,* ed 3, St. Louis, 1986, Mosby.

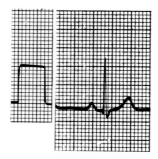

2. The room should be comfortably warm, quiet, pleasant, and not crowded with medical instruments, which may make the patient apprehensive.
3. The electrocardiograph (and patient) should be positioned away from wires, cords, and any other source of AC interference.
4. The bed or examining table must be wide enough so that the patient may rest comfortably with the extremities well supported; otherwise, muscle tension or tremors may cause artifacts.

Preparation of Patient

The quality of the record obtained is influenced by scrupulous attention to fundamental rules regarding the preparation of the patient. The medical assistant who is confident, but emphatic, will make it easier for the patient to relax, both mentally and physically.

1. Explain the nature and purpose of the electrocardiograph to the patient. Tactfully help the patient realize that full cooperation (that is, relaxing and not talking, moving, or chewing gum) will help produce a reading that will help the physician diagnose the patient's condition (when applicable).

2. Ensure the patient that no shock or other sensation will be felt.
3. Have the patient remove any jewelry that would interfere with the electrode placement or come in contact with the electrolyte.
4. Have the patient remove shoes and clothing from the forearms, lower legs, and chest; women may roll knee-hi stockings down. A patient gown should be put on with the opening in the front.
5. Help the patient assume a recumbent position on the table with arms at the sides and legs not touching. The extremities must be well supported on the table.
6. Place a cover over the patient with arms and lower legs exposed. Protecting the patient from cold or any other discomfort is very important. A small pillow can be placed under the head.
7. Locate and mark the six chest locations on the patient. (You can use a felt tip pen and wash the markings off after the procedure with an alcohol sponge.) The patient gown over a woman's chest can be adjusted so as not to expose the breasts and cause possible embarrassment and apprehension and still allow you to adequately locate and record the chest lead positions.
8. Inquire if the patient has any questions before you begin the recording.

Application of Electrodes and Connection of Lead Wires

1. Expose the patient's arms and legs.
2. Attach one end of each rubber strap to each electrode (Figure 16-9, *A*). Disposable electrodes, when used properly, may be used for acceptable EKGs. Prepare the skin and carefully follow manufacturer's usage instructions according to the type of electrode selected.
3. Using the side of the electrode, gently scrub the skin on the fleshy part of the right arm. The area rubbed should not be much larger than the size of the electrode and should be slightly reddened by the rubbing. (If there is lotion or cream on the skin, remove it with an alcohol sponge before the electrolyte and electrode are applied.)
4. Place a small amount of electrolyte gel or paste, about the size of a pea, on the electrode (Figure 16-9, *B*).
5. Place the electrode on this area; pull the rubber strap around, and fasten it to the electrode. The electrode must not be pressing against the table or other body parts. The electrode must not be fastened too loosely or too tightly. Try to move the electrode about once secured in place. If it slips or slides on the limb, it is too loose and must be tightened; if the skin is pinched on either side of the electrode, the strap is too tight and must be loosened.
6. Using a gauze square, wipe away any excess gel or paste from around the electrode.
7. Follow this same procedure to apply the electrodes to the left arm and to the right and left legs over the flesh part of the lower leg, not over the bone. By applying the electrodes to the fleshy areas on the limbs, the chance of

undesirable muscle artifacts is minimized. Also use equal amounts of gel or paste on each electrode. Always follow the same pattern when applying electrodes to ensure consistency.

8. When using presaturated electrolyte pads rather than a gel or paste, run the skin with the pad or a piece of gauze, then place it on the skin. The electrode is to be placed directly in top of the pad (Figure 16-9, *C* and *D*).
9. *If taking an EKG on a patient who has a cast, amputation, or prosthesis, place the electrode above the affected area. The electrode for the other extremity must then be placed in the same location opposite the first. For example, if the patient has a cast extending from the knee to the ankle on the right leg, place the electrode on the inside of the upper right leg. The electrode for the left leg must then be placed on the inside of the upper left leg. If the electrodes are not placed in this manner (that is, if one electrode is placed on the upper part of the right limb above the cast and the other electrode is placed on the fleshy part of the lower left leg), the electric vector would be changed, and abnormal results would occur on the EKG.*
10. Leave the chest electrode unattached but not touching a direct surface, *or* position it on the first chest position using the electrolyte of choice.
11. Firmly connect the patient cable lead wires to the proper electrodes so that the lead wire connector faces the patient's feet. Each wire is alphabetically coded: RA, right arm; LA, left arm; RL, right leg; LL, left leg; and C, chest. In addition, each lead wire is color coded to provide additional identification for the operator. It is very important that the lead wires are connected and arranged to follow the contour of the body without placing any strain on the electrodes so that the possibility of AC artifacts is minimized (Figure 16-10).
12. Plug the patient cable into the patient cable jack on the machine. Make sure that it is pushed all the way in.
13. Before beginning the recording, routinely check that all connections are secure, verify that the patient cable is supported on the table or over the patient's abdomen to prevent pulling of the cable, and see if the patient has any questions.

Recording the Electrocardiogram (Figure 16-11)

Limb leads

1. Set the lead switch to STD (standard).
2. Turn recorded switch to ON. (Some machines require a warm-up period before recording. Check the instruction manual to determine if this is the case for the equipment you are using.)
3. Turn recorder switch to RUN.
4. Center the baseline by turning the centering dial or position control knob.

Figure 16-9 A, *Attach rubber strap to electrode.* B, *Place small amount of electrolyte gel on electrode.* C, *Apply presaturated electrolyte pad and electrode to arm.* D, *Apply electrolyte pad, electrode, and rubber strap to arm.*

A
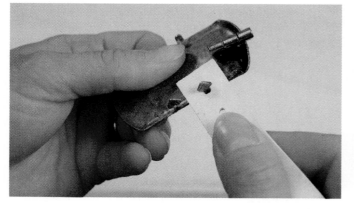

C
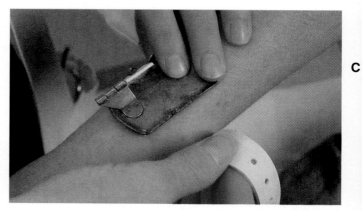

B
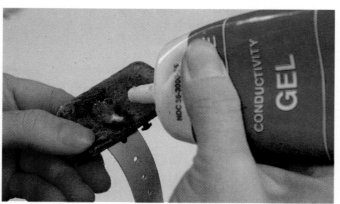

D
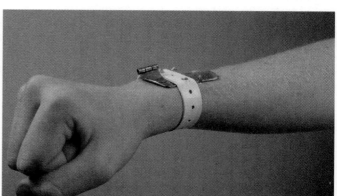

Figure 16-10 *Application of electrodes and connection to unit in correct positions.*
Courtesy The Burdick Corporation, Milton, Wisc.

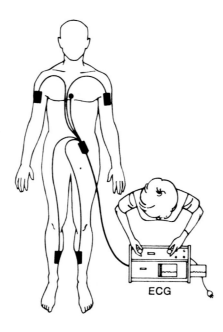

Figure 16-11 *Single-channel electrocardiograph. Can be used in the manual mode or in the automatic mode. When used in automatic mode, the EK-10 records a complete 12-lead EKG in just 38 seconds.*
Courtesy The Burdick Corporation, Milton, Wisc.

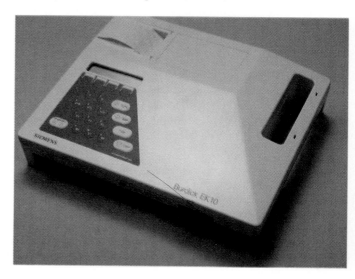

5. Check the standardization; quickly depress and release the standardization button several times while the lead selector is on STD and the recorder switch is on RUN. The height of the standardization measurement should be 10 mm or two large squares from the baseline.
6. Turn the lead selector switch to Lead I.
7. Mark the identification code for the lead immediately after it is selected, unless the machine does this automatically.
8. Run for a few heartbeats; depress the standardization button quickly if the physician requires proof of standardization for each lead. This standardization mark should be inserted between the T wave (or U wave when present) of one complex and the P wave of the next complex.
9. Record at least 8 to 10 inches. This provides ample tracing of the lead.
10. Turn lead selector to Lead II.
11. Repeat steps 7, 8, and 9.
12. Turn the lead selector to Lead III and repeat steps, 7, 8, and 9.

Augmented Leads—aV$_R$, aV$_L$, aV$_F$.

13. Turn the lead selector to lead aV$_R$, mark the identification code, inset a standardization mark if required, and record 5 to 6 inches (see steps 7 and 8).
14. Turn the lead selector to lead aV$_L$, and repeat step 13.
15. Turn the lead selector to lead aV$_F$, and repeat step 13.
16. Turn the machine off.

Chest leads

17. Leave the limb electrodes and patient cable wires in place.
18. Position the chest electrode over the first chest position, V$_1$, applying the electrode with gel *or* paste *or* presaturated electrolyte pad in the same manner used for the limbs.
19. Turn the lead selector to STD, the recorder switch to RUN, and depress the standardization button.

20. Turn the recorder switch to OFF to prevent excessive movement of the stylus.
21. Turn the lead selector switch to V.
22. Turn the recorder switch to ON.
23. Mark the identification code for the lead, and insert standardization marks as described in step 8, when required.
24. Record 5 to 6 inches.
25. Turn the recorder switch to OFF.
26. Move the chest electrode to the next position. Start again with step 21; repeat until all the chest leads have been recorded (that is, leads V$_1$ through V$_6$).
27. When all the leads have been recorded satisfactorily, turn the lead selector to STD and the recorder switch to OFF and unplug the power cord.
28. Disconnect the lead wires, unfasten the rubber straps, and remove the electrodes from the patient.
29. Wipe any electrolyte from the patient's skin.
30. Assist the patient as needed. Provide further instructions as indicated.
31. Label the recording with patient's name, date, and your initials.
32. Clean all equipment, and return it to the proper storage area.
33. Wash your hands.
34. Record the procedure.
35. Mount the recording, using the preferred mount as indicated by the physician; record the required information on the mount. Sign your name to the mounted EKG.
36. Give the mounted EKG to the physician for review and interpretation.

   Throughout the recording of the EKG, make sure that the stylus stays on the same baseline (Figure 16-12). Use the position control knob if any adjustment is necessary. Constantly watch for the appearance of any artifact. If an artifact does occur, determine the cause, and correct the problem (refer to pages 531 to 532).

Figure 16-12 *Electrocardiograph paper and recording.*

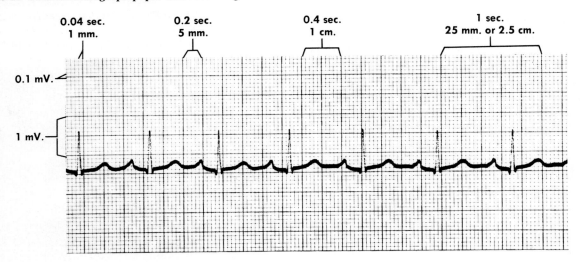

Mounting an Electrocardiogram

Mounting the EKG is important so that the recording can be protected, easily seen by the physician, and inserted into the patient's medical record after the physician has reviewed and interpreted it. A variety of commercially prepared mounts are available for use, or the recording can be mounted on a plain piece of paper.

CLEANING ELECTRODES

All of the suction cup–type electrodes must be wiped clean immediately after each EKG is completed to prevent residual buildup and subsequent contact problems. Use only alcohol or soap and water to clean electrode surfaces, since, polishes, commercial cleaners and other such items if used can cause artifacts in the EKG tracing. Also, never use a scrub brush to clean the electrode surfaces, because the metal plating is very thin and can be scraped away, thus rendering the electrodes useless.

PHONE-A-GRAM: THE COMPUTERIZED EKG

For over 2000 years, physicians from Hippocrates to Lannëc and Einthoven and many others have sought to improve diagnostic accuracy. By 1979 a computer-assisted EKG analysis program was developed. Phone-A-Gram is an example of a computerized EKG service providing all the necessary equipment and a second opinion for the diagnosis of a patient's condition.

It includes a portable automatic EKG transmitter (a standard model, a scout model, or the stripchart recorder model), all the auxiliary equipment, and a personal hookup into the national network (Data Center), which receives, converts, processes, analyzes, and prints out all EKG information for ready reference.

All EKG transmitting units are compact, portable, single-channel units with features of automatic lead switching and standardization across all 12 leads. The *standard model* is a battery-powered portable unit, but it does not provide a stripchart. Like the standard model, the *scout model* is used in conjunction with a conventional electrocardiograph to produce an on-site tracing as the EKG is being transmitted.

Prepare the patient is prepared for the EKG in the usual manner, but all six chest lead electrodes must be applied to the patient's chest before you begin to record the EKG.

A standard telephone is used to dial the Data Center. The telephone handset is placed on the Phone-A-Gram unit, and the EKG is transmitted at the push of a button. The unit picks up signals from the patient and transmits them over the telephone to the Data Center for interpretation.

AUTOMATIC ELECTROCARDIOGRAPHS

The newer electrocardiographs have fewer operating controls and are much easier to use. With these new machines you *don't* have to adjust controls such as position, sensitivity, heat, paper speed, run, and lead markers. You just set one switch to select the format that you want to record. Different *positions* on the electrocardiograph set it at different speeds and sensitivities. On Hewlett-Packard's models many different formats can be selected. Some electrocardiographs have a complete alphanumeric keyboard through which you can enter a wide range of patient data, including the patient's name, the requesting physician, name of the facility, and the operator's initials on the EKG record. Other three-channel electrocardiographs can be operated manually or automatically by the push of a touch pad.

DIGITAL ELECTROCARDIOGRAPH FACSIMILE

Facsimile transmission of medical data is becoming an accepted practice for accessing offsite diagnostic expertise in a timely manner (Figure 16-13). For instance, emergency rooms or private physicians may require quick, expert EKG diagnoses. Direct digital EKG fax transmits directly from the cardiograph to a fax machine and produces a faxed ECG copy of near-original quality. It eliminates the traditional intermediate step of copying the ECG report and sending via the traditional fax machine. A two-way, direct-digital EKG fax enhancement provides comments added by the physician, as well as a signature to be faxed back to the originating cardiograph. Physicians can receive the EKG anywhere there is a fax machine. An internal modem and a software upgrade of the system are required.

AMBULATORY CARDIAC MONITORING (MONITORING)

Ambulatory cardiac monitoring, frequently referred to as monitoring (named after the inventor), is a continuous recording of the electrical activity of the patient's heart (an EKG) for 24 to 48 hours (Figure 16-14). By means of a special monitor, the activity of the patient's heart can be recorded during unrestricted activity, rest, and sleep for

Figure 16-13 *Portable Burdick E560 interpretive electrocardiograph.*
Equipment courtesy The Burdick Corp., Schaumburg, Ill.

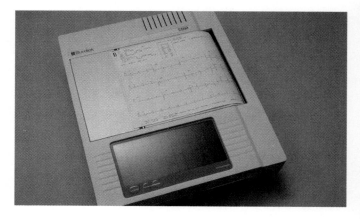

Figure 16-14 *Ambulatory cardiac monitor.*

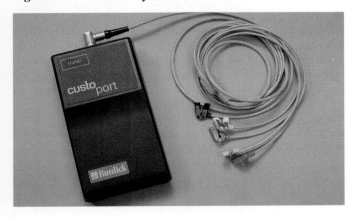

future observation and study. Newer monitor models have a compact built-in computer that performs a wide range of sophisticated EKG recording functions. Ambulatory cardiac monitoring is done to correlate the activity of the patient with his or her heart activity and specifically for the following reasons:

1. To detect any cardiac rhythm disturbances and correlate them with patient symptoms of chest pain, palpitations, dizziness, syncope, or fatigue.
2. To assess the effectiveness of antiarrhythmic medication therapy.
3. To assess the function of a new or old pacemaker.

To record the activity of the heart, special electrodes are applied to the patient's chest. Lead wires are then attached to the electrodes. The lead wires are connected to a cable that is then connected to the portable monitor. The portable monitor, about the size of a small cassette recorder, is placed in a leather holder bag that is worn by the patient on a belt around the waist or over the shoulder. A diary is kept by the patient while the monitor is worn. The patient's activities, along with the time of day, are to be recorded in the diary. Special notation is to be made of any stressful or significant event or any chest pain, palpitations, dizziness, or syncope, along with the time of day and the activity in which the patient is involved. Most of the monitors available have what is referred to as an "event marker." This is a button which is to be pressed briefly at the time the patient experiences any unusual occurrence as just described. In addition, the patient is to record the event and the time of day in the diary. The monitors also have a clock that provides accurate time monitoring on the EKG recording. Explain the procedure to the patient and provide instructions for the care of the monitor.

At the end of the prescribed time period, the patient returns to the physician's office to have the electrodes removed and to turn in the monitor and diary. The monitor or tape (depending on the brand of equipment used) is then processed by a computer, and the EKG tracing, along with the interpretation, is generated. This report can then be matched and compared with the patient's diary. Times of recorded chest pain, palpitations, dizziness, syncope, or any other unusual occurrence are matched with the EKG to see if any abnormal heart rhythm was present at the same time (see also Common Rhythms discussed previously). Some equipment can store all of the data on a hard disk of a computer and also on diskettes. Other systems include an interface unit that provides immediate review of data via an LCD screen while it transfers the complete 24-hour record to a computer diskette for remote analysis.

PROCEDURE AND PATIENT CARE FOR MONITORING

There are a variety of monitors on the market. The manufacturer's directions must be followed explicitly, since the units are not interchangeable and they operate differently. The following procedure presents the general guidelines that you use to prepare the patient for ambulatory cardiac monitoring. Make sure that you read the manufacturer's operating instructions thoroughly before starting any form of operation. In that way you will be able to use your equipment efficiently for the patient's welfare.

Equipment

Five disposable electrodes (sensors)
Lead wires and cable
Monitor (recorder) with a new battery, leather holder bag, and belt for the patient's waist or shoulder harness
Alcohol sponges
Gauze
Razor and blade (if the patient's skin has to be shaved)
Skin rasp (a rough material somewhat like sandpaper)
Nonallergenic adhesive tape
Patient diary for the unit that you are using
Interface unit and printer

PROCEDURE AND PATIENT CARE FOR MONITORING—cont'd

PROCEDURE	RATIONALE

1. Wash your hands. **Use appropriate personal protective equipment (PPE) as dictated by facility.**

2. Assemble and prepare equipment. Review the operating instructions if necessary. Insert a fully charged, new battery into the monitor. Make sure the poles on the battery are positioned correctly.

Only a new fully charged alkaline battery guarantees a 24-hour monitoring period.

3. Identify the patient and explain the procedure. Give the patient the following instructions about caring for the monitor and assure him or her that he or she will not experience any electrical shock from the monitor.
   a. Maintain good contact of the electrodes with the skin.

The electrodes and monitor must be kept dry.

   b. *Do not* bathe or shower with the monitor on under any circumstances.
   c. Unplug the EKG connector when changing clothes. An acoustic signal indicates that the device is disconnected.
   d. *Do not* take the monitor out of the carrying case and *do not* handle the monitor.
   e. *Do not* touch or move the electrodes during the monitoring time. This will help to avoid any artifacts from being recorded.
   f. Maintain the diary properly. You must stress the need to record significant symptoms and events and to record the day's events in the diary (for example, when the patient is awake, takes meals, takes medication, is under stress, smokes, exercises, has a bowel movement).
   g. If any pain or discomfort is experienced, press the event marker button briefly and record the time and the type of pain or discomfort in the diary.
   h. Minimize the use of electrical devices such as shavers and electronic toothbrushes and do not use an electric blanket.

These may cause an interference with an EKG recording.

   i. Call the physician's office if the electrodes become loose or detached or if the recorder stops or malfunctions.

The electrical energy is coming from the patient and is being recorded by the monitor.

4. Have the patient remove clothes from the waist up. A patient gown may be put on with the opening in the front.

Provide for the comfort of the patient.

5. Have the patient lie down on the examining table.

6. Prepare the patient's skin for electrode placement.
   a. Shave the patient's chest if necessary in the areas where the electrodes will be placed.
   b. Thoroughly cleanse skin where the electrodes will be placed with an alcohol sponge.

Skin preparation is recommended to avoid EKG signals with artifacts.
Clean skin to remove any oil.

   c. Allow skin to dry thoroughly.
   d. Using the skin rasp (fine abrasive), with medium pressure rub the skin 3 or 4 times to remove the dead skin layer from the areas where the electrodes will be placed.

PROCEDURE AND PATIENT CARE FOR MONITORING—cont'd

PROCEDURE	RATIONALE
7. Remove the protective backing from the electrode and apply it to the chest position (Figure 16-15, *A* and *B*). The electrodes have an adhesive backing that secures the electrodes to the skin. There is gel in the center of the back of the electrode to provide good conduction of the electrical impulses from the heart monitor. Press on the electrode's adhesive ring first. Avoid pressing the center "gel cap." Repeat until all five electrodes are applied.	*Pressing the center "gel cap" might cause the gel to move out onto the adhesive ring and then it may not stay in place.*
8. Attach the lead wires to the electrodes.	
9. Place a strip of adhesive tape over the wire just below each electrode.	*The tape helps to avoid tension and pressure on the electrodes.*
10. Attach the EKG cable connector to the monitor.	
11. Follow the start-up procedure for the system that you are using by following the directions given in the Operator's Guide. Examine the EKG printout and assess it with the criteria given with the system that you are using. Visually judge the quality of the EKG. If you do not get satisfactory results, check the placement of each electrode.	*The Start Up Procedure for each system determines if the monitor is functioning correctly and recording an adequate EKG.*
12. Most systems will then automatically switch over to monitoring.	
13. Record the start time in the Patient Diary (Figure 16-16).	
14. Have the patient redress.	
15. Put the recorder in the holder bag and attach it to the patient's belt or to a shoulder harness (Figure 16-17). Make sure that the belt or harness is adjusted properly so that it does not pull or strain on the lead wires or cable connector.	*The holder bag supports and protects the monitor. Pulling or putting tension on the lead wires and electrodes must be avoided to ensure a reliable recording. The electrodes must not be detached from the skin.*

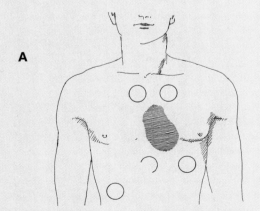
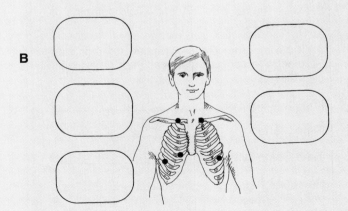

Figure 16-15 **A,** *Suggested electrode (sensor) placement for Holter Monitoring.* **B,** *Electrodes are applied to the patient's chest. Lead wires connect the electrodes to a cable connector attached to the monitor. Adhesive tape is placed over the lead wire just below the electrode.*
Courtesy The Burdick Corporation, Schaumburg, Ill.

PROCEDURE AND PATIENT CARE FOR MONITORING—cont'd

Burdick Custo-Kit

PATIENT DIARY

For Holter Electrocardiogram

Burdick

A Siemens Company
Milton, Wisconsin
800-777-1777

Reorder #097019

To The Patient:

Your physician needs to know more about your heart than he can learn from an EKG taken in his office. For this reason he has requested that you wear a **"Holter"** (named after Dr. Norman J. Holter) **Recorder** for a 24 hour period. This compact device records your heartbeat for 24 hours. When the test is complete the recorder will be returned for final printout and analysis by your physician.

This test is very valuable as it allows your physician to determine how your heart performs during the everyday situations you experience. This test is very common and the fact that your physician has ordered it **DOES NOT** mean that there is a problem with your heart. It is merely another useful tool in acquiring an accuate diagnosis. Try not to alter your daily routine because of this test. Your physician is trying to learn how **Your** heart responds to **Your** lifestyle.

What to Do During The Test

1. Keep an accurate diary. Indicate activities such as walking, running, sleeping, sexual activity, urinating, etc. Indicate symptoms such as pain (specify location), shortness of breath, dizziness, etc.

2. Do not tamper with the recorder.

3. Keep the recorder dry and avoid bumping or dropping it.

4. If the recorder stops or malfunctions or if an electrode comes loose, call your physician's office.

Impedance Value _____

Time Started _____

Time Completed _____

Recorder # _____
Medications:

TIME	ACTIVITY	SYMPTOMS

Figure 16-16 *CUSTO-MEGA ambulatory EKG patient diary.*
Courtesy Burdick, Inc., Schaumburg, Ill.

PROCEDURE AND PATIENT CARE FOR MONITORING—cont'd

PROCEDURE

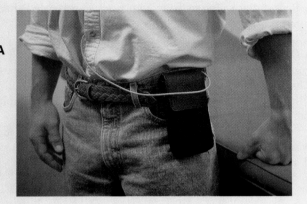

A

RATIONALE

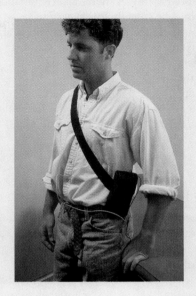

B

Figure 16-17 A *and* **B,** *The monitor is placed in a holder bag that is worn on a belt around the patient's waist or on a shoulder harness.*

16. Remind the patient of the special instructions that must be followed (review step 3 on page 540).

17. Answer any questions that the patient may have.

18. Give the diary to the patient and review the instructions for maintaining this record.

19. Inform the patient when to return to have the monitor removed. The patient is not to remove the monitor. It is to remain in place until the scheduled time for removal.

20. Wash your hands.

21. Record the procedure in the patient's chart.

Charting example:
> *Nov. 7, 19____, 1 p.m.*
> *Monitor applied.*
> *Monitoring commenced at 12:45 pm. Patient to return Nov. 8 at 1 p.m. to have the monitor removed. Special instructions for care of the monitor and dairy record provided.*
> *J.A. Lee, CMA*

TREADMILL STRESS TEST

The *treadmill stress test* is used for noninvasive cardiac evaluation to aid physicians in patient diagnosis and prognosis with EKGs taken under controlled exercise stress conditions. During this test of increased stress and work, abnormal electrocardiographic tracings (that do not appear during an EKG taken when the patient is resting) may appear.

The stress test helps the physician to determine an appropriate exercise program for the patient. It is also used to assess cardiac function after heart surgery, to diagnose heart disorders, and to diagnose the possible cause of chest pain. It is an evaluation to aid physicians in patient diagnosis and prognosis with electrocardiographic tracings (that do not appear during an EKG taken when the patient is resting).

The stress test helps the physician to determine an appropriate exercise program for the patient. It is also used to assess cardiac function following heart surgery, to diagnose heart disorders, and to diagnose the possible cause of chest pain.

The test is done in the presence of a physician, and the patient is constantly monitored. Systems used record and monitor the patient's EKG while it is being monitored by the physician (Figure 16-18).

PATIENT PREPARATION

The following information must be provided to the patient before the test is performed. An explanation of the test is given to help reduce any anxiety the patient may experience and to gain the patient's cooperation.

- Get adequate sleep the night before the test.
- Do not eat, smoke, or drink caffeinated beverages for 4 hours before the test. A light meal (without coffee, tea, or alcohol) may be eaten before that time.
- Wear comfortable clothing and flat walking shoes, preferably with rubber soles, for the test. To facilitate application of the EKG electrodes, wear a shirt that opens in the front.
- There should be no pain during or as a result of the stress test. If excessive fatigue, chest pain, or breathing difficulties occur during the test, the physician will have the test stopped.

Report any complaints experienced following the test to the physician.

PROCEDURE

- Electrodes are applied and a baseline EKG is recorded.
- Vital signs are taken.
- The patient is asked to walk on a treadmill or pedal a bicycle at prescribed rates.
- During the exercises, heart activity is monitored, and the blood pressure is taken at the end of each testing interval.
- At the end of the test, the patient is asked to rest while monitoring continues until the vital signs and the EKG return to normal.
- The electrodes are removed, and the skin cleansed of any electrolyte solution or gel used.

POST-TEST INSTRUCTIONS TO THE PATIENT

- Rest for several hours.
- Avoid extreme temperature changes.

- Avoid stimulants.
- Do not take a hot shower or bath for at least 2 hours.
- Discuss the results and your feelings with the physician. Report if any physical symptoms were experienced after the test.

On very rare occasions, complications, including an MI or a fatal cardiac arrhythmia, may occur. Appropriate emergency equipment must always be available in the test room. This equipment should include antiarrhythmia drugs, a defibrillator, an Ambu bag, an airway, and intubation equipment (an endotracheal tube and laryngoscope).

An assistant must stand near the patient during the test in case the patient becomes dizzy, faints, or falls. In these situations support must be provided immediately.

Figure 16-18 *The treadmill stress test.*

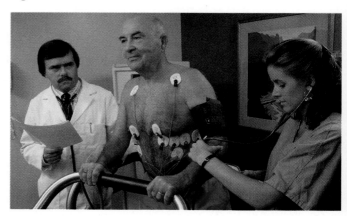

CONCLUSION

Having completed the unit on electrocardiography, you should have acquired a basic understanding of the technique for taking EKGs and the importance of this vital diagnostic procedure. After you have practiced the procedures and are ready to demonstrate your skills and knowledge attained, arrange with your instructor to take a performance test.

REVIEW OF VOCABULARY

The following are EKG reports received in the physician's office from a consulting cardiologist's office. These are presented to expose the medical assistant to ways in which the interpretation reports of the patient's EKG may be written. Normal and abnormal EKG findings are given.

PATIENT NO. 1:
EKG OF 12-12-93 showed frequent PVCs (premature ventricular contractions). Rhythmic strip showed numerous PVCs.

PATIENT NO. 2:
The patient's EKG showed normal sinus tachycardia of 145, with right axis; P pulmonale was noted inferior laterally; there were ST-T wave changes consistent with ischemia; no significant change since the reading on 9-30-87.
Gary Greaves, MD

PATIENT NO. 3:
INTERPRETATION:
   Rate: 75
   Rhythm: sinus
   P waves: normal
   P-R interval: normal
   Position: Intermediate heart
   QRS waves: deep SV_{1-5}
   T waves: normal
CONCLUSION: Intermediate heart within normal limits.
J. Dobbins, MD
PATIENT NO. 4:
INTERPRETATION:
   Rate: 60
   Rhythm: sinus
   P waves: normal
   P-R interval: 0.16
   Position: horizontal heart
   QRS waves: deep SV_{1-4}
   T waves: normal
CONCLUSION: Horizontal heart within normal limits.
Sally Eaton, MD
PATIENT NO. 5:
INTERPRETATION:
   Rate: 108
   Rhythm: sinus tachycardia
   P waves: normal
   P-R interval: 0.18
   Position: normal axis
   QRS waves: deep SV_{1-4}
   T waves: normal

CONCLUSION: Within normal limits except for mild sinus tachycardia.
Carol Overkamp, MD
PATIENT NO. 6:
INTERPRETATION:
   Rate: 52
   Rhythm: sinus bradycardia
   P waves: notched
   P-R interval: 0.16
   Position: left axis deviation
   QRS waves: Deep Q_1, aV_L, V_{5-6} with
   T waves: low T waves
CONCLUSION: Sinus bradycardia, left atrial enlargement, and left ventricular hypertrophy.
Erik Evans, MD
PATIENT NO. 7:
INTERPRETATION:
   Rate: 60
   Rhythm: sinus
   P waves: notched
   P-R interval: 0.18
   Position: horizontal heart
   QRS waves: slurred St_1, aV_L, V_{5-6} with
   T waves: low T waves
CONCLUSION: Horizontal heart with left atrial enlargement, left anterior hemiblock, and old anterolateral myocardial damage.
John Dunn, MD

CASE STUDY

The following case study illustrates cardiovascular disease in a patient being evaluated for *cataract extraction* and *lens implantation*. Read and discuss the italicized terminology.

HISTORY: The patient is a 91-year-old white female who is scheduled for outpatient left *cataract extraction and lens implantation*. She has *bilateral cataracts*, and her vision is so poor now that she is unable to play bingo or read.

PAST MEDICAL HISTORY: She was hospitalized from 1/23/xx to 1/29/xx with the following *diagnosis*:

1. *Coronary atherosclerotic heart disease, hypertensive heart disease, valvular heart disease* with *aortic stenosis, congestive heart failure* and *left bundle branch block* and resultant *cardiac arrest; defibrillation* was successful. Subsequent *electrocardiographic* studies revealed *myocardial infarction* with extensive damage of *myocardium* and continued *arrhythmia*.

2. History of *hypertension*.
3. Borderline elevated *TSH*.
4. *S/P* bilateral *mastectomies* for carcinoma.

ELECTROCARDIOGRAPHY WITH INTERPRETATION
Sinus rhythm, rate 80; *PR:24; QRS:.09*
There is left axis deviation. There are minimal nonspecific St-T wave changes. Q waves in the inferior leads compatible with, although not diagnostic of prior inferior wall MI. No change from previous study.

REVIEW QUESTIONS

1. Draw and label the waves, intervals, and segments of an EKG. Explain what each component signifies.
2. Explain what is happening in the heart during the process of depolarization and repolarization.
3. List eight abnormalities that may be detected on the EKG.
4. Mr. Perry Bloom is having an EKG done and wants to know if the record will pick up his heart sounds and what each of the little squares on the EKG paper mean. State and explain the answer that you give to this patient.
5. The physician expects you to monitor the recording of Mr. Bloom's EKG. List three items that you will look for.
6. During the recording of Max Sugar's EKG, he continually coughs and moves his hand to cover his mouth. What type of artifact would you expect to see on the record?
7. When recording Ms. Lillian Bell's EKG, the stylus continually wanders off the baseline. Describe the actions you would take to try to remedy this situation.
8. Explain to Ms. Maurine McArthur how and why the physician in your office can read her EKG taken on another machine by a different physician in another city.
9. Mrs. D. Bernstrom wants to know why you have to put that "gooey paste" on her body when you are applying the electrodes. State your reply to this patient.
10. Mrs. Sara Pace wants to know how you can tell if your EKG machine is working properly and what all those "funny little" waves on the EKG paper mean. What would you tell her?
11. State what the purposes for which the following items on the electrocardiograph are used:
    a. The STD button
    b. The position control knob
    c. The lead selector knob
    d. The recorder switch
12. In the process of recording Mr. Dan Orlando's EKG, you suddenly notice that there is no tracing on the paper. What could cause this, and how would you remedy the situation?
13. Mrs. Colette Kelly's EKG tracing is very light and hard to distinguish. What could cause this, and how would you remedy the situation?
14. Illustrate identification codes for each of the 12 leads on a standard EKG.
15. List eight instructions that you should give to a patient who will be wearing a monitor.

PERFORMANCE TEST

In a skills laboratory, the medical assistant student will demonstrate skills in performing the following activities without reference to resource materials. For these activities the student will need five different individuals to play the role of the patient. Time limits for the performance of these skills are to be assigned by the instructor (also see page 52).

1. Prepare the patient for an EKG.
2. Locate the six chest lead positions on at least five different individuals; then apply the electrodes and lead wires and record the EKGs of these individuals.
3. Mount the recordings obtained in No. 2.
4. Correctly care for the equipment after use.
5. Apply a monitor to a patient.
6. Give the patient instructions to follow when wearing a Monitor.

The student is expected to perform these activities with 100% accuracy.

Common Emergencies and First Aid

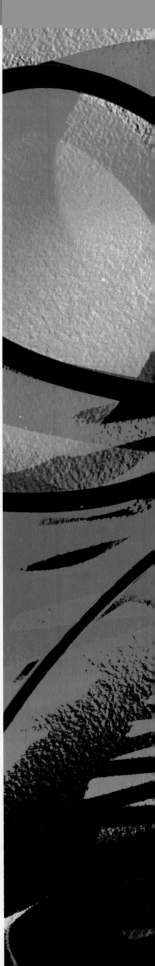

COGNITIVE OBJECTIVES

On completion of Unit Seventeen, the medical assistant student should be able to:

1. Define first aid and the related terminology presented in this unit.
2. State what factors constitute a medical emergency.
3. List four fundamental rules and general procedures to follow in a medical emergency.
4. Explain how to administer cardiopulmonary resuscitation (CPR).
5. Explain how to give first aid treatment for a victim who is choking.
6. List six common warning signals of a heart attack.
7. Discuss the 911 emergency telephone system.
8. State the purpose of a poison control center.
9. Define and list eight signs and symptoms of a cerebral vascular accident (CVA).
10. List five types of shock and the usual causes of each.
11. List at least 10 signs and symptoms of shock.
12. Differentiate between arterial, venous, and capillary bleeding.
13. List four methods used to control severe bleeding.
14. Explain what is meant by the pressure point method, and list the seven pressure points used to control severe bleeding.
15. Differentiate between a superficial burn (first-degree), a partial-thickness burn (second-degree), and a full-thickness burn (third-degree).
16. Explain what is meant by the rule of nines in reference to burns.
17. Differentiate between hypoglycemia (insulin reaction) and hyperglycemia (diabetic coma) by stating the signs, symptoms, and causes of each.
18. List common symptoms of undiagnosed diabetes.
19. Explain when you should and should not induce vomiting when the victim has ingested a poisonous substance.
20. State and describe the first aid treatment for all the emergency situations discussed in this unit.
21. List at least 15 items that should be included in a first aid kit.

TERMINAL PERFORMANCE OBJECTIVES

On completion of Unit Seventeen, the medical assistant student should be able to:

1. Demonstrate the proper first aid care to be used for all the medical emergencies presented in this unit.
2. Demonstrate the proper application of a tourniquet.
3. Locate the seven pressure points, and demonstrate how to use them to control severe bleeding.
4. Make appropriate decisions regarding care when given an example of an emergency.

The student is expected to perform these objectives with 100% accuracy.

The consistent use of universal precautions is required by all health care professionals in all health care settings as a method of infection control. It is assumed that these precautions are used in all of the following procedures. Review Unit One if you have any questions on methods to use as the methods/techniques will not be repeated in detail in each procedure presented in the unit.

Be sure to consult the latest guidelines issued by the Centers for Disease Control and Prevention and consult with infection control practitioners when needed to identify specific precautions that pertain to your particular work situation.

When someone is injured or suddenly becomes ill, there is a critical period—before medical help is obtained—that is of the utmost importance to the victim. What you do or don't do during that time can mean the difference between life and death. For serious conditions, the victim *must* receive medical attention because first aid is not meant to resolve serious problems.

First aid is the immediate and temporary care given the victim of an accident or sudden illness until the services of a physician can be obtained. It is the help that *you* can provide in emergencies until trained medical emergency personnel or a physician takes over. You owe it to yourself, the patients under the care of your physician-employer, your family, and the general public to know and understand the simple procedures that can be rendered quickly and intelligently in an emergency.

Antidote (an′ ti-dot)—An agent used to counteract a poison.

Biologic death—The condition that results when the brain has been deprived of oxygenated blood for a period of 6 minutes or more and irreversible damage has probably occurred.

Clinical death—The state that results when breathing and circulation have stopped.

Concussion (kon-kush′un)—The injury that results from a violent blow or shock.

Concussion of the brain—A short or prolonged altered state of consciousness caused by a blow or fall. May be followed by dizziness, nausea, weak pulse, and transient amnesia.

Contusion (kon-too′zhun)—A bruise, indicating injury to tissues without breakage in the skin. Discoloration appears because of blood seepage under the surface of the skin.

Epinephrine (ep″i-nef′rin)—A hormone produced by the adrenal glands. Epinephrine can be administered parenterally, topically, or by inhalation. It is used as an emergency heart stimulant, to relieve symptoms in allergic conditions, and to counteract the lethal effects of anaphylactic shock.

Tourniquet (toor′ni-ket)—A constricting device used to compress an artery or vein to stop excessive bleeding.

Additional terms are defined under their respective topics in this unit.

First aid is more than a dressing or a cold compress. The victim suddenly has new problems and needs. Both the emotional and physical needs of the victim must be cared for. Your contributions include offering well-chosen words of encouragement, a willingness to help, the uplifting effect of your evident capabilities and calmness, and the performance of temporary physical care to alleviate pain or a life-threatening situation.

It may be your responsibility to deal with an emergency before the physician or other emergency teams arrive. If you are familiar with the procedures for emergency care and can exercise good judgment, remain calm, and avoid panicking others, you can administer care in an orderly manner and thereby render great service to the patient and the physician. Whether you are in the physician's office, at home, or on the street, *you must take prompt action.*

Each year more than 1 million Americans die from sudden death. In many cases of sudden death, especially death from heart attacks, the victim could have been saved if the early warning signs of heart attack were known, if someone close to the victim could have performed cardiopulmonary resuscitation (CPR), or if the victim had been transported quickly to a hospital or received first aid or medical attention at the scene of sudden illness or injury. *Time* is of the essence in any medical emergency in which breathing and heartbeat have ceased. Within 4 to 6 minutes after the heart stops, brain damage begins. Thus the importance of your knowledge and quick actions in a medical emergency cannot be overemphasized. **Know what constitutes an emergency, whom to call for help, and what to do.** An emergency exists when life is threatened, when situations develop that endanger a person's physical and/or psychologic well-being, or when pain and suffering occur.

When an emergency occurs in the physician's office, notify the physician. If the physician is not in the office and is not expected momentarily, call for a nearby physician; if none can be reached for immediate help, call the local emergency medical services (EMS) system, an ambulance, the fire and rescue squad, or the police department. You are *not* to assume the responsibility for making a diagnosis and providing medical treatment, but you *are* expected to make a reasonable judgment (that may require medical knowledge) of the situation and to provide immediate first aid care.

You should perform *only* those procedures that you have been trained to do and, when in the office or health care agency, only with the prior consent of the physician. An office policy should be established between you and the physician as to what should be done in the case of office emergencies and in the case of emergency telephone calls received from patients.

The fundamental rules and general procedures to follow in an emergency are few, but very important.

1. Remain calm, reassure the patient, be empathetic, and do not panic. Act in an orderly, organized manner. Have a reason for what you do; avoid injury to yourself; know the limits of your capabilities; and avoid further injury to the patient.

2. Survey the situation to determine the nature of the emergency. A primary survey includes the ABCs for all emergencies (that is, check the patient for an open airway, for breathing, and for circulation). A secondary survey is done to examine the total body to determine what is wrong.

3. Take immediate steps to remedy the situation. Your responsibilities for the type of care to provide will vary in each situation and depend on the proximity of medical help, the seriousness of the injury or illness, and the immediate environment.

4. Seek medical help if needed and be able to describe the nature of the patient's condition. Think of yourself as a reporter who must obtain concise and relevant information and report it. Seek answers to questions that begin with who, what, when, where, why, and how.

This unit provides important information in concise and convenient form on common emergencies and the first aid treatment to be administered. CPR, care for choking victims, and care for patients in shock are presented first. Other common emergencies are then discussed in alphabetic order. Read and study the contents of this unit carefully, and keep this or other first aid references in a convenient place where they will be on hand for quick reference when needed.

   The purpose of this unit is to provide a review and reference source for first aid treatment to use for common emergencies. It is not intended to be used as a substitute for a certified first aid program of study. It is highly recommended that medical assistants take a certified First Aid and CPR course. Courses are offered by the American Red Cross and at many community colleges. Cardiopulmonary resuscitation courses for basic life support are also provided by the American Heart Association in numerous communities. All medical assistants should then take a refresher course in first aid every few years and in CPR every year.

CARDIOPULMONARY RESUSCITATION FOR CARDIAC ARREST

Cardiopulmonary resuscitation, commonly known as CPR, is a combination of artificial respiration and artificial circulation. CPR should be started immediately by individuals **properly trained** to do so in emergency situations in which cardiac arrest occurs. The performance of CPR is *not recommended unless one has had proper training and practice in the procedure* because serious adverse consequences may result because of faulty technique. Therefore the following information is to serve as a review and reference source *after* you have completed a training course and before you take your next refresher course.

   The goal of CPR is life support. When trained in CPR techniques, you must start life support techniques as quickly as possible and continue them until one of the following has occurred:

1. An effective respiration and pulse are restored to the victim
2. You are completely exhausted and cannot continue CPR
3. Care of the victim is turned over to medical or other properly trained personnel
4. The victim is pronounced dead

Basic and Advanced Life Support

Life support is divided into two systems: basic and advanced life support. Basic life support can be carried out by trained lay and medical persons and includes the following:

Basic ABC Steps

A—Airway opened
B—Breathing restored
C—Circulation restored

Supplementary Techniques

- Positioning—Position the victim properly (for example, in the supine position).

- Jaw thrust maneuver—May be required when the head-tilt alone is unsuccessful for opening the airway. This technique *without* the head-tilt is called the modified jaw thrust maneuver and is the safest to use on a victim who possibly has a neck injury.
- Opening the mouth—At times it may be necessary to force the mouth open for ventilation or to remove foreign bodies or to allow drainage of vomitus or blood.
- Mouth-to-stoma resuscitation—When the victim has had a laryngectomy, he or she breathes through a stoma in the neck; in this case, mouth-to-stoma resuscitation must be performed.
- Adjunctive equipment—To be used only by those trained in its use.

   Advanced life support is to be performed *only* by trained medical personnel and includes the following (Figure 17-1):
- Definitive therapy
   - Diagnosis
   - Drugs
   - Defibrillation
- Cardiac monitoring and stabilization
- Transportation
- Communication

PROCEDURE FOR CARDIOPULMONARY RESUSCITATION

Basic CPR is a simple procedure, as simple as A-B-C: Airway, Breathing, and Circulation. *The following brief review is based on the 1992 standards for CPR. It is to be used only for review purposes. It is not to be used for learning the procedure for performing CPR.*

Airway

If a person has collapsed, determine if he or she is conscious by shaking the shoulder and shouting "Are you all right?" If no response, shout for help. Then open the airway. If the victim is not lying flat on the back, roll him or her over, moving the entire body at one time as a total unit.

Figure 17-1 *Advanced life support being administered to a patient by medical personnel in hospital emergency room.*

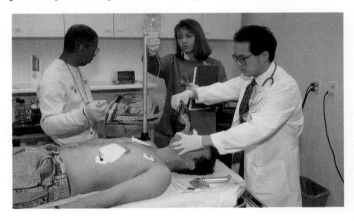

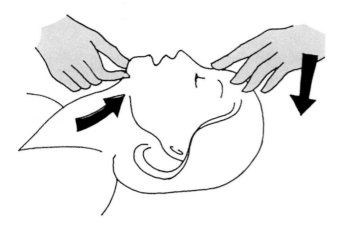

To open the victim's airway, use the head-tilt/chin-lift maneuver. Lift up the chin gently with one hand while pushing down on the forehead with the other to tilt head back. Once the airway is open, place your ear close to the victim's mouth:

- Look—at the chest and abdomen for movement.
- Listen—for sounds of breathing.
- Feel—for breath on your cheek.

If none of these signs is present, the victim is not breathing.

If opening the airway does not cause the victim to begin to breathe spontaneously, you must provide rescue breathing.

Breathing

The best way to provide rescue breathing is by using the mouth-to-mouth technique. Take your hand that is on the victim's forehead and turn it so that you can pinch the victim's nose shut while keeping the heel of the hand in place to maintain head tilt. Your index and middle fingers of your other hand should remain under the victim's chin, lifting up.

Immediately give two full breaths (1.5 to 2 seconds per breath) using the mouth-to-mouth method while maintaining an air-tight seal with your mouth on the victim's mouth. Watch the victim's chest to see that your breath goes in.

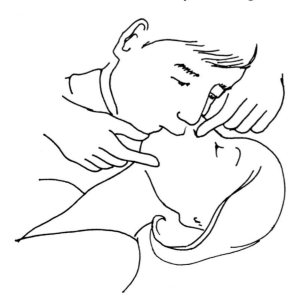

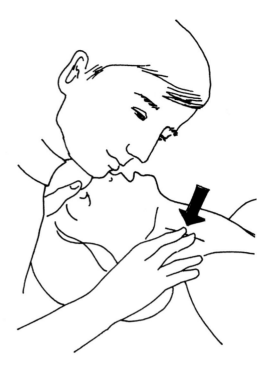

Check Pulse

After giving the two breaths, locate the victim's carotid pulse to see if the heart is beating. To find the carotid artery, take the hand that you are using on the victim's chin and locate the voice box. Slide the tips of your index and middle fingers into the groove beside the voice box. Feel for the carotid pulse. Cardiac arrest can be recognized by absent breathing and an absent pulse in the carotid artery in the neck.

If you cannot find the pulse, you must provide artificial circulation in addition to rescue breathing.

Activate the EMS system. Send someone to call 911 or your local emergency number if this has not already been done. If you are alone and if possible, call the EMS before beginning CPR. If someone is with you, have that person call the EMS system while you begin CPR.

Cardiac Compression

Artificial circulation is provided by external cardiac compression. In effect, when you apply rhythmic pressure on the lower half of the victim's breastbone, you are forcing the heart to pump blood. To perform external cardiac compression properly, kneel at the victim's side near the chest at the level of the victim's shoulders. Locate the notch at the lowest portion of the sternum with the hand that was on the victim's chin. Put your middle finger on this notch and your index finger next to it. Place the heel of the hand that was on the victim's forehead on the lower half of the sternum, close to the index finger of your other hand. Place your other hand on top and parallel to the one that is in position. Be sure to keep your fingers off the chest wall. You may find it easier to do this if you interlock your fingers.

Bring your shoulders directly over the victim's sternum as you compress downward, keeping your arms straight. Depress the sternum about $1^1/2$ to 2 inches for an adult vic-

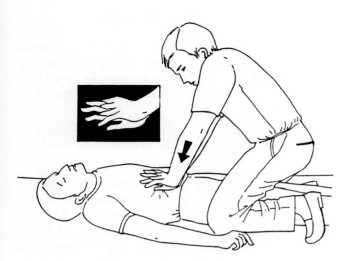

tim. Then relax pressure on the sternum completely. However, *do not* remove your hands from the victim's sternum, but *do* allow the chest to return to its normal position between compressions. Relaxation and compression should be of equal duration.

If you are the only rescuer, you must provide both rescue breathing and cardiac compression. The proper ratio is 15 chest compressions to 2 full, slow breaths. You must compress at the rate of 80 to 100 times per minute when you are working alone since you will stop compressions when you take time to breathe.

When there are two rescuers, position yourselves on opposite sides of the victim, if possible. One of you should be responsible for interposing a breath (1.5 to 2 seconds) after each fifth compression, maintaining an open airway and monitoring the carotid pulse for adequate chest compressions. The other rescuer, who compresses the chest, should use a rate of 80 to 100 compressions per minute.

Continue CPR until advanced life support is available.

CPR FOR INFANTS AND SMALL CHILDREN

Basic life support for infants and small children is similar to that for adults. A few important differences to remember are given below.

Airway

When handling an infant, be careful that you do not exaggerate the backward position of the head tilt. An infant's neck is so pliable that forceful backward tilting might *block* breathing passage instead of opening them.

Breathing

Don't try to pinch off the nose. Cover both the mouth and nose of an infant or *small* child who is not breathing with your mouth. Use small breaths with less volume to inflate the lungs. Give one small breath every 3 seconds for an infant (0 to 1 year) and one small breath every 4 seconds for a child (1 to 8 years). (For a child, a mouth-to-mouth seal should be made with the nose pinched tightly, as is done for adults.)

Check Pulse

The absence of a pulse may be more easily determined by feeling for the brachial pulse for infants (0 to 1 years). Find this pulse by feeling on the inside of the upper arm midway between the elbow and the shoulder. (Locate the carotid pulse for children 1 to 8 years, as you would for an adult.)

Circulation

The technique for cardiac compression is different for infants and small children. Only two fingers are used on an infant, and one hand is used for compression on a child. The other hand may be slipped under the infant to provide a firm support for the back; *or*, for both infant and child, the other hand is used to maintain the head position to maintain an open airway.

For infants, use only the *tips* of two or three fingers to compress the chest. Place the index finger of the hand nearest the infant's legs just under an imaginary line between the nipples where it intersects with the sternum. Compress the chest one fingerbreadth below this intersection, at the location of the middle and ring fingers. Depress the sternum between 1/2 to 1 inch at a fast rate of 100 times a minute. Make sure not to depress the tip of the sternum.

For children 1 to 8 years, use only the *heel* of one hand to compress the chest. Depress the sternum between 1 and 1 1/2 inches, depending on the size of the child. Use the same hand position as for adults. The rate should be 80 to 100 times per minute.

In the case of both infants and small children, breaths should be administered during the relaxation after every fifth chest compression.

CPR for children over 8 years old is the same as for adults.

NECK INJURY

If you suspect the victim has suffered a neck injury, you must not open the airway in the usual manner. If the victim is injured in a diving or automobile accident, you should consider the possibility of such a neck injury. In these cases, the

Rescuers	Ratio of Compressions to Breaths	Rate of Compressions
1	15:2	80 to 100 times/min
2	5:1	80 to 100 times/min

	Part of Hand	Depress Sternum	Rate of Compression
Infants	Tips of 2 fingers	1/2 to 1 inch	At least 100 per minute
Children	Heel of hand	1 to 1 1/2 inches	80 to 100 per minute

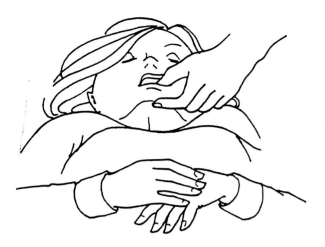

airway should be opened by using a modified jaw thrust, keeping the victim's head in a fixed, neutral position. If the airway remains obstructed, tilt the head slowly and gently until the airway is open.

CHOKING

The urgency of choking cannot be overemphasized. Immediate recognition and proper action are essential. If the victim has good air exchange, or only partial obstruction, and is still able to speak or cough effectively, *do not interfere with his or her attempts to expel a foreign body.* The distress signal for choking is the gesture of clutching the neck between the thumb and index finger. *Prompt action is urgent in every case of choking.*

When you recognize complete airway obstruction by observing the conscious victim's inability to speak, breathe, or cough, the following sequence should be performed quickly on the victim in the sitting, standing, or lying position:

1. Manual thrusts (abdominal or chest) until effective, or the person becomes unconscious.

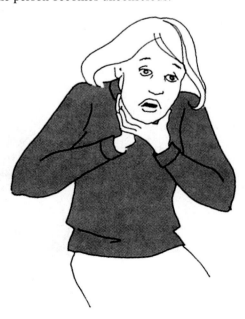

2. Finger sweep if the victim is unconscious.
3. If the victim becomes unconscious, shout for help. Place the victim on the back, face up. Open the airway and attempt to ventilate. If unsuccessful, deliver up to 5 manual thrusts, probe the mouth with the finger, and attempt to ventilate. It may be necessary to repeat these steps. *Be persistent* (Figure 17-2).

MANAGEMENT OF THE OBSTRUCTED AIRWAY
Abdominal Thrusts
Abdominal thrusts for the conscious victim

Abdominal thrusts (subdiaphragmatic abdominal thrusts or abdominal thrusts) is the technique recommended for relieving foreign-body airway obstruction. It may be necessary to repeat the thrust up to 5 times to clear the victim's airway. Never have your hands on the victim's xiphoid process of the sternum or on the lower margins of the victim's rib cage when performing this maneuver (Figure 17-3).

Manual thrusts are a rapid series of thrusts to the upper abdomen or chest that force air from the lungs.

Abdominal thrusts with victim sitting or standing

1. Stand behind the victim; wrap your arms around the waist.
2. Place the thumb side of your fist against the victim's abdomen in the midline slightly below the rib cage well below the tip of the xiphoid process and slightly above the umbilicus.
3. Grasp your fist with your other hand and press it into the victim's abdomen with a *quick upward thrust.*
4. Repeat if necessary.

Figure 17-2 *Lifesaving steps, including abdominal thrusts, for when an infant, child, or adult is choking.*
Courtesy The American National Red Cross.

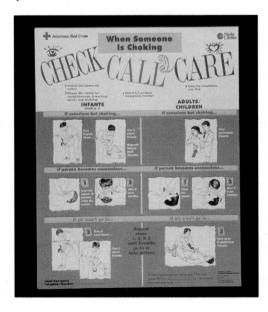

Figure 17-3 *Lifesaving steps, including CPR for the infant, child, and adult.*
Courtesy The American National Red Cross.

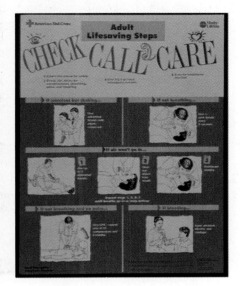

Abdominal thrusts with victim in a lying position

1. Place the victim in a supine position; kneel astride the victim's hips/thighs.
2. Place the heel of your hand in the middle of the abdomen slightly below the rib cage well below the tip of the xiphoid process and slightly above the umbilicus. Place your other hand on top of your bottom hand.
3. Rock forward, having your shoulders directly over the victim's abdomen and press into the abdomen and toward the diaphragm with a *quick upward thrust. Do not* press to either side.

Chest Thrusts

Chest thrusts are to be used *only* when the victim is markedly obese or in the later stages of pregnancy. The downward thrusts will generate effective airway pressures.

Chest thrust with the conscious victim standing or sitting

1. Standing behind the victim, place your arms under the victim's armpits, and encircle the victim's chest.
2. Place the thumb side of your fist on the victim's sternum (breastbone), but not on the xiphoid process.
3. Grasp this fist with your other hand, and press on the victim's sternum with a quick backward thrust.

Chest thrust with the victim in a lying position

1. Place your hands in the same position used for closed chest compression.
2. Exert quick downward thrusts.

Infants and Children

For infants up to 1 year of age, the combination of back blows and 5 chest thrusts continues to be recommended.

Back blows are a rapid series of sharp whacks that are delivered with the heel of the hand over the spine and between the shoulder blades. The blows should be applied quickly, forcefully, and in rapid succession. For a child 1 to 8 years of age, abdominal thrusts are recommended.

Other Causes of Airway Obstruction

An adequate open airway must be maintained at all times in all unconscious patients.

Other conditions that may cause unconsciousness and airway obstruction include stroke, epilepsy, head injury, alcoholic intoxication, drug overdose, diabetes, swelling from infection or trauma, and coma.

Remember:

1. Is the victim unconscious?
2. If so, shout for help, open the airway, and check for breathing.
3. If not breathing, give two breaths.
4. Check carotid pulse.
5. Activate the EMS system: Send someone to call 911 or your local emergency number.
6. If no pulse, begin external cardiac compression by depressing the lower half of the sternum $1^1/_2$ to 2 inches (for adults).
7. Continue uninterrupted CPR until advanced life support is available.

CPR for one rescuer:
  15:2 compressions to breaths at a rate of 80 to 100 compressions a minute (four cycles per minute)
CPR for two rescuers:
  5:1 compressions to breaths at a rate of 80 to 100 compressions a minute

Periodic practice in CPR is essential to ensure a satisfactory level of proficiency. A life may depend on how well you have remembered the proper steps of CPR and how to apply them. You should be sure to have both your skill and knowledge of CPR tested at least once a year. It could mean someone's life.

EMERGENCY MEDICAL SERVICES SYSTEM

Any victim on whom you begin resuscitation must be considered to need advanced life support. He or she will have the best chance of surviving if your community has a total EMS system. This includes an efficient communications alert system, such as 911, with public awareness of how or where to call; well-trained rescue personnel who can respond rapidly; vehicles that are properly equipped; an emergency facility that is open 24 hours a day to provide advanced life support; and an intensive care section in the hospital for the victims. You should work with all interested agencies to achieve such a system.

911: EMERGENCY TELEPHONE SYSTEM

Many communities participate in the nationwide 911 emergency telephone system. To find out if it is in effect in your community, call information in your area.

The 911 telephone system *must be used only in emergency situations when you need help quickly.* Dial 911 only when you or someone nearby needs emergency medical help or an ambulance, when you see a fire or a crime in progress, or when you suspect that a stranger may be in your home or you see him or her trying to enter or leave. Since 911 is a local service in each area, it is not necessary to dial any special access codes before the number. You only need to use three telephone digits—911. You can dial 911 from any type of telephone, including coin-operated public telephones, without any charge (you don't have to put coins into a coin-operated telephone to dial 911). If you are calling for help for someone who does not live in your area, you should call the "O" operator instead of 911. This is because 911 is a *local* service and cannot be used to obtain help outside of your immediate area.

When you dial 911, you reach a specially trained emergency operator. This operator will ask you a few important questions so that the type of help you need will be obtained without delay. Information that you will be asked includes the following:

- What is the emergency?
- Where is the emergency? (Include cross-reference streets when applicable.)
- What is your name and address?

Even if you can't talk, stay on the line. In many communities, the special nature of the 911 system allows the emergency operator to know exactly where you are so that help can come quickly. The emergency operator immediately assesses the problem and by pressing a button, notifies the appropriate public emergency agency. The operator stays on the line to be sure that your problem is handled properly to get the fastest emergency service and to see if other emergency services are necessary. The emergency operator also serves to keep the caller calm while waiting for help to arrive. Callers who are disconnected after dialing 911 can be called right back and, in even greater emergencies, the operator can trace the location of the phone.

Remember to stay calm and don't hang up. The emergency operator should hang up before you do. Often people panic in an emergency situation. They may give the operator information in a hurried fashion and hang up to go back to the emergency scene before the operator has obtained adequate and correct information. When this happens, the proper help may not be able to reach you in an adequate time to meet the needs of the situation. In some communities your line can be left open until the proper type of emergency help arrives. This would allow special instructions to be given for the emergency while you wait for help to arrive and if necessary, to determine your address if you are unable to give it.

Remember, 911 must be used only to report "real" emergencies. It must not be used for every call that you may have to make to the police department, the fire department, or an ambulance service (Figure 17-4).

Figure 17-4 *How to get medical help fast.*
Courtesy The American National Red Cross.

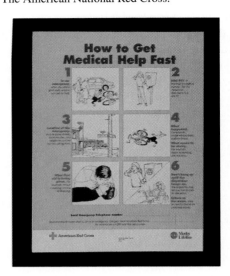

HEART ATTACK: SIGNALS AND ACTIONS FOR SURVIVAL*

There are many causes of sudden death: poisoning, drowning, suffocation, choking, electrocution, and smoke inhalation. But the most common cause is heart attack. Everyone should know the usual early signals of heart attack and have an emergency plan of action. Early treatment often means the difference between life and death.

The most *common signal* of a heart attack is:

- Uncomfortable pressure, squeezing, fullness or pain in the center of the chest behind the breastbone, which may spread to the shoulder, neck, jaw, or arms (the pain may not be severe)

Other signals may be

- Sweating
- Nausea, and maybe vomiting
- Shortness of breath *or*
- A feeling of weakness
- Apprehension

Sometimes these signals subside and return.

Actions

1. Recognize the "signals."
2. Stop activity and sit or lie down.
3. *Act at once if pain lasts for 2 minutes or more*—call the local emergency rescue service, usually 911, or go to the nearest hospital emergency room with 24-hour service.

SHOCK

Shock, a state of collapse or a depressed condition of the circulatory system, occurs when the vital organs of the body are deprived of circulating blood flow necessary to sustain their normal cellular activity. It is a physiologic reaction of the

*Reprinted by permission of the American Heart Association.

body to severe injury or insult. Circulatory collapse may occur following hemorrhage, severe trauma, dehydration, massive infection, severe burns, surgery, increased peripheral resistance, decreased cardiac output, drug toxicity, pain, fear, or emotional distress.

Shock may be immediate or delayed, slight or severe, even fatal. Every injury is accompanied by some degree of shock and should be treated promptly.

TYPES OF SHOCK

Shock may be divided into five basic types. The exact cause of shock is not always the same for every patient.

Traumatic Shock

Traumatic shock is the direct result of extracellular fluid loss (for example, with extensive contusions or the loss of plasma from large burned areas).

Hemorrhagic or Hypovolemic Shock

Hemorrhagic or hypovolemic shock is produced by a decrease in the circulating blood volume. The blood loss may be external or internal (into a body cavity where it is no longer accessible to the circulatory system).

Cardiogenic Shock

Cardiogenic shock is the result of conditions that interfere with the heart's function as a pump. This may be a result of cardiac failure, secondary to myocardial infarction, coronary thrombosis, or certain disorders of the rate and rhythm of the heart.

Septic Shock

Septic shock results from bacterial infection. It may occur when there is massive infection of traumatized tissue or when toxic tissue products are absorbed. Gram-negative shock is a form of septic shock caused by infection with the gram-negative bacteria (see Unit Six).

Neurogenic Shock

Neurogenic shock is the result of loss of peripheral vascular tone with subsequent dilation of the blood vessels, decreased heart rate, and a drop in the blood pressure to the point at which the supply of oxygen carried to the brain by the blood is insufficient. The patient then faints; thus this type of shock is frequently called fainting (syncope).

Anaphylactic Shock

Another type of shock is called *allergic* or *anaphylactic shock*. See "Allergic Reaction" on page 556.

SIGNS AND SYMPTOMS OF SHOCK

Five "Ps" denote the outstanding signs and symptoms of shock.

1. Prostration (extreme exhaustion; lack of energy)
2. Pallor (paleness)
3. Perspiration
4. Weak, rapid, and irregular pulse
5. Pulmonary deficiency

These vary in intensity, depending on the patient's condition and the injury or cause.

The most outstanding signs and symptoms of severe shock or the later stages of shock include the following:

1. The pulse is weak, rapid, and irregular.
2. Respirations increase in rate and are shallow.
3. Blood pressure is lowered—less than 90 mm Hg systolic.
4. The skin is markedly pale and may feel cold to the touch and moist with perspiration.
5. The lips, nailbeds, tips of the fingers, and lobes of the ears may be bluish (cyanosis).
6. The face may appear pinched and without expression.
7. The eyes may stare and often lose their characteristic luster.
8. The pupils may be dilated, especially in the late stages.
9. Occasionally the patient may be unusually anxious, restless, or excited.
10. When conscious, the patient appears disinterested in the surroundings and complains little of pain, although he or she may be groaning.
11. Later the patient may become apathetic and unresponsive. Eyes are sunken with a vacant expression.
12. If untreated, the patient eventually loses consciousness, vital signs drop, and death may occur.

FIRST AID CARE

In any emergency situation, routinely evaluate the situation for the possibility of shock and take measures to prevent it. The following objectives for preventing or treating shock should be met:

1. Improve circulation of blood; control bleeding when necessary.
2. Ensure an open airway and an adequate supply of oxygen.
3. Maintain normal body temperature, and keep the patient at rest.
4. Obtain medical assistance as and when required.

When treating a patient in shock:

1. Do a quick primary survey of the situation. Ensure the ABCs of all emergencies; that is, maintain an open airway, and check for breathing and circulation. Be prepared to give CPR if necessary.
2. Control severe bleeding if present.
3. Position the patient in a supine (lying) position with the lower extremities elevated 8 to 12 inches, *except* when there is a head injury, if breathing difficulty is thereby increased, if the patient complains of pain when this is attempted, or if the patient is vomiting. Keep a patient with a head injury lying flat, or prop the head and shoulders up slightly.
4. Keep the patient warm, but do not overheat.
5. Loosen tight clothing.
6. Do not move the patient unnecessarily.
7. Avoid disturbing the patient with noise and questions.
8. Do not give anything by mouth. When the patient has very dry lips and/or mouth, soak 4 × 4 gauze squares in water. Have the patient suck on them. This helps to relieve some of the dryness.

9. When necessary, administer oxygen, but only with the consent and directions of the physician.
10. Provide constant, kindly, tactful encouragement and extreme gentleness when caring for the patient.
11. Call the physician or hospital promptly when the patient is going into or is in the state of shock.
12. Arrange for ambulance transport as indicated. Do not attempt to move the patient alone without explicit instructions from the physician unless the immediate surroundings would cause further harm to the patient.

ABDOMINAL PAIN

All abdominal pain should be investigated, especially unusual pain that occurs rather suddenly and is accompanied by fever. Treatment varies with the cause of pain. For pain caused by trauma, keep the patient lying flat if possible, in case of internal bleeding. For pain caused from metabolic or pathologic causes, keep the patient in a comfortable position until medical help arrives or the patient is transported to the hospital. The patient may flex the knees if moving the legs doesn't cause pain. Flexing the knees allows the abdominal muscles to relax. For any abdominal pain:

- Keep the patient quiet and warm. Keep activity to a minimum.
- Do not apply heat.
- Do not give food, liquids, or laxatives.
- Place an emesis basin nearby in case the patient vomits.
- Check the patient frequently.
- Be empathetic.

Pathologic processes causing acute abdominal emergencies are inflammation, hemorrhage, perforation, obstruction, and ischemia (lack of adequate blood supply). These medical emergencies require immediate care by a physician because most often they require surgical intervention, although some may be treated medically.

ALLERGIC REACTION (ANAPHYLACTIC REACTION) DRUGS

Usually in an anaphylactic reaction or in any type of drug overdose reaction, the airway, breathing, and circulation will become impaired because of the effects of drugs on the central nervous system. Thus a primary survey (the ABCs) must be done.

A = *Airway*
Ensure that the airway is open.
B = *Breathing*
After you ensure that the airway is open, make sure that the breathing is spontaneous; in other words, make sure that the patient is breathing on his or her own.
C = *Circulation*
Check for a pulse beat. The best place to check the pulse rate is at the carotid artery.

When any of these areas requires stabilization, do nothing else except stabilize the ABCs and call or send for medical help. A secondary survey should also be made to ensure that the patient has no additional injury. This is a quick head-to-toe check to observe for any obvious bleeding or injury that may require immediate attention. It is necessary to stay with the patient until medical help arrives to ensure the ABCs. Oxygen and epinephrine should be available for administration on the physician's order. Usually 4 to 8 L of oxygen is administered by mask or nasal cannula, and 0.1 to 0.5 mg epinephrine 1:1000 IU is administered subcutaneously.

Constantly monitor the level of consciousness and vital signs, and maintain an adequate airway and ventilation.

Positioning the patient is also very important. Frequently when a patient goes into anaphylaxis, a lying position cannot be tolerated. Usually the patient must be in a sitting or a semi-Fowler position to expand the lungs and breathe more easily. Monitor the vital signs carefully, approximately every 2 or 3 minutes, note the skin color, and again monitor the airway. An oropharyngeal airway may be used at times to allow more air to get into the air passageways. When there is not a reversal within a reasonable time, rapid transport to the hospital is necessary.

You should encourage patients with known allergies to wear a MedicAlert bracelet or necklace.

ASPHYXIA

Asphyxia may occur whenever there is an interference with the normal exchange of oxygen and carbon dioxide between the lungs and outside air. A common cause is obstruction of the airway caused by foreign bodies, by the tongue, or by edema of the tissues, as seen in burns or inflammatory processes of the air passages. Drowning, electric shock, inhalation of smoke and poisonous gases, trauma to or disease of the lungs, bronchi, and trachea, or allergic reactions can all cause asphyxia. Basically the patient is apneic (not breathing). Immediate treatment is essential. Follow the ABCs—check for an open airway, breathing, and circulation. Open the airway if necessary, and give artificial ventilation. Remove the underlying cause whenever possible. When there is absence of both breathing and heartbeat, give CPR immediately. Have oxygen available; it may be given when the patient is having difficulty breathing, and also is frequently administered after breathing resumes to treat the resultant hypoxia. Send for medical help or call the physician.

HUMAN, ANIMAL, SNAKE, AND INSECT BITES AND STINGS

BITES

Injuries caused from animal or human bites may cause punctures, lacerations, or even avulsions, as the person attempts to pull away from the animal or human (see Unit Six for types of wounds). Human bites have a high potential for infection because of the high bacterial count in the human mouth. The danger of animal bites is rabies. Bites on the face, neck, or head are considered most serious and require immediate medical attention.

HUMAN AND ANIMAL BITES

The first aid care for human and animal bites is a thorough washing with soap and water for 5 minutes and copious rinsing under running water. An antibiotic ointment may be applied to the wound and then covered with a sterile or clean dressing. Keep the patient quiet, and avoid movement of the affected part until attended by the physician. Report animal bites to the police or health department, because the animal should be kept for observation for rabies. Collect information from the patient for the possibility of rabies. If the animal is not found and it is believed that the animal was rabid, treatment for rabies will be administered. Also treatment against tetanus will be given.

COMMON INSECT BITES

Bites from ants, mosquitoes, and chiggers can be cared for by washing the affected parts with soap and water, applying a paste made from baking soda and a little water, or applying calamine lotion. Cover the site to keep it clean. When swelling is present, cover the area with a cloth saturated with ice water or a cold pack.

TICK BITES

Don't try to tear an embedded tick lose. Cover it with heavy oil (mineral or salad) or petroleum jelly to close the tick's breathing pores. Frequently this will disengage the tick at once; if not, allow the oil or jelly to remain in place for 30 minutes. If the tick does not disengage after this time, remove it with tweezers (close to the head of the tick), working slowly and gently, and in a counterclockwise direction, so that all parts are removed. Wash the area with soap and water for 5 minutes. Apply an antibiotic ointment if one is available. Do not touch the tick with your hands, because ticks can transmit several diseases. If the skin area becomes inflamed and swollen, if the patient develops a fever or flulike symptoms, or if you suspect Lyme disease, the physician *must* be notified.

SEVERE REACTIONS TO BITES FROM SPIDER, JELLYFISH, OR INSECT OR MARINE ANIMAL OF UNKNOWN ORIGIN

Maintain an open airway; give CPR, and treat for shock when necessary.

For jellyfish and other marine life, rub the affected area with sand and soak it in salt water. Apply a baking soda paste if available.

Keep the affected part immobile and below the individual's heart level. The victim should lie quietly and be covered with a blanket to maintain warmth. Wash the wound and apply ice wrapped in a towel or plastic bag or cold compresses to prevent spread of the poison and to prevent and reduce swelling. Summon the physician, or have the victim taken to a hospital emergency room at once.

Antivenins can be given by professionals for black widow spider bites and for a scorpion sting.

SNAKE BITES

There has been much controversy in the past few years regarding the care of a victim of a snake bit. The current recommended care follows.

- Wash the wound with soap and water, blot dry, and apply a dressing (preferably sterile) and bandage.
- Immobilize the area.
- Keep the affected area lower than the victim's heart level.
- Get medical attention as soon as possible. Call the nearest physician or hospital to notify them to prepare antivenom serum.
- If possible, carry the victim who must be transported. If the victim must walk, have her or him walk slowly. Rapid movement must be avoided.
- If professional help cannot be obtained within 30 minutes, you should suction the wound using the suction cup from a snakebite kit.

Regardless of what you have heard, **DO NOT** apply ice, cut the wound, or apply a tourniquet.

STINGS OF BEES, WASPS, HORNETS

Snap the barb off with your finger, then with tweezers try to remove the stinger. Run cold water over and around the sting, or apply ice in a towel or plastic bag around it to relieve pain and slow the absorption of the venom. A victim of massive stings should be seen by a physician. If an allergic reaction develops, the victim must be immediately seen by the physician.

SEVERE BLEEDING (HEMORRHAGE)

Three types of bleeding can be observed from open wounds. Spurting of bright red blood from a wound indicates arterial bleeding; continuous flow of dark red blood indicates capillary bleeding. Arterial bleeding is the most serious, requiring immediate control and medical intervention after the initial control to prevent severe shock or death. Generally, venous bleeding is easier to control than arterial bleeding, because there is less pressure on the blood flow in the veins than in the arteries. However, venous bleeding may also be life-threatening, especially if several large veins are involved. Capillary bleeding is easily controlled by first aid measures and the body's own clotting mechanisms.

Immediate action is imperative for any wound accompanied by severe bleeding because shock, loss of consciousness, and even death may occur from a rapid loss of blood in a short time.

OBJECTIVES OF WOUND CARE

- To control the bleeding immediately
- To protect the wound from contamination and infection (as feasible; in emergency situations where sterile dressings are not available, you must use materials on hand, even if not sterile. It is more important to save the person's life by controlling the bleeding than it is to worry about preventing infection.

- To treat for shock
- To obtain medical attention

FOUR METHODS TO CONTROL SEVERE BLEEDING

The following methods are listed in order of preference (Figure 17-5).

Direct Pressure

Place a sterile dressing (or the cleanest cloth item on hand) over the wound site and apply hard, firm, direct pressure. This is usually effective in controlling severe bleeding. In the absence of dressing or cloth materials, apply direct pressure with the hand or fingers, but only until a compress is obtained. If a dressing becomes saturated with blood, do not remove it, but place additional dressings directly over the saturated one and continue firm, direct pressure.

Elevation

Elevate a limb above the person's heart level in conjunction with direct pressure, unless there is evidence of a fracture. Elevation helps reduce blood pressure within the limb, thus slowing down blood loss from the wound.

Pressure Bandage

A bandage applied to control bleeding is called a pressure bandage. Cover the dressing that you have placed on the wound with a roller bandage using overlapping turns. Tie or tape the bandage in place. If blood soaks through, add more dressings and bandage over them.

Pressure Points

When severe bleeding is not controlled with direct pressure and elevation of an affected limb, the pressure point method can be applied in conjunction with the first two methods. The pressure point method compresses the blood vessel supplying blood to the wound against an underlying bone or muscle tissue in an effort to close it off and reduce the amount of blood flowing through the vessel to the wound site. This method will control bleeding in all but a few circumstances. The exact position of the pressure point must be known and located quickly; otherwise significant blood loss will result. The seven pressure points follow (really fourteen, because there is one on each side of the body) (Figure 17-6).

Temporal artery. Compression on the temporal artery may be used to control superficial wounds of the forehead or the frontal part of the scalp.

Facial artery. Upward and outward compression of the facial artery against the jawbone with two or more fingers may be used to control bleeding in the facial region.

Carotid artery. Compression of the carotid artery in the neck against underlying muscle tissue may be used to control *only* serious hemorrhaging in the head. When this pressure point is used, extreme care must be taken to avoid obstruct-

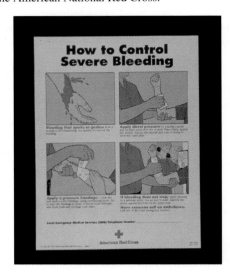

Figure 17-5 *How to control severe bleeding.*
Courtesy The American National Red Cross.

ing the person's airway. *Do not* apply pressure dressings around the neck.

Subclavian artery. Downward compression with the fingers on the subclavian artery just behind the collar bone (the clavicle) may be used to control bleeding in the arm and upper shoulder regions.

Brachial artery. Compression of the brachial artery against the bone with the fingers applied midway between the shoulder and elbow on the inside of the arm may be used to control bleeding from the arm, hand, and fingers.

Femoral artery. Compression of the femoral artery (in the center of the groin area) against the pelvic bone with the heel of the hand may be used to control bleeding from the leg.

Radial artery. Compression of the radial artery on the anterior side of the wrist on the thumb side may be used to control severe bleeding from the hand or fingers.

Compression of the ulnar artery (on the little finger, anterior side of the wrist) should be used in conjunction with compression of the radial artery when there is profuse hemorrhaging from the hand. If bleeding does not stop with compression on the radial and ulnar arteries, apply pressure to the brachial artery to control the bleeding.

TOURNIQUET

The use of a tourniquet is no longer recommended as standard first aid practice by the American Red Cross. The procedure is presented here to be used only in very extreme cases that comply with medical practice in your locality.

The use of a tourniquet is dangerous and should be used only as a last resort to control severe, life-threatening hemorrhage when direct pressure, elevation, pressure bandage, and pressure point methods fail to control the bleeding. The

Figure 17-6 *Location of pressure points.*
From Parcel G, Rinear C: *Basic emergency care of the sick and injured*, ed 4, St. Louis, 1990, Mosby.

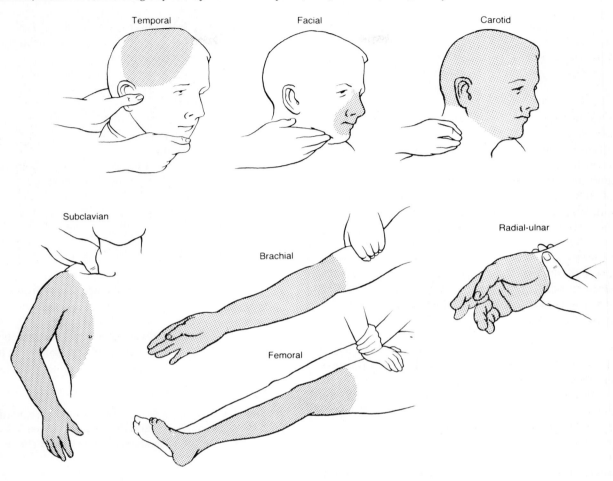

dangers of nerve damage, blood vessel damage, and tissue damage exist when a tourniquet is applied; thus, a tourniquet must be avoided unless a life could be lost. In essence, the decision to apply a tourniquet is a decision to risk the loss of the person's limb to save life. After the application of a tourniquet, it is imperative that the person be attended to by a physician. The following directions *must* be observed when a tourniquet is applied (Figure 17-7).

1. Use appropriate materials at least 2 inches wide such as a stocking, a cloth, a folded triangular bandage, or a blood pressure cuff, if available.
2. Apply the tourniquet just above the wound, or just above a joint when the wound is in or below a joint area.
3. Wrap the tourniquet material around the limb twice, and secure it with a knot.
4. Insert a strong stick or similar object between the two loops and twist this object to tighten the tourniquet until bleeding stops. Tourniquets must be applied tightly enough to stop the bleeding; if applied too loosely, bleeding will increase.
5. Wrap the ends of the tourniquet material around the stick or similar object, and tie it in place.

Figure 17-7 *Procedure for application of tourniquet.*
From Parcel G, Rinear C: *Basic emergency care of the sick and injured*, ed 4, St. Louis, 1990, Mosby.

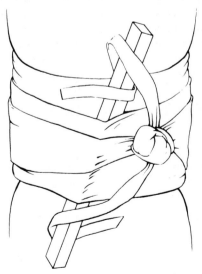

6. Make a written note of the time of application and the location of the tourniquet, and attach this to the person's clothing, or mark this information on the person. Frequently people will mark a large TK (for tourniquet) on the injured person's forehead with lipstick when at the scene of the accident.
7. *Never release* a tourniquet once it has been applied. A tourniquet must be removed only by a physician, who can provide supportive treatment for shock.
8. Elevate the limb slightly if this will not cause further injury.
9. Treat for shock, and give first aid for other injuries as required.
10. Transport the person immediately to receive medical attention.

AMPUTATION

In cases of amputation, the amputated part should be kept cool and moist, if possible, and taken with the victim to the physician. With the advent of microsurgery, amputated limbs can frequently be reattached successfully, providing there is minimal tissue damage to the surrounding tissues.

FURTHER WOUND CARE

For capillary bleeding, direct pressure and the application of ice wrapped in a towel or plastic bag are useful. Remember that ice is not effective in controlling severe bleeding.

In all cases when caring for bleeding wounds, provide reassurance and emotional support to the victim, and remain calm. If possible, estimate how much blood was lost because this will help the physician treat the person and determine if fluid replacement is necessary. However, remember that even an ounce of blood can discolor large numbers of dressings; and a cup of blood poured on the floor or gown covers a fairly large area, because when blood first comes from the vessels it is thin, and a small amount looks like a lot. Also observe the actual bleeding—is it a minimal, moderate, or heavy flow? This information will aid the physician, in addition to guiding your decision for the use of a tourniquet.

When bleeding stops, bandage the dressings firmly in place. Do not remove the initial dressings, because blood clots may be disturbed and bleeding resumed. Leave the cleaning and treatment of the wound to the physician.

PREVENTION OF CONTAMINATION AND INFECTION

To prevent infection, avoid touching the wound with an unsterilized dressing or your unscrubbed hands if possible. Do not disturb or remove the initial dressing placed over the wound.

BURNS

Burns are wounds caused by body contact with fire (dry heat), steam and scalding water (moist heat), electricity, chemicals, radiation (sun or nuclear rays), or lightning. Each year thousands of burns occur, many of which could have been prevented, and many of which are fatal in both the young and old. Burns involving over one third to one half of the body are often fatal, especially in children. Theories on the treatment for burns have undergone many changes over the years; many remedies were advocated and later rejected. Current thought on the matter can best be summed up by following the three Bs and the three Cs.

> *B = burn*
> Stop the burning.
> *B = breathing*
> Check the breathing.
> *B = Body examination*
> Examine where and how extensively the body has been burned, and assess any associated injuries.

> *C = cool*
> Cool the burn.
> *C = cover*
> Cover the burn.
> *C = carry*
> Carry the burn patient to the nearest medical treatment facility.

In addition, current treatment practices *condemn* the application of greasy substances, ointments, powders, or antiseptics to a burned area.

CLASSIFICATION OF BURNS

Burns are classified as first, second, and third degree, depending on the depth of the wound; they are also classified according to the percentage of body surface involved (Figures 17-8 and 17-9).

DEPTH OF WOUND

First-degree burns, also called *superficial burns*, involve only the outer layers of the skin. The skin is reddened without blister formation and is painful. The best example is a sunburn. *Second-degree burns*, also referred to as *partial-thickness burns*, involve deeper layers of the epidermis, are painful, and usually form blisters. *Third-degree burns*, also called *full-thickness burns*, are the most serious, destroying all layers of the skin, including the hair follicles and the sebaceous and sweat glands. Nerves are destroyed; thus the wound is painless. Muscles, blood supply, and bones may also be destroyed in third-degree burns.

BODY SURFACE

The percentage of total body surface involved usually determines the severity of the burn. The body surface is divided into areas by the rule of nines. Each arm is 9%, each leg is 18%, the front or back of the trunk is 18%, and the head and neck are 9% of the total body surface.

A first-degree burn that involves more than 20% of total body surface, involves the face and airway, or impairs the person when walking or wearing clothes should receive medical attention. Any second- or third-degree burn involving more than 20% of the total body surface or the feet, hands, or

Figure 17-8 A, *Cross-section showing structures of skin;* **B,** *classification of burns by degree.*
From Parcel G, Rinear C: *Basic emergency care of the sick and injured*, ed 4, St. Louis, 1990, Mosby.

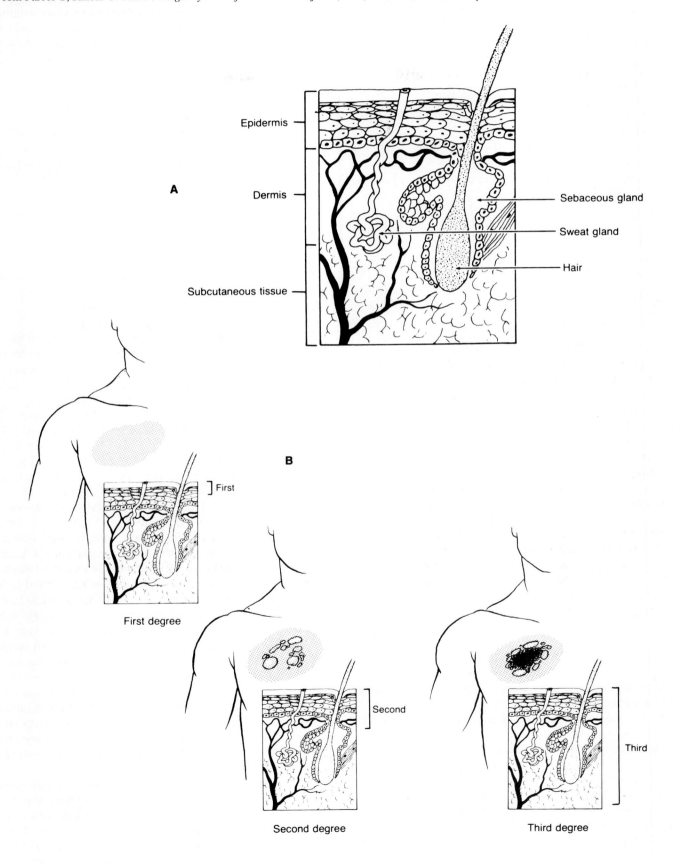

A

Epidermis

Dermis

Subcutaneous tissue

Sebaceous gland

Sweat gland

Hair

B

First

First degree

Second

Second degree

Third

Third degree

Figure 17-9 *Classification of burns by body surface area.*
From Parcel G, Rinear C: *Basic emergency care of the sick and injured,* ed 4, St. Louis, 1990, Mosby.

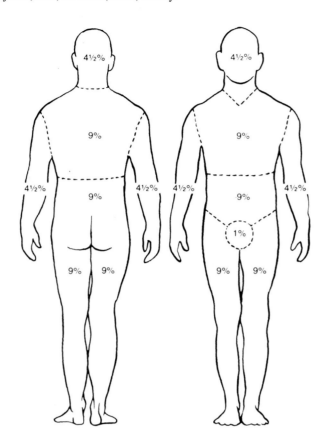

genitalia is considered a serious burn in need of medical attention. When more than 40% of total body surface is burned, it is considered a *severe burn.*

FIRST AID TREATMENT FOR BURNS
Objectives for Care of First Degree (Superficial) Burns

- To relieve pain
- To prevent the formation of blisters

First-Degree Burn Care

1. Immediately submerge the burned part in cool water, or place cold compresses directly on the burn.
2. Continue this treatment until pain has subsided when the cold is discontinued.
3. Apply a dry sterile dressing if the burn is in an area that will be irritated by clothing.
4. When running water is available, it is best to place the burned part under cold running water for 20 minutes. The reason is that, even though the top layers of the skin are cooled within a few minutes, the underlying tissue is still very heated, and the burn continues to cause tissue damage up to periods of 20 minutes after the initial burn.

5. For *small* superficial burns and burns with *small* open blisters that do not require medical attention, wash with soap and water, keep the area clean, and apply an antibiotic ointment to help prevent infection.

Objectives for Treating Second- and Third-Degree Burns (Partial- and Full-Thickness Burns):

1. Treat the person for shock
2. Prevent infection
3. Relieve pain

Second-Degree (Partial-Thickness) Burn Care

1. Immediately submerge the burned part in cold water for 1 to 2 hours, *or* place under running water for 20 minutes.
2. *Do not* break blisters or remove tissue.
3. Cover with a dressing or clean cloth that has been wrung out in cool water.
4. Apply a dry dressing and loosely bandage in place.

Third-Degree (Full-Thickness) Burn Care

1. Stop the burning; check for breathing; remove the burning agent. Remove any smoldering clothing; certain synthetics retain heat. Remove any jewelry on the burned area. Clothing and jewelry retain heat and also can become constricting as edema develops. Do a quick body assessment to determine the extent and severity of the burn.
2. Keep the person lying down with the head a little lower than the legs and hips, unless there is a chest or head injury, or if the person has difficulty breathing in this position.
3. Keep burned feet or legs elevated.
4. Keep burned hands above the level of the victim's heart.
5. Cool and cover the wound. Cover the burned areas with sterile dressings if available, or a cloth or sheet. Pour copious amounts of cool water (**NOT** ice water), or saline, if available, onto the material covering the wound. Continue pouring cool water onto the material periodically because the burn continues to heat the water up to the material. If clean material is not available, water may be poured directly onto the wound. Do not use ice or ice water because this causes critical body heat loss. When the wound is cooled, wrap the person for transport to a medical facility. *Never open any blisters.* Covering the wound prevents moving air from reaching the wound, lessens pain, and reduces contamination, helping to prevent infection.
6. If adjoining surfaces of skin are burned, separate them with gauze or cloth to keep them from sticking together (such as between the toes or fingers, ears and head, arms and chest).

7. For *chemical burns*, wash immediately with *copious* amounts of cool running water for at least 5 minutes (Figure 17-10). Remove any clothing that was in contact with the chemical. If the chemical is on the face or eyes, flush the face and eyes with a gentle flow of cool water for at least 15 minutes (Figure 17-11). Remove contact lenses if the victim is wearing them. Try to find out what chemical caused the burn so that you can tell the personnel at the emergency department where the victim will be taken. Also see the above steps. NOTE: *Never* flush a phosphorus burn with any type of solution, including water, as this could cause tissue sloughing. Instead, *soak* the affected area in water.

8. For facial burns prop the victim up and observe for signs of difficult breathing. Air passages could swell and cause breathing to be impaired or stopped. If you suspect a burned airway or burned lungs, continually monitor the victim's breathing.

9. If possible while awaiting transport for the person, take the pulse, respiration, and blood pressure to assess impending shock.

10. Keep the patient warm and resting quietly. Chilling must be avoided to prevent additional discomfort and loss of energy.

11. Constantly provide emotional support for the patient.

12. Inform the patient before transfer is undertaken.

WHAT *NOT* TO DO ABOUT BURNS

- *Don't* pull clothing over the burned area—cut it away if necessary.
- *Don't* try to remove any pieces of cloth or bits of debris or dirt that are stuck to the burn.
- *Don't* try to clean the burn; *don't* use iodine or other antiseptics on it; and *don't* open any blisters that may form on the burn.
- *Don't* use grease, butter, ointment, salve, petroleum jelly, or any type of medication on *any* burn.
- *Don't* breathe on a burn, and *don't* touch it with anything except a sterile or clean dressing.
- *Don't* apply ice directly to second-degree (partial-thickness) or third-degree (full-thickness) burns.
- *Don't* use absorbent cotton on burns.
- *Don't* change the dressings that were initially applied to the burn until directed to do so by a physician.

CEREBRAL VASCULAR ACCIDENT (STROKE)

A cerebral vascular accident (CVA), also called a stroke, is a disorder of the blood vessels of the brain. It results in a lack of blood supply to parts of the brain. Main causes of a CVA include a cerebral thrombus or a cerebral embolus, a ruptured artery and a cerebral hemorrhage, compression of cerebral arteries (as from edema or tumors), and arterial spasms (Figure 17-12). The symptoms and effects of a CVA vary greatly. It can be slight or severe, temporary or permanent, depending on

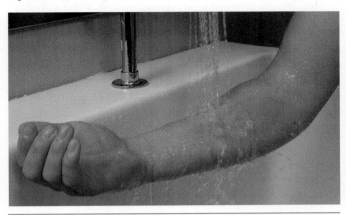

Figure 17-10 *For chemical burns, wash immediately with copious amounts of cool running water for at least 5 minutes.*

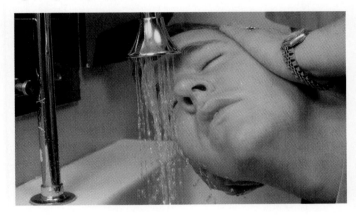

Figure 17-11 *If chemical gets on face, flush face and eyes with a gentle flow of cool water.*

the cause, location, and extent of the damage in the brain. Signs and symptoms of a CVA include the following:

- Dizziness, mental confusion, headache, and poor coordination
- Difficulty in speaking or loss of speech
- Loss of bladder and bowel control
- Paralysis or weakness usually on only one side of the body
- Loss of vision, especially in one eye
- Difficulty in breathing and in swallowing
- Unequal size of the pupils
- Loss of consciousness

First Aid Measures for a Cerebral Vascular Accident

1. Loosen all constricting clothing, especially around the neck. This may help to improve breathing and circulation to the head.

2. Maintain an open airway.

3. Position the victim on the affected side so that secretions will drain from the mouth and thus prevent aspiration of saliva and mucus.

Figure 17-12 *Cerebral vascular accident (CVA) can be caused by a cerebral thrombus or embolus, or from a ruptured artery and also from a cerebral hemorrhage.*
From Ingalls AJ, Salerno MC: *Maternal and child health nursing*, ed 7, St. Louis, 1991, Mosby.

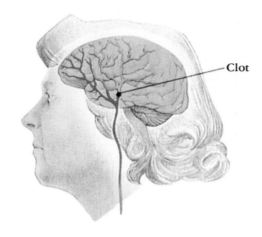

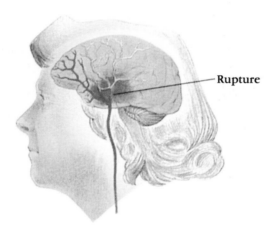

4. Keep the victim calm and provide reassurance that care is being provided.
5. If conscious, the victim may sit up or have the head elevated. This will help to lessen blood pressure in the head.
6. Do not give fluids unless the victim is able to swallow and is fully conscious. Discontinue all fluids if the victim vomits.
7 Seek medical attention as soon as possible. The victim will usually need to be hospitalized.
8. Be prepared to administer CPR if required.

CHEST PAIN

Chest pain can be associated with heart disease, lung disease, pain in the muscle fibers of the chest wall, and a few other conditions. It can be serious. It is advisable to treat all patients with chest pain as if they are heart patients. First aid measures include the following:

1. Observe the symptoms.
2. Keep the patient quiet and warm. Allow the patient to rest. Frequently the patient finds it easier to breathe when in a semisitting or upright position. Do not have the patient walk any distance.
3. Loosen all tight clothing.
4. Administer 4 to 6 liters of oxygen (if you are in the office and have prior directions and permission from the physician).
5. Contact the physician. When the physician cannot be reached, call the EMS system in your community, or an ambulance, or the fire department.
6. Stay with the patient until medical help arrives.
7. If the patient is conscious, inquire if she or he has any medication with her or him that is used for attacks of chest pain. The usual medication is nitroglycerin tablets, which are taken sublingually. You may give them to the patient with the patient's consent.
8. When feasible, obtain pertinent information from the patient. Use the PQRST method:
   P = provoking
   What provoked the pain? Was the patient doing any physical activity, experiencing emotional upset or excitement, or just sitting quietly?
   Q = quality of pain
   Is it a sharp pain, prolonged oppressive pain, or unusual discomfort?
   R = radiation of pain
   Where, if at all, does the pain radiate to? Is it in the center of the chest? Is it in the chest wall? Does it radiate to the abdomen or to the neck or to the left arm?
   S = severity
   How severe is the pain—mild, moderate, or severe?
   T = time
   When did the pain start? How long does it last? How frequently does it recur?
9. Keep an emesis basin handy in case the patient vomits.
10. At times it may be necessary to start rescue breathing if breathing stops or CPR if there is no breathing and no pulse.
11. If in the physician's office, you may connect the patient to the electrocardiograph and record a few tracings for the physician to interpret. Leads II and V_1 are considered the monitoring leads.
12. Remain calm; offer emotional support and reassurance to the patient, because most patients will be anxious and frightened.

CONVULSIONS

Convulsions are the involuntary spasms or contractions of muscles caused by an abnormal stimulus to the brain, or by changes in the chemical balance in the body. The primary effort in first aid for convulsions is to protect the patient from causing harm to the body during the convulsion.

1. Move items that may cause harm to the patient. Ask curious onlookers to remove themselves from the immediate area.
2. Loosen clothing around the neck and in any other area where it is constricting.
3. Place a padded bite block between the teeth to protect against biting of the tongue. *Do not* insert a bite block when force is required to get it in place. If an appropriate bite block is not available, one can be made by wrapping and taping a couple of pieces of gauze around two tongue blades.
   Some suggest not to put anything between the patient's teeth. Check with the physician for his or her preference and policy.
4. Do not restrain the patient's movements except to prevent injury. Protect the head at all times.
5. When movement has ceased, keep the patient lying down and allow him or her to rest.
6. Ensure an open airway.
7. If bleeding from a bitten tongue, excessive saliva, or vomit is present, turn the patient's head to one side to prevent aspiration of these excretions.
8. After all seizure activity has ceased, allow the patient to rest or sleep in a quiet, comfortable place until he or she is sufficiently oriented to time and place and capable of moving without weakness.

Anyone who has experienced a seizure (convulsion) should be seen by a physician, although the occurrence of one seizure is not considered an emergency. If convulsive activity is repeated or occurs frequently, medical attention must be sought.

If reporting the convulsion to the physician, it is very important that you describe the convulsive activity; that is, whether the convulsion was generalized or localized, how and where it started, how many convulsions there were, and how long they lasted. The *seizures* associated with epilepsy are a form of convulsion.

EPISTAXIS (NOSEBLEED)

Most nosebleeds are not serious and can be easily controlled. However, excessive bleeding requires medical attention and may require electrocauterization of the ruptured vessels causing the bleeding.

First aid for nosebleeds is relatively simple. Have the patient in a sitting position, and pinch the lower portion of the nose between the thumb and index finger for 5 to 10 minutes. When this does not control the bleeding, apply ice packs to the nasal and facial areas. Place a moistened gauze pad gently into the bleeding nostril, leaving one end of the gauze outside so that it can be removed easily, then pinch the nose between the thumb and index finger for 10 minutes. If this does not control the bleeding, medical attention should be obtained.

FAINTING (SYNCOPE)

Fainting is a partial or complete loss of consciousness of limited duration caused by a decreased amount of blood to the brain. A person may feel weak and dizzy, cold, or nauseated; appear pale; perspire; and have numbness or tingling in the hands and feet before fainting; or one may faint suddenly. First aid management for patients who faint follows:

1. Lay the person flat with the head lowered slightly.
2. Ensure an open airway.
3. Loosen tight clothing.
4. Apply cold cloths to the face. These are beneficial because of their stimulating effect.
5. Pass aromatic spirits of ammonia back and forth in front of the person's nose to allow inhalation. Avoid holding them too close to the person's nose.
6. Observe the person carefully, looking for anything unusual.
7. Observe for local weakness of the arms and legs, and locate and count the pulse. These observations may be of great importance if the condition turns out to be something other than a fainting episode.
8. Keep the person resting quietly for at least 10 minutes after full consciousness has been regained.
9. Lower the head between the legs when the person is in a sitting position and begins to feel faint. Stay with the person, and protect against falling should fainting occur.
10. When fainting lasts more than a minute or two, keep the person warm and resting quietly, and summon the physician or transport to the hospital, for the condition may not be a simple episode of fainting. It may, in fact, be a symptom of diabetes, heart disease, epilepsy, stroke, or any one of many diseases.

FOREIGN BODIES IN THE EAR, EYE, AND NOSE

EAR

Foreign bodies lodged in the ear canal are frequently seen in children. *Do not* attempt to remove them. They must be removed by the physician, because of the possibility of injury to the eardrum (tympanic membrane) and ear canal tissue.

If the foreign body in the ear is a live bug or insect, instill a few drops of sterile oil into the ear canal. This will asphyxiate and stop the movement of the intruder.

EYE

Foreign bodies in the eye are irritating and can be harmful because of the possibility of their scratching the eye surface or becoming embedded in the eye tissue.

Instruct the patient not to rub the affected eye.

Wash your hands, and examine the eye by pulling the lower lid down and turning the upper lid back. If the object is on either lid, take a moistened corner of a clean cloth and touch it lightly to try to remove it. Avoid applying any pressure on the eye. If the object is on the eye itself, do not attempt to remove it this way. At times when the object is located under the upper eyelid or on the eye, it may be dislodged by pulling the upper eyelid forward and down over the lower lid; tears may dislodge the object. The eye then may be flushed with clean water (see also Eye Irrigation in Unit Eight.)

When the previous methods do not remove the object, it may be embedded. Cover the closed eye with a dressing, and summon the physician.

NOSE

When the object cannot be removed easily, a physician must be consulted. Instruct the patient to avoid violent nose blowing and probing the nose, because these acts may only push the object deeper or injure the tissues of the nose.

FRACTURES

A fracture is a break in the continuity of a bone. Broad classifications of fractures are *open fracture*—one in which the bone penetrates the skin producing an open wound, and *closed fracture*—one in which there is no break in the skin. Closed fractures are much more common than open fractures. Not all fractures prevent the patient from moving the injured part; therefore never ask the patient to move to determine the presence of broken bones. Movement of a fractured area may cause additional harm and, at times, permanent damage (Figure 17-13).

Figure 17-13 *Types of fractures.*
From Ingalls AJ, Salerno MC: *Maternal and Child Health Nursing,* ed 7, St. Louis, 1991, Mosby.

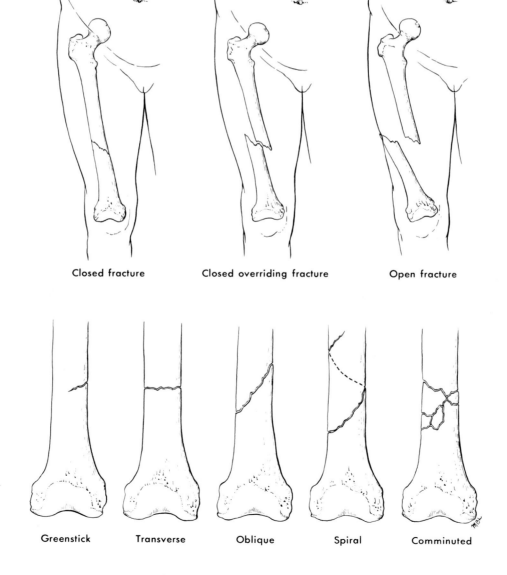

Closed fracture   Closed overriding fracture   Open fracture

Greenstick   Transverse   Oblique   Spiral   Comminuted

First Aid for Fractures

1. Treat for shock and give artificial respiration when necessary; keep the patient warm and quiet.
2. Prevent movement of the injured part and adjacent joints, and do not move the injured part.
3. Elevate affected extremities when possible without disturbing the suspected fracture. This will help reduce hemorrhage, when present, and swelling.
4. Apply an ice bag to the painful area.
5. Never attempt to reduce (set) a fracture. This is the physician's responsibility.
6. Never attempt to push a protruding bone back into place.
7. For an open fracture, in addition to the above:
   a. Control any serious bleeding.
   b. Do not attempt to clean the wound.
   c. Avoid contaminating the wound; do not touch the wound.
   d. Do not replace bone fragments.
   e. Cover the wound with a sterile dressing or clean cloth material, and secure in place with a bandage.
8. To prevent additional trauma when the patient has to be moved or transported, the injured part must be immobilized by applying splints or slings, and bandages. Splints must be long enough to reach beyond the joint above and below the break on both sides. Pad improvised splints to prevent additional pressure or injury, and tie them in place with bandages or strips of material. Make sure that the bandages or splints are not too tight. Normal circulation must not be hindered. Refer to a first aid textbook for additional information on the application of various types of splints.

FRACTURED NECK OR BACK

When there is a suspected neck, back, pelvis, or skull fracture, *do not* attempt to move the patient. Trained medical or ambulance personnel are required. When the patient experiences a numbness or tingling around the shoulders and cannot move the fingers readily, a neck fracture should be suspected.

When there is numbness or tingling in the legs or pain when trying to move the back or neck, or when the feet or toes cannot be moved, a back fracture is suspected.

In either of the above cases, loosen the patient's clothing around the neck and waist. Do not move the patient, and do not let the patient attempt to move, because injury to the spinal cord may occur. Keep the patient warm and quiet, and treat for shock, as indicated. Call for medical help immediately. The patient will need to be transported by ambulance to the nearest hospital.

FRACTURED JAW

When a fractured jaw is suspected, tie a bandage around the chin and over the head to stop movement. Do not manipulate the jaw. Medical attention is required for treatment.

HEAD INJURIES

The severity of head injuries can vary greatly. The patient may appear normal, experience a headache, have a momentary loss of consciousness or lack of memory, be dazed, or be unconscious. Bleeding from the mouth, nose, ears, or scalp may be present; pulse may be rapid and weak; pupils of the eyes may be unequal in size; and pallor, vomiting, or double vision may be present. *In all cases medical attention is imperative.* When the initial symptoms are minor, it must be remembered that even after a period of time, hours or days, the injured person may become drowsy or confused or unconscious as a result of a head injury. A prompt recovery from a state of minor signs and symptoms may not be an indication of the seriousness of the injury. The following steps and precautions should be taken:

1. Assess the patient's physical and mental status. For physical assessment, check for signs as stated above, and take the blood pressure if equipment is available. For mental assessment, when the patient is conscious, check for orientation as to time, place, name, and alertness, and ask the patient to repeat a simple phrase. Talking with the patient is a good way to check the level of consciousness and alertness.
2. Keep the patient at rest in a supine position if the face is ashen and gray, or raise the head and shoulders (together) if the face is flushed. *Never position the patient with the head lower than the rest of the body.*
3. Always ensure an open airway. Be prepared to give artificial respiration when necessary.
4. Control hemorrhage if present.
5. Do not give fluids by mouth.
6. Apply a dressing to a scalp wound, and bandage it in place with a head bandage.
7. Take note of any period of unconsciousness, and record it.
8. Observe and record any changes in the pupils of the eyes.
9. Take and record the blood pressure and the time of any changes (if the equipment is available). When the blood pressure begins to rise and if the pupils begin to dilate or the state of consciousness begins to decrease, this usually indicates an elevation of intracranial pressure.
10. If the patient is unconscious, gently turn the head to one side to prevent aspiration of any blood or mucus that may be present.
11. Keep the patient resting quietly until medical help arrives or the patient is transported to the hospital.

HYPERVENTILATION

Hyperventilation is a common complication of emotional upsets or hysterical situations. It usually affects persons who are anxious, high-strung, and have a history of job or home stress, anxiety from lack of sleep, sudden stoppage of prescribed drugs such as diazepam (Valium), or a history of drug usage that increases sensitivity of the respiratory centers such as high concentrations of salicylate. These individuals usually unknowingly breathe too rapidly, which in turn disturbs the normal balance of carbon dioxide in the blood.

At the outset, individuals may feel a tightness in the chest and have a feeling of air hunger; they feel that they cannot fill the lungs because they can't get enough air. Frequently these individuals become apprehensive, which only leads to increased hyperventilation and at times to syncope (fainting). Palpitation of the heart, abdominal pain, and a feeling of fullness in the throat may also occur.

Immediate first aid treatment is to have the individual breathe into a paper bag held tightly over the mouth and nose for 10 minutes or more to replace the carbon dioxide that has been given off during hyperventilation. Removing the victim from the surroundings is helpful, because frequently people who are trying to help the victim become excited and anxious and unknowingly only promote the victim's anxiety and subsequent hyperventilation. In all cases, the first aider or medical assistant should be the calming influence and provide reassurance to the victim.

When frequent attacks of hyperventilation occur, it is recommended that the victim seek medical attention for treatment of the underlying cause(s).

HYPOGLYCEMIA—DIABETES (INSULIN REACTION) AND HYPERGLYCEMIA (DIABETIC COMA)

Diabetes mellitus is a disorder of carbohydrate metabolism in which the ability to oxidize and use carbohydrates is lost and a subsequent derangement of protein and fat metabolism occurs. This results from disturbances in the normal insulin mechanism, a hormone secreted by the islets of Langerhans in the pancreas.

There is either an insufficiency of insulin or a resistance to the actions of insulin or both. The main types of diabetes are Type I, or insulin-dependent diabetes mellitus (IDDM), formerly called juvenile or childhood onset, in which the body does not produce insulin because of destruction of the insulin-producing beta cells of the pancreas. It is thought to be an autoimmune disease in which the pancreas destroys itself with its own antibodies. There appears to be a genetic tendency toward this type of diabetes. Type II or noninsulin-dependent diabetes, formerly called mature or adult onset diabetes, is frequently diagnosed in people over 40 years old, although it can occur much earlier. In Type II diabetes the person experiences a defect in insulin production *and* a tendency of the cells in the body to resist the action of insulin. It is estimated that in the United States alone there are millions of people who suffer from diabetes but are unaware of their condition. It is therefore very important for all of us to be familiar with the most *common symptoms of diabetes*, which include the following:

- Thirst
- Frequent urination
- Fatigue and weakness
- Apathy
- Hunger

Further symptoms include:

- Blurred vision
- Irritability
- Numbness or tingling in the extremities
- Repeated infections of the urinary tract, skin, or gums
- Itchy skin

Sometimes there are no apparent symptoms, and the condition is only detected when a person has a complete physical examination. The presence of diabetes is confirmed by a fasting blood glucose level. If the blood glucose level is consistently elevated, the person has diabetes.

Adverse conditions can occur when a person with diabetes is undiagnosed or does not follow the therapy prescribed or when there is a disturbance in the normal functions of the body.

Common complications of diabetes include the following:

- Blindness
- Cardiovascular disease
- Cataract formation
- Congenital defects
- Dental caries
- Gangrene
- Glaucoma
- Impotence
- Kidney disease
- Stillbirths and/or miscarriages

Treatment should be obtained and followed diligently. The primary goal of treatment for both types of diabetes is the control of the person's blood glucose levels. Control of blood glucose levels can help to prevent complications and also helps to maximize the individual's general health level.

All persons with diabetes, their immediate families, and persons in the health care professions should know the signs and symptoms and the treatment or immediate first aid for hypoglycemia (formerly called an insulin reaction, in which blood glucose levels fall and there is too much insulin or presence of insulin without food) and hyperglycemia, formerly called diabetic coma (a condition that may develop when there is lack of insulin and the blood glucose level is high in the diabetic patient's system) (Table 17-1). Diabetics should carry a card stating the fact that they are diabetic, their daily insulin or oral hypoglycemic drug dosage, their address, and the name and address of their physician. Many diabetics wear Medic-Alert bracelets or necklaces, which indicate their condition in case of emergency situations requiring treatment.

First Aid for Hypoglycemia (Insulin Reaction)

1. If the patient is conscious, give some form of simple sugar such as hard candy, sugar, or sweetened orange juice. These are easily digested forms of sugar. Do not give candy bars for treatment of hypoglycemia. They contain many times the needed calories and also have proteins and fats that would slow down the absorption of glucose.

TABLE 17-1

Signs and Symptoms of Hypoglycemia (Insulin Reaction) and Hyperglycemia (Diabetic Coma)

	Insulin Reaction	Diabetic Coma
Onset	Sudden	Gradual
Skin	Perspiration, pallor, cold and damp skin (cool and clammy)	Flushed, warm, and dry skin, dry tongue
Behavior	Tremors, restlessness, fatigue, faint feeling, headache, confusion or strange behavior. May seem dazed or slow to respond. May appear irritable or grumpy.	Weakness, drowsiness, lethargy
Gastrointestinal tract	Extreme hunger, nausea	Thirst, nausea, and vomiting
Vision	Double vision	Eyeball tension low
Respiration	Shallow	Difficulty in breathing or air hunger; rapid, deep, gulping respirations
Pulse	Rapid or normal	Rapid, weak
Speech	Slurred	
Breath	No acetone smell	Sweet or fruity odor; smell of acetone
Level of consciousness	May have loss of consciousness	Coma if unattended Apparent confusion and disorientation
Blood glucose	Low (40-70 mg/100 ml)	High (over 200 mg/100 ml)
Urine test	Sugar-absent, or a trace at most Acetone-negative	Sugar-positive in high amounts Acetone-positive

2. Seek medical attention if the patient does not respond readily to Step No. 1. The patient should respond within 15 to 20 minutes, if not sooner.
3. If the patient is unconscious, do not force fluids or food. Call the physician, or get the patient to the hospital immediately.

First Aid for Hyperglycemia (Diabetic Coma)

There is *no adequate first aid* treatment for hyperglycemia or diabetic coma. *Immediate medical treatment is necessary.*

OPEN WOUNDS

Types of wounds include abrasions, avulsions, incisions, lacerations, and puncture wounds. See pages 224 to 227 and Figure 6-31.

First Aid for Minor Wounds

1. Wash your hands thoroughly before treating any wound to minimize the possibility of infection. Don disposable single-use exam gloves.
2. Observe the wound to check for foreign objects, such as pieces of glass, wood, and dirt.
3. Control bleeding (see pages 558 to 560).
4. Gently wash the skin around the wound with soap and water. Wash away from the wound, not toward it.

5. For minor cuts, scratches, and abrasions, wash the wound well with soap and water to remove foreign matter.
   a. Lacerations and incisions may be irrigated with large amounts of water or normal saline. Do not apply an antiseptic unless instructed to do so by the physician.
   b. For puncture wounds, gently squeeze the wound to encourage a small amount of bleeding to help wash out microorganisms. Then wash the wound with soap and water.
   c. Wounds with severe bleeding should not be cleansed.
6. Cover the wound with a sterile dressing, and bandage it in place. Use the cleanest material on hand when sterile dressings are not available.
7. Refer the person to the physician for follow-up care. Tetanus immunization may be required. Lacerations, incisions, and avulsions will require medical attention, because they may have to be sutured.
8. Advise the person to be alert for signs of infection, and if present, to seek medical attention. Signs to watch for are:
   a. Swelling
   b. Excessive redness
   c. Heat and increasing tenderness
   d. Drainage
   e. Red streaks away from the wound
   f. Fever
   g. Excessive pain

POISONING

The symptoms of poisoning vary greatly and depend on the type and amount of substance taken. All types of poisonings are considered emergencies that require immediate attention. The following points should be considered when poisoning is suspected:

1. Look for any physical changes such as an abrupt onset of pain or illness; burns or stains around the mouth or on the face, which would indicate poisoning with a caustic substance; breath odor, which may indicate the type of poison ingested; or depressed consciousness and irregular heartbeat.
2. Observe the surroundings for empty containers, spilled fluids, or containers of substances that would be poisonous if ingested.
3. Obtain information from the person or an observer when possible.

Objectives of First Aid Measures

1. To induce vomiting, except when the person has swallowed corrosive or petroleum products, when the person is unconscious, when the person is convulsing, or if the person ingested substances that could absorb rapidly and produce seizures (such as camphor or strychnine) or cause drowsiness, seizures, or coma (such as cyclic antidepressants).
2. To prevent absorption of the poison.
3. To maintain an open airway, breathing, and vital functions.
4. To obtain medical attention without delay.

NOTE: The old thought that you should dilute or neutralize the poison is very controversial. Many experts believe that it may cause more harm than good, especially if it is done incorrectly. Therefore current recommendations are *not to* dilute or neutralize a poison without expert advice.

First Aid

Speed is essential to stop absorption of a poison. First aid for poisoning depends on the type of poison ingested. It is not possible for the first aider or medical assistant to know exactly what to do for all cases, but general guidelines must be followed.

1. In all cases, monitor the person's vital signs, maintain an open airway, and be prepared to administer cardiopulmonary resuscitation if necessary.
2. Make every effort to determine what, when, and how much was ingested.
3. Obtain specific information to follow. **Most specialists recommend that you** *should not carry out any specific first aid measures without expert advice (this may be analogous to not moving a trauma victim with a potential spine injury).*

Call the physician, the poison control center that is in the nearest city, or the hospital emergency physician. Antidote labels may be on the product ingested, but *caution* must be taken, because the label may be out-of-date and incorrect. Poison control centers are open 24 hours a day and maintain antidote information on several thousand available commercial products. Most states have a poison control center in the major cities. Keep this number on hand with other important telephone numbers.

4. Carry out the specific first aid instructions obtained.
5. When specific directions cannot be obtained, the following may be performed:
   a. If the person is awake and able to swallow, 1 glass of water may be given.
   b. *Do not induce vomiting* if the person (1) is unconscious or in a coma; (2) is having a convulsion; (3) has ingested a petroleum product such as kerosene, lighter fluid, gasoline; (4) has ingested a corrosive substance (for example, strong acids or alkalis). In these situations, if the person can swallow, give 1 glass of water.
6. Poison control centers do not advocate the use of syrup of ipecac without expert advice. They also suggest that activated charcoal be used *only* in the hospital.
   a. If the person has ingested a *noncorrosive* substance and is not unconscious or convulsing, the following may be suggested by the Poison Control Center:
      (1) Give 1 tablespoon of syrup of ipecac, followed by 2 cups of water for children ages 1 to 12 years. For a person over 12 years of age, give 2 tablespoons of syrup of ipecac followed by 2 glasses of water. Keep children active. Repeat the same dose in 15 minutes if vomiting has not occurred. *Repeat only once.* The onset of vomiting will usually occur within 20 to 30 minutes.

   DO NOT give syrup of ipecac if the person has ingested anything that may cause seizures or drowsiness because, by the time the person starts to vomit, he or she also could be having a seizure or be very drowsy, which increases the chance of the person aspirating the vomitus (studies have shown that aspiration happens approximately 50% of the times that vomiting is induced).
      (2) When retching and vomiting begin, place the person's head down with the head lower than the hips. This prevents vomitus from entering the lungs, causing further injury.
      (3) When the poison is unknown, save the vomitus, and take it to the physician or hospital for analysis.
7. It is recommended *not* to dilute poisons taken in capsule or tablet form. The increased fluid in the stomach could speed the rate at which the capsule or tablet dissolves, thereby increasing the rate at which the poison would

be absorbed into the bloodstream. NOTE: The universal antidote of 2 parts burned toast, 1 part milk of magnesia, and 1 part strong tea that was formerly recommended is now believed to be *useless*. Therefore *do not* waste time preparing this mixture for administration.

8. Arrange for transportation of the person to the physician or the hospital. *All cases of poisoning must receive medical attention.*
9. Remain calm at all times. Stay with the person and provide reassurance.

Many poisoning cases are related to drug abuse. To determine the proper first aid care to give in these cases, you should be aware of the characteristics of intoxication for drugs that are commonly abused. See Table 17-2 for selected effects of commonly abused drugs.

POISON CONTROL CENTERS

Poison control centers have been established in many cities across the nation to provide quick and reliable information on possible poisonings or drug-related problems. They provide information on the appropriate first aid and clinical management to use for cases of suspected or known poisoning. Some centers also offer specialized poisoning treatment and consultant services, professional training, and poisoning prevention education for consumers. Many centers are staffed by clinical pharmacists 24 hours a day, every day of the year.

Not all states have poison control centers; some rely on centers in nearby cities. Some states have state-designated centers that are located in 2 or 3 major cities in that state. Other states have poison control centers that are regional centers established by a particular city. These centers are usually financed locally. The centers are usually located at major hospitals or major medical universities. You should post the telephone number of the nearest poison control center near your telephone both at work and at home so that you are able to obtain information as quickly as possible when the need arises.

More information on poison control centers can be obtained from:

The American Association of Poison Control Centers
National Capital Poison Center
Georgetown University Hospital
3800 Reservoir Rd. NW
Washington, D.C. 20007
Telephone: (202) 784-2088

For a list of poison control centers in the United States write to:

Publication Office of Veterinary and Human Toxicology
Comparative Toxicology Laboratories
Kansas State University
Manhattan, Kansas 66506
Telephone: (916) 532-5679

EMERGENCY TRAY/CRASH CART

See Unit Seven, page 261.

FIRST AID KIT

Now is the time to check the first aid kit kept in the office, home, and family automobile. A properly equipped kit, with fresh supplies that are kept replenished after use, is a practical aid in relieving many minor injuries and ailments. It may even be lifesaving before medical help arrives. But, the best time to provide the office, home, or automobile first aid kit is *before* it is needed. The following first aid supplies are suggested:

1. Sterile gauze pads—2 and 4-inch squares
2. Sterile gauze roller bandages
3. Adhesive tape
4. Adhesive dressings in various sizes
5. Absorbent cotton—sterile
6. Triangular bandage
7. Elastic bandage
8. A mild antiseptic and antiseptic wipes
9. Syrup of ipecac
10. Analgesic, such as aspirin and/or acetaminophen
11. Petroleum jelly
12. Calamine lotion
13. Aromatic spirits of ammonia
14. Tweezers
15. A scissors with rounded ends
16. Clinical thermometer (digital thermometer may be used)
17. Flashlight with extra batteries
18. Safety pins
19. Sugar for diabetics
20. Icebag and/or chemical ice pack
21. Disposable single-use exam gloves
22. Airway/mouthpiece
23. First aid book

For automobiles, the American National Red Cross suggests a specially designed compact unit with standardized first aid materials fitted into a case, like blocks. The packet is readily stored, and the supplies do not become easily disarranged. Each packet is clearly labeled, and instructions for use are included. These kits can be obtained at auto supply stores and department stores with contents selected to meet the purchaser's particular needs. Ask your physician about other medications for such things as car sickness, upset stomach, and allergies. Take some road flares for car safety, and a blanket in the car.

Regardless of how well equipped the first aid kit is, its effective use depends on individuals knowing how to give aid properly. A course in first aid, as well as training in CPR, can be an invaluable investment. For additional drugs and supplies that may be kept in the physician's office or clinic for emergency situations, see Emergency Tray in Unit Seven.

TABLE 17-2

Comparison of Selected Effects of Commonly Abused Drugs

Drug category	Physical Dependence	Characteristics of Intoxication
Opiates	Marked	Analgesia with or without depressed sensorium; pinpoint pupils (tolerance does not develop to this action); patient may be alert and appear normal; respiratory depressions with overdose
Barbiturates	Marked	Patient may appear normal with usual dose, but narrow margin between doses needed to prevent withdrawal symptoms and toxic dose is often exceeded and patient appears "drunk," with drowsiness, ataxia, slurred speech, and nystagmus on lateral gaze; pupil size and reaction normal; respiratory depression with overdose
Nonbarbiturate sedatives: glutethimide (Doriden)	Marked	Pupils dilated and reactive to light; coma and respiratory depression prolonged; sudden apnea and laryngeal spasm common
Antianxiety agents ("minor tranquilizers")	Marked	Progressive depression of sensorium as with barbiturates; pupil size and reaction normal; respiratory depression with overdose
Ethanol	Marked	Depressed sensorium, acute or chronic brain syndrome, odor on breath, pupil size and reaction normal
Amphetamines	Mild to absent	Agitation, with paranoid thought disturbance in high doses; acute organic brain syndrome after prolonged use; pupils dilated and reactive; tachycardia, elevated blood pressure, with possibility of hypertensive crisis and CVA; possibility of convulsive seizures
Cocaine	Marked	Paranoid thought disturbance in high doses, with dangerous delusions of persecution and omnipotence; tachycardia; respiratory depression with overdose
Marijuana	Absent	Milder preparations: drowsy, euphoric state with frequent inappropriate laughter and disturbance in perception of time or space (occasional acute psychotic reaction reported); stronger preparations such as hashish: frequent hallucinations or psychotic reaction; pupils normal, conjunctivas injected (marijuana preparations frequently adulterated with LSD, tryptamines, or heroin)
Psychotomimetics: LSD, STP, tryptamines, mescaline, morning glory seeds	Absent	Unpredictable disturbance in ego function, manifest by extreme lability of affect and chaotic disruption of thought, with danger of uncontrolled behavioral disturbance; pupils dilated and reactive to light
Phencyclidine	Unknown	Disinhibition, agitation, confusion, chaotic thought disturbance, unpredictable behavior, hypertension, meiosis, respiratory collapse, cardiovascular collapse, death
Anticholinergic agents	Absent	Nonpsychotropic effects such as tachycardia, decreased salivary secretion, urinary retention, and dilated, nonreactive pupils plus depressed sensorium, confusion, disorientation, hallucinations, and delusional thinking
Inhalants*	Unknown	Depressed senorium, hallucinations, acute brain syndrome; odor on breath; often glassy-eyed appearance

*The term inhalant is used to designate a variety of gases and highly volatile organic liquids, including the aromatic glues, paint thinners, gasoline, some anesthetic agents and amylnitrite. The term excludes liquids sprayed into the nasopharynx (droplet transport required) and substances that must be ignited before administration (such as marijuana). (Courtesy Mosby)

Table 17-2—cont'd

Comparison of Selected Effects of Commonly Abused Drugs

Characteristics of Withdrawal	"Flashback" Symptoms	Masking of Symptoms of Illness or Injury During Intoxication
Rhinorrhea, lacrimation, and dilated, reactive pupils, followed by gastrointestinal disturbances, low back pain, and waves of gooseflesh; convulsions not a feature unless heroin samples were adulterated with barbiturates	Not reported	An important feature of opiate intoxication, due to analgesic action, with or without depressed sensorium
Agitation, tremulousness, insomnia, gastrointestinal disturbances, hyperpyrexia, blepharoclonus (clonic blink reflex), actue brain syndrome, major convulsive seizures	Not reported	Only in presence of depressed sensorium or after onset of acute brain syndrome
Similar to barbiturate withdrawal syndrome, with agitation, gastrointestinal disturbances, hyperpyrexia, and major convulsive seizures	Not reported	Same as in barbiturate intoxication
Similar to barbiturate withdrawal syndrome, with danger of major convulsive seizures	Not reported	Same as in barbiturate intoxication
Similar to barbiturate withdrawal syndrome, but with less likelihood of convulsive seizures	Not reported	Same as in barbiturate intoxication
Lethargy, somnolence, dysphoria, and possibility of suicidal depression; brain syndrome may persist for many weeks	Infrequently reported	Drug-induced euphoria of acute brain syndrome may interfere with awareness of symptoms of illness or may remove incentive to report symptoms of illness
Similar to amphetamine withdrawal	Not reported	Same as in amphetamine intoxication
No specific withdrawal symptoms	Infrequently reported	Uncommon with milder preparations; stronger preparations may interfere in same manner as psychotomimetic agents
No specific withdrawal symptoms; symptoms may persist for indefinite period after discontinuation of drug	Commonly reported as late as 1 year after last dose	Affective response or psychotic thought disturbance may remove awareness of, or incentive to report symptoms of illness
No specific withdrawal symptoms	Occasionally reported	Same as in LSD intoxication
No specific withdrawal symptoms; mydriasis may persist for several days	Not reported	Pain may not be reported as a result of depression of sensorium, acute brain syndrome, or acute psychotic reaction
No specific withdrawal symptoms	Infrequently reported	Same as in anticholinergic intoxication

CONCLUSION

In the event of a sudden illness or an accident that causes trauma to a person, the trained, competent medical assistant should be prepared to properly administer the appropriate first aid treatment and obtain medical assistance as needed. In time of emergencies, prompt action must be taken. It is important that the you remain calm in all cases and provide care in a competent, orderly, and organized manner. Do not perform procedures that you have not been trained to do. To maintain your skills and knowledge in first aid and CPR, it is suggested that you enroll in a refresher course every few years.

REVIEW OF VOCABULARY

The following is a hospital discharge summary received in the office on one of the physician's patients who had been in an accident. After reading this, you should be able to discuss the contents with your instructor. Be prepared to define and explain any medical terms that are used. A medical dictionary, other reference books, and information given in preceding units of this book may be used as references for obtaining definitions or explanations of the contents of this report.

Discharge Summary

PATIENT: Will Nelson
ADMITTED: January 10, 19__
DISCHARGED: February 10, 19__
DISCHARGE DIAGNOSES
1. Multiple facial fractures, including fracture of the maxilla, mandible, nose, and right orbit.
2. Comminuted fracture, left patella.

HISTORY: This 22-year-old man was injured in a head-on motorcycle accident with another motorcycle at about 4:30 p.m. on January 10. The patient was brought to the emergency room of this hospital by ambulance.

PHYSICAL EXAMINATION: At the time of admission, the patient was conscious. He was alert and oriented and aware of his surroundings. Physical examination revealed gross bleeding from mouth and nose. There were multiple contusions and abrasions over the facial area. Blood pressure was 118/60, pulse was 74, respirations 16.

HEENT: The ears were clear. The eyes had marked ecchymotic areas present periorbitally, with diffuse edema in the periorbital area. The fundus on the left was clear. The fundus on the right was not seen. The nose was filled with blood clots, and there was some active bleeding in the nasal area. At the time of admission, this was not delineated clearly. There was a marked amount of blood in the right side of the mouth. The patient was unable to open his mouth because of deviation of the jaw. Neck was supple.

CARDIORESPIRATORY: Chest was clear to auscultation. There was a regular sinus rhythm with no murmurs.

GI: The abdomen was soft, without masses or organs palpable. Bowel sounds were active.

EXTREMITIES: There was ecchymosis and edema over the left knee.

NEUROLOGIC: The patient was conscious. The deep tendon reflexes were within normal limits, and there were no pathologic toe signs elicited.

DIAGNOSTIC DATA: X-ray studies at the time of admission revealed a fracture of the right patella, comminuted, and maxillary and mandibular fractures of the face. CBC at the time of admission revealed a hemoglobin of 12.6 g with a hematocrit of 38%. The hemoglobin on January 26 was down to 10.5 g with a hematocrit of 32% and WBC of 8300 with a normal differential. On February 2, hemoglobin was 11.7 g with hematocrit of 34%. Urinalysis on January 27 was normal. Serum electrolytes were normal on January 13. The chloride was 101 mEq/L. PCO_2 content 30 mEq/L. Potassium 3.5 mEq/L. Sodium 135 mEq/L. Serum osmolality ran from 276 to 282. On January 13, hemoglobin had dropped to 8.6 and 8.7 g, with a packed cell volume of 25% and mean proportional hemoglobin concentration of 34% and 35%. The patient was transfused with two units of blood at that time, and hemoglobin rose, on January 14, to 11.2 g, with a packed cell volume of 32%. X-ray examinations on January 10, at the time of admission, of skull, facial bones, left ribs, and left knee revealed multiple fractures of the facial bones, including the nasal bones and the mandible. There was a fracture of the left patella and, after surgery on January 12, a PA view of the chest (portable) revealed a hazy infiltration in the right upper lung field, resembling pneumonitis. A film of the right hand, on January 12, revealed a very small chip fracture of the palm as described. A portable chest x-ray film, on January 16, revealed the small patch of hazy infiltration in the upper right field, which was probably due to lung contusion. The chest otherwise was unremarkable. On January 14, stereo views of the pelvis revealed a gas pattern, heavy in the visible part of the abdomen. Bony structures were intact. There were no signs of dislocation of the hips. X-ray film of the left arm revealed the elbow and wrist to be intact. Cervical spine was negative, except for a fracture in the mandible as described. Lumbosacral spine showed anterior displacement of L-5 on S-1, and L-1 was wedged very slightly anteriorly. It was not believed that this was a fracture. Water's view of the sinuses revealed multiple facial bone fractures, evident with generalized

REVIEW OF VOCABULARY—cont'd

haziness in the central part. On January 18, AP x-ray films of the facial bones revealed superior fractures of the nasal and maxillary bones, as well as the previously described fractured mandible. There were no specific changes.

HOSPITAL COURSE: On the night of admission, January 10, the patient was taken to the operating room where, under general anesthesia, he first had a tracheostomy by Dr. U. R. Belson. The patient then had a reduction of fracture of the mandible and maxilla with repair of facial lacerations and mucous membrane of the mouth and packing of the right antrium, reduction of nasal bones, and fixation of nasal packing. This was done by Drs. U. R. Belson, B. Beal, and I. B. Tucker. A simultaneous patellectomy was done on the left knee by Dr. P. Adamson. The patient did relatively well in the intensive care unit following surgery, maintained on antibiotics and tracheostomy care. On January 18, the patient was returned to the operating room where, under general anesthesia, Drs. U. R. Belson and I. B. Tucker performed open reduction of the fracture of the facial bones. The patient has continued to do well since that

time on a general basis, requiring constant observation and very close and meticulous care of his tracheostomy site. He has been gradually ambulated from the bed to a wheelchair and ambulation in the room. The cast has been removed from the left leg. Sutures have been removed from his face. The patient was seen in consultation by Dr. I. B. Tucker, concerning the eyes, and he was found to have Berlin's edema from the fractures of the floor and rim of the right orbit. On January 11, the patient also was seen in consultation by Dr. P. Brown concerning advice for maintenance and following of his tracheostomy site and antibiotic therapy. The patient is being discharged today to his home, where he will be under observation by his father, Dr. W. F. Nelson, and will be followed by the physicians, as required, at General Hospital.

Andrew Berger, MD

CASE STUDY

Read the following and discuss the italicized terminology.

On a hot summer afternoon 14-year-old Brooke wanders was stung by an insect on her left lower leg. Initially she complained of a burning, stinging *sensation*. However, within 15 minutes she began to experience *dyspnea* and a feeling of fullness in her *trachea*. This progressed quickly to lightheadedness followed by one episode of *syncope* at which time she was brought to the office for emergency examination.

On arrival she *exhibited signs and symptoms* of *shock*, which soon developed specifically into *cardiogenic and neurogenic shock*. Her pulse was *rapid and thready*. Her leg was examined for remnants of the stinger and it was removed *intact*. An appropriate *antidote* and *epinephrine* were administered, and she began to stabilize from the *acute allergic anaphylactic shock* caused by the inset bite and was transferred to the hospital via ambulance.

She was admitted and observed for 36 hours and then released to be followed in the office in 2 days.

REVIEW QUESTIONS

1. List three factors that determine if a situation is an emergency.
2. As a medical assistant, you are responsible for rendering first aid when the need arises. Define first aid, and state the contributions you can make for the physical and psychologic care of the victim in an emergency situation.
3. List four fundamental rules and procedures to follow in a medical emergency.
4. Mr. Bill Bailey has been experiencing uncomfortable pressure and pain in the center of the chest, shortness of breath, and slight nausea for the past 3 minutes. What medical condition would you suspect him to have? What type of action should be taken for this condition?
5. While having lunch with a friend, she suddenly clutches her neck between her thumb and index finger. What should this indicate to you?
6. Define shock. List and explain the five types of shock. List eight outstanding symptoms of shock.
7. Dave Rubin has just had minor surgery in the physician's office. As you are assisting him after the procedure, you observe that he is very pale and his skin quite cold to the touch. You immediately take his vital signs and find that the pulse is weak and rapid, the blood pressure 92/70, and respirations 34 and shallow. What condition would you suspect that he is experiencing? What must be your immediate actions?

REVIEW QUESTIONS—cont'd

8. Anna Westover is having a severe reaction to penicillin. Describe the first aid treatment that you could provide.

9. Ray Wood is cleaning the windows in your office. By accident, he breaks a window. He comes running to you at the desk. You observe that he is clutching his wrist and that bright red blood is spurting from his wrist, as well as from his hand and fingers. State the type of bleeding this would indicate, the vessel that may be cut, and the first aid treatment that you would administer.

10. List and locate the seven pressure points used to control severe bleeding.

11. State the difference between a first, second, and third degree burn (superficial, partial-, and full-thickness burn).

12. After having blood drawn, Joanne Newman faints. State the first aid treatment that you would provide for this patient.

13. Ann O'Brien, a diabetic patient, is displaying the signs and symptoms of hypoglycemia or an insulin reaction. List six signs and symptoms of hypoglycemia insulin reaction. State the immediate care that you could provide for Ann.

14. List six signs and symptoms of hyperglycemia (diabetic coma).

15. In the case of ingested poisoning, when should you *not* have the victim vomit?

16. When is the use of a tourniquet advisable?

17. List at least 15 items that you would include when compiling supplies for a first aid kit.

PERFORMANCE TEST

In a skills laboratory, with simulations of emergency situations, the medical assistant student will demonstrate skill in performing the following procedures without reference to source materials. The student needs a person to play the role of the patient. Time limits for the performance of each procedure are to be assigned by the instructor (see also page 52.)

1. Demonstrate the proper first aid treatment to be administered to patients who have experienced all the emergency situations given in this unit.

2. Demonstrate how to locate the seven pressure points to be used when controlling severe bleeding.

3. Demonstrate the proper method of applying a tourniquet to a patient's left arm, right leg.

4. Demonstrate on the manikin (if available) the correct method of administering CPR.

The student is to perform these activities with 100% accuracy before passing this unit.

Anatomy and Physiology

COGNITIVE OBJECTIVES

On completion of Unit Eighteen, the medical assistant should be able to:

1. Define and pronounce terms that are new to you by using an English or a medical dictionary.
2. Define the terms that are in bold print or italicized.
3. List and describe the three planes used to describe the body.
4. State the five cavities of the body. List the organs that are located in each cavity.
5. List and locate the nine regions into which the abdominal and pelvic cavities are divided.
6. List and locate the four quadrants of the abdominal region.
7. Describe the functions of muscle cells, red blood cells, epithelial cells, and nerve cells.
8. List the body systems presented in this unit.
9. State the main function(s) of each body system discussed in this unit.
10. Identify the main structures and/or organs in each body system and state the function of each.
11. List, describe, and give examples of the four main shapes of bones.
12. Differentiate between the axial skeleton and the appendicular skeleton. List and identify the bones in each part of the skeleton.
13. Differentiate between tendons and ligaments.
14. Differentiate between voluntary and involuntary muscle, giving examples of each.
15. State the three types of muscle tissue found in the human body.
16. State the two components of the circulatory system. State the makeup of each component.
17. Differentiate between blood plasma and blood serum.
18. Briefly state the function of red blood cells, white blood cells, and platelets.
19. Define anemia and differentiate between the four different types discussed.
20. Differentiate between arteries, capillaries, and veins.
21. Briefly discuss the function of the heart.
22. Briefly discuss the concept of a heart attack or coronary or a myocardial infarction.
23. State where the main groupings of lymph nodes are located.
24. Differentiate between the central nervous system, the peripheral nervous system, and the autonomic nervous system. Briefly state the main functions of each of these divisions of the nervous system.
25. State and briefly discuss the two divisions of the autonomic nervous system.
26. Identify the location and state the function of the accessory organs of the digestive system.
27. Trace the route of food from ingestion to the elimination of waste products of digestion by identifying the anatomic parts of the digestive system.
28. State the difference between inspiration and expiration.
29. State the three processes of respiration.
30. Discuss the structural and functional units of the urinary system.
31. Discuss the processes of ovulation, menstruation, fertilization, implantation, and menopause.
32. Discuss the reasons for and the benefits of hormone replacement therapy (HRT) after menopause in females.
33. State at least one hormone produced by each of the endocrine glands discussed in this unit.
34. List and briefly discuss the five specialized organs of the senses.
35. Differentiate between sebaceous glands and sudiferous glands.
36. Differentiate between the various types of skin lesions discussed.
37. Discuss the difference between basal cell carcinoma of the skin and squamous cell carcinoma. State the most common type of cancer.

TERMINAL PERFORMANCE OBJECTIVES

On completion of Unit Eighteen, the medical assistant student should be able to:

1. Given diagrams of the human body, label the body systems and organs that are presented in this unit.
2. Using an English or a medical dictionary, define terms with which you are unfamiliar and/or that you have not previously learned in your Medical Terminology courses.

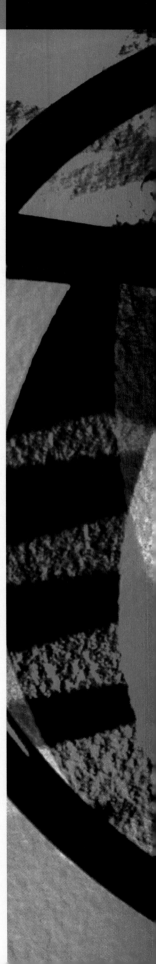

VOCABULARY

Anatomy—The study of body structures and their location. Body structures are organized on four levels (Figure 18-1):

Cells—The smallest unit structures capable of reproducing and maintaining life. Compose all living things.

Tissues—Combinations of similar cells.

Organs—Collections of tissues that work together to perform a particular function.

Body system—Consists of organs that work together to provide a major body function.

Physiology—The study of the functions of the body. Functions are studied according to body systems and the related organs that together accomplish functions necessary to maintain and support life. Eleven major systems compose the human body: skeletal, digestive, respiratory, urinary, reproductive, endocrine, sensory, and integumentary. The following pages discuss the body systems in some detail.

Additional vocabulary terms are presented in the specific sections to which they apply throughout this unit.

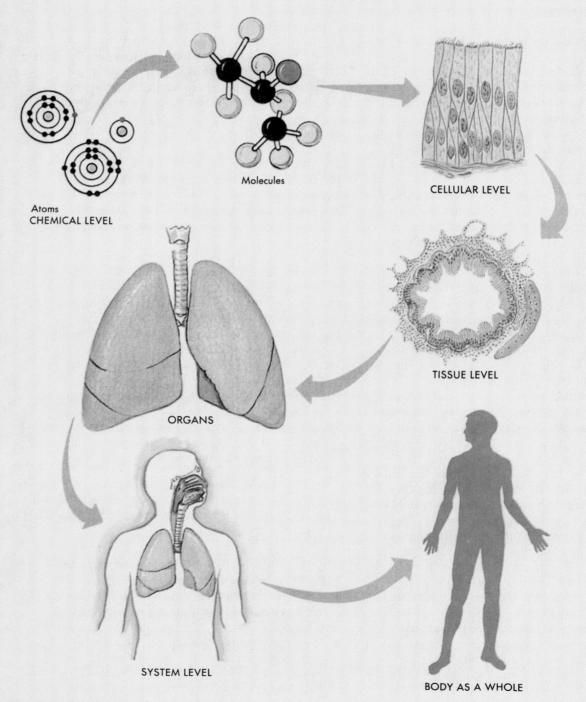

Molecules

CELLULAR LEVEL

Atoms
CHEMICAL LEVEL

TISSUE LEVEL

ORGANS

SYSTEM LEVEL

BODY AS A WHOLE

Figure 18-1 *Structural levels of organization in the body.*
From Thibodeau GA: *Anthony's textbook of anatomy and physiology*, ed 13, St. Louis, 1990, Mosby.

This unit is meant to be a general introduction to anatomy and physiology and must of necessity be brief. It is not offered as a substitute for a textbook on anatomy and physiology, but it is intended to supplement such textbooks, of which there are many excellent ones available.

BODY PLANES

Structures of the body can be located and described in relation to planes that divide the body. Three planes used to describe the body are as follows (Figure 18-2):

- *The coronal plane.* The coronal plane separates the front and back of the body.
- *The transverse plane.* The transverse plane divides the upper and lower body.

- *The sagittal plane.* The sagittal plane divides the body into right and left sides.

The location of organs is described in relation to these planes. For example, an organ or growth may be below (inferior) or above (superior) the transverse plane. It may be close to (medial) or away from (lateral) the sagittal plane. It may be in front of (anterior or ventral) or behind (posterior or dorsal) the coronal plane. Other terms for location include close to (proximal) or away from (distal) a point where one organ attaches to another.

BODY CAVITIES

There are five cavities in the human body (Figure 18-3).

Figure 18-2 *Directions and planes of the body.*
From Thibodeau GA: *Anthony's textbook of anatomy and physiology*, ed 13, St. Louis, 1990, Mosby.

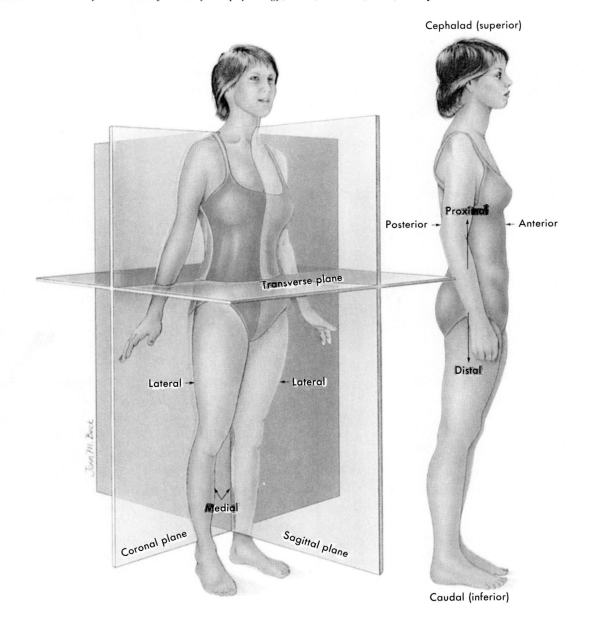

Cephalad (superior)

Posterior — Proximal — Anterior

Transverse plane

Distal

Lateral — — Lateral

Medial

Coronal plane

Sagittal plane

Caudal (inferior)

Figure 18-3 *Locations and subdivisions of the major body cavities.*

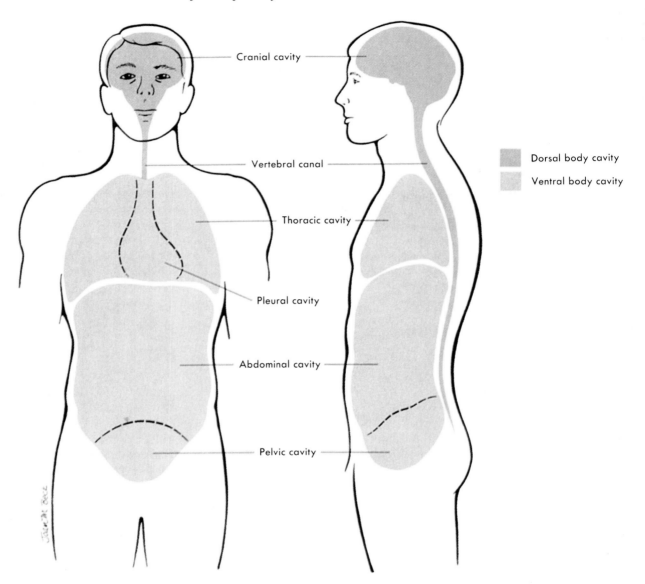

Cavity	Organs	Cavity	Organs
1. Thoracic	Right and left lung		Kidneys
	Heart		Ureters
	Trachea		Adrenal glands
	Right and left bronchi	**3. Pelvic**	Reproductive organs
	Thymus gland		Urinary bladder
	Esophagus		Sigmoid colon
	Major blood vessels		Rectum
	Various lymph nodes and nerves	**4. Cranial**	Brain
2. Abdominal	Stomach		Ventricles
	Gallbladder		Pineal gland (pineal body)
	Pancreas		Pituitary gland
	Liver	**5. Spinal**	Spinal cord
	Intestines		Nerves
	Spleen		

BODY REGIONS

For ease in locating body areas and organs, locations within the abdominal and pelvic cavities are described in terms of nine regions (Figure 18-4). The abdomen is also sometimes sectioned into four quadrants to describe the site of pain or some other diagnostic finding (Figure 18-5, *A* and *B*). An imaginary line passing vertically and a line passing horizontally through the umbilicus divides the abdomen into the right and left upper quadrants, and the right and left lower quadrants.

THE CELLULAR BASIS OF HUMANS

Before 1838, little was known of the minute structure of the human body. Aristotle's notions of humors and other superstitions prevailed. In 1838, however, Schleiden and Schwann published a description of cell structure that established the fact that all organic bodies were composed of definite units of material called cells, which were arranged in characteristic patterns in different animals and plants.

Figure 18-4 *The nine regions of the abdominopelvic cavity showing the most superficial organs.*
From Thibodeau GA: *Anthony's textbook of anatomy and physiology,* ed 13, St. Louis, 1990, Mosby.

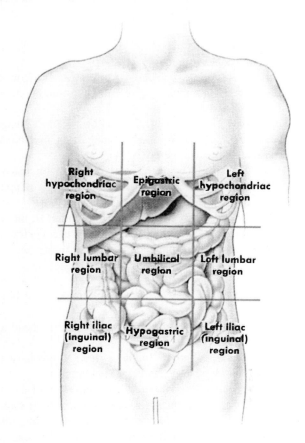

Right hypochondriac region

Epigastric region

Left hypochondriac region

Right lumbar region

Umbilical region

Left lumbar region

Right iliac (inguinal) region

Hypogastric region

Left iliac (inguinal) region

CELLS

Cells arise from cells. The origin of the human body is the gamete (ovum) of the female ♀ that has been fertilized by the gamete (sperm) of the male ♂. Thus the fertilized ovum is a human individual in the one-cell stage of development. This cell, called a zygote, splits into two cells, and these resulting daughter cells divide into four. This process continues until the developing individual is an intricate mass of many cells.

In the early stages of development, the cells all look alike. As development proceeds, however, these cells begin to take on special characteristics and look differently from those nearby. This change is called *differentiation* of the cell. Thus, from cells that are at one stage alike, there arise specialized cells known as muscle cells, epithelial cells, connective tissue cells, blood cells, and many others.

CELLULAR FUNCTIONS

This change in structure of the cells is the outward manifestation of profound changes in the functions of the cell. In the stage preceding differentiation, the cells carry on all the processes of life. They take in food, eliminate waste, respond to stimuli, move, and reproduce their kind. Now, with differentiation, special functions become highly developed in certain cells. *Muscle cells* specialize in contraction and hence are foremost in producing movement. *Nerve cells* develop the ability to receive and transmit stimuli and hence play a special part in making the individual aware of his world. *Epithelial cells* specialize in producing secretions and perform certain protective functions. *Red blood cells* (RBCs) transmit to all parts of the body the gases necessary for life.

Homeostasis is the tendency of a cell or the whole organism to maintain a state of balance. Molecules pass into and out of the cell to maintain this balance. The cells of the body constantly adjust to preserve a balance of fluids, temperature, oxygen, electrolytes, and nutrients.

TISSUES

As development proceeds, like cells become organized into masses known as tissues and grouped in arrangements that permit them to carry on effectively their specialized functions. Thus a group of muscle cells form *muscle tissue* in certain parts; the *connective tissue* cells mass together in structures known as bones, ligaments, cartilage, and soft tissue such as fat and blood cells; *epithelial tissue* covers the body, forms glands, and lines the surface of cavities and organs; and *nervous tissue,* composed largely of specialized cells called neurons, is found in the eyes, ears, brain, spinal cord, and peripheral nerves. Nervous tissue transmits communications.

ORGANS AND SYSTEMS

Beyond these simple groupings of like cells in tissue arrangements there are more complex groupings in the body into coordinated organizations known as organs and systems.

Figure 18-5 *Division of the abdomen into four quadrants. A, Photo showing surface outlines of right upper quadrant (RUQ) (1); left upper quadrant (LUQ) (2); right lower quadrant (RLQ) (3); left lower quadrant (LLQ) (4). B, Diagram showing relationship of internal organs to the four abdominopelvic quadrants.*
From Thibodeau GA: *Anthony's textbook of anatomy and physiology,* ed 13, St. Louis, 1990, Mosby.

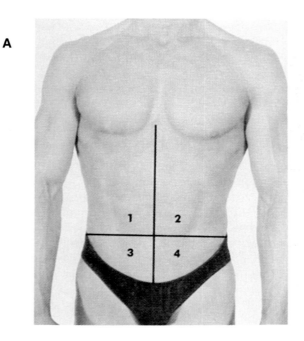

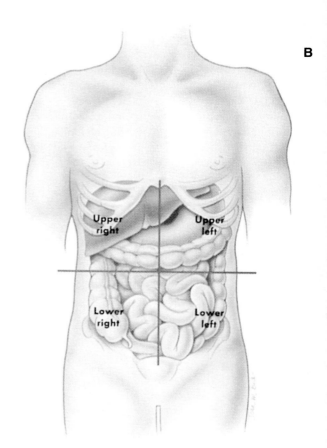

Each organ is unique in size, shape, appearance, and placement in the body. Each organ can be identified by the type and pattern of tissues that compose it. Examples of organs are the heart, the lungs, the brain, and the kidneys. At the system level, varying numbers and types of organs are arranged and work together to perform complex functions of the body.

Thus epithelial cells, connective tissue cells, muscle cells, nerve cells, and blood cells may all coordinate in a mass effort to perform a highly specialized function such as breathing, which is carried on by the organs comprising the respiratory system.

THE SKELETAL SYSTEM

Skeletons of animals vary widely in their design. In some the skeleton is on the outside of the animal, such as that of the lobster; in others it is enclosed within soft parts, such as that of humans. In some animals the skeleton serves as a protection against enemies (note the remarkable case of the oyster), but in humans its **function** is primarily that of support, mechanical leverage, and movement (Figure 18-6).

Other functions of the skeletal system are to provide shape to the body, to provide protection for the internal organs, to store minerals, and to produce blood cells.

TYPES OF BONES

The two major types of bone tissue are compact (dense) and cancellous (loosely packed or spongy).

SHAPES OF BONES

The four main shapes of bones are:

1. *Long bones.* These bones are longer than wide. Examples of long bones are the femur, humerus, radius, ulna, tibia, and fibula.
2. *Short bones.* These bones have similar width and length. Examples of short bones include the tarsals, metatarsals, carpals, and metacarpals.
3. *Flat bones.* These bones have two layers with space in between. Examples include the cranium, ribs, scapula, and sternum.
4. *Irregular bones.* These are bones that do not fit into the other categories. Examples include the vertebrae, mandible, patella, ilium, and the ossicles in the ear.

MAJOR GROUPS OF BONES

The skeletal system consists of two major group of bones (Table 18-1).

1. Axial skeleton—Includes the 80 bones of the head and trunk.
2. Appendicular skeleton—Includes the 126 bones of the pelvis, shoulders, arms, and legs (extremities).

There are normally 206 bones in the human body (Table 18-1). The skeleton is composed of bones and strong bands, called **ligaments,** that hold the bones together in joints. Ligaments attach bones to other bones in joints. **Tendons** join bones to muscles. Bones may have **cartilage,** a fibrous connective tissue, on some surfaces. Cartilage has some flexibility and is avascular, whereas bone is rigid and is very vascular.

Figure 18-6 A, *Skeletal system.*
From LaFleur M, Starr W: *Exploring medical language: a student-directed approach*, ed 2, St. Louis, 1989, Mosby.

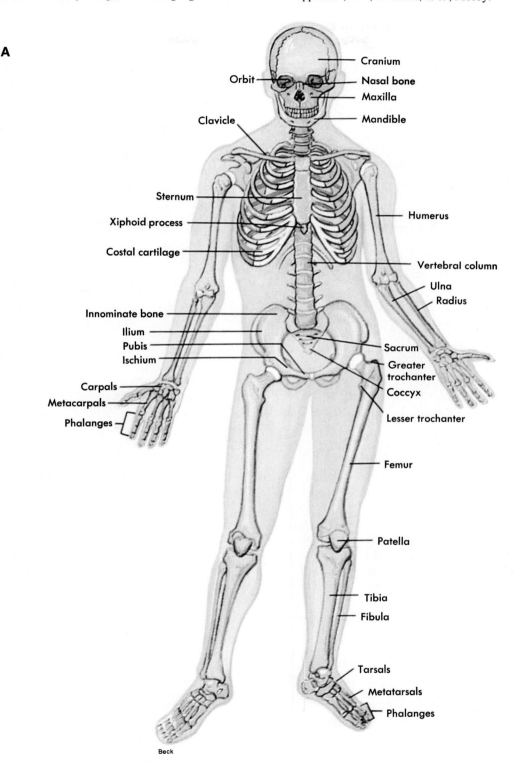

A

Cranium
Orbit
Nasal bone
Maxilla
Mandible
Clavicle
Sternum
Xiphoid process
Costal cartilage
Humerus
Vertebral column
Ulna
Radius
Innominate bone
Ilium
Pubis
Ischium
Sacrum
Greater trochanter
Coccyx
Lesser trochanter
Carpals
Metacarpals
Phalanges
Femur
Patella
Tibia
Fibula
Tarsals
Metatarsals
Phalanges

Beck

Figure 18-6—cont'd B, *Skeletal system.*
From LaFleur M, Starr W: *Exploring medical language: a student-directed approach*, ed 2, St. Louis, 1989, Mosby.

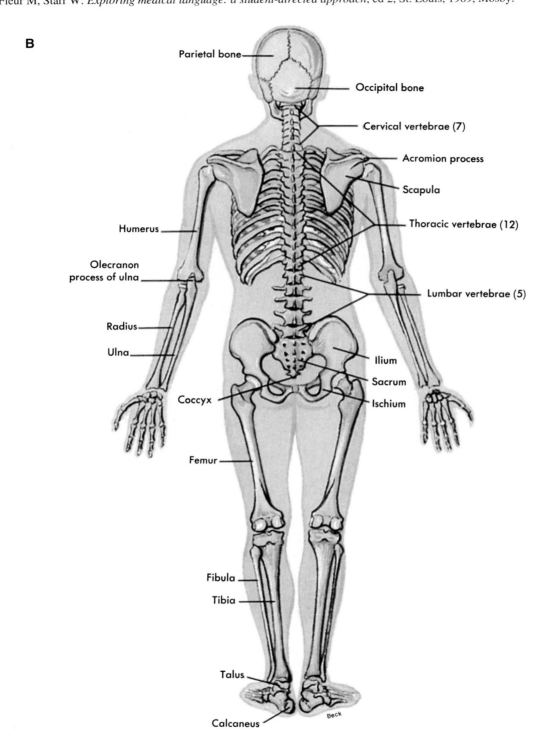

TABLE 18-1

Axial and Appendicular Skeletons

Class	Name of bone	Single	Paired
Axial skeleton—80 bones			
Skull	Frontal	1	
	Parietal		2
	Occipital	1	
	Temporal		2
	Sphenoid	1	
	Ethmoid	1	
Face	Nasal		2
	Lacrimal		2
	Maxilla		2
	Turbinate		2
	Zygoma		2
	Palatine		2
	Vomer	1	
	Mandible	1	
Vertebral column	Cervical	7	
	Thoracic	12	
	Lumbar	5	
	Sacrum (5 fused)	1	
	Coccyx (4)	1 unit	
Thorax	Ribs		24
	Sternum	1	
Miscellaneous	Ossicles of ears (3 pairs)		6
	Hyoid	1	
Appendicular Skeleton—126 bones			
Upper extremity	Clavicle		2
	Scapula		2
	Humerus		2
	Radius		2
	Ulna		2
	Carpals		16
	Metacarpals		10
	Phalanges of fingers and thumbs		28
Lower extremity	Hip (3 fused—illium, ischium, pubis)		2
	Femur		2
	Patella		2
	Tibia		2
	Fibula		2
	Tarsals		14
	Metatarsals		10
	Phalanges of toes		28
Total			206

Axial Skeleton

Skull and ribs. Balanced on top of the first cervical vertebra is the skull. The *skull* presents two chief parts: the facial bones and the rounded cranium, which contains the brain.

In the skeleton (see Figure 18-6) the spine is seen as the central axis. In the thoracic region 12 pairs of *ribs* reach laterally and forward, enclosing the *thorax* as they join the *breastbone (sternum)* in the front. The first seven pairs of ribs are called true ribs and attach to the sternum through *costochondral junctions* (costal cartilages).

The next five pairs of ribs are called false ribs. The costal cartilage of pairs eight, nine, and ten attach to the cartilage of the rib above each and then to the costal cartilage of pair number seven, which attaches to the sternum.

The eleventh and twelfth ribs remain unattached to bone at their forward (anterior) ends where they are embedded in muscles and other soft parts. They are called floating ribs and attach only to the spine in the back.

The trunk. The bones of the trunk are the vertebrae, sternum, ribs, scapulae, clavicles, and pelvis. The backbone of the adult consists of 26 segments, or vertebrae (Figure 18-7). Each segment has a bony ring posteriorly with spikes or projections on three sides for muscle attachments. The vertebral bodies are separated by pads of fibrocartilage called **intevertebral disks.** The backbone has four normal forward and backward curves in the *sagittal plane,* which sometimes become exaggerated through injury, disease, or poor posture.

Figure 18-7 *The spinal column from three views.*
From Thibodeau GA: *Anthony's textbook of anatomy and physiology,* ed 13, St. Louis, 1990, Mosby.

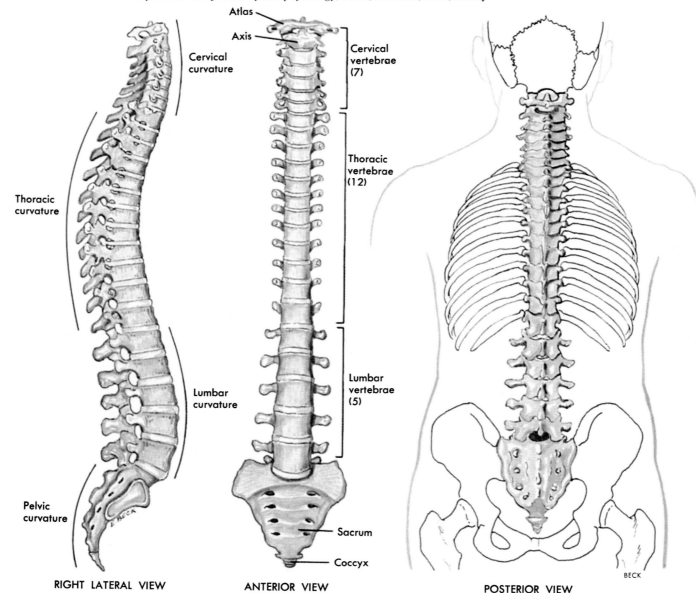

RIGHT LATERAL VIEW   ANTERIOR VIEW   POSTERIOR VIEW

The vertebrae are divided into groups as follows: the top seven are called the cervical, the next 12 are called the thoracic, or dorsal, and the next five the lumbar vertebrae. The next section, the sacrum, is formed from five vertebrae fused together into one solid bone. The coccyx, or lower tip of the spine, is made up of four small segments comprising a short tailbone that has very little flexibility. The vertebral column supports the head and trunk; the intevertebral disks between the vertebrae permit a variety of spinal motions and ease the jolts during walking or falling.

The spinal cord passes downward from the brain through the bony rings of the vertebrae, which serve as a protection for its delicate and important structure.

The sternum, or breastbone, a flat, bladelike bone, forms the front boundary of the upper part of the trunk.

The sternum is divided into three parts:
* Manubrium (top)
* Body
* Xiphoid process (the sharp tip at the bottom)

The **ribs** form the sides of the chest cavity. They are narrow, flat bones arranged in pairs. There are 12 on each side, and they articulate with the spine at the back. They curve around forward like hoops of a barrel and attach to the sternum in front, except for the last two pairs, which are called *floating ribs*. The forward (anterior) ends of the upper 10 pairs of ribs are composed of *cartilage (costochondral junctions),* which resembles bones but is not as hard as bone. The spaces between the ribs are occupied by intercostal muscles. Thus the dorsal spine, arteries, veins, and nerves, sternum, and ribs form what is known as the bony cage around the heart and lungs.

Appendicular Skeleton

Pelvis. The **pelvis** is the lower part of the main bony framework of the body. It is formed by two large, flat irregular bones that spread outward at the top and narrow down at the lower edges in front. Each bone arises from three cartilage segments, the ilium, ischium, and pubis in the infant; at adulthood they form a single bone on each side of the pelvis. They are joined to the sacrum at the *sacroiliac joints* in the back. Each side of the pelvis has a large hollow or socket below the flaring portion to receive the upper end of the thighbone, the femur, which fits into this socket, the acetabulum, forming the hip joint. The pelvis of a female is relatively larger and wider than that of a male. The size and shape of the female pelvis are significant in the birth of a baby. If the pelvis is too small to permit the baby to pass through, an abdominal operation known as a cesarean section becomes necessary. The pelvis can be measured and ultrasound sonograms can be obtained to determine whether or not it is sufficiently wide to allow the baby's head to pass through during birth. Most of the male organs of reproduction are on the outside of the body, whereas those of the female are more protected, inside the pelvis or pelvic cavity.

The upper extremities. You may find it helpful to refer frequently to Figure 18-6 during the remaining discussion of the skeleton.

Shoulder girdle. Above and in front of the rib cage and extending outward on either side, at right angles to the sternum (breastbone), are two long bones known as the *clavicles,* or collarbones. Their medial ends are joined to the breastbone at the *sternoclavicular joints.* The lateral ends of the collarbones join the shoulder blades (*scapulae*) at the *acromioclavicular joints* at the tops of the shoulders. The scapulae are triangular, rather flat bones, placed just back of the shoulder joints.

Together the clavicles and the scapulae form the shoulder girdle.

Arms. The single long bone of the upper arm, or *brachium,* is called the *humerus.* Its upper end articulates with the *scapula* in the *scapulohumeral* (or *glenohumeral*) *joint.* The lower end articulates with the two long bones of the forearm, the *radius* and *ulna,* to form the *elbow joint.*

The longer of the two forearm bones is the *ulna.* It has a deep notch or saddle near its *proximal* end, where the lower end of the humerus rides in the elbow joint. If you place your elbow and forearm on the table, with your palm upward, in *supination,* the second long bone in the forearm, the *radius,* lies to the thumb side of the forearm, and parallels the ulna. Next, turn your palm to face downward on the table, in *pronation.* The *distal* half of the radius can be seen to cross over the ulna, to assume an x relationship to the ulna. This is accomplished by the radius rotating on its long axis at the elbow and rolling over the ulna at the wrist, while the ulna remains stationary. This allows the hand to be placed in a number of different positions by supination or pronation of the forearm. It can be readily seen that the ulna does not change position at the elbow or wrist, thereby lending stability to the whole forearm and hand structure during an almost 180-degree change of position of the wrist and hand. This knowledge is of great importance when one attempts to position the forearm properly for x-ray studies.

Wrists and hands. Eight small, irregular *carpal bones* form the wrist. They are placed in two rows of four each and allow about 80 degrees of *palmar (volar)* flexion of the wrist. Deviation (turning) of the wrist toward the ulnar (little finger) side is about 45 degrees; deviation toward the radial (thumb) side only about 15 degrees. Rotary motion (*circumduction*) of the hand describes a full circle when you combine the movements of deviation, flexion, extension, pronation, and supination of the wrist, as in dialing a telephone (see Figure 15-13).

Distal to the eight carpal bones are the five *metacarpals.* These are elongated bones, slender in the middle, and enlarged somewhat at each end. They are slightly concave (curved inward; rounded and somewhat hollowed out) on the palmar side, lending a shallow saucerlike contour to the palm.

The fingers each have *three phalanges,* whereas the thumbs each have only two. The many joints in the wrist and hand, as well as the powerful forearm muscles activating them, make the hand a very useful prehensile (adapted for grasping) mechanism on the end of a long, highly mobile and muscular upper extremity. Small muscles within the hand, called the *intrinsic* muscles of the hand, control fine movements of pinching—positioning the digits for grasping, adducting and abducting the digits as in typing or playing the piano, and pill-rolling movements as in identifying or manipulating small objects such as coins, pencils, tube caps, or bobby pins. Patients who have suffered strokes or have severe arthritis of the hands may have great difficulty buttoning clothing if they have intrinsic muscle weakness.

The lower limbs. The *femur* is the longest and strongest bone in the body. The ball-shaped head, or upper end, of this bone fits into the hip socket, or *acetabulum*. Roman anatomists named the hip socket *acetabulum* because of its resemblance to a vinegar cruet, in which vinegar (*acetum*) was served. The *thigh* is that portion of the lower limb between the hip and the knee; therefore the femur is commonly called the thighbone.

The **leg** is that portion of the lower extremity reaching from the knee to the ankle. There are two long bones in the leg. The larger of the two is the *tibia* ("tube" or "flute"). The long, slender bone toward the outer side of the leg is called *fibula* because it resembles a clasp or pin. The tibia, or shinbone, is the chief weight-bearing bone in the leg, whereas the fibula serves almost exclusively for calf muscle attachments.

The upper end of the tibia has two broad plateaus, slightly cupped, which receive the rounded condyles of the lower femur, forming the knee joint. Condyles are the large, rounded bulges at the distal end of each femur. There is one condyle on the medial surface and one condyle on the lateral surface of each femur (see Figure 18-6). Strong ligaments and fascial (sheets of connective tissue) bands on all sides of the knee help support this heavy weight–bearing joint.

The *patella* (kneepan or **kneecap**) is the largest *sesamoid* bone (resembling a sesame seed) in the body and is found in the front of the knee joint. It is covered by the heavy quadriceps tendon, which continues below the patella, as the patellar ligament, to insert into the front of the upper tibia.

The ankle and foot. The lower ends of tibia and fibula are slightly enlarged and are called the medial (tibial) and lateral (tibular) *malleoli* (diminutive of *malleus,* hammer). They are the bony prominences readily felt and seen on either side of the ankle. The large notch between them is the *ankle mortise,* into which the *talus* fits, completing the ankle joint. The talus is the uppermost of the tarsals—one of the bones of the ankle.

The hindfoot and midfoot contain seven tarsal bones. The forefoot includes five metatarsals and 14 phalanges of the toes. As in the four fingers of the hand, we find three phalanges in each of the four lesser toes. The great toe resembles the thumb in that it has only two phalanges. Big toes may be surgically transplanted to replace amputated thumbs.

The largest tarsal is the heel bone, called *calcaneus* or *os calcis.* It makes the first contact with the ground when we are walking or jogging. The tarsal bones join the metatarsal bones or instep bones to form a longitudinal arch extending from heel to toe. Arches are architecturally sound, giving more

supporting strength per given amount of material than any other type of structural construction. The arches created by the bones form a highly stable base (for example, as in standing or walking). Strong leg muscle tendons and strong ligaments hold the foot bones in their arched position. If these weaken, it will cause the arches to flatten—a condition commonly referred to as flatfeet or fallen arches. Toward the distal ends of the metatarsals, there is a transverse arch crossing the forefoot from side to side. These arches sometimes flatten out when supporting muscles and ligaments become overstressed by excess body weight or improper footwear. A shoe with a pointed toe or one that is too narrow or too short may cause disfiguring enlargement of the great toe joint, creating a *bunion.* Diseases such as poliomyelitis, spastic muscle imbalance, or birth defects such as clubfoot may seriously deform the feet.

FUNCTIONAL DIFFERENCES AND CHANGES

Although the structures of the lower and upper extremities have some similarity, their functional uses are quite different. The hip joint is more stable than the shoulder but has less free range of motion. The knee can endure much greater stresses than the elbow can while moving in a flat plane of flexion and extension. The forearm can rotate almost 180 degrees in combined pronation and supination, whereas the leg has very little ability to rotate or to accommodate to rotational stresses. The foot, built strongly to support the body weight, lacks the dexterity and suppleness of the hand.

The skeleton is not a dead and static affair. In youth, bones are more readily altered in shape than in mature years. Cells within bones are constantly functioning in response to stresses placed on them. An example of this occurs when a bone is broken and healing occurs during the next few weeks. But even in maturity the bone cells are active and are always responsive to the physical and chemical forces that play on them. They are collectively a large reservoir of calcium and other minerals that may be drawn on under conditions of stress such as pregnancy or malnutrition.

HEMATOPOIESIS

Bones also serve a very important function in making blood cells. The ends of long bones contain red bone marrow. RBCs, some types of white blood cells (WBCs), and platelets are produced in the ends of long bones. The formation and development of blood cells is called *hematopoiesis.* In the center cavity of the shaft of long bones there is yellow bone marrow. The fatty tissue of the yellow marrow provides stored energy.

THE MUSCULAR SYSTEM

There are more than 600 muscles in the human body, (Figure 18-8) the function of which are to:
- Aid in movement
- Provide and maintain posture
- Protect internal organs

Figure 18-8 *A, Muscular system.*
From LaFleur M, Starr W: *Exploring medical language: a student-directed approach*, ed 2, St. Louis, 1989, Mosby.

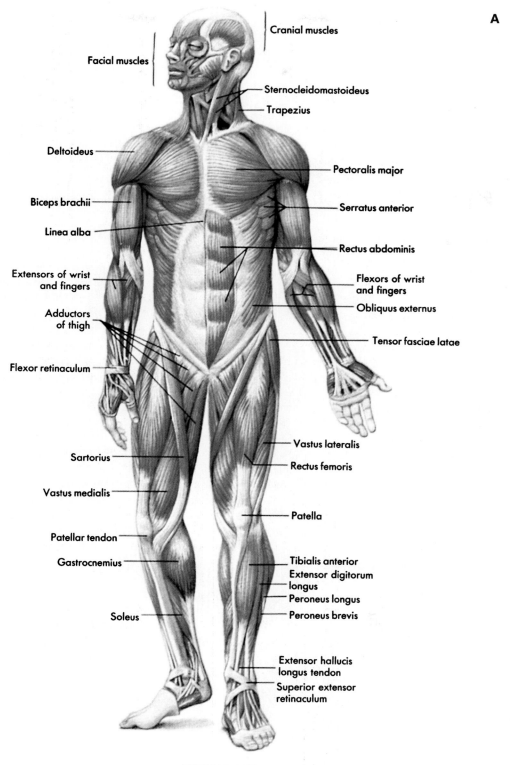

A

Cranial muscles

Facial muscles

Sternocleidomastoideus

Trapezius

Deltoideus

Pectoralis major

Serratus anterior

Biceps brachii

Linea alba

Rectus abdominis

Extensors of wrist and fingers

Flexors of wrist and fingers

Obliquus externus

Adductors of thigh

Tensor fasciae latae

Flexor retinaculum

Vastus lateralis

Sartorius

Rectus femoris

Vastus medialis

Patella

Patellar tendon

Gastrocnemius

Tibialis anterior

Extensor digitorum longus

Peroneus longus

Peroneus brevis

Soleus

Extensor hallucis longus tendon

Superior extensor retinaculum

ANTERIOR VIEW

Figure 18-8—cont'd B, *Muscular system.*
From LaFleur M, Starr W: *Exploring medical language: a student-directed approach*, ed 2, St. Louis, 1989, Mosby.

B

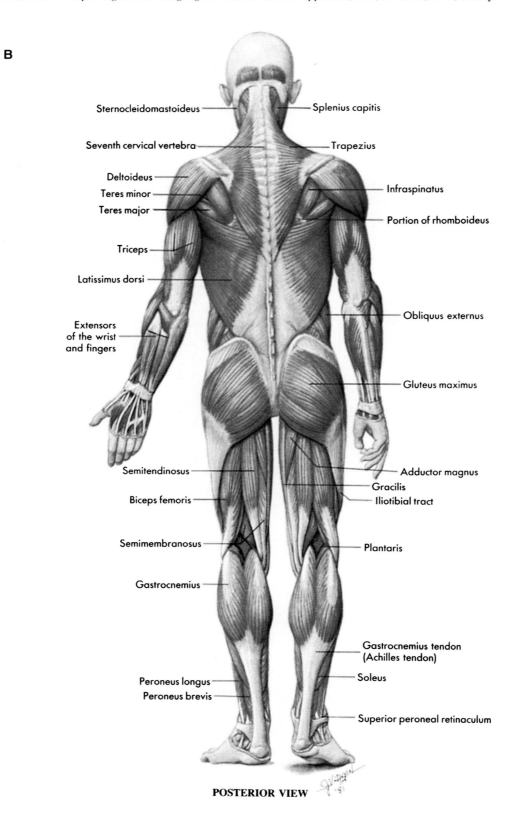

Sternocleidomastoideus — — Splenius capitis

Seventh cervical vertebra — — Trapezius

Deltoideus — — Infraspinatus
Teres minor —
Teres major — — Portion of rhomboideus

Triceps —

Latissimus dorsi —

— Obliquus externus

Extensors
of the wrist
and fingers —

— Gluteus maximus

Semitendinosus — — Adductor magnus
— Gracilis
Biceps femoris — — Iliotibial tract

Semimembranosus — — Plantaris

Gastrocnemius —

— Gastrocnemius tendon
(Achilles tendon)
Peroneus longus — — Soleus
Peroneus brevis —

— Superior peroneal retinaculum

POSTERIOR VIEW

- Provide movement of blood, food, and waste products through the body
- Open and close body openings
- Produce heat

TYPES OF MUSCLES

There are three different kinds of muscle found in the body. One is the extensive distribution of muscle masses over the skeleton, providing power for movement and giving form and substance to the extremities. These are the **skeletal** muscles. Another is a special kind of muscle that forms the heart walls. This is **cardiac** muscle. The third, **smooth muscle** or **visceral muscle,** differs from the preceding two. It is found in the eye, the walls of the alimentary canal, blood vessels, and various ducts and channels that transmit fluids; and it even comprises the bulk of an organ, the womb (uterus). Skeletal muscle is called **voluntary** because it can contract under voluntary control. Smooth muscle is called **involuntary** because its contractions are not under voluntary control. It is controlled instead by reflexes and portions of the nervous system below the centers of conscious control. Skeletal muscle is called **striated** because it shows parallel striped markings under the microscope, and smooth muscle is called **nonstriated** since it lacks these markings.

Skeletal Muscle

Skeletal muscles generally attach to bones and commonly to two bones. Skeletal muscles usually produce their effects on parts at some distance from the muscle mass. Thus the power shown in the foot when one runs or rises on the toes is located in the calf of the leg. It is transmitted to the foot through structures called *tendons,* which attach muscles to bones. If the strong movement in the ankle had to be accomplished by muscle masses located there, the ankle would be many times its present size, and the presence of the muscles there would of course limit movement itself.

Bodily line is determined by skeletal formation, by fat underneath the skin, and by the size and contour of muscles. Notice, for example, the curves of the arm that reflect underlying muscles, the lateral and medial enlargement of the calf in the leg, the margins of the trunk, and the crescentic (a crescent-shaped structure) roll of the neck. It is an interesting and important fact that a person's postures are expression of muscular action.

Cardiac Muscle

The second variety of muscle, *cardiac,* forms the walls of the heart. The primary function of cardiac muscle is for contraction of the heart. The left ventricle wall in the heart is much thicker than the right wall. There is reason for this striking difference. The left ventricle pumps blood over the entire body against a high resistance or pressure. The right ventricle supplies blood a shorter distance to the lungs against a lower resistance or pressure, and its walls are therefore not as thick as those of the left ventricle. Most persons appreciate from their own experiences that working a muscle increases its size and strengthens it. The heart is a muscle, and the greater work done by the left side produces a larger muscle than the one on the right side. The heart muscle is kept strong by physical activity in precisely the same way that other muscles are maintained in strength.

Smooth or Visceral Muscle

Smooth or visceral muscle, which is *not* under voluntary control, comprises important parts of the walls of all blood vessels except the tiny capillaries. It is found in the walls of all hollow organs or tubes and hence in the whole length of the digestive tract. It also forms the main part of the iris of the eye, and its movements there dilate and constrict the pupil.

It is not so important for you to know the names of the muscles as it is to know the kinds of things muscles do. The muscles of the face are used when we laugh or smile or frown. Muscles control the movements of the eyes and open and close the lids. They move the lips and tongue and jaw. Large, flat muscles extend like bands along the shoulders and on either side of the backbone. We stimulate the nerves and circulation of blood in these muscles when we rub a back. Muscles furnish support for the abdominal organs and hold the uterus in place. They are indispensable to the breathing process for the heartbeat, and in moving food along the digestive canal.

THE CIRCULATORY SYSTEM

Two components of the circulatory system are the cardiovascular system (CVS) and the lymphatic system (Figure 18-9). The CVS consists of the heart and blood vessels. The lymphatic system consists of lymphatic vessels, lymph nodes, lymph, and specialized organs such as the spleen and thymus.

Circulation in humans exhibits several distinctive characteristics. The heart in the thorax hangs from several large vessels and rests on the *diaphragm,* the muscle that separates the chest from the abdominal cavity.

The vessels usually lie in protected places. The large vessels of the arm, lying in the armpit, pass downward on the inner side of the arm. In the lower extremity they are disposed toward the midline, and at the knee they pass behind the joint.

Food materials and oxygen must be delivered to all parts of the body. Waste materials must be collected and carried to the organs through which our bodies rid themselves of waste. These two functions are performed by means of the blood itself, the blood vessels, the lymphatics, and the heart. In addition to pumping blood, the circulatory system carries warmth to the tissues and hormones, enzymes, various chemicals, protective immune bodies, and other substances to all parts of the body.

THE BLOOD

The amount of blood in the body of an adult varies with weight. If one weighs 132 pounds (60 kg), the amount will be 4 quarts (3.8 L). The color varies from bright to dark red, depending on the amount of oxygen or carbon dioxide present in the red cells. It is half cells and half liquid, although it

Figure 18-9 A, *Circulatory system.*
From LaFleur M, Starr W: *Exploring medical language: a student-directed approach,* ed 2, St. Louis, 1989, Mosby.

A

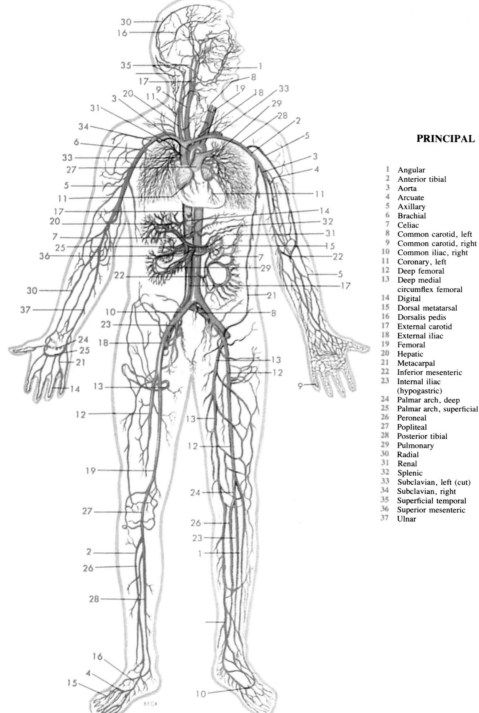

PRINCIPAL VEINS AND ARTERIES

1	Angular	1	Anterior tibial
2	Anterior tibial	2	Axillary
3	Aorta	3	Basilic
4	Arcuate	4	Brachial
5	Axillary	5	Cephalic
6	Brachial	6	Cervical plexus
7	Celiac	7	Colic
8	Common carotid, left	8	Common iliac, left
9	Common carotid, right	9	Digital
10	Common iliac, right	10	Dorsal venous arch
11	Coronary, left	11	External jugular
12	Deep femoral	12	Femoral
13	Deep medial circumflex femoral	13	Great saphenous
14	Digital	14	Hepatic
15	Dorsal metatarsal	15	Inferior mesenteric
16	Dorsalis pedis	16	Inferior sagittal sinus
17	External carotid	17	Inferior vena cava
18	External iliac	18	Brachiocephalic, left
19	Femoral	19	Internal jugular, left
20	Hepatic	20	Internal jugular, right
21	Metacarpal	21	Lateral thoracic
22	Inferior mesenteric	22	Median cubital
23	Internal iliac (hypogastric)	23	Peroneal
24	Palmar arch, deep	24	Popliteal
25	Palmar arch, superficial	25	Portal
26	Peroneal	26	Posterior tibial
27	Popliteal	27	Pulmonary
28	Posterior tibial	28	Subclavian, left
29	Pulmonary	29	Superior mesenteric
30	Radial	30	Superior sagittal sinus
31	Renal	31	Superior vena cava
32	Splenic		
33	Subclavian, left (cut)		
34	Subclavian, right		
35	Superficial temporal		
36	Superior mesenteric		
37	Ulnar		

Figure 18-9—cont'd B, *Circulatory system.*
From LaFleur M, Starr W: *Exploring medical language: a student-directed approach*, ed 2, St. Louis, 1989, Mosby.

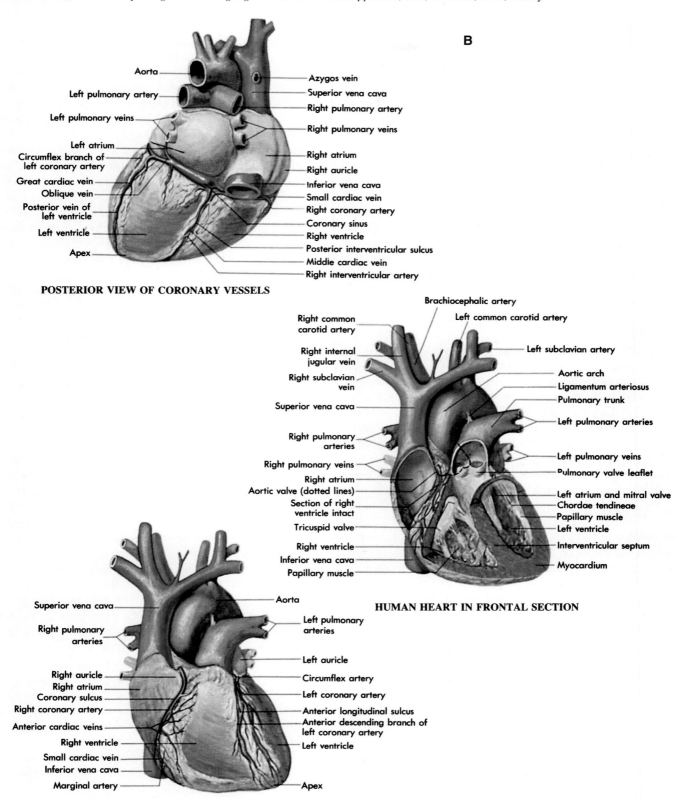

B

POSTERIOR VIEW OF CORONARY VESSELS

HUMAN HEART IN FRONTAL SECTION

ANTERIOR VIEW OF CORONARY VESSELS

appears all liquid until something causes it to clot. The liquid part is known as the *blood plasma;* it is light yellow in color, transparent, and almost entirely water. Dissolved in this liquid are food materials, salt, protective substances, and waste materials. *Blood serum* is blood plasma from which the fibrinogen and all clotting elements, the platelets, and the red and white cells have been removed by permitting the blood to stand until it clots. The blood picks up waste materials from all parts of the body. It also contains those substances made by the endocrine glands called *hormones* and certain other substances that aid in body resistance to disease. There are three kinds of cells or corpuscles in the blood—RBCs, WBCs, and platelets (also see Unit Thirteen).

Red Blood Cells

The *RBCs (erythrocytes)* are the most numerous and get their color from an iron compound called *hemoglobin.* Hemoglobin combines with the oxygen breathed into the lungs, and the red cells are a bright or darker red, depending on the amount of oxygen they have absorbed. The RBCs are made in the red marrow of the bones, are released into the bloodstream, and live for about 4 months.

White Blood Cells

The *WBCs (leukocytes),* some of which are formed in the red bone marrow and some of which are formed in the lymph nodes and spleen, are larger than the RBCs but fewer in number. There is about one white blood cell to every 600 or 700 red cells. The white cells can move through the walls of the blood vessels and are part of the body's protection against infection. When infectious organisms enter the body, these white cells are attracted in great numbers and surround and destroy the invading organisms. The pus in wounds is comprised of dead and living white cells.

Platelets

In addition to red and white cells, the blood contains small cells called *platelets.* These cells, also called *thrombocytes,* are important in the process of blood clot formation. They are formed in red bone marrow.

When blood vessels are injured, the blood is exposed to substances that cause it to clot. The clot acts as a plug or cork, and the bleeding stops. There is a normal time for the clotting of blood, and if the blood does not clot within that time, there may be a deficiency of one or more of the presently recognized *blood factors* responsible for clotting.

Conditions Affecting the Blood

Loss of large amounts of blood is called *hemorrhage.* Hemorrhage may also be caused by many conditions. There may be a decreased number or altered function of platelets when the clot will form but will not retract. Capillaries may be weak, and hemorrhage result. Many infections, allergies, and certain diseases may be the cause of these conditions.

A *thrombus* is a blood clot within the walls of a blood vessels. If a thrombus becomes loosened from the blood vessel and travels in the bloodstream, it is called an *embolus.* A loosened blood clot may block circulation at some vital point and cause death.

Anemia is a condition characterized by an insufficient concentration of *hemoglobin,* which carries oxygen in the blood, or a reduction of the number of RBCs. Often both situations exist.

Different types of anemia have different causes. *Pernicious anemia* involves inadequately developed RBCs. It results from poor absorption of vitamin B_{12}, which is needed in the formation of RBCs. *Iron-deficiency anemia* involves an inadequate amount of hemoglobin caused by a shortage of iron. *Sickle-cell anemia* is an inherited disorder in which the RBCs become crescent or sickle shaped if subjected to low levels of blood oxygen, and are unable to supply sufficient oxygen to the body tissues. It is caused by an abnormal type of hemoglobin(s). This disease causes severe pain and premature death. *Aplastic anemia* is caused by disease of the bone marrow or destruction of the bone marrow by certain agents, especially chemicals. This condition is frequently fatal.

The number of blood cells and the amount of hemoglobin can be estimated in the laboratory. The RBCs usually number 4,500,000 to 5,000,000 per cubic millimeter of blood. The WBCs usually number between 5000 and 9000 per cubic millimeter of blood. The term *leukocytosis* is applied to the condition in which there are more than this number present, as in the presence of infections. *Leukopenia* is an abnormally low white blood cell count.

THE CARDIOVASCULAR SYSTEM
Blood Vessels

The blood is carried through the body in a network of tubes of various sizes called *arteries, veins,* and *capillaries.* The arteries carry the blood away from the heart through the *aorta,* the largest artery, and its branches. The aorta resembles a large tube and divides into smaller tubes to carry the blood to all parts of the body. The walls of the arteries are somewhat elastic. The smallest division of the arteries, the arterioles, join a network of very tiny tubes called *capillaries,* which bring the blood to venules, the smallest veins, then to similar divisions of the *veins,* the blood vessels that bring the blood back to the heart. The blood is emptied into the right atrium of the heart by two large veins known as the *superior* and *inferior venae cavae.* The superior vena cava brings the blood from the upper part of the body, and the inferior vena cava brings the blood back to the heart from the lower part of the body (from below heart level). Like the aorta, the two large veins divide into many branches. Many of them contain little flaps or folds called *valves,* which prevent the blood from flowing back into the capillaries.

With the exception of the pulmonary artery to the lungs, blood in the arteries is oxygenated. Except for the pulmonary veins from the lungs, blood in veins is deoxygenated.

Pulse and Pressure in the Arteries

The heart pumps the blood through the blood vessels. You can feel the force of the heart contraction over certain arteries that lie fairly close to the skin. If you put a finger over these arteries, you can feel the wave of pressure caused by each heartbeat. Counting the number of waves for a minute is called *taking the pulse.* Pulse is usually counted at the wrist, the side of the neck, or the temple because these arteries are easily accessible. As arteries become older, their walls may become harder and less elastic. A condition that is popularly called hardening of the arteries (*arteriosclerosis*) sometimes develops. The pressure within arteries is called the *blood pressure* and is higher in adults than in children. Weight, exercise, and emotional disturbances influence blood pressure. Pressure greatly above or below normal for any age has great medical significance. It can be measured by an apparatus known as the *sphygmomanometer.* Measurement of blood pressure should always be included in any complete physical examination. Also see Unit Two.

The Heart

The heart is a hollow muscular organ, about the size of the person's fist, that pumps blood through the body. It is located in the left lower part of the chest cavity and is divided into two sides, the left and the right, by a solid wall called the *septum.* Each of these sides is divided into two chambers. Deoxygenated blood is brought from the upper and lower parts of the body by the superior and inferior venae cavae and emptied into the *right atrium,* which is the upper right chamber; it then passes into the *right ventricle,* which is the lower right chamber (see Figures 16-1 and 18-9, *B*). The opening between these chambers is provided with flaps that create a valve (the *tricuspid valve*) that prevents blood from flowing backward from the right ventricle to the right atrium. As the heart contracts, it pumps blood from the right ventricle through the *pulmonary valve* into the pulmonary artery and to the lungs, where the blood gives off carbon dioxide and picks up oxygen that is brought in from the air we breathe. The blood in the right side of the heart is dark red in color, having left most of its oxygen in the cells of the body in exchange for carbon dioxide. Picking up oxygen in the lungs and giving up carbon dioxide to be exhaled, the blood again becomes bright red and flows back to the heart through the four pulmonary veins into the *left atrium,* the upper chamber on the left side of the heart. Between the left atrium and the left ventricle, there is another set of flaps that form a valve (the *mitral valve*) that keeps the blood from flowing backward when the heart contracts. Blood passes into the *left ventricle* and is then pumped out through the aorta to the body. Blood is kept from flowing backward from the aorta to the ventricle by the *aortic valve.* Failure of any of the valves of the heart may cause the heart to pump inefficiently and lead to heart failure.

For the heart to pump efficiently, valves must function properly, and there must be continuous supply of blood to provide oxygen and nutrients to it. The two coronary arteries, which arise from the aorta just beyond the aortic valve, serve this function.

Specialized heart tissue called the *conduction system* is also required for the heart to beat effectively to maintain life. See Unit Sixteen for more information on the conduction system and the heartbeat.

Heart disease. The heart is enclosed in a thin sac called the *pericardium.* The muscular part of the heart is called the *myocardium;* the inner lining of the heart, the *endocardium. Pericarditis, myocarditis,* and *endocarditis* are forms of heart disease caused by infection or inflammation of these structures.

If the coronary arteries become severely narrowed, insufficient blood reaches the heart muscle. Narrowing and occlusion of these arteries because of deposition of fatty substances (*atherosclerosis*) is called *coronary artery disease* and is a leading cause of death throughout the world.

When insufficient quantities of blood reach the heart muscle, severe chest pain, called *angina pectoris,* may result. Individuals suffering from this condition are said to have *coronary insufficiency.* If the supply is seriously impaired, some of the heart muscle may actually die. This is called a *heart attack,* or a *myocardial infarction coronary.*

Some individuals with a heart attack have a clot or thrombus in their coronary arteries. The term *coronary thrombosis* is used to describe this condition.

Physiology of Blood Pressure

There are many factors that influence blood pressure. The most obvious is the *force* of the pumping action of the heart muscle. If the *volume* of blood in the system decreases, as with sudden hemorrhage, the blood pressure falls. If the *volume* of blood returning to the heart increases, as in raising the patient's feet and lowering the head, the blood pressure rises. If the *resistance* offered by the small blood vessels is increased as in arteriosclerosis, atherosclerosis, or chronic (sticky, gummy, or thick) nephritis; if blood becomes abnormally viscous; if the patient is consistently overweight; or if arterial walls lose their elasticity, the heart has to pump harder to maintain blood pressure high enough to deliver necessary elements to all body tissues. If a prolonged state of high blood pressure (*hypertension*) exists, the heart may become seriously overburdened and fail.

Through a system of nerve and chemical and hormonal controls, the body has the ability to respond to chemical sensors in the walls of the aorta and carotid arteries in and certain centers in the brain. Strong emotions such as love, hate, fear, anger, or sadness and stimuli from our special sense organs of sight, sound, smell, or touch can trigger alarm reactions, which sharply affect blood pressure.

The valves in our veins and the so-called reservoirs in the liver, spleen, other viscera, and the muscles exert some mechanical control over circulating blood volume and pressure. Exercise increases blood pressure temporarily, and rest tends to lower it.

Normal *systolic* (when the heart muscle contracts) blood pressure varies with individuals. It is said to be somewhat less than 100 millimeters of mercury (mm Hg) at birth and gradually rises throughout childhood, reaching about 120 mm Hg in healthy young adults. *Diastolic* pressure (when the heart is resting between contractions) averages about 80 mm Hg in most adults.

Drugs that speed up heart rate or increase stroke volume, or inhibit these activities can affect blood pressure in a matter of seconds. Changes in blood (oxygen or carbon dioxide concentrations) can stimulate brain centers to act automatically to adjust heart and respiration rates and blood pressure.

The method of taking blood pressure is described in detail in Unit Two. The complex subject of the physiology of blood pressure is discussed at length and in understandable terms in other references.*

THE LYMPHATIC SYSTEM

In addition to the arterial and venous systems, which circulate blood throughout the body, there is a third part to the circulatory system, called the **lymphatic system** (Figure 18-10). It is a system comprised of *capillary channels* that convey *lymph* and *interstitial* fluid (extracellular fluid filling spaces between most of the cells, bathing most tissues) from all parts of the body into the *lymph channels,* which finally reach the larger *lymphatic ducts.* These ducts empty into the venous system of the body at the right and left sides of the neck where the subclavian veins join the internal jugular veins.

There is no distinct pumping mechanism such as the heart to move fluid along the lymphatic system. Instead, the lymphatic vessels and ducts are equipped with *semilunar valves,* which permit flow only in one direction, toward the junctions of the *internal jugulars* and the *subclavian veins,* right and left.

The entire right upper extremity, the right side of the head and neck, and the right thoracic region are drained by the *right lymphatic system.* The remainder of the entire body is drained by the *lymphatic capillaries* leading into the *thoracic duct* and finally into the *left internal jugular* and *subclavian veins.* It is also important to know that the drainage from the intestinal tract of the *chyle,* containing absorption products after digestion of food, makes it way into the *cisterna chyli* just below the *diaphragm.* From there it enters the *thoracic duct* and finally reaches the bloodstream at the *left internal jugular/left subclavian* juncture.

The force that slowly moves the lymphatic fluid toward the heart is supplied by skeletal muscle action involved in breathing, coughing, and sneezing, or in any muscle action that may increase intraabdominal pressure such as straining to do muscular work. Elevation of any of the extremities above heart level lowers pressure in the extremity and promotes both *lymphatic* and *venous* drainage toward the right side of the heart. For this reason, injured arms or legs must be kept elevated above heart level as much as possible to minimize swelling.

Lymph Nodes and Lymph Glands

In the lymphatic systems there are additional structures called *lymph glands* or *nodes.* These seem to serve as delaying or fil-

tering stations where the lymph is subjected to "search and seizure" of foreign materials such as bacteria or foreign proteins, which may be destroyed by phagocytic WBCs before they can do harm to the whole individual. Phagocytes are cells that engulf and destroy bacteria or other foreign microorganisms and particles (also see Unit Five).

Lymph nodes are usually round in shape, about the size of a pea or bean, and are found in groupings at the *inguinal, femoral,* and *axillary* regions. There is a chain of nodes along each side of the *neck* that may be readily palpated during inflammations of the sinuses, teeth, or throat. Lymph channels in the skin are often seen as inflamed, reddish streaks when an acute infection involves tissues drained by those parts of the lymphatic system. There are chains of lymph nodes in the *abdomen* and in the *chest,* which may become involved in the spread of cancer or disease such as *tuberculosis.*

The *thymus gland* is located behind the breastbone and is much larger in children than in adults. Although some of its functions are not quite clear, it is well known that this gland is very important in creating cells capable of recognizing foreign substances in the body. These cells are called *lymphocytes* and are important in the body's ability to fight off infection.

Several large glandular organs such as the thymus, liver, pancreas, spleen, adrenals, prostate, kidneys, and thyroid are also richly supplied with lymphatic capillaries. Thus cancers or infections of glands such as the breast, the pancreas, or the prostate frequently spread, or *metastasize,* to distant places by way of the lymphatic channels and nodes, as well as by the blood vessels.

Summary of Function

In summary, the lymphatic system is important as a rich source of *lymphocytes* (a type of WBC) as a protection against infection and is involved in the overall function of the immune system, which plays a critical role in protecting the body against disease (also see Unit Five).

It is also a collecting system that returns intercellular body fluids containing valuable salts, water, and proteins to the bloodstream. Products of food digestion are extracted from the gut by *lacteals* and delivered by the lymphatics to the bloodstream. Unfortunately, when its protective abilities cannot cope successfully with infection or cancer, the lymphatic system can become a route for spread of infection or cancer to other parts of the body, resulting in death if treatment is not successful in stopping the progress of the disease.

THE NERVOUS SYSTEM

The nervous system is one of the most complex and least understood body systems. New discoveries are made continuously about the capabilities of the nervous system. The functions of the nervous system are to sense, interpret, and respond to internal and external environmental changes to maintain a steady state in the body (homeostasis). There is excitation, conduction, and integration.

*From Thibodeau GA: *Textbook of anatomy and physiology,* ed 13, St. Louis, 1990, Mosby, Chapter 15.

Figure 18-10 A, *Lymphatic system.*
From LaFleur M, Starr W: *Exploring medical language: a student-directed approach*, ed 2, St. Louis, 1989, Mosby.

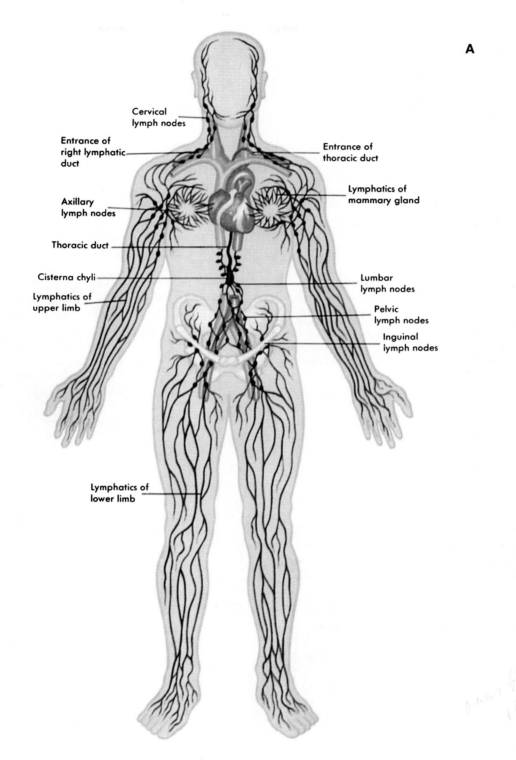

LYMPHATIC SYSTEM

Figure 18-10—cont'd   B, *Lymphatic system.*
From LaFleur M, Starr W: *Exploring medical language: a student-directed approach*, ed 2, St. Louis, 1989, Mosby.

B

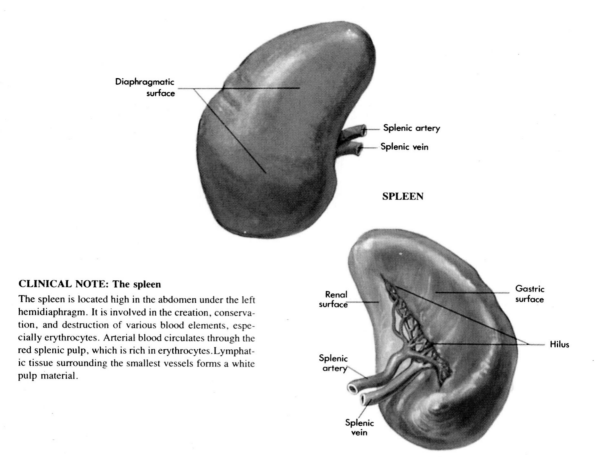

SPLEEN

CLINICAL NOTE: The spleen
The spleen is located high in the abdomen under the left hemidiaphragm. It is involved in the creation, conservation, and destruction of various blood elements, especially erythrocytes. Arterial blood circulates through the red splenic pulp, which is rich in erythrocytes. Lymphatic tissue surrounding the smallest vessels forms a white pulp material.

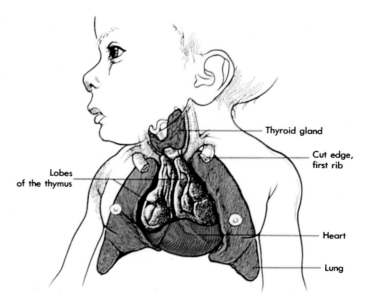

LOCATION AND GROSS ANATOMY OF THYMUS

Excitation operates through the function of specialized cells arranged to form structures that pick up particular messages from the environment (Figure 18-11). The papillae of the tongue are taste receptors. The ending of the auditory nerve is an elaborate receptor for picking up sound vibrations transmitted to the inner ear. The eye is one of the most highly developed of the sensory receptors, with numerous parts that direct light rays on the retina, which contains filaments of the optic nerve. Touch receptors are in the skin. These are the more obvious receptors, but in addition there are sense organs that pour into central stations messages of excitation from internal parts. It may be said then that from the environment and from the organism itself constantly arise excitations that bring to central stations a vast amount of information regarding the surrounding world and the state of the organism itself.

The **conduction** pathways, or nerves, pass to and from the cord and brain. The structure known as a **nerve** is composed of fibers that are extensions of nerve cells in the cord and brain or nerve cell masses outside the cord, known as *ganglia.* Those fibers carrying stimuli toward the brain are called *afferent* fibers, and those leading away from the brain and spinal cord are called *efferent* fibers. The cell bodies of efferent nerves are within the cord or brain, whereas those of afferent nerves are in the spinal sensory ganglia on each side of the cord or in the brain.

The brain is a highly developed center. It serves to **integrate** messages received from both the external and the internal environment. Some of these messages are handled automatically by *internuncial* fibers in the cord, which complete a simple reflex arc without the stimulus reaching the brain for a decision. This is the pattern of the simple knee-jerk reflex over which we have no conscious control. Bundles or strands of **nerve fibers** gathered together outside of the spinal cord or brain are called *peripheral nerves*, whereas organized pathways of nerve fibers within the brain or the spinal cord are called *tracts*. Peripheral nerves characteristically have mixtures of afferent and efferent fibers side by side. Tracts in the brain or spinal cord, however, are purely afferent or purely efferent, depending on their specific function of transmitting stimuli either toward the brain or away from it.

The nervous system is divided into two major divisions: the central nervous system (CNS) and the peripheral nervous system (PNS) (Figure 18-11, *C*).

THE CENTRAL NERVOUS SYSTEM (CNS)

The CNS is made up of the brain and the spinal cord. It functions as the coordinator of the body's full nervous system and contains the nerves that control connections between impulses coming to and from the brain and the rest of the body. The CNS plays a crucial role in maintaining a healthy, normally functioning body.

The Brain

The brain weighs about 3 pounds (1.4 kg) in the adult and reaches its full growth at about the twentieth year (Figure 18-

11, *D*). It is a delicate structure, and the bones of the skull serve as a protection from injury. It is covered by three membranes called **meninges.** The meninges include the dura mater ('hard mother'), a tough outer covering; the arachnoid ('like a spider web'), a very delicate membrane; and the pia mater ('tender mother'), richly supplied with blood vessels. The dura is firmly attached to the inner table of the skull. The pia is next to the brain, and the arachnoid lies between the dura and the pia mater. There are potential spaces between these membranes. Between the arachnoid and the pia the *subarachnoid space* is filled with clear, watery fluid that acts as a cushion all about the brain and cord.

The cerebrum. The outer portion, or *cortex* of the brain, is called the *cerebrum* and is made up of a convoluted (rolled together; a fold of the brain) layer of millions of nerve cells termed *gray matter*. Afferent (incoming) fibers transmit messages from all parts of the body to the cells of the cerebrum; decisions are made, and efferent (outgoing) fibers carry messages away from the brain to some muscle group, organ, or gland for appropriate response. The inner portion of the brain is composed of *white matter* made up of nerve fibers that communicate with the nerve cells in the gray matter (see Figure 18-11, D).

Control centers. The cerebrum is the largest part of the brain. It contains the control centers for the five special senses of sight, hearing, touch, smell, and taste. It also controls speaking, learning, thinking, and remembering. It sets in motion many acts we do voluntarily, as well as those that take place without our thinking about them, such as right or left handedness, consciousness, performance of skills, display of emotions, and the integration of our various activities.

Cerebellum. The back part of the brain is known as the *cerebellum*. It controls the coordination of muscular activities. It has direct connections with the cerebrum and coordinates thought and action with the sights, sounds, and other stimuli received from our environment.

Medulla. The connection between the brain and the spinal cord is through the *spinal bulb,* or *medulla*. The medulla is beneath the cerebellum, and its lower end is the beginning of the spinal cord. It controls our breathing and the action of the heart and blood vessels (see Figure 18-11, *C*; Table 18-2).

Spinal Cord. The spinal cord extends down through the length of the thoracic spine. It is covered by extensions of the three membranes, the meninges, covering the brain. The space between the two inner membranes is filled with the same clear fluid that surrounds the brain, *cerebrospinal fluid* (CSF). Afferent messages come along the nerves from the body to the spinal cord and up to the cerebrum. The cerebrum in turn sends efferent messages back through the cord to nerves that go out to all parts of the body.

Figure 18-11 *A, Nervous system.*
From LaFleur M, Starr W: *Exploring medical language: a student-directed approach*, ed 2, St. Louis, 1989, Mosby.

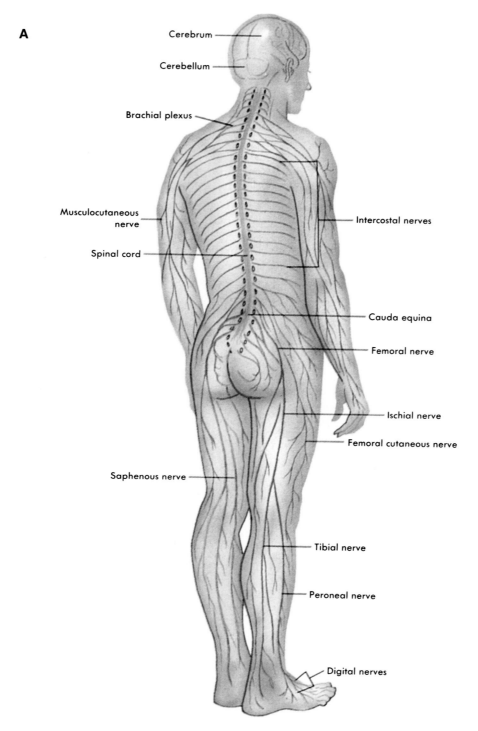

SIMPLIFIED VIEW OF NERVOUS SYSTEM

Figure 18-11—cont'd *B, Nervous system.*
From LaFleur M, Starr W: *Exploring medical language: a student-directed approach*, ed 2, St. Louis, 1989, Mosby.

ANATOMY OF CEREBELLUM

B

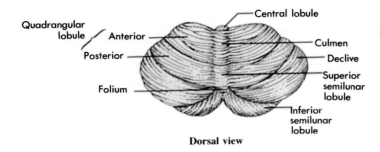

Dorsal view

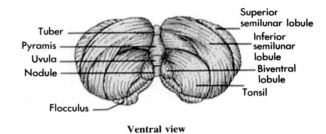

Ventral view

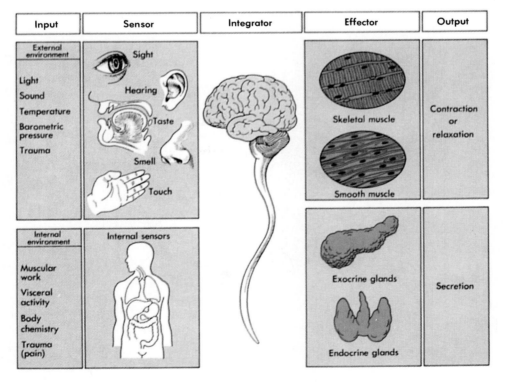

COMPONENTS OF NERVOUS SYSTEM

Figure 18-11—cont'd *C, divisions of the nervous system; D, parts of the brain with major lobes outlined.*
C and D from Gerdin, J: *Health careers today*, St. Louis, 1991, Mosby.

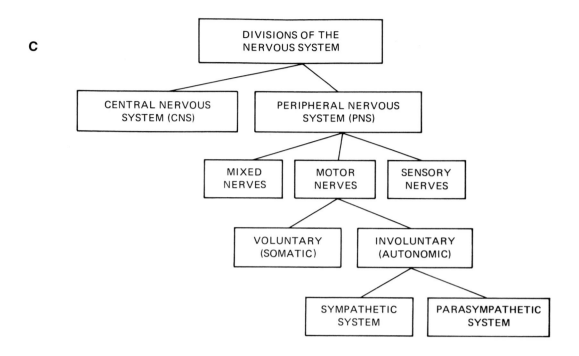

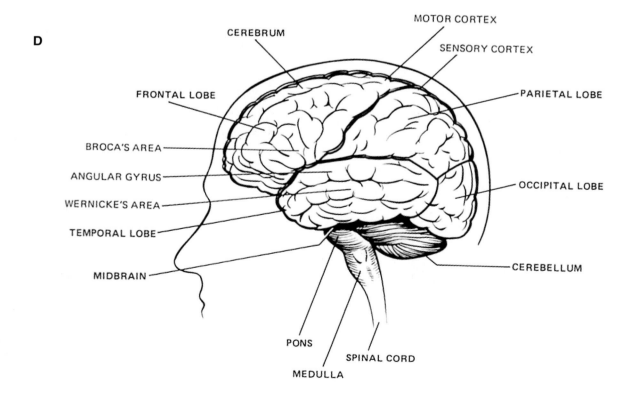

THE PERIPHERAL NERVOUS SYSTEM

The peripheral nervous system consists of 12 pairs of cranial nerves and 31 pairs of spinal nerves (Table 18-2) reaching all parts of the body. The cranial nerves originate in the brain, and the spinal nerves emerge from the spinal cord. The spinal cord nerves can act independently from the brain in some reflex reactions such as is seen in response to an injury of the foot. The organs of the peripheral nervous system contain sensory (afferent) and motor (efferent) neurons. Efferent nerves are classified as voluntary (somatic) or involuntary (autonomic).

Cranial Nerves

The 12 pairs of cranial nerves, designated I to XII, come directly off the underside of the brain and leave the skull through various foramina (openings). They are named in order as follows: I, olfactory; II, optic; III, oculomotor; IV, trochlear; V, trigeminal; VI, abducens; VII, facial; VIII, acoustic, with two parts, a vestibular branch and a cochlear or auditory branch; IX, glossopharyngeal; X, vagus; XI, spinal accessory; and XII, hypoglossal.

Peripheral Nerves

The 31 pairs of peripheral nerves attach to the spinal cord. They leave the spinal canal in pairs, through the foramina (an opening or passageway) in each side of the vertebral column. They do not have individual names but are designated by the vertebral level at which they leave the spinal canal. There are eight cervical pairs, 12 thoracic, five lumbar, five sacral, and one pair of coccygeal nerves (Table 18-3).

Nerve Damage

When nerve pathways are interrupted, the nerve fibers separated from the cell body degenerate. Destruction of a cell body, as in poliomyelitis, also results in degeneration of the nerve pathway. A cut nerve in the arm causes loss of function of the nerve beyond the cut end and results in paralysis of the muscles and loss of sensation in the skin areas supplied by that nerve. If the spinal cord is severely damaged by a fracture or dislocation of the neck, paralysis and sensory loss to arms and legs and the entire body below the neck may result. This is called *quadriplegia*. Damage to the spinal cord in the thoracic region may result in paralysis and sensory loss from the waist down, known as *paraplegia*. Quadriplegia and paraplegia may also be accompanied by loss of *sphincter* control of bladder and bowels, and the patient is said to be incontinent of urine or feces.

AUTONOMIC NERVOUS SYSTEM

Thus far we have been describing in simplified terms the *central nervous system* (CNS), including the brain and the spinal cord. We have also considered briefly the *peripheral nervous system*, which consists of 12 paired cranial nerves and 31 paired spinal nerves. There is another part of the peripheral nervous system. It is probably older developmentally, but in some respects less well known than the systems we have been discussing. It is composed of ganglia (a group of nerve cell bodies) lying outside the cord, with nerves connecting it with the viscera (internal organs within a body cavity, especially the abdominal organs), various

TABLE 18-2

Functions of the Brain

Brain part	Function
Cerebrum	
Frontal lobe	Personality, behavior, memory, reasoning, emotion
Broca's area	Speech
Sensory cortex	Sensations of heat and pain
Motor cortex	Control of movement
Angular gyrus	Written language
Wernicke's area	Understanding written or spoken language
Parietal lobe	Understanding speech, choosing words
Temporal lobe	Hearing, understanding speech and printed words, memory of music and visual scenes
Occipital lobe	Vision and its interpretation
Cerebellum	Coordination of voluntary movement, balance
Brain stem	
Pons	Breathing, relaying impulses between cerebrum and medulla
Medulla	Control of involuntary movements, heartbeat, blood pressure, respiration, swallowing
Midbrain	Visual and auditory reflex
Diencephalon	
Hypothalamus	Regulation and coordination of activity of the autonomic nervous system. Control of hormone secretion and appetite
Thalamus	Transfer of sensory impulses to the sensory areas of the cerebral cortex

TABLE 18-3

Functions of the Peripheral Nervous System

Cranial Nerve Function

Nerve	Function
I. Olfactory	Smell (S)
II. Optic	Vision (S)
III. Oculomotor	Raise eyelid, move eye, focus lens, control pupil size (M)
IV. Trochlear	Rotate eyes (M)
V. Trigeminal	Facial and head sensation; control muscles in floor of mouth for chewing (B)
VI. Abducens	Move eyes laterally (M)
VII. Facial	Taste in anterior of mouth; control facial expression (B)
VIII. Acoustic (auditory)	Hearing and balance (S)
IX. Glossopharyngeal	Taste, swallowing (B)
X. Vagus	Control muscles of speech, swallowing, and of thorax and abdomen; feeling from pharynx, larynx, and trachea (B)
XI. Spinal accessory	Move neck and back muscle (M)
XII. Hypoglossal	Move tongue (M)

Spinal Nerve Function

	Nerve	Areas Controlled
C1-C8	Cervical (8 pair)	Neck and head movement, elevation of shoulders, movement of arms, hands, diaphragmatic breathing
T1-T12	Thoracic (12 pair)	Intercostal muscles of respiration, abdominal contractions
L1-L5	Lumbar (5 pair)	Leg movement
S1-S5	Sacral (5 pair)	Sphincter muscles of anus and urinary meatus; foot movement

S, Sensory; M, motor; B, sensory and motor functions.

glands, and the spinal cord. The functions of this part of the nervous system relate to breathing, digestion, excretion, circulation and blood pressure, sweating or lack of it, functions of the glands of internal secretion, focusing of the eyes, salivation or dryness of the mouth, and all such automatic functions. The autonomic system operates without voluntary control, although it is continually influenced by cerebral function. It functions to maintain or quickly restore homeostasis by regulating the heartbeat, smooth muscle contraction (for example, in blood vessels, bronchial tubes, the stomach, gallbladder, intestines, urinary bladder, spleen, eye, and hair follicles), and glandular secretions (for example, the sweat glands, lacrimal glands, digestive glands, including the liver, pancreas, salivary and gastric glands, and the adrenal medulla).

The two divisions of the autonomic nervous system are:

1. The sympathetic system
2. The parasympathetic system

Sympathetic System

Under normal conditions this system maintains normal functioning of cardiac muscle, smooth muscle, and glands (see previous paragraph for examples of each of these) and maintains normal blood pressure. Under *stress conditions* this system acts like an emergency system and prepares the body for maximum energy expenditure by producing the "fight or flight" syndrome of reactions. Examples of changes resulting in this reaction include stronger, faster heartbeat; dilated bronchi; dilated blood vessels in skeletal muscles; increased blood sugar levels; and secretion of epinephrine from the adrenal glands.

Parasympathetic System

This system functions in response to normal everyday situations. It dominates control of most visceral effectors *most* of the time. For example, the parasympathetic system stimulates digestion of food and slows the heart rate, whereas the sympathetic system inhibits digestion and increases the heart rate.

For example, fear may stop digestion, cause evacuation of bowels or bladder, accelerate the heart, contract some structures, and increase the output of some glands such as the adrenals. The act of lying, feelings of guilt, or fear of detection can cause abnormal deviations on a *polygraph,* recording sudden changes in blood pressure, pulse rate, respirations, and other psychologically induced electric responses by the patient. Keep in mind, however, that a polygraph is simply a recording device for various bodily functions. It is not an infallible "lie detector," as it has been termed, and like all laboratory tests it requires an experienced expert to make proper evaluation of polygraph recordings.

THE DIGESTIVE SYSTEM

The digestive system, also called the gastrointestinal (GI) system, (Figure 18-12) is a tubular conduit about 26 to 30 feet long within which our food is digested and from which our supplies of water and nutrients are absorbed into the bloodstream.

The digestive system extends from the *mouth,* where food and fluids are taken in, to the *rectum* and *anus,* where unabsorbed waste, undigested materials, and bacteria are expelled.

The functions of the digestive system include the ingestion, digestion, and absorption of water and nutrients and the elimination of waste products that were not absorbed.

ORGANS IN THE DIGESTIVE PROCESS

The main organs of the digestive system form a tube often referred to as the alimentary canal or the GI tract. They include the following:
- Mouth
- Oropharynx
- Esophagus
- Stomach
- Small intestine: duodenum, jejunum, and ileum
- Large intestine: cecum, colon (ascending, transverse, descending, and sigmoid colon) (Figure 18-12, *C*)
- Rectum
- Anal canal and anus

Accessory Organs of Digestion

The following organs that aid in the process of digestion include the following:
- Salivary glands: parotid, submandibular, sublingual
- Tongue
- Teeth
- Liver
- Gallbladder
- Pancreas

Teeth. Food is cut and ground into fine particles by the *teeth,* which are rooted firmly in sockets in the upper and lower jawbones. The *root* is that portion of the tooth extending into the body socket. The *crown* extends above the gum, and the *neck* is the slightly narrowed part between the crown and the root. A tooth is composed of *dentin* and contains a

central pulp cavity that encloses the *pulp, blood vessels,* and *nerves. Enamel* protects the crown, and *cement* covers the root. Dentin, enamel, and cement are harder than bone. The front and side teeth are shaped for tearing and cutting, and the back teeth are shaped for grinding. The first set of 20 teeth is temporary and later is replaced by the 32 permanent teeth. The last upper and lower teeth on each side of the mouth are the so-called wisdom teeth and often do not erupt through the gums before the 25th year. They are commonly crowded for space or grow in a wrong direction and may become troublesome and painful.

Liver. The liver is the largest gland in the body, weighing about 3 to 4 pounds (1.5 kg). It is one of the most vital organs in the body and has a variety of functions.

The liver produces bile, a bitter-tasting alkaline fluid that contains no digestive enzymes but does contain bile salts, blood pigments, and other materials. Bile serves to alkalinize the strongly acid material coming into the duodenum from the stomach. It further serves to saponify, or emulsify, the fatty materials in our food. This action divides the fatty substances into fine droplets, exposing them more completely to the fat-digestive enzymes coming from the pancreas and from glands in the intestinal walls.

The liver is a major storage area for sugar in the form of *glycogen,* a ready fuel-energy source for muscle activity. It is the major site for *synthesis* (creation or formation) of *proteins* we need for growth and cell repair everywhere in the body. The liver also modifies many drugs, as well as metabolic products occurring naturally in the body, into forms that can be excreted by the kidneys.

The liver stores the fat-soluble vitamins (A, D, E, and K) and vitamin B_{12}. It also breaks down many of the toxins taken into body, including alcohol. It destroys old RBCs, reprocesses the products, and synthesizes blood proteins. The liver produces cholesterol, coagulation products, and antibodies.

Gallbladder. Some of the bile is stored in the *gallbladder,* where it is concentrated. The presence of acid and fatty food in the duodenum stimulates the gallbladder to eject some of its contents into the *common hepatic duct* and on into the duodenum immediately after a meal. Because bile is concentrated in the gallbladder, it is common for gallstones to form in this pouch, a condition called *cholelithiasis.* These stones may cause obstruction of the flow of bile, backing it up into the liver and causing an obstructive jaundice or yellow color to appear in the whites of the eyes and in the skin of patients with severe obstruction. The gallbladder, like the appendix, is a fairly common site of infection and abscess formation, occasionally requiring emergency surgery and antibiotic therapy.

Pancreas. The *pancreas* is situated behind the stomach. It contains two distinctly different kinds of cells, exocrine and endocrine. Exocrine cells and glands release secretions into a duct. Endocrine glands secrete hormones directly into the blood. Pancreatic juice, which aids in food digestion, is

Figure 18-12 A, *Digestive system.*
From LaFleur M, Starr W: *Exploring medical language: a student-directed approach*, ed 2, St. Louis, 1989, Mosby.

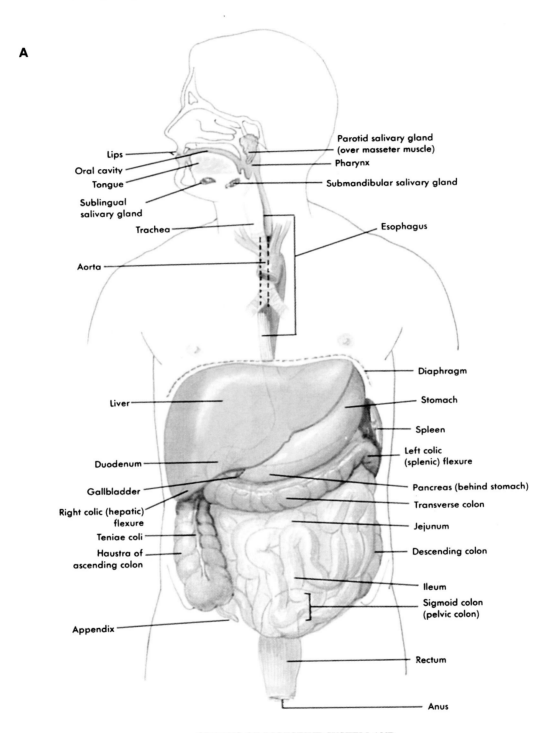

A

Lips
Oral cavity
Tongue
Sublingual
salivary gland
Trachea
Aorta

Parotid salivary gland
(over masseter muscle)
Pharynx
Submandibular salivary gland

Esophagus

Liver

Duodenum

Gallbladder

Right colic (hepatic)
flexure
Teniae coli
Haustra of
ascending colon

Appendix

Diaphragm
Stomach
Spleen
Left colic
(splenic) flexure
Pancreas (behind stomach)
Transverse colon
Jejunum
Descending colon
Ileum
Sigmoid colon
(pelvic colon)
Rectum
Anus

**ORGANS OF DIGESTIVE SYSTEM AND
SOME ASSOCIATED STRUCTURES**

Figure 18-12—cont'd B, *Digestive system.*
From LaFleur M, Starr W: *Exploring medical language: a student-directed approach*, ed 2, St. Louis, 1989, Mosby.

B

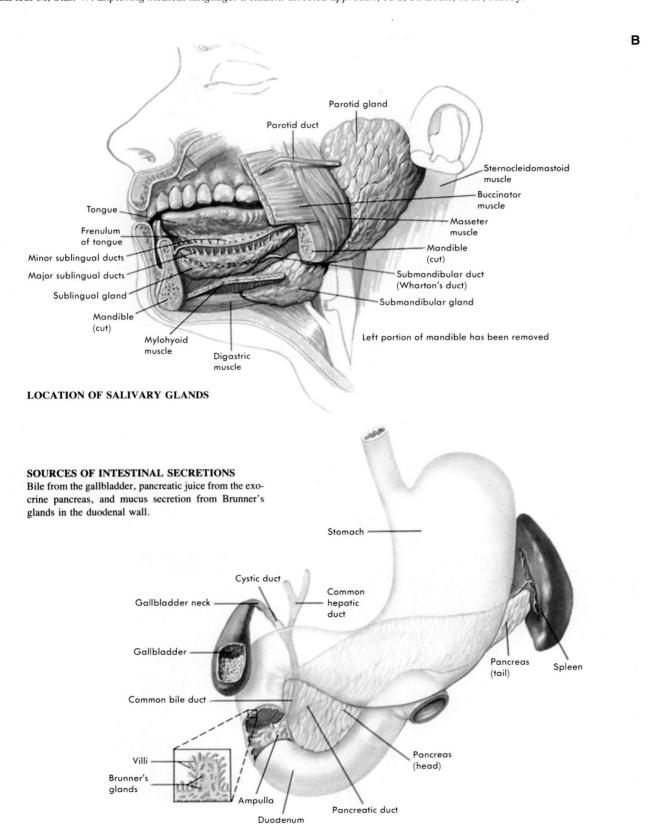

LOCATION OF SALIVARY GLANDS

SOURCES OF INTESTINAL SECRETIONS
Bile from the gallbladder, pancreatic juice from the exocrine pancreas, and mucus secretion from Brunner's glands in the duodenal wall.

A-22

Figure 18-12—cont'd C, *Digestive system.*
From LaFleur M, Starr W: *Exploring medical language: a student-directed approach*, ed 2, St. Louis, 1989, Mosby.

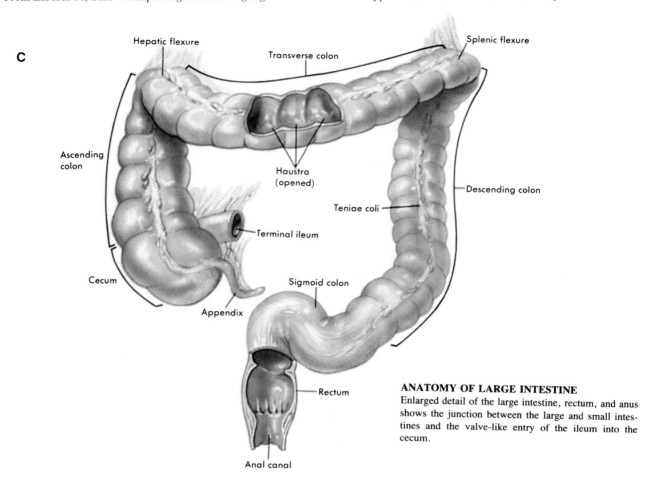

ANATOMY OF LARGE INTESTINE
Enlarged detail of the large intestine, rectum, and anus shows the junction between the large and small intestines and the valve-like entry of the ileum into the cecum.

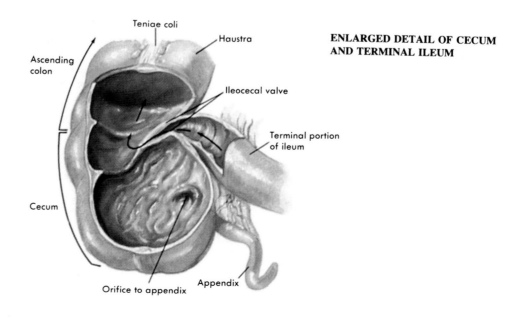

ENLARGED DETAIL OF CECUM AND TERMINAL ILEUM

secreted by *exocrine* cells that empty their products into the ducts of the pancreas. The *endocrine* cells, in the *islands of Langerhans,* secrete two opposing hormones that pass directly through blood capillary walls into the general circulation. The two kinds of endocrine cells in the islands of Langerhans are called alpha and beta cells. *Alpha cells* secrete *glucagon,* which tends to raise blood glucose levels. *Beta cells* secrete *insulin,* which lowers the blood glucose, thus maintaining a normally fluctuating blood glucose level between 60 and 120 mg/dl.

PROCESSING OF FOOD

The **tongue,** having on its surface many *taste buds* and being muscular in structure, mixes the food with *saliva* containing *ptyalin,* a starch-digesting enzyme. Stimulation of taste buds on the tongue and pleasant food odors in the nose increase the flow of saliva into the mouth. When the bolus of food has been thoroughly chewed to a semiliquid consistency, the tongue pushes it backward into the **pharynx.** From there it moves down the **esophagus** to the **stomach,** a pouchlike enlargement of the gut, just under the left leaf of the *diaphragm.*

The stomach is very muscular, enabling it to enlarge and contract freely. It moves the food toward the small intestine and churns it vigorously. Gastric juices containing *hydrochloric acid* and additional digestive *enzymes* poured out by glands in the stomach wall are mixed with the food for *protein* digestion. Food may remain in the stomach a few minutes or several hours until it is partially liquefied. It then passes through the *pylorus,* the lower portion of the stomach, which opens into the first segment of the **small intestine**, the *duodenum,* so named because its length is about 12 fingerbreaths.

The greatest amount of digestion and absorption of food takes place in the *small intestine.* It contains digestive juice that comes from its walls. In addition, the *pancreas* contributes protein-digesting and starch-digesting enzymes through the pancreatic duct, and the *liver* and *gallbladder* send *bile* through their common duct into the duodenum (see functions of bile discussed under Liver, page 605).

Through the action of these juices, digestion proceeds as food moves through the small intestine in a wavelike motion by contractions of involuntary smooth muscles in the intestinal walls. This movement is called *peristalsis.* It usually takes over 5 hours for food to traverse the small intestine, which is about 20 feet long. The small intestine has a mucosal lining with many folds. These folds are covered with tiny fingerlike projections called *villi,* which greatly increase the mucosal surface area and facilitate *absorption.* Digested carbohydrates and proteins, vitamins, salts, water, and some fats are absorbed into blood capillaries in the villi and carried by the *portal vein* to the *liver.* Lacteals in the villi absorb most of the digested fats and carry them as a milky lymphatic substance called *chyle* upward through the *cisterna chyli* and the *thoracic duct* to reach the bloodstream at the *left subclavian vein.*

The divisions of the small intestine are the *duodenum,* the *jejunum,* and the *ileum.* Food that has not been digested in the small intestine moves into the **large intestine** at the *ileocecal valve.* The *appendix* is attached to the *cecum* near the ileocecal junction. It is similar to the other parts of the gut in general structure but is much smaller. It has no specific digestive function but may create an emergency surgical problem if it becomes inflamed or gangrenous. The appendix is sometimes classified as an accessory digestive organ because of its location.

The **colon** is a major site for reabsorption of essential fluids and salt. It is divided into four parts: the *ascending colon* in the right side of the abdomen; the *transverse colon,* which passes from the *hepatic flexure,* just under the liver on the right, across the abdomen to the *splenic flexure* on the left; from there it goes down the left side of the abdomen as the *descending colon* to reach the *sigmoid* or S-shaped flexure in the pelvis. The **rectum** and the **anus** mark the termination of the digestive tract.

Through the use of various imaging methods, it is possible to discover whether food is going through the intestine normally and to locate growths or other conditions that interfere with peristalsis. Inflamed and irritated areas sometimes develop on the inside of the stomach and the intestine. These areas of irritation can become localized ulcerations of the mucosa, resulting in *gastric ulcers, duodenal ulcers, ileitis,* or *ulcerative colitis,* depending on the exact location in the entire alimentary or GI tract.

THE RESPIRATORY SYSTEM

Respiration is a process in which oxygen, a gas needed by body cells, is made available, and waste gas, carbon dioxide, is removed from the blood (Figure 18-13). The lungs and circulation cooperate in this function. Air enters the lungs by *inspiration* or inhaling and is expelled from the lungs by *expiration* or exhaling. Oxygen in the inhaled air passes into the blood from the air sacs in the lungs and is carried to the body cells. Carbon dioxide passes into the blood from the body cells, is carried to the air sacs in the lungs, and leaves the body in the exhaled air.

Three functions of the respiratory system include:
1. Exchange of gases between the blood and the lungs
2. Exchange of air between the lungs and the ambient air
3. Help in maintaining the oxygen-carbon dioxide balance in the blood

Three processes of respiration include:
1. External respiration, or ventilation, brings oxygen into the lungs.
2. Internal respiration exchanges oxygen and carbon dioxide between the blood and the body cells.
3. Cellular respiration changes acid produced during metabolism into harmless chemicals in the cells.

The voluntary and involuntary nervous systems control respiration. The rate and depth of the breaths are regulated chemically. If the concentration of gases in the blood changes, the brain adjusts respiratory rate and depth to counteract the changes (also see Unit Two).

Figure 18-13 A, *Respiratory system.*
From LaFleur M, Starr W: *Exploring medical language: a student-directed approach*, ed 2, St. Louis, 1989, Mosby.

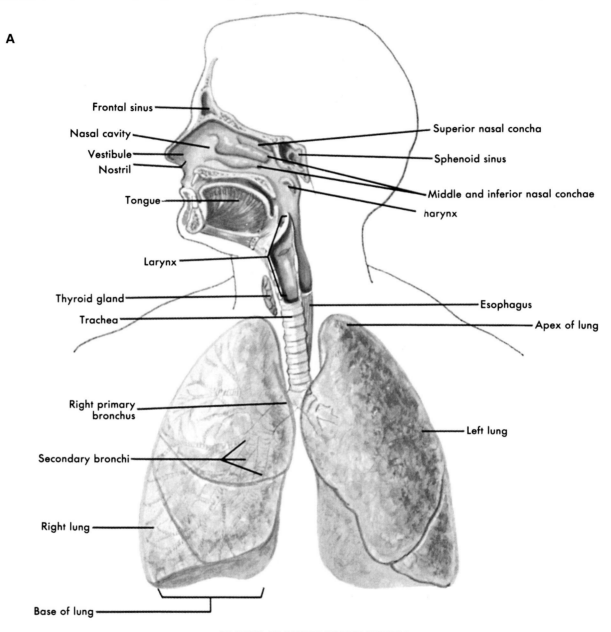

**ORGANS OF RESPIRATORY SYSTEM
AND ASSOCIATED STRUCTURES**

Figure 18-13—cont'd B, *Respiratory system.*
From LaFleur M, Starr W: *Exploring medical language: a student-directed approach*, ed 2, St. Louis, 1989, Mosby.

B

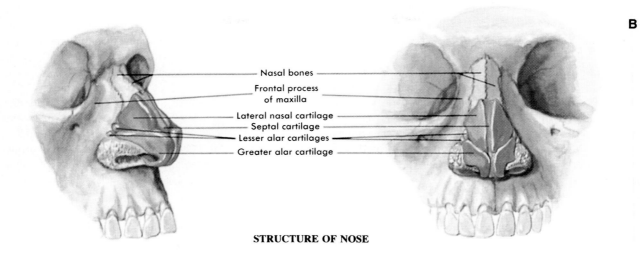

Nasal bones
Frontal process of maxilla
Lateral nasal cartilage
Septal cartilage
Lesser alar cartilages
Greater alar cartilage

STRUCTURE OF NOSE

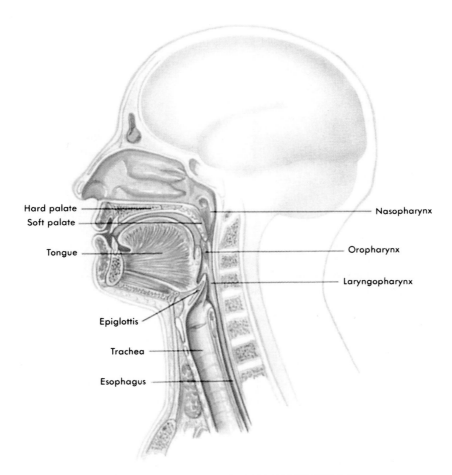

Hard palate
Soft palate
Tongue
Epiglottis
Trachea
Esophagus
Nasopharynx
Oropharynx
Laryngopharynx

STRUCTURES OF NASAL PASSAGES AND THROAT

ORGANS OF RESPIRATION

The organs of respiration are the nose, the pharynx, the larynx, the trachea, the bronchi, and the lungs. The first five serve as passageways to and from the lungs. They warm and moisten the air and catch particles of dust and dirt.

Nose

The *nose* is formed by bone and cartilage and is divided into two cavities by a cartilaginous partition called the *septum.* The nasal cavities open into the upper part of the throat and at the upper end contain the openings to the *sinuses* and *tear ducts.* Three small bones, the *turbinates* or conchae, project into each nasal cavity. The nasal cavities are lined with mucous membrane. The nasal septum and mucous membranes have a rich blood supply. Nosebleeds often occur as a result of a direct blow to the nose. Tiny hairs at the outer entrance act as filters to remove the dust from the inhaled air. The nose is also the organ of smell; the endings of the nerves of smell, or the *olfactory nerves,* are found in the mucous membrane.

Eustachian tubes, adenoids, and tonsils.
The *eustachian tubes,* connected with the middle ears for equalization of air pressure, open into the space behind the nasal cavities. In the center of the rear wall is a mass of lymph tissue called the *adenoids.* This mass is usually much larger in children than in adults and sometimes seriously interferes with breathing. If the mass gets large and becomes infected, it may be necessary to remove it by surgery. The *tonsils* are usually removed during the same procedure, known as *tonsillectomy* and *adenoidectomy.*

Pharynx, larynx, and vocal cords.
The **pharynx** is a tube-shaped structure behind the nose and mouth that serves as a passageway for both air and food. Air passes through the pharynx to the *larynx* and, in the act of swallowing, muscles lift the pharynx to receive the food and press it down into the esophagus. That part of the pharynx behind the mouth is called the throat. The tonsils lie at the back of the throat. The **larynx,** or **voice box,** is a boxlike structure that lies in front of the esophagus at the upper part of the neck and is moved by the muscles attached to it. In the act of swallowing, a small lid, the epiglottis, closes down over the upper end to shut out food. Inside this triangular box are two folds of mucous membrane, the **vocal cords,** extending from front to back. There is a space between these folds that changes in shape to become wider in breathing and narrower in speaking. The vibrations of these cords as air passes over them produce the sound of speaking or singing. When the cords vibrate slowly, the voice is lower in pitch. If they vibrate rapidly, the pitch becomes higher. Voices differ because of differences in the length of the vocal cords and the size of the voice box. Vibrations are produced by the air breathed out, and the voice becomes louder and stronger if we force air out rapidly or in large amounts. If the air passages are blocked in any way, the voice is usually affected. When the vocal cords become inflamed, the voice becomes hoarse.

Trachea.
The trachea, or windpipe, is in front of the esophagus. It is a tube held rigid by rings of cartilage and lined with mucous membrane filled with cilia, tiny hairlike processes. These processes move constantly to wave the mucus back and up into the throat and thus prevent dust and foreign material from entering the lungs. The upper end of the trachea joins the lower end of the larynx. At the lower end, the trachea divides into two branches called bronchi.

Bronchi.
The *bronchi* are the divisions of the trachea that enter the right and left lungs and divide into many branches that grow smaller and thinner-walled until they end in the *air sacs,* the *alveoli.* The smallest branches of the bronchi are called *bronchioles.* Capillaries in the walls of the alveoli exchange oxygen and carbon dioxide by the process of diffusion.

Lungs.
The lungs are two cone-shaped organs that lie in the chest cavity, or rib cage. They are composed of spongy material containing the many small branches of the bronchi, numerous blood vessels, nerves, and air sacs. They are capable of holding 7 or 8 pints (3.3 to 3.8 L) of air. A thin membrane, called the *pleura,* covers each lung and also lines the chest cavity. These two membranes are separated by a fluid that keeps the surfaces moist so that they move smoothly against each other with the motion of the lungs in breathing. If these surfaces become inflamed or rough, they rub against each other and cause pain with every breath. This condition is known as *pleurisy.* Sometimes an abnormal amount of fluid forms, and if the amount becomes so great that it interferes with breathing, it has to be withdrawn. This condition is known as *pleural effusion.* There is usually no air between the lung and the chest wall. If a defect in the chest wall or lung develops, a collection of air between the chest wall and the lining of the lung is formed. This is called a *pneumothorax.*

THE URINARY SYSTEM

The organs of the urinary system include the two kidneys, two ureters, one bladder, and one urethra (Figure 18-14). The two primary functions of the urinary system are:

- To regulate the chemical composition of body fluids
- To remove body wastes by filtering blood

The urinary system filters about 192.21 quarts (180 L) of fluid daily. On the average, 1.05 to 1.59 quarts (1 to 1.5 L) of urine is formed and excreted daily to remove waste products. Also see Unit Twelve.

KIDNEYS

The basic structural unit of the urinary system is the kidney. The *kidneys* are two bean-shaped organs located in the upper back part of the abdomen on either side of the backbone slightly above the waist. They are embedded in cushions of fat that help keep them in place.

Each kidney is about the size of a fist, about 4 inches (10 cm) long and 2 inches (5 cm) wide, and weighs about 5 ounces (150 g). The kidney has three layers (Figure 18-14, *B*):

Figure 18-14 A, *Urinary system.*
From LaFleur M, Starr W: *Exploring medical language: a student-directed approach*, ed 2, St. Louis, 1989, Mosby.

A

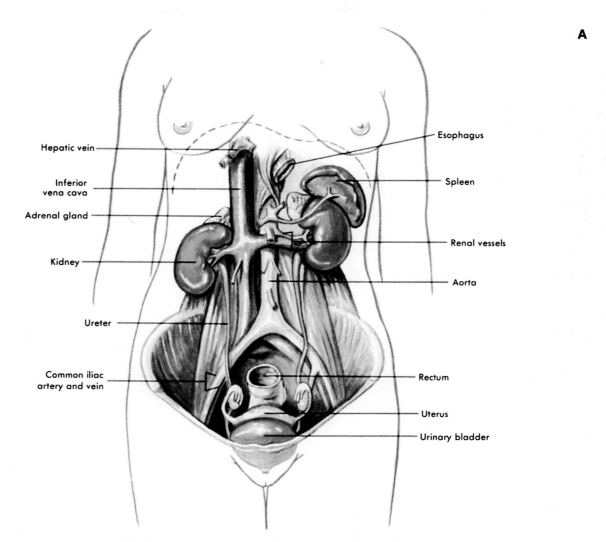

URINARY SYSTEM AND SOME ASSOCIATED STRUCTURES

Figure 18-14—cont'd   B, *Urinary system.*
From LaFleur M, Starr W: *Exploring medical language: a student-directed approach*, ed 2, St. Louis, 1989, Mosby.

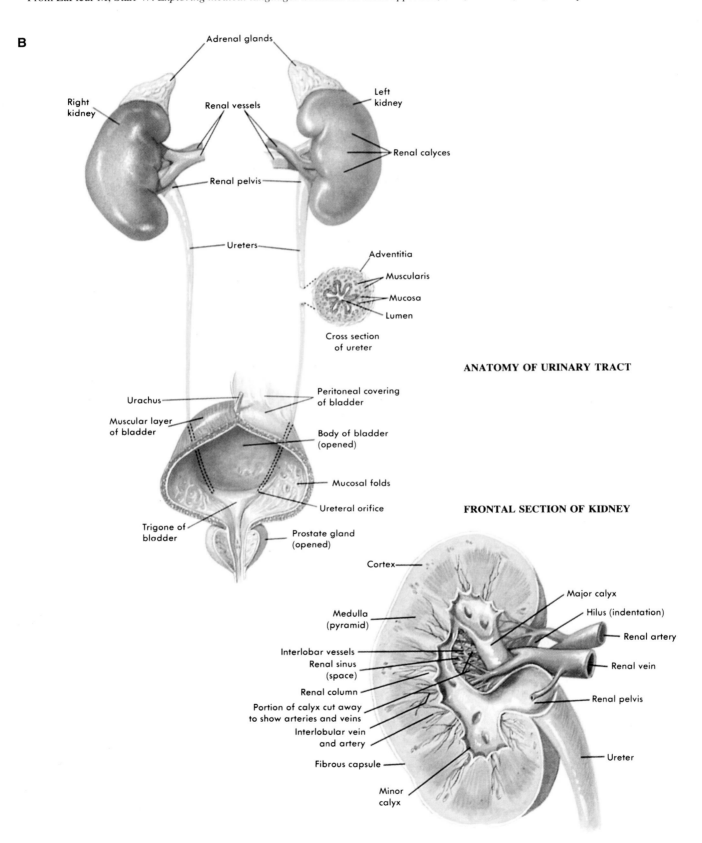

B

Adrenal glands

Right kidney

Renal vessels

Left kidney

Renal calyces

Renal pelvis

Ureters

Adventitia

Muscularis

Mucosa

Lumen

Cross section of ureter

ANATOMY OF URINARY TRACT

Urachus

Peritoneal covering of bladder

Muscular layer of bladder

Body of bladder (opened)

Mucosal folds

Ureteral orifice

FRONTAL SECTION OF KIDNEY

Trigone of bladder

Prostate gland (opened)

Cortex

Major calyx

Medulla (pyramid)

Hilus (indentation)

Renal artery

Interlobar vessels

Renal sinus (space)

Renal vein

Renal column

Portion of calyx cut away to show arteries and veins

Renal pelvis

Interlobular vein and artery

Fibrous capsule

Ureter

Minor calyx

- The *cortex,* the outer layer, is composed of soft, granular, reddish-brown tissue
- The *medulla,* the middle layer, is a deep red color.
- The *renal pelvis* is the funnel-shaped, innermost structure that collects urine as it is formed. Urine passes through the renal pelvis into the ureter, then to the bladder. Each kidney is encased in a tough, white, fibrous capsule. On the medial (toward the midline) side of each kidney is a small area called the *hilum,* through which structures such as the lymph vessels, nerves, and renal artery enter the kidney and the renal vein and ureter leave the kidney.

The kidneys help maintain the state of homeostasis in the internal environment (environment within the body) by selectively excreting or reabsorbing various substances according to the needs of the body. The functional unit of the kidney is the nephron unit. This is where the formation of urine occurs. Each kidney contains about one million microscopic nephron units working together to selectively retain or excrete the substances passing through them in the blood.

The kidneys remove from the blood those salts, poisons, proteins, wastes, and water that are eliminated from the body as urine (also see Unit Twelve).

URETERS AND URINARY BLADDER

The urine is carried away from the kidneys by two tubes called the *ureters.* The ureters are about 10 inches (25 cm) long and contract to move the urine down into the *bladder.* The bladder lies in the pelvic cavity behind the pubic bone. It is in front of the rectum in the male and in front of the vagina and the neck of the uterus in the female. It is hollow and muscular and acts as a reservoir for the urine, normally holding about a pint. When it become full, pressure causes a desire to empty the contents. To prevent a constant leakage of urine, the opening into the urethra is provided with a tight, circular muscle, or *sphincter,* that normally is contracted and relaxes only during the act of *urination.*

URETHRA

The *urethra* is the narrow passageway from the bladder that ends in the outer opening through which urine is voided. This opening, called the urinary meatus, is at the end of the penis of the male and between the clitoris and the opening of the vagina in the female. The urethra is approximately 7 to 8 inches long in a male and about 1 to 1½ inches long in a female.

Factors Affecting Urination

Involuntary urination, or *incontinence,* is caused by lack of bladder control, which may in turn be caused by lack of consciousness, injury to the nerves that control the bladder, weak sphincter muscle, bladder disease, or substances in the urine that cause irritation. Nervousness and the sight and sound of water sometimes cause a desire to urinate. If the bladder cannot be emptied normally, it is sometimes necessary to draw the urine out by a catheter. A catheter is a hollow, flexible rubber tube that is inserted through the urethra into the bladder to allow urine to drain out of the bladder.

THE REPRODUCTIVE SYSTEM

The reproductive organs differ in the male and female and in general begin to function at the time of puberty (Figure 18-15). In boys, this development usually begins at about the age of 13 to 15 years, but in girls is it usually a year or two earlier. The growth of the organs of reproduction causes increased changes in general body growth and in the emotions. This period of change is called *puberty.*

THE MALE REPRODUCTIVE SYSTEM

The male reproductive system consists of the testes, epididymis, vas deferens, two seminal vesicles, one ejaculating duct, prostate gland, urethra, and penis (Figure 18-15, *A*). The **testes** are two oval glands suspended in and covered by the baglike sac known as the *scrotum.* The testes serve two main functions: to make male reproductive cells called *spermatozoa* (sperm) and to secrete *testosterone,* the principal male hormone.

Adjacent to each testis is a 20-foot, tightly coiled tube called the **epididymis.** Sperm are stored here while they mature. Spermatozoa are carried from the testes to the epididymis, then through a narrow tube to the ejaculatory duct into the **urethra** and to the outside of the body. During an operation called a *vasectomy,* which is performed to cause sterility, the vas deferens is cut.

Before reaching the urethra within the **penis, the epididymis, the seminal vesicles, the prostate, and Cowper's gland** contribute secretions that provide a vehicle for the spermatozoa. This fluid is discharged from the body during ejaculation and is called semen or seminal fluid. The largest of the glands is the *prostate gland,* which lies at the base of the bladder. This gland sometimes becomes enlarged and hard in later life and presses against the urethra, interfering with the passage of urine. Sometimes this gland becomes inflamed, a condition known as *prostatitis.* In older men, this gland must often be removed surgically, either because it has increased in size or because it has developed cancer.

Sometimes the *epididymis* becomes infected and extremely swollen and painful, a condition called *epididymitis.*

The **penis** consists of the shaft, a passageway for urine and semen called the **urethra,** and the *glans.* The glans is highly sensitive and is located at the end of the penis. At the tip of the glans is the opening to the urethra. It is covered by a fold of skin, the *prepuce* or foreskin, that is often removed for hygienic or religious reasons (*circumcision*). During sexual stimulation, or under a variety of conditions involving involuntary reflexes, the penis may become engorged with blood, enlarged, hardened, and erect.

THE FEMALE REPRODUCTIVE SYSTEM

The female reproductive system (Figure 18-15, *B* and *C*) contains the **ovaries,** which are two almond-shaped glands that lie near the back wall of the pelvic cavity and produce the female sex cells known as *ova* (eggs). Each cell is contained in a little sac, and when the egg or ovum is fully developed, the sac bursts and the ovum is discharged into the pelvic cavity. The ovaries also secrete two important

Text continues on page 620.

Figure 18-15 *A to C, Reproductive systems. D, Menstrual cycle. Diagram illustrating the inter-relationships among the cerebral, hypothalamic, pituitary, ovarian, and uterine functions throughout a usual 28-day cycle. The variations in basal body temperature are also illustrated at the bottom.*

A to C from LaFleur M, Starr W: *Exploring medical language: a student-directed approach*, ed 2, St. Louis, 1989, Mosby.

A

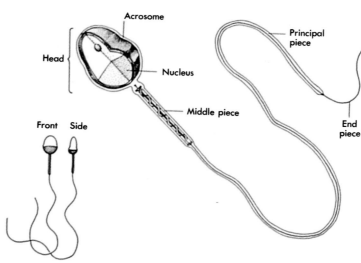

Rectum

Seminal vesicle and duct

Fat

Bulbourethral (Cowper's) gland and duct

Anus

Vas deferens

Epididymis

Testis

Urinary bladder

Symphysis pubis

Prostatic urethra

Prostate gland

Urogenital diaphragm

Membranous urethra

Cavernous bodies of penis

Spermatic cord

Cavernous urethra

Glans penis

Fossa navicularis

Prepuce (foreskin)

Scrotum

**MALE REPRODUCTIVE ORGANS AND
ASSOCIATED STRUCTURES**

Acrosome

Head

Nucleus

Middle piece

Front   Side

Principal piece

End piece

ANATOMY OF A SPERM

Figure 18-15—cont'd B, *Female reproductive system.*

B

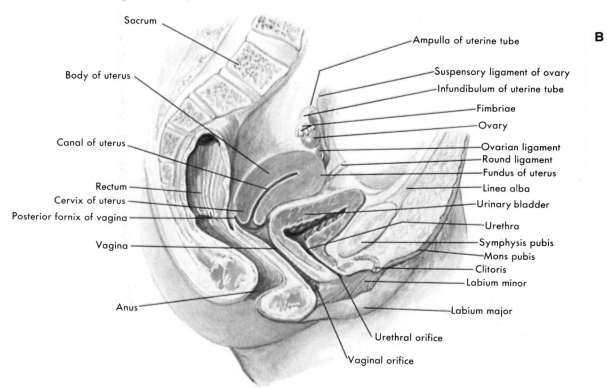

Sacrum

Body of uterus

Canal of uterus

Rectum

Cervix of uterus

Posterior fornix of vagina

Vagina

Anus

Ampulla of uterine tube

Suspensory ligament of ovary

Infundibulum of uterine tube

Fimbriae

Ovary

Ovarian ligament

Round ligament

Fundus of uterus

Linea alba

Urinary bladder

Urethra

Symphysis pubis

Mons pubis

Clitoris

Labium minor

Labium major

Urethral orifice

Vaginal orifice

**FEMALE REPRODUCTIVE ORGANS AND
ASSOCIATED STRUCTURES**

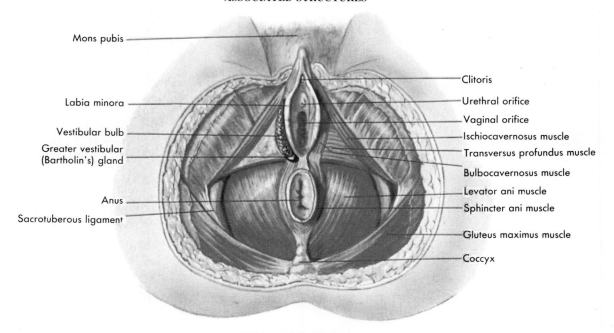

Mons pubis

Labia minora

Vestibular bulb

Greater vestibular
(Bartholin's) gland

Anus

Sacrotuberous ligament

Clitoris

Urethral orifice

Vaginal orifice

Ischiocavernosus muscle

Transversus profundus muscle

Bulbocavernosus muscle

Levator ani muscle

Sphincter ani muscle

Gluteus maximus muscle

Coccyx

FEMALE PERINEUM

Figure 18-15—cont'd   C, *Female reproductive system.*

CLINICAL NOTE: Female reproductive system
Immense structural changes occur within the uterus during pregnancy. However, if fertilization does not take place, then the endometrial lining is shed cyclically under hormonal control in the phenomenon of menstruation.

C

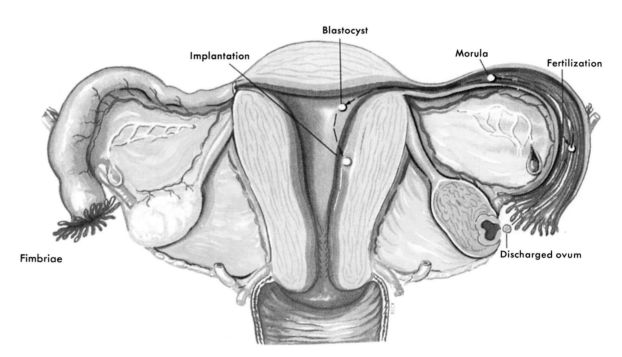

**APPEARANCE OF UTERUS AND UTERINE TUBES
FROM FERTILIZATION TO IMPLANTATION**
Fertilization occurs in the outer third of the uterine tube.
Development reaches the blastocyst stage after the
embryo has entered the uterus.

Figure 18-15—cont'd *D, Menstrual cycle. Diagram illustrating the inter-relationships among the cerebral, hypothalamic, pituitary, ovarian, and uterine functions throughout a usual 28-day cycle. The variations in basal body temperature are also illustrated at the bottom.*

D from Thibodeau GA: *Anthony's textbook of anatomy and physiology,* ed 13, St. Louis, 1990, Mosby.

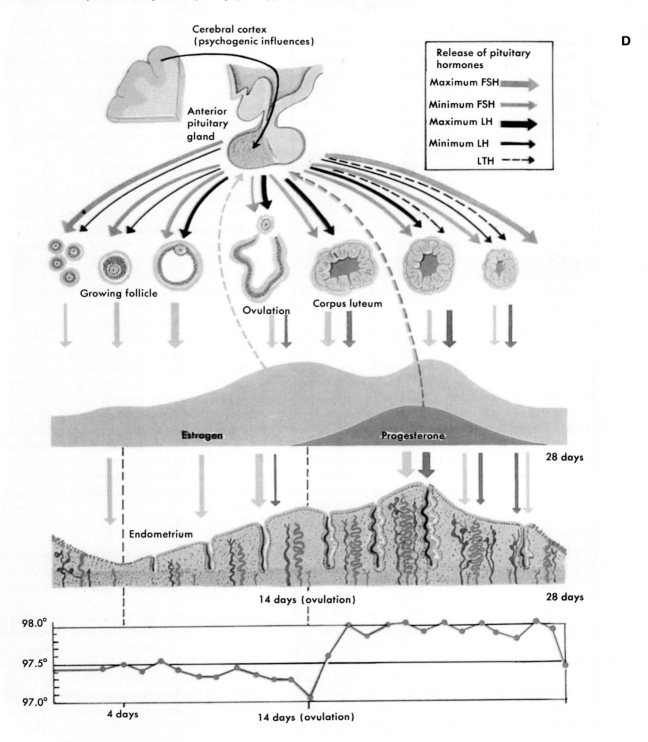

hormones: *estrogen* and *progesterone*. These are the principal female hormones and influence changes in menstruation and the growth of a fertilized ovum during pregnancy and changes seen during menopause. During adult life the ovaries contain many eggs in various stages of development, and one is released approximately every 28 days. This process, which is called *ovulation*, usually occurs 14 days before the next menstrual period begins. Ovulation begins at puberty and continues at regular intervals until late middle age when, during *menopause, menstruation* gradually ceases. There are two uterine tubes, also known as the **fallopian tubes.** They carry the ova from the ovaries to the uterus. The upper ends are near the ovaries and are provided with little fringes that catch the ovum as it leaves the ovary. The ovum passes into the tube and, if it is not fertilized within 24 to 36 hours, does not survive. *Fertilization* takes place in the distal third of either fallopian tube when a male sperm cell penetrates the ovum. An impregnated ovum passes down into the uterus and becomes attached to the uterine wall. This is called *implantation*. If, as occasionally happens, the impregnated ovum remains in the tube, its growth distends and may rupture the tube. This causes bleeding that may be fatal and necessitates an immediate surgical procedure. This condition is called a *tubal* or an *ectopic pregnancy*.

The **uterus** is a hollow, pear-shaped organ that is muscular and capable of great expansion. The lower part tapers to a narrow neck, the *cervix*, which extends into the vagina. The uterus is supported by ligaments and is easily tilted forward and backward. During pregnancy it enlarges upward into the abdominal cavity.

The **vagina** is the canal that lies between the bladder and the rectum. It surrounds the lower end of the uterus and opens into the *vulva*, on the outside of the body. Its inner surface is moistened by fluid secreted by glands within its walls. The vagina changes considerably under the influence of the female hormones at puberty. After menopause, when the ovaries produce less estrogen, the vaginal mucosa becomes thin and less elastic and produces less secretion.

The **vulva (the external genitals)** (Figure 18-15, *B*) consists of the labia, the clitoris, and the hymen. The **labia** are two sets of liplike folds at the opening of the vagina. The **clitoris** is a small body containing many nerves and blood vessels; it is located at the upper meeting point of the labia majora and labia minora. Like the glans of the penis, it is very sensitive and subject to engorgement and enlargement during sexual stimulation. The **hymen** is a fold of mucous membrane and fibrous tissue at the entrance of the vagina. It may be ruptured during sexual intercourse and is completely obliterated after childbirth. In addition, the hymen may be torn or perforated at an earlier time in a young woman's life (for example, during physical exercise). Thus the presence of the hymen *is not* a reliable indicator of the woman's virginity as was once thought. The pubic area (*pudendum*) consists of the external genitals and the *mons veneris*, the rounded fatty pad covered with skin and hair (*pubes*) above the clitoris and over the bone called the **pubis**, or **pubic bone** and the *symphysis pubis*, the cartilaginous joint between the pubic bones. The space between the vaginal orifice and the anus is called the **perineum.**

The **breasts**, or **mammary glands**, are an important part of the reproductive process in the female. They are present but undeveloped in the male. These two glands are located on the outer surface of the chest, are composed of milk ducts and fat, contain many blood vessels, and open into the *nipples* through many small canals. They secrete the milk that nourishes the child after it is born. Careful examination of the breasts for masses, retractions of the skin, or a blood discharge from the nipples must be performed monthly in all women. Any of these may be early signs of cancer of the breast. See Unit Four for the Breast Self-Examination.

Menstruation

Through the influence of pituitary and ovarian hormones, the lining of the adult uterus is prepared during each menstrual cycle to receive a fertilized ovum. If fertilization does not occur, a portion of the lining of the uterus is discarded as a bloody discharge, a process called *menstruation* (Table 18-4 and Figure 18-15, *D*). In some women this occurs every 28 days, whereas in others it is irregular. If a fertilized ovum nestles in the lining of the uterus, it produces hormones that keep the uterine lining from being discarded. The fertilized ovum is thus able to grow on the inner surface of the uterus. As the embryo grows, a complex series of events eventually leads to a connection between the uterus and the embryo called the **placenta.** The embryo is connected to the placenta by an **umbilical cord.**

During menstruation many women feel cramping sensations and varying degrees of discomfort. The severity of this discomfort (menstrual cramps or *dysmenorrhea*) is highly variable among different women and for an individual woman may vary from month to month. Severe, prolonged, or incapacitating menstrual pain is sufficient reason for a medical evaluation.

Menopause

The ovaries cease to ovulate when a women is about 45 to 54 years old, although the age varies in individuals. This is called the menopause, and menstruation ceases at this time. The average age in the United States for the onset of menopause is currently 51.4 years. It is a difficult period for some women because, as estrogen levels decrease, certain annoying and disturbing symptoms may appear in the form of a feeling of alternate heat and cold, a flushing and perspiring face (hot flashes), dizziness, headache, and mental depression that sometimes becomes serious. Also the vagina becomes dry and itchy, sometimes causing pain during intercourse. Breasts may lose some of their fullness and tend to sag.

More serious health hazards are also associated with menopause, the most common being an increased risk for heart disease and a loss of bone density that could result in osteoporosis.

To cope with and reduce some of the risks that reduced levels of estrogen can produce, *hormone-replacement therapy*

TABLE 18-4

Menstrual Cycle

Day	Hormone Activity	Change in System
1	Pituitary secretes follicle stimulating hormone (FSH)	Follicle cells mature and produce estrogen
	Pituitary secretes luteinizing hormone (LH)	Promotes estrogen production
2 3 4 5 6 7 8 9 10 11 12 13	Estrogen increases	Uterine lining begins to thicken; secondary sexual characteristics are maintained
14	Pituitary secretes FSH & LH	Mature follicle ruptures causing release of ovum* (ovulation), follicle of ovary becomes corpus luteum
15 16 17 18 19 20 21 22 23	Corpus luteum secretes progesterone and estrogen	Lining of uterus becomes more vascular; secretions of pituitary inhibited
24		Corpus luteum degenerates if ovum not fertilized
25 26	Progesterone and estrogen secretion decreases	Blood vessels to uterine lining constrict; tissues disintegrate and slough
27 28		Menses begin and last about 5 days

From Gerdin J: Health careers today, St. Louis, 1991, Mosby.
*If the ovum is fertilized after leaving the ovary, it is implanted in the rich uterine wall. The corpus luteum continues to secrete progesterone throughout the pregnancy to maintain the uterine wall and inhibit the secretion of pituitary hormones.

(HRT) is frequently given to help the individual through this period of physical and mental adjustment. Today there are many products that aid in the menopausal period, and women should have very little difficulty during this period if properly attended by good medical advice. Usually a combination of estrogen and progestin (a form of progesterone) is recommended by the specialists. HRT lowers the risk of heart disease and osteoporosis and helps to reduce vaginal dryness and hot flashes. Despite the benefits for some, HRT does have potential side effects and risks for some women such as spotting or menstrual-like flows and gallbladder disease. However, many studies and researchers state that the benefits of HRT outweigh the risks and that the risks subside 1 year after women stop HRT.

THE ENDOCRINE SYSTEM

The primary functions of the endocrine system are to monitor and coordinate body activities (Figure 18-16). Remarkable advances have been made in the knowledge about several glands in the body that have to do with vital occurrences of growth, development, and function. These glands are grouped into a system known as the endocrine system. The primary functions of the endocrine system are to monitor and coordinate body activities. The glands involved are the pineal, pituitary, thyroid, parathyroids, thymus, pancreas, adrenals, ovaries, testes, and the placenta during pregnancy. The secretions from these glands are released directly into the bloodstream and are called hormones.

Hormones are chemical messengers. Each type of hormone moves through the blood to its own target cells, which react specifically to it. Hormones direct many body processes, including growth, metabolism, and reproductive functions. Hormones regulate the body's reaction to stress and maintain the internal environment (environment within the body). This is known as homeostasis. The amount of hormones in the blood is monitored through a negative-feedback mechanism, which stimulates more secretion when needed. In addition, the autonomic nervous system controls and stimulates the secretion of the hormones of the adrenal gland.

PINEAL GLAND

The pineal gland is a small pea-sized gland located in the midline behind the third ventricle of the brain. It produces the hormone melatonin. Melatonin regulates the release of substances in the hypothalamus of the brain that influence secretion of the pituitary gonadotropins, or sex hormones. It is believed that melatonin inhibits the activity of the ovaries and the luteinizing hormone secretion. Thus it influences the menstrual cycle and onset of puberty. The hypothalamus secretes neurohormones that regulate the pituitary gland.

PITUITARY GLAND

The *pituitary gland* (the hypophysis) is often referred to as the "master gland" because the hormones that it produces regulate the secretion of other glands. It is located at the base of the brain and is divided into an anterior and posterior lobe. The *anterior lobe* of this gland produces a number of very important hormones that are released into the blood and regulate many important body functions. One hormone controls the thyroid gland, another the reproductive glands, and yet another the adrenal glands. Two hormones control growth and development of the breasts during pregnancy. The *posterior pituitary lobe* secretes at least two hormones. One controls the elimination of water by the kidney, whereas the other causes contractions of the uterus during childbirth. Pituitary hormones can be prescribed for individuals who do not produce them. For example, growth hormones can be given to promote growth in some types of dwarfs. Another pituitary hormone, *oxytocin,* is commonly given to pregnant women to induce labor or to contract the uterus after childbirth.

THYROID GLAND

The *thyroid gland* is located in the neck below the voice box. It regulates the metabolic activity of the individual. This gland frequently produces either too much (hyperthyroidism) or too little (hypothyroidism) thyroid. *Hyperthyroidism* is characterized by nervousness, weight loss, and a fast pulse. *Hypothyroidisn* is characterized by sluggishness, weight gain, and a slow pulse. If the thyroid gland enlarges, the condition is known as a *goiter*. A goiter may be present with overproduction or underproduction of thyroid hormone.

PARATHYROID GLANDS

The *parathyroid glands* are small, round bodies, usually four in number. They are usually embedded or attached to the posterior portion of the thyroid gland. The parathyroid glands control calcium levels in the blood by secreting *parathyroid hormone*. Excessive secretion of this hormone causes an elevation of blood calcium levels (*hypercalcemia*), whereas underproduction of the hormone causes low calcium levels (*hypocalcemia*). This latter condition, if severe, results in *tetany*, a condition characterized by excessive muscular contraction.

THYMUS GLAND

The thymus gland (see Figure 18-10, *B*) is a small gland located above the heart and beneath the sternum in the thoracic cavity. It secretes a hormone called *thymosin*. Both the thymus and thymosin play an important role in the development of the immune system. The thymus reaches maximum development during puberty. Its immunologic function decreases with age.

PANCREAS

The *pancreas,* which was discussed under the digestive system, is a gland located behind the stomach. In addition to its digestive function, it secretes the hormone *insulin*. Lack of insulin results in *diabetes mellitus,* whereas too much insulin can cause the blood glucose to become too low. This is called *hypoglycemia*.

ADRENAL GLANDS

There are two *adrenal glands,* which are located above the kidneys. These glands are divided into two sections. The outer section, known as the *adrenal cortex,* produces *cortisone,* which is an important hormone in adapting to stressful situations. The inner part of the gland is called the *adrenal medulla* and produces two closely related hormones called *epinephrine* and *norepinephrine*. These hormones are important in maintaining blood pressure and increasing the heart rate during stressful situations. Cortisone and a wide variety of drugs related to it are used in medicine for treatment of allergic, arthritic, and inflammatory disorders. Epinephrine, also known commercially as Adrenalin, is used in medical emergencies and should be available in every physician's office.

Figure 18-16 A, *Endocrine system.*
From LaFleur M, Starr W: *Exploring medical language: a student-directed approach*, ed 2, St. Louis, 1989, Mosby.

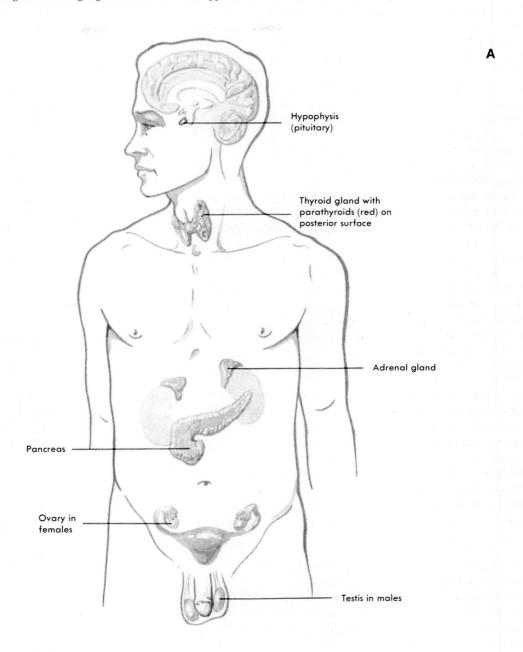

A

Hypophysis
(pituitary)

Thyroid gland with
parathyroids (red) on
posterior surface

Adrenal gland

Pancreas

Ovary in
females

Testis in males

Figure 18-16—cont'd   B, *Endocrine system.*
From LaFleur M, Starr W: *Exploring medical language: a student-directed approach*, ed 2, St. Louis, 1989, Mosby.

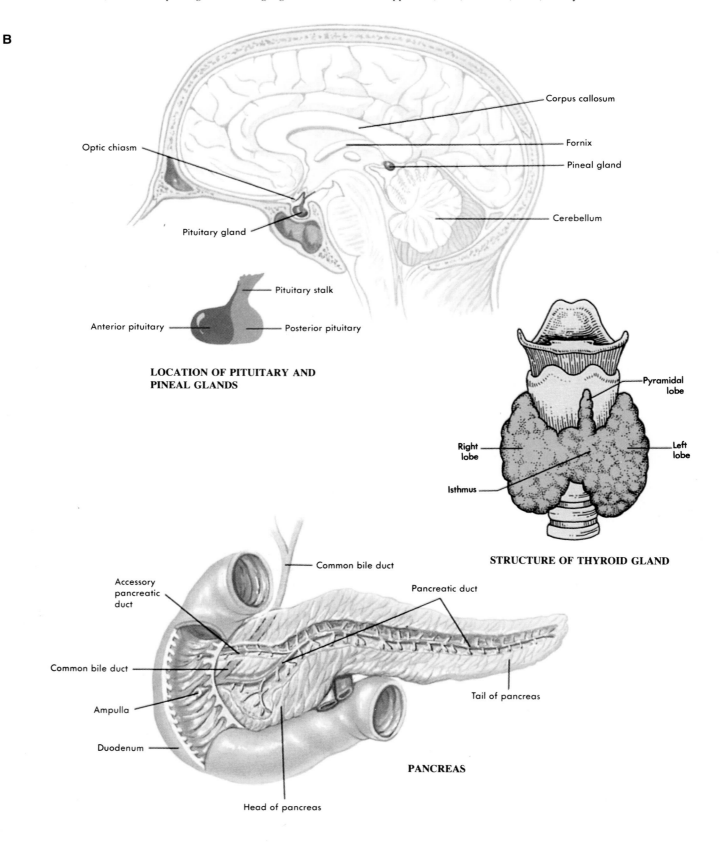

B

LOCATION OF PITUITARY AND
PINEAL GLANDS

STRUCTURE OF THYROID GLAND

PANCREAS

OVARIES

The *ovaries* and the two important female hormones, estrogen and progesterone, were described in the discussion of the female reproductive system. Estrogen is the main feminizing hormone and causes female sexual characteristics to develop at puberty. Estrogen and progesterone enable normal reproductive functions and are important in regulating the normal menstrual cycle.

PLACENTA

During pregnancy the *placenta* serves as a temporary endocrine body. It produces *chorionic gonadotropins,* estrogens, and progesterone. A woman's urine or blood is tested for the presence of the human chorionic gonadotropin (HCG) hormone to determine the presence of a pregnancy.

TESTES

The *testes* were described in the discussion of the male reproductive system. The male hormone, testosterone, causes male sexual development and promotes growth of a beard, male bone and muscular development, and deepening of the voice.

THE SENSORY SYSTEM

The sensory system (also called special senses) consists of *receptors* in specialized cells and organs that perceive changes (*stimuli*) in the internal and external environment (Figure 18-17, *A* and *B*). Stimuli cause nervous impulses that are sent to the brain for interpretation. Environmental stimuli are perceived with the senses of vision, hearing, touch, taste, smell, position, and balance. Specialized organs of the senses include the ear, eye, tongue, nose, and skin.

THE EAR

The ear is the organ of hearing and is divided into the external, middle, and inner ear (Figure 18-17 *A* and *B*). *Cartilage* forms the external ear and performs much the same function as the shell behind the band in the outdoor bandstand, serving to collect the sound waves and send them inward. The canal leading from the external to the middle ear is provided with glands that secrete a waxy substance that prevents many foreign objects from reaching the eardrum. The *eardrum* (or tympanic membrane) is a thin membrane that separates the external ear canal from the cavity of the middle ear. One end of a tiny bone known as the *malleus* (hammer) is fastened to the inner side of the eardrum. The other end of the malleus joins another small bone called the *incus* (anvil), which in turn is joined to a third bone known as the *stapes* (stirrup). The inner end of the stapes fits into the *oval window* between the middle ear and the inner ear.

The *eustachian tube* leads from the middle ear to the throat, and the *mastoid* (air cells in the mastoid process of the temporal bone) is located just behind the middle ear. The *inner ear* or *labyrinth,* consisting of the vestibule, cochlea, and semi-circular canals, is a cavity containing fluid that catches the sound waves that strike the tympanic membrane or eardrum and are carried by the chain of three small bones

across the middle ear. These sound waves are passed to the *cochlear nerve* and carried to the hearing center of the brain. Deafness may be the result of injury to the hearing center, the cochlear (auditory) nerve, or the tympanic membrane (eardrum) or to poor vibration of the chain of small bones across the middle ear.

Each inner ear also contains three *semicircular canals* filled with fluid and communicating through the *vestibular nerve* to inform us of changes in position of the head. These passages control the sense of balance. When this system is not working properly, we become dizzy and nauseated and lose our sense of balance.

The cochlear (auditory) nerve and the vestibular (balance) nerve join together to form the *vestibulocochlear* (eighth) cranial nerve.

THE EYE

The structure and function of the eye resemble that of a camera, except that the images of objects are permanently registered on the camera film, whereas those registered in the eye are constantly changing. The eyeball lies in the eye socket and is protected by the eyebrows, the lids, and the lashes. It is connected at the back with the *optic* (second cranial) *nerve,* which communicates with the seeing center in the brain. The movements of the eyeballs are controlled by six muscles that work in pairs in opposition to each other. They are innervated by the third, fourth, and sixth cranial nerves. Muscles in the lids control opening and shutting and are innervated by the third and the seventh cranial nerves. The *conjunctiva* is the thin, transparent mucous membrane that lines the lids and covers the anterior surface of the eyeball. The *tear* (lacrimal) *glands* open on the underside of the upper lids and secrete a fluid that keeps the eyes moist. The excess is usually carried away by the lacrimal ducts into the nose, except at times of oversecretion in emotional upsets and in inflammation of the conjunctiva when the tears spill out over the cheeks.

The eyeball is divided into two chambers separated by the *lens.* The chamber in front of the lens is small and filled with watery fluid, called *aqueous humor.* The chamber behind the lens is much larger and contains a thicker fluid, *vitreous humor.* The outer layer of the eyeball is the *sclera,* or the white of the eye. It is a touch-sensitive layer and is transparent over the front of the eyeball. The transparent section is called the *cornea.* The cornea permits light to enter the eye. It is part of the focusing system of the eye. The next layer, the *vascular tunic (middle coat),* contains many blood vessels and the pigment that gives color to the eye. This vascular tunic, associated with the scleral portion of the eye, is called the *choroid.* The choroid is the vascular coat between the sclera and retina. The pigmented section over the front of the eyeball is called the *iris.* The iris has an opening in the center, the *pupil.* The pupil varies in size with the amount of light admitted, contracting to shut out bright light and enlarging in dim light. It is like the opening in the shutter of a camera. The *lens* is a transparent body behind the pupil. The inner surface of the eyeball is the *retina.* The retina contains the nerve fibers of the optic nerve and cells sensitive to light. The light

Figure 18-17 *Special senses.* **A,** *Hearing.*
From LaFleur M, Starr W: *Exploring medical language: a student-directed approach*, ed 2, St. Louis, 1989, Mosby.

A

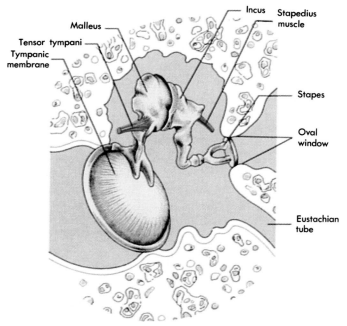

Semicircular canals

Incus

Vestibular nerve

Facial nerve

Cochlear nerve

Cochlea

Round window

Eustachian tube

Malleus

Stapes at oval window

Tympanic membrane

External auditory canal

GROSS ANATOMY OF THE EAR IN FRONTAL SECTION

Malleus

Incus

Stapedius muscle

Tensor tympani

Tympanic membrane

Stapes

Oval window

Eustachian tube

IMPEDENCE-MATCHING COMPONENTS OF INNER EAR

Figure 18-17—cont'd *Special senses.* **B,** *sight.*
From LaFleur M, Starr W: *Exploring medical language: a student-directed approach,* ed 2, St. Louis, 1989, Mosby.

B

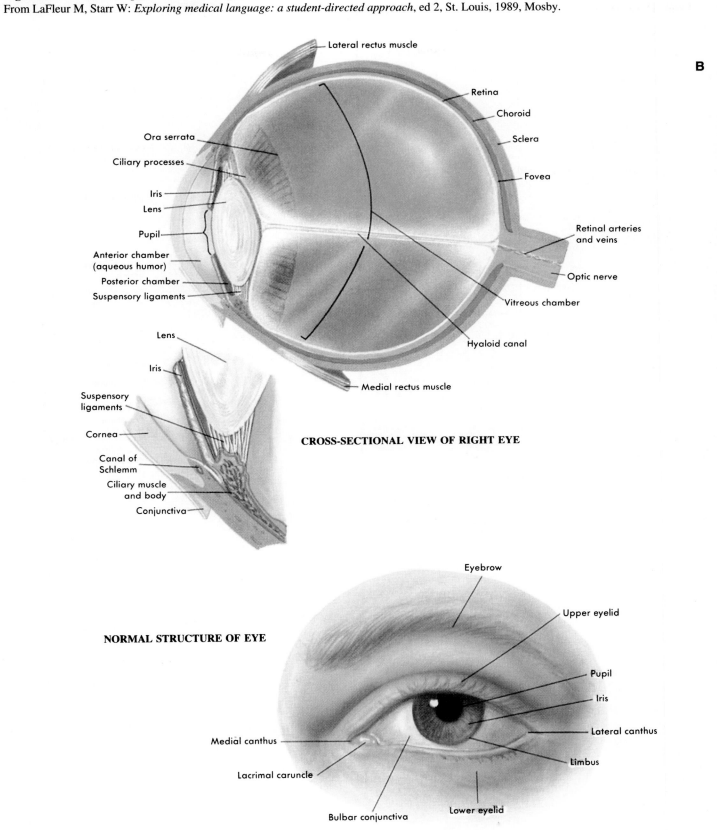

CROSS-SECTIONAL VIEW OF RIGHT EYE

NORMAL STRUCTURE OF EYE

Figure 18-17—cont'd *Special senses.* **C,** *Skin: protection and touch.*
From LaFleur M, Starr W: *Exploring medical language: a student-directed approach*, ed 2, St. Louis, 1989, Mosby.

C

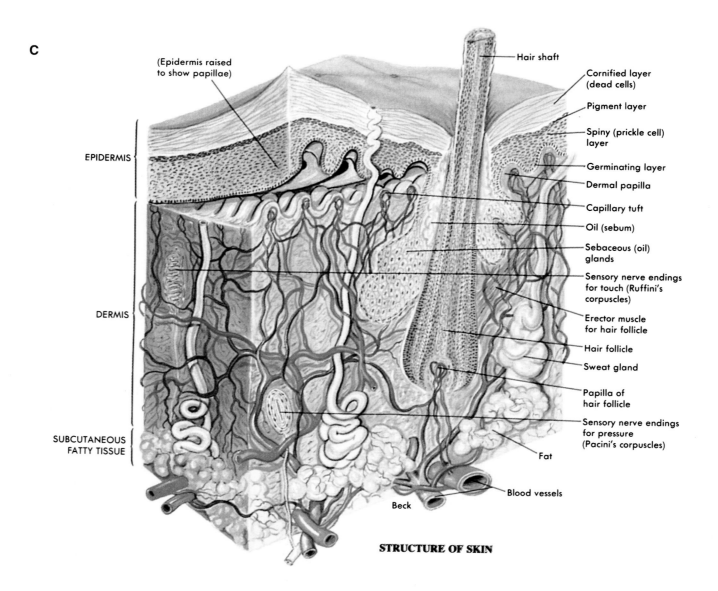

STRUCTURE OF SKIN

rays are brought to a focus by the lens, and the image it produces is transmitted to the retina and carried by the optic nerve to the seeing center in the brain. The retina in each eye receives the image from a slightly different angle. The sensation aroused by the two images combine in the brain if they have fallen on corresponding points of the retina of the two eyes and give depth to the image. To make the image points identical, the eyes must coordinate perfectly. The ability to see objects at different distances is known as *accommodation* and is accomplished when the curves of the surfaces of the lens are changed. Rays of light are bent as they enter the eye through the lens to make them focus on the retina (see Figure 18-17, *B*).

OTHER SPECIAL SENSES

In addition to hearing and sight, humans have three other special senses: taste, smell, and touch. The last includes general sensations of heat, cold, pain, pressure, size, and texture of objects. Although these senses are no less important to us, from a clinical standpoint their abnormal functions are not encountered in office practice with great frequency. Therefore they are described only briefly in this text. For additional information the student is referred to other, more complete anatomic works listed on page 633.

THE INTEGUMENTARY SYSTEM

The integumentary system is composed of the skin and accessory structures. **Accessory structures** of the system include the hair, nails, specialized glands, and nerves. The **main function** of the integumentary system is to protect the other body systems from injury and infection. A **second function** is to help the body maintain homeostasis by regulating temperature, retaining body fluids, and eliminating wastes. The skin also helps to perceive the environment with sensory receptors. The skin stores energy and vitamins and produces vitamin D from sunlight.

STRUCTURES OF THE INTEGUMENTARY SYSTEM
Skin

The skin (Figure 18-17, *C*) is the largest organ in the body. It varies in thickness from $1/50$ inch (0.5 mm) thick in the eyelids to $1/4$ inch (6.3 mm) in the soles of the feet. The skin often shows the presence of other body system disorders, including anemia, respiratory disorders, liver disorders, cancer, and shock.

The *epidermis*, or cuticle, is the outermost layer of the skin and is composed of a surface of dead cells with an underlying layer of living cells. There are no blood vessels in the epidermis. Some oil (*sebaceous*) and the sweat (*sudiferous*) glands, as well as hair follicles, open onto the epidermis. Melanocytes, which produce melanin, are located in this layer. Melanin is the pigment that gives skin its color.

The *dermis,* or corium, is called the "true" skin. The dermis contains the blood vessels, nerves, and glands.

The innermost layer of the skin is called the *subcutaneous* layer. Fatty (*adipose*) tissue of the subcutaneous layer cushions and insulates the body's organs.

The nerve endings in the skin allow it to be sensitive to environmental stimuli. Skin senses pain, pressure, touch, and changes in temperature.

Hair and Hair Follicles

Skin normally has hair (*pilus*) in all areas except the soles of the feet, palms of the hands, and on the lips. Some hair serves to block foreign particles from entering the body through structures such as the nose and eyes. Each hair root originates in the dermis. The visible portion is called the shaft. The hair *follicle* is the tubular cavity in the dermis that encloses the hair and from which the hair grows. One or two oil (sebaceous) glands are attached to each hair follicle. A tiny muscle (arrector pili) is attached to the hair shaft, which causes "goosebumps" and the hair to "stand on end" in response to cold or fear. Hair color is inherited and depends on the amount of melanin in the cells. Hair texture is also genetically determined.

Glands

The **three types of glands** in the skin are the oil glands (sebaceous), sweat glands (sudoriferous), and ceruminous glands of the ear canal.

Oil or *sebaceous* glands are located everywhere in the skin except the palms of the hands and the soles of the feet. Sebum, or oil, causes the skin to be soft and waterproof.

Sudoriferous or sweat glands originate mainly in the dermis, and sometimes in the subcutaneous layer of the skin. Some (apocrine) are attached to hair follicles, and others (eccrine) empty directly onto the skin through pores. Apocrine glands are located in areas such as under the arms (axilla), the breasts, and pubic area. There are about 3 million sudoriferous glands in the skin. Sudoriferous glands help regulate the body temperature and excrete body wastes. The skin loses at least 500 ml of water each day; more water is lost through sweating caused by exercise or heat.

Ceruminous glands are located only in the auditory canal of the ear. These glands secrete wax that helps to protect the ear from infection and prevents entry of foreign bodies.

Nails

The **function** of nails is to protect fingers and toes from injury. Fingernails and toenails are formed from dead, keratinized epidermal cells. The root or area of nail growth is covered by skin at the area of attachment to finger or toe. The crescent-shaped white area near the root is the *lunula*.

ASSESSMENT

Dermatology is the study of skin. *Dermatitis* is the general term for inflammation of the skin. Skin disorders are usually uncomfortable and unattractive, but not life threatening.

Skin lesions can usually be seen with visual inspection. The size, shape, texture, and color of a lesion often help reveal its cause (Table 18-5). A *biopsy* or culture may be used to identify the causative organism.

The uppermost part of the dermis is composed of *papillae,* or ridges. The papillae form regular patterns in the fingers, palms of the hands, and soles of the feet where the skin is thick. On the fingertips and toes, the patterns are unique. The patterns may also be linked to disorders like Down's syndrome.

SUN AND SKIN CANCER

The skin defends against the damaging ultraviolet radiation of the sun by producing melanin. Melanin accumulates in the cells of the skin and causes a tan. But the skin is easily damaged by excessive sunlight. It causes damage to cells of the dermis and loss of moisture that results in wrinkled, dry, and tough skin. Sunburn is actually a first-degree burn. A more serious second-degree burn can result if blisters form. Newer skin products contain para-aminobenzoic acid (PABA), which is effective in blocking the ultraviolet rays of the sun.

Ultraviolet rays in sunlight may also change the DNA structure in skin cells. Such changes may lead to mutations in the cells, or skin cancer.

Basal cell carcinoma is the most common type of skin cancer. It appears as waxy, pearly growth or red, scaly patches. It most often appears on the face, arms, and hands.

Squamous cell carcinoma is the second most common type. It spreads more quickly than basal cell and also appears on areas on skin most often exposed to the sun. This cancer looks like red, scaly patches.

Melanoma is the third and most serious form of skin cancer. It is most often caused by exposure to the sun. It appears as a brown or black molelike growth on the back, legs, or torso. If not treated early, melanoma may be fatal.

Although skin cancer is the most common form of cancer, it is also the most treatable, particularly if diagnosed early. Treatments include surgical removal, freezing affected tissue (cryotherapy), and use of radiation. Early signs of skin cancer include a spot or growth that does not heal or a mole or birthmark that changes color, size, thickness, or texture.

TABLE 18-5

Skin Lesions

Lesion	Description	Possible Cause	Illustration
Abrasion (ah-bra' zhun)	Scraped-away skin; red, swollen, closed	Trauma	
Angioma (an-je-o'mah)	Red central body with radiating branches	Liver disease, Vitamin B deficiency	
Atrophy (at'-ro-fe)	Thinning of skin surface; paperlike, translucent	Aging	
Bulla (bul'ah)	Vesicle more than 0.5 cm diameter	Blister	
Cicatrix (sik'ah-triks)	Tissue formed in healing process; white, red, or pink scar	Healed wound or healed surgical incision	
Crust	Dry pus, lymph, or blood covering injury; secondary skin lesion	Scab on abrasion, eczema	
Cyst	Sac of fluid or dead cells, solid to touch	Plugged oil gland	

Table 18-5—cont'd

Skin Lesions

Lesion	Description	Possible Cause	Illustration
Desquamation (des-kwah-ma'shun)	Sloughing (shedding) scales or excessive epithelial cells	Psoriasis	
Ecchymosis (ek-ih-mo'sis)	Large area of purpura, bruise	Trauma, vasculitis	
Erosion	Loss of part of epidermis leaving moist, depressed area	Rupture of blister	
Excoriation	Loss of epidermis leaving crusted area and dermis exposed	Scratch, abrasion	
Fissure	Deep groove in skin, crack	Athlete's foot	
Hemangioma (he'man"je-o'mah)	Benign tumor composed of blood vessels	Birthmark, or nevus (ne'vus)	
Incision	Cut into skin, edges regular	Surgery	
Keloid (ke'loid)	Progressively enlarging scar	Burn	
Laceration	Cut into skin, edges irregular	Trauma	
Lichenification (li"ken-if-ih-ka'shun)	Thick, rough epidermis with skin markings resembling lichen	Dermatitis	
Macule (mak'ule)	Discolored spot on skin; not raised or depressed	Measles, mononucleosis, freckles	
Nodule (nod'ule)	Solid area, deeper in skin than papule; may be in any layer of skin	Lipoma	

Table 18-5—cont'd

Skin Lesions

Lesion	Description	Possible Cause	Illustration
Papule (pap'ule)	Raised, solid area, less than 1 cm diameter	Warts, moles, pimples	
Patch	Flat, irregular-shaped macule greater than 1 cm diameter	Vitiligo (vit-ih-li'go), port-wine marks	
Petechiae (peh'te'ke-i)	Form of purpura; hemorrhages, appearing as tiny dots below skin	Aplastic anemia, scurvy	
Plaque (plak)	Firm, elevated papule greater than 1 cm in diameter	Psoriasis	
Purpura (pur'pu-rah)	Hemorrhage in capillaries of dermis discoloring skin	Contact allergies, scurvy	
Pustule (pus'tule)	Pus-filled, raised area; white, yellow, greenish-yellow	Pimples, acne	
Scale	Flaky, irregular skin of silver, white, or tan	Psoriasis, dermatitis	
Tumor	Solid, elevated mass greater than 2 cm in diameter	Benign or malignant growth	
Ulcer	Open sore; may bleed or have discharge	Bedsore	
Venous star	Bluish, spiderlike webs	Pressure in peripheral veins	
Vesicle	Raised, fluid-filled pouch; specific location	Burns, scabies, shingles, chickenpox	
Wheal	Flat or rounded, white or red elevation; shifts location	Allergic reaction, urticaria (hives)	

CONCLUSION

You have now completed the unit on Anatomy and Physiology. When given diagrams of the human body by your instructor, you should be able to accurately label body systems and organs that are presented in this unit.

CASE STUDY

The importance of understanding anatomy and physiology is most evident in the final component of the patient's health history, the review of systems. It serves as verification that all relevant data have been obtained and groups together symptoms by relationship. Read the headings for a review of systems and discuss the underlined terminology and possible symptoms for each category.

Cranial Cavity
  EENT-Eyes
  Ears
  Nose
  Throat
  Neck

Breast
Thoracic cavity
  Cardiovascular-lymphatic
  Respiratory
  Abdominal cavity
  Gastrointestinal
  Pelvic cavity
  Urinary tract
  Genital tract
Musculoskeletal
Cerebrospinal
Integumentary
Endocrine

REVIEW QUESTIONS

1. Define anatomy and physiology.
2. List the five cavities in the human body.
3. State the main functions of the skeletal system.
4. List five functions of muscles.
5. Differentiate between the cardiovascular system and the lymphatic system.
6. State the main functions of the nervous system.
7. Discuss the difference between the central nervous system and the peripheral nervous system.
8. List the main functions of the digestive tract.
9. List six accessory organs of the digestive tract.
10. List the three divisions of the small intestine.
11. List the four parts of the colon.
12. State which is the largest organ in the body; the largest bone.
13. State where bile is produced and where it is stored. Briefly discuss the functions of bile.
14. List three functions of the respiratory tract.
15. State the name of the functional unit of the kidney. (Where is urine produced?)
16. State two primary functions of the urinary system.
17. State where sperm are produced in the male and where ova are produced in the female.
18. Discuss the difference between menstruation and menopause.
19. State the advantage of HRT for women after menopause.
20. State which endocrine gland is commonly referred to as the master gland and why it is referred to as the master.
21. List the five specialized organs of the senses.

SUGGESTED READINGS

Thibodeau GA: *Anthony's textbook of anatomy and physiology*, ed 13, St. Louis, 1990, Mosby.
Seeley RR, Stephens TD, Tate P: *Anatomy and physiology*, ed 2, St. Louis, 1992, Mosby.

Nutrition

COGNITIVE OBJECTIVES

On completion of Unit Nineteen, the medical assistant student should be able to:

1. Define the vocabulary terms listed in this unit.
2. List the five main nutrients (excluding water) and give three food examples for each.
3. List the five food groups.
4. Identify the main functions of protein, carbohydrates, and fats.
5. Identify the dietary sources of vitamins and minerals.
6. List five benefits of increasing fiber in your diet.
7. Briefly describe the therapeutic diets.
8. State the difference between a full liquid diet and a clear liquid diet.

TERMINAL PERFORMANCE OBJECTIVES

On completion of Unit Nineteen, the medical assistant student should be able:

1. Given the dietary guidelines and the Food Guide Pyramid, write a nutritious sample food plan for a five-day period.
2. Given the therapeutic diets (excluding BRAT), write a sample one-day food plan for each.

NUTRITION AND YOUR HEALTH

The keys to healthful eating are moderation, balance, and variety. Nutrition scientists know that what you eat directly affects your long-term health. Dietary factors contribute substantially to premature death and preventable illnesses in the United States. For example, overweight to obesity, largely self-induced conditions, increase the risk for heart disease, various types of cancer, diabetes, stroke, and early death (Table 19-1).

Numerous scientific studies continually demonstrate that the typical American diet has:

- Too many calories
- Too much cholesterol
- Too much fat, especially saturated fat
- Not enough complex carbohydrates
- Not enough fiber

VOCABULARY

Calorie—The amount of energy required to raise the temperature of 1 kg of water 1° C.

Digestion—The mechanical and chemical breakdown of food into substances small enough to be absorbed and used by body cells to maintain life.

Food labeling—Nutritional information, including mandatory reporting of total calories, calories from fat, total fat, saturated fat, cholesterol, sodium, total carbohydrate, dietary fiber, sugars, protein, vitamins A and C, calcium, and iron.

Uniform definitions—Nutrition language describing a food's nutrition content such as "light," "low-fat," and "high-fiber" to ensure the same meaning for any product on which they appear.

Nutrient—A substance derived from food that provides the body with nourishment. Nutrients are essential for life and are responsible for particular body functions. Nutrients needed by the body include proteins, fats, carbohydrates, vitamins, and minerals.

Nutrition—The science of the study of all of the processes involved with the taking in of food and drink and how they are used for normal body functioning and maintenance of health. The processes involved are ingestion, digestion, and absorption of nutrients and the elimination of waste products.

Obesity—Mildly obese: 20% to 40% above one's ideal weight; moderately obese: 41% to 100% above one's ideal weight; severely obese: 100% above one's ideal weight (see page 49 for the suggested weights for adults)

RDAs (Recommended Daily Allowances)—The RDAs are defined as "...the levels of intake of essential nutrients that, on the basis of scientific knowledge, are judged by the Food and Nutrition Board to be adequate to meet the known nutrient needs of practically all healthy persons." The U.S. RDAs are averaged and rounded figures and are used by food manufacturers in labeling their products.

TABLE 19-1

Relationship Between Overweight and Disease Risk

Disease	Increased Risk (20%-30% Overweight)	(40% Overweight)
Heart disease		
Male	32	95
Female	39	107
Cancer		
Male		
Prostate	37	39
Colon	26	73
Female		
Breast	16	53
Cervix	51	139
Endometrium	85	442
Ovary	0	63
Diabetes		
Male	156	419
Female	234	690
Stroke		
Male	17	127
Female	16	52

Other
Chances of suffering from arthritis, gallstones, gout, and premature death also increase for both males and females.
Obesity
High percentage of body fat increases the low-density lipoproteins and increases total blood cholesterol.

Courtesy American Cancer Society, San Francisco, Calif.

You are often involved in the health education of patients with special dietary needs. It is important to understand nutritional requirements, help patients choose a variety of foods from the five food groups (Figure 19-1, *A* and *B*), and be supportive of the need for patients to make behavioral changes to bring their diets into balance.

DIGESTION

Digestion is the physical and chemical changes that food undergoes in the body to make it absorbable. Some foods that are already absorbable include water, minerals, and certain carbohydrates in fruits. In others, the cooking process initiates the chemical changes before food enters the body.

The digestive process is controlled by the nervous and hormonal systems. Digestive fluids are inhibited by strong emotion, which interferes with digestion. Food attractively served in pleasant surroundings with cheerful conversation enhances proper digestion.

METABOLISM

Metabolism is the series of chemical processes that occurs when your body changes air, food, and other materials into substances needed to function properly. The chemical balance in your body and the rate of your metabolism differ from those of others. There are two types of metabolic disorders that affect the digestive system. One is caused by poor nutrition, or eating and drinking the wrong kinds and amounts of foods. The second one is genetic and inherited from your parents; however, rarely does an individual inherit a specific disease that predisposes him or her to become and stay obese.

NUTRIENTS

There are six main classifications of nutrients required by the body to maintain health: proteins, fats, carbohydrates, vitamins, minerals, and water. These components are discussed according to composition, sources, function, and caloric requirements.

Figure 19-1 A, *Food guide pyramid: a guide to daily food choices.*
A courtesy U.S. Department of Agriculture/U.S. Department of Health and Human Services.

A

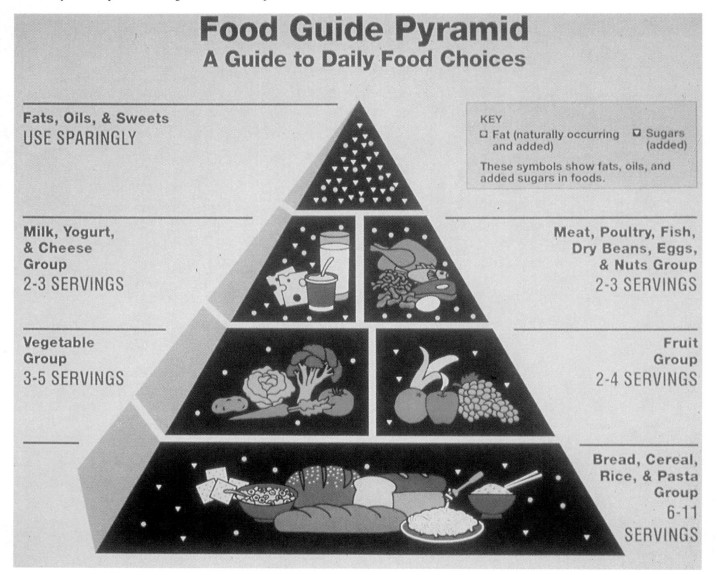

PROTEINS
Composition

Proteins are often thought of as the building blocks of our body. They are found in every living cell. Proteins are composed of chains of approximately 20 *amino acids*, nine of which are called *essential amino acids*. To function and survive, the body needs the nine essential amino acids contained in complete proteins. The remaining amino acids can be synthesized by the body.

Sources

The essential amino acids must be obtained from the food we eat and are obtained from foods referred to as *complete proteins*. The best food sources of complete proteins are meat, milk, cheese, eggs, and fish. Foods that do not contain all of the essential amino acids are called *incomplete protein foods*. Examples of these foods include legumes (dry beans

and peas, soy bean curd [tofu]), grains, nuts, and seeds. A combination of various sources of incomplete protein foods provides an adequate amount of the amino acids needed for protein synthesis (for example, peanut butter on wheat bread).

Function

The main functions of protein include the following:

1. Promotes growth, repair, and maintenance of musculoskeletal and other body tissues.
2. Serves as a framework for bones, muscles, blood, hair, and fingernails.
3. Helps to regulate some body processes by serving as a component of hormones and enzymes.
4. Helps to maintain the acid-base balance in the body.
5. Serves as a source of energy (four calories for every gram of protein consumed).

Figure 19-1—cont'd B, *serving sizes and suggested number of servings.*
B Adapted from Gerdin J: *Health careers today,* St. Louis, 1991, Mosby.

RECOMMENDED DAILY SERVINGS OF THE BASIC FOOD GROUPS

B

Group	Food Sources	Number of Daily Servings
Milk or equivalents	Cheese, ice cream, buttermilk, yogurt, cottage cheese	2 (Adult) 4 (Teenager) 3 (Child)
Meat or equivalents	Meat, fish, eggs , poultry, dried beans, peas, nuts	2 (Adult) 2 (Teenager)
Vegetables and fruits	Dark green or yellow vegetables, citrus fruits, tomatoes	2 (Adult) 4 (Teenager) 4 (Child)
Breads and cereals	Enriched or whole grain, grits, macaroni, noodles, rice, spaghetti	4 (Adult) 4 (Teenager) 4 (Child)
Sweets and alcohol	Candy, wine, etc.	Provides calories only, no nutrients

Serving sizes

Food	Portion Equaling One Serving	Food	Portion Equaling One Serving
Milk	1 cup	Potato	1 (medium)
Buttermilk	1 cup	Raw fruit or vegetables	1 cup
Yogurt	1 cup	Juice	1/2 cup
Cheddar cheese	1 1/2 slices (1 1/2 oz)	Cooked fruit or vegetables	1/2 cup
Pudding	1 cup	Bread	1 slice
Ice cream	1 3/4 cup	Cereal	1 cup
Lean meat, fish, poultry	2 oz.	Noodles, corn meal, rice, grits	1 (small)
Cheddar cheese	2 slices (2 oz)	Muffin, roll, biscuit	1 (small)
Eggs	2	Cracker, saltine	5
Dried beans or peas	1 cup	Oatmeal	1/2 cup
Peanut butter	4 tablespoons		
Cottage cheese	1/2 cup		

Caloric Requirements

Nutritionists recommend that 12% to 15% of our daily caloric requirement be derived from protein sources. Excess protein, like excess calories from any source, are stored as fat. Disease and injury affecting the musculoskeletal system may require additional protein intake.

FATS

Fats (lipids) are composed of fatty acids in various combinations with glycerin. These fatty acids can be classified as either saturated or unsaturated. It is their chemical structure that makes them different.

Saturated fat. Saturated fat comes from animal sources (meats, lard, eggs, and dairy products) and plants (coconut oil, palm oil, and palm kernel oil). Products such as commercial cookies, nondairy whipped toppings and creamers, and commercial cake mixes contain hidden saturated fat (Figure 19-2). Saturated fat can increase the level of cholesterol in the blood. (For the amounts of both found in some common foods, see Table 19-2.) Too much cholesterol in the blood is associated with an increased risk of heart disease. No more than *10%* of daily calorie intake should come from saturated fats. Reducing fat intake also reduces the risk for cancer of the breast, colon, and prostate and the occurrence of obesity.

TABLE 19-2

Cholesterol and Saturated Fat Content of Selected Foods

Food (Amount)	Cholesterol (mg)	Saturated Fat (mg)
Lamb, 3 oz.	85	3000-9000
Pork, 3 oz.	55-75	3500-9200
Beef, 3 oz.	55-75	2200-6000
Poultry (light meat), 3 oz.	60	1000
Poultry (dark meat), 3 oz.	85	4000
Liver, 3 oz.	372	2500
Fish, 3 oz.	40-60	1000-1700
Shrimp, 3 oz.	90	400
Egg, 1 large	252	1700
Whole milk, 1 cup	34	4700
Lowfat milk, 1 cup	22	2700
Nonfat milk, 1 cup	5	—
Half and half, $1/2$ cup	26	7800
Cottage cheese, $1/2$ cup	15-23	1800-4900
Most cheeses, 1 oz.	16-30	4000-6000
Yogurt, 1 cup	5-20	500-4200
Ice cream $1/2$ cup	30	6500
Ice milk, $1/2$ cup	13	1900
Peanut butter, 1 Tbsp	—	1500
Butter, 1 Tbsp	34	6500
Margarine, 1 Tbsp	—	2100
Mayonnaise, 1 Tbsp	7	2000
Sour cream, 1 Tbsp	8	4600
Olive oil, 1 Tbsp	—	1500
Corn oil, 1 Tbsp	—	1400
Cottonseed oil, 1 Tbsp	—	3400
Salad dressing, (Italian), 1 Tbsp	—	1600
Chocolate, 1 oz.	5	8400

Figure 19-2 *Where's the fat? Hidden fat is found in products such as chocolate cake, nondairy whipped toppings, cookies, and milk. Visible fat is seen on meats, oils, and butter.*

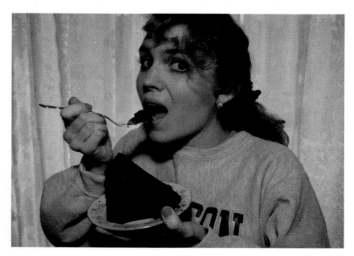

Unsaturated fat. The two types of unsaturated fats are polyunsaturated and monounsaturated fats.

Polyunsaturated fat includes vegetable oils and fish oils (Omega-3 fatty acids). Unsaturated fat is usually liquid at room temperature. The process of hydrogenation can convert some unsaturated fat into solid fat for cooking purposes. The production of margarine is an example of hydrogenation.

Monounsaturated fat, the more beneficial unsaturated fat because it lowers cholesterol levels and LDLs, includes olive oil, canola oil, and peanut oil (Tables 19-3 and 19-4). Olive and canola oils are the oils that are recommended for use if you must use oil.

Function

The functions of fat in the body include the following:

1. Provides a concentrated source of energy (that is, every gram of fat provides nine calories)
2. Helps to satisfy our appetite

TABLE 19-3

A Basic Primer on Fats in the Diet

On average, people in the United States eat about 37% of their total calories as fat. Many nutrition authorities have suggested it is best to restrict fat intake to no more than 30% of total calories, limiting saturated fatty acids to about a third of this amount. Limiting cholesterol is also important to your health. A basic definition of these terms and dietary suggestions follow.

Fat	Fat is the most concentrated source of food energy (calories). Each gram of fat supplies about 9 calories, compared with about 4 calories in a gram of protein or carbohydrates. In addition to providing energy, fat aids in the absorption of certain vitamins. Some fats provide linoleic acid, an essential fatty acid which is needed by everyone in small amounts. Butter, margarine, shortening and oil are obvious sources of fat. Well-marbled meats, poultry skin, whole milk, cheese, ice cream, nuts, seeds, salad dressings and some baked products also provide a good deal of fat.
Cholesterol	Cholesterol is not a fat, but a fat-like substance, found in the body cells of humans and animals. It is needed to form hormones, cell membranes and other body substances. The body is able to make the cholesterol it needs for these functions. Cholesterol is not needed in the diet. Cholesterol is present in all meat, poultry and fish, in milk and milk products and in egg yolks. It is not found in foods of plant origin such as fruits, vegetables, nuts, grains and seeds.
Fatty acids	Fatty acids are the basic chemical units in fat. They may be either "saturated," "monounsaturated" or "polyunsaturated." All dietary fats are made up of mixtures of these fatty acid types. **Saturated fatty acids** are found largely in fats of animal origin, including whole milk, cream, cheese, butter, meat and poultry. They are also found in large amounts in some vegetable oils, including coconut and palm. **Monounsaturated fatty acids** are found in fats of both plant and animal origin. Olive and peanut oil are the most common examples, along with most margarines and hydrogenated vegetable shortening. **Polyunsaturated fatty acids** are found largely in fats of plant origin including sunflower, corn, soybean, cottonseed and safflower oils. Some fish are also good sources.
To your health...	Eating a diet high in fat—especially saturated fatty acids—and cholesterol causes elevated blood cholesterol levels in many people. High blood cholesterol levels increase the risk of heart disease. Reducing fat is an especially good idea for those people who are limiting calories. Not only do fats provide more than twice the calories of proteins and carbohydrates, but they also contain few vitamins and minerals.
Moderation is the key	Eliminating all fats is not good for you either. For example, milk, meat, poultry, fish, and eggs all contribute fat, saturated fat, and cholesterol to your diet; but they also provide essential nutrients such as calcium, iron and zinc. So the key is moderation. Focus on a balanced overall diet and avoid too much fat when possible by using lower fat dairy products and lean meats and reducing the amount of fats added at the table.

Table 19-3—cont'd

A Basic Primer on Fats in the Diet

How does your diet score?   Do the foods you eat provide more fat than is good for you? Answer the questions below, then see how your diet stacks up.

How often do you eat:

	Seldom or never	1-2x per week	3-5x per week	Almost daily
Fried, deep-fat fried or breaded foods?	❏	❏	❏	❏
Fatty meats such as bacon, sausage, luncheon meats and heavily marbled steaks and roasts?	❏	❏	❏	❏
Whole milk, high-fat cheeses and ice cream?	❏	❏	❏	❏
High-fat desserts such as pies, pastries and rich cakes?	❏	❏	❏	❏
Rich sauces and gravies?	❏	❏	❏	❏
Oily salad dressings or mayonnaise?	❏	❏	❏	❏
Whipped cream, table cream, sour cream and cream cheese?	❏	❏	❏	❏
Butter or margarine on vegetables, dinner rolls and toast?	❏	❏	❏	❏

Take a look at your answers. Several responses in the last two columns mean you may have a high fat intake. Perhaps it's time to cut back.

Cutting back on fat   Here are 15 tips to help you avoid too much fat, saturated fat and cholesterol in your diet:

1. Steam, boil or bake vegetables; or for a change, stir fry in a small amount of vegetable oil.
2. Season vegetables with herbs and spices rather than with sauces, butter or margarine.
3. Try lemon juice on salads or use limited amounts of oil-based salad dressing.
4. To reduce saturated fat, use margarine instead of butter in baked products and, when possible, use oil instead of shortening.
5. Try whole-grain flours to enhance flavors of baked goods made with less fat and cholesterol-containing ingredients.
6. Replace whole milk with skim or lowfat milk in puddings, soups and baked products.
7. Substitute plain lowfat yogurt, blender-whipped lowfat cottage cheese or buttermilk in recipes that call for sour cream or mayonnaise.
8. Choose lean cuts of meat.
9. Trim fat from meat before and/or after cooking.
10. Roast, bake, broil or simmer meat, poultry or fish.
11. Remove skin from poultry before cooking.
12. Cook meat or poultry on a rack so the fat will drain off. Use a non-stick pan for cooking so added fat will be unnecessary.
13. Chill meat or poultry broth until the fat becomes solid. Spoon off the fat before using the broth.
14. Limit egg yolks to one per serving when making scrambled eggs. Use additional egg whites for larger servings.
15. Try substituting egg whites in recipes calling for whole eggs. For example, use two egg whites in place of each whole egg in muffins, cookies and puddings.

For more information about fats and oils in your diet, contact:

The U.S. Department of Agriculture, Human Nutrition Information Service, Room 360, 6505 Belcrest Road, Hyattsville, Md. 20782 and ask for a list of relevant publications.

The American Heart Association, National Center, 7320 Greenville Avenue, Dallas, Tex. 75231 or call your local American Heart Association office.

Your local county extension agent or public health nutritionist or dietitians in hospitals and other community agencies.

Courtesy the Worldview Quarterly, Nestle USA, Inc., Washington, D.C.

TABLE 19-4

Effects of Fats on Blood Lipids

Type of Fat	Effects on Blood Lipids	Sources
Saturated	Increases total cholesterol Increases (LDLs) low-density lipoproteins	Most red meats Lard Butter Hydrogenated shortenings Stick margarine Plant fats • Coconut oil • Palm oil Palm kernel oil Animal fats Milk products with high butterfat
Polyunsaturated (vegetable)	Decreases total cholesterol Decreases LDLs Decreases (HDLs) high-density lipoproteins May decrease the functions of the immune system Risks may outweigh the benefits	Safflower oil Sunflower oil Corn oil Soybean oil Cottonseed oil Sesame oil Soft margarine
Polyunsaturated (fish)	Decreases total cholesterol Decreases LDLs Increases HDLs Decreases triglycerides Retards plaque formation Reduces the body's tendency to form blood clots which can trigger a heart attack	Cold-water fish • Mackerel • Salmon • Tuna • Trout • Anchovy • Herring
Monounsaturated	Decreases total cholesterol Decreases LDLs May reduce blood pressure May reduce blood sugar	Canola oil Peanut oil, peanuts Peanut butter Olives, olive oil Almonds Pecans Cashews Avocados

3. Helps in making food taste good

4. Stores the fat-soluble vitamins

5. Aids in transporting the fat-soluble vitamins (A, D, E, and K)

6. Helps to keep our skin healthy

7. Is used for tissue building but most of the fat is stored for future energy needs

8. Gives us stamina

9. Provides insulation for the body against low temperatures

Sources

Because currently there is so much talk about the disadvantages of fat (lipids) in the diet, some people are beginning to think that fat is not needed in their diet, but it is. Fat plays an important role in body functions and health. The problem is that most people eat too much fat. It is estimated that fat accounts for up to 42% of the daily calories in the average American diet. About 95% of the fat that is ingested is absorbed and used *or* stored in the body. Approximately 15% of the average person's body weight is fat. In addition to eating foods containing fat, the body converts some protein and carbohydrates into fat.

Another area of concern is that about 50% of the fat that we eat is "hidden" fat. It is often not visible when we look at the food. For example, when you look at a piece of chocolate cake, you don't see little fat bubbles oozing out. What you do see is a nice, moist, crumbly texture of a product that may be very tasty to you. Other sources of hidden fats are snack foods, cookies, crackers, nondairy whipped toppings, nondairy creamers, and cereals. Many of these contain tropical oils (palm, coconut, and palm kernel oils), which are saturated fats. Many food items are labeled with the percentage of fat content. An example is 2% milk. Many people think that in the whole gallon of milk there is only 2% fat, which sounds like a low-fat food. What they fail to realize is that the 2% means that the milk is 2% fat by weight not by volume; thus, in reality, in one serving of 2% milk containing 5 g of fat and 120 calories per serving, 37% of the total calories per serving come from fat. See page 655 for the formula for determining the percentage of calories from fat in a food product.

Another example is a bran muffin. We often think muffins are a good source of fiber, and many times they may be, but you must read the label because many packaged muffins are high in fat and sugar and low in fiber. If you read the label, you may see that the muffin contains eggs, palm oil (both containing fat), honey and sugar (both simple carbohydrates), and processed cake flour, which is low in fiber. That is not to say that you can never have another muffin in your life, but it is suggested that you be aware of the contents of the food you eat so you can make more responsible choices, maintaining a diet of a *variety* of foods, even if you do indulge at times.

Caloric Requirements

It is suggested that we reduce our fat consumption so that fat makes up *only* 30% of our daily calorie requirement. Many health experts suggest that a recommendation of 20% would be a better goal. These experts realize, however, that this is not very feasible, considering the dietary habits of Americans and the various foods available—unless the individual makes a very concerted effort.

CHOLESTEROL
Composition

Cholesterol is an odorless, soft, fatlike substance found in body cells of animals and humans.

Function

It is an important component for a healthy body because it is essential for the functioning of body systems such as the nervous system. It is also essential for the formation of cell membranes and many hormones, including the sex hormones, and other substances, such as bile salts and nerve fibers.

Sources

Cholesterol comes from two sources—from our own bodies and from food that comes from animal sources. There is *no* cholesterol in foods from plant sources. In addition, it is thought that *saturated fats* found in animal fats and other sources contribute to the formation of cholesterol in the body, thereby increasing the body's normal supply and contributing to a high blood serum cholesterol level.

Cholesterol is transported to and from the body cells by compounds called lipoproteins. There are several types of lipoproteins that are classified according to their size and density. The types of main concern are the *high-density lipoproteins (HDLs)* and the *low-density lipoproteins (LDLs)*. The HDLs are commonly referred to as the "good guys" or "good cholesterol." The LDLs are commonly referred to as the "bad guys" or "bad cholesterol." The LDLs are the major carrier of cholesterol in the bloodstream. They contain 60% to 70% of the serum cholesterol. The HDLs contain 20% to 30% of the serum cholesterol. The *higher* the level of HDLs in the bloodstream, the *lower* the *risk* for cardiovascular disease. The LDLs carry cholesterol to blood vessels, where it is deposited. This leads to a narrowing of the blood vessels, thereby increasing the risk for heart disease. HDLs carry cholesterol away from the arteries and back to the liver for processing and removal, thereby helping to decrease the risk for heart disease.

Increased levels of serum cholesterol, associated with atherosclerosis, increase the risk for heart disease. On the other hand, it appears that *unsaturated* fats help to reduce the amount of cholesterol in the blood (see Table 19-1). When choosing foods, it is very important to look at the content of saturated fat present in addition to the amount, if any, of cholesterol (see Table 19-3) because, even if the food is low in cholesterol but high in saturated fat, our bodies will turn the saturated fat into cholesterol. In some foods there may be no or low amounts of cholesterol but high levels of saturated fat. Chocolate is a good example. In one ounce of chocolate there is only 5 mg of cholesterol *but* 8400 mg (or 8.4 g) of saturated fat; thus, even though the level of cholesterol is very low, the high amount of saturated fat will be changed into cholesterol and affect the cholesterol levels in our bloodstream.

Caloric Requirements

Our body produces all of the cholesterol needed for the functions it performs, primarily in the liver and the small intestine; thus it isn't necessary to eat more. Most recommend that the daily intake of cholesterol be limited to 300 mg or less (Table 19-5). See Table 13-2 for a blood lipid profile.

CARBOHYDRATES
Composition

Carbohydrates are the most abundant and economical sources of energy. All simple sugars and all substances that can be converted into simple sugars by hydrolysis are carbohydrates.

Function

Carbohydrates provide the main source of energy for all body functions. There are four calories for every gram of carbohydrate. They are also necessary for the metabolism of other nutrients. In the body, carbohydrates are either absorbed for immediate use or stored in the form of glycogen. They can also be manufactured in the body from some components of fat and from some amino acids.

TABLE 19-5

The First Step in Eating Right is Buying Right
A Guide to Choosing Low Saturated–Fat, Low-Cholesterol Foods

Following a low-saturated fat, low-cholesterol diet is a balancing act: getting the variety of foods necessary to supply the nutrients you need without too much saturated fat and cholesterol or excess calories. One way to ensure variety—and with it, a well-balanced diet—is to select foods each day from each of the following food groups. Select different foods from within groups, especially foods low in saturated fat (the left column). The amount and size of each portion should be adjusted to reach and maintain your desirable weight. As a guide, the recommended daily number of portions is listed for each food group.

	Choose	Go Easy On	Decrease
Meat, Poultry, Fish and Shellfish (Up to 6 ounces a day)	*Lean cuts* of meat with fat trimmed; such as: • Beef — Round, sirloin, chuck, loin • Lamb — Leg, arm, loin, rib • Pork — Tenderloin, leg (fresh), shoulder (arm or picnic) • Veal (all trimmed cuts except ground) Poultry without skin Fish Shellfish		"Prime" grade Fatty cuts of meat, such as: • Beef — Corned beef brisket, regular ground, short ribs • Pork — Spareribs, blade roll, fresh Goose, domestic Duck Organ meats Sausage, bacon Regular luncheon meats Frankfurters Caviar, roe
Dairy Products 2-3 servings for women who are pregnant or breastfeeding	Skim milk, 1% milk, low-fat buttermilk, low-fat evaporated or nonfat milk Low-fat yogurt Low-fat soft cheeses, like cottage, farmer, pot Cheeses labeled no more than 2 to 6 g of fat an ounce	2% milk Yogurt Part-skim ricotta Part-skim or imitation hard cheeses, like part-skim mozzarella "Light" cream cheese "Light" sour cream	Whole milk, such as regular, evaporated, condensed Cream, half and half, most nondairy creamers, imitation milk products, whipped cream Custard style yogurt Whole-milk ricotta Neufchatel Brie Hard cheeses, like swiss, American mozzarella, feta, cheddar, muenster Cream cheese Sour cream
Eggs (No more than 3 egg yolks a week)	Egg whites Cholesterol-free egg substitutes		Egg yolks
Fats and Oils Use sparingly	Unsaturated vegetable oils: corn, olive, peanut, rapeseed (canola oil), safflower, sesame, soybean Margarine; or shortening made from unsaturated fats listed above: liquid, tub, stick, diet	Nuts and seeds Avocados and olives	Butter, coconut oil, palm oil, palm kernel oil, lard, bacon fat Margarine or shortening made from saturated fats listed above

Table 19-5—cont'd

The First Step in Eating Right is Buying Right
A Guide to Choosing Low–Saturated Fat, Low-Cholesterol Foods

	Choose	Go Easy On	Decrease
Breads, Cereals, Pasta, Rice (6 to 11 servings a day)	Breads, like white, whole wheat, pumpernickel, and rye breads; pita; bagel; English muffin; sandwich buns; dinner rolls; rice cakes Low-fat crackers, like matzo, bread sticks, rye krisp, saltines, zwieback Hot cereals, most cold dry cereals	Store-bought pan-cakes, waffles, bis-cuits, muffins, corn-bread	Croissant, butter rolls, sweet rolls, danish pastry, doughnuts Most snack crackers, such as cheese crackers, butter crackers, those made with saturated oils Granola-type cereals made with satu-rated oils Pasta and rice prepared with cream, but-ter or cheese sauces; egg noodles
Dried Peas and Beans (2 to 3 servings)	Pasta, like plain noodles, spaghetti, macaroni Any grain rice Dried peas and beans, like split peas, black-eyed peas, chick peas, kidney beans, navy beans, lentils, soy-beans, soybean curd (tofu)		
Fruits and Vegetables (2 to 4 servings of fruit and 3 to 5 servings of vegeta-bles a day)	Fresh, frozen, canned or dried fruits and vegeta-bles		Vegetables prepared in butter, cream or sauce
Sweets and Snacks (Use sparingly)	Low-fat frozen desserts, like sherbet, sorbet, Italian ice, froxzen yogurt, popsicles Low-fat cakes, like angel food Low-fat cookies, like fig bars, gingersnaps Low-fat candy, like jelly beans, hard candy Low-fat snacks like plain popcorn, pretzels Nonfat beverages like car-bonated drinks, juices, tea, coffee	Frozen desserts, like ice milk Homemade cakes, cookies, and pies using unsaturated oils sparingly Fruit crisps and cob-blers	High-fat frozen desserts, such as ice cream, frozen tofu High-fat cakes, like most store-bought, pound, and frosted cakes Store-bought pies Most store-bought cookies Most candy, like chocolate bars High-fat snacks, such as chips, buttered popcorn High-fat beverages, like frappes, milk-shakes, floats, and eggnogs

Table 19-5—cont'd

The First Step in Eating Right is Buying Right
A Guide to Choosing Low–Saturated Fat, Low-Cholesterol Foods

Choose	Go Easy On	Decrease

Label Ingredients
Go easy on products that list any fat or oil first or that list many fat and oil ingredients. The following lists clue you in to names of saturated fat ingredients (decrease) and unsaturated ingredients (go easy on).

	Go Easy On	Decrease
	Carob, cocoa	Cocoa butter
	Oils, like corn, cotton- seed, olive, safflower, sesame, soybean or sunflower oil	Animal fat, like bacon, beef, chicken, ham, lamb, meat, port or turkey fats, butter, lard
	Nonfat dry milk, non- fat dry milk solids, skim milk	Coconut, coconut oil, palm or palm kernel oil
		Cream
		Egg and egg-yolk solids
		Hardened fat or oil
		Hydrogenated vegetable oil
		Milk chocolate
		Shortening or vegetable shortening
		Vegetable oil (could be coconut, palm kernel or palm oil)

Sources

Carbohydrates are present, at least in small quantities, in most foods. The chief sources are the sugars (simple carbohydrates) and the starches (complex carbohydrates).

Sources of simple sugars include the following:
* *Refined sugars* such as white and brown sugar, honey, and syrup
* *Naturally occurring sugars* as found in fruits and vegetables. Like fats, much of the sugar consumed is hidden. Many fail to realize that there is sugar in foods such as canned vegetables and fruits, in ketchup, salad dressings, in cured meat products, and in many other food products.

Sources of complex carbohydrates or starches include the following:
* Vegetables such as broccoli, cabbage, cauliflower, carrots, yams, and potatoes
* Fruits such as citrus fruits and yellow fruits
* Grains such as wheat, rice, oats, corn, breads, and pastas
* Cereals

Complex carbohydrates provide a good source for many vitamins and minerals. In addition, many provide a good source for dietary fiber. Generally, these foods are low in fat (Figure 19-3).

As with fats and proteins, if excessive amounts of carbohydrates are eaten, the body will change them into fats and store them as fat.

Caloric Requirements

It is recommended that *less than 10%* of our total caloric requirements be obtained from *refined* sugars. *Complex carbohydrates should account for 50% to 60%* of our daily caloric requirement. The recommendation for most people is to decrease their intake of refined sugars and increase their intake of naturally occurring sugars and starches.

VITAMINS
Composition

Vitamins are isolated organic substances present in minute quantities in natural foods. They are usually identified by an alphabetic designation, and their functions established.

Vitamins are classified as fat- or water-soluble. Fat-soluble vitamins require bile in the intestinal tract for absorption, and water-soluble vitamins are absorbable in water in the body. The *fat-soluble vitamins* are A, D, E, and K; *water-soluble vitamins* are the B complex, consisting of a number of components, and C.

Function

Vitamins are required by every part of the body and essential to growth, metabolism, health maintenance, and disease prevention. Vitamins work together and with other nutrients and in many energy-producing processes.

Figure 19-4 *Fruits and vegetables in the diet may help prevent certain types of cancer.*

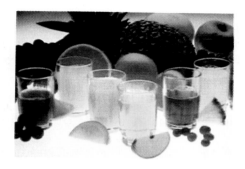

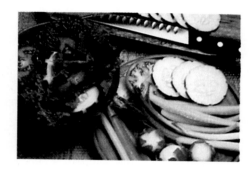

Sources

Sources of fat-soluble vitamins include:

- Vitamin A—Foods of animal origin, dark-green and deep-yellow vegetables
- Vitamin D—Milk, butter, and margarine (especially fortified), fish-liver oil, canned sardines and fish, egg yolks, and liver
- Vitamin E—Wheat germ, soybean, cottonseed, and corn oils
- Vitamin K—Green leafy vegetables, cauliflower, and pork liver

Sources of water-soluble vitamins include:

- Vitamin B_1 (thiamin)—Pork, liver, eggs, enriched cereals, wheat germ, nuts and yeast
- Vitamin B_2 (riboflavin)—Liver, milk, wheat germ, wild rice, almonds, egg whites, and yeast
- Niacin—Liver, halibut, tuna, peanuts, poultry, enriched cereals, and yeast
- B_6 (pyridoxine)—Molasses, wheat bran, wheat germ, soybeans, liver, corn, bananas, prunes, raisins, and yeast
- B_{12} (cyanocobalamin)—Liver, beef, ham, shellfish, milk, and most cheeses
- Folacin (folic acid)—Green leafy vegetables, organ meats, and legumes
- Biotin—Organ meats, egg yolks, and legumes
- Pantothenic acid—Animal products, whole grains, and legumes
- Vitamin C—Citrus fruits, raw strawberries, liver, and raw vegetables (rutabaga, watercress, kale, parsley, turnip greens, broccoli, cauliflower, and peppers).

It is essential to store fresh food properly and use it within a minimum amount of time to preserve nutrients. Short processing techniques lessen the effect cooking has on foods rich in vitamins. The vitamins in food can be destroyed by prolonged heating or temperatures higher than boiling or can readily be destroyed by heat, especially slow cooking.

Caloric Requirements

Vitamins *do not* supply any calories and thus no energy. For the daily minimum requirements of vitamins, see Table 19-6.

MINERALS
Composition

Minerals are inorganic substances that make up nearly 5% of the body and are found primarily in the skeleton. There are two major divisions of minerals, *macrominerals* (also called *major minerals*) and *microminerals* (known as *trace minerals*). Our body needs greater amounts on a daily basis of macrominerals than it does of microminerals. Macrominerals include calcium, phosphorus, magnesium, sodium, potassium, chlorine, and sulfur. The trace minerals include iron, copper, iodine, manganese, cobalt, zinc, molybdenum, fluorine, selenium, chromium, nickel, tin, silicon, and vanadium.

Function

Minerals are needed for a variety of body functions, including the building of strong teeth and bones and the regulation of a number of body processes, including muscle contraction, transmission of messages over the nerves, blood clotting, and protein and red blood cell formation.

Sources

Minerals are essential in the metabolism of body cells. The best way to have the necessary minerals in your body is by eating a variety of foods in a balanced diet of carbohydrates, fat, and protein. However, calcium, phosphorus, iron, iodine, and copper may be deficient unless vegetables and fruit are included. For example, milk is the best source of calcium, but calcium is also present in leafy vegetables. A minute amount of iron is required, but quantities in foods are also minute; therefore effort must be made to ensure the proper requirement.

Caloric Requirements

As with vitamins, minerals *do not* supply any calories and thus no energy. See Table 19-7 for more information on minerals.

WATER
Composition

Water is a vital nutrient needed for life and survival. Most of us could live for a few weeks without food, but all of us would survive for only a few days without water. The average healthy female is composed of 50% water, and the average healthy male is composed of 60% water. Men have more water because they have more muscle tissue, which holds more water. Women have more fat tissue, which holds less water than muscle tissue. The average adult contains 40 to 50 quarts of water.

Body cells contain 40% water; blood, 84%; brain and muscle tissue, 75%; and bone tissue, 22%.

Function

Every cell in the body needs water. It serves as a medium for all chemical reactions in the body. In addition, water:

- Regulates the body temperature.
- Carries oxygen and nutrients to all cells.
- Removes wastes from all cells.
- Lubricates the joints.
- Protects tissues and organs.
- Prevents dehydration.
- Replaces sweat losses during and after exercising or exposure to heat or elevated temperatures.

Water is lost from our body daily through the processes of urination, respiration, defecation and through the skin, whether perspiring or not.

Sources

Water comes from three sources: beverages or other liquids; foods, especially vegetables and fruits; and water formed in the tissues as the result of metabolism.

Requirements

Requirements for the need for water vary with body size, metabolic rate, exercise, climate, type of diet, and other conditions such as pregnancy or illness. It is recommended that individuals drink at least six to eight cups of water daily, since there is some water in foods such as fruits and vegetables and also in other beverages. There is even water in foods such as chicken, cheese, eggs, hamburger, cookies, and crackers. Coffee, tea, and alcohol are *not* good fluids to use to replace water because the caffeine and alcohol act like a diuretic, causing water loss rather than replacement.

The simplest way to determine if you are drinking enough water is to check the color and amount of urine you excrete. If you are urinating only small amounts of urine and if it is dark in color, drink more water. If the urine is pale yellow or clear, it is an indication that normal water balance has occurred.

The Environmental Protection Agency (EPA) regulates the content of tap water. In many locations throughout the country, fluoride is added to the water supply to aid in preventing tooth decay in children. Most water is disinfected with chlorine. Water pipes lined with lead can contaminate the water from the tap. To avoid lead contamination, run the water until it is cold before using it, since lead is more soluble in hot water.

To have your water supply checked and obtain the location of a nearby certified laboratory, contact The Safe Drinking Water Hotline at 1-800-426-4791.

Bottled water may taste better to some people, but it may not be any healthier or safer than your tap water. Minimum standards for both are set by the Food and Drug Administration (FDA).

FIBER
Composition

Fiber is an important element of our diet, although by definition it is not considered a nutrient. Dietary fiber is a complex mixture of cell walls of plants that are resistant to breakdown by the digestive tract. It is the indigestible part of a food.

There are two major types of dietary fiber:

1. *Water-insoluble* fiber includes cellulose, hemicellulose, and lignin. They are not metabolized by intestinal bacteria and *do not* readily dissolve in water.
2. *Soluble* fiber includes gums, mucilages, and pectins. These substances readily swell or dissolve when put in water.

Function

Dietary fiber in the diet is required because of the important roles it plays in bowel function. It is recommended for people who suffer from conditions such as irritable bowel syndrome (IBS), diverticular disease, constipation, or hemorrhoids. Some of the functions of fiber are as follows:

1. Fiber promotes increased chewing, which is good for the teeth.
2. Food sources of fiber are lower in fat than animal food sources, and most people need to decrease their intake of fat.
3. Fiber food sources increase a person's intake of vitamins.
4. Fiber food sources have less additives than processed foods.
5. Insoluble fiber promotes normal elimination by providing bulk for stool formation and thus hastening the passage of the stool through the colon.
6. Insoluble fiber helps to satisfy appetite by creating a feeling of fullness. It also aids weight control.
7. Fiber in the diet also helps to control weight because the foods have fewer calories than other food sources.
8. Soluble fiber may play a role in reducing the level of cholesterol in the blood.
9. Soluble fiber is thought to slow down the release of carbohydrates from their source; it holds onto the sugar and releases it more slowly so that we derive the benefits of the sugar for a longer period of time.
10. Fiber is thought to be protective against heart disease, gallbladder disease, hiatal hernia, varicose veins, appendicitis, diabetes, breast and colon cancer, constipation, and diverticulosis because of some of the proceeding functions (Table 19-8).
11. Food sources rich in fiber are usually less expensive than foods from other sources.

Sources

The main sources of dietary fiber come from grain products, fruits, and vegetables (Table 19-9). Dietary fiber *is not* found in animal products such as milk meats.

Text continues on page 651.

TABLE 19-6

Vitamin Facts

Vitamin	U.S RDA*	Best Dietary Sources	Functions
A (carotene)	5000 IU/day	Formation and maintenance of skin, hair and mucous membranes; helps us see in dim light; bone and tooth growth	Yellow or orange fruits and vegetables, green leafy vegetables, fortified oatmeal, liver, dairy products
B_1 (thiamine)	1.5 mg/day	Helps body release energy from carbohydrates during metabolism; growth and muscle tone	Fortified cereals and oatmeals, meats, rice and pasta, whole grains, liver
B_2 (riboflavin)	1.7 mg/day	Helps body release energy from protein, fat and carbohydrates during metabolism	Whole grains, green leafy vegetables, organ meats, milk and eggs
B_6 (pyridoxine)	2 mg/day	Helps build body tissue and aids in metabolism of protein	Fish, poultry, lean meats, bananas, prunes, dried beans, whole grains, avocados
B_{12} (cobalamin)	6 μg/day	Aids cell development, functioning of the nervous system and the metabolism of protein and fat	Meats, milk products, seafood
Biotin	0.3 mg/day	Involved in metabolism of protein, fats and carbohydrates	Cereal/grain products, yeast, legumes, liver
Folate (folacin, folic acid)	0.4 mg/day	Aids in genetic material development and involved in red blood cell production	Green leafy vegetables, organ meats, dried peas, beans and lentils
Niacin	20 mg/day	Involved in carbohydrate, protein and fat metabolism	Meat, poultry, fish, enriched cereals, peanuts, potatoes, dairy products, eggs
Pantothenic Acid	10 mg/day	Helps in the release of energy from fats and carbohydrates	Lean meats, whole grains, legumes, vegetables, fruits
C (ascorbic acid)	60 mg/day	Essential for structure of bones, cartilage, muscle and blood vessels. Also helps maintain capillaries and gums and aids in absorption of iron	Citrus fruits, berries, and vegetables—especially peppers
D	400 IU/day	Aids in bone and tooth formation; helps maintain heart action and nervous system	Fortified milk, sunlight, fish, eggs, butter, fortified margarine
E	30 IU/day	Protects blood cells, body tissue and essential fatty acids from harmful destruction in the body	Fortified and multi-grain cereals, nuts, wheat germ, vegetable oils, green leafy vegetables
K†		Essential for blood-clotting functions	Green leafy vegetables, fruit, dairy and grain products

IU, International units; mg - milligrams; μg, micrograms.
* For Adults and Children over age 4.
† There is no U.S. RDA for vitamin K; however the Recommended Dietary Allowance is 1 μg/kg of body weight.

Table 19-6—cont'd

Vitamin Facts

Deficiency Symptoms*	Results of Toxicity	Processing Tips
Night blindness, dry and scaly skin, frequent fatigue	Toxic in high doses, but beta-carotene is nontoxic	Serve fruits and vegetables raw and keep covered and refrigerated. Steam veggies; broil, bake, or braise meats.
Heart irregularity, fatigue, nerve disorders, mental confusion	Nontoxic, as high doses are excreted by the kidneys	Don't rinse rice or pasta before and after cooking. Cook in minimal water.
Cracks in corners of mouth, skin rash, anemia	No toxic effects reported	Store foods in containers that light cannot enter; cook vegetables in minimal water; roast or broil meats.
Convulsions, dermatitis, muscular weakness, skin cracks, anemia	Long-term megadoses may cause nerve damage in hands and feet	Serve fruits raw or cook for shortest time in little water; roast or boil meats.
Anemia, nervousness, fatigue, and, in some cases, neuritis and brain degeneration	No toxic effects reported	Roast or broil meat and fish.
Nausea, vomiting, depression, hair loss, dry, scaly skin	No toxic effects reported	Storage, processing, and cooking do not appear to affect this vitamin.
Gastrointestinal disorders, anemia, cracks on lips	Some evidence of toxicity in large doses	Store vegetables in refrigerator and steam, boil, or simmer in minimal water.
Skin disorders, diarrhea, indigestion, general fatigue	Nicotinic acid form should be taken only under doctor's care	Roast or broil beef, veal, lamb, and poultry. Cook potatoes in minimal water.
Fatigue, vomiting, stomach stress, infections, muscle cramps	No toxic effects reported	Eat fruits and vegetables raw.
Swollen or bleeding gums, slow wound healing, fatigue/depression, poor digestion	Intakes of 1g or more can cause nausea, cramps and diarrhea	Do not store or soak fruits and vegetables in water. Refrigerate juices and store only 2-3 days.
In children: rickets and other bone deformities. In adults: calcium loss from bones.	High intakes may cause diarrhea and weight loss	Storage, processing, and cooking do not appear to affect this vitamin.
Muscular wasting, nerve damage, anemia/reproductive failure	Relatively nontoxic	Store in air-tight containers away from light.
Bleeding disorders in newborn infants and those on blood-thinning medications	Nontoxic as found in food	Store in air-tight containers away from light.

Courtesy the Food and Drug Administration, the American Institute for Cancer Research and the United States Department of Agriculture/Human Nutrition Information Service and Worldview Quarterly, Nestle USA, Inc., Washington, D.C. Vitamins D, E, and K are fat-soluble; all the rest are water-soluble.

* *Many of the symptoms outlined under this heading can also be attributed to problems other than vitamin deficiency. If you have these symptoms and they persist, consult your doctor.*

TABLE 19-7

Summary of Water and the Major Minerals

Name	RDA or Minimum Requirements	Major Functions	Best Dietary Sources	Deficiency Symptoms	Results of Toxicity	Most at Risk for Deficiency
Water	1 ml/kcal burned*	Medium for chemical reactions, removal of waste products, perspiration to cool the body	As such and in foods	Thirst, muscle weakness, poor endurance	Probably only in mental disorders, headache, blurred vision, convulsions	Infants with a fever, elderly in nursing homes
Sodium	500 mg	A major ion of the extracellular fluid, nerve transmission	Table salt, processed foods	Muscle cramps	High blood pressure in susceptible individuals	People severely restricting sodium to lower blood pressure (250-500 mg/day)
Potassium	2000 mg	A major ion of intracellular fluid, nerve transmission	Vegetables, fruits, milk	Irregular heartbeat, loss of appetite, muscle cramps	Slowing of the heartbeat, seen in kidney failure	Use of potassium-wasting diuretics, poor diets seen in poverty and alcoholism
Chloride	700 mg	A major ion of the extracellular fluid, acid production in stomach	Table salt, some vegetables	Convulsions in infants	High blood pressure in susceptible people when combines with sodium	No one, probably, if infant formula manufacturers control product quality adequately
Calcium	800 mg (1200 mg ages 11-24)	Bones, teeth, blood clotting, nerve transmission, muscle contractions, cell regulation	Dairy products, canned fish, leafy vegetables, tofu, fortified orange juice	Poor intake probably increased the risk for osteoporosis	Very high intakes may cause a form of kidney stones in susceptible people	Women in general especially those who consume few dairy products
Phosphorus	Men: 350 mg	Bones, teeth, metabolic compounds such as ATP, ion of intracellular fluid	Dairy products, processed foods, soft drinks	Probably none; poor bone maintenance possible	Induces high levels of parathyroid hormone in kidney failure; poor bone mineralization if calcium intakes are low	Elderly consuming very nutrient-poor diets, total vegetarians? alchoholism?
Magnesium	Women: 280 mg	Bones, enzyme function, nerve and heart function	Wheat bran, green vegetables, nuts, chocolate	Weakness, muscle pain, poor heart function	Causes weakness in kidney failure	People on thiazide diuretics
Sulfur	None	Part of vitamins and amino acids, drug detoxification, acid-base balance	Protein foods	None	None likely	No one who meets their protein needs

Adapted with permission from Wardlaw, I: Perspectives in Nutrition, St. Louis, 1993, Mosby.
Just an approximation; best to keep urine volume greater than 1 L (4 cups).

TABLE 19-8

Types, Sources, and Functions of Fiber

Water-insoluble fiber	Gums	Pectins	Function
	Oatmeal Oat products Dried beans Barley	Apples Squash Citrus fruits Cauliflower Green beans Cabbage Dried peas Carrots Strawberries Potatoes	• Binds with cholesterol-containing bile acids in gut preventing reabsorption • Decreases blood cholesterol • Delays glucose absorption and gastric emptying • Protective against heart disease and diabetes

Water-insoluble fiber	Celluloses	Hemicelluloses	Function

	Whole wheat
	  products
	Bran
	Cabbage
	Green beans
	Broccoli
	Brussels
	  sprouts
	Peppers
	Apples
		Bran
		Cereals
		Whole grains
		Brussels sprouts
		Mustard greens
			• Absorbs water
			• Increases stool volume
			
			• Decreases stool transit time
			• Dilutes concentration of bile acids
			• Protective against colon and breast cancer, constipation, and diverticulosis

NOTE: Serving sizes: $1/2$ cup beans, legumes, barley, rice
$3/4$ cup cereals, oatmeal, oat bran
1 slice whole grain bread
1 medium fruit

Recommended Amounts of Fiber Intake

The National Cancer Institute recommends 20 to 30 g of fiber per day with an upper limit of 35 g. According to government surveys, average dietary intake of fiber varies from 12 to 17 g. Therefore for most people an increase in their fiber intake is recommended. Eating a variety of foods that contain dietary fiber is the best way to get an adequate amount. See Table 19-8 for a list of foods and the fiber content. The serving sizes used on the list are only estimates of the amounts of food you might eat. The amount of the nutrient in a serving depends on the weight of the serving. For example, $1/2$ cup of a cooked vegetable contains more fiber than $1/2$ cup of the same vegetable served raw, because a serving of a cooked vegetable weighs more. Therefore the cooked vegetable may appear on the list whereas the raw form does not. In this example, the raw vegetable provides dietary fiber—but just not enough in a $1/2$ cup serving to be significant source of dietary fiber. A selected serving size in Table 19-7 contains at least 2 g of dietary fiber.

To retain dietary fiber in foods, serve fruits and vegetables with edible skins and seeds and use whole-grain flours. Cooking can reduce some of the dietary fiber in a food.

SALT AND SODIUM

Table salt contains sodium and chloride—both are essential in the diet. However, most Americans eat more salt and sodium than they need. Food and beverages containing salt provide most of the sodium in our diets, much of it added during processing and manufacturing.

In populations with diets low in salt, high blood pressure is less common than in populations with diets high in salt. Other factors that affect blood pressure are heredity, obesity, and excessive drinking of alcoholic beverages.

TABLE 19-9

Sources of Dietary Fiber

Food	Selected Serving Size*	Food	Selected Serving Size*
BREADS, CEREALS, AND OTHER GRAIN PRODUCTS		Prunes, dried:	
Bagel, whole-wheat	1 medium	Cooked, unsweetened	1/2 cup
Biscuit, whole-wheat	1 medium	Uncooked	1/4 cup
Breads, multigrain, pumpernickel rye, white and whole-wheat blend, whole wheat, or whole-wheat with raisins	2 regular slices	Raisins	1/4 cup
		Raspberries, raw or frozen, unsweetened	1/2 cup
Bulgur, cooked or canned	2/3 cup	Strawberries, frozen, unsweetened	1/2 cup
English muffin, whole-wheat	1	Tangelo, raw	1 medium
Muffins, bran or whole-wheat	1 medium		
Oatmeal:		**VEGETABLES**	
Instant, fortified, prepared	2/3 cup	Artichoke, globe (french), cooked	1 medium
Regular or quick, cooked`	2/3 cup	Beans, green or lima, cooked	1/2 cup
Pita bread, whole-wheat	1 small	Beets, cooked	1/2 cup
Ready-to-eat bran cereals	1 ounce	Broccoli, cooked	1/2 cup
Rolls:		Brussels sprouts, cooked	1/2 cup
Multigrain	1 large	Cabbage, cooked	1/2 cup
Whole-wheat	1 medium	Carrots, cooked	1/2 cup
		Okra, cooked	1/2 cup
FRUITS		Parsnips, cooked	1/2 cup
Apples:		Peas, green, cooked	1/2 cup
Dried, cooked, unsweetened	1/2 cup	Potato, boiled, with skin	1 medium
Raw	1 medium	Snow peas, raw or cooked	1/2 cup
Applesauce, unsweetened	1/2 cup	Spinach, cooked	1/2 cup
Apricots, dried:		Squash, winter, cooked, mashed	1/2 cup
Cooked, unsweetened	1/2 cup	Sweet potato, baked or boiled	1 medium
Uncooked	1/4 cup	Tomatoes, stewed	1/2 cup
Banana, raw	1 medium		
Blackberries, raw or frozen, unsweetened	1/2 cup	**MEAT, POULTRY, FISH, AND ALTERNATES**	
Blueberries, frozen, unsweetened	1/2 cup	**Dry Beans, Peas, and Lentils**	
Dates, chopped	1/4 cup	Beans; black-eyed peas (cowpeas), calico, chickpeas (garbanzo beans), lima, mexican, pinto, red kidney, or white; cooked	1/2 cup
Fruit mixture, dried	1/4 cup		
Guava, raw	1		
Kiwifruit, raw	1 medium	Lentils, cooked	1/2 cup
Mango, raw	1/2 medium	Peas, split, green or yellow, cooked	1/2 cup
Nectarine, raw	1 medium		
Orange, raw	1 medium	**Nuts and Seeds**	
Peaches, dried:		Almonds or chestnuts, roasted	2 tablespoons
Cooked, unsweetened	1/2 cup	Peanut butter	2 tablespoons
Uncooked	1/4 cup	Pine nuts (pignolias)	2 tablespoons
Pears:		Pumpkin or squash seeds, hulled, roasted	2 tablespoons
Canned, juice-pack	1/2 cup	Sesame seeds	2 tablespoons
Dried, cooked, unsweetened	1/2 cup	Sunflower seeds, hulled, unroasted	2 tablespoons
Dried, uncooked	1/4 cup		
Raw	1 medium		

A selected serving size contains at least 2 g of dietary fiber.

The daily value for sodium is 2400 mg. It is wise for most people to eat less salt and sodium because they usually need much less than they eat and reduction will benefit those people whose blood pressure rises with salt intake. See Table 19-10 for the amount of sodium found in some foods.

ALCOHOL

Alcoholic beverages supply calories but little or no nutrients. Drinking them has no net health benefit, is linked with many health problems, is the cause of many accidents, and can lead to addiction. Their consumption is not recommended. If adults elect to drink alcoholic beverages, they should consume them in moderate amounts (see box).

CALORIES

Calories *are not* food, but rather the amount of energy that can be derived from protein, fat, and carbohydrate in food.

Technically, a calorie is a unit of heat. One calorie is the amount of heat required to raise the temperature of 1 kg of water 1° Celsius.

The amount of energy that can be obtained from a food can be calculated by measuring the amount of heat units or calories in that food using the following measurements.

- 1 g of protein provides four calories
- 1 g of carbohydrate provides four calories
- 1 g of fat provides nine calories

Note that the fat in a food provides a little more than double the number of calories provided by protein and carbohydrates. This is important to keep in mind when trying to reduce or increase the number of total calories in a diet. When more calories are taken in than the body requires for its energy needs, the excess calories converted and stored as body fat. Also, the body is more efficient at converting fat (versus protein or carbohydrate) that is ingested into fat. The following demonstrates how the amount of calories consumed affects weight gain.

1 pound of body weight = approximately 3500 calories
Daily caloric requirement for Mr. B. = 2000 calories

If You Drink Alcoholic Beverages, Do So in Moderation

Some people should *not* drink alcoholic beverages:
- *Women who are pregnant or trying to conceive.* Major birth defects have been attributed to heavy drinking by the mother while pregnant. However, there is no conclusive evidence that an occasional drink is harmful.
- *Individuals who plan to drive or engage in other activities that require attention or skill.* Most people retain some alcohol in the blood 3 to 5 hours, after even moderate drinking.
- *Individuals using medicines, even over-the-counter kinds.* Alcohol may affect the benefits or toxicity of medicines. Also, some medicines may increase blood alcohol levels or increase the adverse effect of alcohol on the brain.
- *Individuals who cannot keep their drinking moderate.* This is a special concern for recovering alcoholics and people whose family members have alcohol problems.
- *Children and adolescents.* Use of alcoholic beverages by children and adolescents involves risks to health and other serious problems.

Heavy drinkers are often malnourished because of low food intake and poor absorption of nutrients by the body. Too much alcohol may cause cirrhosis of the liver, inflammation of the pancreas, damage to the brain and heart, and increased risk for many cancers.

Some studies have suggested that moderate drinking is linked to lower risk for heart attacks. However, drinking is also linked to higher risk for high blood pressure and hemorrhagic stroke.

Advice for today: If you drink alcoholic beverages, do so in moderation; and don't drive.
If you don't drink, don't start.

What's Moderate Drinking?

Women: No more than 1 drink a day
Men: No more than 2 drinks a day

Count as a drink:
- 12 ounces of regular beer
- 5 ounces of wine
- 1½ ounces of distilled spirits (80 proof)

Some of the Scientific Bases for These Guidelines:
- *The Surgeon General's Report on Nutrition and Health,* 1988, Public Health Service, U.S. Department of Health and Human Services.
- *Diet and Health: Implications for Reducing Chronic Disease Risk,* 1989, National Research Council, National Academy of Sciences.
- *Recommended Dietary Allowances,* ed 10, 1989, National Research Council, National Academy of Sciences.
- *Food Guide Pyramid,* 1992.

Daily caloric intake for Mr. B. = 3000 calories
Excess number of daily caloric intake = 1000 calories
Excess number of calories for 1 week = 1000
calories × 7 days = 7000 calories
7000 extra calories ÷ 3500 calories/pound = 2 pounds

Therefore Mr. B. has just gained 2 pounds in 1 week.

The same formula can be applied to determine weight loss (that is, if you want to lose 2 pounds you would have to eat 7000 calories less or burn off 7000 extra calories by increased activity).

TABLE 19-10

Sodium Content of Foods

Food	Sodium (mg)	Food	Sodium (mg)
Fresh fruit, 1/2 C or med.	2	Chips—10	220
Canned or frozen fruit	2	Pretzels, 10 rings	336
Fresh vegetables, 1/2 C	1-5		
Naturally high sodium veg. carrots, celery,		Hot cereal, 1/2 C	1
beets, spinach, kale, swiss chard	30-45	Instant hot cereal, 1/2 C	280
Canned veg., 1/2 C	250-280	Dry cereal, 1 C	165-340
Frozen veg., 1/2 C	5-15	Rice, pasta, cooked with no salt	1
(except naturally high)		Seasoned rice and pasta mixes, 1/2 C	600
Sauerkraut, 1/2 C	750	Bread, 1 slice	170
		Crackers, 4	120-200
Milk, yogurt, 1 C	120		
Buttermilk, 1 C	225	Vegetable oils	tr
Natural cheese, 1 oz.	175	Butter or margarine, 1 t	50
Processed cheese, 1 oz.	400	Bottled salad dressing, 1 T	200
Fresh meat, fish, poultry, 3 oz.	75	Canned soups, 1/2 can	600
Shellfish, 3 oz.	150	Salt, sea salt, seasoned salt, 1 t	2300
Ham, 3 oz.	675	MSG. 1 t	500
Luncheon meats, 3 oz.	1170	Baking soda, 1 t	820
Frankfurter, 1	540	Baking powder, 1 t	330
Frozen dinners	1100	Soy sauce, 1 t	365
		Worcestershire sauce, 1 T	315
Dried beans, 1/2 C cooked	15	Catsup, 1 T	200
		Bouillon cube, 1 cube	960
Canned baked beans, 1/2 C	450	Olive, 4 green	325
		4 ripe	130
Unsalted nuts, 1/2 C	1	Pickle, dill	903
Salted nuts, 1/2 C	230	Herbs and spices	tr
Peanut butter, 2 T	200		

Sodium Content of Nonprescription Drugs

Drug	Sodium Content per dose
Alka-Seltzer (2 tablets)	935 mg
Bromo-Seltzer	717 mg
Fleet's Enema	250-300 absorbed
Metamucil instant mix	250 mg
Rolaids (2 tablets)	70 mg
Vicks' Formula 44 (2 t)	105 mg

To determine the number of calories in a cracker that is labeled as follows, use the following calculations.

I cracker = I g of protein, 4 g of carbohydrate, and 3 g of fat

I g of protein × 4 calories = 4 calories

4 g of carbohydrates × 4 calories = 16 calories

3 g of fat × 9 calories = 27 calories

TOTAL CALORIES = 4 + 16 + 27 = 47 calories

This means that in each cracker labeled as above there are 47 calories, the majority of which come from fat.

Formula for Determining the Percentage of Calories in a Food Supplied from Fat

1. Grams of fat × 9 = "Fat" calories

2. $\frac{fat\ calories}{total\ calories} \times 100$ = percentage of calories from fat

Using the values given for the cracker, this equation would be:

1. 3 × 9 = 27

2. $\frac{27}{47} \times 100 = \frac{2700}{47}$ = 57.4% of the calories in this cracker are supplied from fat.

Also see Table 19-11

To find the maximum amount of fat you can eat every day according to the American Heart Association's recommendation that no more than 30% of your daily calorie intake should be obtained from fat, follow these recommended steps:

Step 1: Multiply your ideal weight by 15 if you are moderately active, or by 20 if you are very active.

Step 2: From that total, subtract the following according to your age:

25 to 34, subtract 0

35 to 44, subtract 100

45 to 54, subtract 200

55 to 64, subtract 300

65 and older, subtract 400

This will give you your recommended daily calories. This is *only approximate*: ask your physician for guidance.

Step 3: Find your recommended calories intake on the chart below and read across to determine your daily fat allowance.

Daily Calories	Maximum Grams of Saturated Fat	Maximum Grams of Total Fat
1200	13	40
1400	16	47
1600	18	53
1800	20	60
2000	22	67
2200	24	73
2400	27	80
2600	29	37
2800	31	93
3000	33	100

DAILY CALORIC REQUIREMENTS

Daily caloric requirements vary and depend on the following.

1. Age: Generally young people need more calories than older people.

2. Sex: Generally men need more calories than women.

3. Body frame: The larger the body frame, the more calories are needed to maintain the weight.

4. Weight: Heavier people need more calories than lighter people to maintain their weight.

5. Percentage of body fat: Women have more body fat (average 19% to 24%) than men (average 12% to 17%).

6. Activity level: The more active a person, is the more calories will be burned and needed to maintain body weight.

7. Basal metabolic rate: The basal metabolic rate is the amount of energy (calories) needed when the body is at rest to maintain basic body activities such as temperature, respiration, circulation, muscle tone, and peristalsis. This is a special test performed with the person at rest in a comfortable environment 14 to 18 hours after the last meal was eaten.

It is recommended that the consumption of fat in the diet be reduced so that fat makes up only 30% or less of a person's daily caloric requirement.

Empty calorie is a term used to denote calories obtained from a food source that provides energy but very little other nutritional value. For example, the calories obtained from alcohol and sugar are thought of as being empty calories.

DIETARY GUIDELINES FOR AMERICANS

The Food Nutrition Board, a division of the National Academy of Sciences, a nongovernmental agency, publishes *Recommended Dietary Allowances,* known as RDA. It includes the following.

1. *Median heights and weights and recommended energy intake*

2. *RDA*

3. *Estimated safe and adequate daily dietary intakes*

TABLE 19-11

Fat in Foods

Low Fat (0%-20% of Calories)	High Fat (over 20% of Calories)
Fresh fruits and vegetables, fruit and vegetable juices, dried fruit	Olives, avocado, coconut, french fries, hash browns, potato chips
Most breads and cereals, noodles, pasta, matzoh, barley, bulgur, corn tortillas, popcorn (air popped), soda crackers, rye wafers, water crackers, Wasa and Ak Mak crackers, pretzels	Cornbread, biscuits, muffins, waffles, pancakes, granola, croissant, soft rolls, wheatgerm, flour tortillas, popcorn (oil popped), donuts, pastries, snack chips, snack crackers
Nonfat milk, nonfat dry milk, buttermilk, nonfat yogurt, low-fat yogurt, low-fat cottage cheese, sherbet, ice milk, frozen yogurt	Whole milk, low-fat milk, creamed cottage cheese, all cheeses, ice cream, whipping cream, half and half, nondairy creamer, lard, butter, margarine, oils, sour cream, cream cheese, tofu
Legumes, egg whites, cod, halibut, sole, flounder, red snapper, shrimp, scallops, squid, abalone, clams, crab, lobster, mussles, oyster, tuna in water, light meat of chicken and turkey (without skin), ham, Canadian bacon, veal, flank steak, round steak	Whole eggs, salmon, trout, swordfish, anchovies, sardines, mackerel, tuna in oil, dark meat of chicken and turkey, light meat of chicken and turkey (with skin), beef, pork, lamb, bacon, sausages, hot dogs, salami, cold cuts, organ meats, nuts, seeds, soybeans, commercial refried beans
Broths, bouillon, most soups, spices, herbs, sugar, jam, jellies, applesauce, apple butter, tomato sauces, mustard, ketchup, salsa, soy sauce, horseradish	Creamed soups, salad dressings, custard, mayonnaise, chocolate, candy bars, pies, cakes

4. *Estimated sodium, chloride, and potassium minimum requirements of healthy persons*

The detailed data are grouped by age and sometimes by sex and used primarily by health professionals.

A simplified version of the RDAs intended more for the use of consumers has been developed by the FDA and is called the U.S. Recommended Daily Allowances or U.S. RDA.

FOOD LABELING

Through the Department of Health and Human Services and the Food Safety and Inspection Service of the U.S. Department of Agriculture, the food industry is required to put a nutrition label on certain food products (Figure 19-4). The purpose of the label is "to help consumers choose more healthful diets and offer an incentive to food companies to improve the nutritional qualities of their products."

Food labels entitled "Nutrition Facts" must contain the following information:

Mandatory components
- Total calories
- Calories from fat
- Total fat

Dietary Guidelines for Americans

Eat a variety of foods.
Maintain healthy weight.
Choose a diet low in fat, saturated fat, and cholesterol.
Choose a diet with plenty of vegetables, fruits, and grain products.
Use sugars only in moderation.
Use salt and sodium only in moderation.
If you drink alcoholic beverages, do so in moderation.

- Saturated fat
- Cholesterol
- Sodium
- Total carbohydrate
- Dietary fiber
- Sugars
- Protein
- Vitamin A
- Vitamin C
- Calcium
- Iron

unit nineteen Nutrition **657**

Figure 19-3 *Food label. Read food labels and note if the food has a high content of sugars and/or salt.*
Courtesy Aetna Health Plans, San Bruno, Calif.

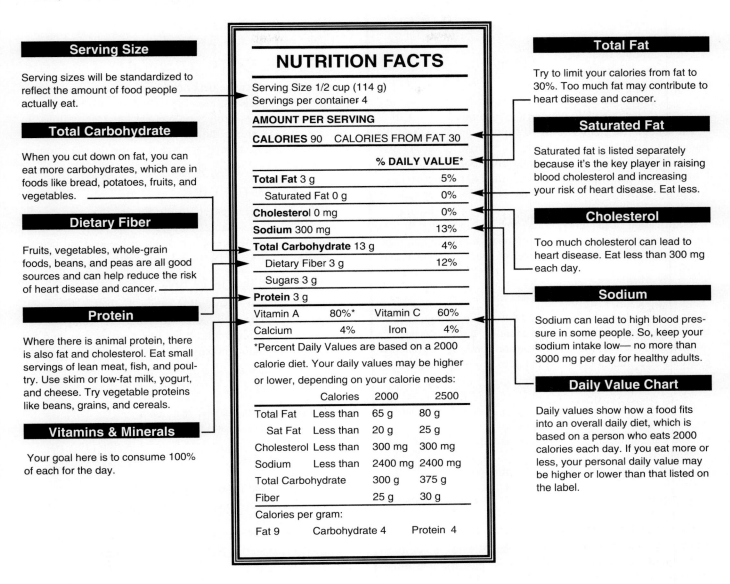

Serving Size

Serving sizes will be standardized to reflect the amount of food people actually eat.

Total Carbohydrate

When you cut down on fat, you can eat more carbohydrates, which are in foods like bread, potatoes, fruits, and vegetables.

Dietary Fiber

Fruits, vegetables, whole-grain foods, beans, and peas are all good sources and can help reduce the risk of heart disease and cancer.

Protein

Where there is animal protein, there is also fat and cholesterol. Eat small servings of lean meat, fish, and poultry. Use skim or low-fat milk, yogurt, and cheese. Try vegetable proteins like beans, grains, and cereals.

Vitamins & Minerals

Your goal here is to consume 100% of each for the day.

Total Fat

Try to limit your calories from fat to 30%. Too much fat may contribute to heart disease and cancer.

Saturated Fat

Saturated fat is listed separately because it's the key player in raising blood cholesterol and increasing your risk of heart disease. Eat less.

Cholesterol

Too much cholesterol can lead to heart disease. Eat less than 300 mg each day.

Sodium

Sodium can lead to high blood pressure in some people. So, keep your sodium intake low— no more than 3000 mg per day for healthy adults.

Daily Value Chart

Daily values show how a food fits into an overall daily diet, which is based on a person who eats 2000 calories each day. If you eat more or less, your personal daily value may be higher or lower than that listed on the label.

NUTRITION FACTS

Serving Size 1/2 cup (114 g)
Servings per container 4

AMOUNT PER SERVING

CALORIES 90   CALORIES FROM FAT 30

% DAILY VALUE*

Total Fat 3 g	5%
Saturated Fat 0 g	0%
Cholesterol 0 mg	0%
Sodium 300 mg	13%
Total Carbohydrate 13 g	4%
Dietary Fiber 3 g	12%
Sugars 3 g	
Protein 3 g	

Vitamin A	80%*	Vitamin C	60%
Calcium	4%	Iron	4%

*Percent Daily Values are based on a 2000 calorie diet. Your daily values may be higher or lower, depending on your calorie needs:

	Calories	2000	2500
Total Fat	Less than	65 g	80 g
Sat Fat	Less than	20 g	25 g
Cholesterol	Less than	300 mg	300 mg
Sodium	Less than	2400 mg	2400 mg
Total Carbohydrate		300 g	375 g
Fiber		25 g	30 g

Calories per gram:

Fat 9   Carbohydrate 4   Protein 4

No More False Claims

Now when you see words and health claims on food products, they will actually mean something. Here's a list of the most commonly used buzz words, along with their new government definitions:

Fat Free — Less than 0.5 g of fat per serving

Low Fat — 3 g of fat (or less) per serving.

Lean — Less than 10 g of fat, 4 g of saturated fat, and 95 mg of cholesterol per serving.

Light (Lite) — 1/3 less calories or no more than 1/2 the fat of the higher-calorie, higher fat-version; or no more than 1/2 the sodium of the higher-sodium version

Cholesterol Free — Less than 23 mg of cholesterol and 2 g (or less) of saturated fat per serving.

- Voluntary components
- Calories from saturated fat
- Polyunsaturated fat
- Monounsaturated fat
- Potassium
- Soluble fiber
- Insoluble fiber
- Sugar alcohol
- Other carbohydrate
- Other essential vitamins and minerals

The amount of grams are listed to the right of each of the names of these nutrients and the "% Daily Value" is also listed. This clarifies misinterpretations about foods with a high number. An example is a food with 140 (mg) of sodium, which represents less than 6% of the Daily Value for sodium, which is 2400 mg.

Modification in the amount and type of food ingested may be needed for some medical conditions to aid in the treatment process. The following are examples of special diets that may be used.

CLEAR LIQUID DIET

A clear liquid diet may be required before the patient has certain laboratory tests or other examinations. It may also be recommended after episodes of diarrhea or vomiting. It generally provides little nutritional value but does provide needed fluids and relieves thirst.

Foods Recommended

- Clear soups such as broth or bouillon
- Clear coffee, tea, or carbonated beverages (as allowed and tolerated)
- Clear fruit juices, such as apple or cranberry
- Plain, flavored gelatin and popsicles
- Hard, clear candies

FULL LIQUID DIET

A full liquid diet may be used for a patient who cannot tolerate or chew solid foods, who has acute gastritis and infections, or for patients before and after surgery.

Foods Recommended

- All liquids allowed on the clear liquid diet
- Milk, milkshakes
- Strained fruit and vegetable juices
- Creamed soups, strained soups
- Ice creams, custards, puddings

MECHANICAL SOFT DIET/DENTAL SOFT DIET

A mechanical or dental soft diet may be required for patients who have difficulty chewing because of sore gums or lack of teeth and for those who have difficulty in swallowing.

Foods Recommended

- Chopped or ground meats and vegetables
- Soups

- All liquids
- Casseroles
- Canned fruits
- Well-cooked vegetables
- Tender meats such as baked chicken or turkey

HIGH-FIBER DIET

A high-fiber diet may be beneficial for a patient who has constipation, diverticulosis, diabetes, irritable bowel syndrome, and for everyone as protection against these conditions. In addition, it may aid in the prevention of heart disease and breast and colon cancer (also see the previous section on fiber, page 647).

Food Recommended

- All foods with increased emphasis on fiber-rich foods, which include vegetables and fruits, especially raw fruits and vegetables, legumes, whole-grain breads, and cereals (see Tables 19-8 and 19-9).

LOW-RESIDUE OR LOW-FIBER DIET

A low-residue diet, also called a low-fiber diet, is recommended for patients with indigestion, diarrhea, colitis, ileitis, as well as for patients who have had a colostomy and for those having radiation therapy.

Foods Recommended

- Eggs
- Lean beef, chicken, turkey, veal, lamb
- Refined flour, breads and rolls, rice, noodles, spaghetti
- Cooked cereals
- Cooked vegetables
- Fruit juices
- Canned or stewed fruits; bananas are allowed
- Soups BUT NO creamed soups or any milk products
- Desserts *without* milk, milk products, nuts, or seeds

These foods must **NOT** be fried or cooked with milk or milk products and must **NOT** he highly seasoned.

LOW-FAT DIET

A low-fat diet is generally recommended for a patient who has liver, gallbladder, or pancreatic disease. It is also highly recommended for everyone to reduce the risk of heart disease and cancer of the colon, prostate, and breast, as well as obesity. An average, healthy adult should strive for no more than 30 to 50 g of fat per day. A patient for whom a low-fat diet is prescribed should strive to consume less than this amount daily.

Foods Recommended (Figure 19-5)

- Up to 5 ounces of meat per day—baked, broiled, roasted, or steamed. It must *not* be fried or served with gravy. All visible fat must be removed before cooking.
- Fruits
- Vegetables—but no fried vegetables
- Skim milk, low fat or nonfat yogurt, and low fat cheeses
- Ice milk—chocolate, strawberry, vanilla

Figure 19-5 *A low-fat dinner.*
From Wardlaw, GM: *Perspectives in nutrition*, ed 2, St. Louis, 1993, Mosby.

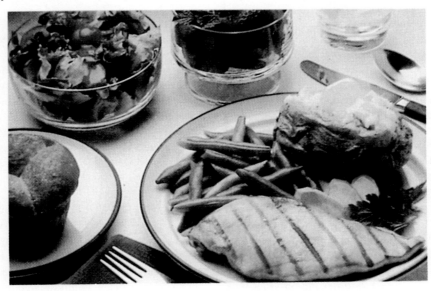

- Whole grain breads (nonfat)
- Cold cereals, cooked cereals, soda crackers
- Unbuttered popcorn
- Plain angel food cake, vanilla wafers, ladyfingers, graham crackers, arrowroot cookies
- Pudding made with skim milk as well as rise pudding and tapioca
- Fruit whips made with gelatin or egg whites
- Fats (strictly limited)—measured amounts of margarine, salad dressings, vegetable oils. Generally only 3 servings per day of either 1 teaspoon or 1 tablespoon depending on the fat.

SODIUM RESTRICTED/LOW SODIUM/SALT-FREE/NO ADDED SALT/LOW-SALT DIETS

A diet with varied amounts of sodium/salt is used for patients with high blood pressure, congestive heart failure (CHF), fluid retention, renal disease, and cirrhosis.

The amount of sodium should be specified. Sodium is found in most foods naturally so that a salt-free or no-salt diet is technically impossible (see Table 19-11).

Mild Restriction

4000 to 5000 mg of sodium per day (174 to 216 mEq)
- Limited use of foods high in sodium
- 1/2 teaspoon of table salt is allowed each day

Moderate Restriction

2000 mg of sodium per day (87 mEq)
- Omit foods with a high sodium content
- 1/2 teaspoon of table salt is allowed each day or the equivalent in prepared foods

2000 mg of sodium per day (45 mEq)
- Omit canned or processed foods containing salt
- No salt is allowed in preparation of food or at the table

Strict Restriction

500 mg of sodium per day (22 mEq)
- Omit canned or processed foods containing salt
- No salt is allowed in preparation of food or at the table
- Low-sodium bread must be used rather than regular bread
- Omit vegetables containing high amounts of natural sodium such as sauerkraut, pickles, celery, frozen corn, frozen mixed vegetables, frozen vegetables in sauce, frozen peas, frozen lima beans

Severe Restriction

250 mg of sodium per day
- THIS DIET IS NOT RECOMMENDED, BUT IT COULD BE USED FOR SHORT TERM OR TESTS ONLY.
- The same restrictions as outlined for the 500 mg/day are to be followed. In addition, limit protein foods and use low-sodium milk in place of regular milk.

When a patient is placed on a sodium-restricted diet, instructions must be given to read *all* the labels on a food for the sodium content.

Food Recommended for a 1000-mg (1 g) Sodium Diet

- Plain, unprocessed foods, including fresh fruits and vegetables or those processed without added sodium
- Whole or skim milk
- Unsalted cheddar cheese and cottage cheese
- Unsalted breads, crackers, cooked cereals, dry cereals, rice, noodles

- Unsalted popcorn
- Flour (but not if self-rising flour)
- Unsalted nuts
- Unsalted margarine, oils, and butter
- Fresh or frozen meats
- Fresh fish (no shellfish or canned fish)

REDUCED-CALORIE DIET

A reduced-calorie diet is used for patients needing to lose weight or to aid in maintaining a desirable weight.

Foods Recommended

In general, all of the basic five food groups should be included with smaller servings. Low-fat foods are often encouraged.

DIABETIC DIET

A diabetic diet is ordered as part of the treatment program for a patient who has diabetes mellitus. Many factors, including the patient's activity level and insulin dosage, have to be considered. The physician works with a dietitian and provides the patient with a diet to include a set amount of grams of protein, fat, and carbohydrates. Food exchange lists are provided for patients so that they can select various foods and the correct amount from the basic five food groups.

PEPTIC ULCER (GASTRIC AND DUODENAL) DIET

The pain experienced with a gastric ulcer is increased with eating. The pain experienced with a duodenal ulcer is frequently relieved by eating. Diets used for patients with ulcers have changed significantly in the past decade. The bland, low-fat, low-fiber diets with frequent small feedings of milk or cream had no scientific basis and thus have been discontinued. Also, it is now known that milk protein stimulates acid secretion, thereby interfering with ulcer healing and related pain. Currently an ulcer diet restricts only those

foods that have been shown to interfere with the healing process.

Recommendations

- Eat small-to-moderate servings at mealtime to avoid gastric distention.
- Avoid caffeine-containing foods (coffee, tea, colas, chocolate), decaffeinated coffee, all alcohol, and black or red pepper. These foods are known to increase gastric acid secretion.
- Some individuals must avoid gas-producing foods because they have a tendency to cause distress. Examples include carbonated beverages, onions, brussel sprouts, cauliflower, and cabbage.

BRAT

The acronym BRAT stands for a special diet comprised of *bananas, rice, applesauce, and toast.* Is it often prescribed for patients recuperating from gastrointestinal problems with symptoms of nausea, vomiting, and diarrhea.

PATIENT TEACHING

The physician, dietitian, and/or the medical assistant must work with the patient and possibly the family to individualize any diet recommended for therapy. Nutritional assessments should be done. Find out what the patient usually eats and likes, and then see how small changes can be made to fit his or her needs. The patient needs to know how to select the right foods, incorporating as many family and cultural favorites as possible. The patient may need instruction in reading a food label so that informed decisions can be made regarding food choices. Standard diet forms are not generally used anymore because they often confused the patient with too much information and thus the patient did not pay attention to any of the recommendations.

CONCLUSION

You have now completed the unit on Nutrition. Given your knowledge of dietary guidelines and therapeutic diets, you should be able to identify an appropriate food plan for patients requiring a standard diet to patients requiring any one of the special therapeutic diets.

CASE STUDY

Many diseases and illnesses, including the recovery period from injuries and trauma, require proper nutrition.

To properly understand nutrition labeling, you must be familiar with its terminology. Read the following and discuss the italicized terminology.

The *NLEA* and *FDA* developed the guidelines for mandatory and voluntary nutrition labeling. Required *dietary components* include *calories* from *fat* and identify *saturated fat* from *total fat*. These elements are carefully monitored in patients on a weight reduction program.

Cholesterol, produced naturally by our body and from food from animal sources, and *sodium,* much of which is added during processing and manufacturing, must be closely monitored in daily diets to achieve the proper levels for patients treated for *hypertension*.

The function of *fiber* affects teeth (chewing some fiber-rich foods can help reduce tartar), vitamin consumption, elimination by providing bulk for stool formation, and appetite satisfaction, as well as weight control. Often diets high in fiber are prescribed for *gastrointestinal ailments*.

Complex carbohydrates from vegetables, fruits, and grains provide a good source for many *vitamins* such as *A* and *C*, and the minerals, *calcium* and *iron*, are essential in diabetic conditions.

Protein to promote growth, repair, and maintenance of body tissues is essential in musculoskeletal repair.

REVIEW QUESTIONS

1. Using the dietary guidelines and the Food Guide Pyramid, write a sample menu/food plan for the next 3 days.
2. List the five main nutrients (excluding water) and give three food examples for each.
3. Explain the difference between HDL and LDL.
4. List the fat-soluble vitamins and the water-soluble vitamins, stating foods that are a good source of these vitamins.
5. Explain the difference between a full liquid diet and a clear liquid diet.
6. List five benefits of increasing the fiber in your diet.
7. Explain why water is so important to the body.

Special Vocabulary

PART 1: VOCABULARY USED WHEN RECORDING INFORMATION OBTAINED FROM THE REVIEW OF SYSTEMS

The following vocabulary lists *some* of the terms that an examiner may use when recording the *subjective* findings of the review of systems (ROS) of a patient. Terms are presented in the order in which they appear in the patient's ROS and under the body part or system for which they are used in describing ROS findings (see also Unit Two).

Eyes

Photophobia (fo″to-fo′be-ah)—An abnormal visual intolerance to light

Ears

Tinnitus (ti-ni′tus)—A ringing or buzzing noise in the ears.

Nose

Coryza (ko-ri′zah)—A head cold; an acute inflammation of the nasal mucous membrane with a profuse discharge.

Epistaxis (ep″i-stak′sis)—A nosebleed; hemorrhage from the nose. Many episodes of epistaxis are caused by the rupture of the small vessels over the anterior part of the cartilaginous nasal septum.

Respiratory

Asthma (az′mah)—Recurrent attacks of difficulty in breathing (dyspnea) with wheezing that is caused by spasms in the bronchial tubes.

Expectoration (ek-spek″to-ra ′shun)—The coughing up, expulsion, or spitting out of material (mucus, sputum, or phlegm) from the throat, trachea, bronchi, or lungs.

Hemoptysis (he-mop′ti-sis)—The spitting and/or coughing up of blood from the respiratory tract caused by bleeding in any part of the respiratory tract. In true hemoptysis, sputum is frothy with air bubbles and bright red. (Hemoptysis must not be confused with *hematemesis,* in which a dark red–or black-colored substance is ejected from the gastrointestinal tract.)

Hyperventilation (hi′per-ven″ti-la ′shun)—Abnormal deep and prolonged breathing; increase in the inspiration and expiration of air resulting from an increase in the depth or rate of respirations or both. This results especially with depletion of carbon dioxide. This condition is often associated with emotional tension or acute anxiety situations.

Cardiovascular (CV)

Palpitation (pal″pi-ta′shun)—An unusually strong, rapid, or irregular heartbeat, usually over 120 beats per minute (nor-mal heart rate varies between 60 to 100 beats per minute). Palpitation is often the result of strong exertion, nervousness, excitement, or the taking of certain medications. Palpitations may also result from a variety of heart disorders.

Peripheral edema—(pe-rif′er-al)—Pertaining to the periphery, which means the surface or outward structures; (e-de′mah)—An abnormal accumulation of fluid in the intercellular spaces of the body.

Varicosity (var″i-kos′i-te)—Pertaining to a varicose condition; distended, swollen veins.

Gastrointestinal

Anorexia (an″o-rek′se-ah)—Loss of appetite. Anorexia can be caused by illness, emotional upsets, or unattractive food.

Colic (kol′ik)—Pertaining to the colon; abdominal pain caused by spasmodic contractions of the intestinal tract.

Constipation (kon″sti-pa-shun)—Difficult elimination of fecal material from the intestinal tract; often the infrequent passage of waste material that is hard to eliminate easily results in the passage of unduly dry and hard fecal material.

Diarrhea (di″ah-re′ah)—The rapid movement of fecal material through the intestine, the feces having more or less fluid consistency; primarily a result of increased peristalsis in the intestinal tract.

Distention (dis-ten′ shun)—The state of being stretched out, or distended.

Dysphagia (dis-fa′je-ah)—Difficulty in swallowing.

Flatus (fla′tus)—Air or gas in the gastrointestinal tract.

Hemorrhoid (hem′o-roid); also called *piles*—A dilated blood vessel in the anus that may bleed, cause discomfort or pain, and itch.

Jaundice (jawn′dis); also called *icterus* (ik′ter-us)—A symptom of different disorders of the gallbladder, liver, and blood characterized by yellowness of the skin, mucous membranes, and whites of the eyes caused by excessive bilirubin in the blood and deposition of bile pigments.

Melena (me-le′nah)—Black fecal material; blood pigments darken the feces.

Genitourinary (GU)

Enuresis (en″u-re′sis)—The involuntary excretion of urine, especially at night during sleep; bedwetting; most commonly seen in children with physical or emotional problems.

Frequency—(fre′kwen-se)—The need to urinate frequently.

Hesitancy—Dysuria caused by nervous inhibition or obstruction in the vesical outlet.

Incontinence (in-kon′ti-nens)—The inability to refrain from the urge to urinate. This may occur in times of stress, anxiety, or anger; after surgery; or because of obstructions that prevent the normal emptying of the urinary bladder, spasms of the bladder, irritation caused by injury or inflammation of the urinary tract, damage to the spinal cord or brain, or the development of a fistula (an abnormal tubelike passage) between the bladder ant the vagina or urethra. The word also may refer to fecal incontinence caused by nervous disorders or weakening of the anal sphincter.

Nocturia (nok-tu're-ah)—Excessive urination at night.

Potency (po'ten-se)—The ability of a male to have sexual intercourse.

Renal colic (re'nal kol'ik)—Spasms accompanied by pain that radiates from the kidney region around to the abdomen and into the groin. Renal colic is experienced during movement of a stone in the ureter.

Retention (re-ten'shun)—The process of urine accumulating in the bladder because of the individual's inability to urinate.

Urgency—The immediate need to urinate.

Urination (u"ri-na'shun); also called *micturition* (mik "tu-rish'un)—Voiding; the act of passing urine from the body.

Venereal (ve-ne're-al) *disease*—A disease that is transmitted by sexual contact and intercourse. Venereal disease is now more commonly referred to as *sexually transmitted disease*. Abbreviations used are VD and STD.

Female Reproductive

Abortion (ah-bor'shun)—The termination of a pregnancy before the fetus is capable of surviving outside of the uterus. In lay terminology, *abortion* refers to a deliberate interruption of pregnancy by various methods, and *miscarriage* refers to the natural loss of the fetus (*spontaneous abortion*).

Dyspareunia (dis"pah-ru'ne-ah)—Difficult or painful genital sexual intercourse in women.

Gravida (grav'i-dah)—A pregnant woman. During the first pregnancy the woman would be referred to as Gravida I (*primigravida*), and so on with each succeeding pregnancy.

Leukorrhea (loo"ko-re' ah)—An abnormal yellow or white mucus discharge from the cervix or vaginal canal. Leukorrhea may be a symptom of pathologic changes in the vagina and endocervix.

Menarche (me-nar'ke)—The beginning of the menstrual functions in a woman.

Menopause (men'o-pawz)—The period in a woman's life at which the menstrual cycles decrease and gradually stop; the period when menstruation and the ability to have a child cease because the ovaries stop functioning. Menopause is often referred to as *the change of life* and also called the *climacteric*.

Parous (pa'rus)—Having borne at least one child. For example, if a woman has one live child and is now pregnant for the second time, she would be referred to as Gravida II, Para I (see **gravida**).

Endocrine

Goiter (goi'ter)—An enlargement of the thyroid gland.

Skin

Allergy (al'er-je)—An abnormal condition of individual hypersensitivity to substances (*allergens*) that are usually harmless. Allergens, substances capable of inducing hypersensitivity, can be almost any substance in the environment. Examples of allergens to which people become sensitive include dust, animal hairs, plant and tree pollens, mold spores, soaps, detergents, cosmetics, dyes, foods, feathers, plastics, and even some valuable medicines. When the allergen is in contact with or enters the body, it sets off a chain of events that brings about the allergic reaction. The allergen itself is not directly responsible for the allergic reaction. An allergy does not develop on the first contact with the allergen, but can develop on the second contact or even years later, after repeated contact with the allergen. Signs and symptoms of allergies include sneezing, stuffed up and running nose, watery eyes, itching, coughing, shortness of breath, wheezing, rashes, skin eruptions, slight local edema, and mild to severe anaphylactic shock, which can be fatal unless treated.

Mole (mol)—A discolored blemish or growth on the skin; also called a *nevus*.

Ulcer (ul'ser)—An open sore or lesion on the surface of the skin or mucous membranes of the body, produced by the sloughing of dead inflammatory tissues.

Musculoskeletal

Atrophy (at'ro-fe)—A wasting away and decrease in size of a normal tissue or organ.

Dislocation (dis"lo-ka'shun)—The displacement of a bone from its normal position in a joint.

Fracture (frak'chur)—A break in the continuity of a bone. Broad classifications of fractures are *open fracture,* in which the bone penetrates the skin, producing an open wound; and *closed fracture,* in which there is no break in the skin.

Spasm (spazm)—An involuntary sudden movement or contraction of a muscle or group of muscles, commonly accompanied by pain and varying from mild twitches to severe convulsions. Spasms may be **clonic,** in which muscles alternate between contacting and relaxing; or **tonic,** in which the contraction of the muscle is sustained. Tonic spasms are the more severe type, because they are caused by diseases that affect the brain or central nervous system, such as rabies or tetanus.

Tetany (tet'ah-ne)—A continuous tonic spasm of a muscle without distinct twitching. The spasms are usually sudden, periodic, or recurrent; and they involve the extremities.

Neurologic

Convulsion (kun-vul'shun)—Involuntary spasms or contractions of muscles caused by an abnormal stimulus to the brain or by changes in the chemical balance of the body.

Paralysis (pah-ral'i-sis)—A state caused by damage to parts of the nervous system resulting in impairment or loss of motor function in a part or parts of the body.

Paresthesia (par"es-the'ze-ah)—An abnormal sensation experienced without an objective cause. Examples include a burning, tingling, or numb feeling.

Tremor (trem'or)—An involuntary quivering or trembling movement of the body or limbs caused by alternate contractions of opposing muscles. Tremors may have a psychologic or a physical cause or both.

Vertigo (ver'ti-go)—A sensation of dizziness (that is, rotation of oneself or of external objects in one's surroundings).

PART 2: VOCABULARY USED IN RECORDING PHYSICAL FINDINGS

The following vocabulary lists *some* of the terms that an examiner may use in recording the *objective* findings of the physical examination of a patient. Each term is presented under the body part or system for which it is used when describing the findings of the physical examination. The order in which the body part or system is presented follows the usual sequence that examiners follow in performing a physical examination.

Skin

Abrasion (ah-bra'zhun)—A scrape on the surface of the skin or on a mucous membrane (for example, a skinned knee).

Avulsion (a-vul' shun)—A piece of soft tissue that is torn loose or left hanging as a flap.

Contusion (kon-too'zhun)—A bruise; an injury to the tissues without skin breakage. In a contusion blood seeps into the surrounding tissues from the injured and broken blood vessels, causing pain, tenderness, swelling, and discoloration of the surface skin.

Cyanosis (si"ah-no'sis)—A bluish discoloration of mucous membranes and skin

Ecchymosis (ek"i-mo'sis)—A round or irregular nonelevated hemorrhagic spot on mucous membranes or skin. The appearance is that of a blue-black or purplish patch changing to yellow or greenish brown. An ecchymosis is *larger* than a patechia.

Erythema (er"i-the'mah)—A redness of the skin caused by capillary congestion in the lower layers of the skin. Erythema is present in any inflammatory process, infection, or injury of the skin.

Jaundice (jawn'dis)—See ROS vocabulary.

Laceration (las "e-ra'shun) A tear or jagged-edged wound of body tissue.

Petechia (pe-te'ke-ah)—A tiny, round, nonraised, purplish-red spot caused by submucous or intradermal hemorrhage. Later a petechia will turn blue or yellow. Small red patches.

Purpura (per'pu-rah)—Purpura is a hemorrhagic disease of obscure cause. It is characterized by the escape or discharge of blood from vessels into tissues under the skin and through mucous membranes, producing small red patches and bruises on the skin.

Turgor (tur'gor)—The condition of normal tension or fullness in a cell.

Ulcer (ul'ser)—See under ROS vocabulary.

Urticaria (ur"ti-ka're-ah)—Also called *hives*. An inflammatory reaction of the skin characterized by the appearance of slightly elevated red or pale patches that are often itchy.

Eyes

Acuity (ah-ku'i-te)—Clearness, sharpness, or acuteness of vision.

Adnexa (ad-nek'sah)—Accessory organs of the eye.

Arcus senilis (ar'kus seni-lis)—An opaque white ring partially surrounding the margin of the cornea, usually seen in people 50 years old or older. This condition often occurs bilaterally and is a result of fat granules depositing in the cornea or lipoid degeneration.

Fundus (fun'dus) (of the eye)—The back portion of the interior of the eye. The physician can observe this part of the eye by looking into or through the pupil of the eye with an ophthalmoscope.

Nystagmus (nis-tag'mus)—The constant, involuntary, rhythmic movement of the eyeball in any direction.

Papilledema (pap"il-e-de'mah)—Edema and inflammation of the optic nerve, usually caused by intracranial pressure as a result of a brain tumor pressing on the optic nerve.

Ptosis (to'sis)—A drooping of the upper eyelids caused by paralysis.

Ears

Cerumen (se-roo'men)—Earwax.

Tympanic (tim-pan'ik) membrane; also called *eardrum*—A thin membrane that separates the middle ear from the outer ear.

Nose

Nares (na'rez)—The external openings into the nasal cavity; the nostrils.

Nasal septal defect—A deviation of the bone and cartilage that divides the nasal cavity so that one part of the nasal cavity is larger than the other. On occasion this may produce difficulty in normal breathing, prevent normal drainage from infected sinuses, and interfere with the normal flow of mucus from the sinuses when one has a cold.

Neck

Supple (sup'l)—Easily movable.

Respiratory System

Fremitus (frem'i-tus)—A vibration or tremor felt through the chest wall, usually during palpation.

Tactile fremitus—A vibration felt when a person speaks.

Tussive fremitus—A vibration felt when a person coughs.

Vocal fremitus—A vibration heard during auscultation of the chest wall when a person speaks.

Friction rub; also called *rub*—A sound heard during auscultation that is produced when two serous membrane surface rub together.

Rale (rahl)—An abnormal respiratory sound heard when the physician auscultates the chest. A rale indicates a pathologic condition. There are many types of rales. Examples include a *dry rale,* which is a whistling or squeaky sound as heard in a person who has bronchitis or asthma; a *moist rale,* which is produced by fluid in the bronchial tubes; and a *crepitant rale,* which is a dry, crackling sound heard in the early stages of pneumonia when the person completes an inspiration.

Resonance (rez′o-nans)—The quality of sound heard when the physician is examining the chest wall by percussion.

Rhonchus (rong′kus) (pl. *rhonchi*)—A dry rale in the bronchus or a rattling in the throat.

Rub—See under friction rub.

Sputum (spu′tum)—The mucous secretion that comes from the lungs, bronchi, and trachea and that is ejected from the mouth. *Saliva* is not the same as sputum; saliva is secreted from the salivary glands in the mouth.

Stridor (stri′dor)—A harsh, shrill respiratory sound heard during inspirations in individuals who have laryngeal obstruction.

Cardiovascular System (CVS)

Bruit (bru′e)—A blowing sound heard over an aneurysm during auscultation of the cardiovascular system.

Congestion (kon-jes′chun)—An abnormal accumulation of blood in a body part.

Ecchymosis—See under Skin.

Engorgement (en-gorj′ment)—A distention of a body part with blood.

Erythema—See under Skin.

Gallop (gal′op)—A disordered rhythm of the heart heard during auscultation. In a gallop rhythm, three or four extra sounds are heard during the diastolic phase; the sounds are related to atrial contraction.

Infarction (in-fark′shun)—A localized area of deficiency of blood in a part causing death to the cells. This is caused by blockage of arterial blood supply to the area. With reference to the heart, the term *myocardial infarction* is used. This pertains to the death of the cells in the myocardial layer of the heart caused by the lack of blood supply to the area.

Ischemia (is-ke′me-ah)—The deficiency of blood in a body part. Ischemia may be caused by an obstruction in a blood vessel such as from a clot or cholesterol deposits, or by a functional constriction.

Murmur (mer′mer)—A sound heard during auscultation that is cardiac or vascular in origin, especially a periodic sound of short duration. This sound may be heard over the aortic valve, over the apex of the heart, or over an artery; all of these indicate possible disease in the particular area.

Petechia—See under Skin.

Purpura—See under Skin.

Resuscitation (re-sus″i-ta′shun)—The act of restoring life or consciousness to a person whose respirations have stopped and who is thought to be dead.

Rub; also called *friction rub*—See under Respiratory System.

Pericardial rub—A rub associated with inflammation of the pericardium. When this condition is present during auscultation, the physician will hear a grating or scraping sound with the heartbeat.

Thrill (thril)—A vibration that is felt by the physician when palpating the area over the heart, either during diastole or systole.

Abdomen

Ascites (ah-si′tez)—An abnormal excessive accumulation of serous fluid in the peritoneal cavity that may cause abdominal distention. Ascites can be caused by a variety of conditions, some of which are tumors, kidney and heart disease, inflammation of the abdominal cavity, and cirrhosis of the liver.

Contour (kon′toor)—The outline or shape, as of the abdomen.

Distention—See under ROS vocabulary.

Flaccid—See under Musculoskeletal System.

Hernia (her′ne-ah)—An abnormal projection or protrusion of an organ or tissue or part of an organ through the wall of the cavity in which it is normally contained.

Protuberant (pro-tu′ber-ant)—With reference to the abdomen, an area that projects out or is prominent beyond the usual surface abdominal area.

Scaphoid (skaf′oid)—In reference to the abdomen, appearing as having a hallowed anterior wall; boat-shaped.

Rigidity—See under Musculoskeletal System.

Gastrointestinal System

Caries (ka′re-ez, kar′ez)—The decay of teeth or bone.

Distention (dis-ten′shun)—See under ROS vocabulary.

Fissure (fish′er)—A slit or cracklike sore. For example, an anal fissure is a lineal ulcer at the border of the anus.

Fistula (fis′tu-lah)—An abnormal tubelike passage from a tube, organ, or cavity to another cavity or organ or from an internal organ to a free body surface.

Hemorrhoid (hem′or-roid)—A varicose (enlarged) vein in the mucous membrane just outside (external hemorrhoid) or inside (internal hemorrhoid) the rectum. Also called piles, these enlarged veins may be painful and itchy and may bleed.

Peristalsis (per″i-stal′sis)—A wavelike movement by which tubular organs and the alimentary canal propel their contents. Peristalsis is an involuntary movement seen in tubes that have both circular and longitudinal layers of smooth muscle fibers.

Reproductive System

Adnexa (ad-nek′sah)—Accessory organs of the uterus (ovaries, uterine tubes, and ligaments).

Atrophy (at′roo-fe)—A decrease in size of organs or tissues after having reached full functional development. Atrophy is seen in the female reproductive organs after menopause.

Gravida—See under ROS vocabulary.

Introitus (in-tro′itus)—The opening into a body cavity or canal, as the opening into the vagina.

Involution (in″vol-lu′shun)—The retrogressive change in the size and the vital processes of organs and tissues after they have fulfilled their functions, such as seen after menopause or in the reduction in size of the uterus after birth.

Parous—See under ROS vocabulary.

Musculoskeletal System (MS)

Crepitation (krep″i-ta′shun)—A crackling, grating sound produced by movement of the ends of a fractured bone.

Exostosis (ek″sos-to′sis)—A new bony growth arising and projecting from the surface of a bone, characteristically capped by cartilage.

Flaccid (flak-sid)—Relaxed, soft, weak, flabby; applied especially to muscles that lack muscular tone.

Gait (gat)—The style or manner in which a person walks.

Kyphosis (ki-fo′sis); also called *hunchback*—When viewing a person from the side, the examiner sees an abnormal convexity in the curvature of the thoracic spine.

Lordosis (lor-do′dis)—An abnormal forward curvature of the lumbar spine.

Protuberance (pro-tu′ber-ans)—A part that projects or is prominent beyond the usual surface area.

Rigidity (ri-jid′i-te)—A state of being stiff or inflexible.

Scoliosis (sko″le-o′sis)—A lateral curvature of the vertebral column that usually consists of two curves, one in the opposite direction from the first.

Supple (sup′ l)—Flexible, limber, or easily bent.

Extremities

Claudication (klaw″di-ka′shun)—Limping, lameness.

Intermittent claudication—A severe pain, tension, and weakness in the calf muscles that occurs after walking is begun and that subsides when walking stops and the limb has been resting. This condition is seen in patients with occlusive arterial disease in the limbs.

Clubbing (klub′ing)—A process or result of rapid reproduction of the soft tissue on the ends of the fingers and toes, as seen in adults with long-standing pulmonary disease.

Edema (e-de′mah)—An abnormal accumulation of fluid in the body's intercellular spaces. It can be local or general.

Passive congestion (kon-jes′chun)—An abnormal accumulation of blood in an area on the body.

Ulcer (ul′ser)—See under ROS vocabulary.

Varicosity (var′i-ko′i-te) (pl. *varicosities*)—The condition of being varicose; a swollen, distended, enlarged, and twisted vein.

General

cachexia (kah-kek′se-ah)—A general state of ill health, wasting away, and malnutrition, as seen in many chronic diseases.

Dehydration (de″hi-dra′shun)—The condition that results when water output exceeds water intake; the excessive loss of water from the tissues or body.

Diaphoresis (di″ah-fo-re′sis)—Perspiration.

Emaciation (e-ma″se-a′shun)—A condition in which the body is extremely thin and wasting away. Emaciation is generally caused by extreme malnutrition or diseases of the gastrointestinal tract.

Fingerbreadth (fin′ger-bredth)—The width of the finger from side to side, used when measuring the width of something such as lesion, or when measuring the distance between two areas (for example, "two fingerbreadths from the umbilicus)."

Lethargic (leth′ar′gic)—The state of being indifferent, drowsy, or sluggish.

Patulous (pat′u-lus)—The state of being open, spread apart widely, or distended.

Tenderness (ten′der-nes)—A sensitivity to touch or pressure.

Summary of Studies Used for Diagnosing Conditions Affecting Body Organs and Systems

A history and physical examination are the preliminary steps; then individual or combined studies as outlined may be requested.

1. Heart
   a. Chest X-ray studies
   b. Electrocardiogram
   c. Serum enzyme levels
   d. Cardiac catheterization
   e. Angiogram
   f. Echocardiography (ultrasonography)
   g. Radioisotope and radionuclide techniques
   h. Cardiac scan
   i. Treadmill stress test (see Figure 16-8)
   j. Magnetic Resonance Imaging (MRI)
2. Vascular system
   a. Angiography
   b. Venous pressure measurement
   c. Funduscopic examination
   d. Arteriography
   e. Cerebral angiogram
   f. Ultrasound techniques
   g. Splenoportography
   h. Bone marrow studies
   i. Lymph node biopsy
   j. Aortography
   k. Radionuclide studies (bone marrow scan)
   l. Arterial catheterization
   m. Digital radiography
   n. Positron Emission Tomography (PET)
3. Respiratory system and chest
   a. Pulmonary function tests
   b. Spirometry
   c. X-ray studies
   d. Bronchoscopy
   e. Bronchogram
   f. Tomography
   g. CT scan (computed tomography)
   h. Magnetic Resonance Imaging (MRI)
   i. Lung perfusion
   j. Lung ventilation
4. Gastrointestinal (GI) system
   a. Upper GI series
   b. Barium enema
   c. Sigmoidoscopy
   d. Fecal occult blood test
   e. Gastric analysis
   f. Gastroscopy
   g. Esophagoscopy
   h. CT scan
   i. Magnetic resonance imaging (MRI)
   j. Colonoscopy
5. Liver, gallbladder, and pancreas
   a. Laboratory tests, such as bilirubin blood levels, bromosulphalein (BSP), serum amylase and lipase for pancreatic disease, and tests for chronic malabsorption
   b. Biopsy of the liver
   c. Liver scan
   d. Abdominal x-ray films
   e. Cholecystogram
   f. Cholangiogram
   g. CT scan
   h. Magnetic Resonance Imaging (MRI)
   i. Hepatobiliary scan
6. Kidney and genitourinary system
   a. Cultures
   b. Urinalysis
   c. Blood urea nitrogen and creatinine blood tests
   d. Renal biopsies
   e. Cystogram
   f. Retrograde cystourethrogram
   g. Intravenous pyelogram (IVP)
   h. Kidney, ureter, bladder (KUB), x-ray film
   i. Catheterization
   j. Cystoscopy
   k. Seminal fluid examination
   l. Aortogram
   m. Excretion urogram
   n. Vasogram
   o. Ultrasonography
   p. Kidney scan
   q. Magnetic Resonance Imaging (MRI)
7. Female genital organs
   a. Pelvis examination
   b. Pap smear
   c. Cultures

d. Pregnancy test

e. Dilation and curettage (D&C) for endometrial biopsy (surgery)

f. Laparoscopy (surgery)

g. Hematocrit blood test

h. Biopsy of the cervix

i. X-ray studies, such as abdomen for fetus, hysterosalpingogram

j. Ultrasonography

k. CT scan

l. Magnetic Resonance Imaging (MRI)

8. Breast
   a. Mammography
   b. Thermography
   c. Xeroradiography
   d. Biopsy
   e. Physical examination (palpation and inspection)
   f. Self-examination for lumps, pain, or discharge from the nipple

9. Skin
   a. Physical examination for rash, lesion, pain, itching, and appearance
   b. Incisional biopsies
   c. Excisional biopsies
   d. Laboratory tests—culturing purulent lesions, smears, blood tests
   e. Diagnostic skin tests for allergies and tuberculosis

10. Eye
    a. Visual field defects (focal areas of blindness)
    b. Physical examination and history to determine presence of
       (1) Pain
       (2) Blurring of vision
       (3) Papilledema as seen through the ophthalmoscope
       (4) Photophobia (uncomfortable sensitivity to light)
       (5) Infections
       (6) Nystagmus (flickering eye movements)—may be caused by a variety of central nervous system lesions
    c. Clinical tests
       (1) Eye charts or machines for testing visual acuity
       (2) Visual field tests
       (3) Funduscopic examination with the ophthalmoscope
       (4) Tonometry
       (5) Tests for refractive errors (myopia or hyperopia)

11. Bones and joints
    a. Observation of pain, decreased mobility, deformity, and fractures
    b. Physical examination
    c. X-ray films (for example, of fractures, tumors, joints, skull, sinus cavities, teeth)

d. Blood serum tests—calcium, phosphorus, alkaline phosphatase, sedimentation rate, rheumatoid factor (latex fixation titer), and uric acid levels

e. Whole blood test—red blood cell count

f. Cultures—for diagnoses of acute arthritis and osteomyelitis

g. Biopsy—to diagnose bone tumors

h. Arthrography

i. Diskography

j. Myelography

k. Pelvimetry

l. Bone scan

m. Magnetic Resonance Imaging (MRI)

12. Skeletal muscle
    a. Physical examination, to observe atrophy, weakness
    b. Laboratory tests, such as for the enzyme aldolase and creatine phosphokinase (CPK)
    c. Electromyography
    d. Muscle biopsy
    e. Ultrasonography

13. Central nervous system
    a. Physical examination—neurologic examination of the motor and sensory systems
    b. Lumbar puncture to examine the cerebrospinal fluid and the pressure of the fluid; chemical, serologic, and culture tests may be performed
    c. Angiogram
    d. Skull x-ray films
    e. Electroencephalogram (EEG)
    f. Pneumoencephalogram
    g. CT scan
    h. Brain scan
    i. Cerebral angiogram
    j. Echoencephalogram (ultrasonography)
    k. Myelogram
    l. Positron Emission Tomography
    m. Magnetic Resonance Imaging (MRI)

14. Mental illness
    a. Physical examinations
    b. Screening laboratory tests
    c. X-ray studies of the chest and skull
    d. Electroencephalogram
    e. Psychologic assessment, such as personality inventory and intelligence testing

15. Endocrine system
    a. Measurement of hormones—either hypersecretion or hyposecretion.
    b. Laboratory measurements—presence of glucose in blood or urine, glucose tolerance test, measurements of the presence of hormones in blood or urine, and measurement of calcium and phosphorus levels (for the status of the parathyroid glands) in the blood and urine

c. Radionuclide studies—thyroid scan

d. CT scan

e. Magnetic Resonance Imaging (MRI)

16. Infectious diseases

    a. Physical examination and history—often physical examination of lesions is sufficient for diagnosis (for example, rash of measles or chickenpox, swelling of parotid glands in mumps, pus draining from an abscess)

    b. Laboratory studies

       (1) Culture and sensitivity tests on throat, urine, sputum, purulent lesions, blood, and cerebrospinal fluid specimens

       (2) Smears—for determining gonorrhea and meningitis

       (3) White blood count and differential

       (4) Urinalysis

       (5) Gram stain

    c. Immunologic tests

       (1) Serology tests, tests for antibodies in the patient's blood serum, such as for syphilis and viral infections

       (2) Skin tests, such as the purified protein derivative (PPD) or the Tine test for tuberculosis

    d. Radiologic tests

    e. Gallium scans

    f. White blood cell nuclear medicine scan

    g. Ultrasound examinations

    h. CT scan

17. Immunologic diseases

    a. Skin tests—used for diagnosing allergies, such as the patch and scratch tests

    b. Laboratory tests—varied blood tests often specific for the type of disease and the body organ or system that is affected, such as the tests used in diagnosing rheumatoid arthritis and systemic lupus erythematosus (SLE)

Common Medical Terminology/ Combining Word Parts

In this appendix the basic elements of medical word-making are presented. A scientific vocabulary that conveys complex ideas and descriptions is needed. Our medical traditions and word sources have been commonly taken from Greek and Latin writings.

Learning a medical vocabulary becomes a matter of memorizing a few score Greek and Latin prefixes, suffixes, and word roots and combining them systematically to make thousands of precise terms.

When studying, the student should have at hand a good medical dictionary. Spelling, pronunciation, word structure, and usage need to be verified constantly if one is to build a medical vocabulary.

The base word we call the *root*; the combining modified (or affix) we call the *prefix* when it is placed *before* the root, or the *suffix* when we place it *after* the root. Thus in the foregoing sentence, *pre-* and *suf-* are prefixes to *-fix. Ophthalmo-* (eye) and *-scope* (instrument for viewing) become *ophthalmoscope,* an instrument for examining the eye. *Oto-* (ear) and *-scope* become *otoscope,* an instrument for examining the ear. Combining the suffix *itis,* meaning inflammation, with the base words *tonsilla, peritoneum, otos,* and *osteon,* we get *tonsillitis, peritonitis, otitis,* and *osteitis.*

Prefixes and suffixes give special meaning to the ideas the roots express. In English we have, for example, *before*hand, handi*ness* and handi*craft.* Memorize the following commonly used prefixes, word elements, and suffixes. Get the feel of their usage in medical-word, construction.

Prefixes and Word Elements	Prefixes and Word Elements	Common Usage Examples*
a-, an-	without	absent *a*plasia
ab-	away from	*ab*duct
ad-	to, at	*ad*hesive
aden/o	gland	*aden*osis
albo/o	white	*alb*icans
album-	white,	albumin *alb*uminuria
alveolo-	alveoli	*alveolo*tomy
ana-,/an-	up, too much, backward	*ana*phylaxis
angi/o	blood vessel	*angi*ogram
ankyl/osis	bent, crooked, adhesion	*anky*losis
ante-	before	*ante*febrile
antero-	in front of, before	*antero*grade
anti-	against, opposed to	*anti*biotic, *anti*body
aort/o	aorta	*aort*itis
appendic/o	appendix	*appendic*itis
arteri/o	artery	*arterio*sclerosis
arthr/o	joint	*arthr*opathy
audi/o	hearing	*audi*ogram
auto-	self	*auto*graft
bacteri/o	bacteria	*bacteri*uria
bi-	two	*bi*lateral
blast-	germ cell	*blast*oma
blenno-: see muco-		
blephar/o	eyelid	*blephar*oplasty
brady-	slow	*brady*cardia
bronch/o	bronchus	*bronch*itis
bucc/o	cheek	*bucc*al
burs/o	bursa	*burs*itis
cardi/o	heart	electro*cardi*ogram
cephal/o	head	*cephal*ogram

Prefixes and Word Elements	Common Usage	Examples*
cerebr/o	cerebrum	cerebropathy
cervic/o	neck, cervix	cervical; cervicitis
cheil/o	lip	cheiloplasty
cholecyst-	gallbladder	cholecystectomy
chondr/o	cartilage	chondritis
coccuscoccus	(bacterium)	streptococcus
col/o	colon	colostomy
colp/o	vagina	colpostenosis
cost/o	rib	costovertegral
crani/o	cranium	craniotomy
cyan/o	blue	cyanosis
cyst/o	bladder	cystocele
cyto-	cell	cytoplasm
dacry/o	tears	dacryagogic
dacryocyst/o	lacrimal sac	dacryocystdacryocystitis
dent/o	tooth	dentalgia
derm-	skin	dermal
dermat/o	skin	dermatology
dextr/o	to the right side	dextrocardia
dia-	through	diaphragm
diplo-	double	diplopia
dis-	to separate	disarticulate
doch/o	duct	choledochetomy
duoden/o	duodenum	duodenoscopy
dys-	difficult, painful	dyspnea
ec. ex-	out of, away from	ectopy, excrete
ecto-	outside	ectopic
electro-	electric in nature	electrocardiogram
emesis	vomit	hematemesis
encephal/o	brain, or enclosed within the head	encephalogram
endo-	within, inside of	endocardium
enter/o	intestine	enterocolitis
epi-	on, over	epidermis, epidural
erythr/o	red	erythrocyte
esophag/o	esophagus	esophagitis
esthesia	sensation	anesthesia
eti-	causation	etiology
ex/o	outside	exocardia
extra-	outside of	extradural, extraperitoneal
gastro-	stomach	gastroenteritis
gen/o	producing	ginesis
gingiv/o	gums	gingivitis
gloss/o	tongue	glossitis
glyc/o	sugar	glycogen
gyne-, gyneco	women	gynecology
hemat/o	blood	hematemesis
hemi-	one half	hemiplegia
hem/o	blood	hemotoma
hepat/o	liver	hepatitis
hidr/o	sweat	hidrosis
hist/o	tissue	histology
hydr/o	water	hydrotherapy
hyper-	over, excessive, increased	hyperalimination, hyperesthesia, hypertrophy

Prefixes and Word Elements	Common Usage	Examples*
hyp/o	under, below less	hypotension hypodermic hypogastric
hyster/o	uterus	hysterectomy
iatro	physician, medicine	iatrogenic
im- (replaces in- before *b, m* or *p*)	negative prefix, not	imbalance
in-	negative prefix, *not*	inoperable
in-	in, into	inclusion
infra-	below	infrapatellar
inter-	(contrast between, among)	intercostal

intra-	within, inside of (separate the
	  the double a with a hyphen)
		ntra-articular, intramusculare
		  intravenous

intro-	into, within	introspection
intus-	in, into	intussusception
ipsi-	self, the same	ipsilateral
ir-	not	irregular, irreversible
ir-	in, into	irradiate
ir/o, irid/o	iris	iridocele
isch- (pronounced *isk*)	to suppress	ischemia
ischi/o (pronounced *iskee [o]*)	ischium	ischiectomy, ischiodynia
iso-	equal, alike	isotonic
juxta-	near	juxta-articular, juxtaposition
kal-, kali-	potassium (K⁺)	kalemia
karyo-	nucleus	karyocyte
kerat/o	horny tissue,	kertosis, cornea keratitis
keto-	carbonyl group (*through German, from Latin* acetum, vinegar)	ketogenic, ketosis
kilo-	one thousand	kilogram, kilometer, kilovolt
kine-, kinesi/o	movement	kinesiology
labio-	lip (compare *labium*, lip, and *labrum*, edge or lip)	labioplasty
lacrima, lacrimo-	tears	lacrimatory
lact/o	milk	lactigenous
lalo-	speech; babbling	lalognosis, laloplegia, lalorrhea
lamell/a	thin leaf or plate	lamelliform (a little lamina)
lamin/a	thin plate or layer	laminectomy
lapar/o	abdomen	laparotomy
laryng/o	larynx	laryngitis
lepto-	delicate, slender, thin	leptocyte, leptomeninges
leuko-, leuco-	white (*leuko-* is preferred)	leukocyte, leukemia (o omit- ted before vowel)
levo-	to the left side	levocardia, levorotation
lip/o	fat, lipid	lipase, lipotropic
litho	stone, calculus	lithonephritis
lob/o	lobe	lobectomy
lymphaden/o	lymph gland	lymphadenopathy
lympho-	lymph	lymphoblast, lymphosarcoma
macro-	large, abnormal	lymacroscopic, longmacrocyte
malacia	softening	cerebromalacia
mamm/o	breast	mammogram
mast/o	breast	mastectomy
melan/o	black	melanoma
mening/o	meninges	meningeal
meso-	middle, intermediate, mesentery	mesoderm, mesoappendix
metr/o	uterus	metroptosis
micro-	small (in Greek originally *short*)	microscopic, microcyte

Prefixes and Word Elements	Common Usage	Examples*
mito-	thread, threadlike, mitosis	*mito*chondria, *mito*genesis
mon/o	one, single	*mono*blast, *mono*cular
mortem	deathpost	*mortem*
muco- (Latin), *myxo-* and *blenno-* (Greek)	mucus	*muco*sa, *muco*purulent, *myxo*ma, *myxo*rrhea, or *blenno*rrhea
multi-	many, much	*multi*factorial, *multi*form
my-; see *myo-*		
mycet-, mycl/o	fungus	*myco*logy, *myco*bacterial
mycet-, mycl/o, myelo-	marrow, often specifically spinal cord	*myelo*blastoma, *myelo*cele, *myelo*cyte
mylo	muscle	*my*atrophy or *myo*atropy, *myo*cardial, *myo*tonia
myring/o	eardrum	*myring*oplasty
nas/o	nose	*naso*pharyngitis
natal	birth	*natal*ity
natr/i	sodium (Na$^+$)	*natr*emia
necr/o	death	*necr*osis
neo-	new	*neo*natal, *neo*plastic
nephr/o	kidney	*nephr*itis, *nephr*ostomy
neur/o	nerve or nervous *system*	*neur*ectomy, *neuro*der matitis, *neuro*fibroma
non-	without; not	*non*union
normo-	normal, usual	*normo*blast, *normo*calcemia
nos/o	disease	*noso*comia, *noso*logy
oculo-	eye	*oculo*facial, oculomotor
odont/o	teeth	*odont*algia, *odonto*blast
olig/o	few, scanty	*olig*uria
oncl/o	mass, bulk, tumor	*onc*ology
onych/o	nails	*onycho*dystrophy, *ony* chogryphosis, *onych*omycosis
oo- (Greek); *ov/i, ov/o* (Latin)	egg, ovum	*oo*genesis, *ovi*parous, *ov*oid
oophor/o	ovary	*oophor*ectomy
ophthalm/o	eye	*ophthalm*oscope
orchi/o	testes	*orchi*oplasty
orchid/o	testes	*orchid*ectomy
orth/o	straight, normal, correct	*orth*opedic
ost-, osteo-	bone	*ost*ectomy, *osteo*malacia
ot/o	ear	*ot*oscope
ox/o, oxy	oxygen	*oxy*genation
pan-	all	*pan*carditis, *pan*hysterosalp ingo-oophorectomy
para-	beyond, beside, apart, accessory to	*para*-appendicitis, *para*colitis
partum	birth	post*partum*
ped-	child; foot	*ped*iatrics; *ped*al
peri-	around	*peri*anal, *peri*osteum
phagia	swallowing	dys*phagia*
pharyng/o	pharynx	*pharyng*itis
phasia	speech	dys*phasia*
phleb/o	vein	*phleb*itis
phobia	fear	acro*phobia*
phon/o	sound	*phono*cardiogram, *phono*myogram
phot/o	light (the radiation)	*photo*meter

Prefixes and Word Elements	Common Usage	Examples*
phren-, phrenic	diaphragm, mind, of the phrenic nerve	*phren*ectomy or *phrenic*ectomy
phys-, physio-	nature, or physical things	*phys*iology, *phys*iatry, *physio*therapy
pilo-	hair	*pilo*nidal
plegia	paralysis	para*plegia*
pneumato-, pneumo-, pneumon-	lungs, air in lungs, breath	*pneumo*encephalogram, *pneumon*ia
post-	after	*post*partum
pre-	before	*pre*natal
proct/o	rectum	*proct*oscope
prostat/o	prostate gland	*prostat*ectomy
pseud/o	false	*pseudo*ankylosis
pulm/o	lung; air or gas	*pulm*onary
py/o	pus	*pyo*cyst
pyel/o	kidney pelvis	*pyel*ogram
quadri-, quadru-	four	*quadri*ceps *quadri*plegia
radi/o	x radiation, radius bone, shortwave radiation	*radio*active, *radio*carpal, *radio*thermy
recto-	rectum	*recto*cele, *recto*sigmoid
ren/o	kidney	*ren*al
retin/o	retina	*retin*itis
retro-	backward, behind	*retro*cecal, *retro*bulbar
rhin/o	nose, noselike	*rhin*itis
sacr/o	sacrum	*sacro*coccygeal, *sacro*iliac
salping/o	tube or auditory	(uterine *salping*ectomy, *salpingo*pharyngeal
sangui-	blood	*sangui*neous
sarc/o	flesh	*sarc*oidosis, *sarc*oma
scler/o	hard	*scler*edema, *sclero*derma
semi-	half, partly	*semi*coma, *semi*flexion
sinistr/o	left side; left	*sinistr*aural, *sinistro*manual
spleno- (lien/o)	spleen	*spleno*megaly, *lien*ectomy
spondyl/o	vertebra, vertebrae, spinal column	*spondyl*itis, *spondyl*olysis
staped/o	stapes	*staped*ectomy
staphyl/o	resembling a bunch *of grapes*	*staphyl*ococcus
sten/o	narrow, contracting	*sten*osis
stere/o	solid, three-*dimensional*	*stere*ognosis, *stere*ogram
stomat/o	mouth	*stomat*itis
sub-	under, near, almost	*sub*acute, *sub*clinical, *sub*ungual
supra-	above	*supra*renal
sym-, syn, sys, sy-	together, union or association	*sym*physis, *syn*apse, *syn*drome
synov/io	synovial	*synov*itis
tachy-	swift, rapid	*tachy*cardia
teno- (less used: tendo-, tendon-, tenonto-)	tendon	*teno*plasty (*tendino*plasty, *tendo*plasty), *teno*desis, *teno*tomy
tetra-	four	*tetra*basic, *tetra*logy
therm/o	heat	*therm*al, *thermo*meter
thorac/o, thoracico	chest	*thoraco*centesis, *thorac*algia,
thromb/o	clot, thrombus	*thromb*ectomy, *thrombo*embolism
thyr/o	thyroid	*thyro*tomy

Prefixes and Word Elements	Common Usage	Examples*
tomo-	a cutting, a section	*tomography*
trache/o	trachea	*tracheostomy*
trans-	through, across	*transfusion*
tri-	three	*triceps*
tympan/o	tympanic membrane or eardrum	*tympanitis*
ungu/o	nail	*unguinal*
uni	one	*unilateral*
ureter/o	ureter	*ureteritis*
urethr/o	urethra	*urethritis*
urin/o, ur/o	urine	*urinalysis, urinometer*
vas/o	vessel, a duct	*vasoconstriction, vasectomy*
ven/o	vein	*venogram*
xanth/o	yellow	*xanthelasma, xanthochromia*
xer/o	dry; dryness	*xeroderma, xerography*
xiph-, xiphi, xipho- (swordlike)	xiphoid process	*xiphisternal, xiphocostal*
zoo- (pronounced zo-o, not zu)	animal	*zoonosis*
zyg/o	yoked, joined	*zygopophysis, zygote*

Suffixes	Common Usage	Examples*
-ac	pertaining to	cardi*ac*
-al	pertaining to	or*al*
-algia	pain	arthr*algia*
-ase	an enzyme	amyl*ase*
-centesis	puncture and aspiration of	pare*centesis*, amnio*centesis*, amthro*centesis*
-cele	hernia, cavity, tumor	hydro*cele*, recto*cele*
-clasis	breaking	osteo*clasis*
-clysis	to wash out	hypodermo*clysis*
-desis	binding	arthro*desis*
-dynia	pain	cephalo*dynia*
-ectasis	dilation, distention	colp*ectasis*
-ectomy	excision of organ or part	anappend*ectomy*, gastr*ectomy*
-emia	blood condition	hypervol*emia*, septic*emia*
-gnosis	knowledge	dia*gnosis*
-gram	recorded; written	electrocardio*gram*
-graphy	making a graphic tracing or recording	electrocardio*graphy*
-ia	state; condition; disease	card*ia*
-iac	pertaining to	cardi*ac*
-iasis	condition of; process or its result	cholelith*iasis*
-itis	inflammation	gingiv*itis*, gloss*itis*
-logy	word, reason, science, study of	patho*logy*, etio*logy*, embryo*logy*
-lysis	dissolution, releasing, freeing	hemo*lysis*
-megaly	enlarged	hepato*megaly*
-meter	measures	phygmomano*meter*
-odynia	pain condition	ophthalmo*dynia* (same as ophthalgia)
-oid	resembling, like	lip*oid*
-ologist	specialist; expert in the study of	cardi*ologist*
-ology	study of science	cardi*ology*
-oma	tumor	aden*oma*

Prefixes and Word Elements	Common Usage	Examples*
-opia, opsia	vision	diplopia, hemianopsia
-ose	carbohydrate (sugars, starches, and celluloses)	glucose, cellulose
-osis	process, disease, abnormal increase	hepatosis
-para	bring forth (woman who has borne viable young)	multipara, nullipara, primipara
-pathy	disease	neuropathy, myopathy, osteopathy
-penia	abnormal reduction in number	erythropenia, leukopenia, neutropenia
-pexy, -pexia	surgical fixation of an organ, suspension	nephropexy
-plasty	shaping or formation of	surgical arthroplasty, mammaplasty or rhinoplasty
-pnea	breathing	dyspnea
-ptosis	drooping; sagging	nephroptosis
-ptysis	cough up	hemoptysis
-rrhage, -rrhagia	a bursting forth, excessive flow	hemorrhage, menorrhagia, metrorrhagia
-rrhaphy	surgical repair by suture	herniorrhaphy, tenorrhaphy
-rrhea	flow, discharge	dysmenorrhea
-scope	instrument for observing	otoscope, ophthalmoscope, bronchoscope, arthroscope, sigmoidoscope, laryngoscope
-scopy	examination of	gastroscopy
-sect	act of cutting, sectioning	dissect
-stomy	(mouth) surgical creation of an opening of a viscus for drainage or for communication from one viscus to another	colostomy, tracheostomy, gastrojejunostomy
-tome	instrument for cutting	myringotome, osteotome
-tomy	act of cutting, incising	tracheotomy, gastrotomy
-trophy	nutrition, as it has to do with vitality and growth	atrophy, hypertrophy
-uria	urine condition	dysuria, anuria, oliguria

As you study, find these words in the medical dictionary and include them in your vocabulary. Also note that the terminal vowel of some prefixes, usually o but often i or even a, is dropped when the root word begins with a vowel, such as hypesthesia, kalemia, and laminectomy.

Summary of Pediatric Immunization Recommendations

Notes on IMMUNIZATION SCHEDULES

A. Can give any and all of these vaccines simultaneously, at separate anatomic sites. Can start immunizations at age 6 weeks even for premature and/or low-birth-weight infants who are otherwise well.

B. For any of these vaccines, if delay occurs between doses, regardless of the length, the series does not have to be restarted; pick up the schedule where it left off.

C. Intervals between doses in the series should not be less than those indicated as immunologic response can be compromised.

D. Two Hib-conjugate vaccines are approved for use in infants less than 12 months of age: HibTITER and PedvaxHIB. As these brands are not known to be interchangeable in infants under age 12 months, use only one brand on each infant. Record brand used on the child's personal immunization record. Any Hib conjugate vaccine (including ProHIBIT) *can* be used for children 15 months of age and older, regardless of any brand used earlier.

E. Alternative age for first MMR dose for some measles epidemic or hyperendemic counties only: MMR at age 12 months (*on or after* the first birthday). No repeat MMR at 15 months needed if first dose given at ≥ 12 months.

F. Some of these immunizations are required for school/child care center entry. A child may be exempted from these requirements because of (a) a permanent or temporary medical reason (an explanatory letter from the physician stating reason and time period of exemption is required), or (b) because of a parent/guardian's personal or religious beliefs. Parent/guardian must sign exemption affidavit at school.

G. Normally, oral polio vaccine (OPV) is used. For immunocompromised infants or children and infants or children with immunocompromised persons in the household, use inactivated polio vaccine (IPV).

H. Hepatitis B vaccine:

(1) Infants, children, and adults who are household contacts of a hepatitis B carrier, not known to have serologic evidence of prior or current hepatitis B infection, if they have not already received it, should get the 3-dose Hep B vaccine series (2nd and 3rd doses given 1 month and 6 months, respectively, after the first).

(2) Children who are in households of immigrants or refugees from areas of high hepatitis B endemicity (such as Africa, East Asia, or the Pacific Islands) should get the 3-dose Hep B vaccine series if they haven't already done so, if resources allow it.

(3) The same is true for adolescents (age 11 years and older) and teenagers who are injecting drug users, have more than one sex partner every 6 months, or are in communities where injecting drug use, teenage pregnancy, and/or sexually transmitted diseases are common, if resources allow it.

I. Current limitations on use of Immunization Branch-supplied vaccines:

(1) MMR: Second MMR dose available only for (a) children 4-5 years old in kindergarten or who will enter kindergarten, and (b) college/university entrants (freshman, undergraduate transfer or graduate school entrant). These restrictions are relaxed during outbreaks. Providers using MMR vaccine from other sources can take advantage of any visit by school chidlren ages 6-18 years and college/university students to give the second MMR dose if not already received.

(2) Hepatitis B vaccine available for:

a) Persons in households of hepatitis B-infected (HBsAg-positive) pregnant women or new mothers, including newborns.

b) All infants under age 12 months. If infant starts vaccine series but does not complete it before age 12 months. If infant starts vaccine series but does not complete it before age 12 months, the series can be finished with Immunization Branch-supplied vaccine, even though he/she is now over age 12 months.

(3) IPV: Available only for immunocompromised vaccinees or vaccinees in households with immunocompromised

Adapted from Immunization Branch, California State Department of Health Services—Effective November, 1992.

Children Beginning Immunization In Infancy

Age: Vaccine:	At Birth	6 weeks- 2 months	4 months	6 months	12 months	15 months	4-6 years, before school entry	14-16 years
DTP/DTaP		DTP #1 (whole cell)	DTP #2 (whole cell)	DTP #3 (whole cell)		DTaP or DTP #4 (whole cell or acellular) (can be at age 18 months)	DTaP or DTP #5 (whole cell or acellular)	Td
POLIO (OPV OR IPV)		Polio #1	Polio #2			Polio #3 (can be at age 18 months)	Polio #4	
MMR						MMR #1 (12 months in some areas; not before 1st birthday)	MMR #2 (less preferred alternative: middle school entry)	
HIB HibTITER		HibTITER #1	HibTITER #2	HibTITER #3		HibTITER #4 (or can use PedvaxHIB or ProHIBIT)		
or PedvaxHIB		PedvaxHIB #1	PedvaxHIB #2		PedvaxHIB #3 (or can use ProHIBIT)			
HEPATITIS B Option 1	Hep B #1	Hep B #2		Hep B #3 (any time between ages 6 and 18 months)				
or Option 2		Hep B #1	Hep B #2		Hep B #3 (any time between ages 6 and 18 months)			

1. HIB:

(a) *If infant starts at age 7-11 months, give 2 doses of either HibTITER or PedvaxHIB 2 months apart (don't intermix these two vaccines) and third dose (can be hibTITER, PedvaxHIB or ProHIBIT) at age 15 months.*

(b) *If infant starts at age 12-14 months, give first dose (HibTITER or PedvaxHIB). Give second (and last) dose (HibTITER, PedvaxHIB or ProHIBIT) at age 15 months.*

(c) *If child starts at age 15 months-4 years give just one dose (HibTITER, PedvaxHIB or ProHIBIT).*

2. Hep B:

(a) *Third option with one Hep B vaccine (Engerix-B): 4 doses, at birth and ages, 1, 2, and 12 months.*

(b) *Infants of HBsAg-positive mothers need 3 Hep B vaccine doses, at birth (also give 0.5 ml HBIG at this time), age 1 to 1 1/2 months, and age 6 months. All doses are 0.5 ml for these infants. Other susceptible household contacts of HBsAg-positive mother: 3-dose hepatitis B vaccine series, with second and third doses 1 and 6 months after first dose, respectively. See package insert for dosage, which varies with age and vaccine used.*

Children Beginning Immunization At or After Age 15 months But Before Age 7 Years

Visit/Age[a]	Vaccine Doses
Ist visit	DTP[b] #1, POLIO #1, MMR #1, HIB[c]
6-8 weeks after Ist visit	DTP,[b] POLIO #2
4-8 weeks after 2nd visit	DTP[b] #3
6-12 months after 3rd visit	DTaP or DTP #4, POLIO #3
Age 4-6 years (before school entry)	DTaP or DTP #5,[d] POLIO #4,[d] MMR #2
Age 14-16 years	Td

[a] *If immunization started before age 15 months, give first two doses of polio and first three DTP doses per this schedule and give MMR at 15 months. Follow Hib schedule in footnote of table for children beginning immunication in infancy.*
[b] *DTaP should* not *be used for these doses.*
[c] *Immunologically normal children age 5 years and older do not need Hib vaccine.*
[d] *The USPHs and the AAP consider DTaP or DTP #5 and POLIO #4 necessary unless the DTaP or DTP #4 and POLIO #3 were given after the 4th birthday. California's school entry law, which is a minimally acceptable standard rather than an optimum recommendation, does not require these doses unless DTaP or DTP #4 and POLIO #3 were given before the* second *birthday. Physicians and clinics should follow the USPHS/AAP recommendation.*

Children Beginning Immunization At Ages 7-17 Years

Visit	Vaccine Doses
Ist visit	Td #1, POLIO #1, MMR #1
6-8 weeks after Ist visit	Td #2, POLIO #2, MMR #2
6-12 months after 2nd visit	Td #3, POLIO #3
10 years after 3rd Td	Td

For adolescents and teenagers at high risk, a 3-dose Hepatitis B vaccine series also is recommended. See package insert for dosage.

VALID CONTRAINDICATIONS

Vaccine(s)	Condition
All	1. Acutely ill; e.g., appears to have marked fever and/or appears sick.
MMR, MR Influenza	2. *Anaphylactic* allergy to eggs (collapse, shock, tongue or mouth and throat swelling, hypotension, respiratory distress, hives)—Do *not* give measles and mumps-containing vaccines or influenza vaccine.
MMR, MR, OPV	3. *Anaphylactic* allergy to neomycin (see No. 2 for symptoms/signs)—Do not give measles, mumps or rubella-containing vaccines or OPV.
OPV, IPV	4. *Anaphylactic* allergy to streptomycin (cf. above for symptoms/signs)—Do not give OPV, IPV.
Hepatitis B	5. *Anaphylactic* allergy to yeast.
Virtually all inactivated vaccines	6. *Anaphylactic* allergy to thimerosal (a preservative used in vaccines, contact lens cleaning solutions, etc.). Some preparations (e.g. MSD's Pneumovax) do not contain thimerosal.
MMR, MR, OPV, IPV	7. Pregnancy (of vaccinee)—Do not give measles, mumps, or rubella-containing vaccines. Give OPV only if at high risk of exposure.
MMR, MR	8. Immune globulin or blood transfusion within past 3 months—Do not routinely give measles, mumps or rubella-containing vaccines until 3 months have passed. However, if exposure risk high, can give MMR/MR within 3 months.
MMR, MR, OPV	9. Immunodeficiency or immunosuppression—Do not give measles, mumps, or rubella-containing vaccines or OPV. Also, do not give OPV if any other household member is immunodeficient or immunosuppressed. (See guide for HIV-infected children below.)
DTP, DTaP	10. Serious reaction to prior DTP or DTaP dose; i.e., a. Immediate anaphylactic reaction b. Encephalopathy within 7 days (major alteration in consciousness, persisting seizures or unresponsiveness, without recovery within 24 hours, convulsions lasting more than a few hours) c. Precautions—not absolute contraindications; i.e., can consider more DTaP or DTP if there is a high incidence of pertussis locally: (1) Temp ≥ 105° F (≥40° C) within 48 hours with no other cause (2) Collapse or shock-like state (hypotonic hyporesponsive episode) within 48 hours (3) Convulsion(s) with or without fever within 3 days* (4) Persistent inconsolable crying for ≥ 3 hours, within 48 hours
DTP, DTaP	11. Uncontrolled epilepsy, infantile spasms, progressive encephalopathy. Consider DT instead.*

Acetaminophen Note: If/when DTaP/DTP/DT given to infant/child with convulsion history or with convulsion history in parents or siblings, advise parent to give acetaminophen (15 mg/kg) on returning home from IZ clinic and again every 4-6 hours for 24 hours. DTaP preferred over DTP for 4th and 5th doses in these children.

Schedule for DT for Infants and Children Who Cannot Take DTP/DTaP

Infants under age 1 year—3 doses at 4-8 week intervals: a fourth dose 6-12 months after the third, and a fifth dose at age 4-6 years, just before school entry. If fourth dose given after fourth birthday, the fifth dose is not necessary.
Children ages 1-6 years—2 doses 4-8 weeks apart, a third dose 6-12 months after the second, and a fourth dose at age 4-6 years, just before school entry. If third dose given after fourth birthday, the fourth dose is not necessary.

Immunizing Children with HIV Infection

Vaccine	Known Asymptomatic	Symptomatic
DTaP, DTP/DT/Td	Yes	Yes
OPV	No	No
IPV	Yes	Yes
MMR	Yes	Yes, consider
HIB	Yes	Yes
Hepatitis B	Yes	Yes
Pneumococcal	Yes	Yes
Influenza	Optional	Yes

NON-CONTRAINDICATIONS

Immunizations generally can be given in these situations:

1. Lack of physical exam or measurements of temperature, even for infants.
2. Mild acute illness. A moderate or severe acute illness is reason to postpone immunizations, but minor illnesses, such as mild upper-respiratory infections (URI), low-grade fever (101°F, oral or rectal, if measured, although temperature measurement is not a routine prerequisite for immunization) or mild diarrhea, are not contraindications for immunization if infant/child appears otherwise well.
3. Mild to moderate local reaction (soreness, redness, swelling) or mild to moderate fever after prior dose of same vaccine.
4. Prematurity.
5. Allergy to ducks, chickens, or feathers.
6. Allergy to penicillin or other antibiotic (except anaphylactic allergy to neomycin or streptomycin). Also, non-anaphylactic allergy to eggs.
7. "Allergies" in general, or relatives with allergies.
8. Currently taking antibiotics or other medicine (except immunosuppressive therapy).
9. Convalescent phase of illness-past febrile stage.
10. Recent exposure to infectious illness, including varicella.
11. Tuberculosis, or tuberculosis in family. Also TB skin test not a prerequisite for measles or other vaccines.
12. Convulsions in siblings or parents.*
13. Mother or other household contact is pregnant.
14. Breastfeeding.
15. Concurrent or recent doses of other vaccines (Exceptions: DTP/DTaP and influenza should be given ≥3 days apart. OPV, if not given on the same day as MMR/MR, should be given ≥1 month later).
16. Prior history of immunization with or illness due to one or two of its three components is not a contraindication to MMR.
17. Do not require negative pregnancy test, enrollment in family planning program, to be on contraception, or to be within 2 weeks of last menses. Can immunize childbearing-age woman with MMR or MR if she states she is not pregnant and does not plan pregnancy in next 3 months.
18. Family history of SIDS, allergies, adverse reactions to vaccines.
19. History of prematurity or low birth weight.
20. Injection site reaction or fever (temp. <105°F) after prior DTP or DTaP dose.
21. Stable neurologic condition (including well-controlled convulsions*), resolved or corrected neurologic disorder. Can give DTP or DTaP.

See acetominophen note, valid contraindications column.

Timing Restrictions Between Different Vaccines

MMR/MR and OPV: Can give on same day, but if not given on same day and MMR given first, wait 4 weeks before giving OPV. If OPV given first, give MMR at any time afterwards. No restrictions exist between the different inactivated vaccines or between inactivated and live vaccines.

MMR/MR and TB skin test: Can give TB skin test before or on same day as MMR, but if ≥ 1 day has passed after giving MMR/MR wait 4-6 weeks before giving TB skin test.

MMR/MR and IG (or any other immune globulin preparation): Give MMR/MR either at least 2 weeks before IG or at least 3 months after giving IG. If exposure risk increased, drop this restriction for MMR/MR.

Routes of Vaccine Administration

OPV: Oral
DTaP, DTP/DT/Td: IM
MMR/MR: SC

IPV: SC
Influenza: IM
Pneumococcal: IM or SC

TETANUS PROPHYLAXIS IN WOUND MANAGEMENT

Prior Tetanus Doses	Clean, Minor Wounds		Other Wounds [1]	
	Td[2]	TIG[3]	Td[2]	TIG[3]
Uncertain, or <3	Yes	No	Yes	Yes
3 or more	No[4]	No	No[5]	No

1. E.g., Wound contaminated with dirt, feces, soil, etc.; puncture wound; avulsion; wound resulting from missle, crushing, burn, or frostbite; wound extends into muscle.
2. Substitute DTP or DTaP for children under age 7 years.
3. TIG-Tetanus Immune Globulin.
4. Yes, if ≥ 10 years since last dose.
5. Yes, if ≥5 years since last dose.

VACCINE STORAGE AND HANDLING

1. DTaP/DTP/DT/Td, Hib; Hep B, Influenza, Pneumococcal—Store at 36°-46°F (refrigerate but do not freeze—check refrigerator periodically). Do not store in door.
2. MMR, MR-Store at 35°—46°F (refrigerator). *Do not allow to warm up or be exposed to light before use.*
3. OPV—Store in freezer. May be stored in refrigerator for up to 30 days if unopened. Do *not* allow to warm up to room temperature before use.

Glossary

Abdominal pulse—Abdominal aorta pulse.

Abdominal respirations—The inspiration and expiration of air by the lungs accomplished primarily by the abdominal muscles and diaphragm.

Accelerated respirations—More than 25 respirations per minute, after 15 years of age.

Acetonuria (as″e-to-nu′re-ah) or ketonuria (ke″to-nu′re-ah)—The presence of acetone or ketone in the urine.

Acrotism (ak′ro-tizm)—Apparent absence of pulse.

Addiction (ah-dik′shun)—An acquired physiologic and/or psychologic dependence on a drug with tendencies to increase its use.

Agglutination (ah-gloo″tin-na′shun)—A clumping together of cells, as of blood cells or bacteria. An example is when red blood cells (RBC) clump together as a result of an incompatible blood transfusion.

Agranulocyte (a-gran′ u-lo-sit″)—A white blood cell (WBC) with a clear or non granular cytoplasm. There are two types, monocytes and lymphocytes.

Albuminuria (al-bu″mi-nu′re-ah)—The presence of serum albumin in urine.

Allergen (al-er-jen)—Any substance that induces hypersensitivity.

Allergy (al′er-je)—An unusual and increased sensitivity (hypersensitivity) to specific substances that are ordinarily harmless.

Alternating pulse—Alternating weak and strong pulsations.

AMA—American Medical Association.

Amplify (am′pli-fi)—To enlarge, to extend.

Anaerobic Culturette culture collection system—This system offers the same basic properties of the Culturette, plus a standardized and dependable anaerobic environment for transport of anaerobic bacteria. The transport medium once released maintains an anaerobic environment for up to 48 hours. Many laboratories request that the anaerobic culture system be used when taking a wound culture. (See also Culturette.)

Anaphylactic (an″ah-fi-lak′tik) **shock**—An intense state of shock brought on by hypersensitivity to a drug, foreign toxin, or protein. Early symptoms resemble an allergic reaction, then increase in severity rapidly to dyspnea, cyanosis, and shock. This can be fatal if emergency measures are not taken immediately (see also Unit Seventeen, Allergic Reactions to Drugs).

Anaphylaxis (an″ah-fi-lak′sis)—An unusual or hypersensitive reaction of the body to foreign protein and other substances; frequently caused by drugs, foreign serum (for example, tetanus), and insect stings and bites.

Anemia (ah-ne′me-ah)—There is a variety of forms of anemia, but broadly speaking it is a lack of red blood cells in the circulating blood or a reduction of hemoglobin or both. Anemia is thought of as a symptom of a disease or disorder; it is not a disease.

Anesthesia (An″es-the′ze-ah)—The loss of sensation or feeling.

Anisocytosis (an-i″-so-si-to′sis)—A state of abnormal variations in the size of red blood cells in the blood.

Anoscope (an′no-skop)—A speculum or endoscope inserted into the anal canal for direct visual examination.

Antidote (An′ti-dot)—An agent used to counteract a poison.

Antiseptic (an′ti-sep′ tik)—A substance capable of inhibiting the growth or action of microorganisms, without necessarily killing them; generally safe for use on body tissues.

Anuria (ah-nu′re-ah)—The absence of urine.

Apnea (ap-ne′ah)—Cessation or absence of breathing.

Applicator—A slender rod of glass or wood with a pledget of cotton on one end used to apply medicine or to take a culture from the body.

Arrhythmia (ah-rith′me-ah)—A variation from the normal or an irregular rhythm of the heartbeat.

Arthritis (ar-thri′ tis)—Inflammation of a joint.

Artificial respiration—Artificial methods to restore respiration in cases of suspended breathing.

Asepsis (a-sep′sis)—The absence of all microorganisms causing disease; absence of contaminated matter.

Aspiration/needle biopsy—Removal of material from internal organ by means of hollow needle inserted through the body wall and into affected tissue.

Atopy (at″o-pe)—A hypersensitive state that is subject to hereditary influences, such as hay fever, asthma, and eczema.

Atrium (a′tre-um)—One of the upper chambers of the heart. The right atrium receives deoxygenated blood from the body, whereas the left atrium receives oxygenated blood from the lungs. (The plural is **atria.**)

Auricle (aw′ri-kl)—The outer projection of the ear; also known as the pinna (pin′nah).

Bactericide (bak-ter′i-sid)—A substance capable of destroying bacteria but not spores.

Bacteriology (bak-te″re-ol′o-je)—The study of bacteria.

Bacteriolysis (bak-te″re-ol′i-sis)—The destruction of bacteria.

Bacteriostatic (bak-te″re-o-stat′ik)—A substance that inhibits the growth of bacteria.

Bacteriuria (bak-te″re-u′re-ah)—The presence of bacteria in urine.

Band-form Granulocyte—A granular WBC in a stage of development.

Benign (be-nin) **hypertension**—Hypertension of slow onset that is usually without symptoms.

Bigeminal (bi-jem′in-al) **pulse**—Two regular beats followed by a longer pause. It has the same significance as an irregular pulse.

Bimanual (bi-man′u-al)—With both hands, as bimanual palpation.

Biochemistry (bi″o-kem′s-tre)—The study of chemical changes occurring in living organisms.

Biologic death—The condition that results when the brain has been deprived of oxygenated blood for a period of 6 minutes or more, and irreversible damage has probably occurred.

Biopsy (bi′op-se)—Removal of tissue from the body for examination.

Biopsy (bi′op-se) **forceps**—Two-pronged instruments of varying sizes and shapes used to remove tissue from the body for examination.

Biot respiration—Irregularly alternating periods of apnea and hyperpnea; occurs in meningitis and disorders of the brain.

Blood culture—Used in the diagnosis of specific infectious diseases. Blood is withdrawn from a vein and placed in or upon suitable culture media; then it is determined whether or not pathogens grow in the media. If organisms do grow, they are identified by bacteriologic methods.

Blood dyscrasia (dis-kra′ze-ah)—An abnormal or diseased condition of the blood.

BNDD—Bureau of Narcotics and Dangerous Drugs (a federal government agency of the DEA).

Bowel movement—The elimination/excretion of fecal material from the intestinal tract.

Bradycardia (brad-i-kay′di-a)—Slow heart action; extremely slow pulse, generally below 60 beats per minute.

Bronchoscope (brong′ko-skop)—An endoscope designed specifically for passage through the trachea to allow visual examination of the interior of the tracheobronchial tree.

Bronchoscopy (bron-kos′ ko-pi)—Internal inspection of the tracheobronchial tree with the use of a bronchoscope; used for diagnostic or treatment purposes. For diagnosis, the physician will inspect the interior of the bronchi and may obtain a sample of secretions or a biopsy of tissue; for treatment, foreign bodies or mucus plugs that may be causing an obstruction to the air passages can be located and removed.

Bursitis (bur-si ′tis)—Inflammation of a bursa. The most commonly affected is the bursa of the shoulder.

Canthus (kan′thus)—The inner canthus is the angle of the eyelids near the nose; the outer canthus is the angle of the eyelids at the outside corner of the eyes.

Cardiac (kar′de-ak) **arrest**—Sudden and often unexpected cessation of the heartbeat. Permanent damage of vital organs and death are probable if treatment is not given immediately.

Cassette (kah-set′)—A light-proof aluminum or bakelite container with front and back intensifying screens, between which x-ray film is placed when used for x-ray examinations.

Cautery (kaw′ter-e)—A hot instrument used to cut or destroy tissue, causing hemostasis at the time.

Cerumen (se-roo′men)—Ear wax secreted by the glands of the external auditory meatus.

Chemotherapy (ke″mo-ther′ah-pe)—The use of drugs (chemicals) to treat disease; a type of therapy used for cancer patients in which powerful drugs are used to interfere with the reproduction of the fast-multiplying cancer cells.

Cheyne-Stokes (chan-stoks) **respiration**—Respirations gradually increasing in rapidity and volume, until they reach a climax, then gradually subsiding and ceasing entirely for from 5 to 50 seconds, when they begin again. These are often a sign of impending death. Cheyne-Stokes respirations may be observed in normal persons (especially the aged) during sleep or during visits to higher altitudes.

Clinical death—The state that results when breathing and circulation have stopped.

Colicky—Acute intermittent abdominal pain usually caused by spasmodic contractions.

Concussion (kon-kush′un)—The injury that results from a violent blow or shock.

Concussion of the brain—A violent disturbance of the brain caused by a blow or fall.

Conduction (kon-duk′shun)—The passage or conveyance of energy, as of electricity, heat or sound.

Conjunctiva (kon″junk-ti ′vah)—The delicate membrane lining the eyelids and reflected onto the front of the eyeball.

Constant fever—High fever with a variation not exceeding 1 or 2 degrees F (0.06° or 1.2° C) between morning and evening temperatures.

Constipation (kon-sti-pa′shun)—A condition in which the waste material in the intestine is too hard to pass easily, or in which bowel movements are so infrequent that discomfort results.

Contact dermatitis—Dermatitis caused by an allergic reaction resulting from contact of the skin with various substances such as poison ivy, or chemical, physical, and mechanical agents.

Contaminated, contamination (kon-tam″i-na′shun)—The act of making unclean, soiling, or staining, especially the introduction of disease germs or infectious material into or on normally sterile objects.

Contraindication (kon″tra-in″di-ka′shun)—Condition in which the use of certain drugs or treatments should be withheld or limited.

Contusion (kon-too′zhun)—A bruise, indicating injury to tissues without breakage in the skin. Discoloration appears because of blood seepage under the surface of the skin.

Cross-tolerance—Cross-tolerance can develop when tolerance to one drug increases the body's tolerance to drugs in the same category. For example, a tolerance to one depressant drug leads to a tolerance of other depressant drugs.

Crude drug—An unrefined drug.

Culture (kul ′tur)—The reproduction or growth of microorganisms or of living tissue cells in special laboratory media (the material on which the organisms grow) conducive to their growth. Various types of cultures follow.

Culture medium—A commercial preparation used for the growth of microorganisms or other cells. (Types of culture media are described in Unit Six.)

Culturette—A commercially prepared bacterial culture collection/transport system, consisting of a sterile plastic tube with applicator. Modified Stuart's transport medium is held in a glass ampule at the bottom end, to assure stability of medium at the time of use. Transport medium is released only after the sample is taken, by crushing the ampule. A moist environment (not immersion) is maintained up to 72 hours to preserve the specimen.

Culturette II culture collection system—This is identical to the Culturette, with the exception that the plastic tube contains two applicators and the ampule contains twice the medium (1 ml).

Cumulative action of a drug—A drug accumulates in the body; it is eliminated more slowly than it is absorbed.

Cystoscope (sist′o-skop)—A hollow metal tube instrument (endoscope) designed specifically for passing through the urethra into the urinary bladder to permit internal inspection. The bladder interior is illuminatd by an electric bulb at the end of the cystoscope. Special lenses and mirrors allow the bladder mucosa to be examined for calculi (stones), inflammation, or tumors.

Cystoscopy (sis-tos′kop-i)—Internal examination of the bladder with a cystoscope. Samples of urine for diagnostic purposes can be obtained by passing a catheter through the cystoscope into the bladder or beyond, up into the ureters and kidneys. Also, radiopaque dyes may be injected through the cystoscope into the bladder or up into the ureters when taking x-ray films of the urinary tract.

Cytology (si-tol′o-je)—The study of the structure and function of cells.

DEA—Drug Enforcement Administration. This is the federal law enforcement agency charged with the responsibility of combating drug diversion.

Debridement (da-bred-ment′)—The process of removing foreign material and devitalized tissue.

Defibrillation (de-fi″bri-la ′shun)—The application of electrical impulses to the heart to stop heart fibrillation.

Density—The quality of being dense or impenetrable.

Dermatitis (de″mah-ti′ tis)—Inflammation of the skin.

Detail—The sharpness of the radiograph image.

Diaphragmatic respiration—Performed mainly by the diaphragm.

Diarrhea (di-a-re′a)—Rapid movement of fecal material through the intestine, resulting in poor absorption, producing frequent, watery stools.

Digital (dij′ti-al)—The use of a finger to insert into a body cavity, such as the rectum, for palpating the tissue.

Dilute—To weaken the strength of a substance by adding something else.

Disinfectant (dis″in-fek′tant)—A substance capable of destroying pathogens, but usually not spores; generally not intended for use on body tissue, because it is too strong.

Diuresis (di″u-re-′sis)—An abnormal, increased secretion of urine as seen in diabetes mellitus, diabetes insipidus, or when drinking large amounts of fluid; this can be artificaly produced by drugs with diuretic properties.

Don—To put an article on, such as gloves or a gown.

Drug idiosyncrasy (id″e-o-sing′krah-se)—An unusual or abnormal response or susceptibility to a drug that is peculiar to the individual.

Drug tolerance—The decreased susceptibility to the effects of a drug after continued use. In this case an increased dosage would be required to produce the desired effects, as the initial dose would be ineffective.

Dysplasia (dis-pla′ze-ah)—An abnormal development of tissue.

Dyspnea (disp-ne′ah)—Labored or difficult breathing.

Dysuria (dis-u′re-ah)—Painful or difficult urination.

Electrocardiograph (e-lek″tro-kar′de-o-graf″)—The instrument used in electrocardiography.

Electrolyte (e-lek′ tro-lit)—Substances that separate into their component atoms when dissolved in water. They play an important part in maintaining fluid balance and a normal acid-base balance, and in the functions of cells in the body. EXAMPLES: sodium, potassium, calcium, magnesium, chloride, and bicarbonate.

Electrophoresis (e-lek″tro-fo-re′sis)—A laboratory method used to diagnose certain diseases by analyzing the plasma protein content.

Endoscope (en′do-skop)—A specially designed instrument made of metal, rubber, or glass that is used for direct visual examination of hollow organs or body cavities. All endoscopes have similar working elements, even though the design will vary according to its specific use. The viewing part (scope) is a hollow tube fitted with a lens system that allows viewing in a variety of directions. Each endoscope has a light source, power cord, and power source; examples include bronchoscope, cystoscope, proctoscope, and sigmoidoscope.

Endoscopy (en-dos′ko-pi)—Visual examination of internal cavities of the body with an endoscope (e.g., a proctoscope, bronchoscope, cystoscope, gastroscope, and laryngoscope).

Enema (en′e-mah)—The introduction of a solution into the rectum; for an x-ray examination of the colon, a radiopaque solution is administered by enema.

Enuresis (en″u-re′sis)—The involuntary excretion of urine, especially at night during sleep; bedwetting; most frequently seen in children with either physical or emotional problems.

Epinephrine (ep″i-nef′rin)—A hormone produced by the adrenal glands. Epinephrine can be administered parenterally, topically, or by inhalation. It is used as an emergency heart stimulant, to relieve symptoms in allergic conditions, and to counteract the lethal effects of anaphylactic shock.

Erythrocytosis (e-rith″ro-si-to′sis)—Increased numbers of red blood cells (erythrocytes).

Essential hypertension (idiopathic or primary hypertension)—Hypertension that develops in the absence of kidney disease. Its cause is unknown. About 85% to 90% of the cases of hypertension are in this category.

Eupnea (up-ne′ah)—Easy or normal respiration.

Excisional biopsy—Removal of an entire small lesion.

Excreta (ek-skre′tah)—Waste material excreted or eliminated from the body. Feces, urine, perspiration, and also mucus and carbon dioxide (CO_2) can be considered excreta.

Excrete—To eliminate useless matter, such as feces and urine.

Excretion (ek-skre′shun)—The elimination of waste materials from the body. Ordinarily, what is meant by excretion is the elimination of feces, but it can refer to the material eliminated from any part of the body.

Excruciating pain—Torturing, extreme pain, often intractable.

Exfoliative cytology—Microscopic examination of cells desquamated (shedding) from a body surface as a means of detecting malignant change.

Expectorate—The ejection of sputum and other materials from the air passages.

Exquisite pain—Intense pain to which an individual is extremely sensitive.

External auditory meatus (me-a′-tus)—The canal or passage leading from the outside opening of the ear to the eardrum. Also called the external acoustic meatus.

External ear—Includes the auricle, or pinna, and the external auditory meatus.

FDA—Food and Drug Administration (a federal government agency).

Febrile (feb′rile) pulse—A full, bounding pulse at the onset of a fever, becoming feeble and weak when the fever subsides.

Feces (fe′sez)—Body waste excreted from the intestine; also called stool, excreta, or excrement.

Fever—Pyrexia, or elevation of body temperature above normal, 98.6° F (Fahrenheit) or 37° C (centigrade or Celsius) registered orally. Some classify it as:

Low   99° to 101° F
             (37.2° to 38.3° C)
Moderate   101° to 103° F
             (38.3° to 39.5° C)
High   103° to 105° F
             (39.5° to 40.6° C)

- **Crisis**—Sudden drop of a high temperature to normal or below; generally occurs within 24 hours.
- **Intermittent fever**—Variations with alternate rises and falls, with the lowest often dropping below 98.6° F. An intermittent fever reaches the normal line at intervals during the course of an illness (e.g., a.m. 98° F, p.m. 101° F).
- **Onset**—Beginning of a fever.
- **Remittent fever**—Variations in temperature but always above 98.6° F (37° C), a persistent fever that has a day-time variation of 2° F (1.2° C) or more (e.g., a.m. 100° F, p.m. 103° F; a.m. 99° F, p.m. 102.4° F).

Fibrillation (fi″bri-la′shun)—A cardiac arrhythmia characterized by rapid, irregular, and ineffective electrical activity in the heart. Ventricular fibrillation is a common cause of cardiac arrest.

Fixation of a smear—Spraying with or immersing a slide into a special solution, or drying the slide over a flame, or air drying to harden and preserve the bacteria for future microscopic examination.

Flatulence (flat′u-lens)—Excessive formation of gases in the stomach or intestine.

Flatus (fla′tus)—Air or gas in the stomach or intestine.

Fluoroscope (floo′ro-skop″)—An instrument that is used during x-ray examinations for visual observation of the internal body structures by means of x-rays. The body part that is to be viewed is placed between the x-ray tube and a fluorescent screen. As x-rays pass through the body, shadowy images of the internal organs are projected on the screen.

Fluoroscopy (floo″or-os′ko-pe)—Visual examination by means of a fluoroscope.

Forced respiration—Voluntary hyperpnea.

Formicant (for′mi-kant′) pulse—A small, febble pulse.

Frequency—The need to urinate frequently.

Fungicide (fun′ji-sid)—A substance that destroys fungi.

Gastroscopy (gas ′tros′ ko-pi)—Internal inspection of the stomach with a gastroscope.

Gelatin culture—A culture of bacteria on gelatin.

Germicide (jer′mi-sid)—A substance that is capable of destroying pathogens.

Glucosuria (gloo″ko-su ′re-ah) or **glycosuria** (gli ″ko-su ′re-ah)—Abnormally high sugar content in urine.

Granulocyte (gran ′u-lo-sit ″)—A white blood cell (WBC) having granules in its cytoplasm. These types of WBCs are neutrophils, basophils, and eosinophils.

Guaiac (gwi ′ak) test—The preferred chemical test to determine the presence of occult blood in feces.

Guarding—A reflex usually related to abdominal pain; the action of muscles tensing, knees drawn up and/or hand placed over a part to prevent examination and/or protect against increasing pain.

Habituation—Emotional dependence on a drug due to repeated use, but without tendencies to increase the amount of the drug.

Hanging drop culture—A culture in which the bacteria are inoculated into a drop of fluid on a coverglass, and then mounted into the depression on a concave slide.

Health—The state of mental, physical, and social well-being of an individual, and not merely the absence of disease.

Hematuria (hem″ah-tu″re-ah)—The presence of blood in urine.

Hemoglobin (he″mo-glo′bin)—A protein in a red blood cell that carries oxygen and carbon dioxide. The pigment in hemoglobin is what gives the blood its red color. The protein in hemoglobin is globin; the red pigment is heme. For the body to make hemoglobin, it must have iron, which is derived from the food we eat.

Hemolysis (he-mol ′i-sis)—The destruction of red blood cells with the release of hemoglobin into the plasma.

Hemoptysis (he-mop′-ti-sis)—Coughing up blood as a result of bleeding from any part of the respiratory tract. The appearance of the secretion in true hemoptysis is bright red and frothy with air bubbles.

HHS—Health and Human Services (a federal government agency).

Histology (his-tol ′ o-je)—The study of the microscopic form and structure of tissue.

Hyperbilirubinemia (hi″per-bil″i-roo″bi-ne′me-ah)—Increased or excessive levels of bilirubin in the blood.

Hypercalcemia (hi″per-kal-se′me-ah)—Increased or excessive levels of calcium in the blood.

Hypercholesterolemia (hi′per-ko-les″ter-ol-e′ me-ah)—Excessive levels of cholesterol in the blood.

Hyperchromia (hi′per-kro′me-ah)—An abnormal increase of the hemoglobin levels in red blood cells.

Hypercythemia (hy′ per-si-the′me-ah)—An excessive number of red blood cells in the circulating blood.

Hyperemia (hi′per-e′me-ah)—An excessive amount of blood in a part.

Hyperglycemia (hi″per-gli-se′me-ah)—Excessive amounts of glucose in the blood.

Hyperkalemia (hi″per-kah-le′me-ah)—An excessive level of potassium in the blood.

Hypernatremia (hi′per-na-tre′me-ah)—An excessive amount of sodium in the blood.

Hyperoxemia (hi″per-ok-se′me-ah)—A condition in which the blood is excessively acidic.

Hyperpnea (hy″perp-ne′ah)—Increase in rate and depth of breathing.

Hyperproteinemia (hi″per-pro″te-i-ne′me-ah)—An excessive amount of protein the blood.

Hypertension (hi′per-ten ′shun)—High blood pressure; a condition in which patient has higher blood pressure than normal for his or her age; (e.g., systolic pressure consistently above 160 mm Hg and a diastolic pressure above 90 mm Hg).

Hyperventilation—Increase of air in the lungs above the normal amount; abnormally prolonged and deep breathing, usually associated with acute anxiety or emotional tensions.

Hypo (hi′po)—A word part meaning an abnormal decrease or deficient amounts. If you replace this word element and definition for the word element "hyper" in all of the preceding terms (except in hyperemia and hyperoxemia), the correct meaning will be defined.

Hypotension (hi′po-ten′shun)—A decrease of systolic and diastolic blood pressure to below normal; for example, below 90/50 is considered low blood pressure.

Hypothermia (hi′po-ther′me-ah)—Low body temperature.

Hypoxemia (hi′ pok-se ′ me-ah)—A deficient amount of oxygen (O_2 in the blood.

Hypoxia (hi-pok′se-ah)—Reduced amounts of oxygen to the body tissues.

Immunization (im″u-ni-za′shun)—The process of rendering a person immune (protected from or not susceptible to a disease) or of becoming immune; frequently called vaccination or inoculation. A process by which a person is artifically prepared to resist infection by a specific pathogen.

Immunosuppressive agents—Drugs that inhibit the formation of antibodies to antigens that may be present.

Incisional biopsy—Incision into and removal of part of a lesion.

Incontinence (in-kon′ti-nens)—The inability to refrain from the urge to urinate. This may occur in times of stress, anxiety, anger, postoperatively, or from obstructions that prevent the normal emptying of the urinary bladder, spasms of the bladder, irritation caused by injury or inflammation of the urinary tract, damage to the spinal cord or brain, or from the development of a fistula (an abnormal tube-like passage) between the bladder and the vagina or urethra.

Incubation (in″ku-ba′shun) period—The interval of time between the invasion of a pathogen into the body and the appearance of the first symptoms of disease.

Incubation (in″ku-ba′shun)—When pertaining to bacteriology, this term refers to the period of culture development.

Induration (in″du-ra′shun)—An abnormally hard spot; a process of hardening.

Infection (in-fek′shun)—A condition caused by the multiplication of pathogenic microorganisms that have invaded the body of a susceptible host.
- **Acute**—rapid onset, severe symptoms, and usually subsides within a relatively short period of time.
- **Chronic**—Develops slowly, milder symptoms; lasts for a long period of time.
- **Latent**—Dormant or concealed; pathogen is everpresent in the host, but symptoms are present only intermittently, often in response to a stimulus. At other times the pathogen is dormant.
- **Localized**—retricted to a certain area.
- **Generalized**—systemic; involving the whole body.

Infectious mononucleosis—Also called glandular fever, it is an acute infectious disease, caused by the Epstein-Barr virus.

Inoculate (i-nok″u-lat)—In microbiology, this refers to introducing infectious matter into a culture medium in an effort to produce growth of the causative organism.

Insufflator (in′suf-fla-tor)—An instrument, device, or bag used for blowing air, powder, or gas into a cavity.

Intermittent pulse—A pulse in which occasional beats are skipped.

Intractable—Unmanageable, not controllable with conventional means, that is, rest, heat, medication.

Ionizing (i″on-i-zing)—Radiant energy given off by radioactive atoms and x-rays.

irradiate (i-ra″de-at)—To treat with radiant energy.

Irradiation (i-ra″de-a′shun)—Exposure to radiation; the passage of penetrating rays through a substance or object.

Irregular pulse—A pulse with variation in force and frequency; an excess of tea, coffee, tobacco, or exercise may cause this.

Ischemia (is-ke′me-ah)—A deficient amount of blood in a body part due to an obstruction or a functional constriction of a blood vessel.

Isocytosis (i″so-si-to′sis)—A state in which cells are equal in size, especially equality of size of red blood cells.

Labored breathing—Dyspnea or difficult breathing; respiration that involves active participation of accessory inspiratory and expiratory muscles.

Laryngeal (lar-in′je-al) **mirror**—An instrument used to view the pharynx and larynx consisting of a small rounded mirror attached to the end of a slender (metal or chrome plate) handle.

Laryngoscope (lar-in′go-skop)—An endoscope used to examine the larynx. It is equipped with mirrors and a light for illumination of the larynx.

Leukemia (lu-ke′me-ah)—A malignant disease of various types that is classified clinically as acute or chronic, depending on the character and duration of the disease; myeloid, lymphoid, or monocytic, depending on the cells involved. This disease affects the tissues of the lymph nodes, spleen, and/or bone marrow. Symptoms include an uncontrolled increase of white blood cells, accompanied by a decrease in red blood cells and platelets. This results in anemia and an increased tendency to infection and hemorrhage. Other classical symptoms include pain in bones and joints, fever, and swelling of the liver, spleen, and lymph nodes. The precise cause is unknown.

Leukocytosis (lu″ko-si-to′sis)—An increased number of circulating white blood cells.

Leukopenia (lu″ko-pe′ne-ah)—A deficient number of circulating white blood cells.

Lienteric stool—Feces containing much undigested food.

Ligate (li′gat)—To apply a ligature.

Ligature (lig′ ah-tur)—A suture; material used to tie off blood vessels to prevent bleeding, or to constrict tissues.

Light therapy or phototherapy (fo′ to-ther′ah-pe)—The use of light rays in the treatment of disease processes. By custom, this includes the use of ultraviolet and infrared or heat rays (radiation).

Lysis—Gradual decline of a fever.

Macrocyte (mak′ro-sit)—The largest type of red blood cell; seen in cases of pernicious anemia (vitamin B_{12} deficiency) and folic acid deficiency.

Macroscopic (mak-ro-skop′ ik) **examination**—An examination in which the specimen is large enough to be seen by the naked eye.

Malignant (mah-lig′nant) **hypertension**—Hypertension that differs from other types in that it is a rapidly developing hypertension and may prove fatal if not treated immediately after symptoms develop, before damage is done to the blood vessels. This type occurs most often in persons in their twenties or thirties.

Mayo stand (mo′o)—A stand with a flat metal tray used to hold sterile supplies during an aseptic procedure.

Medical microbiology—The study and identification of pathogens, and the development of effective methods for their control or elimination.

Melena (me-le′nah)—Darkening of stool by blood pigments.

Microcyte (mik′kro-sit)—An abnormally small red blood cell, found in cases of iron deficient anemia and thalassemia.

Microorganism (mi-kro-or′gan-ism)—A minute living body not perceptible to the naked eye, especially a bacterium or protozoon; these are viewed with a microscope.

Microscopic (mi-kro-skop′ik) **examination**—An examination in which the specimen is visible only with the aid of a microscope.

Miotic (mi-ot′ik)—A medication that causes the pupil of the eye to contract.

Modality (mo-dal′i-te)—Therapeutic agents used in physical medicine and physical therapy.

Mononucleosis (mon″o-nu″kle-o′sis)—An abnormal increase of the mononuclear white blood cells in the blood.

Mydriatic (mid″re-at′k)—A medication that causes the pupil of the eye to dilate.

Myocardial infarction (MI) (mi″o-kar ′de-al in-fark ′shun)—The formation of ischemic necrosis in the heart muscle due to an interference of blood supply to the area.

Myocardium (mi″o-kar′de-um)—The heart muscle.

Nasal speculum (na′zl spek′u-lum)—A short, funnel-like instrument used to examine the nasal cavity.

necrosis (ne-kro′-sis)—The death of a cell or a group of cells because of injury or disease.

Negative culture—A culture made from suspected material that fails to reveal the suspected microorganism.

Normal flora—Microorganisms that normally reside in various body locations such as in the vagina, intestine, urethra, upper respiratory tract, and on the skin. These microorganisms are nonpathogenic and do not cause any harm (they may become pathogenic and cause harm if they are introduced into a body area in which they do not normally reside).

Objective symptom—A symptom that is apparent to the observer; also called a sign, for example, rash, swelling.

Obstipation (ob′sti-pa′shun)—Extreme constipation caused by an obstruction.

Occult blood—Obscure or hidden from view.

Occult blood test—A microscopic or a chemical test performed on a specimen to determine the presence of blood not otherwise detectable. Stool is tested when intestinal bleeding is suspected, but there is no visible evidence of blood in the stool.

Ocular (ok′u-lar)—Pertaining to the eye.

Oliguria (o″i-gu′ re-ah)—Scanty amounts of urine.

Ophthalmic (of-thal′mik)—Pertaining to the eye.

Ophthalmology (of″thal-mol′o-je)—The study and science of the eye and its diseases.

Ophthalmoscope (of-thal′mo-skop)—An instrument used for examining the interior parts of the eye. It contains a perforated mirror and lens. When the ophthalmoscope is turned on and brought close to the eye, it sends a narrow, bright beam of light through the lens of the eye. By looking through the lens of the instrument, the physician is then able to examine the interior parts of the eye, including the lens, anterior chamber, rentinal structures, and blood vessels, to detect any possible disorders. Many ophthalmoscopes come with an interchangeable otoscope, throat illuminator head, or nasal illuminator head.

Oral examination—Examination pertaining to the mouth.

Orthopnea (or″thop-ne′ah)—Severe dyspnea in which breathing is possible only when the patient sits or stands in an erect positon.

Orthostatic (or″tho-stat′ik) hypotension—Hypotension occurring when a patient assumes an erect position.

Oscilloscope (o-sil′o-skop)—An instrument for visualizing the shape or wave form of sound waves, as in ultrasonography; or of electric currents, as when monitoring heart action and other body functions.

Otic (o′ tik)—Pertaining to the ear.

Otology (o-tol′o-je)—The study and science of the ear and its diseases.

Otoscope (o′to-skop)—An instrument used for visual examination of the external ear canal and eardrum.

Pacemaker (pas′mak-er)—The pacemaker of the heart is the sinoatrial node located in the right atrium.

Papanicolaou smear or test (pap″ah-nik″o-la ′oo)—A smear examined microscopically to detect cancer cells from body excretions (urine and feces), secretions (vaginal fluids, sputum or prostatic fluid), or tissue scrapings (as obtained from the stomach or uterus); most commonly done on a cervical scraping to detect abnormal or cancerous cells in the mucus of the uterus and cervix. This test is often referred to as a Pap smear or test.

Parasite (par′ah-sit)—An organism that lives on or in another organism, known as the host, from which it gains its nourishment (e;g;, fungi, bacteria, and single-celled, and multi-celled animals).

Pathogen (path′o-jen)—A disease-producing substance or microorganism.

Pathogenic (path′o-jen′ic)—Pertaining to a disease-producing microorganism or substance.

- **Pathogenic microorganism**—One that produces disease in the body.
- **PDR**—*Physician's Desk Reference,* a book on drugs.

Pelvic examination—Examination of the external and internal female reproductive organs.

Percussion (per-kush ′un) hammer—A small hammer with a triangular-shaped rubber head used for percussion.

Pericarditis (per″i-kar-di′tis)—Inflammation of the pericardium, the fibroserous sac enveloping the heart.

Phagocytosis (fag″o-si-to′sis)—The process by which white blood cells destroy and engulf or ingest harmful microorganisms.

Physical signs—Objective manifestations of disease that are apparent on a physical examination; observable changes representing alterations resulting from a disease or dysfunction in the body (see also sign).

Placebo (plah-se′bo)—An inactive substance resembling and given in place of a medication for its psychologic effects to satisfy the patient's need for the drug; it hopefully will produce the same effect as the real medication through psychological means. A placebo may be used experimentally.

Poikilocytosis (poi″ki-lo-si-to′sis)—The presence of red blood cells in the blood that show abnormal variations in their shape.

Polycythemia (pol″e-si-the′me-ah)—An abnormal increased amount of red blood cells or hemoglobin.

Polyuria (pol″e-u′re′ah)—Excessive excretion of urine.

Positive culture—A culture that reveals the suspected microorganism.

Positive findings—Evidence of disease or body dysfunction.

Postoperative (post-op′er-ah-tiv)—Pertaining to the period of time following surgery.

Postural hypotension—Hypotension occurring upon suddenly arising from a recumbent position or when standing still for a long period of time.

Preoperative (pre-op′er-ah-tiv)—Pertaining to the time preceding surgery.

Proctoscope (prok′to-skop)—A specially designed tubular endoscope that is passed through the anus to permit internal inspection of the lower part of the large intestine.

Prodrome—An early symptom, indicating the onset of a disease, such as an achy feeling before having the flu.

Prognosis—A statement made by the physician indicating the probable or anticipated outcome of the disease process in a patient; usually stated simply as *good, fair, poor,* or *guarded.*

Prophylaxis (pro″fi-lak ′sis)—Prevention of disease.

Proteinura (pro″te-in-u′re-ah)—An abnormal increase of protein in urine.

Psoriasis (so-ri′ah-sis)—A chronic inflammatory recurrent skin disease characterized by scaly red patches on the body surfaces. The lesions are seen most often on knees, elbows, scalp, and fingernails. Other areas frequently affected are the chest, abdomen, palms of the hands, soles of the feet, and backs of the arms and legs. The cause is unknown, although a hereditary factor is suggested.

Pulse deficit—The apical rate is greater than the radial pulse rate.

Pulse pressure—The difference between the systolic and the diastolic blood pressure.

EXAMPLE: IF BP is 120/80,

$$120 = \text{systolic pressure}$$
$$\underline{- 80} = \text{diastolic pressure}$$
$$40 = \text{pulse pressure}$$

A pulse pressure consistently over 50 points or under 30 points is considered abnormal.

Pure culture—A culture of a single microorganism.

Pure drug—A refined drug; one that has been processed to remove all impurities.

Pyuria (pi-u′re-ah)—The presence of pus in the urine.

Qualitative tests—Used for screening purposes. These tests provide an indication as to whether or not a substance is present in a specimen in abnormal quantities. A qualitative test does not determine the exact amount of a substance present in a specimen. Color charts are usually used to interpret qualitative tests. Sometimes they are called semi-quantitative tests. Results are reported in terms such as trace, small amount, moderate, large amount, or 1+, 2+, 3+ or simply as positive or negative.

Quantitative tests—More precise tests. They determine accurately the amount of a specific substance that is present in a specimen. A high level of skill is required to perform these tests on sophisticated equipment. Results are reported in units such as grams (g) per 100 milliliters (ml), or milligrams (mg) percent, or milligrams per deciliter (dl).

Radiating—Diverting from a common central point; for example, gallbladder pain begins in the right upper quadrant of the abdomen, and it is diverted from that central point to the right flank and right scapular area.

Radiation (ra″de-a′shun)—Electro-magnetic waves of streams of atomic particles capable of penetrating and being absorbed into matter. Examples of electromagnetic waves are x-rays, gamma rays, ultraviolet rays, infrared rays, and rays of visible light. Atomic particles are alpha and beta particles.

Radiogram (ra′de-o-gram″)—A picture of internal body structures produced by the action of gamma rays or x-rays on a special film.

Radiograph (ra′de-o-graf″) or roentgenograph (rent′gen-o-graf) or roentgenogram (rent′gen-o-gram″)—The film or photographic record produced by radiography.

Radiography (ra″de-og′rah-fe)—The taking of radiograms.

Radioisotope (ra″de-o-i′so-top)—A radioactive form of an element consisting of unstable atoms that emit rays of energy or streams of atomic particles. Radioisotopes occur naturally, as in the case of radium, or can be created artificially, as in the case of cobalt.

Radiologist (ra″de-ol′o-jist)—A physician specialist in the study of radiology.

Radiolucent (ra″de-o-lu-sent)—That which permits the partial or complete passage of radiant energy such as x-rays. Dense objects appear white on the x-ray film because they absorb the radiation. An example of this is bone.

Radionuclide (ra″de-o-nu′klid)—A radioactive substance.

Radiopaque (ra-do-o-pak′)—That which is impenetrable by x-rays and other forms of radiant energy; matter that obstructs the passage of radiant energy, such as lead which is frequently used as a protective device.

Rales (rahls)—An abnormal bubbling sound heard on auscultation of the chest; often classified as either moist or crackling and dry.

Rebound tenderness—A sensation of pain felt when pressure applied on a body part is released.

Regular pulse—The rhythm of the pulse rate is regular.

Renal hypertension—Hypertension resulting from kidney disease.

Reservoir (rez′er-vwrar)—The source in which pathogenic microorganisms grow and from which they leave to spread and cause disease.

Resistance (re-zis′tans)—The ability of the body to resist disease or infection because of its own defense mechanisms.

Reticulocyte (re-tik′u-lo-sit)—A nonnucleated immature red blood cell. Generally, of all the red blood cells in the circulating blood, less than 2% are reticulocytes.

Rhythm strip—A rhythm strip is an EKG recording of a single lead that is used to determine the rhythm of the heartbeat such as a fast, slow, regular, or irregular rhythm, and certain types of ventricular fibrillation. It is also used to determine if the patient is in any type of heart block, such as third-degree heart block. The rhythm strip gives a one-dimensional picture of the beating of the heart which determines only the rhythm of the heartbeat in contrast to the 12-lead EKG, which can slow damage to the heart and other conditions. Data from the rhythm strip can be a useful "screening" tool because frequent runs of arrhythmias can be more easily observed. The rhythm strip can also be used to confirm the basic assessment made on the 12-lead EKG. Currently for the rhythm strip most practitioners will record lead V1, and possibly Leads V2 and V5, although one could record any lead that is desired. Rhythm strips are frequently recorded from a continuous cardiac monitor in intensive care units in the hospital and by paramedics when they are in the field in emergency situations.

Roentgenologic (rent-gen-ol′oj-ik)—Pertaining to an examination with the use of x-ray film (radiographs).

Saliva (sah-li′vah)—The enzyme-containing secretion of the salivary glands in the mouth.

Secondary hypertension—Hypertension that is traceable to known causes such as a pheochromocytoma (tumor of the adrenal gland), hardening of the arteries, kidney disease, or obstructions to kidney blood flow. Approximately 10% to 15% of the cases of hypertension are secondary. Patients with secondary hypertension can often be cured if the underlying cause can be eliminated.

Sepsis (sep′sis)—A morbid state or condition resulting from the presence of pathogenic microorganisms.

Septicemia (sep″ti-se′me-ah)—A condition in which there are bacteria or toxins in the blood.

Serologic (se-ro-loj′ik) test—A laboratory test involving the examination and study of blood serum.

Serum (se′rum)—The clear, straw-colored liquid portion obtained after blood clots; it consists of plasma minus fibrinogen, which is removed in the process of clotting.

Side effect—A response in addition to that for which the drug was used, especially an undesirable result.
  • **Untoward effect**—An undesirable side effect.

Sigmoidoscope (sig-moy′do-skop)—A tubular endoscope used to examine the interior of the sigmoid colon.

Sign—Sometimes called a physical sign; any objective evidence (apparent to the observer) representing disease or body dysfunction. Signs may be observed by others or revealed when the physician performs a physical examination; examples include swollen ankles, a distended rigid abdomen, elevated blood pressure, and decreased sensation.

Sims vaginal speculum—A form of bivalve speculum used in the examination of the vagina and cervix.

Slow pulse—A pulse between 40 and 60 beats per minute, often found among the elderly and among athletes at rest.

Smear (smer)—Material spread thinly across a slide or culture medium with a swab, loop, or another slide in preparation for microscopic study.

Smear culture—A culture prepared by smearing the specimen across the surface of the culture medium.

Specimen (spec'i-men)—A small part or sample taken to show kind and quality of the whole, as a specimen of urine, blood, or other body excretions, or a small piece of tissue for macroscopic and microscopic examination.

Speculum (spek'u-lum)—An instrument used for distending or opening a body cavity or orifice to allow visual inspection; a bivalve speculum is one having two parts or valves.

Spore (spor)—A reproductive cell, usually unicellular, produced by plants and some protozoa, and possessing thick walls to withstand unfavorable environmental conditions. Bacterial spores are resistant to heat and must undergo a prolonged exposure to extremely high temperatures to be destroyed.

Sprain (spran)—A joint injury in which some fibers of a supporting ligament are ruptured, but continuity of the ligament remains intact. There may also be damage to the associated muscles, tendons, nerves, and blood vessels.

Sputum (spu'-tum)—A mucous secretion from the trachea, bronchi, and lungs, ejected through the mouth, in contrast to saliva, which is the secretion of the salivary glands.

Stab culture—A bacterial culture made by thrusting a needle inoculated with the microorganisms under examination deep into the culture medium.

Stabbing pain—Deep, sharp, intermittent pain.

Sterile (ster'il)—Free from all microorganisms.

Sterile field—A work area prepared with sterile drapes (coverings) to hold sterile supplies during a sterile procedure.

Sterile setup—Specific sterile supplies used in a specific sterile procedure.

Stertorous (ste'to-rus) respirations—Characterized by a deep snoring sound with each inspiration.

Stethoscope—An instrument used in auscultation to amplify the sounds produced by the lungs, heart, intestines, and other internal organs; also used when taking a blood pressure reading.

Stock supply—A large supply of medications kept in the physician's office or pharmacy.

Stool (stool)—Body waste material discharged from the large intestine; synonym: feces, bowel movement.

Strain (stran)—An overexertion or overstretching of some part of a muscle.

Streak culture—A bacterial culture in which the infectious material is implanted in streaks across the culture media.

Subjective symptoms—Symptoms of internal origin that are apparent or perceptible only to the patient; examples include pain, dizziness (vertigo).

Suture (soo'cher)—Various types and sizes of absorbable and nonabsorbable materials used to close a wound with stitches.

Swab (swob)—A small piece of cotton or gauze wrapped around the end of a slender stick used for applying medications, cleansing cavities, or obtaining a piece of tissue or body secretion for bacteriological examination; synonym: cotton-tipped applicator.

Symmetry (sim'et-ri)—Correspondence in form, size, and arrangement of parts on opposite sides of the body.

Symptom—Any subjective evidence of disease or body dysfunction; a change in the physical or mental state of the body that is perceptible or apparent only to the individual; examples include anorexia, nausea, headache, pain, itching.

Syndrome—A combination of symptoms resulting from one cause or commonly occurring together to present a distinct clinical picture; an example is the dumping syndrome, which consists of nausea, weakness, varying degrees of syncope, sweating, palpitation, and sometimes diarrhea and a feeling of warmth. This may occur immediatley after eating in patients who have had a partial gastrectomy.

Tachycardia (tak"y-kar 'di-a)—A pulse of 170 or more beats per minute; abnormal rapidity of heart action.

Tendinitis (ten'di-ni ' tis)—Inflammation of a tendon; one of the most common causes of acute pain the shoulder.

Thready pulse—A pulse that is very fine and scarely perceptible, as seen in syncope (fainting).

Threshold—The level that must be exceeded for an effect to be produced; the level of pain that an individual can tolerate without external intervention. Threshold is unique to each individual, and the overall physiopsychologic makeup of an individual must be considered when evaluating pain.

Thrombocyte (throm' bo-sit)—A blood platelet.

Thrombocythemia (throm"bo-si-the'me-ah)—An increased number of platelets in the circulating blood.

Thrombocytopenia (throm"bo-si'to-pe 'ne-ah)—A decreased number of platelets in the circulating blood.

Tissue culture—The growing of tissue cells in artifical nutrient media.

Tongue blade—A flat, thin, smooth piece of wood or metal with rounded ends approximately 6 inches long; also called a tongue depressor. It is used for pressing tissue down to permit a better view when examining the mouth and throat. In addition, it may be used for application of ointments to the skin.

Tonometer (ton-nom'e-ter)—An instrument used to measure tension or pressure, especially intraocular pressure.

Tourniquet (toor'ni-ket)—A constricting device used to compress an artery or vein to stop excessive bleeding or to prevent the spread of snake venom.

Toxicity (tok-sis' i-te)—The nature of exerting harmful effects on a tissue or organism. The level at which a drug becomes toxic to the body. Minor or major damage may result.

Toxin (tok'sin)—A poisonous substance produced by pathogenic bacteria and some animals and plants. The toxins produced by bacteria include toxic enzymes, exotoxins, and endotoxins. Toxins in the body cause antitoxins to form, which provide a means for establishing immunity to certain diseases.

Transfer forceps—A type of instrument (forcep) that is kept in a chemical disinfectant or germicide and used for transferring or handling sterile supplies and equipment.

Transient—Fleeting, brief, passing, coming and going.

Tuning fork—A steel, two-pronged, forklike instrument used for testing hearing; the prongs give off a musical note when struck.

Tympanic (tim-pan ′ik) **membrane (TM)**—The eardrum; it serves as the membrane that separates the external auditory meatus from the middle ear cavity.

Type culture—A culture that is generally agreed to represent microorganisms of a particular species.

Unequal pulse—A pulse in which some beats are strong and others are weak; pulse in which rates are different in symmetrical arteries.

Unit-dose—A system that supplies prepackaged, premeasured, prelabeled, individual portions of a medication for patient use.

Uremia (u-re′me-ah)—A toxic condition in which there are substances in the blood that should normally be eliminated in the urine.

Urgency—The need to urinate immediately.

Urination (u″ri-na′shun), voiding, micturition (mik″tu-rish ′un)—The act of passing urine from the body.

Urine (u′rine)—The fluid containing certain waste products and water that is secreted by the kidneys, stored in the bladder, and excreted through the urethra.

Urobilinogen—A colorless compound formed in the intestines by the reduction of bilirubin.

USP-NF—United States Pharmacopeia-National Formulary, a drug book listing all official drugs authorized for use in the United States.

Vaccination (vak″si-na′shun)—The introduction of weakened or dead microorganisms (inoculation) into the body to stimulate the production of antibodies and immunity to a specific disease.

Venipuncture (ven″i-pungk′tur)—Puncturing a vein to collect a blood specimen or to administer a medication.

Venous pulse—A pulse in a vein, especially one of the large veins near the heart such as the internal and external jugular. Venous pulse is undulating and scarcely palpable.

Ventricle (ven′tri-kl)—One of the lower chambers of the heart. The right ventricle receives deoxygenated blood from the right atrium and pumps this blood through the pulmonary arteries to the lungs; the left ventricle receives oxygenated blood from the left atrium and pumps this blood out through the aorta to all body tissues.

Vesicle (ves′i-kl)—A circular, blisterlike elevation on the skin containing fluid.

Viable (vi′ah-bl)—Able to maintain an independent existence.

Virulence (vir′u-lens)—The degree of ability of a pathogen to produce disease.

Vitamin K—A vitamin that is essential for the formation of prothrombin and the normal clotting of blood. A deficiency may result in hemorrhage because of a prolonged prothrombin time.

Voltage (vol-tij)—The electromotive force measured in volts (the units of force for electricity to flow).

Wheal (hwel)—A temporary, more or less round, elevation on the skin that is white in the center and often accompanied by itching.

Index

A

Abbreviations
  medical, 66-69, 262-263
  prescription, 259
ABCs; *see* Airway; Breathing; Circulation
Abdomen
  abbreviations related to, 67, 262
  examination of, during pregnancy, 131
  terms related to, 66
Abdominal cavity, 580
  quadrants of, 581, 582
Abdominal pain, first aid for, 556
Abdominal pulse, 31
Abdominal respiration, 33
Abdominal thrusts, 552-553
Abduction, 510
ABO blood groups, 462
ABO system, 452
Abrasion, 223, 226
  first aid for, 569
  identification of, 630
Abscess, 204
  incision and drainage of, materials for, 220
Absorbable sutures, 210
AC; *see* Alternating current
Accelerated respirations, 33
Accommodation of eye, 629
Accucheck III system, use of, 439-442
AccuMeter Cholesterol Test, 447-449
Ace bandage, 233
Acetabulum, 587, 588
Acetest, 394, 395
Acetone in urine, tests for, 391, 394
Acetonuria, 381, 391
Acid, ingestion of, first aid for, 570;
    see also specific acid
Acquired immune deficiency syndrome,
    2, 368; *see also* HIV disease
  broadened definition of, 13-14
  employees with, 12
  body fluids from patient with, mucous
      membrane or conjunctival
      exposure to, 11-12
  other diseases in, 12
Acquired immunity, 174, 176
Acromioclavicular joints, 587
Activated charcoal, poisoning and, 570
Active immunity, 174
Acuity, visual; *see* Visual acuity
Acute infection, 170
Addiction, 249
Additive interactions of drugs, 272
Adduction, 510
Adenoidectomy, 612
Adenoids, respiration and, 612
Adhesive skin closures, 211-212
Adhesive tape, 232
Administered medication, 258
Adnexa, bimanual palpation of, 105
Adolescents, examinations for, 135
Adrenal cortex, 622
Adrenal glands, endocrine system and, 622
Adrenal medulla, 622
Adrenalin; *see* Epinephrine
Adson dressing forceps, 213
Adult onset diabetes, 568-569
Adulteration, 249
Aerobe, 338
Aerobic, 338

Aerosol, 2, 261
Afferent fibers, 599
Age and drug dosage and action, 271
AggBand-form granulocyte, 416
Agglutination, 416
Agranulocyte, 416
AIDS; *see* Acquired immune deficiency
        syndrome
AIDS antibody test, 15
Air conduction test of hearing, 119
Air hunger, hyperventilation and, 568
Air sacs, 612
Airway
  in allergic reaction to drugs, 556
  in cardiopulmonary resuscitation, 549-550
      for infants and small children, 551
  obstructed, management of, 552-553
Albuminuria, 381, 391
Albustix test, 389
Albuterol, 261
Alcohol, 653
Alimentary canal, 605
Alkali, ingestion of, first aid for, 570
Allergens, 299, 300
Allergic reactions
  to drugs, 556
  to local anesthetics, 207
Allergic shock, 555
Allergies, 299-305
  diagnosis and treatment of, 299-300
  drug, 272
  to latex gloves, 7
  patch test to diagnose, 300-301
  scratch test to diagnose, 300, 302-303
  signs and symptoms of, 299
  testing for, sterile syringes for, 283
Allergy tests, diagnostic, and intradermal skin
        tests, 299-309
Allis clamp, 219
Allis tissue forceps, 213
Alpha cells, 609
Alpha-fetoprotein blood test for pregnant
        woman, 133
Alternating current (AC), 532
Alternating current interference, electrocardio-
        gram and, 531, 532
Alternating pulse, 31
Alveoli, 612
AMA; *see* American Medical Association
Ambu bag, 13
Ambulatory cardiac monitoring, 538-543
American Association of Poison Control
        Centers, 571
American Heart Association, 549, 640
American Hospital Formulary Service, 251
American Medical Association, 249
  Drug Evaluations, 250
American Red Cross, 558, 571
Ames Seralyzer Blood Chemistry Analyzer, 437
Amino acids, 636
Amniocentesis, 133-134
Amphetamines, 253, 572-573
Amplify, definition of, 525
Ampule, 278
Amputation, first aid and, 560
Amubulatory cardiac monitoring, electrocar-
        diography and, 538-543
Anaerobic Culturette culture collection
        system, 339

Analgesic, 253
Anaphylactic reaction to drugs, 556
Anaphylactic shock, 249, 555
Anaphylaxis, 300
Anatomic selection of injection sites, 278-283
Anatomy, 578
  and physiology, 577-633
Anemia, 416, 594
  in pregnancy, 131
  screening for, and copper sulfate, 434
Aneroid manometer, 39
Anesthesia, 204
  local, 207
      materials for administering, 219-220
  for minor surgery, 207
Anesthetic, 254
  local, allergic reaction to, 207
Angina pectoris, 595
Angiocardiogram, 473
Angiogram, 473
Angioma, identification of, 630
Angiotensin-converting enzyme inhibitors, 253
Animal bites, first aid for, 556-557
Animal reservoirs for disease, 172
Animal Ultralente insulin, 291
Animals, skeletons of, 582
Anisocytosis, 416
Ankle joint, 588
  and foot, bandage-wrapping techniques for,
      235
Ankle mortise, 588
Anoscope, 82
  Hirschman, 78
Antacid, 253
Antagonistic interactions of drugs, 272
Anthelmintics, 253
Antianginal drug, 253
Antianxiety agents, 572-573
Antiarrhythmic agent, 253
Antiarthritic preparation, 254
Antibiotic, 253
Antibody test
  HIV or AIDS, 15
  p24, 14
Anticholinergic agents, 572-573
Anticoagulant, 253
Anticonvulsant, 253
Antidepressant, 253
Antidiabetic agents, 253
Antidiarrheal agent, 253
Antidote, 254, 548
  universal, poisoning and, 571
Antidote labels, poisoning and, 570
Antiemetic, 254
Antifungal agent, 254
Antigen test, p24, 14
Antigen-antibody reaction, 174
Antihistamine, 254
Antihypertensive, 254
Antiinflammatory agent, 254
Antineoplastic agent, 254
Antiseptic agents, 170, 254
  for sterilization, 198
Antitoxins, 176
Antitussive, 254
Ants, bites from, first aid for, 557
Anuria, 381, 384
Anus, 605, 609
Aorta, 594

Aortic valve, 595
Apical pulse, 29
Aplastic anemia, 594
Apnea, 33
Apocrine glands, 629
Apothecary equivalents, 269, 270
Appendicular skeleton, anatomy and physiology of, 582, 585, 587-588
Appendix, 605, 609
Applanation tonometry, 126
Applicator, 82
Aprons as protective equipment, 8-9
Aqueous humor, 625
Arachnoid, 599
Arches, fallen, 588
Arm
   anatomy and physiology of, 587
   of microscope, 331
   Tubegauz bandaging of, 239
Arrector pili, 629
Arrhythmia, 31, 525, 527
   electrocardiogram and, 530-531
Arterial bleeding, 557
Arterial wall, condition of, 29
Arteries, 594-595
   determining pulse rate at, 32
   walls of, elasticity of, blood pressure and, 36
Arteriogram, 473
Arterioles, 594
Arteriosclerosis, 595
Arthritis, 496
Arthrogram, 473
Artifacts, electrocardiogram and, 531-532
Artificial active immunity, 174
Artificial passive immunity, 176
Artificial respiration, 33
Ascending colon, 609
Asepsis, 170, 204
   medical, 168-201
   surgical, 184, 186
      and minor surgery, 202-246
      principles and practices of, 203-204
Aseptic technique; *see* Surgical asepsis
Asphyxia, first aid for, 556
Aspiration, fine-needle, 204
Aspiration/needle biopsy, 204
   of breast, materials for, 222
Assessment in POMR, 63
Astigmatism, 120
Astringent, 254
Asymptomatic HIV disease, 13
Ataractics, 256
Atherosclerosis, 595
   increased levels of serum cholesterol and, 642
ATI Instrument Protectors for sterilization, 188, 190
ATI Steriline bags for sterilization, 188, 190
Atopy, 300
Atrial arrhythmia, electrocardiogram and, 530
Atrial fibrillation, 29
   electrocardiogram and, 530
Atrial rate, electrocardiogram and, 529
Atrial rhythm, electrocardiogram and, 529
Atrial tachycardia, paroxysmal, electrocardiogram and, 530
Atrioventricular bundle, 528
Atrioventricular node, 528
Atrium, 525, 526, 527, 595
Atrophy, identification of, 630
Atropine, sinus tachycardia and, 529
Attenuated vaccines, 174
Audiometer, hearing examination using, 119
Auditory meatus, external, 312

Augmented leads, electrocardiogram and, 532-533, 537
Auricle, 312, 526
Auscultation in physical examination, 60
Auscultation method of measuring blood pressure, 40-41
Auscultatory gap, 41
Authorized personnel to fill out medical records, 64
Autoclave, 190-193
Autoclave indicator tape, 193, 194
Autoclaving, 188-197
Automatic electrocardiographs, electrocardiography and, 538
Automation in clinical laboratory, 452-467
Automobiles, first aid kit for, 571
Autonomic nervous system, 603-605
   heartbeat and, 528
AV node; *see* Atrioventricular node\par
Avulsion, 223, 226
   first aid for, 569
Axial skeleton, anatomy and physiology of, 582, 585, 586-587
Axillary temperature, procedure for taking, 25
Axillary temperature readings, contraindications to, 22
AZT; *see* Zidovudine

B

Bacillus(bacilli), 223
   causing disease, 171
Back, fractured, first aid for, 567
Back blows in management of obstructed airway in children, 553
Backbone, 586
Backhaus towel clamps, 213
Bacteria, 171
   life cycle of, sterilization and, 189
   in urine, 403
Bacterial culture and sensitivity testing, 363
Bactericidal agents for sterilization, 198
Bactericide, 170
Bacteriology, 323, 338
Bacteriology smears, 361
Bacteriolysis, 338
Bacteriostatic, 170
Bacteriuria, 381, 391, 403
   detection and semiquantitation of, 403, 407-408
Balance, sense of, inner ear and, 625
Bandage pressure in controlling severe bleeding, 558
Bandage scissors, 212, 219
Bandages, 232-239
   application of, 234-239
   basic wrapping techniques for, 234-237
   materials for, 232-234
   purposes of, 232
   roller, 232-233
   types of, 233
   Tubegauz, 234
      application of, 237-239
Barbiturates, 572-573
Barrier precautions, 6-7
Basal cell carcinoma, 630
Baseline in electrocardiogram, 528
   wandering, 531-532
Baseline shift, electrocardiogram and, 531-532
Basic food groups, recommended daily servings of, 635, 637
BE; *see* Barium enema
Bee stings, first aid for, 557
Benadryl, 261
Bence Jones protein in urine, 408
Bence Jones Protein Test, 408

Beta cells, 609
Beta-2 microglobulin test, 14
Beta-adrenergic blockers, 254
Big E eye chart, 120
Bigeminal pulse, 31
Bile, 605, 607, 609
Bili-Labstix test, 388
Bilirubin in urine, 391
   tests for, 391, 394-395
Bilirubinuria, 391
   tests for, 391, 394-395
Bimanual, definition of, 77
Bimanual palpation of uterus and adnexa, 105
Binaurals of stethoscope, 40
Biochemistry, 338
Biohazard labels, 4, 340
Biologic death, definition of, 548
Biologic strips to monitor sterilization process, 194
Biopsy, 204
   aspiration/needle, 204
      of breast, materials for, 222
   cervical, materials for, 220-221
   endometrial, 221
      materials for, 222
   excisional, 204
   fine-needle aspiration, 204
   incisional, 204
   punch, 204
   of skin lesions, 629
      materials for, 222
   vulvar, materials for, 222
Biopsy forceps, 82, 212
   cervical, 213
   punch, 219
Biopsy instruments for minor surgery, 213
Biopsy punch, 213
Biopsy specimens, tissue, materials for removing, 220
Biotin, 646, 647-648
Biot's respiration, 33
Bipolar leads, electrocardiogram and, 532
Bites, first aid for, 556-557
Black widow spider bites, antivenins for, 557
Bladder, 612, 615
   cancer of, 114-115
Bleeding, severe, first aid for, 557-560
Block anesthesia, 207
Blood
   amount of, in body of adult, 591-594
   as barrier to disease and infection, 174
   circulatory system and, 591-594
   clotting of, 594
   components, functions, and formation of, 416-418
   conditions affecting, 594
   culture of, 338
   dyscrasia of, 416
   examinations of, types of, 454-461
   occult, 347
   specimens of, handling of, 11-12
   thickness of, blood pressure and, 36
   in urine, 391
   viscosity of, blood pressure and, 36
   volume of, in blood vessels, blood pressure and, 36
Blood agar culture media, 363
Blood banking, 323
Blood and body substance precautions, universal, 1-17
Blood cells, red, 588, 594
Blood chemistries, 437-448
Blood glucose meters, 437, 438, 442-445
Blood glucose, tests for, 437-448
   Accucheck III system, 439-442

Blood glucose, tests for—cont'd
    Chemstrip bG, 439-442
    One Touch Blood Glucose Meter, 442-445
    Reflotron Plus System, 438
Blood groups and types, 452
Blood lipids, effects of fats on, 638, 641
Blood plasma, 594
Blood pressure, 33, 35-41
    abnormal readings of, 37
    in arteries, 594-595
    child's, measuring, 153
    diastolic, 33, 35
    factors determining, 35-36
    high, 36; see also Hypertension
    instruments for measuring, 39-40
    measuring, 40-45
    normal readings and values for, 36
        long-term maintenance to achieve, 39
        variations in, 36-37
    orthostatic, 36, 41, 45
    patient history and, 37-38
    physiology of, 595-596
    recommended action after measurement of, 38
    systolic, 33, 35
    vocabulary related to, 36
Blood samples
    obtaining, 418-432
    venous, 418-421
Blood serum, 594
Blood tests, 433-436
    alpha-fetoprotein, for pregnant woman, 133
    fasting, 421
    Guthrie, to diagnose phenylketonuria, 156, 157-158
    patient preparation for, 421
    during prenatal physical examination, 131
Blood urea nitrogen, 437
Blood vessels
    cardiovascular system and, 594
    peripheral resistance of, to blood flow, blood pressure and, 36
    volume of blood in, blood pressure and, 36
Bloodborne pathogen standard, federal, 5
Bloodborne pathogens, 2
BNDD; see Bureau of Narcotics and Danger Drugs
Body
    cavities of, 579-580
    defenses of, against disease and infection, 173-177
    planes of, 579
    regions of, 581
    structural levels of organization in, 578
Body fluid and blood precautions, 6
Body fluids
    from AIDS patients, mucous membrane or conjunctival exposure to, 11-12
    handling of, 11
    spills of, cleaning, 3
Body mechanics, 510-512
Body substance, 2
Body substance and blood precautions, universal, 1-17
Body system, 578
    abbreviations related to, 67, 262
Body temperature, 19-28
    changes in, 20
    child's, measuring, 143
    equipment needed to take, 22
    graph demonstrating changes in, 21
    infant's, taking, 27
    infrared radiation measurement of, 20, 22, 27-28, 30-31
    methods and procedures for, 22
    normal, 19

Body temperature—cont'd
    taking, contraindications to forms of, 22
    variations in, 19-20
Body tube of microscope, 331
Bone conduction test of hearing, 120
Bone marrow, 588
Bone marrow scan, 482
Bone scan, 482
Bone(s), 582-585
Books on drugs, official, 250-251
Borderline hypertension, 36
Boucheron and Toynbee ear specula used with otoscope, 79
Bowel movement, 347
Bracelet, Medic-Alert; see Medic-Alert bracelet or necklace
Brachial artery
    checking for pulse at, in cardiopulmonary resuscitation of infants, 551
    compression of, in controlling severe bleeding, 558, 559
    determining pulse rate at, 32
    to measure blood pressure, 41
Brachium, 587
Bradycardia, 31
    sinus, electrocardiogram and, 530
Brain, 599
    anatomy and physiology of, 599-602
    cancer of, 114-115
    concussion of, definition of, 548
    functions of, 603
Brain scan, 482
Brand name of drug, 248, 250
BRAT, 660
Breasts, 620
    aspiration (needle) biopsy of, materials for, 222
    cancer of, 114-115
    examination of, during pregnancy, 131
    self-examination of, 91-94
Breastbone, 586, 587
Breathing
    in allergic reaction to drugs, 556
    in cardiopulmonary resuscitation, 550
    for infants and small children, 551
Broad-spectrum drugs, 249
Broken glassware, handling of, 12-13
Bronchi, respiration and, 612
Bronchioles, 612
Bronchodilator, 254
Bronchogram, 473
Bronchoscope, 82
Bronchoscopy, 77
Buccal route of drug administration, 266
Bulla, identification of, 630
BUN; see Blood urea nitrogen
Bundle
    atrioventricular, 528
    of His, 528
Bunion, 588
Burdick E500 interpretive electrocardiogram, portable, 538
Bureau of Narcotics and Danger Drugs, 249
Burns, 560-563
Bursitis, 496

C

Calcaneus, 588
Calcium, 646, 649, 661
Calcium channel blockers, 254
Calorie(s), 634, 653
    calculating number of, 655
    empty, 655
    formula for determining percentage of, supplied from fat, 655
    nutrition and, 653-655

Camphor, ingestion of, first aid for, 570
Cancellous bone, 582
Cancer
    bladder, 114-115
    brain, 114-115
    breast, 114-115
        breast self-examination to detect, 91-94
    cervical, 114-115
        screening for, 99
    colon, screening for, 99, 108
    colorectal, 114-115
    common sites for, 112
    endometrial, 114-115
    examinations to detect, recommendations for, 113
    facts about, 112
    lung, 116-117
    major sites of, 114-117
    mouth, 116-117
    nutrition guidelines for prevention of, 113
    oral, 116-117
    ovary, 116-117
    pancreas, 116-117
    prostate, 116-117
        screening for, 99
    skin, 116-117
        sun and, 630
    stomach, 116-117
    testicular, 116-117
    warning signals of, 113
Candidiasis, 13
    smear for, 367
Canes, use of, 517-518
Cannula, nasal, for oxygen administration, 264, 265
Canthus, 312
Capillaries, 594
Capillary bleeding, 557
Caplets, 260
Capsules, 260
Carbohydrates
    calories supplied by, 642, 653
    complex, 645, 661
    nutrition and, 642-645
    simple, 645
Carbon dioxide, respiration and, 609
Carcinoma, 630; see also Cancer
Cardiac arrest, 525
    cardiopulmonary resuscitation for; see Cardiopulmonary resuscitation
Cardiac compression in cardiopulmonary resuscitation, 550-551
Cardiac cycle, 527-529
Cardiac monitoring, ambulatory, 538-543
Cardiac muscle, anatomy and physiology of, 591
Cardiac output, blood pressure and, 36
Cardiac profile, 462, 467
Cardiac scan, 482
Cardiogenic agent, 255
Cardiogenic shock, 555
Cardiopulmonary resuscitation (CPR), 12-13, 549-553
    activating EMS system and, 550
    airway in, 549-550
    basic ABC steps in, 549
    basic and advanced life support in, 549
    breathing in, 550
    cardiac compression in, 550-551
    checking pulse in, 550
    for children, 551
    courses in, 549, 571
    head-tilt in, 549
    for infants, 551
    jaw thrust maneuver in, 549
    modified jaw thrust maneuver in, 549
    mouth-to-stoma resuscitation in, 549

Cardiopulmonary resuscitation (CPR)—cont'd
   positioning victim in, 549
   procedure for, 549-551
   supplementary techniques of, 549
   in victim with possible neck injury, 551-552
Cardiovascular system, 591
   anatomy and physiology of, 594-596
   disease of, urine findings in, 392-393
   terms related to, 66
Care plans, 62
Carotene, 647-648
Carotid artery
   checking for pulse at, in cardiopulmonary
      resuscitation, 550, 551
   compression of, in controlling severe
      bleeding, 558, 559
Carpal bones, 587
Cartilage, 582
   costal, 586
   of ear, 625
Cartridge, drug, 278
Cassette, 471
Casts, 240-243
   in urine, 403, 405
Category-specific precautions, 6
Cathartic, 255
Catheter, emptying bladder with, 615
Causative agents, infectious process and, 169-173
Cause of infectious process, 171-172
Cautery, 204
CBC; *see* Complete blood count
CD4 cells, 14
Cecum, 608, 609
Cells, 578
   types of, 581
   in urine sediment, 401, 403, 404
Cellular basis of humans, 581-582
Cellular respiration, 609
Cement of tooth, 605
Centigrade degrees, conversion to Fahrenheit
      degrees and, 22, 23
Centigrade thermometers, reading, 22
Central nervous system
   anatomy and physiology of, 599-602, 603
   abbreviations related to, 67, 262
Centrifuged urine sediment, microscopic exami-
      nation of, 395, 400-403
Centrifuges, 334
Cerebellum, anatomy and physiology of,
      599, 601
Cerebral angiogram, 473
Cerebral vascular accident, first aid for, 563-564
Cerebrospinal fluid, 599
Cerebrum, anatomy and physiology of, 599
Cerumen, 312
Ceruminous glands, 629
Cervical biopsy, materials for, 220-221
Cervical biopsy forceps, 213
Cervical biopsy punch forceps, 79
Cervical cancer, screening for, 99
Cervical nerves, 603
Cervical smear, 103
Cervical vertebrae, 587
Cervicitis, 368
Cervix, 620
   cancer of, 114-115
Cesarean section, 587
Charcoal, activated, poisoning and, 570
Chemical barriers to disease and infection,
      173-174
Chemical burns, first aid for, 563
Chemical disinfection, 198, 199
Chemical examination of urine using reagent
      strips, 385, 387-388
Chemical name of drug, 248, 250

Chemical sterilization, 197, 198
Chemical sterilization indicators, 192-194
Chemicals, safety rules for handling, 329
Chemistry, clinical, 323
Chemistry analyzers, urine, for use with reagent
      strips, 388-390
Chemotherapy, 249
Chemstrip bG, use of, 439-442
Chest
   abbreviations related to, 67, 262
   circumference
      of child, measuring, 143
      of infant, measuring, 155
   pain in, first aid for, 564
Chest leads, electrocardiogram and, 533, 537
Chest thrusts, 553
Chestpiece of stethoscope, 40
Cheyne-Stokes respiration, 33
Chief complaint, 55
Chiggers, bites from, first aid for, 557
Childhood, physical growth during, general
      trends in, 138, 139, 143; *see also*
      Children
Childhood onset diabetes, 568-569
Children; *see also* Infants; Pediatric examinations
   AAP guidelines for health supervision
      of, 137
   cardiopulmonary resuscitation for, 551
   height and weight of, measuring, 139
   injections in, 159, 160
   management of obstructed airway in, 553
   pain rating scales for, 144
   physical growth patterns of, recording, 143
Chlamydia, 368
   culture for, during prenatal physical
      examination, 131
Chlamydia trachomatis direct specimen test,
      370-371
Chloride, 649
Chlorine in tap water, 650
Chocolate, amount of saturated fat in, 642
Choking, 552
Cholangiogram, intravenous, 473
Cholecystogram, 473
Cholelithiasis, 605
Cholesterol, 661
   nutrition and, 637-642
Cholesterol content of selected foods, 637, 638
Cholesterol free, food labeling and, 657
Chorionic gonadotropin, human, 126, 625
   urine tests for, 408
Chorionic villi sampling, 133
Choroid, 625
Chyle, 609
Cicatrix, identification of, 630
Cidex for chemical sterilization, 198
Circular turn during bandaging, 234, 235
Circulation
   in allergic reaction to drugs, 556
   in cardiopulmonary resuscitation for infants
      and small children, 551
Circulatory system, anatomy and physiology
      of, 591-596
Circumcision, 615
Circumduction of hand, 587
Circumduction, 510
Cisterna chyli, 596, 609
Cisternogram, 482
Clamps
   Allis, 219
   towel, 213
Clavicles, 586, 587
Clean-catch urine specimen, 343
   collecting, 344-346

Cleaning
   of patient care areas, 3, 11
   ultrasonic, 198-199
   of uniforms and clothing, 4
Clear liquid diet, 658
Clinical chemistry, 323
Clinical death, definition of, 548
Clinical laboratory, 2
Clinical Laboratory Improvement
      Amendments of 1988, 338
Clinistix test, 389
Clinitek 10 analyzer for urine, 389-390
Clinitest, 389, 391, 394
Clitoris, 620
Closed fracture, first aid for, 566-567
Clostridium perfringens, 223
Clostridium tetani, 223
Clothing, uniforms and, cleaning, 4
Clotting of blood, 594
CNS; *see* Central nervous system
Coarse-focusing knob of microscope, 332
Cobalamin, 647-648
Cocaine, 572-573
Cocci causing disease, 171
Coccygeal nerves, 603
Coccyx, 587
Cochlea of labyrinth, 625
Cochlear nerve, 625
Cold
   dry, 502
   moist, 502-503
Cold packs, chemical, 502
Colicky pain, 66
Collarbones, 587
Colloidal solution, 260
Colon, 609
   bacillus in, 223
   cancer of, screening for, 99, 108
Color Tool pain rating scale, 144
Color vision, testing, 124-125
Colorectal cancer, 114-115
Colposcopy, 99, 221-222
Colyte prep, 118
Coma, diabetic; *see* Diabetic coma\par
Combistix test, 388, 389
Common carotid artery, determining pulse rate
      at, 32
Communications of hazards to employees, 4-5
Compact bone, 582
Compazine, 261
Complete blood count, 418
   hematology test, 449-452
Complex carbohydrates, 645, 661
Compliance with Universal Precautions, 5
Comprehensive Drug Abuse Prevention and
      Control Act, 251
Compress, use of, 501
Compression cuffs, recommended widths of, 40
Computed tomography, 476-477
Computerized EKG, electrocardiography
      and, 538
Conchae, 612
Concussion, 548
Conduction, 496
Conduction pathways, nervous system and,
      596, 599
Conduction system of heart, 527, 595
   cardiac cycle and, 528
Conduction time, electrocardiogram and, 529
Condyles, 588
Condyloma, 368
Confidentiality of medical records, 64
Congenital immunity, 174
Conjunctiva, 312, 625

Conjunctival exposure to body fluids from AIDS patients, 11-12
Connective tissue, 581
Consent, informed
    for IUD insertion, 223
    for minor surgery, 213, 214
Constipation, 347
Contact dermatitis, 300
Contact lenses, removal of, chemical burn and, 563
Contaminated, definition of, 2, 170
Contaminated laundry, 2
    handling of, 4
Contaminated sharps, 2
Contaminated waste, 3
Contamination, 170
Contraceptive, 255
Contractions, premature ventricular, electrocardiogram and, 530
Contraindication, 249
Contrast medium radiologic techniques, 472-473
Controlled substances, storage and handling of, 259-260
Controlled Substances Act of 1970, 251
Controlled substances inventory and prescriber's record, 264
Controls, engineering, 2
Contusion, definition of, 548
Convulsions, first aid for, 564-565
Copper sulfate relative density test, 434-436
Copper-T 380A intrauterine device, 222-223
Corium, 629
Cornea, 625
Coronal plane, 579
Coronary arteries, 595
Coronary artery disease, 595
Coronary insufficiency, 595
Coronary thrombosis, 595
Coronary vessels, anatomy and physiology of, 593
Corrections of medical records, 64-65
Cortisone, 622
Cost containment for laboratory tests, 324
Costal cartilages, 586
Costochondral junctions, 586, 587
Cowper's gland, 615
CPR; *see* Cardiopulmonary resuscitation
Cradle position for carrying infant, 153
Cramps, menstrual, 620
Cranial cavity, 580
Cranial nerves, anatomy and physiology of, 603
Cravat bandage, 233
Crescentic roll of neck, 591
Cross-tolerance, 249
Crown of tooth, 605
Crude drug, 249
Crust, identification of, 630
Crutches, 513-517
Cryosurgery, 221, 222
Cryosurgery unit and probe, 212
Cryotherapy, 501-503
    in treatment of skin cancer, 630
Cryptococcosis, 13
Crystals in urine, 403, 406
CSF; *see* Cerebrospinal fluid
CT scan; *see* Computed tomography
Cuff of sphygmomanometer, 40
Culture, 338
    blood, 338
    to detect gonorrhea, 367, 370
    gelatin, 338
    for gonorrhea and chlamydia during prenatal physical examination, 131
    handling of, 11
    hanging drop, 338
    nasopharyngeal, 354, 357

Culture,—cont'd
    negative, 338
    positive, 338
    pure, 338
    smear, 338
    stab, 338
    streak, 338
    throat, 354, 355-357
    tissue, 338
    type, 338
    vaginal, collection of, 363, 366-370
    wound, 358
        dressing change with, 228-232
Culture and sensitivity testing, bacterial, 363
Culture collection systems, 339
Culture medium, 339, 363
    inoculating, 364-365
Culture plate methods for bacteriuria testing, 407
Culture strip method for bacteriuria testing, 407
Culturette, 339
Culturette II culture collection system, 339
Cumulative action of drug, 249, 272
Curettage, endocervical, 221, 222
Curettes, 212
Cuticle, 629
CVA; *see* Cerebral vascular accident
CVS; *see* Cardiovascular system
Cyanocobalamin, 646
Cyclic antidepressants, poisoning by, first aid for, 570
Cyst
    identification of, 630
    incision and drainage of, materials for, 220
    sebaceous, 204
Cystoscope, 82
Cystoscopy, 77
Cytology, 324, 339
    exfoliative, 353
Cytology smears, 358-360
Cytomegalovirus, 14
    in AIDS patients, 12
Cytotoxins, 255

D

Daily caloric requirements, nutrition and, 655
Data base in POMR, 63
ddC; *see* Zalcitabine
DEA; *see* Drug Enforcement Administration
Deafness, 625
Death
    biologic, 548
    clinical, 548
Debridement, 496
Decongestant, 255
Decontamination, 2
    of work surfaces and equipment, 3, 11
Defibrillation, definition of, 525
Definite hypertension, 37
Delivery, expected date of, pregnancy table for, 132
"Delta" hepatitis, 16
Deltoid muscle, injection into, 160, 279, 280
Density, 471
Dental soft diet, 658
Dentin of tooth, 605
Department of Health and Human Services, 249, 251
Depolarization, cardiac cycle and, 527
Dermatitis, 300, 629
    contact, 300
Dermatology, 629-630
Dermis, 629
Descending colon, 609
Desquamation, identification of, 631
Detail, 471
Detergents, 2

Development, motor, guideposts in, 136
Dextrose 50%, 261
Dextrostix, 437
Diabetes, 568-569
Diabetes mellitus, 568-569, 622
    diet for patient with, 660
Diabetic coma, first aid for, 568-569
Diabetic diet, 660
Diagnosis, abbreviations related to, 67, 262
Diagnostic allergy tests and intradermal skin tests, 299-309
Diagnostic data, 61
    for inflammatory process, 177
Diagnostic plan in POMR, 63
Diagnostic procedures
    organizing recording of, 325-328
    reasons for, 325
Diagnostic studies, 61
Diagnostic tests, prenatal physical examination and, 131-133
Diagnostic and therapeutic procedures, 325-328
Diaper test to diagnose phenylketonuria, 156, 409
Diaphragm, 591, 596, 609
    of stethoscope, 40
Diaphragmatic respiration, 33
Diarrhea, 347
Diastix test, 389
Diastole, cardiac cycle and, 527
Diastolic blood pressure, 33, 35, 595-596
Diastolic sounds, 41
Diathermy, 497
Diazepam, sudden stoppage of, hyperventilation and, 567
Dietary guidelines for Americans, 655-656
Differential culture media, 363
Differential diagnosis, 62
Differential white cell count, 450
Differentiation of cell, 581
Digestion, 634
    nutrition and, 635
    organs of, 605-609
Digestive system, anatomy and physiology of, 605-609
Digital, definition of, 77
Digital electrocardiograph facsimile, electrocardiography and, 538
Digital radiography, 477-479
Digitalis, 530
Digoxin, 261
Diluent, 260
Dilute, 249
Dilution and neutralization of poisons, 570-571
Diphtheria antitoxin, 176
Diphtheria and tetanus toxoid, 159
    and pertussis toxoids, guide for use of, 178
Diplococci causing disease, 171
Dipstick tests of urine, 396-399
Direct digital EKG fax, 538
Direct pressure in controlling severe bleeding, 558
Direct transmission of disease, 172
Disabilities, physical, and therapy, 519-521
Disc-plate method for sensitivity test, 363
Discharge summary, 62
Disease
    body's defenses against, 173-177
    risk of, relationship between overweight and, 634, 635
Disinfectants, 170
    for sterilization, 198
Disinfection, 170, 186
    chemical, 198, 199
    procedures for, 198-199
Diskogram, 473
Dispensed medication, 258
Disposable bags for sterilization, 188, 190

Disposable thermometers, 20, 21
Disposable urine collector, 155, 156
Disposal of waste, 5
Dissecting scissors, 212
Distance visual acuity
    examination of, 120-121
    measuring, 122-123
Diuresis, 343
Diuretic, 255
Dizziness, inner ear and, 625
Documentation, medical records and, 64-65
Don, definition of, 204
Donning and removing sterile gloves, 207,
    209-210
Doriden; *see* Glutethimide\par
Dorsal vertebrae, 587
Dorsal-recumbent position, 84-85
Dorsalis pedis artery, determining pulse rate
    at, 32
Dorsiflexion, 510
Dorsogluteal intramuscular injection, 279, 280
Dorsogluteal muscle, injection into, 160
Dosage of drugs
    calculation of, 268-270, 271
    and drug action, factors influencing, 270-272
    parenteral, 249
Down's syndrome, patterns of papillae and, 630
Drainage
    incision and, of abscess or cyst, materials
        for, 220
    terms to describe, 223
Drainage/secretion precautions, 6
Draping, gowning, and positioning patient for
    physical examination, 84-91
Dressings, 227-232
    change of, with wound culture, 228-232
    materials for, 227, 232
    purposes of, 227
    spray-on, 232
Drug Enforcement Administration, 249, 251-252
Drug idiosyncrasy, 249, 272
Drug screen urine specimen, 343
Drug therapy for HIV-positive people, 15
Drug tolerance, 249
Drugs
    actions of, types of, 272
    administered, 258
    administration of, 265-270, 272
        pharmacology and, principles of, 247-298
    allergic reaction to, 556
    allergies to, 272
    classification of, 252
        based on actions or effects on body,
            253-256
    commonly abused, effects of, 571, 572-573
    controlled, storage and handling of, 259-260
    cumulative action of, 249
    dispensed, 258
    dosage of
        and action of, factors influencing,
            270-272
        calculation of, 268-270, 271
    emergency tray of, 261
    for injection, 276
    interaction of, 272
    labeling of, 261
    legal classification of, 251-252
    liquid, 278
        terms to describe, 260-261
    names of, 248, 250
    nonprescription, 252
    outdated, discarding, 258-259
    patient education on use of, 272-273
    pharmacology and, 248-252
    powdered, reconstitution of

Drugs—cont'd
    for injection, 276
    for insulin injection, 295
    prescribed, 258
    prescription, 252
        top 50, 257
    pure, 249
    references and official books on, 250-251
    solid, terms to describe, 260
    sources of, 248
    standards and laws governing use of, 251
    storage and handling of, 258-259, 261
    tolerance of, and drug dosage and action, 271
Dry heat sterilization, 198
Dry heat sterilization indicator labels, 193, 194
Duodenal ulcer, 609
Duodenal ulcer diet, 660
Duodenum, 609
Dura mater, 599
Dysmenorrhea, 620
Dysplasia, 339
Dyspnea, 33
Dysuria, 381, 384

E
Ear(s)
    abbreviations related to, 67, 262
    anatomy of, 311
    external, 312
    gross anatomy of, in frontal section, 626
    instillations into, 310, 313-314
    irrigation of, 310-311, 314-316
    sensory system and, 599, 625
    vocabulary referring to, 66
Ear specula used with otoscope, 79
Eardrum, 625
    thermometers measuring body temperature
        using, 20, 22, 27-28, 30-31
Earpieces of stethoscope, 40
Ecchymosis, identification of, 631
Eccrine glands, 629
Echocardiography, 479
Echoencephalogram, 479
Ectoparasites causing disease, 172
Ectopic pregnancy, 620
EDTA, 419
Educative plan in POMR, 63
EECG; *see* Echoencephalogram
EEG; *see* Electroencephalogram
Efferent fibers, 599
Efferent nerves, 603
Ejaculating duct, 615
EKG; *see* Electrocardiogram
Elastic bandages, 233
Elastic gauze bandage, 233
Elastic tape, 232
Elbow joint, 587, 588
    bandage-wrapping techniques for, 236
Electric vision testing devices, 121
Electrical impulse of cardiac cycle, 528
Electrocardiogram, 519, 529-538
    alternating current interference and, 532
    application of electrodes and, 535, 536
    artifacts and, 531-532
    atrial arrhythmias in, 530
    atrial fibrillation and, 530
    augmented leads and, 532-533
        application of, 537
    baseline shift and, 531-532
    bipolar leads and, 532, 533
    chest leads and, 533
        application of, 537
    cleaning electrodes and, 538
    common rhythms in, 529-531
    computerized, electrocardiography and, 538

Electrocardiogram,—cont'd
    connection of lead wires and, 535, 536
    cycle of, electrocardiography and, 527-529
    definition of, 524-525
    electrocardiography and, 529-538
    equipment for obtaining, 533
    interpretation of, 529-532
    intervals of, 527, 528
    limb leads and
        application of, 535-537
        standard, 532, 533
    mounting, 538
    normal, 527, 529
    paroxysmal atrial tachycardia and, 530
    portable Burdick E500 interpretive, 538
    precordial leads and, 533
    premature atrial contractions and, 530
    premature ventricular contractions and, 530
    preparation and procedure for obtaining, 533-
        538
    recording, 535-537
    sinus rhythms in, 529-530
    somatic tremor and, 531
    suggested codes for marking leads and,
        533, 534
    ventricular arrhythmias in, 530-531
    ventricular fibrillation and, 531
    ventricular tachycardia and, 530
    wandering baseline and, 531-532
Electrocardiogram electrodes and
    electrolytes, 532
Electrocardiogram leads, 532-533, 537
Electrocardiogram paper, 529, 530, 537
Electrocardiograph, 525
    automatic, electrocardiography and, 538
    single-channel, 535, 536
    standardizing, 533, 534
Electrocardiograph room, preparation of, 533-534
Electrocardiography, 524-546
    ambulatory cardiac monitoring and, 538-543
    automatic electrocardiographs and, 538
    cardiac cycle and, 527-529
    case study in, 545
    cognitive objectives of, 524
    computerized EKG and, 538
    digital electrocardiograph facsimile and, 538
    EKG cycle and, 527-529
    electrocardiogram and, 529-538
    monitoring and, 538-543
    Phone-A-Gram and, 538
    terminal performance objectives of, 524
    treadmill stress test and, 543-544
Electrocauterization, materials for, 222, 223
Electrodes, electrocardiogram, 532
    application of, 535, 536
Electrodiagnostic examinations, 519
Electroencephalogram (EEG), 519
Electrolytes, 416
    electrocardiogram electrodes and, 532
Electronic thermometers, 20, 21
Electrophoresis, 416
Electrotherapy, using galvanic and faradic
    currents, 518-519
Elevation in controlling severe bleeding, 558
ELISA test, 15
Elixirs, 261
Embolus, 594
Embryo, 620
Emergencies
    common, and first aid; *see* First aid, common
        emergencies and
    office, office policy for, 548
Emergency drug tray, 261
Emergency medical services (EMS) system, 553-
    554

Emergency tray crash cart, 571
Emetic, 255
Emotional condition of patient and drug dosage
        and action, 271
Employees; *see* Hospital employees
Empty calorie, 655
EMS system; *see* Emergency medical services
        system\par
Emulsion, 260
Enamel of tooth, 605
Endocarditis, 595
Endocardium, 526, 595
Endocervical curettage, 221, 222
Endocervical smear, 103
Endocrine cells of pancreas, 605, 609
Endocrine system, anatomy and physiology
        of, 622-625
Endometrial biopsy, 221, 222
Endometrial suction curette, 212
Endometrium, cancer of, 114-115
Endoscope, 82
Endoscopic examination, 99, 109-111, 118
Endoscopy, 77
Enema, 471
Engineering controls, 2
Enrichment culture media, 363
Enteric precautions, 6
Entry(ies)
        means of, of etiologic agent, 172
        in medical records, 64
Enuresis, 343
Envelope wrap, opening, 205-206
Enzyme-Linked ImmunoSorbent Assay, 15
Eosinophils and basophils, 450
Epidermis, 629
Epididymis, 615
Epididymitis, 615
Epiglottis, 612
Epilepsy, seizures associated with, 565
Epinephrine, 261, 622
        in allergic reaction to drugs, 556
        definition of, 548
        sinus tachycardia and, 529
Epistaxis, first aid for, 565
Epithelial cells, 581
        in urine, 403, 404
Epithelial tissue, 581
Equipment
        decontamination of, 3
        for injections, 273-276
        for neurologic examination, 118
        for physical examinations, 78-82
        for taking temperature, 22
        handling of, 9-11
        personal protective, 7-9
        reusable, handling of, 12
        safety rules for handling, 329
        sterile, storing, 195
Erect position, 91
Erosion, identification of, 631
Erythrocytes, 594
Erythrocytosis, 416
Escherichia coli, 223
Esophagus, 609
Essential amino acids, 636
Essential hypertension, 36
Estrogens, 255, 620-621, 625
        combination of, with progestin, 621
Ethanol, 572-573
Etiologic agent, 171-172
Eupnea, 33
Eustachian tube, 625
        respiration and, 612
Event marker, ambulatory cardiac monitoring
        and, 539
Eversion, 510

Examination; *see also* Test(s)
        abdomen, during pregnancy, 131
        breast, 91-94
                during pregnancy, 131
        chemical, of urine using reagent strips, 385,
                387-388
        endoscopic, 99, 109-111, 118
        eye, 120-126
        gynecologic, 91, 98
        hearing, 119-120
        neurologic, 118, 119
        obstetric, 126-134
        ophthalmoscopic, 125
        oral, 78
        pediatric, 134-163
                general points for, 135, 138-139
        pelvic, 78
                and Pap smear, 98-99, 100-105
                during pregnancy, 131
        physical; *see* Physical examination
        rectal, 99, 106-108
        vaginal, 98-99
                during pregnancy, 131
Excisional biopsy, 204
Excitation, nervous system and, 596, 599
Excoriation, identification of, 631
Excreta, 347
Excrete, 347
Excretion, 347
Excruciating pain, 66
Exercises, therapeutic, 505-510
Exfoliative cytology, 353
Exocrine cells of pancreas, 605, 609
Expected date of delivery, pregnancy table
        for, 132
Expectorant, 255
Expectorate, 353
Expiration, respiration and, 609
Exposure, occupational, 2
Exposure incident, 2
Exposure time for steam sterilization, 192
Exquisite pain, 66
Extension, 510
External auditory meatus, 312
External ear, 312
External eye examinations, 120-125
External respiration, 31, 609
Extremities
        examination of, vocabulary referring to, 66
        lower; *see* Lower extremity
        upper; *see* Upper extremity
Eye(s), 627
        abbreviations related to, 67, 262
        anatomy of, 311, 312
        examination of, 120-126
        instillations and irrigations of, 310-321
        sensory system and, 599, 625-629
        terms related to, 66
Eye chart, Snellen, 120-121
        measuring distance visual acuity using, 122-
                123
Eyeball, 625
Eyebrows, 625
Eyedrops, instillation of, 316-317
Eyelashes, 625
Eyelids, 625
Eyepiece of microscope, 330
Eyewear, protective, masks and, 8

F

Face, bones of, 585
Face mask, 8
        for oxygen administration, 264-265
Face shields, 8

Facial artery
        compression of, in controlling severe
                bleeding, 558, 559
        determining pulse rate at, 32
Facial burns, first aid for, 563
Facsimile, digital electrocardiograph, electro-
        cardiography and, 538
Fahrenheit degrees, conversion to centigrade
        degrees and, 22, 23
Fahrenheit thermometers, reading, 22
Fainting
        first aid for, 565
        hyperventilation and, 568
Fallen arches, 588
Fallopian tubes, 620
False ribs, 586
Family history, 55
Fasting urine specimen, 342
Fat, 637, 638, 642
        calories supplied by, 638, 639, 653
        cutting back on, 640
        definition of, 639
        effects of, on blood lipids, 638, 641
        foods high in, 656
        foods low in, 656, 658, 659
        formula for determing percentage of calories
                supplied from, 655
        hidden, 637, 638
        monounsaturated, 638
        nutrition and, 637-642
        polyunsaturated, 638
Fat-free, food labeling and, 657
Fat-soluble vitamins, 645, 646
Fatty acids, 639
        omega-3, 638
FDA; *see* Food and Drug Administration
Febrile pulse, 31
Feces, 347
Federal regulation, Universal Precautions as, 5
Female reproductive system
        abbreviations related to, 67, 262
        anatomy and physiology of, 615-621
Femoral artery
        compression of, in controlling severe
                bleeding, 558, 559
        determining pulse rate at, 32
Femur, 587, 588
Fertilization, 620
        appearance of uterus and uterine tubes from,
                to implantation, 618
Fever, 20, 21
Fiber, 650-652, 661
Fiberglass cast application, 242
Fiberglass tape measure, 79
Fiberoptic flexible sigmoidoscope, 82
Fibrillation, 525
        atrial, 29
                electrocardiogram and, 530
        ventricular, electrocardiogram and, 531
Fibula, 588
Fight or flight reaction, sympathetic system
        and, 604
Figure-eight turn during bandaging, 234, 235
Fine-focusing knob of microscope, 332
Fine-needle aspiration biopsy, 204
Fingernails, integumentary system and, 629
Fingers, 587
Fingertip skin puncture
        using a lancet, 427-428
        using a Penlet, 429
First aid, 547
        common emergencies and, 547-576
        courses in, 549, 571
First aid kit, 571
First morning urine specimen, 342
First-degree burns, first aid for, 560, 562

Fissure, identification of, 631
Fixation of smear, 339
Flat bones, 582
Flatfeet, 588
Flatulence, 347
Flatus, 347
Flexion, 510
Floating ribs, 586, 587
Flora, normal, 170
Fluids, body; *see* Body fluids
Fluoride in tap water, 650
Fluoroscope, 471
Fluoroscopy, 471, 472
Focusing of microscope, 333
Foerster sponge forceps, 213
Folacin, 647-648
Folate, 647-648
Folic acid, 646, 647-648
Follow-up prenatal visits, 133
Food, processing of, digestive system and, 609
Food and Drug Administration, 249, 251
Food, Drug and Cosmetic Act of 1938, 251
Food guide pyramid, 635, 636-637
Food labeling, 656-660, 661
    definition of, 634
Food Nutrition Board of National Academy of
        Sciences, 655
Food Safety and Inspection Service of U.S.
        Department of Agriculture, food
        labeling and, 656
Foot
    anatomy and physiology of, 588
    and ankle, bandage-wrapping techniques
        for, 235
Football position for carrying infant, 153
Foramina of skull, 603
Forced respiration, 33
Forceps
    biopsy, 82, 212
    for minor surgery, 212-213
    punch, cervical biopsy, 79
    punch biopsy, 219
    transfer, 204
    types of, 212-213
Forearm, 587, 588
Foreign bodies
    in ear, first aid for, 565-566
    in eye, first aid for, 565-566
    in nose, first aid for, 566
    in subcutaneous tissues, materials for
        removing, 220
Foreskin of penis, 615
Formicant pulse, 31
Fowler's position, 90, 91
Fracture
    of back, first aid for, 567
    closed, first aid for, 566-567
    first aid for, 566-567
    of jaw, first aid for, 567
    of neck, first aid for, 567
    open, first aid for, 566-567
Frankel head band and mirror set, 80
Frequency, 343
Fruits, nutrition and, 645, 646
Full liquid diet, 658
Full-thickness burns, first aid for, 560, 562-563
Fungi causing disease, 171
Fungicide, 170

G

Gaits, crutch-walking, types of, 515-517
Gallbladder, 609
    digestive system and, 605
Gallstones, 605
Gamete, 581

Gamma globulin to produce immunity, 176
Ganglia, 599, 603
Gas bacillus, 223
Gas sterilization, 198
Gasoline, ingestion of, first aid for, 570
Gastric juices, 609
Gastric ulcer, 609
Gastric ulcer diet, 660
Gastrointestinal infections, signs and
        symptoms of, 177
Gastrointestinal system
    abbreviations related to, 67, 262
    anatomy and physiology of, 605-609
    as barrier to disease and infection, 174
    disease of, urine findings in, 392-393
    terms related to, 66
Gastroscopy, 77
Gauze, 232-233
Gauze bandage, elastic, 233
Gelatin culture, 338
Generalized infection, 170
    signs and symptoms of, 176-177
Generic name of drug, 248, 250
Genital warts, 368
Genitourinary infections, signs and symptoms
        of, 177
Genitourinary system, vocabulary referring to, 66
German measles, stages of infection with, 173
German measles vaccine, guide for use of, 179
Germicidal agents for sterilization, 198
Germicide, 170
GI system; *see* Gastrointestinal system
Gland(s)
    adrenal, endocrine system and, 622
    apocrine, 629
    ceruminous, 629
    Cowper's, 615
    eccrine, 629
    lacrimal, 625
    mammary, 620
    oil, 629
    parathyroid, endocrine system and, 622
    pineal
        endocrine system and, 622
        location of, 624
    pituitary
        endocrine system and, 622
        location of, 624
    prostate, 615
    salivary, 605
    sebaceous, 629
    skin, integumentary system and, 629
    sudoriferous, 629
    sweat, 629
    tear, 625
    thymus, 596
        endocrine system and, 622
    thyroid
        endocrine system and, 622
        tructure of, 624
Glans of penis, 615
Glass thermometers, 20, 21
    care of, after each use, 27
    reading, 22
Glasses, safety, as protective eyewear, 8
Glassware
    broken, handling of, 12-13
    safety rules for handling, 329
Glenohumeral joint, 587
Gloves
    for handling laboratory specimens, 12
    latex, sensitivity or allergy to, 7
    as protective equipment, 7-8
    sterile, donning and removing, 207, 209-210
Glucagon, alpha cells and, 609

Glucose in urine, 391
    Tes-Tape test for, 395, 400
    tests for, 391, 394, 395
Glucose control solution, use of, 441-442
Glucosuria, 381, 391
Glutaraldehyde for chemical sterilization, 198
Glutethimide (Doriden), 572-573
Gluteus medius intramuscular injection, 279, 280
Glycogen, 605
Goggles as protective eyewear, 8
Goiter, 622
Golytely prep, 118
Gonadotropin, chorionic, human, 126
    urine tests for, 408
Gonorrhea, 369
    culture for, during prenatal physical
        examination, 131
    smears and cultures to detect, 367, 370
Goosebumps, 629
Gowning, positioning, and draping patient for
        physical examination, 84-91
Gowns as protective equipment, 8-9
Gram stain, 361-362
Granulocyte, 416
Graves vaginal speculum, 80
Gray matter, 599
Growth(s)
    physical; *see* Physical growth
    small, materials for removing, 220
Growth hormone, 622
Guaiac test, 347
Guarding pain, 66
Guidelines for Adolescent Preventive
        Services, 135
Guthrie blood test to diagnose phenylketonuria,
        156, 157-158
Gynecologic examination, 91, 98
Gynecology, 91

H

Habituation, 249
Haemophilus b polysaccharide vaccine, 159
Hair, 629
Hair follicles, integumentary system and, 629
Halsted mosquito forceps, 213
Hammer, percussion, 80, 83
Hand, anatomy and physiology of, 587-588
Hand lotion, handwashing and use of, 6-7
Handling and storage of drugs, 258-259, 261
Handwashing, 6-7
    medical asepsis and, 177
    procedure for, 184-185, 186
Hanging drop culture, 338
Hardening of arteries, 595
Harrison Narcotic Act of 1914, 251
Hazards, communications of, to employees, 4-5
HBV; *see* Hepatitis B virus
HCG; *see* Human chorionic gonadotropin
HDLs; *see* High-density lipoproteins
Head
    bandage-wrapping techniques for, 237
    circumference of
        of child, measuring, 143
        of infant, measuring, 155
Head band and mirror set, 80
Head-tilt/chin-lift maneuver in cardiopulmonary
        resuscitation, 549, 550
Healing process, stages of, 226
Health, 54
    nutrition and, 634-635
Health care during pregnancy, 126-127
Health history and physical examinations, 53-75
Health issues, employee, 11-13
Health supervision of children, AAP guidelines
        for, 137

Hearing examination, 119-120
Heart
    abbreviations related to, 67, 262
    cardiovascular system and, 595
    conduction system of, 527, 528, 595
    in frontal section, 593
    pumping action of, blood pressure and, 36
    workings of, 525, 526-527
Heart attack, 595
    signals and actions for survival of, 554
Heart disease, 595
    increased risk for, menopause and, 620
Heart murmurs, heart sounds and, 529
Heart rate, production of, 528
Heart sounds during cardiac cycle, 529
Heartbeat
    control of, cardiac cycle and, 528
    variations in rhythm of, 29; *see also* Pulse
Heat
    dry, 499-500; *see also* Thermotherapy
    local applications of; *see* Thermotherapy
    moist, 500-501; *see also* Thermotherapy
    and moisture in steam sterilization, 189
Heating pad, electric, use of, 499
Heel bone, 588
Height and weight, physical measurements
        of, 41, 46-47
    of children, 139
Helper cells, 14
Hema-Combistix test, 388
Hemangioma, identification of, 631
Hemastix test, 389
Hematocrit, 450
    screening for, and copper sulfate, 434
Hematology, 323, 415-469
    blood chemistries, 437-448
    blood components, functions, and
            formation, 416-418
    blood groups and types, 452
    blood tests, 433-436
    complete blood count, 449-452
    venipuncture technique, 433-436
Hematopoiesis, skeletal system and, 588
Hematuria, 381, 391
Hemoccult slide test on stool specimen, 349-352
Hemoglobin, 416, 449-450, 594
Hemolysis, 416
Hemoptysis, 353
Hemorrhage, 594
    first aid for, 557-560
Hemorrhagic shock, 555
Hemostatic agent, 255
Hemostatic forceps, 213
Hemostats, types of, 213
Hepatic flexure, 609
Hepatitis, 15-16
    "delta," 16
    non-A, non-B, 16
Hepatitis A, 15
Hepatitis B, 15-16
Hepatitis B vaccine, 159
Hepatitis C, 16
Hepatitis D, 16
Hepatitis E, 16
Hepatobiliary scan, 482
Herpes, 369
Herpes simplex, 14
Herpes simplex viruses, 371-373
HHS; *see* Department of Health and Human
        Services
High-density lipoproteins (HDLs), 642
High-fiber diet, 658
Hilum of kidney, 615
Hip joint, 587, 588
Hirschman anoscope, 78
His, bundle of, 528

Histology, 324, 339
History, 55-58
    assisting with, 58-59
    family, 55
    health, physical examinations and, 53-75
    medical, past, and drug dosage and
            action, 271
    past, 55
    patient
        abbreviations related to, 67
        pediatric, 140-142
            during pregnancy, 126-127
    and physical examination, 54-61
    preprinted forms for, 56-57
    of present illness, 55
    of present pregnancy, 127, 131
    social and occupational, 55
HIV; *see* Human immunodeficiency virus
HIV antibody test, 15
HIV dementia, 14
HIV disease, 13; *see also* Acquired immune
        deficiency syndrome
    signs and symptoms of, 14-15
HIV infection, diagnosis of, 15
HIV-positive people, drug therapy for, 15
HIVID; *see* Zalcitabine
Hoarseness of voice, 612
Hodgkin's disease, 114-115
Holter monitoring, 538-543
Homeostasis, 581, 596, 615, 622
Hormone(s), 255, 594, 622
    growth, 622
    parathyroid, 622
    vaginal secretions for evaluation of, 363
Hormone determinations with urine tests, 408
Hormone-replacement therapy (HRT),
            menopause and, 620-621
Hornet stings, first aid for, 557
Hospital departments, abbreviations related
        to, 68, 263
Hospital employees
    with AIDS, 12
    communications of hazards to, 4-5
    health issues for, 11-13
    immunosuppressed individuals as, 12
Host, susceptible, 172-173
Hot water bottle, use of, 499-500
Household system equivalents, 269, 270
HRT; *see* Hormone-replacement therapy\par
HSV; *see* Herpes simplex viruses
Hubbard tank, 501
Human bites, first aid for, 556-557
Human chorionic gonadotropin, 126, 625
    urine tests for, 408
Human immunodeficiency virus
    infections with, 13-15
    transmission of, 14
Human Nutrition Information Service of U.S.
        Department of Agriculture, 640
Human reservoirs for disease, 172
Human Ultralente insulin, 291
Humerus, 587
Hydrochloric acid, gastric juices containing, 609
Hydrotherapy, 503-504
Hymen, 620
Hyperbilirubinemia, 416
Hypercalcemia, 416, 622
Hypercholesteremia, 416
Hyperchromia, 416
Hypercythemia, 416
Hyperemia, 417
Hyperextension, 510
Hyperglycemia, 417
    first aid for, 568-569
Hyperkalemia, 417
Hypernatremia, 417

Hyperopia, 120
Hyperoxemia, 417
Hyperpnea, 33
Hyperproteinemia, 417
Hypertension, 36, 37, 595, 651-653, 661
    detection and evaluation of, 37-38
    diagnosis of, 37
    long-term management of, 39
    myths about, 39
    patient history and evaluation of, 37-38
    recommended action for, 38
    salt and, 651-653, 661
    terms related to, 36
Hyperthyroidism, 622
Hyperventilation, 33
    first aid for, 567-568
Hypnotic agent, 255
Hypo, 417
Hypocalcemia, 622
Hypoglycemia, 622
    first aid for, 568-569
Hypophysis, 622
Hypotension, 36, 37
Hypotensive agents, 254
Hypothermia, 496
Hypothyroidism, 622
Hypovolemic shock, 555
Hypoxemia, 417
    signs and symptoms of, 264
Hypoxia, 33
Hysterosalpingogram, 473

I

Ice collars, 502
Ice massage, 503
Icon Strep A test, 358
Ictotest, 389, 394-395
IDDM; *see* Insulin-dependent diabetes mellitus
Idiosyncrasy, drug, 249, 272
Ileitis, 609
Ileocecal valve, 609
Ileum, 608, 609
Illiterate people, measuring distance visual
        acuity in, 123
Illness, present, history of, 55
Illuminator of microscope, 332-333
Immune deficiency syndrome, acquired; *see*
        Acquired immune deficiency
        syndrome
Immune response, phases of, 174, 175
Immune sera, 176
Immune system, 174-176
Immunity, 172, 174, 176
Immunization consent forms, 161-163
Immunizations, 159, 170
    recommended schedule for, 139
Immunochemistry, 324
Immunosuppression, individuals with, as hospital
        employees, 12
Immunosuppressive agents, 255, 353
Implant, subdermal, 260
    for drug administration, 267
Implantation, 620
    appearance of uterus and uterine tubes from
            fertilization to, 618
Impression of patient's condition, 61-62
Inactivated vaccines, 174
Incident, exposure, 2
Incision, 223, 226
    and drainage of abscess or cyst, materials
            for, 220
    first aid for, 569
    identification of, 631
Incisional biopsy, 204
Incontinence, 343, 603, 615
Incubation, 170, 339

Incus, 625
Indicators, chemical sterilization, 192-194
Indirect transmission of disease, 172
Induced immunity, 174
Induration, 300
Infants; *see also* Children
    cardiopulmonary resuscitation for, 551
    carrying, techniques for, 153
    chest circumference of, measuring, 155
    head circumference of, measuring, 155
    length of, measuring, 154-155
    management of obstructed airway in, 553
    obtaining urine specimen from, 155, 156
    temperature of, taking, 27
    weight of, measuring, 154
Infarction, myocardial, definition of, 525
Infection, 170
    body's defenses against, 173-177
    HIV, 13-15
    in open wounds, signs of, 569
    opportunistic, in AIDS patients, 12
    signs and symptoms of, 176-177
    types of, 170
Infection control, 168-201
Infection control systems, 5-6
Infectious materials, potentially, 2
Infectious mononucleosis, 417
Infectious process and causative agents, 169-173
Infectious waste, handling of, 11
Infiltration anesthesia, 207
Inflammation, signs and symptoms of, 176
Inflammatory pelvic disease, 369
Inflammatory response, 176
Inflation bulb of sphygmomanometer, 40
Influenza vaccine, guide for use of, 178
Information, statistic, medical records
        providing, 65
Informed consent
    for IUD insertion, 223
    for minor surgery, 213, 214
Infrared radiation, application of, 499
Infrared radiation temperature measurement,
        20, 22, 27-28, 30-31
Infrared tympanic thermometry, 20, 22, 27-28,
        30-31
Inhalants, 572-573
Inhalation route of drug administration, 266
Inherited immunity, 174
Injections, 273-295
    administration of, supplies and equipment
        for, 273-276
    anatomic sites for, 278-283
    body areas to avoid with, 273
    in child, 159, 160
    dangers and complications associated
        with, 273
    insulin, 284, 294-295
    intradermal; *see* Intradermal injections
    intramuscular; *see* Intramuscular injections
    medications and diluents for, 276
    needles for, selection of size of, 276,
        278, 279
    parenteral, angles of insertion for, 283
    reasons for, 273
    reconstitution of powdered drug for, 276
    skin cleansing before, 276
    subcutaneous, 279-280, 282
        administration of, 293-294
    syringes for, selection of size of, 276,
        278, 279
Injector, Tubex, using, 284, 285
Inoculate, 339
Insect in ear, 565
Insect bites and stings, first aid for, 556-557
Inspection in physical examination, 59, 60

Inspiration, respiration and, 609
Instillation
    of drug, 266
    ear, 310, 313-314
    eye, 311
    of eye ointment, 318
    of eyedrops, 316-317
Instrument Protectors for sterilization, 188, 190
Instruments
    biopsy, for minor surgery, 213
    inspection of, before sterilization, 188
    for minor surgery, 212-213
    for physical examinations, 78-82
    sanitizing, 187
    wrapping, for sterilization, 188, 189, 191
Insufflator, 80, 82
Insulin, 622
    beta cells and, 609
Insulin injections, 284, 294-295
    sites and factors influencing absorption
        of, 284, 294
Insulin preparations and concentrations, 284, 291
Insulin reaction, first aid for, 568-569
Insulin syringes, 274
Insulin-dependent diabetes mellitus (IDDM),
        568-569
Integrated medical record, 328
Integration, nervous system and, 596, 599
Integumentary system, 629-632
Intercostal muscles, 587
Intermittent fever, 21
Intermittent pulse, 31
Internal eye examinations, 125-126
Internal respiration, 31, 609
International certificates of vaccination, 180-183
Internuncial fibers, 599
Interstitial fluid, 596
Intervertebral disks, 586, 587
Interview, patient, assisting with, 58-59
Intestinal secretions, sources of, 607
Intractable pain, 66
Intradermal injections, 280-283
    administration of, 303-305
    in child, 159
Intradermal skin tests, diagnostic allergy tests
        and, 299-309
Intramuscular injections, 278-279
    administration of, 286-291
    in child, 159, 160
    Z-tract technique for, 292
Intrauterine device, insertion of, 222-224
Intrinsic muscles of hand, 588
Inunction route of drug administration, 266
Inventory, controlled substances, 264
Inversion, 510
Involuntary muscle, 591
Involuntary urination, 603, 615
Iodine compounds, 472-473
Ionizing, 471
Iontophoresis, 519
Ipecac, 261
    syrup of, poisoning and, 570
Iris, 625
Iris scissors, 212, 219
Iron, 646, 661
Iron-deficiency anemia, 594
Irradiate, 471
Irradiation, 471
Irregular bones, 582
Irregular pulse, 31
Irrigation
    of drug, 266
    ear, 310-311, 314-316
    of eyes, 311, 318-319
Ischemia, 417

Ishihara plates for color vision testing, 125
Islands of Langerhans, 609
Isoelectric line in electrocardiogram, 528
IUD; *see* Intrauterine device
IVAC thermometer, 20, 22

J

Jackknife or proctologic position, 86
Jaw, fractured, first aid for, 567
Jaw thrust maneuver in cardiopulmonary
        resuscitation, 549
Jejunum, 609
Jellyfish bites, first aid for, 557
Juvenile onset diabetes, 568-569

K

Kaposi's sarcoma, 13
Kelly forceps, 219
Kelly hemostatic forceps, 213
Kelly proctoscope, 81
Keloid, identification of, 631
Kerosene, ingestion of, first aid for, 570
Keto-Diastix test, 389
Ketone bodies in urine, 391
Ketostix test, 389
Kidney
    anatomy of, 382, 383, 612-615
    disease of, urine findings in, 392-393
Kidney function profile, 467
Kidney scan, 482
Kidney, ureter, bladder test, 480
Kilograms and pounds, conversion of, 47, 48
Kilovoltage, effect of on images, 485
Kitchen cleanser, washing electrocardiogram
        electrodes with, 531
Kling bandage, 233
Knee joint, 588
    bandage-wrapping techniques for, 235
Knee-chest position, 87
Knee-jerk reflex, 599
Kneecap, 588
Knobs of microscope, 332
Korotkoff sounds, 41
Kovorkian biopsy forceps, 212
Kovorkian curette, 212
KUB; *see* Kidney, ureter, bladder test

L

Label(s)
    biohazard, 340
    warning, 4
Labeling
    drug, 261
    food; *see* Food labeling
    proper, for blood sample, 421
Labia, 620
Labophot microscope, 330
Laboratory coats as protective equipment, 8-9
Laboratory orientation, 322-336
Laboratory report records, 326-327
Laboratory reports, filing, in patient's medical
        record, 325
Laboratory request form to order pregnancy
        test, 127
Laboratory safety, 329
Laboratory specimens, handling of, 11-12
Laboratory tests
    abbreviations related to, 68, 262-263
    cost containment for, 324
Laboratory
    clinical, 2
    labeling of specimens for, 324
    typical, 323-324
Labored breathing, 33
Labstix test, 388

Labyrinth, 625
Laceration, 223, 226
    first aid for, 569
    identification of, 631
    suturing, materials for, 220
Lacrimal glands, 625
Lacteals, 596
Large intestine, 605, 608, 609
Laryngeal mirror, 80, 82
Laryngoscope, 78, 82
Larynx, respiration and, 612
Lasix, 261
Latent infection, 170
Latex gloves, sensitivity or allergy to, 7
Laundry, contaminated, 2
    handling of, 4
Laws governing use of drugs, 251
Laxative, 255
LDLs; *see* Low-density lipoproteins
Lead, contamination of tap water with, 650
Lead wires, application of, for electrocardiogram, 535, 536
Leads, electrocardiogram, 532, 534, 537
Lean, food labeling and, 657
Left lateral position, 88-89
Left lower quadrant, 582
Left upper quadrant, 582
Leg, 588
    lower, bandage-wrapping techniques for, 235
    Tubegauz bandaging of, 239
Legal classification of drugs, 251-252
Length of infant, measuring, 154-155
Lens of eye, 625, 629
Lente insulin, 291
Leukemia, 116-117, 417
Leukocytes, 594
    in urine, 391
Leukocytosis, 417, 594
Leukoencephalopathy, multifocal, progressive, 14
Leukopenia, 417, 594
Lichenification, identification of, 631
Lie detector, 605
Lienteric stool, 347
Lifting techniques, 510-512
Ligaments, 582
Ligate, 204
Ligature, 204
Light, food labeling and, 657
Light source of microscope, 332
Light therapy, 496
Lighter fluid, ingestion of, first aid for, 570
Limb leads, electrocardiogram and, 532, 533, 535-537
Liniment, 261
Linoleic acid, 639
Lipids, 637-642
    blood, effects of fats on, 638, 641
Lipoproteins, 642
Liquid culture media, 363
Liquid drugs, terms to describe, 260-261
Lite, food labeling and, 657
Lithotomy position, 84-85
Liver, 609
    digestive system and, 605
    disease of, urine findings in, 392-393
Liver function profile, 467
Liver scan, 482
LLQ; *see* Left lower quadrant
Local action of drug, 272
Local anesthesia, 207
    materials for administering, 219-220
Local anesthetics, allergic reaction to, 207
Localized infection, 170
    signs and symptoms of, 176
Lofstrand (Canadian) crutch, 513

Long bones, 582
Lotions, 261
    hand, handwashing and use of, 6-7
Low fat, food labeling and, 657
Low-sodium diet, 659-660
Low-cholesterol foods, choosing, 642, 643-645
Low-density lipoproteins, 642
Low-fat diet, 658-659
Low-fiber diet, 658
Low-residue diet, 658
Low-salt diet, 659-660
Low-saturated foods, choosing, 642, 643-645
Lower extremity(ies)
    anatomy and physiology of, 588
    bones of, 585
    range-of-motion exercises for, 508
Lozenges, 260
LSD, 572-573
Lubb dupp heart sound, 529
Lumbar nerves, 603
Lumbar puncture, 373-376
Lumbar vertebrae, 587
Lung(s)
    abbreviations related to, 67, 262
    cancer of, 116-117
    respiration and, 612
Lung perfusion, 482
Lung ventilation, 482
Lunula of nails, 629
LUQ; *see* Left upper quadrant
Lyme disease, tick bites and, 557
Lymph channels, 596
Lymph glands, 596
Lymph nodes, 596
Lymphangiogram, 473
Lymphatic ducts, 596
Lymphatic system, 591
Lymphocytes, 450, 596
Lymphoid tissue as barrier to disease and infection, 174
Lymphoma, non-Hodgkin's, 13, 114-115
Lysocytosis, 417

M

Macrocyte, 417
Macrominerals, 646
Macroscopic, 339
Macule, identification of, 631
Magnesium, 649
Magnetic resonance imaging, 477
Major minerals, 646
Male reproductive system, anatomy and physiology of, 615, 616-619
Malignant hypertension, 36
Malleoli, 588
Malleus, 625
Mammary glands, 620
Mammography, 474
Mantoux test
    to diagnose tuberculosis, 283, 306
    during prenatal physical examination, 131
Marijuana, 572-573
Masks and protective eyewear, 8
Massage, 505
Materials
    for office surgeries, 218-222
    identification of, in laboratory, 329
    potentially infectious, 2
    suture, 207, 210-212
Mature onset diabetes, 568-569
Mayo scissors, 212
Mayo stand, 204
Measles, German
    stages of infection with, 173
    vaccine against, guide for use of, 179
Measles vaccine, 179

Measles-mumps-rubella vaccine, 159
Meatus, auditory, external, 312
Mechanical soft diet, 658
Media; *see* Culture media
Medic-Alert bracelet or necklace
    allergic reaction to drugs and, 556
    diabetes and, 568
Medical abbreviations, 66-69, 262-263
Medical asepsis, 168-201
Medical assistant
    and laboratories, liaison and responsibilities of, 324-325
    minor surgery assistance provided by, 215-218
    responsibilities of
        during physical examination, 83-84
        during prenatal examinations, 134
        during radiologic procedures, 486-490
Medical history, past, and drug dosage and action, 271
Medical microbiology, 169, 170, 323, 339
Medical records, 53-54
    and documentation, 64-65
    filing laboratory reports in, 325
    integrated, 328
    management of, 64-65
    problem-oriented, 328
    retention of, 65
    source-oriented, 325
    statistic information provided by, 65
Medication; *see* Drugs
Medium, culture; *see* Culture media
Medulla
    of brain, anatomy and physiology of, 599
    of kidney, 615
Melanin, 629, 630
Melanocytes, 629
Melanoma, 116-117, 630
Melatonin, 622
Melena, 347
Membrane, tympanic, 312
Meninges, 599
Menopause, 603, 620-621
Menstrual cramps, 620
Menstruation, 603, 619, 620, 621
Mensuration in physical examination, 60
Mercury manometer, 39
Mercury spill kit, 11
Mercury spills, 11
Mescaline, 572-573
Metabolism, nutrition and, 635
Metacarpals, 587
Metal sigmoidoscope, 82
Metastasis of cancer by lymphatic system, 596
Metatarsals of toes, 588
Metazoa causing disease, 172
Metric system equivalents, 269, 270
Metricide for chemical sterilization, 198
Metzenbaum blunt blade scissors, 219
Metzenbaum scissors, 212
Microbiology, medical, 169, 170, 323, 339
Microcyte, 417
Microglobulin test, beta-2, 14
Microminerals, 646
Microorganisms, 169, 339
Microscope, 330-334
Microscopic, 339
Microscopic agents, methods to control, 186-198
Microscopic examination of urine sediment, 395, 400-403
Microstix tests, 389
Microstix-3 reagent strip for bacteriuria testing, 407-408
Microtainer system, 433
Middeltoid intramuscular injection, 279, 280
Midstream urine specimen, 343

Midstream urine specimen,—cont'd
    collecting, 344-346
Mild hypertension, 36
Milk, 2%, amount of fat in, 642
Milliamperage, effect of on images, 485
Miltex fiberglass tape measure, 79
Miltex tuning forks, 79
Minerals, 646, 649, 661
Minor surgery, 207, 210-224
    anesthesia for, 207
    assisting with, 215-218
    informed consent for, 213, 214
    instruments used for, 212-213
        care of, 213
    listing of procedures for, 207
    materials for, 218-222
    preparing patient for, 213-215
    surgical asepsis and, 202-246
Minor tranquilizers, 572-573
Miotic agent, 255, 312
Mirror, laryngeal, 80, 82
Mitral valve, 595
Modality, 496
Moisture and heat in steam sterilization, 189
Monilial vaginitis, smear for, 367
Monitoring, ambulatory cardiac, electrocardio-
        graphy and, 538-543
Monocytes, 450
Monoject safety syringes, 276, 277-278
Mononucleosis, 417
Monounsaturated fat, 638
Mons veneris, 620
Monunsaturated fatty acids, 639
Morning glory *seeds*, 572-573
Mosquito bites, first aid for, 557
Mosquito forceps, 219
Motor development, guideposts in, 136
Motor neurons, 603
Mouth, 605
    cancer of, 116-117
Mouth-to-mouth resuscitation, 550
Mouth-to-stoma resuscitation, 549
Movement, bowel, 347
MRI; *see* Magnetic resonance imaging
Mucous membrane exposure to body fluids from
    AIDS patients, 11-12
Mucous membranes as barrier to disease and
    infection, 173
Multifocal leukoencephalopathy, progressive, 14
Multiphasic tests, 462
Multiple-dose containers, 276
Multiple-glass test, 343
Multiple-glass urine specimen, 343
Multistix 10 SG reagent strips for urinalysis, 387
Multistix tests, 388, 389
Mumps vaccine, guide for use of, 179
Muscle cells, 581
Muscle relaxant, 255
Muscle tissue, 581
Muscles, 588-591
Muscular system, anatomy and physiology of,
    588-591
Musculoskeletal system
    abbreviations related to, 67, 262
    terms related to, 66
Mycobacterium avium complex, 14
Mycology, 323
Mydriatic agent, 255, 312
Myelogram, 473
Myocardial infarction, 525, 595
Myocarditis, 595
Myocardium, 525, 526, 595
Myopia, 120

N

Nails, integumentary system and, 629
Names, drug, 248, 250
Narcan, 261
Narcotic agent, 255
Nasal cannula for oxygen administration,
    264, 265
Nasal passages, 611
Nasal speculum, 81, 83
Nasopharyngeal cultures, 354, 357
National Academy of Sciences, Food Nutrition
    Board of, 655
National Cancer Institute, 651
National Childhood Vaccine Injury Act of
    1988, 159
Natural immunity, 174
Near visual acuity, measuring, 124
Neck injury, possible, cardiopulmonary
        resuscitation and, 551-552
Neck
    crescentic roll of, 591
    fractured, first aid for, 567
    of tooth, 605
    vocabulary referring to, 66
Necrosis, 170
Needle biopsy, 204
    of breast, materials for, 222
Needle holder, 219
    for minor surgery, 213
Needles, 211
    for injections, 274
        selection of, 276, 278, 279
    and other sharps, handling of, 11
    suture materials and, 207, 210-212
    syringes and, wrapping, for steam
        sterilization, 191
Needlesticks, 11-12
    preventing, guidelines for, 283-284
Negative culture, 338
Negative findings, 54
Nephron, anatomy of, 383
Nephron unit, 615
Nerve block anesthesia, 207
Nerve cells, 581
Nerve damage, peripheral nervous system
    and, 603
Nerve fibers, 599
Nerve(s), 596-605
    cochlear, 625
    cranial, 603
    efferent, 603
    integumentary system and, 629
    olfactory, 612
    peripheral, 603
    spinal, 603
    vestibular, 625
Nervous system
    anatomy and physiology of, 596-605
    autonomic; *see* Autonomic nervous system
    central; *see* Central nervous system
    peripheral; *see* Peripheral nervous system
Nervous tissue, 581
Neurogenic shock, 555
Neurologic examination, 118, 119
Neurologic pinwheel, 80
Neurological examination, vocabulary
        referring to, 66
Neurons, 581, 603
Neutralization and dilution of poisons, 570-571
Neutrophils, 450
Niacin, 647-648
Nikon microscopes, 330
911 emergency telephone system, 554
Nines, rule of, burns and, 560-562
Nipples, 620

Nitrite in urine, 391
Nitrite test for bacteriuria testing, 407
Nitroglycerin tablets, chest pain and, 564
Nitroglycerin, 261
N-Multistix test, 388
No added salt diet, 659-660
Nodule, identification of, 631
Non-A, non-B hepatitis, 16
Non-English speaking people, measuring
        distance visual acuity in, 123
Non-Hodgkin's lymphoma, 13, 114-115
Nonabsorbable sutures, 210-211
Nonadhering dressings, 227
Nonbarbiturate sedatives, 572-573
Noninsulin-dependent diabetes, 568-569
Nonprescription drugs, 252
Nonstriated muscle, 591
Norepinephrine, 622
Normal flora, 170
Normal sinus rhythm, 529
Nose
    respiration and, 612
    structure of, 611
    terms related to, 66
Nosebleed, 612
    first aid for, 565
Nosepiece of microscope, 330-331
Notes, progress, 62
NPH insulin, 291
Nuclear medicine, 481-482; *see also* Radiology
Numeric Scale for rating pain, 144
Nutrients, 634
    nutrition and, 635-650
Nutrition, 634-661
Nutrition facts, food labeling and, 656-660

O

Obesity, definition of, 634
Objective findings in POMR, 63
Objectives of microscope, 330-331
    use of, 333
Objects Chart for eye examination, 120
Obstetric examinations and record, 126-134
Obstipation, 347
Obstructed airway, management of, 552-553
Occult blood, 347
Occult blood test, 347
Occupational exposure, 2
Ochsner-Kocher hemostatic forceps, 213
Ocular, definition of, 312
Office policy for office emergencies, 548
Office surgery, materials for, 218-222
Official books on drugs, 250-251
Oil glands, 629
Ointment, 261
    eye, instillation of, 318
Olfactory nerves, 612
Oliguria, 381, 384
Omega-3 fatty acids, 638
One Touch Blood Glucose Meter, use of,
    442-445
Open fracture, first aid for, 566-567
Open wounds, 223, 226
    first aid for, 569
Operating scissors, 212
Ophthalmic, 312
Ophthalmology, 312
Ophthalmoscope, 81, 83
Ophthalmoscopic examination, 125
Opiates, 572-573
Opportunistic infections in AIDS patients, 12
Optic nerve, 629
Optiphot microscope, 330
Oral cancer, 116-117
Oral examination, 78

Oral route of drug administration, 266
Oral temperature, procedure for taking, 23-24
Oral temperature readings, contraindications to, 22
Organisms, pathogenic, terms to describe, 223
Organs, 578
  anatomy and physiology of, 581-582
Orthopnea, 33
Orthostatic blood pressure, 36, 41, 45
Orthostatic hypertension, 36
Os calcis, 588
Oscilloscope, 471, 525
Osteoporosis, increased risk for, menopause and, 620
Otic, 312
Otology, 312
Otoscope, 79, 83, 312
  ear examination using, 119
Oucher pain rating scale, 144
Oval window, 625
Ovaries, 615
  cancer of, 116-117
  endocrine system and, 625
Overweight
  complications of, 41
  relationship between disease risk and, 634, 635
Ovulation, 603
Ovum, 581, 615
Oxygen
  administration of, 264-265
  respiration and, 609
Oxytocin, 622

P

P wave, cardiac cycle and, 527, 529
p24 antibody test, 14
p24 antigen test, 14
P-R interval, 527, 529
Pacemaker, 525
  of heart, 528
Packages, sterile, opening, 204-206
PACs; *see* Premature atrial contractions
Pain, 65, 66
  abdominal, first aid for, 556
  chest, first aid for, 564
Pain rating scales for children, 144
Pain threshold, 66
Palmar flexion of wrist, 587
Palpation
  in physical examination, 59, 60
  of uterus and adnexa, bimanual, 105
Palpation method for measuring blood pressure, 41
Pancreas, 609
  anatomy and physiology of, 624
  cancer of, 116-117
  digestive system and, 605-609
  disease of, urine findings in, 392-393
  endocrine system and, 622
Pancreatic juice, 605-609
Pantothenic acid, 646, 647-648
Papanicolaou smear, 78, 366
  pelvic examination and, 98-99, 100-105
  during prenatal physical examination, 131
Papanicolaou test, 78, 366
Paper, electrocardiogram, 529, 530, 537
Paper waste, handling of, 11
Papillae of dermis, 630
PAPNET, 99
Papule, identification of, 632
Para-aminobenzoic acid (PABA), skin protection and, 630
Paraplegia, 603
Parasites, 347
  causing disease, 171-172

Parasites,—cont'd
  in urine, 403
Parasitology, 323
Parasympathetic system of autonomic nervous system, 604-605
Parathyroid glands, endocrine system and, 622
Parathyroid hormone, 622
Parenteral, 249
Parenteral dosage, 249
Parenteral injections, angles of insertion for, 283
Parenteral route of drug administration, 266
Paroxysmal atrial tachycardia, electrocardiogram and, 530
Parrafin wax hand bath, 504
Partial-thickness burns, first aid for, 560, 562
Passive immunity, 174, 176
Past medical history, 55
  and drug dosage and action, 271
PAT; *see* Paroxysmal atrial tachycardia
Patch
  identification of, 632
  skin, 260
  transdermal, for drug administration, 267
Patch test to diagnose allergies, 300-301
Patella, 588
Patella reflex, eliciting, 119
Patellar ligament, 588
Pathogenic, definition of, 170, 339
Pathogens, 169, 339
  bloodborne, 2
  terms to describe, 223
Patient care areas, cleaning of, 3, 11
Patient diary, ambulatory cardiac monitoring and, 541, 542
Patient history; *see* History
Patient teaching, nutrition and, 660
Patient(s)
  AIDS, body fluids from, mucous membrane or conjunctival exposure to, 11-12
  condition of, impression of, 61-62
  education of, about drug use, 272-273
  gowning, positioning, and draping, for physical examination, 84-91
  post-test instructions to, treadmill stress test and, 543-544
  preparation of
    for electrocardiogram, 534-535
    for minor surgery, 213-215
PDR; *see* Physician's Drug Reference
Pediatric examinations, 134-163; *see also* Children
  general points for, 135, 138-139
Pediatric patient history, 140-142
Pediatrics, 134
Peel-down packages, opening, 205
Peg bandage, 233
Pelvic cavity, 580
Pelvic disease, inflammatory, 369
Pelvic examination, 78
  and Pap smear, 98-99, 100-105
Pelvis
  anatomy and physiology of, 586, 587
  examination of, during pregnancy, 131
Penis, 615
Penlet, skin puncture using, 429, 430
Peptic ulcer diet, 660
Percussion in physical examination, 59, 60
Percussion hammer, 80, 83
Pericarditis, 525, 595
Pericardium, 526, 595
Perineum, 620
  female, 617
Peripheral nerves, 599
  anatomy and physiology of, 603
Peripheral nervous system
  anatomy and physiology of, 603

Peripheral nervous system—cont'd
  functions of, 603, 604
Peripheral resistance of blood vessels to blood flow, blood pressure and, 36
Peristalsis, 609
Permanent protection of medical records, 64
Pernicious anemia, 594
Personal history of present pregnancy, 127, 131
Personal protective equipment, 7-9
PET; *see* Positron emission tomography
Petechiae, identification of, 632
pH of urine, 390
Phagocytes, 596
Phagocytosis, 174, 417
Phalanges
  of fingers, 587
  of toes, 588
Pharmaceutical preparations, 258
  terms related to, 260-261
Pharmacology, 248
  and drug administration, principles of, 247-298
  and drugs, 248-252
Pharynx, 609
  respiration and, 612
Phencyclidine, 572-573
Phenistix test, 389
  to diagnose phenylketonuria, 156, 408
Phenylketonuria, 155-156, 159
  urine tests to diagnose, 408-409
Phone-A-Gram, electrocardiography and, 538
Phonophoresis, 519
Phosphorus, 649
Phosphorus burns, first aid for, 563
Phycology, 323
Physiatrics, 496 *see also* Physical therapy
Physiatrists, 496
Physical barriers to disease and infection, 173-174
Physical condition of patient and drug dosage and action, 271
Physical examination, 59-61
  abbreviations related to, 67, 262
  complete, 95-98
  general instructions and responsibilities for medical assistant during, 83-84
  gowning, positioning, and draping patient for, 84-91
  health history and, 53-75
  history and, 54-61
  instruments used for, 78-82
  prenatal, and diagnostic tests, 131-133
  routine and special, preparing for and assisting with, 76-167
  special, 61
  thorough, essentials of, 60-61
Physical findings, recording, vocabulary used for, 65-66
Physical growth
  during childhood
    general trends in, 138, 139, 143
    patterns of, recording, 143
  patterns in, 139, 143
    in boys, 145-148
    in girls, 149-152
Physical measurements, 18-52
  of height and weight, 41, 46-47
Physical medicine, 496; *see also* Physical therapy
Physical sign, 54
Physical therapy, 495-523
  body mechanics and, 510-512
  and cold applications (cryotherapy), 498, 501-503
  conditions benefiting from, 520-522
  and heat applications (thermotherapy), 498-501

Physical therapy,—cont'd
    physical disabilities and, 519-521
Physician's Drug Reference, 249, 250
Physiology, definition of, 578
Physiotherapists, 496
Pia mater, 599
Pill-rolling movement of fingers, 588
Pills, 260
Pilus, 629
Pinching movement of fingers, 588
Pineal gland, 622, 624
Pinion head of microscope, 332
Pinwheel, neurologic, 80
Pitocin, 261
Pituitary gland, 622, 624
PKU; *see* Phenylketonuria
Placebo, 249
Placenta, 620, 625
Plain splinter forceps, 213
Plain-tipped forceps, 212, 213, 219
Plan in POMR, 63
Plaque, identification of, 632
Plasma, 417
Plaster of Paris cast application, 240-241
Platelets, 588, 594
Pleura, 612
Pleural effusion, 612
Pleurisy, 612
Pneumocystis carinii pneumonia, 13
Pneumonia
    Pneumocystic carinii, 13
    stages of infection with, 173
Pneumothorax, 612
Poikilocytosis, 417
Poison control centers, 570, 571-573
Poisoning, first aid for, 570-571
Poisons, dilution and neutralization of, 570-571
Poker Chip pain rating scale, 144
Polio vaccine, trivalent oral, 159
Poliomyelitis vaccine, guide for use of, 178-179
Polycythemia, 417
Polygraph, 605
Polyunsaturated fat, 638
Polyunsaturated fatty acids, 639
Polyuria, 381, 384
POMR; *see* Problem-oriented medical record
Popliteal artery, determining pulse rate at, 32
Portals of exit of pathogens, 172
Positioning, gowning, and draping patient for
        physical examination, 84-91
Positive culture, 338
Positive findings, 54
Positron emission tomography, 475-476
Postoperative, definition of, 204
Postpartum visit, 6 weeks', 134
Postprandial urine specimen, 343
Postural hypertension, 36
Posture; *see* Body mechanics
Potassium, 649
Potentially infectious materials, 2
Potentiating interactions of drugs, 272
Pounds and kilograms, conversion of, 47, 48
Powdered drug, reconstitution of
    for injection, 276
    for insulin injection, 295
Powders, 260
PQRST method, chest pain and, 564
Precordial leads, electrocardiogram and, 533
Pregnancy, 126
    ectopic, 620
    health care during, 126-127
    patient history during, 126-127
    present, personal history of, 127, 131
    radioimmunoassay tests to diagnose, 408
    tubal, 620

Pregnancy,—cont'd
    weight gain during, 131
Pregnancy table for expected date of delivery,
        132
Pregnancy tests, 126
    laboratory request form to order, 127
    urine for, 408, 409, 410-411
Premature atrial contractions, 530
Premature ventricular contractions, 530
Prenatal physical examination and diagnostic
        tests, 131-133
Prenatal records, 128-130
Prenatal visits, follow-up, 133
Preoperative, definition of, 204
Prepuce of penis, 615
Preschoolers, measuring distance visual acuity
        in, 122-123, 124
Prescribed medication, 258
Prescription drugs, 252
    top 50, 257
Prescription pads, 258
Prescriptions, 252, 256, 258
    abbreviations and symbols used in, 259
Present illness, history of, 55
Pressure
    blood; *see* Blood pressure
    direct, in controlling severe bleeding, 558
    pulse, 31, 35
    for steam sterilization, 189-190
Pressure bandage in controlling severe
        bleeding, 558
Pressure control valve of sphygmomanometer, 40
Pressure indicators of sphygmomanometer, 40
Pressure points in controlling severe bleeding,
        558, 559
Primary diagnosis, 61
Probe(s)
    cryosurgery unit and, 212
    for minor surgery, 213
Problem list in POMR, 62, 63
Problem-oriented medical record, 62-64, 328
Problem-Oriented System, 62
Proctoscope, 81, 83
Proctoscopy, 99, 109-111, 118
Prodrome, 54, 78
Progestasert intrauterine device, 222, 223
Progesterone, 603, 621, 625
Prognosis, 54, 62
Progress notes in POMR, 62, 63
Progressive multifocal leukoencephalopathy, 14
Pronation, 510
    arm placed in, 587
Prone position, 90
Prophylaxis, 249
Propranolol, sinus bradycardia and, 530
Prostate gland, 615
    cancer of, 116-117
        screening for, 99
Prostatitis, 615
Protection of medical records, permanent, 64
Protective equipment, personal, 7-9
Protective eyewear, masks and, 8
Protein, 636-637, 661
    calories supplied by, 653
    digestion of, gastric juices and, 609
    synthesis of, glycogen and, 605
    in urine, 381, 391
Proteinuria, 381, 391
Protozoa causing disease, 172
Protozoology, 323
Provisional diagnosis, 61-62
Psoriasis, 496
Psychedelic agent, 255
Psychotomimetics, 572-573
PT; *see* Physical therapy

Ptyalin, 609
Puberty, 615
Pubic bone, 620
Pubis, 620
Publication Office of Veterinary and Human
        Toxicology, 571
Pudendum, 620
Puerperium, 126
Puff tonometry, 126
Pulmonary valve, 595
Pulp of tooth, 605
Pulse, 28-31
    in arteries, 594-595
    checking, in cardiopulmonary
            resuscitation, 550
        for infants and small children, 551
    child's, measuring, 143
    radial, taking, 34
Pulse deficit, 29, 31
Pulse pressure, 31, 35
Pumping action of heart, blood pressure and, 36
Punch, biopsy, 213
Punch biopsy, 204
Punch biopsy forceps, 219
    for cervical biopsy, 79
Puncture, 223, 226
    lumbar, 373-376
Puncture wounds, first aid for, 569
Pupil, 625
Pure culture, 338
Pure drug, 249
Purpura, identification of, 632
Purulent drainage, 223
Pus, 594
Pustule, identification of, 632
PVCs; *see* Premature ventricular contractions
Pyelogram, 473
Pylorus, 609
Pyridoxine, 646, 647-648
Pyuria, 381, 403

Q

QDR; *see* Quality Digital Radiography
QRS complex, cardiac cycle and, 527, 529
QRS wave, cardiac cycle and, 527, 529
Q-T interval, cardiac cycle and, 528, 529
QTEST Strep A test, 358
Quadrants of abdomen, 581, 582
Quadriceps tendon, 588
Quadriplegia, 603
Qualitative tests on urine, 381
Quality assurance in hematologic tests, 445-446
Quality control, 328-329
Quantitative tests on urine, 381

R

R wave, cardiac cycle and, 529
Rabies, animal bites and, 556, 557
Radial artery
    compression of, in controlling severe
            bleeding, 558, 559
    determining pulse rate at, 32
Radial pulse, taking, 34
Radiating pain, 66
Radiation, 471
Radiation therapy, 480-481
Radiograph, 471
    preparation of patient and assisting with,
            489-490
Radiography, 471
Radioimmunoassay tests to diagnose pregnancy,
        408
Radioisotope, 471
Radiologic procedures, 470-471

Radiologic procedures,—cont'd
  medical assistant responsibilities during, 486-490
Radiologist, 471
Radiology, diagnostic, and radiation therapy and nuclear medicine, 470-523
Radiolucent, 471
Radionuclide, 471
Radiopaque, 471
Radius, 587
Rales, 33
Random urine specimen, 342
Range-of-motion exercises, 506-508
Ratchet of forceps, 212
RBCs; *see* Red blood cells
RDAs; *see* Recommended Daily Allowances; Recommended Dietary Allowances
Reagent strips
  chemical examination of urine using, 385, 387-388
  urine chemistry analyzers for use with, 388-390
Reagent tests for urinalyses, 388
Reagents, safety rules for handling, 329
Rebound tenderness, 66
Recommended Daily Allowances, 634, 656
Recommended daily servings of basic food groups, 635, 637
Recommended Dietary Allowances, 655-656
Reconstitution of powdered drug
  for injection, 276
  for insulin injection, 295
Recording of blood sample, proper, 421
Records
  for controlled substances prescriptions, 264
  laboratory report, 326-327
  medical, 53-54
  obstetric, 126-134
  prenatal, 128-130
Rectal biopsy punch, 213
Rectal examination, 99, 106-108
Rectal route of drug administration, 266
Rectal temperature, 20
  infant's, taking, 27
  procedure for taking, 26
Rectal temperature readings, contraindications to, 22
Rectum, 605, 609
Recurrent turn during bandaging, 237
Red blood cells, 581, 588, 594
  stained, examination of, 452
  in urine, 401, 403, 404
Red bone marrow, 588
Red cell count, 449
Reduced-calorie diet, 660
References on drugs, 250-251
Reflex, patella, eliciting, 119
Reflotron Plus System, 437, 438
Refraction, 125
Refractometer to determine specific gravity of urine, 384-385
Regular insulin, 291
Regular pulse, 31
Regulated waste, 2
Relative density test, copper sulfate, 434-436
Relaxant, muscle, 255
Remittent fever, 21
Removing and donning sterile gloves, 207, 209-210
Renal hypertension, 36
Renal pelvis, 615
Repolarization, cardiac cycle and, 527
Reproductive system
  anatomy and physiology of, 615-621
  female, 615-621
    abbreviations related to, 67, 262

Reproductive system—cont'd
  male, 615, 616-619
  terms referring to, 66
Reservoir, 170, 172
Resistance, 170
Resistance level of body, 173
Respiration, 31-33, 609
  child's, measuring, 143
  rate of; *see* Respiratory rate
Respiratory rate, 32
  taking, 35
  variations in, 33
Respiratory system
  anatomy and physiology of, 609-612
  as barrier to disease and infection, 173
  vocabulary referring to, 66
Respiratory tract specimens, 353-358
Resuscitation
  cardiopulmonary; *see* Cardiopulmonary resuscitation
  mouth-to-mouth, 550
  mouth-to-stoma, 549
Retention of medical records, 65
Reticulocyte, 417
Retina, 599, 625, 629
Retractors for minor surgery, 213
Reusable equipment, handling of, 12
Review of systems, 55
Rh factor; *see* Rhesus factor
Rhesus factor, 452
Rhythm strip, definition of, 525
Rhythms, electrocardiogram and, 529-531
Riboflavin, 646, 647-648
Ribs, anatomy and physiology of, 586, 587
Rickettsiae causing disease, 171
Rickettsiology, 323
Right lower quadrant, 582
Right upper quadrant, 582
Ring-handle forceps, 213
RLQ; *see* Right lower quadrant
Rochester-Pean hemostatic forceps, 213
Roentgenologic, definition of, 78
Roller bandages, 232-233
  wrapping, 234
Root of tooth, 605
Rosenbaum chart for testing near vision, 124
Rotation, 510
Routine and special physical examinations, preparing for and assisting with, 76-167
Rubella, stages of infection with, 173
Rubella vaccine, guide for use of, 179
Rubeola vaccine, guide for use of, 179
Rule of nines, burns and, 560-562
Rule out, definition of, 62
RUQ; *see* Right upper quadrant

S

SA; *see* Sinoatrial node
Sacral nerves, 603
Sacroiliac joints, 587
Sacrum, 587
Safe Drinking Water Hotline, 650
Safety, laboratory, 329
Safety glasses as protective eyewear, 8
Safety rules for laboratory, 329
Safety-Lok syringe, 274
  procedure for using, 275
Sagittal plane, 579, 586
Salicylate, hyperventilation and, 567
Saliva, 353, 609
Salivary glands, 605, 607
Salt, nutrition and, 651-653
Salt-free diet, 659-660
Sampling, chorionic villi, 133-134
Sanguineous drainage, 223

Sanitization, 186
Sanitizing instruments, 187
Sarcoma, Kaposi's, 13
Saturated fat content of selected foods, 637, 638, 642
Saturated fatty acids, 639
Saturated steam for steam sterilization, 190
Scale
  identification of, 632
  weighing infant on, 154
Scalpel blade and handle, 219
Scalpels for minor surgery, 212
Scapulae, 586, 587
Scapulohumeral joint, 587
Schedule I drugs, 251
Schedule II drugs, 251
Schedule III drugs, 251
Schedule IV drugs, 251
Schedule V drugs, 251
Scissors, types of, 212, 219
Sclera, 625
Scorpion sting, antivenins for, 557
Scratch test to diagnose allergies, 300, 302-303
Screening
  streptococcus, 358
  urine toxicology, 343
Scrotum, 615
Sebaceous cyst, 204
Sebaceous glands, 629
Secondary diagnosis, 61
Secondary hypertension, 36
Second-degree burns, first aid for, 560, 562
Secretion/drainage precautions, 6
Secretions, vaginal, for hormone evaluation, 363
Sedative, 256
  nonbarbiturate, 572-573
Sediment, urine, centrifuged, microscopic examination of, 395, 400-403
Seizures, first aid for, 564-565
Selective action of drug, 272
Selective culture media, 363
Semen, 615
Semi-Fowler's position, 90, 91
Semicircular canals of labyrinth, 625
Semilente insulin, 291
Semilunar valves, 596
Seminal fluid, 615
Seminal vesicles, 615
Senses, special, 625-629
Sensitivity to latex gloves, 7
Sensitivity testing, culture and, bacterial, 363
Sensors, electrocardiogram, 532
Sensory neurons, 603
Sensory system, anatomy and physiology of, 625-629
Sepsis, 170
Septic shock, 555
Septicemia, 417
Serologic, 339
Serology, 323
Serosanguineous drainage, 223
Serous drainage, 223
Serrated forceps, 212, 213
Serum, 417, 418
  immune, 176
Serum pregnancy test, 126
Serum separator tube, 419
Sesamoid bone, 588
Sex and drug dosage and action, 271
Sexually transmitted diseases, 368-369
Shaft of penis, 615
Sharps
  contaminated, 2
  needles and, handling of, 11
Shields, face, 8
Shinbone, 588

Shock, 554-556
  anaphylactic, 249
Short bones, 582
Shoulder girdle
  anatomy and physiology of, 587
  bandage-wrapping techniques for, 236
ShowerSafe waterproof cast and bandage
    cover, 243
Sick-child visits, 155
Sickle-cell anemia, 594
Side effect, 249
Sigmoid flexure, 609
Sigmoidoscopes, 82, 83
Sigmoidoscopy, 99, 109-111, 118
Sign(s), 54, 78
  of infection, 176-177
  of inflammation, 176
  warning, 4
Simple carbohydrates, 645
Simple Descriptive Scale for rating pain, 144
Sims' or left lateral position, 88-89
Sims vaginal speculum, 83
Single-channel electrocardiograph, 535, 536
Single-use solutions, 276
Sinoatrial node, 528
Sinus arrhythmia, 530
Sinus bradycardia, 530
Sinus rhythm, 529-530
Sinus tachycardia, 529
Sinuses, 612
Sitting position, 90, 91
Skeletal muscle, anatomy and physiology of, 591
Skeletal system
  anatomy and physiology of, 582-588
  functional differences and changes in, 588
  major groups of bones in, 582-585
Skeleton
  of animals, 582
  appendicular; see Appendicular skeleton
  axial; see Axial skeleton
Skin
  antiseptics for, 254
  as barrier to disease and infection, 173
  biopsy of, materials for, 222
  cancer of, 116-117
    sun and, 630
  cleansing, before injection, 276
  integumentary system and, 629
  lesions of, 629, 630-632
  preparation of, before minor surgery,
      216, 219
  structure of, 628
    burns and, 560, 561
  touch receptors in, 599
  vocabulary referring to, 66
Skin closures, adhesive, 211-212
Skin patch, 260
Skin tests, intradermal, diagnostic allergy tests
    and, 299-309
Skull
  anatomy and physiology of, 585, 586
  foramina of, 603
Slow pulse, 31
Small growths, materials for removing, 220
Small intestine, 605, 609
Smear, 339
  bacteriology, 361
  for candidiasis, 367
  cervical, 103
  for cytology studies, 358-360
  to detect gonorrhea, 367, 370
  endocervical, 103
  fixation of, 339
  for monilial vaginitis, 367
  Papanicolaou, 78, 366

Smear,—cont'd
  pelvic examination and, 98-99, 100-105
  during prenatal physical examination, 131
  for trichomoniasis vaginitis, 363-364
  vaginal, 363, 366-370
Smear culture, 338
Smell
  in physical examination, 60
  sense of, 629
Smooth muscle, anatomy and physiology of, 591
Snake bites, first aid for, 556-557
Snellen Big E chart, 120
Snellen eye chart, 120-121
  measuring distance visual acuity using,
      122-123
SOAP notes, 63
Social and occupational history, 55
Sodium, 649, 651-653
Sodium content of foods, 653, 654
Sodium hypochlorite for disinfection, 3
Sodium-restricted diet, 659-660
Solid culture media, 363
Solid drugs, terms to describe, 260
Soluble fiber, 650
Solutes, 260
Solutions, 260
  sterile, pouring, 207, 208
Somatic tremor, electrocardiogram and, 531
Sonnenschein nasal speculum, 81
Source or reservoir of etiologic agent, 172
Source-oriented medical record, 325
Spansules, 260
Special examinations, 61
  and routine physical examinations, preparing
      for and assisting with, 76-167
Special senses, 625-629
Specimen(s), 339-342
  caring for, handling, transporting, and
      storing, 340-342
  collecting and handling, 337-379
  instructions to patient and special preparation
      for, 339-340
  labeling, for laboratory, 324
  laboratory, handling of, 11-12
  respiratory tract, 353-358
  sputum, 353-355
  stool, collection of, 346, 347-352
  tissue biopsy, materials for removing, 220
  urine; see Urine specimens
Speculum, 83
  ear, used with otoscope, 79
  nasal, 81, 83
  vaginal, 80
    Sims, 83
Sperm, 581, 615, 616
  in urine, 403
Sphincter control of bladder and bowels,
    loss of, 603
Sphygmomanometers
  to measure blood pressure, 39-40, 595
  parts of, 40
Spider bites, first aid for, 557
Spills
  cleaning up, 3
  mercury, 11
  universal, 11
Spinal bulb, 599
Spinal cavity, 580
Spinal column, anatomy and physiology of, 586
Spinal cord, anatomy and physiology of, 587, 599
Spinal nerves, 603
Spiral turn during bandaging, 234, 235
Spiral-reverse turn during bandaging, 237
Spirilla causing disease, 171
Spleen, anatomy and physiology of, 598

Spleen scan, 482
Splenic flexure, 609
Sponge forceps, 213
Spore, 170
Spot urine specimen, 342
Sprain, 496
Spray, 261
Spring of stethoscope, 40
Spring-handle forceps, 213
Sputum, 339
Sputum specimens
  collection of, 353-354
  laboratory requisition for, 355
Squamous cell carcinoma, 630
ST segment, cardiac cycle and, 528, 529
Stab culture, 338
Stabbing pain, 66
Stage of microscope, 331
Stain, Gram, 361-362
Stand of microscope, 331
Standards, drug, 251
Standing position, 91
Stapes, 625
Staphylococci, 223
  causing disease, 171
Starches, 645
Statistic information, medical records
      providing, 65
Steam sterilization, 188-197
  critical factors in, 189-190
  general procedures for, 190-194
  insufficient, causes of, 194-197
Steam sterilizer
  positioning loads in, 190-192
  removing loads from, 193
Sterile, definition of, 170
Sterile field, 204
Sterile gloves, donning and removing, 207,
      209-210
Sterile packages, opening, 204-206
Sterile solutions, pouring, 207, 208
Sterile supplies
  handling, 204-207
  storing, 195
Sterile technique; see Surgical asepsis
Steriline bags for sterilization, 188, 190
Sterilization, 168-201
  chemical; see Chemical sterilization
  dry heat, 198
  gas, 198
  inspecting instruments before, 188
  methods for, 187
  preparation of materials for, 188
  problems encountered in, 195
  steam, 188-197; see also Steam sterilization
  ultrasonic, 198-199
  wrapping instruments and supplies for,
      188, 189, 191
Sterilize, definition of, 2
Sterilometer-Plus, 192-193, 194
Sterilo-meters, 193, 194
Steri-Strip, 212
Sternoclavicular joints, 587
Sternum, 586, 587
Steroids, 261
Sterotactic Mammotest machine, 474
Stertorous respiration, 33
Stethoscope, 40, 83
Stimulant, 256
Stings, first aid for, 556-557
Stock supply, 249
Stomach, 609
  cancer of, 116-117
Stool, 339, 346, 347

Stool specimens
    collection of, 346, 347-352
    Hemoccult slide test on, 349-352
Storage
    and handling of drugs, 258-259, 261
    of sterile supplies, 195
STP, 572-573
Strain, 496
Streak culture, 338
Streptococci, 223
    causing disease, 171
Streptococcus screening, 358
Stress, sympathetic system and, 604
Stress test, treadmill, electrocardiography
        and, 543-544
Striated muscle, 591
Stroke, first aid for, 563-564
Strychnine, ingestion of, first aid for, 570
Styptic agent, 256
Subarachnoid space, 599
Subclavian artery, compression of, in controlling
        severe bleeding, 558, 559
Subcutaneous injections, 279-280, 282
    administration of, 293-294
    in child, 159
Subcutaneous tissues, foreign bodies in, materials
        for removing, 220
Subdermal implants, 260
    for drug administration, 267
Subdiaphragmatic abdominal thrusts in manage-
        ment of obstructed airway, 552
Subjective findings in POMR, 63
Subjective symptom, 54, 78
Sublingual route of drug administration, 266
Substage of microscope, 331
Substances, controlled; *see* Controlled substances
Suction curette, endometrial, 212
Sudoriferous glands, 629
Sugars, 645
Sulfa preparations, 256
Sulfur, 649
Summary, discharge, 62
Sun, skin cancer and, 630
Sunburn, 630
    first aid for, 560
Superficial burns, first aid for, 560
Superheated steam for steam sterilization, 190
Superior vena cava, 594
Supination, 510
    arm placed in, 587
Supine position, 90
Supplies
    handling of, 9-11
    for injections, 273-276
    sterile
        handling, 204-207
        storing, 195
Suppositories, 260
Surface anesthesia, 207
Surgery
    abbreviations related to, 263
    minor; *see* Minor surgery
Surgical asepsis, 184, 186
    background of, 203
    and minor surgery, 202-246
    principles and practices of, 203-204
Surgical studies, abbreviations related to, 68
Surgical terms, abbreviations related to, 263
Susceptible host, 172-173
Suspension, 260
Suture(s), 204
    absorbable, 210
    for lacerations, materials for, 220
    materials for
        and needles, 207, 210-212
        nonabsorbable, 210-211

Suture(s)—cont'd
    prepackaged, 210
    removal of, 224, 225
Suture needles, 211
Suture scissors, 212, 219
Swab, 339
Swaged needles, 211
Swallowing, 612
Sweat glands, 629
Symbols, 69
    medical, 263
    prescription, 259
Symmetry, 54, 78
Sympathetic system of autonomic nervous
        system, 604
Symphysis pubis, 620
Symptomatic HIV disease, 13
Symptoms, 54, 78
    of infection, 176-177
    of inflammation, 176
    subjective, 78
Syncope
    first aid for, 565
    hyperventilation and, 568
Syndrome, 54, 78
Synergistic interactions of drugs, 272
Syphilis, 369
Syringes
    for injection, 273-274
        selection of, 276, 278, 279
    Monoject safety, 276, 277-278
    and needles, wrapping, for steam
        sterilization, 191
    parts of, 274
    Safety-Lok, 274
        procedure for using, 275
    sterile, for allergy testing, 283
    types of, 274
Syrup, 261
    of ipecac, poisoning and, 570
System action of drug, 272
Systems
    anatomy and physiology of, 581-582
    review of, 55
Systole, cardiac cycle and, 527
Systolic blood pressure, 33, 35, 595
Syva MicroTrak HSVI/HSV2 Direct Specimen
        Identification/Typing Test, 372-373

T

T cell count, 14
T cells, levels of, in AIDS, 14
T wave, cardiac cycle and, 527, 529
T4 cells, 14
Table salt, 651-653
Tablets, 260
Tachycardia, 31, 529, 530
Tailbone, 587
Talus, 588
Tanning, melanin and, 630
Tap water, content of, 650
Tape, adhesive and elastic, 232
Tape measure, fiberglass, 79
Tapotement, 505
Tarsals, 588
Taste, sense of, 599, 629
Taste buds, 609
Taylor percussion hammer, 80
TDA; *see* Therapeutic drug assays
Tear ducts, 612
Tear glands, 625
Teeth
    digestive system and, 605
    wisdom, 605
Temperature
    body; *see* Body temperature

Temperature—cont'd
    for steam sterilization, 189-190
Temporal artery
    compression of, in controlling severe
        bleeding, 558, 559
    determining pulse rate at, 32
Tenaculum, uterine, 212
Tenderness, rebound, 66
Tendinitis, 496
Tendons, 582, 591
Tentative diagnosis, 61-62
Tes-Tape test for glucose in urine, 395, 400
Testes, 615
    cancer of, 116-117
    endocrine system and, 625
Testosterone, 615, 625
Testpack Strep A test, 358
Tests; *see also* Examination
    allergy
        diagnostic, and intradermal skin tests,
            299-309
        sterile syringes for, 283
    bacterial culture and sensitivity, 363
    Bence Jones Protein, 408
    blood; *see* Blood tests
    Chlamydia trachomatis direct specimen,
        370-371
    to diagnose HIV infection, 15
    diagnostic, 177
        prenatal physical examination and,
            131-133
    guaiac, 347
    of health status of HIV-positive patient, 14
    hearing, 119, 120
    Hemoccult slide, on stool specimen, 349-352
    laboratory, abbreviations related to, 262-263
    Mantoux, to diagnose tuberculosis, 283, 306
    nitrite, for bacteriuria testing, 407
    occult blood, 347
    Papanicolaou, 78, 366
    patch, to diagnose allergies, 300-301
    for phenylketonuria, 409
    pregnancy, 126
        laboratory request form to order, 127
        urine for, 408, 409, 410-411
    radioimmunoassay, to diagnose pregnancy,
        408
    reagent, for urinalyses, 388
    scratch, to diagnose allergies, 300, 302-303
    skin, intradermal, diagnostic allergy tests
        and, 299-309
    Syva MicroTrak HSVI/HSV2 Direct
        Specimen Identification/Typing,
        372-373
    tine tuberculin, 306-308
    urine
        for glucose, 391, 394-395, 400
        normal values for, 412-413
        qualitative and quantitative, 381
Tetanus antitoxin, 176
Tetanus bacillus, 223
Tetanus and diphtheria toxoids, guide for use of,
        178
Tetany, 622
Therapeutic drug assays, 437
Therapeutic plan in POMR, 63
Thermography, 475
Thermometer sheaths, 20, 21
Thermometers, 20-22
    glass; *see* Glass thermometers
Thermoscan, 27, 28
Thermotherapy, 498-501
Thiamine, 646, 647-648
Thigh, 588
Thighbone, 588
Third-degree burns, first aid for, 560, 562-563

Thoracic cavity, 580
Thoracic duct, 596, 609
Thoracic nerves, 603
Thoracic vertebrae, 587
Thorax, 585, 586
Thready pulse, 31
Threshold, pain, 66
Throat, 611, 612
Throat cultures, 354, 355-357
Thrombocytes, 417, 594
Thrombocythemia, 417
Thrombocytopenia, 417
Thrombosis, coronary, 595
Thrombus, 594
Thumb, 587
Thumb forceps, 213
Thymosin, 622
Thymus gland, 596, 598, 622
Thyroid gland, 622, 624
Thyroid scan, 482
Tibia, 588
Tick bites, first aid for, 557
Time for steam sterilization, 189
Timed urine specimen, 343
Tincture, 260
Tine tuberculin test, 306-308
    during prenatal physical examination, 131
Tischler cervical biopsy punch forceps, 79
Tissue, 578
    anatomy and physiology of, 581
    biopsy specimens of, materials for
        removing, 220
    blood and lymphoid, as barrier to disease
        and infection, 174
    handling of, 11
    subcutaneous, foreign bodies in, materials
        for removing, 220
Tissue culture, 338
Tissue forceps, 213, 219
Titmus II Vision Tester, 121
TK mark for tourniquet, 560
Toe, great, 588
Toenails, integumentary system and, 629
Tolerance, drug, 249
    and drug dosage and action, 271
Tomography, 475
Tongue, taste buds of, 609
Tongue blade, 83
Tonometers, 81, 83
Tonometry, 126
Tonsillectomy, 612
Tonsils, respiration and, 612
Tooth-tipped forceps, 212-213, 219
Topical anesthesia, 207
Total Solids Meter, 384
Touch, sense of, 629
Touch receptors in skin, 599
Tourniquet, 548
    in controlling severe bleeding, 558-560
Towel clamps, 213
Toxemia in pregnancy, 131
Toxicity, 249
Toxin, 170
Toxoids, 174, 176
    guide for use of, 178-179
Toxoplasmosis, 14
Trace minerals, 646
Trachea, respiration and, 612
Traction, various types of, 504-505
Tracts, 599
Trade name of drug, 248, 250
Tranquilizers, 256
    minor, 572-573
Transdermal patch, 260
    for drug administration, 267

Transfer forceps, 204
Transient pain, 66
Transmission
    HIV, 14
    means of, of etiologic agent, 172
Transverse colon, 609
Transverse plane, 579
Traumatic shock, 555
Treadmill stress test, electrocardiography and,
        525, 543-544
Tremor, somatic, electrocardiogram and, 531
Trendelenburg position, 89-90
Triangular bandages, 233
Trichomoniasis vaginitis, smear for, 363-364
Tricuspid valve, 595
Trivalent oral polio vaccine, 159
Troches, 260
True solution, 260
Trunk, anatomy and physiology of, 586-587
Tryptamines, 572-573
Tubal pregnancy, 620
Tubegauz, 234
    application of, 237-239
Tuberculin reaction, interpreting, 306
Tuberculin syringe, 274
Tuberculin test, tine, 306-308
Tuberculosis, 305-308
    lymph nodes in chest and, 596
    Mantoux test for, 283
    tests for, during prenatal physical
        examination, 131
Tubes, placement of, in centrifuge, 334
Tubex injector, using, 284, 285
Tubing of stethoscope, 40
Tumor, identification of, 632
Tuning forks, 79, 83
    for hearing examination, 119
Turbinates, 612
24-hour urine specimen, 343
Tympanic membrane, 312, 625
Tympanic thermometry, infrared, 20, 22,
        27-28, 30-31
Type culture, 338

U

Ulcer, 609
    identification of, 632
Ulcer diet, 660
Ulcerative colitis, 609
Ulna, 587
Ultrasonic cleaning and sterilization
        procedures, 198-199
Ultrasound
    diagnostic, 479-480
    for pregnant woman, 134
    therapeutic, 498
Ultraviolet light, 497
Umbilical cord, 620
Unalterable entries in medical records, 64
Underweight, 41
Unequal pulse, 31
Uniform definitions, 634
Uniforms and clothing, cleaning, 4
Unit-dose, 249
*United States Pharmacopeia-National
        Formulary*, 249, 250
Universal antidote, poisoning and, 571
Universal blood and body substance
        precautions, 1-17
Universal precautions, 2
    compliance with, 5
Universal spill kit, 11
Universal spills, 11
Unopette system, 429-432
Unsaturated fat, 637, 638, 642

Untoward effect, 249
Upper extremities
    anatomy and physiology of, 587
    bones of, 585
    range-of-motion exercises for, 506-507
Upright position for carrying infant, 153
Uremia, 417
Ureters, 612, 615
Urethra, 612, 615
Urethritis, 369
Urgency, 343
Urinalysis, 323, 380-414
    categories of, 381-382
    laboratory requisitions for, 403
    during prenatal physical examination, 131
    reagent tests for, 388-389
    routine, 381-403
        controls for, 395
    standard procedures for, 382
Urinary bladder, urinary system and, 612, 615
Urinary meatus, 615
Urinary system
    anatomy and physiology of, 612-615
    factors affecting urination and, 615
    formation of, 380-381
Urination, 343, 615
Urine, 339
    acetone in, tests for, 391, 394
    artifacts in, 403, 407
    bacteria in, 403
    bilirubin in, 391
        tests for, 391, 394-395
    blood in, 391
    casts in, 403, 405
    centrifuged sediment of, microscopic exami-
        nation of, 395, 400-403
    chemical examination of, using reagent strips,
        385, 387-388
    chemistry analyzers for, for use with reagent
        strips, 388-390
    crystals in, 403, 406
    Dipstick testing of, 396-399
    epithelial cells in, 403, 404
    formation of, 615
    glucose in, 391
        Tes-Tape test for, 395, 400
        tests for, 391, 394, 395
    hormone determinations using, 408
    ketone bodies in, 391
    leukocytes in, 391
    nitrite in, 391
    normal, components of, 380-381
    odor of, 384
    pH of, 390
    physical characteristics and measurements
        of, 383-385
    pregnancy test using, 408, 409, 410-411
    profile of, in different diseases, 392-393
    protein in, 391
    protein determinations for, 408
    qualitative and quantitative tests on, 381
    quantity of, 384
    red blood cells in, 401, 403, 404
    sediment in, atlas of, 402
    specific gravity of, 384
        procedure for determining, 384-385,
            386-387
    spermatozoa in, 403
    terms related to, 343, 381, 384, 391
    tests of
        to diagnose phenylketonuria, 408-409
        normal values for, 412-413
    urobilinogen in, 391
    white blood cells in, 403, 404
    yeast and parasites in, 403

Urine collector, disposable, 155, 156
Urine specimens
    collection of, 342-346
        general facts relating to, 343-344
    obtaining, from infant, 155, 156
    types of, 342-343
Urine toxicology screening, 343
Urinometer to determine specific gravity of urine, 386-387
Uristix tests, 388, 389
Urobilinogen, 347
    in urine, 391
Urobilistix test, 389
Urogram, 473
U.S. Adopted Name Council, 250
U.S. Department of Agriculture
    Food Safety and Inspection Service of, food labeling and, 656
    Human Nutrition Information Service of, 640
U.S. Department of Health and Human Services, food labeling and, 656
USP-NF; *see United States Pharmacopeia-National Formulary*
Uterine tenaculum, 212
Uterine tubes, appearance of, from fertilization to implantation, 618
Uterus, 620
    appearance of, from fertilization to implantation, 618
    bimanual palpation of, 105

V

Vaccination, 170
    international certificates of, 180-183
Vaccine, 256
    attenuated, 174
    common, 159
    guide for use of, 178-179
    inactivated, 174
    to prevent hepatitis B, 15
Vacutainer system, 419-420
Vacuum tubes, frequently used, 420
Vagina, 620
Vaginal examinations, 98-99
    during pregnancy, 131
Vaginal route of drug administration, 266
Vaginal secretions for hormone evaluation, 363
Vaginal smears and culture collection, 363, 366-370
Vaginal speculum, 80
    Sims, 83
Vaginitis, 369
    monilial, smear for, 367
Valium; *see Diazepam*
Valves
    heart, 526, 595
    of veins, 594
Vas deferens, 615
Vascular tunic, 625
Vasectomy, 615
Vasoconstrictor, 256
Vasodilator, 256
Vastus lateralis intramuscular injection, 160, 279, 281, 282
Vegetables, nutrition and, 645, 646
Veins, 594
Venipuncture, 417
    using a syringe and needle, 422-425
    using Vacutainer evacuated blood, 426-427
Venipuncture technique, 421-427
Venipuncture tips, 422
Venous bleeding, 557
Venous blood sample, 418-421
Venous pulse, 31
Venous star, identification of, 632
Ventilation devices as protective equipment, 9

Ventrescreen Strep A enzyme immunoassay, 358
Ventricle, 525, 526, 527, 595
Ventricular arrhythmia, 530-531
Ventricular contractions, premature, 530
Ventricular fibrillation, 531
Ventricular rate, 529
Ventricular rhythm, 529
Ventricular tachycardia, 530
Ventrogluteal muscle, injection into, 160, 279, 280
Venules, 594
Vertebrae, 586, 587
Vertebral bodies, 586
Vertebral column, bones of, 585, 587
Vesicle, 300
    identification of, 632
Vestibular nerve, 625
Vestibule of labyrinth, 625
Vestibulocochlear cranial nerve, 625
Viable, 339
Vials, 276, 278
Villi
    chorionic, sampling of, 133-134
    of small intestine, 609
ViraPap, 99
Virology, 323
Virulence, 170
Viruses
    causing disease, 171
    herpes simplex, 371-373
Viscera, 603
Visceral muscle, anatomy and physiology of, 591
Vision, color, testing, 124-125; *see also* Visual acuity
Vision testing devices, electric, 121
Visual acuity, 120
    distance, 120-123
    near, measuring, 124
Visual fields, testing, 124
Vital signs, 19-41
    in children, measuring, 143, 153
Vitamin(s), 256, 646, 647-648, 661
    nutrition and, 645-646
Vitamin K, 417, 646, 647-648
Vitreous humor, 625
Vocal cords, 612
Voice box, 612
Voltage, 471
Voluntary muscle, 591
Vomiting, inducing, poisoning and, 570
von Hochstetter's site for intramuscular injection, 279, 281
Vulva, 620
    biopsy of, materials for, 222

W

Walkers, 518
Wampole 2-minute slide test to diagnose pregnancy, 410-411
Wandering baseline, electrocardiogram and, 531-532
Warning labels, 4
Warning signs, 4
Wartenberg neurologic pinwheel, 80
Warts, genital, 368
Wasp stings, first aid for, 557
Waste, 2-3
    contaminated, 3
    handling and disposing of, 5, 11
    infectious, handling of, 11
    regulated, 2
Water, nutrition and, 646-650
Water-insoluble fiber, 650
Water-soluble vitamins, 645, 646
WBC; *see* White blood cell count; White blood cells

Weight
    of children, measuring, 139
    desirable, 49
    dosages of drugs and, 268-270, 271
    drug action and, 271
    gain of, during pregnancy, 131
    and height, measuring, 41, 46-47
    of infant, measuring, 154
Well-child visits, 135-155
Wen, 204
Western Blot test, 15
Wet steam for steam sterilization, 190
Wheal, 300, 632
Wheelchairs, 512-513
White blood cell count, 450
White blood cell scan, 482
White blood cells, 588, 594
    abnormal, 450-452
    in urine, 403, 404
White matter, 599
Windpipe, 612
Wisdom teeth, 605
Wong-Baker Faces Pain Rating Scale, 144
Work surfaces, decontamination of, 3, 11
World AIDS Day, 15
Wounds, 224, 226-227
    culture of, 358
        dressing change with, 228-232
    first aid for, 569
Wrapping techniques for bandages, basic, 234-237
Wrists
    anatomy and physiology of, 587-588
    bandage-wrapping techniques for, 236

X

X-ray film
    processing of, 490-491
    reports, and records, ownership of, 491
X-ray film studies
    abbreviations related to, 68, 263
    position of patient for, 482-485
X-ray materials, storage of, 491
X-rays, 471-479
Xeroradiography, 474

Y

Yeast in urine, 403
Yellow bone marrow, 588
Yeoman biopsy forceps, 82

Z

Zalcitabine, 15
Zidovudine for HIV-positive people, 15
Zoonosis, 172
Zygote, 581
Z-tract technique for intramuscular injection, 292